The Biomedical Engineering Handbook
Third Edition

Medical Devices and Systems

D1477773

The Electrical Engineering Handbook Series

Series Editor
Richard C. Dorf
University of California, Davis

Titles Included in the Series

The Handbook of Ad Hoc Wireless Networks, Mohammad Ilyas

The Avionics Handbook, Cary R. Spitzer

The Biomedical Engineering Handbook, Third Edition, Joseph D. Bronzino

The Circuits and Filters Handbook, Second Edition, Wai-Kai Chen

The Communications Handbook, Second Edition, Jerry Gibson

The Computer Engineering Handbook, Vojin G. Oklobdzija

The Control Handbook, William S. Levine

The CRC Handbook of Engineering Tables, Richard C. Dorf

The Digital Signal Processing Handbook, Vijay K. Madisetti and Douglas Williams

The Electrical Engineering Handbook, Third Edition, Richard C. Dorf

The Electric Power Engineering Handbook, Leo L. Grigsby

The Electronics Handbook, Second Edition, Jerry C. Whitaker

The Engineering Handbook, Third Edition, Richard C. Dorf

The Handbook of Formulas and Tables for Signal Processing, Alexander D. Poularikas

The Handbook of Nanoscience, Engineering, and Technology, William A. Goddard, III, Donald W. Brenner, Sergey E. Lyshevski, and Gerald J. Iafrate

The Handbook of Optical Communication Networks, Mohammad Ilyas and Hussein T. Mouftah

The Industrial Electronics Handbook, J. David Irwin

The Measurement, Instrumentation, and Sensors Handbook, John G. Webster

The Mechanical Systems Design Handbook, Osita D.I. Nwokah and Yidirim Hurmuzlu

The Mechatronics Handbook, Robert H. Bishop

The Mobile Communications Handbook, Second Edition, Jerry D. Gibson

The Ocean Engineering Handbook, Ferial El-Hawary

The RF and Microwave Handbook, Mike Golio

The Technology Management Handbook, Richard C. Dorf

The Transforms and Applications Handbook, Second Edition, Alexander D. Poularikas

The VLSI Handbook, Wai-Kai Chen

The Biomedical Engineering Handbook
Third Edition

Edited by
Joseph D. Bronzino

Biomedical Engineering Fundamentals

Medical Devices and Systems

Tissue Engineering and Artificial Organs

DATE DUE FOR RETURN

6/7/11

This book may be recalled before the above date.

The Biomedical Engineering Handbook
Third Edition

Medical Devices and Systems

Edited by

Joseph D. Bronzino

Trinity College
Hartford, Connecticut, U.S.A.

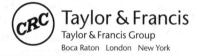

Taylor & Francis
Taylor & Francis Group
Boca Raton   London   New York

A CRC title, part of the Taylor & Francis imprint, a member of the
Taylor & Francis Group, the academic division of T&F Informa plc.

Published in 2006 by
CRC Press
Taylor & Francis Group
6000 Broken Sound Parkway NW, Suite 300
Boca Raton, FL 33487-2742

International Standard Book Number-10: 0-8493-2122-0 (Hardcover)
International Standard Book Number-13: 978-0-8493-2122-1 (Hardcover)
Library of Congress Card Number 2005056892

Library of Congress Cataloging-in-Publication Data

Medical devices and systems / edited by Joseph D. Bronzino.
    p. cm. -- (The electrical engineering handbook series)
  Includes bibliographical references and index.
  ISBN 0-8493-2122-0
  1. Medical instruments and apparatus--Handbooks, manuals, etc. I. Bronzino, Joseph D., 1937- II. Title. III. Series.

R856.15.B76 2006
610.28--dc22   1005009315   2005056892

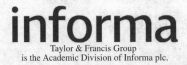

Taylor & Francis Group
is the Academic Division of Informa plc.

Visit the Taylor & Francis Web site at
http://www.taylorandfrancis.com

and the CRC Press Web site at
http://www.crcpress.com

Introduction and Preface

During the past five years since the publication of the Second Edition — a two-volume set — of the *Biomedical Engineering Handbook*, the field of biomedical engineering has continued to evolve and expand. As a result, this Third Edition consists of a three volume set, which has been significantly modified to reflect the state-of-the-field knowledge and applications in this important discipline. More specifically, this Third Edition contains a number of completely new sections, including:

- Molecular Biology
- Bionanotechnology
- Bioinformatics
- Neuroengineering
- Infrared Imaging

as well as a new section on ethics.

In addition, all of the sections that have appeared in the first and second editions have been significantly revised. Therefore, this Third Edition presents an excellent summary of the status of knowledge and activities of biomedical engineers in the beginning of the 21st century.

As such, it can serve as an excellent reference for individuals interested not only in a review of fundamental physiology, but also in quickly being brought up to speed in certain areas of biomedical engineering research. It can serve as an excellent textbook for students in areas where traditional textbooks have not yet been developed and as an excellent review of the major areas of activity in each biomedical engineering subdiscipline, such as biomechanics, biomaterials, bioinstrumentation, medical imaging, etc. Finally, it can serve as the "bible" for practicing biomedical engineering professionals by covering such topics as a historical perspective of medical technology, the role of professional societies, the ethical issues associated with medical technology, and the FDA process.

Biomedical engineering is now an important vital interdisciplinary field. Biomedical engineers are involved in virtually all aspects of developing new medical technology. They are involved in the design, development, and utilization of materials, devices (such as pacemakers, lithotripsy, etc.) and techniques (such as signal processing, artificial intelligence, etc.) for clinical research and use; and serve as members of the health care delivery team (clinical engineering, medical informatics, rehabilitation engineering, etc.) seeking new solutions for difficult health care problems confronting our society. To meet the needs of this diverse body of biomedical engineers, this handbook provides a central core of knowledge in those fields encompassed by the discipline. However, before presenting this detailed information, it is important to provide a sense of the evolution of the modern health care system and identify the diverse activities biomedical engineers perform to assist in the diagnosis and treatment of patients.

Evolution of the Modern Health Care System

Before 1900, medicine had little to offer the average citizen, since its resources consisted mainly of the physician, his education, and his "little black bag." In general, physicians seemed to be in short supply, but the shortage had rather different causes than the current crisis in the availability of health care professionals. Although the costs of obtaining medical training were relatively low, the demand for doctors' services also was very small, since many of the services provided by the physician also could be obtained from experienced amateurs in the community. The home was typically the site for treatment and recuperation, and relatives and neighbors constituted an able and willing nursing staff. Babies were delivered by midwives, and those illnesses not cured by home remedies were left to run their natural, albeit frequently fatal, course. The contrast with contemporary health care practices, in which specialized physicians and nurses located within the hospital provide critical diagnostic and treatment services, is dramatic.

The changes that have occurred within medical science originated in the rapid developments that took place in the applied sciences (chemistry, physics, engineering, microbiology, physiology, pharmacology, etc.) at the turn of the century. This process of development was characterized by intense interdisciplinary cross-fertilization, which provided an environment in which medical research was able to take giant strides in developing techniques for the diagnosis and treatment of disease. For example, in 1903, Willem Einthoven, a Dutch physiologist, devised the first electrocardiograph to measure the electrical activity of the heart. In applying discoveries in the physical sciences to the analysis of the biologic process, he initiated a new age in both cardiovascular medicine and electrical measurement techniques.

New discoveries in medical sciences followed one another like intermediates in a chain reaction. However, the most significant innovation for clinical medicine was the development of x-rays. These "new kinds of rays," as their discoverer W.K. Roentgen described them in 1895, opened the "inner man" to medical inspection. Initially, x-rays were used to diagnose bone fractures and dislocations, and in the process, x-ray machines became commonplace in most urban hospitals. Separate departments of radiology were established, and their influence spread to other departments throughout the hospital. By the 1930s, x-ray visualization of practically all organ systems of the body had been made possible through the use of barium salts and a wide variety of radiopaque materials.

X-ray technology gave physicians a powerful tool that, for the first time, permitted accurate diagnosis of a wide variety of diseases and injuries. Moreover, since x-ray machines were too cumbersome and expensive for local doctors and clinics, they had to be placed in health care centers or hospitals. Once there, x-ray technology essentially triggered the transformation of the hospital from a passive receptacle for the sick to an active curative institution for all members of society.

For economic reasons, the centralization of health care services became essential because of many other important technological innovations appearing on the medical scene. However, hospitals remained institutions to dread, and it was not until the introduction of sulfanilamide in the mid-1930s and penicillin in the early 1940s that the main danger of hospitalization, that is, cross-infection among patients, was significantly reduced. With these new drugs in their arsenals, surgeons were able to perform their operations without prohibitive morbidity and mortality due to infection. Furthermore, even though the different blood groups and their incompatibility were discovered in 1900 and sodium citrate was used in 1913 to prevent clotting, full development of blood banks was not practical until the 1930s, when technology provided adequate refrigeration. Until that time, "fresh" donors were bled and the blood transfused while it was still warm.

Once these surgical suites were established, the employment of specifically designed pieces of medical technology assisted in further advancing the development of complex surgical procedures. For example, the Drinker respirator was introduced in 1927 and the first heart-lung bypass in 1939. By the 1940s, medical procedures heavily dependent on medical technology, such as cardiac catheterization and angiography (the use of a cannula threaded through an arm vein and into the heart with the injection of radiopaque dye) for the x-ray visualization of congenital and acquired heart disease (mainly valve disorders due to rheumatic fever) became possible, and a new era of cardiac and vascular surgery was established.

Following World War II, technological advances were spurred on by efforts to develop superior weapon systems and establish habitats in space and on the ocean floor. As a by-product of these efforts, the development of medical devices accelerated and the medical profession benefited greatly from this rapid surge of technological finds. Consider the following examples:

1. Advances in solid-state electronics made it possible to map the subtle behavior of the fundamental unit of the central nervous system — the neuron — as well as to monitor the various physiological parameters, such as the electrocardiogram, of patients in intensive care units.
2. New prosthetic devices became a goal of engineers involved in providing the disabled with tools to improve their quality of life.
3. Nuclear medicine — an outgrowth of the atomic age — emerged as a powerful and effective approach in detecting and treating specific physiologic abnormalities.
4. Diagnostic ultrasound based on sonar technology became so widely accepted that ultrasonic studies are now part of the routine diagnostic workup in many medical specialties.
5. "Spare parts" surgery also became commonplace. Technologists were encouraged to provide cardiac assist devices, such as artificial heart valves and artificial blood vessels, and the artificial heart program was launched to develop a replacement for a defective or diseased human heart.
6. Advances in materials have made the development of disposable medical devices, such as needles and thermometers, as well as implantable drug delivery systems, a reality.
7. Computers similar to those developed to control the flight plans of the *Apollo* capsule were used to store, process, and cross-check medical records, to monitor patient status in intensive care units, and to provide sophisticated statistical diagnoses of potential diseases correlated with specific sets of patient symptoms.
8. Development of the first computer-based medical instrument, the computerized axial tomography scanner, revolutionized clinical approaches to noninvasive diagnostic imaging procedures, which now include magnetic resonance imaging and positron emission tomography as well.
9. A wide variety of new cardiovascular technologies including implantable defibrillators and chemically treated stents were developed.
10. Neuronal pacing systems were used to detect and prevent epileptic seizures.
11. Artificial organs and tissue have been created.
12. The completion of the genome project has stimulated the search for new biological markers and personalized medicine.

The impact of these discoveries and many others has been profound. The health care system of today consists of technologically sophisticated clinical staff operating primarily in modern hospitals designed to accommodate the new medical technology. This evolutionary process continues, with advances in the physical sciences such as materials and nanotechnology, and in the life sciences such as molecular biology, the genome project and artificial organs. These advances have altered and will continue to alter the very nature of the health care delivery system itself.

Biomedical Engineering: A Definition

Bioengineering is usually defined as a basic research-oriented activity closely related to biotechnology and genetic engineering, that is, the modification of animal or plant cells, or parts of cells, to improve plants or animals or to develop new microorganisms for beneficial ends. In the food industry, for example, this has meant the improvement of strains of yeast for fermentation. In agriculture, bioengineers may be concerned with the improvement of crop yields by treatment of plants with organisms to reduce frost damage. It is clear that bioengineers of the future will have a tremendous impact on the qualities of human life. The potential of this specialty is difficult to imagine. Consider the following activities of bioengineers:

- Development of improved species of plants and animals for food production
- Invention of new medical diagnostic tests for diseases

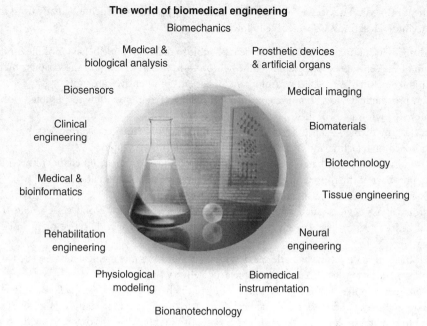

The world of biomedical engineering

Biomechanics

Medical &
biological analysis

Prosthetic devices
& artificial organs

Biosensors

Medical imaging

Clinical
engineering

Biomaterials

Biotechnology

Medical &
bioinformatics

Tissue engineering

Rehabilitation
engineering

Neural
engineering

Physiological
modeling

Biomedical
instrumentation

Bionanotechnology

FIGURE 1   The World of Biomedical Engineering.

- Production of synthetic vaccines from clone cells
- Bioenvironmental engineering to protect human, animal, and plant life from toxicants and pollutants
- Study of protein–surface interactions
- Modeling of the growth kinetics of yeast and hybridoma cells
- Research in immobilized enzyme technology
- Development of therapeutic proteins and monoclonal antibodies

   Biomedical engineers, on the other hand, apply electrical, mechanical, chemical, optical, and other engineering principles to understand, modify, or control biologic (i.e., human and animal) systems, as well as design and manufacture products that can monitor physiologic functions and assist in the diagnosis and treatment of patients. When biomedical engineers work within a hospital or clinic, they are more properly called clinical engineers.

Activities of Biomedical Engineers

The breadth of activity of biomedical engineers is now significant. The field has moved from being concerned primarily with the development of medical instruments in the 1950s and 1960s to include a more wide-ranging set of activities. As illustrated below, the field of biomedical engineering now includes many new career areas (see Figure 1), each of which is presented in this handbook. These areas include:

- Application of engineering system analysis (physiologic modeling, simulation, and control) to biologic problems
- Detection, measurement, and monitoring of physiologic signals (i.e., biosensors and biomedical instrumentation)
- Diagnostic interpretation via signal-processing techniques of bioelectric data
- Therapeutic and rehabilitation procedures and devices (rehabilitation engineering)
- Devices for replacement or augmentation of bodily functions (*artificial organs*)

- Computer analysis of patient-related data and clinical decision making (i.e., medical informatics and artificial intelligence)
- Medical imaging, that is, the graphic display of anatomic detail or physiologic function
- The creation of new biologic products (i.e., *biotechnology* and *tissue engineering*)
- The development of new materials to be used within the body (biomaterials)

Typical pursuits of biomedical engineers, therefore, include:

- Research in new materials for implanted artificial organs
- Development of new diagnostic instruments for blood analysis
- Computer modeling of the function of the human heart
- Writing software for analysis of medical research data
- Analysis of medical device hazards for safety and efficacy
- Development of new diagnostic imaging systems
- Design of telemetry systems for patient monitoring
- Design of biomedical sensors for measurement of human physiologic systems variables
- Development of expert systems for diagnosis of disease
- Design of closed-loop control systems for drug administration
- Modeling of the physiological systems of the human body
- Design of instrumentation for sports medicine
- Development of new dental materials
- Design of communication aids for the handicapped
- Study of pulmonary fluid dynamics
- Study of the biomechanics of the human body
- Development of material to be used as replacement for human skin

Biomedical engineering, then, is an interdisciplinary branch of engineering that ranges from theoretical, nonexperimental undertakings to state-of-the-art applications. It can encompass research, development, implementation, and operation. Accordingly, like medical practice itself, it is unlikely that any single person can acquire expertise that encompasses the entire field. Yet, because of the interdisciplinary nature of this activity, there is considerable interplay and overlapping of interest and effort between them. For example, biomedical engineers engaged in the development of biosensors may interact with those interested in prosthetic devices to develop a means to detect and use the same bioelectric signal to power a prosthetic device. Those engaged in automating the clinical chemistry laboratory may collaborate with those developing expert systems to assist clinicians in making decisions based on specific laboratory data. The possibilities are endless.

Perhaps a greater potential benefit occurring from the use of biomedical engineering is identification of the problems and needs of our present health care system that can be solved using existing engineering technology and systems methodology. Consequently, the field of biomedical engineering offers hope in the continuing battle to provide high-quality care at a reasonable cost. If properly directed toward solving problems related to preventive medical approaches, ambulatory care services, and the like, biomedical engineers can provide the tools and techniques to make our health care system more effective and efficient; and in the process, improve the quality of life for all.

Joseph D. Bronzino
Editor-in-Chief

Editor-in-Chief

Joseph D. Bronzino received the B.S.E.E. degree from Worcester Polytechnic Institute, Worcester, MA, in 1959, the M.S.E.E. degree from the Naval Postgraduate School, Monterey, CA, in 1961, and the Ph.D. degree in electrical engineering from Worcester Polytechnic Institute in 1968. He is presently the Vernon Roosa Professor of Applied Science, an endowed chair at Trinity College, Hartford, CT and President of the Biomedical Engineering Alliance and Consortium (BEACON) which is a nonprofit organization consisting of academic and medical institutions as well as corporations dedicated to the development and commercialization of new medical technologies (for details visit www.beaconalliance.org).

He is the author of over 200 articles and 11 books including the following: *Technology for Patient Care* (C.V. Mosby, 1977), *Computer Applications for Patient Care* (Addison-Wesley, 1982), *Biomedical Engineering: Basic Concepts and Instrumentation* (PWS Publishing Co., 1986), *Expert Systems: Basic Concepts* (Research Foundation of State University of New York, 1989), *Medical Technology and Society: An Interdisciplinary Perspective* (MIT Press and McGraw-Hill, 1990), *Management of Medical Technology* (Butterworth/Heinemann, 1992), *The Biomedical Engineering Handbook* (CRC Press, 1st ed., 1995; 2nd ed., 2000; Taylor & Francis, 3rd ed., 2005), *Introduction to Biomedical Engineering* (Academic Press, 1st ed., 1999; 2nd ed., 2005).

Dr. Bronzino is a fellow of IEEE and the American Institute of Medical and Biological Engineering (AIMBE), an honorary member of the Italian Society of Experimental Biology, past chairman of the Biomedical Engineering Division of the American Society for Engineering Education (ASEE), a charter member and presently vice president of the Connecticut Academy of Science and Engineering (CASE), a charter member of the American College of Clinical Engineering (ACCE) and the Association for the Advancement of Medical Instrumentation (AAMI), past president of the IEEE-Engineering in Medicine and Biology Society (EMBS), past chairman of the IEEE Health Care Engineering Policy Committee (HCEPC), past chairman of the IEEE Technical Policy Council in Washington, DC, and presently Editor-in-Chief of Elsevier's BME Book Series and Taylor & Francis' *Biomedical Engineering Handbook*.

Dr. Bronzino is also the recipient of the Millennium Award from IEEE/EMBS in 2000 and the Goddard Award from Worcester Polytechnic Institute for Professional Achievement in June 2004.

Contributors

Joseph Adam
Premise Development
 Corporation
Hartford, Connecticut

P.D. Ahlgren
Ville Marie Multidisciplinary
 Breast and Oncology Center
St. Mary's Hospital
McGill University
Montreal, Quebec, Canada
and
London Cancer Centre
London, Ontario
Canada

William C. Amalu
Pacific Chiropractic and
 Research Center
Redwood City, California

Kurt Ammer
Ludwig Boltzmann Research
 Institute for Physical
 Diagnostics
Vienna, Austria
and
Medical Imaging Research Group
School of Computing
University of Glamorgan
Pontypridd, Wales
United Kingdom

Dennis D. Autio
Dybonics, Inc.
Portland, Oregon

Raymond Balcerak
Defense Advanced Research
 Projects Agency
Arlington, Virginia

D.C. Barber
University of Sheffield
Sheffield, United Kingdom

Khosrow Behbehani
The University of Texas at
 Arlington
Arlington, Texas
and
The University of Texas
Southwestern Medical Center
Dallas, Texas

N. Belliveau
Ville Marie Multidisciplinary
 Breast and Oncology Center
St. Mary's Hospital
McGill University
Montreal, Quebec, Canada
and
London Cancer Centre
London, Ontario, Canada

Anna M. Bianchi
St. Raffaele Hospital
Milan, Italy

Carol J. Bickford
American Nurses Association
Washington, D.C.

Jeffrey S. Blair
IBM Health Care Solutions
Atlanta, Georgia

G. Faye Boudreaux-Bartels
University of Rhode Island
Kingston, Rhode Island

Bruce R. Bowman
EdenTec Corporation
Eden Prairie, Minnesota

Joseph D. Bronzino
Trinity College
Biomedical Engineering Alliance
 and Consortium (BEACON)
Harford, Connecticut

Mark E. Bruley
ECRI
Plymouth Meeting, Pennsylvania

Richard P. Buck
University of North Carolina
Chapel Hill, North Carolina

P. Buddharaju
Department of Computer Science
University of Houston
Houston, Texas

Thomas F. Budinger
University of California-Berkeley
Berkeley, California

Robert D. Butterfield
IVAC Corporation
San Diego, California

Joseph P. Cammarota
Naval Air Warfare Center
Aircraft Division
Warminster, Pennsylvania

Paul Campbell
Institute of Medical Science
  and Technology
Universities of St. Andrews
  and Dundee
and
Ninewells Hospital
Dundee, United Kingdom

Ewart R. Carson
City University
London, United Kingdom

Sergio Cerutti
Polytechnic University
Milan, Italy

A. Enis Çetin
Bilkent University
Ankara, Turkey

Christopher S. Chen
Department of Bioengineering
Department of Physiology
University of Pennsylvania
Philadelphia, Pennsylvania

Wei Chen
Center for Magnetic Resonance
  Research
and
The University of Minnesota
  Medical School
Minneapolis, Minnesota

Victor Chernomordik
Laboratory of Integrative and
  Medical Biophysics
National Institute of Child Health
  and Human Development
Bethesda, Maryland

David A. Chesler
Massachusetts General Hospital
Harvard University Medical
  School
Boston, Massachusetts

Vivian H. Coates
ECRI
Plymouth Meeting, Pennsylvania

Arnon Cohen
Ben-Gurion University
Be'er Sheva, Israel

Steven Conolly
Stanford University
Stanford, California

Derek G. Cramp
City University
London, United Kingdom

Barbara Y. Croft
National Institutes of Health
Kensington, Maryland

David D. Cunningham
Abbott Diagnostics
Process Engineering
Abbott Park, Illinois

Ian A. Cunningham
Victoria Hospital
The John P. Roberts Research
  Institute
and
The University of Western Ontario
London, Ontario, Canada

Yadin David
Texas Children's Hospital
Houston, Texas

Connie White Delaney
School of Nursing and Medical
  School
The University of Minnesota
Minneapolis, Minnesota

Mary Diakides
Advanced Concepts Analysis, Inc.
Falls Church, Virginia

Nicholas A. Diakides
Advanced Concepts Analysis, Inc.
Falls Church, Virginia

C. Drews-Peszynski
Technical University of Lodz
Lodz, Poland

Ronald G. Driggers
U.S. Army Communications and
  Electronics Research,
  Development and Engineering
  Center (CERDEC)
Night Vision and Electronic
  Sensors Directorate
Fort Belvoir, Virginia

Gary Drzewiecki
Rutgers University
Piscataway, New Jersey

Edwin G. Duffin
Medtronic, Inc.
Minneapolis, Minnesota

Jeffrey L. Eggleston
Valleylab, Inc.
Boulder, Colorado

Robert L. Elliott
Elliott-Elliott-Head Breast Cancer
  Research and Treatment Center
Baton Rouge, Louisiana

K. Whittaker Ferrara
Riverside Research Institute
New York, New York

J. Michael Fitzmaurice
Agency for Healthcare Research
  and Quality
Rockville, Maryland

Ross Flewelling
Nellcor Incorporation
Pleasant, California

Michael Forde
Medtronic, Inc.
Minneapolis, Minnesota

Amir H. Gandjbakhche
Laboratory of Integrative and
  Medical Biophysics
National Institute of Child Health
  and Human Development
Bethesda, Maryland

Israel Gannot
Laboratory of Integrative and
  Medical Biophysics
National Institute of Child Health
  and Human Development
Bethesda, Maryland

Leslie A. Geddes
Purdue University
West Lafayette, Indiana

Richard L. Goldberg
University of North Carolina
Chapel Hill, North Carolina

Boris Gramatikov
Johns Hopkins School
of Medicine
Baltimore, Maryland

Barton M. Gratt
School of Dentistry
University of Washington
Seattle, Washington

Walter Greenleaf
Greenleaf Medical
Palo Alto, California

Michael W. Grenn
U.S. Army Communications and
Electronics Research,
Development and Engineering
Center (CERDEC)
Night Vision and Electronic
Sensors Directorate
Fort Belvoir, Virginia

Eliot B. Grigg
Department of Plastic Surgery
Dartmouth-Hitchcock Medical
Center
Lebanon, New Hampshire

Warren S. Grundfest
Department of Bioengineering
and Electrical Engineering
Henry Samueli School of
Engineering and Applied
Science
and
Department of Surgery
David Geffen School
of Medicine
University of California
Los Angeles, California

Michael L. Gullikson
Texas Children's Hospital
Houston, Texas

Moinuddin Hassan
Laboratory of Integrative and
Medical Biophysics
National Institute of Child Health
and Human Development
Bethesda, Maryland

David Hattery
Laboratory of Integrative and
Medical Biophysics
National Institute of Child Health
and Human Development
Bethesda, Maryland

Jonathan F. Head
Elliott-Elliott-Head Breast Cancer
Research and Treatment Center
Baton Rouge, Louisiana

William B. Hobbins
Women's Breast Health Center
Madison, Wisconsin

Stuart Horn
U.S. Army Communications and
Electronics Research,
Development and Engineering
Center (CERDEC)
Night Vision and Electronic
Sensors Directorate
Fort Belvoir, Virginia

Xiaoping Hu
Center for Magnetic Resonance
Research
and
The University of Minnesota
Medical School
Minneapolis, Minnesota

T. Jakubowska
Technical University of Lodz
Lodz, Poland

G. Allan Johnson
Duke University Medical Center
Durham, North Carolina

Bryan F. Jones
Medical Imaging Research Group
School of Computing
University of Glamorgan
Pontypridd, Wales
United Kingdom

Thomas M. Judd
Kaiser Permanente
Atlanta, Georgia

Millard M. Judy
Baylor Research Institute and
MicroBioMed Corp.
Dallas, Texas

Philip F. Judy
Brigham and Women's Hospital
Harvard University Medical
School
Boston, Massachusetts

G.J.L. Kaw
Department of Diagnostic
Radiology
Tan Tock Seng Hospital
Singapore

J.R. Keyserlingk
Ville Marie Multidisciplinary
Breast and Oncology Center
St. Mary's Hospital
McGill University
Montreal, Quebec, Canada
and
London Cancer Centre
London, Ontario
Canada

C. Everett Koop
Department of Plastic Surgery
Dartmouth-Hitchcock Medical
Center
Lebanon, New Hampshire

Hayrettin Köymen
Bilkent University
Ankara, Turkey

Luis G. Kun
IRMC/National Defense
University
Washington, D.C.

Phani Teja Kuruganti
RF and Microwave Systems Group
Oak Ridge National Laboratory
Oak Ridge, Tennessee

Kenneth K. Kwong
Massachusetts General Hospital
Harvard University Medical
School
Boston, Massachusetts

Z.R. Li
South China Normal University
Guangzhou, China

Richard F. Little
National Institutes of Health
Bethesda, Maryland

Chung-Chiun Liu
Electronics Design Center and
    Edison Sensor Technology
    Center
Case Western Reserve University
Cleveland, Ohio

Zhongqi Liu
TTM Management Group
Beijing, China

Jasper Lupo
Applied Research Associates, Inc.
Falls Church, Virginia

Albert Macovski
Stanford University
Stanford, California

Luca T. Mainardi
Polytechnic University
Milan, Italy

C. Manohar
Department of Electrical &
    Computer Engineering
University of Houston
Houston, Texas

Joseph P. McClain
Walter Reed Army Medical Center
Washington, D.C.

Kathleen A. McCormick
SAIC
Falls Church, Virginia

Dennis McGrath
Department of Plastic Surgery
Dartmouth-Hitchcock Medical
    Center
Lebanon, New Hampshire

Susan McGrath
Department of Plastic Surgery
Dartmouth-Hitchcock Medical
    Center
Lebanon, New Hampshire

Matthew F. McKnight
Department of Plastic Surgery
Dartmouth-Hitchcock Medical
    Center
Lebanon, New Hampshire

Yitzhak Mendelson
Worcester Polytechnic Institute
Worcester, Massachusetts

James B. Mercer
University of Tromsø
Tromsø, Norway

Arcangelo Merla
Department of Clinical Sciences
    and Bioimaging
University "G.d'Annunzio"
and
Institute for Advanced Biomedical
    Technology
Foundation "G.d'Annunzio"
and
Istituto Nazionale Fisica della
    Materia
Coordinated Group of Chieti
Chieti-Pescara, Italy

Evangelia Micheli-Tzanakou
Rutgers Unversity
Piscataway, New Jersey

Robert L. Morris
Dybonics, Inc.
Portland, Oregon

Jack G. Mottley
University of Rochester
Rochester, New York

Robin Murray
University of Rhode Island
Kingston, Rhode Island

Joachim H. Nagel
University of Stuttgart
Stuttgart, Germany

Michael R. Neuman
Michigan Technological
    University
Houghton, Michigan

E.Y.K. Ng
College of Engineering
School of Mechanical and
    Production Engineering
Nanyang Technological University
Singapore

Paul Norton
U.S. Army Communications and
    Electronics Research,
    Development and Engineering
    Center (CERDEC)
Night Vision and Electronic
    Sensors Directorate
Fort Belvoir, Virginia

Antoni Nowakowski
Department of Biomedical
    Engineering,
Gdansk University of Technology
Narutowicza
Gdansk, Poland

Banu Onaral
Drexel University
Philadelphia, Pennsylvania

David D. Pascoe
Auburn University
Auburn, Alabama

Maqbool Patel
Center for Magnetic Resonance
    Research
and
The University of Minnesota
    Medical School
Minneapolis, Minnesota

Robert Patterson
The University of Minnesota
Minneapolis, Minnesota

Jeffrey L. Paul
Defense Advanced Research
    Projects Agency
Arlington, Virginia

A. William Paulsen
Emory University
Atlanta, Georgia

John Pauly
Stanford University
Stanford, California

I. Pavlidis
Department of Computer Science
University of Houston
Houston, Texas

P. Hunter Peckham
Case Western Reserve University
Cleveland, Ohio

Joseph G. Pellegrino
U.S. Army Communications and
    Electronics Research,
    Development and Engineering
    Center (CERDEC)
Night Vision and Electronic
    Sensors Directorate
Fort Belvoir, Virginia

Philip Perconti
U.S. Army Communications and
    Electronics Research,
    Development and Engineering
    Center (CERDEC)
Night Vision and Electronic
    Sensors Directorate
Fort Belvoir, Virginia

Athina P. Petropulu
Drexel University
Philadelphia, Pennsylvania

Tom Piantanida
Greenleaf Medical
Palo Alto, California

T. Allan Pryor
University of Utah
Salt Lake City, Utah

Ram C. Purohit
Auburn University
Auburn, Alabama

Hairong Qi
ECE Department
The University of Tennessee
Knoxville, Tennessee

Pat Ridgely
Medtronic, Inc.
Minneapolis, Minnesota

E. Francis Ring
Medical Imaging Research Group
School of Computing
University of Glamorgan
Pontypridd, Wales
United Kingdom

Richard L. Roa
Baylor University Medical Center
Dallas, Texas

Peter Robbie
Department of Plastic Surgery
Dartmouth-Hitchcock Medical
    Center
Lebanon, New Hampshire

Gian Luca Romani
Department of Clinical Sciences
    and Bioimaging
University "G. d'Annunzio"
and
Institute for Advanced
    Biomedical Technology
Foundation "G.d'Annunzio"
and
Istituto Nazionale Fisica della
    Materia
Coordinated Group of Chieti
Chieti-Pescara, Italy

Joseph M. Rosen
Department of Plastic Surgery
Dartmouth-Hitchcock Medical
    Center
Lebanon, New Hampshire

Eric Rosow
Hartford Hospital
and
Premise Development
    Corporation
Hartford, Connecticut

Subrata Saha
Clemson University
Clemson, South Carolina

John Schenck
General Electric Corporate
    Research and Development
    Center
Schenectady, New York

Edward Schuck
EdenTec Corporation
Eden Prairie, Minnesota

Joyce Sensmeier
HIMSS
Chicago, Illinois

David Sherman
Johns Hopkins School of Medicine
Baltimore, Maryland

Robert E. Shroy, Jr.
Picker International
Highland Heights, Ohio

Stephen W. Smith
Duke University
Durham, North Carolina

Nathan J. Sniadecki
Department of Bioengineering
University of Pennsylvania
Philadelphia, Pennsylvania

Wesley E. Snyder
ECE Department
North Carolina State University
Raleigh, North Carolina

Orhan Soykan
Corporate Science and
    Technology
Medtronic, Inc.
and
Department of Biomedical
    Engineering
Michigan Technological
    University
Houghton, Michigan

Primoz Strojnik
Case Western Reserve University
Cleveland, Ohio

M. Strzelecki
Technical University of Lodz
Lodz, Poland

Ron Summers
Loughborough University
Leicestershire, United Kingdom

Christopher Swift
Department of Plastic Surgery
Dartmouth-Hitchcock Medical
    Center
Lebanon, New Hampshire

Willis A. Tacker
Purdue University
West Lafayette, Indiana

Nitish V. Thakor
Johns Hopkins School of Medicine
Baltimore, Maryland

Roderick Thomas
Faculty of Applied Design and
    Engineering
Swansea Institute of Technology
Swansea, United Kingdom

P. Tsiamyrtzis
Department of Statistics
University of Economics and
    Business Athens
Athens, Greece

Benjamin M.W. Tsui
University of North Carolina
Chapel Hill, North Carolina

Tracy A. Turner
Private Practice
Minneapolis, Minnesota

Kamil Ugurbil
Center for Magnetic Resonance
    Research
and
The University of Minnesota
    Medical School
Minneapolis, Minnesota

Michael S. Van Lysel
University of Wisconsin
Madison, Wisconsin

Henry F. VanBrocklin
University of California-Berkeley
Berkeley, California

Jay Vizgaitis
U.S. Army Communications and
    Electronics Research,
    Development and Engineering
    Center (CERDEC)
Night Vision and Electronic
    Sensors Directorate
Fort Belvoir, Virginia

Abby Vogel
Laboratory of Integrative and
    Medical Biophysics
National Institute of Child Health
    and Human Development
Bethesda, Maryland

Wolf W. von Maltzahn
Rensselaer Polytechnic Institute
Troy, New York

Gregory I. Voss
IVAC Corporation
San Diego, California

Alvin Wald
Columbia University
New York, New York

Chen Wang
TTM International
Houston, Texas

Lois de Weerd
University Hospital of
    North Norway
Tromsø, Norway

Wang Wei
Radiology Department
Beijing You An Hospital
Beijing, China

B. Wiecek
Technical University of Lodz
Lodz, Poland

M. Wysocki
Technical University of Lodz
Lodz, Poland

Martin J. Yaffe
University of Toronto
Toronto, Ontario, Canada

Robert Yarchoan
HIV and AIDS Malignancy
    Branch
Center for Cancer Research
National Cancer Institute (NCI)
Bethesda, Maryland

M. Yassa
Ville Marie Multidisciplinary
    Breast and Oncology Center
St. Mary's Hospital
McGill University
Montreal, Quebec, Canada
and
London Cancer Centre
London, Ontario, Canada

Christopher M. Yip
Departments of Chemical
    Engineering and Applied
    Chemistry
Department of Biochemistry
Institute of Biomaterials and
    Biomedical Engineering
University of Toronto
Toronto, Ontario, Canada

E. Yu
Ville Marie Multidisciplinary
    Breast and Oncology Center
St. Mary's Hospital
McGill University
Montreal, Quebec, Canada
and
London Cancer Centre
London, Ontario, Canada

Wen Yu
Shanghai RuiJin Hospital
Shanghai, China

Yune Yuan
Institute of Basic Medical Science
China Army General Hospital
Beijing, China

Jason Zeibel
U.S. Army Communications and
    Electronics Research,
    Development and Engineering
    Center (CERDEC)
Night Vision and Electronic
    Sensors Directorate
Fort Belvoir, Virginia

Yi Zeng
Central Disease Control of China
Beijing, China

Xiaohong Zhou
Duke University Medical Center
Durham, North Carolina

Yulin Zhou
Shanghai RuiJin Hospital
Shanghai, China

Contents

SECTION I   Biomedical Signal Analysis

Banu Onaral

1   Biomedical Signals: Origin and Dynamic Characteristics;
Frequency-Domain Analysis
Arnon Cohen **1**-1

2   Digital Biomedical Signal Acquisition and Processing
Luca T. Mainardi, Anna M. Bianchi, Sergio Cerutti **2**-1

3   Compression of Digital Biomedical Signals
A. Enis Çetin, Hayrettin Köymen **3**-1

4   Time-Frequency Signal Representations for
Biomedical Signals
G. Faye Boudreaux-Bartels, Robin Murray **4**-1

5   Wavelet (Time-Scale) Analysis in Biomedical
Signal Processing
Nitish V. Thakor, Boris Gramatikov, David Sherman . . . **5**-1

6   Higher-Order Spectral Analysis
Athina P. Petropulu **6**-1

7   Neural Networks in Biomedical Signal Processing
Evangelia Micheli-Tzanakou **7**-1

8   Complexity, Scaling, and Fractals in Biomedical Signals
Banu Onaral, Joseph P. Cammarota **8**-1

9   Future Directions: Biomedical Signal Processing and
Networked Multimedia Communications
Banu Onaral **9**-1

SECTION II Imaging

Warren S. Grundfest

10 X-Ray
   Robert E. Shroy, Jr., Michael S. Van Lysel,
   Martin J. Yaffe **10**-1

11 Computed Tomography
   Ian A. Cunningham, Philip F. Judy **11**-1

12 Magnetic Resonance Imaging
   Steven Conolly, Albert Macovski, John Pauly, John Schenck,
   Kenneth K. Kwong, David A. Chesler, Xiaoping Hu,
   Wei Chen, Maqbool Patel, Kamil Ugurbil **12**-1

13 Nuclear Medicine
   Barbara Y. Croft, Benjamin M.W. Tsui **13**-1

14 Ultrasound
   Richard L. Goldberg, Stephen W. Smith, Jack G. Mottley,
   K. Whittaker Ferrara **14**-1

15 Magnetic Resonance Microscopy
   Xiaohong Zhou, G. Allan Johnson **15**-1

16 Positron-Emission Tomography (PET)
   Thomas F. Budinger, Henry F. VanBrocklin **16**-1

17 Electrical Impedance Tomography
   D.C. Barber **17**-1

18 Medical Applications of Virtual Reality Technology
   Walter Greenleaf, Tom Piantanida **18**-1

SECTION III Infrared Imaging

Nicholas A. Diakides

19 Advances in Medical Infrared Imaging
   Nicholas Diakides, Mary Diakides, Jasper Lupo,
   Jeffrey L. Paul, Raymond Balcerak **19**-1

20 The Historical Development of Thermometry
   and Thermal Imaging in Medicine
   E. Francis Ring, Bryan F. Jones **20**-1

21 Physiology of Thermal Signals
    David D. Pascoe, James B. Mercer, Lois de Weerd **21**-1

22 Quantitative Active Dynamic Thermal IR-Imaging and
    Thermal Tomography in Medical Diagnostics
    Antoni Nowakowski **22**-1

23 Thermal Texture Maps (TTM): Concept, Theory, and
    Applications
    Zhongqi Liu, Chen Wang, Hairong Qi, Yune Yuan, Yi Zeng,
    Z.R. Li, Yulin Zhou, Wen Yu, Wang Wei **23**-1

24 IR Imagers as Fever Monitoring Devices: Physics,
    Physiology, and Clinical Accuracy
    E.Y.K. Ng, G.J.L. Kaw **24**-1

25 Infrared Imaging of the Breast — An Overview
    William C. Amalu, William B. Hobbins, Jonathan F. Head,
    Robert L. Elliott **25**-1

26 Functional Infrared Imaging of the Breast:
    Historical Perspectives, Current Application, and
    Future Considerations
    J.R. Keyserlingk, P.D. Ahlgren, E. Yu, N. Belliveau,
    M. Yassa **26**-1

27 Detecting Breast Cancer from Thermal Infrared Images by
    Asymmetry Analysis
    Hairong Qi, Phani Teja Kuruganti, Wesley E. Snyder . . . **27**-1

28 Advanced Thermal Image Processing
    B. Wiecek, M. Strzelecki, T. Jakubowska, M. Wysocki,
    C. Drews-Peszynski **28**-1

29 Biometrics: Face Recognition in Thermal Infrared
    I. Pavlidis, P. Tsiamyrtzis, P. Buddharaju, C. Manohar . . . **29**-1

30 Infrared Imaging for Tissue Characterization and Function
    Moinuddin Hassan, Victor Chernomordik, Abby Vogel,
    David Hattery, Israel Gannot, Richard F. Little,
    Robert Yarchoan, Amir H. Gandjbakhche **30**-1

31 Thermal Imaging in Diseases of the Skeletal and
    Neuromuscular Systems
    E. Francis Ring, Kurt Ammer **31**-1

32 Functional Infrared Imaging in Clinical Applications
    Arcangelo Merla, Gian Luca Romani **32**-1

33 Thermal Imaging in Surgery
    Paul Campbell, Roderick Thomas **33**-1

34 Infrared Imaging Applied to Dentistry
    Barton M. Gratt **34**-1

35 Use of Infrared Imaging in Veterinary Medicine
    Ram C. Purohit, Tracy A. Turner, David D. Pascoe **35**-1

36 Standard Procedures for Infrared Imaging in Medicine
    Kurt Ammer, E. Francis Ring **36**-1

37 Infrared Detectors and Detector Arrays
    Paul Norton, Stuart Horn, Joseph G. Pellegrino,
    Philip Perconti **37**-1

38 Infrared Camera Characterization
    Joseph G. Pellegrino, Jason Zeibel, Ronald G. Driggers,
    Philip Perconti **38**-1

39 Infrared Camera and Optics for Medical Applications
    Michael W. Grenn, Jay Vizgaitis, Joseph G. Pellegrino,
    Philip Perconti **39**-1

SECTION IV   Medical Informatics

Luis G. Kun

40 Hospital Information Systems: Their Function and State
    T. Allan Pryor **40**-1

41 Computer-Based Patient Records
    J. Michael Fitzmaurice **41**-1

42 Overview of Standards Related to the Emerging Health Care
    Information Infrastructure
    Jeffrey S. Blair **42**-1

43 Introduction to Informatics and Nursing
    Kathleen A. McCormick, Joyce Sensmeier,
    Connie White Delaney, Carol J. Bickford **43**-1

44 Non-AI Decision Making
    Ron Summers, Derek G. Cramp, Ewart R. Carson **44**-1

45 Medical Informatics and Biomedical Emergencies: New
Training and Simulation Technologies for First Responders
Joseph M. Rosen, Christopher Swift, Eliot B. Grigg,
Matthew F. McKnight, Susan McGrath, Dennis McGrath,
Peter Robbie, C. Everett Koop **45**-1

SECTION V Biomedical Sensors

Michael R. Neuman

46 Physical Measurements
Michael R. Neuman **46**-1

47 Biopotential Electrodes
Michael R. Neuman **47**-1

48 Electrochemical Sensors
Chung-Chiun Liu **48**-1

49 Optical Sensors
Yitzhak Mendelson **49**-1

50 Bioanalytic Sensors
Richard P. Buck **50**-1

51 Biological Sensors for Diagnostics
Orhan Soykan **51**-1

SECTION VI Medical Instruments and Devices

Wolf W. von Maltzahn

52 Biopotential Amplifiers
Joachim H. Nagel **52**-1

53 Bioelectric Impedance Measurements
Robert Patterson **53**-1

54 Implantable Cardiac Pacemakers
Michael Forde, Pat Ridgely **54**-1

55 Noninvasive Arterial Blood Pressure and Mechanics
Gary Drzewiecki **55**-1

56 Cardiac Output Measurement
   Leslie A. Geddes **56**-1

57 External Defibrillators
   Willis A. Tacker **57**-1

58 Implantable Defibrillators
   Edwin G. Duffin **58**-1

59 Implantable Stimulators for Neuromuscular Control
   Primoz Strojnik, P. Hunter Peckham **59**-1

60 Respiration
   Leslie A. Geddes **60**-1

61 Mechanical Ventilation
   Khosrow Behbehani **61**-1

62 Essentials of Anesthesia Delivery
   A. William Paulsen **62**-1

63 Electrosurgical Devices
   Jeffrey L. Eggleston, Wolf W. von Maltzahn **63**-1

64 Biomedical Lasers
   Millard M. Judy **64**-1

65 Instrumentation for Cell Mechanics
   Nathan J. Sniadecki, Christopher S. Chen **65**-1

66 Blood Glucose Monitoring
   David D. Cunningham **66**-1

67 Atomic Force Microscopy: Probing Biomolecular
   Interactions
   Christopher M. Yip **67**-1

68 Parenteral Infusion Devices
   Gregory I. Voss, Robert D. Butterfield **68**-1

69 Clinical Laboratory: Separation and Spectral Methods
   Richard L. Roa **69**-1

70 Clinical Laboratory: Nonspectral Methods and Automation
   Richard L. Roa **70**-1

71 Noninvasive Optical Monitoring
   Ross Flewelling **71**-1

72 Medical Instruments and Devices Used in the Home
Bruce R. Bowman, Edward Schuck 72-1

73 Virtual Instrumentation: Applications in Biomedical
Engineering
Eric Rosow, Joseph Adam 73-1

SECTION VII Clinical Engineering

Yadin David

74 Clinical Engineering: Evolution of a Discipline
Joseph D. Bronzino 74-1

75 Management and Assessment of Medical Technology
Yadin David, Thomas M. Judd 75-1

76 Risk Factors, Safety, and Management of Medical Equipment
Michael L. Gullikson 76-1

77 Clinical Engineering Program Indicators
Dennis D. Autio, Robert L. Morris 77-1

78 Quality of Improvement and Team Building
Joseph P. McClain 78-1

79 A Standards Primer for Clinical Engineers
Alvin Wald 79-1

80 Regulatory and Assessment Agencies
Mark E. Bruley, Vivian H. Coates 80-1

81 Applications of Virtual Instruments in Health Care
Eric Rosow, Joseph Adam 81-1

SECTION VIII Ethical Issues Associated with the Use of Medical Technology

Subrata Saha and Joseph D. Bronzino

82 Beneficence, Nonmaleficence, and Medical Technology
Joseph D. Bronzino 82-1

83 Ethical Issues Related to Clinical Research
Joseph D. Bronzino 83-1

Index I-1

I

Biomedical Signal Analysis

Banu Onaral
Drexel University

1 Biomedical Signals: Origin and Dynamic Characteristics; Frequency-Domain Analysis
Arnon Cohen 1-1

2 Digital Biomedical Signal Acquisition and Processing
Luca T. Mainardi, Sergio Cerutti, Anna M. Bianchi 2-1

3 Compression of Digital Biomedical Signals
A. Enis Çetin, Hayrettin Köymen 3-1

4 Time–Frequency Signal Representations for Biomedical Signals
G. Faye Boudreaux-Bartels, Robin Murray 4-1

5 Wavelet (Time-Scale) Analysis in Biomedical Signal Processing
Nitish V. Thakor, Boris Gramatikov, David Sherman 5-1

6 Higher-Order Spectral Analysis
Athina P. Petropulu 6-1

7 Neural Networks in Biomedical Signal Processing
Evangelia Micheli-Tzanakou 7-1

8 Complexity, Scaling, and Fractals in Biomedical Signals
Banu Onaral, Joseph P. Cammarota 8-1

9   Future Directions: Biomedical Signal Processing and Networked
         Multimedia Communications
         Banu Onaral **9**-1

BIOMEDICAL SIGNAL ANALYSIS CENTERS on the acquisition and processing of information-bearing signals that emanate from living systems. These vital signals permit us to probe the state of the underlying biologic and physiologic structures and dynamics. Therefore, their interpretation has significant diagnostic value for clinicians and researchers.

The detected signals are commonly corrupted with noise. Often, the information cannot be readily extracted from the raw signal, which must be processed in order to yield useful results. Signals and systems engineering knowledge and, in particular, signal-processing expertise are therefore critical in all phases of signal collection and analysis.

Biomedical engineers are called on to conceive and implement processing schemes suitable for biomedical signals. They also play a key role in the design and development of biomedical monitoring devices and systems that match advances in signal processing and instrumentation technologies with biomedical needs and requirements.

This section is organized in two main parts. In the first part, contributing authors review contemporary methods in biomedical signal processing. The second part is devoted to emerging methods that hold the promise for major enhancements in our ability to extract information from vital signals.

The success of signal-processing applications strongly depends on the knowledge about the origin and the nature of the signal. Biomedical signals possess many special properties and hence require special treatment. Also, the need for noninvasive measurements presents unique challenges that demand a clear understanding of biomedical signal characteristics. In the lead chapter, entitled, "Biomedical Signals: Origin and Dynamic Characteristics; Frequency-Domain Analysis," Arnon Cohen provides a general classification of biomedical signals and discusses basics of frequency domain methods.

The advent of digital computing coupled with fast progress in discrete-time signal processing has led to efficient and flexible methods to acquire and treat biomedical data in digital form. The chapter entitled, "Digital Biomedical Signal Acquisition and Processing," by Luca T. Mainardi, Anna M. Bianchi, and Sergio Cerutti, presents basic elements of signal acquisition and processing in the special context of biomedical signals.

Especially in the case of long-term monitoring, digital biomedical signal-processing applications generate vast amounts of data that strain transmission and storage resources. The creation of multipatient reference signal bases also places severe demands on storage. Data compression methods overcome these obstacles by eliminating signal redundancies while retaining clinically significant information. A. Enis Cetin and Hayrettin Köymen provide a comparative overview of a range of approaches from conventional to modern compression techniques suitable for biomedical signals. Futuristic applications involving long-term and ambulatory recording systems, and remote diagnosis opportunities will be made possible by breakthroughs in biomedical data compression. This chapter serves well as a point of departure.

Constraints such as stationarity (and time invariance), gaussianity (and minimum phaseness), and the assumption of a characteristic scale in time and space have constituted the basic, and by now implicit, assumptions upon which the conventional signals and systems theories have been founded. However, investigators engaged in the study of biomedical processes have long known that they did not hold under most realistic situations and hence could not sustain the test of practice.

Rejecting or at least relaxing restrictive assumptions always opens new avenues for research and yields fruitful results. Liberating forces in signals and systems theories have conspired in recent years to create research fronts that target long-standing constraints in the established wisdom (dogma?) of classic signal processing and system analysis. The emergence of new fields in signals and system theories that address these shortcomings and aim to relax these restrictions has been motivated by scientists who, rather than mold natural behavior into artificial models, seek methods inherently suited to represent reality. Biomedical scientists and engineers are inspired by insights gained from a deeper appreciation for the dynamic richness displayed by biomedical phenomena; hence, more than their counterparts in other disciplines, they more forcefully embrace innovations in signal processing.

One of these novel directions is concerned with time–frequency representations tailored for non-stationary and transient signals. Faye Boudreaux-Bartels and Robin Murray address this issue, provide an introduction to concepts and tools of time–frequency analysis, and point out candidate applications.

Many physiologic structures and dynamics defy the concept of a characteristic spatial and temporal scale and must be dealt with employing methods compatible with their multiscale nature. Judging from the recent success of biomedical signal-processing applications based on time-scale analysis and wavelet transforms, the resolution of many outstanding processing issues may be at hand. The chapter entitled, "Time-Scale Analysis and Wavelets in Biomedical Signals," by Nitish V. Thakor, familiarizes the reader with fundamental concepts and methods of wavelet analysis and suggests fruitful directions in biomedical signal processing.

The presence of nonlinearities and statistics that do not comply with the gaussianity assumption and the desire for phase reconstruction have been the moving forces behind investigations of higher-order statistics and polyspectra in signal-processing and system-identification fields. An introduction to the topic and potential uses in biomedical signal-processing applications are presented by Athina Petropulu in the chapter entitled, "Higher-Order Spectra in Biomedical Signal Processing."

Neural networks derive their cue from biologic systems and, in turn, mimic many of the functions of the nervous system. Simple networks can filter, recall, switch, amplify, and recognize patterns and hence serve well many signal-processing purposes. In the chapter entitled, "Neural Networks in Biomedical Signal Processing," Evangelia Tzanakou helps the reader explore the power of the approach while stressing how biomedical signal-processing applications benefit from incorporating neural-network principles.

The dichotomy between order and disorder is now perceived as a ubiquitous property inherent in the unfolding of many natural complex phenomena. In the last decade, it has become clear that the common threads shared by natural forms and functions are the "physics of disorder" and the "scaling order," the hallmark of broad classes of fractal entities. Biomedical signals are the global observables of underlying complex physical and physiologic processes. "Complexity" theories therefore hold the potential to provide mathematical tools that describe and possibly shed light on the internal workings of physiologic systems. In the next to last chapter in this section, Banu Onaral and Joseph P. Cammarota introduce the reader to basic tenets of complexity theories and the attendant scaling concepts with hopes to facilitate their integration into the biomedical engineering practice.

The section concludes with a brief chapter on the visions of the future when biomedical signal processing will merge with the rising technologies in telecommunication and multimedia computing, and eventually with virtual reality, to enable remote monitoring, diagnosis, and intervention. The impact of this development on the delivery of health care and the quality of life will no doubt be profound. The promise of biomedical signal analysis will then be fulfilled.

1
Biomedical Signals: Origin and Dynamic Characteristics; Frequency-Domain Analysis

1.1	Origin of Biomedical Signals	1-2
1.2	Classification of Biosignals	1-3
1.3	Stochastic Signals	1-5
1.4	Frequency-Domain Analysis	1-7
1.5	Discrete Signals	1-9
1.6	Data Windows	1-11
1.7	Short-Time Fourier Transform	1-12
1.8	Spectral Estimation	1-13
	The Blackman–Tukey Method • The Periodogram • Time-Series Analysis Methods	
1.9	Signal Enhancement	1-15
1.10	Optimal Filtering	1-16
	Minimization of Mean Squared Error: The Wiener Filter • Maximization of the Signal-to-Noise Ratio: The Matched Filter	
1.11	Adaptive Filtering	1-18
1.12	Segmentation of Nonstationary Signals	1-21
	References	1-22

Arnon Cohen
Ben-Gurion University

A signal is a phenomenon that conveys information. Biomedical signals are signals, used in biomedical fields, mainly for extracting information on a biologic system under investigation. The complete process of information extraction may be as simple as a physician estimating the patient's mean heart rate by feeling, with the fingertips, the blood pressure pulse or as complex as analyzing the structure of internal soft tissues by means of a complex CT machine.

Most often in biomedical applications (as in many other applications), the acquisition of the signal is not sufficient. It is required to process the acquired signal to get the relevant information "buried" in it.

This may be due to the fact that the signal is noisy and thus must be "cleaned" (or in more professional terminology, the signal has to be enhanced) or due to the fact that the relevant information is not "visible" in the signal. In the latter case, we usually apply some transformation to enhance the required information.

The processing of biomedical signals poses some unique problems. The reason for this is mainly the complexity of the underlying system and the need to perform indirect, noninvasive measurements. A large number of processing methods and algorithms is available. In order to apply the best method, the user must know the goal of the processing, the test conditions, and the characteristics of the underlying signal. In this chapter, the characteristics of biomedical signals will be discussed [Cohen, 1986]. Biomedical signals will be divided into characteristic classes, requiring different classes of processing methods. Also in this chapter, the basics of frequency-domain processing methods will be presented.

1.1   Origin of Biomedical Signals

From the broad definition of the biomedical signal presented in the preceding section, it is clear that biomedical signals differ from other signals only in terms of the application — signals that are used in the biomedical field. As such, biomedical signals originate from a variety of sources. The following is a brief description of these sources:

1. *Bioelectric signals.* The bioelectric signal is unique to biomedical systems. It is generated by nerve cells and muscle cells. Its source is the membrane potential, which under certain conditions may be excited to generate an action potential. In single cell measurements, where specific microelectrodes are used as sensors, the action potential itself is the biomedical signal. In more gross measurements, where, for example, surface electrodes are used as sensors, the electric field generated by the action of many cells, distributed in the electrode's vicinity, constitutes the bioelectric signal. Bioelectric signals are probably the most important biosignals. The fact that most important biosystems use excitable cells makes it possible to use biosignals to study and monitor the main functions of the systems. The electric field propagates through the biologic medium, and thus the potential may be acquired at relatively convenient locations on the surface, eliminating the need to invade the system. The bioelectric signal requires a relatively simple transducer for its acquisition. A transducer is needed because the electric conduction in the biomedical medium is done by means of ions, while the conduction in the measurement system is by electrons. All these lead to the fact that the bioelectric signal is widely used in most fields of biomedicine.

2. *Bioimpedance signals.* The impedance of the tissue contains important information concerning its composition, blood volume, blood distribution, endocrine activity, automatic nervous system activity, and more. The bioimpedance signal is usually generated by injecting into the tissue under test sinusoidal currents (frequency range of 50 kHz–1 MHz, with low current densities of the order of 20–20 mA). The frequency range is chosen to minimize electrode polarization problems, and the low current densities are chosen to avoid tissue damage mainly due to heating effects. Bioimpedance measurements are usually performed with four electrodes. Two source electrodes are connected to a current source and are used to inject the current into the tissue. The two measurement electrodes are placed on the tissue under investigation and are used to measure the voltage drop generated by the current and the tissue impedance.

3. *Bioacoustic signals.* Many biomedical phenomena create acoustic noise. The measurement of this acoustic noise provides information about the underlying phenomenon. The flow of blood in the heart, through the heart's valves, or through blood vessels generates typical acoustic noise. The flow of air through the upper and lower airways and in the lungs creates acoustic sounds. These sounds, known as coughs, snores, and chest and lung sounds, are used extensively in medicine. Sounds are also generated in the digestive tract and in the joints. It also has been observed that the contracting muscle produces an acoustic noise (muscle noise). Since the acoustic energy propagates through the biologic medium, the bioacoustic signal may be conveniently acquired on the surface, using acoustic transducers (microphones or accelerometers).

4. *Biomagnetic signals.* Various organs, such as the brain, heart, and lungs, produce extremely weak magnetic fields. The measurements of these fields provides information not included in other biosignals

(such as bioelectric signals). Due to the low level of the magnetic fields to be measured, biomagnetic signals are usually of very low signal-to-noise ratio. Extreme caution must be taken in designing the acquisition system of these signals.

5. *Biomechanical signals.* The term biomechanical signals includes all signals used in the biomedicine fields that originate from some mechanical function of the biologic system. These signals include motion and displacement signals, pressure and tension and flow signals, and others. The measurement of biomechanical signals requires a variety of transducers, not always simple and inexpensive. The mechanical phenomenon does not propagate, as do the electric, magnetic, and acoustic fields. The measurement therefore usually has to be performed at the exact site. This very often complicates the measurement and forces it to be an invasive one.

6. *Biochemical signals.* Biochemical signals are the result of chemical measurements from the living tissue or from samples analyzed in the clinical laboratory. Measuring the concentration of various ions inside and in the vicinity of a cell by means of specific ion electrodes is an example of such a signal. Partial pressures of oxygen (pO_2) and carbon dioxide (pCO_2) in the blood or respiratory system are other examples. Biochemical signals are most often very low frequency signals. Most biochemical signals are actually dc signals.

7. *Biooptical signals.* Biooptical signals are the result of optical functions of the biologic system, occurring naturally or induced by the measurement. Blood oxygenation may be estimated by measuring the transmitted and backscattered light from a tissue (*in vivo* and *in vitro*) in several wavelengths. Important information about the fetus may be acquired by measuring fluorescence characteristics of the amniotic fluid. Estimation of the heart output may be performed by the dye dilution method, which requires the monitoring of the appearance of recirculated dye in the bloodstream. The development of fiberoptic technology has opened vast applications of biooptical signals.

Table 1.1 lists some of the more common biomedical signals with some of their characteristics.

1.2 Classification of Biosignals

Biosignals may be classified in many ways. The following is a brief discussion of some of the most important classifications.

1. *Classification according to source.* Biosignals may be classified according to their source or physical nature. This classification was described in the preceding section. This classification may be used when the basic physical characteristics of the underlying process is of interest, for example, when a model for the signal is desired.

2. *Classification according to biomedical application.* The biomedical signal is acquired and processed with some diagnostic, monitoring, or other goal in mind. Classification may be constructed according to the field of application, for example, cardiology or neurology. Such classification may be of interest when the goal is, for example, the study of physiologic systems.

3. *Classification according to signal characteristics.* From point of view of signal analysis, this is the most relevant classification method. When the main goal is processing, it is not relevant what is the source of the signal or to which biomedical system it belongs; what matters are the signal characteristics.

We recognize two broad classes of signals: continuous signals and discrete signals. Continuous signals are described by a continuous function $s(t)$ which provides information about the signal at any given time. Discrete signals are described by a sequence $s(m)$ which provides information at a given discrete point on the time axis. Most of the biomedical signals are continuous. Since current technology provides powerful tools for discrete signal processing, we most often transform a continuous signal into a discrete one by a process known as sampling. A given signal $s(t)$ is sampled into the sequence $s(m)$ by

$$s(m) = s(t)|_{t=mT_s} \quad m = \ldots, -1, 0, 1, \ldots \tag{1.1}$$

TABLE 1.1 Biomedical Signals

Classification	Acquisition	Frequency range	Dynamic range	Comments
Bioelectric				
Action potential	Microelectrodes	100 Hz–2 kHz	10 μV–100 mV	Invasive measurement of cell membrane potential
Electroneurogram (ENG)	Needle electrode	100 Hz–1 kHz	5 μV–10 mV	Potential of a nerve bundle
Electroretinogram (ERG)	Microelectrode	0.2–200 Hz	0.5 μV–1 mV	Evoked flash potential
Electro-oculogram (EOG)	Surface electrodes	dc–100 Hz	10 μV–5 mV	Steady-corneal-retinal potential
Electroencephalogram (EEG)				
Surface	Surface electrodes	0.5–100 Hz	2–100 μV	Multichannel (6–32) scalp potential
Delta range		0.5–4 Hz		Young children, deep sleep and pathologies
Theta range		4–8 Hz		Temporal and central areas during alert states
Alpha range		8–13 Hz		Awake, relaxed, closed eyes
Beta range		13–22 Hz		
Sleep spindles		6–15 Hz	50–100 μV	Bursts of about 0.2–0.6 sec
K-complexes		12–14 Hz	100–200 μV	Bursts during moderate and deep sleep
Evoked potentials (EP)	Surface electrodes		0.1–20 μV	Response of brain potential to stimulus
Visual (VEP)		1–300 Hz	1–20 μV	Occipital lobe recordings, 200-msec duration
Somatosensory (SEP)		2 Hz–3 kHz		Sensory cortex
Auditory (AEP)		100 Hz–3 kHz	0.5–10 μV	Vertex recordings
Electrocorticogram	Needle electrodes	100 Hz–5 kHz		Recordings from exposed surface of brain
Electromyography (EMG)				
Single-fiber (SFEMG)	Needle electrode	500 Hz–10 kHz	1–10 μV	Action potentials from single muscle fiber
Motor unit action potential (MUAP)	Needle electrode	5 Hz–10 kHz	100 μV–2 mV	
Surface EMG (SEMG)	Surface electrodes			
Skeletal muscle		2–500 Hz	50 μV–5 mV	
Smooth muscle		0.01–1 Hz		
Electrocardiogram (ECG)	Surface electrodes	0.05–100 Hz	1–10 mV	
High-frequency ECG	Surface electrodes	100 Hz–1 kHz	100 μV–2 mV	Notchs and slus waveforms superimposed on the ECG

where T_s is the sampling interval and $f_s = 2\pi/T_s$ is the sampling frequency. Further characteristic classification, which applies to continuous as well as discrete signals, is described in Figure 1.1.

We divide signals into two main groups: deterministic and stochastic signals. Deterministic signals are signals that can be exactly described mathematically or graphically. If a signal is deterministic and its mathematical description is given, it conveys no information. Real-world signals are never deterministic. There is always some unknown and unpredictable noise added, some unpredictable change in the parameters, and the underlying characteristics of the signal that render it nondeterministic. It is, however, very often convenient to approximate or model the signal by means of a deterministic function.

An important family of deterministic signals is the periodic family. A periodic signal is a deterministic signal that may be expressed by

$$s(t) = s(t + nT) \tag{1.2}$$

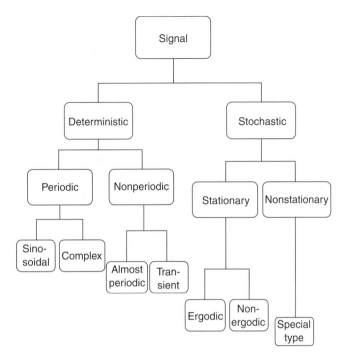

FIGURE 1.1   Classification of signals according to characteristics.

where n is an integer and T is the period. The periodic signal consists of a basic wave shape with a duration of T seconds. The basic wave shape repeats itself an infinite number of times on the time axis. The simplest periodic signal is the sinusoidal signal. Complex periodic signals have more elaborate wave shapes. Under some conditions, the blood pressure signal may be modeled by a complex periodic signal, with the heart rate as its period and the blood pressure wave shape as its basic wave shape. This is, of course, a very rough and inaccurate model.

Most deterministic functions are nonperiodic. It is sometimes worthwhile to consider an "almost periodic" type of signal. The ECG signal can sometimes be considered "almost periodic." The ECG's RR interval is never constant; in addition, the PQRST complex of one heartbeat is never exactly the same as that of another beat. The signal is definitely nonperiodic. Under certain conditions, however, the RR interval is almost constant, and one PQRST is almost the same as the other. The ECG may thus sometimes be modeled as "almost periodic."

1.3   Stochastic Signals

The most important class of signals is the stochastic class. A stochastic signal is a sample function of a stochastic process. The process produces sample functions, the infinite collection of which is called the ensemble. Each sample function differs from the other in it fine details; however, they all share the same distribution probabilities. Figure 1.2 depicts three sample functions of an ensemble. Note that at any given time, the values of the sample functions are different.

Stochastic signals cannot be expressed exactly; they can be described only in terms of probabilities which may be calculated over the ensemble. Assuming a signal $s(t)$, the Nth-order joint probability function

$$P[s(t_1) \leq s_1, s(t_2) \leq s_2, \ldots, s(t_N) \leq s_N] = P(s_1, s_2, \ldots, s_N) \tag{1.3}$$

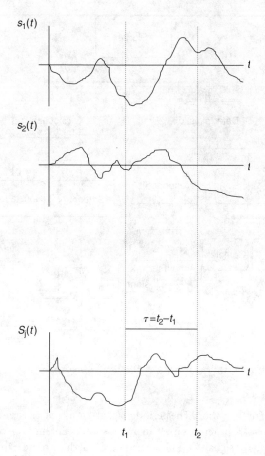

FIGURE 1.2   The ensemble of the stochastic process $s(t)$.

is the joint probability that the signal at time t_i will be less than or equal to S_i and at time t_j will be less than or equal to S_j, etc. This joint probability describes the statistical behavior and intradependence of the process. It is very often useful to work with the derivative of the joint probability function; this derivative is known as the joint probability density function (PDF):

$$p(s_1, s_2, \ldots, s_N) = \frac{\partial^N}{\partial s_1 \partial s_2 \mathrm{L} \partial s_N}[P(s_1, s_2, \ldots, s_N)] \tag{1.4}$$

Of particular interest are the first- and second-order PDFs.

The expectation of the process $s(t)$, denoted by $E\{s(t)\}$ or by m_s, is a statistical operator defined as

$$E\{s(t)\} = \int_{-\infty}^{\infty} sp(s)\,\mathrm{d}s = m \tag{1.5}$$

The expectation of the function $s^n(t)$ is known as the *nth-order moment*. The first-order moment is thus the expectation of the process. The nth-order moment is given by

$$E\{s^n(t)\} = \int_{-\infty}^{\infty} s^n p(s)\,\mathrm{d}s \tag{1.6}$$

Another important statistical operator is the *nth central moment*:

$$\mu_n = E\{(s - m_s)^n\} = \int_{-\infty}^{\infty} (s - m_s)^n p(s)\,ds \tag{1.7}$$

The second central moment is known as the *variance* (the square root of which is the standard deviation). The variance is denoted by σ^2:

$$\sigma^2 = \mu_2 = E\{(s - m_s)^2\} = \int_{-\infty}^{\infty} (s - m_s)^2 p(s)\,ds \tag{1.8}$$

The second-order joint moment is defined by the joint PDF. Of particular interest is the autocorrelation function r_{ss}:

$$r_{ss}(t_1, t_2) = E\{s(t_1)s(t_2)\} = \int_{-\infty}^{\infty} \int_{-\infty}^{\infty} s(t_1)s(t_2)p(s_1, s_2)\,ds_1\,ds_2 \tag{1.9}$$

The cross-correlation function is defined as the second joint moment of the signal s at time t_1, $s(t_1)$, and the signal y at time t_2, $y(t_2)$:

$$r_{sy}(t_1, t_2) = E\{s(t_1)y(t_2)\} = \int_{-\infty}^{\infty} \int_{-\infty}^{\infty} s(t_1)y(t_2)p(s_1, y_2)\,ds_1\,dy_2 \tag{1.10}$$

Stationary stochastic processes are processes whose statistics do not change in time. The expectation and the variance (as with any other statistical mean) of a stationary process will be time-independent. The autocorrelation function, for example, of a stationary process will thus be a function of the time difference $t = t_2 - t_1$ (one-dimensional function) rather than a function of t_2 and t_1 (two-dimensional function).

Ergodic stationary processes possess an important characteristic: Their statistical probability distributions (along the ensemble) equal those of their time distributions (along the time axis of any one of its sample functions). For example, the correlation function of an ergodic process may be calculated by its definition (along the ensemble) or along the time axis of any one of its sample functions:

$$r_{ss}(\tau) = E\{s(t)s(t - \tau)\} = \lim_{T \to \infty} \frac{1}{2T} \int_{-T}^{T} s(t)s(t - \tau)\,dt \tag{1.11}$$

The right side of Equation 1.11 is the time autocorrelation function.

Ergodic processes are nice because one does not need the ensemble for calculating the distributions; a single sample function is sufficient. From the point of view of processing, it is desirable to model the signal as an ergodic one. Unfortunately, almost all signals are nonstationary (and hence nonergodic). One must therefore use nonstationary processing methods (such as, for e.g., wavelet transformation) which are relatively complex or cut the signals into short-duration segments in such a way that each may be considered stationary.

The sleep EEG signal, for example, is a nonstationary signal. We may consider segments of the signal, in which the subject was at a given sleep state, as stationary. In order to describe the signal, we need to estimate its probability distributions. However, the ensemble is unavailable. If we further assume that the process is ergodic, the distributions may be estimated along the time axis of the given sample function. Most of the standard processing techniques assume the signal to be stationary and ergodic.

1.4 Frequency-Domain Analysis

Until now we have dealt with signals represented in the time domain, that is to say, we have described the signal by means of its value on the time axis. It is possible to use another representation for the same signal: that of the frequency domain. Any signal may be described as a continuum of sine waves having different amplitudes and phases. The frequency representation describes the signals by means of the amplitudes and phases of the sine waves. The transformation between the two representations is given by the *Fourier transform* (FT):

$$S(\omega) = \int_{-\infty}^{\infty} s(t)e^{-j\omega t}\, dt = F\{s(t)\} \qquad (1.12)$$

where $\omega = 2\pi f$ is the angular frequency, and $F\{*\}$ is the Fourier operator.

The *inverse Fourier transform* (IFT) is the operator that transforms a signal from the frequency domain into the time domain:

$$s(t) = \frac{1}{2\pi} \int_{-\infty}^{\infty} S(\omega)e^{j\omega t}\, dw = F^{-1}\{S(\omega)\} \qquad (1.13)$$

The frequency domain representation $S(\omega)$ is complex; hence

$$S(\omega) = |S(\omega)|e^{j\theta(\omega)} \qquad (1.14)$$

where $|S(\omega)|$, the absolute value of the complex function, is the amplitude spectrum, and $\theta(\omega)$, the phase of the complex function, is the phase spectrum. The square of the absolute value, $|S(\omega)|^2$, is termed the power spectrum. The power spectrum of a signal describes the distribution of the signal's power on the frequency axis. A signal in which the power is limited to a finite range of the frequency axis is called a band-limited signal. Figure 1.3 depicts an example of such a signal.

The signal in Figure 1.3 is a band-limited signal; its power spectrum is limited to the frequency range $-\omega_{max} \le \omega \le \omega_{max}$. It is easy to show that if $s(t)$ is real (which is the case in almost all applications), the amplitude spectrum is an even function and the phase spectrum is an odd function.

Special attention must be given to stochastic signals. Applying the FT to a sample function would provide a sample function on the frequency axis. The process may be described by the ensemble of spectra. Another alternative to the frequency representation is to consider the correlation function of the process. This function is deterministic. The FT may be applied to it, yielding a deterministic frequency function. The FT of the correlation function is defined as the power spectral density function (PSD):

$$PSD[s(t)] = S_{ss}(\omega) = F\{r_{ss}(\tau)\} = \int_{-\infty}^{\infty} r_{ss}(\tau)e^{-j\omega\tau}\, d\tau \qquad (1.15)$$

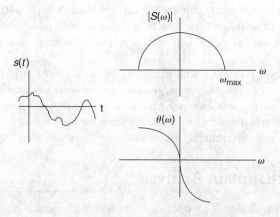

FIGURE 1.3 Example of a signal described in the time and frequency domains.

The PSD is used to describe stochastic signals; it describes the density of power on the frequency axis. Note that since the autocorrelation function is an even function, the PSD is real; hence no phase spectrum is required.

The EEG signal may serve as an example of the importance of the PSD in signal processing. When processing the EEG, it is very helpful to use the PSD. It turns out that the power distribution of the EEG changes according to the physiologic and psychological states of the subject. The PSD may thus serve as a tool for the analysis and recognition of such states.

Very often we are interested in the relationship between two processes. This may be the case, for example, when two sides of the brain are investigated by means of EEG signals. The time-domain expression of such relationships is given by the cross-correlation function (Equation 1.10). The frequency-domain representation of this is given by the FT of the cross-correlation function, which is called the cross-power spectral density function (C-PSD) or the cross-spectrum:

$$S_{sy}(\omega) = F\{r_{sy}(\tau)\} = |S_{sy}(\omega)|e^{j\theta_{sy}(\omega)} \tag{1.16}$$

Note that we have assumed the signals $s(t)$ and $y(t)$ are stationary; hence the cross-correlation function is not a function of time but of the time difference t. Note also that unlike the autocorrelation function, $r_{sy}(\tau)$ is not even; hence its FT is not real. Both absolute value and phase are required.

It can be shown that the absolute value of the C-PSD is bounded:

$$|S_{sy}(\omega)|^2 \le S_{ss}(\omega)S_{yy}(\omega) \tag{1.17}$$

The absolute value information of the C-PSD may thus be normalized to provide the coherence function:

$$\gamma_{sy}^2 \frac{|S_{sy}(\omega)|^2}{S_{ss}(\omega)S_{yy}(\omega)} \le 1 \tag{1.18}$$

The coherence function is used in a variety of biomedical applications. It has been used, for example, in EEG analysis to investigate brain asymmetry.

1.5 Discrete Signals

Assume now that the signal $s(t)$ of Figure 1.3 was sampled using a sampling frequency of $f_s = \omega_s/2\pi = 2\pi/T_s$. The sampled signal is the sequence $s(m)$. The representation of the sampled signal in the frequency domain is given by applying the Fourier operator:

$$S_s(\omega) = F\{s(m)\} = |S_s(\omega)|e^{j\theta_s(\omega)} \tag{1.19}$$

The amplitude spectrum of the sampled signal is depicted in Figure 1.4. It can easily be proven that the spectrum of the sampled signal is the spectrum of the original signal repeated infinite times at frequencies of $n\omega_s$. The spectrum of a sampled signal is thus a periodic signal in the frequency domain. It can be observed, in Figure 1.4, that provided the sampling frequency is large enough, the wave shapes of the spectrum do not overlap. In such a case, the original (continuous) signal may be extracted from the sampled signal by low-pass filtering. A low-pass filter with a cutoff frequency of ω_{max} will yield at its output only the first period of the spectrum, which is exactly the continuous signal. If, however, the sampling frequency is low, the wave shapes overlap, and it will be impossible to regain the continuous signal.

The sampling frequency must obey the inequality

$$\omega_s \ge 2\omega_{max} \tag{1.20}$$

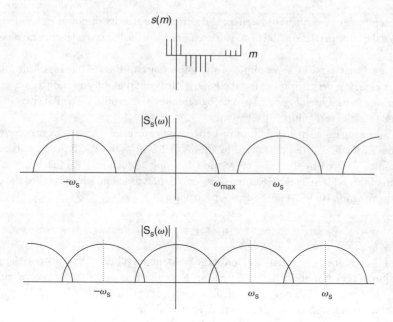

FIGURE 1.4 Amplitude spectrum of a sampled signal with sampling frequency above the Nyquist frequency (upper trace) and below the Nyquist frequency (lower trace).

Equation 1.20 is known as the sampling theorem, and the lowest allowable sampling frequency is called the Nyquist frequency. When overlapping does occur, there are errors between the sampled and original signals. These errors are known as aliasing errors. In practical applications, the signal does not possess a finite bandwidth; we therefore limit its bandwidth by an antialiasing filter prior to sampling.

The discrete Fourier transform (DFT) [Proakis and Manolakis, 1988] is an important operator that maps a finite sequence $s(m)$, $m = 0, 1, \ldots, N - 1$, into another finite sequence $S(k)$, $k = 0, 1, \ldots, N - 1$. The DFT is defined as

$$S(k) = \text{DFT}\{s(m)\} = \sum_{m=0}^{N-1} s(m)e^{-jkm} \tag{1.21}$$

An inverse operator, the inverse discrete Fourier transform (IDFT), is an operator that transforms the sequence $S(k)$ back into the sequence $s(m)$. It is given by

$$s(m) = \text{IDFT}\{S(k)\} = -\sum_{k=0}^{N-1} s(k)e^{jkm} \tag{1.22}$$

It can be shown that if the sequence $s(m)$ represents the samples of the band-limited signal $s(t)$, sampled under Nyquist conditions with sampling interval of T_s, the DFT sequence $S(k)$ (neglecting windowing effects) represents the samples of the FT of the original signal:

$$S(k) = S_s(\omega)|_{\omega=k(\omega_s/N)} \quad k = 0, 1, \ldots, N - 1 \tag{1.23}$$

Figure 1.5 depicts the DFT and its relations to the FT. Note that the N samples of the DFT span the frequency range one period. Since the amplitude spectrum is even, only half the DFT samples carry the information; the other half is composed of the complex conjugates of the first half.

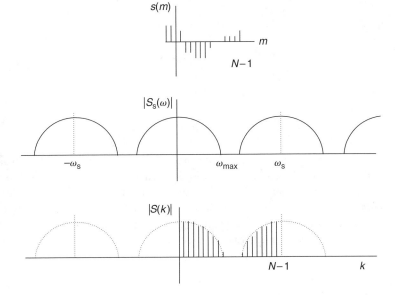

FIGURE 1.5   The sampled signal $s(m)$ and its DFT.

The DFT may be calculated very efficiently by means of the fast (discrete) Fourier transform (FFT) algorithm. It is this fact that makes the DFT an attractive means for FT estimation. The DFT provides an estimate for the FT with frequency resolution of

$$\Delta f = \frac{2\pi f_s}{N} = \frac{2\pi}{T} \tag{1.24}$$

where T is the duration of the data window. The resolution may be improved by using a longer window. In cases where it is not possible to have a longer data window, for example, because the signal is not stationary, zero padding may be used. The sequence may be augmented with zeroes:

$$s_A(m) = \{s(0), s(1), \ldots, s(N-1), 0, \ldots, 0\} \tag{1.25}$$

$$w(t) = 0 \qquad \forall |t| > T/2 \tag{1.25a}$$

The zero padded sequence $s_A(m)$, $m = 0, 1, \ldots, L-1$, contains N elements of the original sequence and $L - N$ zeroes. It can be shown that its DFT represents the samples of the FT with an increased resolution of $\Delta f = 2\pi f_s L - 1$.

1.6   Data Windows

Calculation of the various functions previously defined, such as the correlation function, requires knowledge of the signal from minus infinity to infinity. This is, of course, impractical because the signal is not available for long durations and the results of the calculations are expected at a reasonable time. We therefore do not use the signal itself but the windowed signal.

A window $w(t)$ is defined as a real and even function that is also time-limited:
The FT of a window $W(\omega)$ is thus real and even and is not band-limited.

Multiplying a signal by a window will zero the signal outside the window duration (the observation period) and will create a windowed, time-limited signal $s_w(t)$:

$$s_w(t) = s(t)w(t) \tag{1.26}$$

In the frequency domain, the windowed signal will be

$$S_w(\omega) = S(\omega) * W(\omega) \tag{1.27}$$

where (∗) is the convolution operator. The effect of windowing on the spectrum of the signal is thus the convolution with the FT of the window. A window with very narrow spectrum will cause low distortions. A practical window has an FT with a main lobe, where most of its energy is located, and sidelobes, which cover the frequency axis. The convolution of the sidelobes with the FT of the signal causes distortions known as spectral leakage. Many windows have been suggested for a variety of applications.

The simplest window is the rectangular (Dirichlet) window; in its discrete form it is given by $w(m) = 1$, $m = 0, 1, \ldots, N - 1$. A more useful window is the Hamming window, given by

$$w(m) = 0.54 - 0.46 \cos\left(\frac{2\pi}{N}m\right) \qquad m = 0, 1, \ldots, N - 1 \tag{1.28}$$

The Hamming window was designed to minimize the effects of the first sidelobe.

1.7 Short-Time Fourier Transform

The Fourier analysis discussed in preceding sections assumed that the signal is stationary. Unfortunately, most signals are nonstationary. A relatively simple way to deal with the problem is to divide the signal into short segments. The segments are chosen such that each one by itself can be considered a windowed sample of a stationary process. The duration of the segments has to be determined either by having some a priori information about the signal or by examining its local characteristics. Depending on the signal and the application, the segments may be of equal or different duration.

We want to represent such a segmented signal in the frequency domain. We define the short-time Fourier transform (STFT):

$$\text{STFT}_s(\omega, \tau) = F\{s(t)w(t - \tau)\} = \int_{-\infty}^{\infty} s(t)w(t - \tau)e^{-j\omega t}\, dt \tag{1.29}$$

The window is shifted on the time axis to $t = t$ so that the FT is performed on a windowed segment in the range $t - (T/2) \le t \le t + (T/2)$. The STFT describes the amplitude and phase-frequency distributions of the signal in the vicinity of $t = t$.

In general, the STFT is a two-dimensional, time-frequency function. The resolution of the STFT on the time axis depends on the duration T of the window. The narrower the window, the better the time resolution. Unfortunately, choosing a short-duration window means a wider-band window. The wider the window in the frequency domain, the larger the spectral leakage and hence the deterioration of the frequency resolution. One of the main drawbacks of the STFT method is the fact that the time and frequency resolutions are linked together. Other methods, such as the wavelet transform, are able to better deal with the problem.

In highly nonstationary signals, such as speech signals, equal-duration windows are used. Window duration is on the order of 10–20 msec. In other signals, such as the EEG, variable-duration windows are used. In the EEG, windows on the order of 5–30 sec are often used.

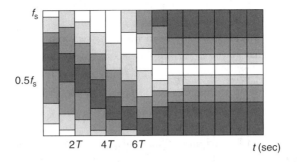

FIGURE 1.6   A spectrogram.

A common way for representing the two-dimensional STFT function is by means of the spectrogram. In the spectrogram, the time and frequency axes are plotted, and the STFT PSD value is given by the gray-scale code or by a color code. Figure 1.6 depicts a simple spectrogram. The time axis is quantized to the window duration T. The gray scale codes the PSD such that black denotes maximum power and white denotes zero power. In Figure 1.6, the PSD is quantized into only four levels of gray. The spectrogram shows a signal that is nonstationary in the time range 0 to 8 T. In this time range, the PSD possesses a peak that is shifted from about 0.6fs to about $0.1f_s$ at time $0.7T$. From time $0.8T$, the signal becomes stationary with a PSD peak power in the low-frequency range and the high-frequency range.

1.8   Spectral Estimation

The PSD is a very useful tool in biomedical signal processing. It is, however, impossible to calculate, since it requires infinite integration time. Estimation methods must be used to acquire an estimate of the PSD from a given finite sample of the process under investigation. Many algorithms for spectral estimation are available in the literature [Kay, 1988], each with its advantages and drawbacks. One method may be suitable for processes with sharp spectral peaks, while another will perform best for broad, smoothed spectra. An a priori knowledge on the type of PSD one is investigating helps in choosing the proper spectral estimation method. Some of the PSD estimation methods will be discussed here.

1.8.1   The Blackman–Tukey Method

This method estimates the PSD directly from its definition (Equation 1.15) but uses finite integration time and an estimate rather than the true correlation function. In its discrete form, the PSD estimation is

$$\hat{S}_{xx}(\omega) = T_s \sum_{m=-M}^{M} \hat{r}_{xx}(m)e^{-j\omega mT_s}$$

$$\hat{r}_{xx}(m) = \frac{1}{N} \sum_{i=0}^{N-i-1} x(m+i)x(i)$$

(1.30)

where N is the number of samples used for the estimation of the correlation coefficients, and M is the number of correlation coefficients used for estimation of the PSD. Note that a biased estimation of the correlation is employed. Note also that once the correlations have been estimated, the PSD may be calculated by applying the FFT to the correlation sequence.

1.8.2 The Periodogram

The periodogram estimates the PSD directly from the signal without the need to first estimate the correlation. It can be shown that

$$S_{xx}(\omega) = \lim_{T \to \infty} E\left\{ \frac{1}{2T} \left| \int_{-T}^{T} x(t)e^{-j\omega t}\, dt \right|^2 \right\} \tag{1.31}$$

The PSD presented in Equation 1.31 requires infinite integration time. The periodogram estimates the PSD from a finite observation time by dropping the lim operator. It can be shown that in its discrete form, the periodogram estimator is given by

$$\hat{S}_{xx}(\omega) = \frac{T_s}{N} |DFT\{x(m)\}|^2 \tag{1.32}$$

The great advantage of the periodogram is that the DFT operator can very efficiently be calculated by the FFT algorithm.

A modification to the periodogram is weighted overlapped segment averaging (WOSA). Rather than using one segment of N samples, we divide the observation segment into shorter subsegments, perform a periodogram for each one, and then average all periodograms. The WOSA method provides a smoother estimate of the PSD.

1.8.3 Time-Series Analysis Methods

Time-series analysis methods model the signal as an output of a linear system driven by a white source. Figure 1.7 depicts this model in its discrete form. Since the input is a white noise process (with zero mean and unity variance), the PSD of the signal is given by

$$S_{ss}(\omega) = |H(\omega)|^2 \tag{1.33}$$

The PSD of the signal may thus be represented by the system's transfer function. Consider a general pole-zero system with p poles and q zeros [ARMA(p, q)]:

$$H(z) = \frac{\sum_{i=0}^{q} b_i z^{-i}}{1 + \sum_{i=1}^{p} a_i z^{-i}} \tag{1.34}$$

Its absolute value evaluated on the frequency axis is

$$|H(\omega)|^2 = \left. \frac{|\sum_{i=0}^{q} b_i z^{-i}|^2}{|\sum_{i=1}^{p} a_i z^{-i}|^2} \right|_{z=e^{-j\omega T_s}} \tag{1.35}$$

Several algorithms are available for the estimation of the model's coefficients. The estimation of the ARMA model parameters requires the solution of a nonlinear set of equations. The special case of $q = 0$, namely, an all-pole model [AR(p)], may be estimated by means of linear equations. Efficient AR estimation

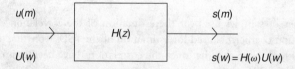

FIGURE 1.7 Time-series model for the signal $s(m)$.

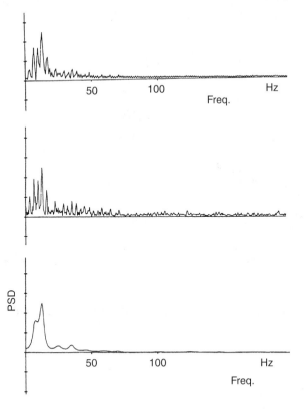

FIGURE 1.8   PSD of surface EMG. (Upper trace) Blackman–Tukey (256 correlation coefficients and 256 padding zeroes). (Middle trace) Periodogram (512 samples and 512 padding zeroes). (Lower trace) AR model ($p = 40$).

algorithms are available, making it a popular means for PSD estimation. Figure 1.8 shows the estimation of EMG PSD using several estimation methods.

1.9   Signal Enhancement

The biomedical signal is very often a weak signal contaminated by noise. Consider, for example, the problem of monitoring the ECG signal. The signal is acquired by surface electrodes that pick up the electric potential generated by the heart muscle. In addition, the electrodes pick up potentials from other active muscles. When the subject is at rest, this type of noise may be very small, but when the subject is an athlete performing some exercise, the muscle noise may become dominant. Additional noise may enter the system from electrodes motion, from the power lines, and from other sources. The first task of processing is usually to enhance the signal by "cleaning" the noise without (if possible) distorting the signal.

Assume a simple case where the measured signal $x(t)$ is given by

$$x(t) = s(t) + n(t) \qquad X(\omega) = S(\omega) + N(\omega) \tag{1.36}$$

where $s(t)$ is the desired signal and $n(t)$ is the additive noise. For simplicity, we assume that both the signal and noise are band-limited, namely, for the signal, $S(\omega) = 0$, for $\omega_{max} \leq \omega, \omega_{min} \geq \omega$. Figure 1.9 depicts the PSD of the signal in two cases, the first where the PSD of the signal and noise do not overlap and the second where they do overlap (for the sake of simplicity, only the positive frequency axis was plotted). We want to enhance the signal by means of linear filtering. The problem is to design the linear filter that will

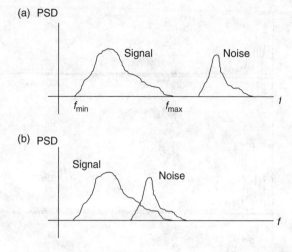

FIGURE 1.9   Noisy signal in the frequency domain (a) nonoverlapping case and (b) overlapping case.

provide best enhancement. Assuming we have the filter, its output, the enhanced signal, is given by

$$y(t) = x(t) * h(t) \qquad Y(\omega) = X(\omega)H(\omega) \tag{1.37}$$

where $y(t) = \hat{s}(t) + n_o(t)$ is the enhanced output, and $h(t)$ is the impulse response of the filter. The solution for the first case is trivial; we need an ideal bandpass filter whose transfer function $H(\omega)$ is

$$H(\omega) = \begin{cases} 1, & \omega_{min} < \omega < \omega_{max} \\ 0, & \text{otherwise} \end{cases} \tag{1.38}$$

Such a filter and its output are depicted in Figure 1.10.

As is clearly seen in Figure 1.10, the desired signal $s(t)$ was completely recovered from the given noisy signal $x(t)$. Practically, we do not have ideal filters, so some distortions and some noise contamination will always appear at the output. With the correct design, we can approximate the ideal filter so that the distortions and noise may be as small as we desire. The enhancement of overlapping noisy signals is far from being trivial.

1.10   Optimal Filtering

When the PSD of signal and noise overlap, complete, undistorted recovery of the signal is impossible. Optimal processing is required, with the first task being definition of the optimality criterion. Different criteria will result in different solutions to the problem. Two approaches will be presented here: the Wiener filter and the matched filter.

1.10.1   Minimization of Mean Squared Error: The Wiener Filter

Assume that our goal is to estimate, at time $t + \xi$, the value of the signal $s(t + \xi)$, based on the observations $x(t)$. The case $x = 0$ is known as smoothing, while the case $\xi > 0$ is called prediction.

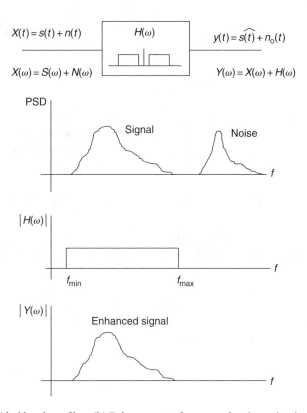

FIGURE 1.10 (a) An ideal bandpass filter. (b) Enhancement of a nonoverlapping noisy signal by an ideal bandpass filter.

We define an output error $\varepsilon(t)$ as the error between the filter's output and the desired output. The expectation of the square of the error is given by

$$E\{e^2(t)\} = E\{[s(t+\xi) - y(t+\xi)]^2\}$$

$$= E\left\{\left[s(t+\xi) - \int_{-\infty}^{\infty} h(\tau)x(t-\tau)\,d\tau\right]^2\right\} \tag{1.39}$$

The integral term on the right side of Equation 1.39 is the convolution integral expressing the output of the filter.

The minimization of Equation 1.39 with respect to $h(t)$ yields the optimal filter (in the sense of minimum squared error). The minimization yields the Wiener–Hopf equation:

$$r_{sx}(\tau + \xi) = \int_{-\infty}^{\infty} h(\eta)r_{xx}(\tau \cdot -\eta)\,d\eta \tag{1.40}$$

In the frequency domain, this equation becomes

$$S_{sx}(\omega)e^{j\omega\xi} = H_{\text{opt}}(\omega)S_{xx}(\omega) \tag{1.41}$$

from which the optimal filter $H_{\text{opt}}(\omega)$ can be calculated:

$$H_{\text{opt}}(\omega) = \frac{S_{sx}(\omega)}{S_{xx}(\omega)}e^{j\omega\xi} = \frac{S_{sx}(\omega)}{S_{ss}(\omega) + S_{nn}(\omega)}e^{j\omega\xi} \tag{1.42}$$

If the signal and noise are uncorrelated and either the signal or the noise has zero mean, the last equation becomes

$$H_{\text{opt}}(\omega) = \frac{S_{ss}(\omega)}{S_{ss}(\omega) + S_{nn}(\omega)} e^{j\omega\xi} \tag{1.43}$$

The optimal filter requires a priori knowledge of the PSD of noise and signal. These are very often not available and must be estimated from the available signal. The optimal filter given in Equation 1.42 and Equation 1.43 is not necessarily realizable. In performing the minimization, we have not introduced a constraint that will ensure that the filter is causal. This can be done, yielding the realizable optimal filter.

1.10.2 Maximization of the Signal-to-Noise Ratio: The Matched Filter

The Wiener filter was optimally designed to yield an output as close as possible to the signal. In many cases we are not interested in the fine details of the signal but only in the question whether the signal exists at a particular observation or not. Consider, for example, the case of determining the heart rate of a subject under noisy conditions. We need to detect the presence of the R wave in the ECG. The exact shape of the wave is not important. For this case, the optimality criterion used in the last section is not suitable. To find a more suitable criterion, we define the output signal-to-noise ratio: Let us assume that the signal $s(t)$ is a deterministic function. The response of the filter, $s(t) = s(t) * h(t)$, to the signal is also deterministic. We shall define the output signal-to-noise ratio

$$\text{SNR}_{\text{o}}(t) = \frac{\hat{s}(t)}{E\{n_{\text{o}}^2(t)\}} \tag{1.44}$$

as the optimality criterion. The optimal filter will be the filter that maximizes the output SNR at a certain given time $t = t_0$. The maximization yields the following integral equation:

$$\int_0^T h(\xi) r_{nn}(\tau - \xi) \, d\xi = a s(t_0 - \tau) \qquad 0 \leq \tau < T \tag{1.45}$$

where T is the observation time and a is any constant. This equation has to be solved for any given noise and signal.

A special important case is the case where the noise is a white noise so that its autocorrelation function is a delta function. In this case, the solution of Equation 1.45 is

$$h(\tau) = \frac{1}{N} s(t_0 - \tau) \tag{1.46}$$

where N is the noise power. For this special case, the impulse response of the optimal filter has the form of the signal run backward, shifted to the time to . This type of filter is called a matched filter.

1.11   Adaptive Filtering

The optimal filters discussed in the preceding section assumed the signals to be stationary with known PSD. Both assumptions rarely occur in reality. In most biomedical applications, the signals are nonstationary with unknown PSD. To enhance such signals, we require a filter that will continuously adjust itself to perform optimally under the changing circumstances. Such a filter is called an adaptive filter [Widrow and Stearns, 1985].

The general description of an adaptive filter is depicted in Figure 1.11. The signal $s(t)$ is to be corrected according to the specific application. The correction may be enhancement or some reshaping. The signal is given in terms of the noisy observation signal $x(t)$. The main part of the system is a filter, and the

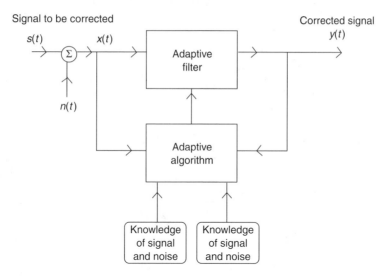

FIGURE 1.11 Adaptive filter, general scheme.

parameters (gain, poles, and zeroes) are controllable by the adaptive algorithm. The adaptive algorithm has some a priori information on the signal and the noise (the amount and type of information depend on the application). It also has a correction criterion, according to which the signal is operating. The adaptive algorithm also gets the input and output signals of the filter so that its performance can be analyzed continuously.

The adaptive filter requires a correction algorithm. This can best be implemented digitally. Most adaptive filters therefore are implemented by means of computers or special digital processing chips.

An important class of adaptive filters requires a reference signal. The knowledge of the noise required by this type of adaptive filter is a reference signal that is correlated with the noise. The filter thus has two inputs: the noisy signal $x(t) = s(t) + n(t)$ and the reference signal $nR(t)$. The adaptive filter, functioning as a noise canceler, estimates the noise $n(t)$ and, by subtracting it from the given noisy input, gets an estimate for the signal. Hence

$$y(t) = x(t) - \hat{n}(t) = s(t) + [n(t) - \hat{n}(t)] = \hat{s}(t) \tag{1.47}$$

The output of the filter is the enhanced signal. Since the reference signal is correlated with the noise, the following relationship exists:

$$N_R(\omega) = G(\omega)N(\omega) \tag{1.48}$$

which means that the reference noise may be represented as the output of an unknown filter $G(\omega)$. The adaptive filter estimates the inverse of this unknown noise filter and from its estimates the noise:

$$\hat{n}(t) = F^{-1}\{\hat{G}^{-1}(\omega)N_R(\omega)\} \tag{1.49}$$

The estimation of the inverse filter is done by the minimization of some performance criterion. There are two dominant algorithms for the optimization: the recursive least squares (RLS) and the least mean squares (LMS). The LMS algorithm will be discussed here.

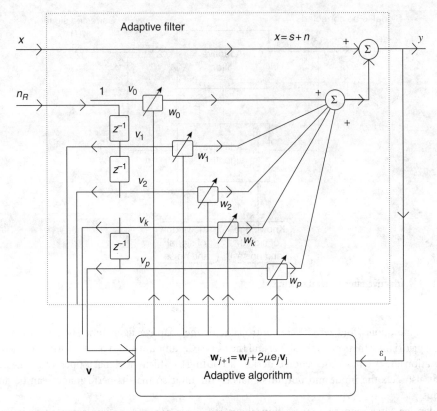

FIGURE 1.12   Block diagram of LMS adaptive noise canceler.

Consider the mean square error

$$E\{\varepsilon^2(t)\} = E\{y^2(t)\} = E\{(s(t) + [n(t) - \hat{n}(t)])^2\}$$

$$= E\{s^2(t)\} + E\{[n(t) - \hat{n}(t)]^2\} \tag{1.50}$$

The right side of Equation 1.50 is correct, assuming that the signal and noise are uncorrelated. We are searching for the estimate $\hat{G}^{-1}(\omega)$ that will minimize the mean square error: $E\{[n(t) - \hat{n}(t)]^2\}$. Since the estimated filter affects only the estimated noise, the minimization of the noise error is equivalent to the minimization of Equation 1.50. The implementation of the LMS filter will be presented in its discrete form (see Figure 1.12).

The estimated noise is

$$\hat{n}_R(m) = \sum_{i=0}^{p} v_i w_i = \mathbf{v}_m^T \mathbf{w} \tag{1.51}$$

where

$$\mathbf{v}_m^T = [v_0, v_1, \ldots, v_p] = [1, n_R(m-1), \ldots, n_R(m-p)]$$

$$\mathbf{w}^T = [w_0, w, \ldots, w_p] \tag{1.52}$$

The vector $\mathbf{w}$ represents the filter. The steepest descent minimization of Equation 1.50 with respect to the filter's coefficients $\mathbf{w}$ yields the iterative algorithm

$$\mathbf{w}_{j+1} = \mathbf{w}_j + 2\mu e_j \mathbf{v}_j \qquad (1.53)$$

where m is a scalar that controls the stability and convergence of the algorithm. In the evaluation of Equation 1.53, the assumption

$$\frac{\partial E\{e_j^2\}}{\partial w_k} \cong \frac{\partial e_j^2}{\partial w_k} \qquad (1.54)$$

was made. This is indeed a drastic approximation; the results, however, are very satisfactory. Figure 1.12 depicts the block diagram of the LMS adaptive noise canceler.

The LMS adaptive noise canceler has been applied to many biomedical problems, among them cancellation of power-line interferences, elimination of electrosurgical interferences, enhancement of fetal ECG, noise reduction for the hearing impaired, and enhancement of evoked potentials.

1.12 Segmentation of Nonstationary Signals

Most biomedical signals are nonstationary, yet the common processing techniques (such as the FT) deal with stationary signals. The STFT is one method of processing nonstationary signals, but it does require, however, the segmentation of the signal into "almost" stationary segments. The signal is thus represented as a piecewise-stationary signal.

An important problem in biomedical signal processing is efficient segmentation. In very highly nonstationary signals, such as the speech signal, short, constant-duration (of the order of 15 msec) segments are used. The segmentation processing in such a case is simple and inexpensive. In other cases such as the monitoring of nocturnal EEG, a more elaborate segmentation procedure is called for because the signal may consist of "stationary" segments with very wide duration range. Segmentation into a priori fixed-duration segments will be very inefficient in such cases.

Several adaptive segmentation algorithms have been suggested. Figure 1.13 demonstrates the basic idea of these algorithms. A fixed reference window is used to define an initial segment of the signal. The duration of the reference window is determined such that it is long enough to allow a reliable PSD estimate yet short enough so that the segment may still be considered stationary. Some a priori information about the signal will help in determining the reference window duration. A second, sliding window is shifted along the signal. The PSD of the segment defined by the sliding window is estimated at each window position. The two spectra are compared using some spectral distance measure. As long as this distance measure remains below a certain decision threshold, the reference segment and the sliding segment are considered close enough and are related to the same stationary segment. Once the distance measure exceeds the decision threshold, a new segment is defined. The process continues by defining the last sliding window as the reference window of the new segment.

Let us define a relative spectral distance measure

$$D_t(\omega) = \int_{\omega_M}^{\omega_M} \left(\frac{S_R(\omega) - S_t(\omega)}{S_R(\omega)} \right)^2 \qquad (1.55)$$

where $S_R(\omega)$ and $S_t(\omega)$ are the PSD estimates of the reference and sliding segments, respectively, and ω_M is the bandwidth of the signal. A normalized spectral measure was chosen, since we are interested in differences in the shape of the PSD and not in the gain.

Some of the segmentation algorithms use growing reference windows rather than fixed ones. This is depicted in the upper part of Figure 1.13. The various segmentation methods differ in the way the PSDs are

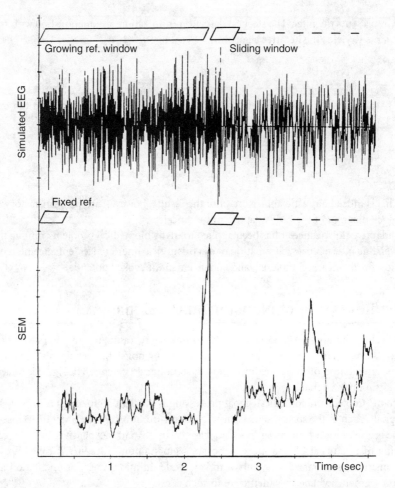

FIGURE 1.13   Adaptive segmentation of simulated EEG. First 2.5 sec and last 2.5 sec were simulated by means of different AR models. (Lower trace) SEM calculated with fixed reference window. A new segment has been detected at $t - 2.5$. (From Cohen, 1986, with permission.)

estimated. Two of the more well-known segmentation methods are the auto-correlation measure method (ACM) and the spectral error measure (SEM).

References

Cohen A. (1986). *Biomedical Signal Processing*. Boca Raton, FL, CRC Press.
Kay S.M. (1988). *Modern Spectral Estimation: Theory and Application*. Englewood Cliffs, NJ, Prentice Hall.
Proakis J.G. and Manolakis D.G. (1988). *Introduction to Digital Signal Processing*. New York, Macmillan.
Weitkunat R. (ed). (1991). *Digital Biosignal Processing*. Amsterdam, Elsevier.
Widrow B. and Stearns S.D. (1985). *Adaptive Signal Processing*. Englewood Cliffs, NJ, Prentice Hall.

2

Digital Biomedical Signal Acquisition and Processing

Luca T. Mainardi
Sergio Cerutti
Polytechnic University

Anna M. Bianchi
St. Raffaele Hospital

2.1 Acquisition 2-2
    The Sampling Theorem • The Quantization Effects
2.2 Signal Processing....................................... 2-6
    Digital Filters • Signal Averaging • Spectral Analysis
2.3 Conclusion 2-22
Defining Terms 2-22
References 2-22
Further Information 2-24

Biologic signals carry information that is useful for comprehension of the complex pathophysiologic mechanisms underlying the behavior of living systems. Nevertheless, such information cannot be available directly from the raw recorded signals; it can be masked by other biologic signals contemporaneously detected (endogenous effects) or buried in some additive noise (exogenous effects). For such reasons, some additional processing is usually required to enhance the relevant information and to extract from it parameters that quantify the behavior of the system under study, mainly for physiologic studies, or that define the degree of pathology for routine clinical procedures (diagnosis, therapy, or rehabilitation).

Several processing techniques can be used for such purposes (they are also called preprocessing techniques); time- or frequency-domain methods including filtering, **averaging**, spectral estimation, and others. Even if it is possible to deal with continuous time waveforms, it is usually convenient to convert them into a numerical form before processing. The recent progress of digital technology, in terms of both hardware and software, makes digital rather than analog processing more efficient and flexible. Digital techniques have several advantages: their performance is generally powerful, being able to easily implement even complex algorithms, and accuracy depends only on the truncation and round-off errors, whose effects can be predicted and controlled by the designer and are largely unaffected by other unpredictable variables such as component aging and temperature, which can degrade the performances of analog devices. Moreover, design parameters can be more easily changed because they involve software rather than hardware modifications.

A few basic elements of signal acquisition and processing will be presented in the following; our aim is to stress mainly the aspects connected with acquisition and analysis of biologic signals, leaving to the cited

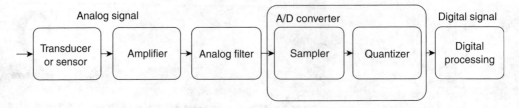

FIGURE 2.1 General block diagram of the acquisition procedure of a digital signal.

literature a deeper insight into the various subjects for both the fundamentals of digital signal processing and the applications.

2.1 Acquisition

A schematic representation of a general acquisition system is shown in Figure 2.1. Several physical magnitudes are usually measured from biologic systems. They include electromagnetic quantities (currents, potential differences, field strengths, etc.), as well as mechanical, chemical, or generally nonelectrical variables (pressure, temperature, movements, etc.). Electric signals are detected by sensors (mainly electrodes), while nonelectric magnitudes are first converted by transducers into electric signals that can be easily treated, transmitted, and stored. Several books of biomedical instrumentation give detailed descriptions of the various transducers and the hardware requirements associated with the acquisition of the different biologic signals [Tompkins and Webster, 1981; Cobbold, 1988; Webster, 1992].

An analog preprocessing block is usually required to amplify and filter the signal (in order to make it satisfy the requirements of the hardware such as the dynamic of the analog-to-digital converter), to compensate for some unwanted sensor characteristics, or to reduce the portion of undesired noise. Moreover, the continuous-time signal should be bandlimited before analog-to-digital (A/D) conversion. Such an operation is needed to reduce the effect of **aliasing** induced by sampling, as will be described in the next section. Here it is important to remember that the acquisition procedure should preserve the information contained in the original signal waveform. This is a crucial point when recording biologic signals, whose characteristics often may be considered by physicians as indices of some underlying pathologies (i.e., the ST-segment displacement on an ECG signal can be considered a marker of ischemia, the peak-and-wave pattern on an EEG tracing can be a sign of epilepsy, and so on). Thus the acquisition system should not introduce any form of distortion that can be misleading or can destroy real pathologic alterations. For this reason, the analog prefiltering block should be designed with constant modulus and linear phase (or zerophase) **frequency response**, at least in the passband, over the frequencies of interest. Such requirements make the signal arrive undistorted up to the A/D converter.

The analog waveform is then A/D converted into a digital signal; that is, it is transformed into a series of numbers, discretized both in time and amplitude, that can be easily managed by digital processors. The A/D conversion ideally can be divided in two steps, as shown in Figure 2.1: the sampling process, which converts the continuous signal in a discrete-time series and whose elements are named samples, and a quantization procedure, which assigns the amplitude value of each sample within a set of determined discrete values. Both processes modify the characteristics of the signal, and their effects will be discussed in the following sections.

2.1.1 The Sampling Theorem

The advantages of processing a digital series instead of an analog signal have been reported previously. Furthermore, the basic property when using a sampled series instead of its continuous waveform lies in the fact that the former, under certain hypotheses, is completely representative of the latter. When this happens, the continuous waveform can be perfectly reconstructed just from the series of sampled

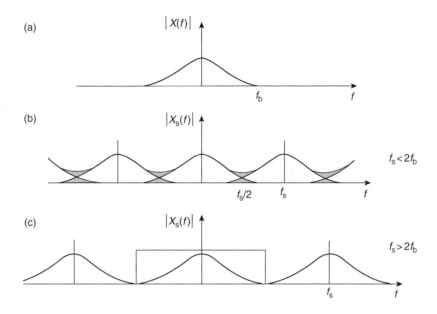

FIGURE 2.2 Effect of sampling frequency (f_s) on a band-limited signal (up to frequency f_b). Fourier transform of the original time signal (a), of the sampled signal when $f_s < 2f_b$ (b), and when $f_s > 2f_b$ (c). The dark areas in part (b) indicate the aliased frequencies.

values. This is known as the sampling theorem (or Shannon theorem) [Shannon, 1949]. It states that a continuous-time signal can be completely recovered from its samples if, and only if, the sampling rate is greater than twice the signal bandwidth.

In order to understand the assumptions of the theorem, let us consider a continuous band-limited signal $x(t)$ (up to f_b) whose Fourier transform $X(f)$ is shown in Figure 2.2a and suppose to uniformly sample it. The sampling procedure can be modeled by the multiplication of $x(t)$ with an impulse train

$$i(t) = \sum_{k=-\infty,\infty} \delta(t - kT_s) \tag{2.1}$$

where $\delta(t)$ is the delta (Dirac) function, k is an integer, and T_s is the sampling interval. The sampled signal becomes

$$x_s(t) = x(t) \cdot i(t) = \sum_{k=-\infty,\infty} x(t) \cdot \delta(t - kT_s) \tag{2.2}$$

Taking into account that multiplication in time domain implies convolution in frequency domain, we obtain

$$X_s(f) = X(f) \cdot I(f) = X(f) \cdot \frac{1}{T_s} \sum_{k=-\infty,\infty} \delta(f - kf_s) = \frac{1}{T_s} \sum_{k=-\infty,\infty} X(f - kf_s) \tag{2.3}$$

where $f_s = 1/T_s$ is the sampling frequency.

Thus $X_s(f)$, that is, the Fourier transform of the sampled signal, is periodic and consists of a series of identical repeats of $X(f)$ centered around multiples of the sampling frequency, as depicted in Figure 2.2b,c.

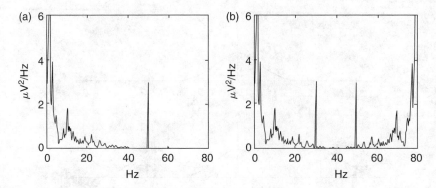

FIGURE 2.3   Power spectrum of an EEG signal (originally bandlimited up to 40 Hz). The presence of 50-Hz mains noise (a) causes aliasing error in the 30-Hz component (i.e., in the b diagnostic band) in the sampled signal (b) if $f_s = 80$ Hz.

It is worth noting in Figure 2.2b that the frequency components of $X(f)$ placed above $f_s/2$ appears, when $f_s < 2f_b$, as folded back, summing up to the lower-frequency components. This phenomenon is known as aliasing (higher component look "alias" lower components). When aliasing occurs, the original information (Figure 2.2a) cannot be recovered because the frequency components of the original signal are irreversibly corrupted by the overlaps of the shifted versions of $X(f)$.

A visual inspection of Figure 2.2 allows one to observe that such frequency contamination can be avoided when the original signal is bandlimited ($X(f) = 0$, for $f > f_b$) and sampled at a frequency $f_s \geq 2f_b$. In this case, shown in Figure 2.2c, no overlaps exist between adjacent reply of $X(f)$, and the original waveform can be retrieved by low-pass filtering the sampled signal [Oppenheim and Schafer, 1975]. Such observations are the basis of the sampling theorem previously reported.

The hypothesis of a bandlimited signal is hardly verified in practice, due to the signal characteristics or to the effect of superimposed wideband noise. It is worth noting that filtering before sampling is always needed even if we assume the incoming signal to be bandlimited. Let us consider the following example of an EEG signal whose frequency content of interest ranges between 0 and 40 Hz (the usual diagnostic bands are δ, 0 to 3.5 Hz; ν, 4 to 7 Hz; α, 8 to 13 Hz; β, 14 to 40 Hz). We may decide to sample it at 80 Hz, thus literally respecting the Shannon theorem. If we do it without prefiltering, we could find some unpleasant results. Typically, the 50-Hz mains noise will replicate itself in the signal band (30 Hz, i.e., the β band), thus corrupting irreversibly the information, which is of great interest from a physiologic and clinical point of view. The effect is shown in Figure 2.3a (before sampling) and Figure 2.3b (after sampling). Generally, it is advisable to sample at a frequency greater than $2f_b$ [Gardenhire, 1964] in order to take into account the nonideal behavior of the filter or the other preprocessing devices. Therefore, the prefiltering block of Figure 2.1 is always required to bandlimit the signal before sampling and to avoid aliasing errors.

2.1.2   The Quantization Effects

The quantization produces a discrete signal, whose samples can assume only certain values according to the way they are coded. Typical step functions for a uniform quantizer are reported in Figure 2.4a,b, where the quantization interval $\triangle$ between two quantization levels is evidenced in two cases: rounding and truncation, respectively.

Quantization is a heavily nonlinear procedure, but fortunately, its effects can be statistically modeled. Figure 2.4c,d shows it; the nonlinear quantization block is substituted by a statistical model in which the error induced by quantization is treated as an additive noise $e(n)$ (**quantization error**) to the signal $x(n)$.

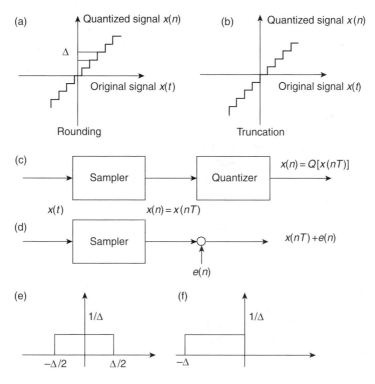

FIGURE 2.4 Nonlinear relationships for rounding (a) and truncation (b) quantization procedures. Description of quantization block (c) by a statistical model (d) and probability densities for the quantization noise $e(n)$ for rounding (e) and truncation (f). Δ is the quantization interval.

The following hypotheses are considered in order to deal with a simple mathematical problem:

1. $e(n)$ is supposed to be a white noise with uniform distribution
2. $e(n)$ and $x(n)$ are uncorrelated

First of all, it should be noted that the probability density of $e(n)$ changes according to the adopted coding procedure. If we decide to round the real sample to the nearest quantization level, we have $-\Delta/2 \leq e(n) < \Delta/2$, while if we decide to truncate the sample amplitude, we have $-\Delta \leq e(n) < 0$. The two probability densities are plotted in Figure 2.4e,f.

The two ways of coding yield processes with different statistical properties. In the first case the mean and variance value of $e(n)$ are

$$m_e = 0 \qquad \sigma_e^2 = \Delta^2/12$$

while in the second case $m_e = -\Delta/2$, and the variance is still the same. Variance reduces in the presence of a reduced quantization interval as expected.

Finally, it is possible to evaluate the signal-to-noise ratio (SNR) for the quantization process:

$$\text{SNR} = 10 \log_{10}\left(\frac{\sigma_x^2}{\sigma_e^2}\right) = 10 \log_{10}\left(\frac{\sigma_x^2}{2^{-2b}/12}\right) = 6.02b + 10.79 + 10 \log_{10}(\sigma_x^2) \qquad (2.4)$$

having set $\Delta = 2^{-2b}$ and where σ_x^2 is the variance of the signal and b is the number of bits used for coding. It should be noted that the SNR increases by almost 6 dB for each added bit of coding. Several forms of quantization are usually employed: uniform, nonuniform (preceding the uniform sampler with a nonlinear block), or roughly (small number of quantization levels and high quantization step). Details can be found in Carassa [1983], Jaeger [1982], and Widrow [1956].

2.2 Signal Processing

A brief review of different signal-processing techniques will be given in this section. They include traditional filtering, averaging techniques, and spectral estimators.

Only the main concepts of analysis and design of digital filters are presented, and a few examples are illustrated in the processing of the ECG signal. Averaging techniques will then be described briefly and their usefulness evidenced when noise and signal have similar frequency contents but different statistical properties; an example for evoked potentials enhancement from EEG background noise is illustrated. Finally, different spectral estimators will be considered and some applications shown in the analysis of RR fluctuations (i.e., the heart rate variability (HRV) signal).

2.2.1 Digital Filters

A digital filter is a discrete-time system that operates some transformation on a digital input signal $x(n)$ generating an output sequence $y(n)$, as schematically shown by the block diagram in Figure 2.5. The characteristics of transformation $T[\cdot]$ identify the filter. The filter will be time-variant if $T[\cdot]$ is a function of time or time-invariant otherwise, while is said to be *linear* if, and only if, having $x_1(n)$ and $x_2(n)$ as inputs producing $y_1(n)$ and $y_2(n)$, respectively, we have

$$T[ax_1 + bx_2] = aT[x_1] + bT[x_2] = ay_1 + by_2 \tag{2.5}$$

In the following, only linear, time-invariant filters will be considered, even if several interesting applications of nonlinear [Glaser and Ruchkin, 1976; Tompkins, 1993] or time-variant [Huta and Webster, 1973; Widrow et al., 1975; Cohen, 1983; Thakor, 1987] filters have been proposed in the literature for the analysis of biologic signals.

The behavior of a filter is usually described in terms of input–output relationships. They are usually assessed by exciting the filter with different inputs and evaluating which is the response (output) of the system. In particular, if the input is the impulse sequence $\delta(n)$, the resulting output, the impulse response, has a relevant role in describing the characteristic of the filter. Such a response can be used to determine the response to more complicated input sequences. In fact, let us consider a generic input sequence $x(n)$ as a sum of weighted and delayed impulses.

$$x(n) = \sum_{k=-\infty,\infty} x(k) \cdot \delta(n-k) \tag{2.6}$$

and let us identify the response to $\delta(n-k)$ as $h(n-k)$. If the filter is time-invariant, each delayed impulse will produce the same response, but time-shifted; due to the linearity property, such responses will be

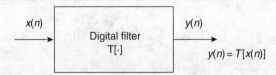

FIGURE 2.5   General block diagram of a digital filter. The output digital signal $y(n)$ is obtained from the input $x(n)$ by means of a transformation $T[\cdot]$ which identifies the filter.

summed at the output:

$$y(n) = \sum_{k=-\infty,\infty} x(k) \cdot h(n-k) \tag{2.7}$$

This convolution product links input and output and defines the property of the filter. Two of them should be recalled: *stability* and *causality*. The former ensures that bounded (finite) inputs will produce bounded outputs. Such a property can be deduced by the impulse response; it can be proved that the filter is stable if and only if

$$\sum_{k=-\infty,\infty} |h(k)| < \infty \tag{2.8}$$

Causality means that the filter will not respond to an input before the input is applied. This is in agreement with our physical concept of a system, but it is not strictly required for a digital filter that can be implemented in a noncausal form. A filter is causal if and only if

$$h(k) = 0 \quad \text{for } k < 0 \tag{2.8a}$$

Even if Equation 2.7 completely describes the properties of the filter, most often it is necessary to express the input–output relationships of linear discrete-time systems under the form of the z-transform operator, which allows one to express Equation 2.7 in a more useful, operative, and simpler form.

2.2.1.1 The z-Transform

The z-transform of a sequence $x(n)$ is defined by [Rainer et al., 1972]

$$X(z) = \sum_{k=-\infty,\infty} x(k) \cdot z^{-k} \tag{2.9}$$

where z is a complex variable. This series will converge or diverge for different z values. The set of z values which makes Equation 2.9 converge is the **region of convergence**, and it depends on the series $x(n)$ considered.

Among the properties of the z-transform, we recall

- The delay (shift) property:

$$\text{If } w(n) = x(n-T) \text{ then } W(z) = X(z) \cdot z^{-T} \tag{2.9a}$$

- The product of convolution:

$$\text{If } w(n) = \sum_{k=-\infty,\infty} x(k) \cdot y(n-k) \text{ then } W(z) = X(z) \cdot Y(z) \tag{2.9b}$$

2.2.1.2 The Transfer Function in the z-Domain

Thanks to the previous property, we can express Equation 2.7 in the z-domain as a simple multiplication:

$$Y(z) = H(z) \cdot X(z) \tag{2.10}$$

where $H(z)$, known as *transfer function* of the filter, is the z-transform of the impulse response. $H(z)$ plays a relevant role in the analysis and design of digital filters. The response to input sinusoids can be

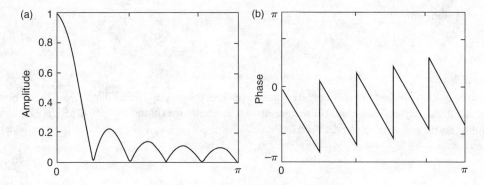

FIGURE 2.6 Modulus (a) and phase (b) diagrams of the frequency response of a moving average filter of order 5. Note that the frequency plots are depicted up to π. In fact, taking into account that we are dealing with a sampled signal whose frequency information is up to $f_s/2$, we have $\omega_{max} = 2\pi f_s/2 = \pi f_s$ or $\omega_{max} = \pi$ if normalized with respect to the sampling rate.

evaluated as follows: assume a complex sinusoid $x(n) = e^{j\omega n T_s}$ as input, the correspondent filter output will be

$$y(n) = \sum_{k=0,\infty} h(k)e^{j\omega T_2(n-k)} = e^{-j\omega n T_s} \sum_{k=0,\infty} h(k)e^{-j\omega k T_s} = x(n) \cdot H(z)|_{z=e^{j\omega T_s}} \qquad (2.11)$$

Then a sinusoid in input is still the same sinusoid at the output, but multiplied by a complex quantity $H(\omega)$. Such complex function defines the response of the filter for each sinusoid of ω pulse in input, and it is known as the frequency response of the filter. It is evaluated in the complex z plane by computing $H(z)$ for $z = e^{j\omega n T_s}$, namely, on the point locus that describes the unitary circle on the z plane ($|e^{j\omega n T_s}| = 1$). As a complex function, $H(\omega)$ will be defined by its module $|H(\omega)|$ and by its phase $\angle H(\omega)$ functions, as shown in Figure 2.6 for a moving average filter of order 5. The figure indicates that the lower-frequency components will come through the filter almost unaffected, while the higher-frequency components will be drastically reduced. It is usual to express the horizontal axis of frequency response from 0 to π. This is obtained because only pulse frequencies up to $\omega_s/2$ are reconstructable (due to the Shannon theorem), and therefore, in the horizontal axis, the value of ωT_s is reported which goes from 0 to π. Furthermore, Figure 2.6b demonstrates that the phase is piecewise linear, and in correspondence with the zeros of $|H(\omega)|$, there is a change in phase of π value. According to their frequency response, the filters are usually classified as (1) low-pass, (2) high-pass, (3) bandpass, or (4) bandstop filters. Figure 2.7 shows the ideal frequency response for such filters with the proper low- and high-frequency cutoffs.

For a large class of linear, time-invariant systems, $H(z)$ can be expressed in the following general form:

$$H(z) = \frac{\sum_{m=0,M} b_m z^{-m}}{1 + \sum_{k=1,N} a_k z^{-k}} \qquad (2.12)$$

which describes in the z domain the following *difference equation* in this discrete time domain:

$$y(n) = - \sum_{k=1,N} a_k y(n-k) + \sum_{m=0,M} b_m x(n-m) \qquad (2.13)$$

When at least one of the a_k coefficients is different from zero, some output values contribute to the current output. The filter contains some feedback, and it is said to be implemented in a recursive form. On the other hand, when the a_k values are all zero, the filter output is obtained only from the current or previous inputs, and the filter is said to be implemented in a *nonrecursive* form.

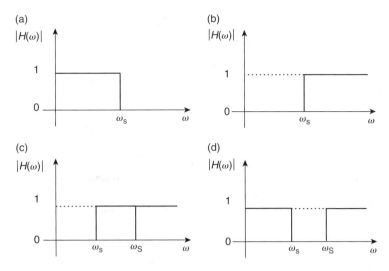

FIGURE 2.7 Ideal frequency-response moduli for low-pass (a), high-pass (b), bandpass (c), and bandstop filters (d).

The transfer function can be expressed in a more useful form by finding the roots of both numerator and denominator:

$$H(z) = \frac{b_0 z^{N-M} \prod_{m=1,M}(z - z_m)}{\prod_{k=1,N}(z - P_k)} \tag{2.14}$$

where z_m are the zeroes and p_k are the poles. It is worth noting that $H(z)$ presents $N - M$ zeros in correspondence with the origin of the z plane and M zeroes elsewhere (N zeroes totally) and N poles. The pole-zero form of $H(z)$ is of great interest because several properties of the filter are immediately available from the geometry of poles and zeroes in the complex z plane. In fact, it is possible to easily assess stability and by visual inspection to roughly estimate the frequency response without making any calculations.

Stability is verified when all poles lie inside the unitary circle, as can be proved by considering the relationships between the z-transform and the Laplace s-transform and by observing that the left side of the s plane is mapped inside the unitary circle [Jackson, 1986; Oppenheim and Schafer, 1975].

The frequency response can be estimated by noting that $(z - z_m)|_{z=e^{j\omega nT_s}}$ is a vector joining the mth zero with the point on the unitary circle identified by the angle ωT_s. Defining

$$\vec{B}_m = (z - z_m)|_{z=e^{j\omega T_s}}$$
$$\vec{A}_k = (z - p_k)|_{z=e^{j\omega T_s}} \tag{2.15}$$

we obtain

$$|H(\omega)| = \frac{b_0 \prod_{m=1,M}|\vec{B}_m|}{\prod_{k=1,N}|\vec{A}_k|}$$
$$\angle H(\omega) = \sum_{m=1,M} \angle\vec{B}_m - \sum_{k=1,N} \angle\vec{A}_k + (N - M)\omega T_s \tag{2.16}$$

Thus the modulus of $H(\omega)$ can be evaluated at any frequency $\omega°$ by computing the distances between poles and zeroes and the point on the unitary circle corresponding to $\omega = \omega°$, as evidenced in Figure 2.8, where a filter with two pairs of complex poles and three zeroes is considered.

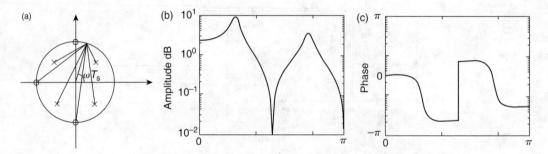

FIGURE 2.8 Poles and zeroes geometry (a) and relative frequency response modulus (b) and phase (c) characteristics. Moving around the unitary circle a rough estimation of $|H(\omega)|$ and $\angle H(\omega)$ can be obtained. Note the zeroes' effects at π and $\pi/2$ and modulus rising in proximity of the poles. Phase shifts are clearly evident in part c closer to zeroes and poles.

To obtain the estimate of $H(\omega)$, we move around the unitary circle and roughly evaluate the effect of poles and zeroes by keeping in mind a few rules [Challis and Kitney, 1982] (1) when we are close to a zero, $|H(\omega)|$ will approach zero, and a positive phase shift will appear in $\angle H(\omega)$ as the vector from the zero reverses its angle; (2) when we are close to a pole, $|H(\omega)|$ will tend to peak, and a negative phase change is found in $\angle H(\omega)$ (the closer the pole to unitary circle, the sharper is the peak until it reaches infinite and the filter becomes unstable); and (3) near a closer pole-zero pair, the response modulus will tend to zero or infinity if the zero or the pole is closer, while far from this pair, the modulus can be considered unitary. As an example, it is possible to compare the modulus and phase diagram of Figure 2.8b,c with the relative geometry of the poles and zeroes of Figure 2.8a.

2.2.1.3 FIR and IIR Filters

A common way of classifying digital filters is based on the characteristics of their impulse response. For finite impulse response (FIR) filters, $h(n)$ is composed of a finite number of nonzero values, while for infinite impulse response (IIR) filters, $h(n)$ oscillates up to infinity with nonzero values. It is clearly evident that in order to obtain an infinite response to an impulse in input, the IIR filter must contain some feedback that sustains the output as the input vanishes. The presence of feedback paths requires putting particular attention to the filter stability.

Even if FIR filters are usually implemented in a nonrecursive form and IIR filters in a recursive form, the two ways of classification are not coincident. In fact, as shown by the following example, a FIR filter can be expressed in a recursive form:

$$H(z) = \sum_{k=0,N-1} z^{-k} = \sum_{k=0,N-1} z^{-k} \frac{(1-z^{-1})}{(1-z^{-1})} = \frac{1-z^{-N}}{1-z^{-1}} \qquad (2.17)$$

for a more convenient computational implementation.

As shown previously, two important requirements for filters are stability and linear phase response. FIR filters can be easily designed to fulfill such requirements; they are always stable (having no poles outside the origin), and the linear phase response is obtained by constraining the impulse response coefficients to have symmetry around their midpoint. Such constrain implies

$$b_m = \pm b_{M-m}^{\cdot} \qquad (2.18)$$

where the b_m are the M coefficients of an FIR filter. The sign $+$ or $-$ stays in accordance with the symmetry (even or odd) and M value (even or odd). This is a necessary and sufficient condition for FIR filters to have linear phase response. Two cases of impulse response that yield a linear phase filter are shown in Figure 2.9.

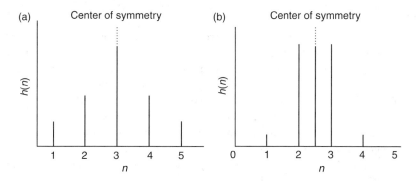

FIGURE 2.9 Examples of impulse response for linear phase FIR filters: odd (a) and even (b) number of coefficients.

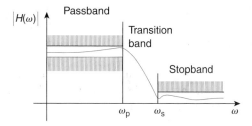

FIGURE 2.10 Amplitude response for a real low-pass filter. Ripples are admitted in both passband and stopband, but they are constrained into restricted areas. Limitations are also imposed to the width of the transition band.

It should be noted that Equation 2.18 imposes geometric constrains to the zero locus of $H(z)$. Taking into account Equation 2.12, we have

$$z^M H(z) = H\left(\frac{1}{z^*}\right) \tag{2.19}$$

Thus, both z_m and $1/z_m^*$ must be zeroes of $H(z)$. Then the zeroes of linear phase FIR filters must lie on the unitary circle, or they must appear in pairs and with inverse moduli.

2.2.1.4 Design Criteria

In many cases, the filter is designed in order to satisfy some requirements, usually on the frequency response, which depend on the characteristic of the particular application the filter is intended for. It is known that ideal filters, like those reported in Figure 2.7, are not physically realizable (they would require an infinite number of coefficients of impulse response); thus we can design FIR or IIR filters that can only mimic, with an acceptable error, the ideal response. Figure 2.10 shows a frequency response of a not ideal low-pass filter. Here, there are ripples in passband and in stopband, and there is a transition band from passband to stopband, defined by the interval $\omega_s - \omega_p$.

Several design techniques are available, and some of them require heavy computational tasks, which are capable of developing filters with defined specific requirements. They include window technique, frequency-sampling method, or equiripple design for FIR filters. Butterworth, Chebychev, elliptical design, and impulse-invariant or bilinear transformation are instead employed for IIR filters. For detailed analysis of digital filter techniques, see Antoniou [1979], Cerutti [1983], and Oppenheim and Schafer [1975].

2.2.1.5 Examples

A few examples of different kinds of filters will be presented in the following, showing some applications on ECG signal processing. It is shown that the ECG contains relevant information over a wide range of frequencies; the lower-frequency contents should be preserved for correct measurement of the slow ST displacements, while higher-frequency contents are needed to correctly estimate amplitude and duration of the faster contributions, mainly at the level of the QRS complex. Unfortunately, several sources of noise are present in the same frequency band, such as, higher-frequency noise due to muscle contraction (EMG noise), the lower-frequency noise due to motion artifacts (baseline wandering), the effect of respiration or the low-frequency noise in the skin-electrode interface, and others.

In the first example, the effect of two different low-pass filters will be considered. An ECG signal corrupted by an EMG noise (Figure 2.11a) is low-pass filtered by two different low-pass filters whose frequency responses are shown in Figure 2.11b,c. The two FIR filters have cutoff frequencies at 40 and 20 Hz, respectively, and were designed through window techniques (Weber–Cappellini window, filter length = 256 points) [Cappellini et al., 1978].

The output signals are shown in Figure 2.11d,e. Filtering drastically reduces the superimposed noise but at the same time alters the original ECG waveform. In particular, the R wave amplitude is progressively reduced by decreasing the cutoff frequency, and the QRS width is progressively increased as well. On the other hand, P waves appear almost unaffected, having frequency components generally lower than 20 to 30 Hz. At this point, it is worth noting that an increase in QRS duration is generally associated with various pathologies, such as ventricular hypertrophy or bundle-branch block. It is therefore necessary to check that an excessive band limitation does not introduce a false-positive indication in the diagnosis of the ECG signal.

An example of an application for stopband filters (**notch filters**) is presented in Figure 2.12. it is used to reduce the 50-Hz mains noise on the ECG signal, and it was designated by placing a zero in correspondence of the frequency we want to suppress.

Finally, an example of a high-pass filter is shown for the detection of the QRS complex. Detecting the time occurrence of a fiducial point in the QRS complex is indeed the first task usually performed in ECG signal analysis. The QRS complex usually contains the higher-frequency components with respect to the other ECG waves, and thus such components will be enhanced by a high-pass filter. Figure 2.13 shows how QRS complexes (Figure 2.13a) can be identified by a derivative high-pass filter with a cutoff frequency to decrease the effect of the noise contributions at high frequencies (Figure 2.13b). The filtered signal (Figure 2.13c) presents sharp and well-defined peaks that are easily recognized by a threshold value.

2.2.2 Signal Averaging

Traditional filtering performs very well when the frequency content of signal and noise do not overlap. When the noise bandwidth is completely separated from the signal bandwidth, the noise can be decreased easily by means of a linear filter according to the procedures described earlier. On the other hand, when the signal and noise bandwidth overlap and the noise amplitude is enough to seriously corrupt the signal, a traditional filter, designed to cancel the noise, also will introduce signal cancellation or, at least, distortion. As an example, let us consider the brain potentials evoked by a sensory stimulation (visual, acoustic, or somatosensory) generally called evoked potentials (EP). Such a response is very difficult to determine because its amplitude is generally much lower than the background EEG activity. Both EP and EEG signals contain information in the same frequency range; thus the problem of separating the desired response cannot be approached via traditional digital filtering [Aunon et al., 1981]. Another typical example is in the detection of ventricular late potentials (VLP) in the ECG signal. These potentials are very small in amplitude and are comparable with the noise superimposed on the signal and also for what concerns the frequency content [Simson, 1981]. In such cases, an increase in the SNR may be achieved on the basis of different statistical properties of signal and noise.

When the desired signal repeats identically at each iteration (i.e., the EP at each sensory stimulus, the VLP at each cardiac cycle), the averaging technique can satisfactorily solve the problem of separating signal

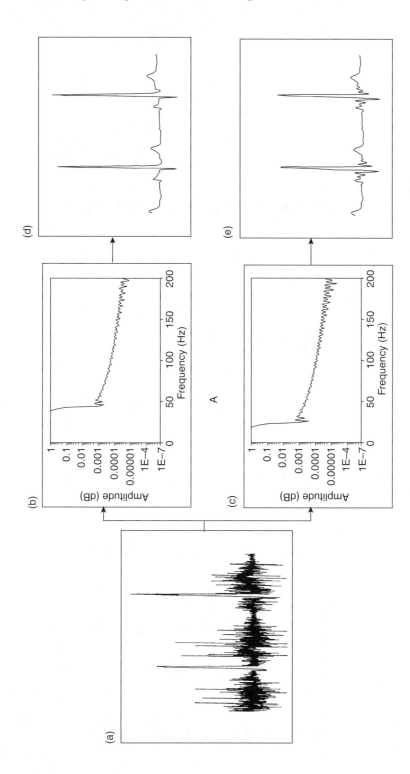

FIGURE 2.11 Effects of two different low-pass filters (b) and (c) on an ECG trace (a) corrupted by EMG noise. Both amplitude reduction and variation in the QRS induced by too drastic low-pass filtering are evidenced.

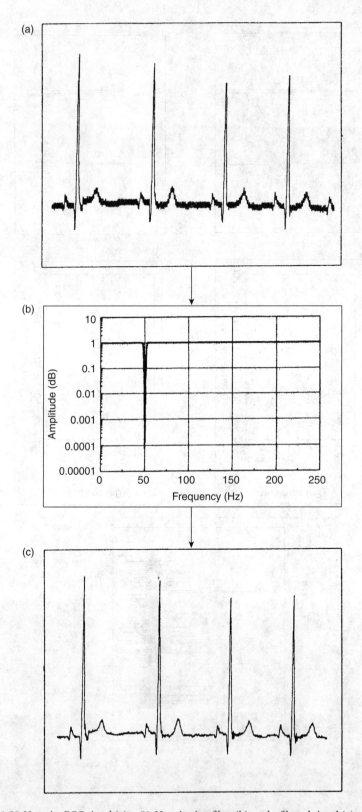

FIGURE 2.12 A 50-Hz noisy ECG signal (a); a 50-Hz rejection filter (b); and a filtered signal (c).

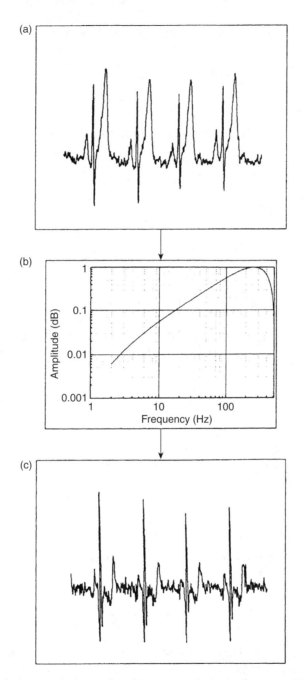

FIGURE 2.13 Effect of a derivative high-pass filter (b) on an ECG lead (a). The output of the filter (c).

from noise. This technique sums a set of temporal epochs of the signal together with the superimposed noise. If the time epochs are properly aligned, through efficient trigger-point recognition, the signal waveforms directly sum together. If the signal and the noise are characterized by the following statistical properties:

1. All the signal epochs contain a deterministic signal component $x(n)$ that does not vary for all the epochs.

2. The superimposed noise $w(n)$ is a broadband stationary process with zero mean and variance σ^2 so that

$$E[w(n)] = 0$$
$$E[w^2(n)] = \sigma^2 \qquad (2.20)$$

3. Signal $x(n)$ and noise $w_i(n)$ are uncorrelated so that the recorded signal $y(n)$ at the ith iteration can be expressed as

$$y(n)_i = x(n) + w_i(n) \qquad (2.21)$$

Then the averaging process yields y_t:

$$y_t(n) = \frac{1}{N} \sum_{i=1}^{N} y_i = x(n) + \sum_{i=1}^{N} w_i(n) \qquad (2.22)$$

The noise term is an estimate of the mean by taking the average of N realizations. Such an average is a new random variable that has the same mean of the sum terms (zero in this case) and which has variance of σ^2/N. The effect of the coherent averaging procedure is then to maintain the amplitude of the signal and reduce the variance of the noise by a factor of N. In order to evaluate the improvement in the SNR (in rms value) in respect to the SNR (at the generic ith sweep):

$$\text{SNR} = \text{SNR}_i \cdot \sqrt{N} \qquad (2.23)$$

Thus signal averaging improves the SNR by a factor of in rms value.

A coherent averaging procedure can be viewed as a digital filtering process, and its frequency characteristics can be investigated. From Equation 2.17 through the z-transform, the transfer function of the filtering operation results in

$$H(z) = \frac{1 + z^{-h} + z^{-2h} + L + z^{-(N-1)h}}{N} \qquad (2.24)$$

where N is the number of elements in the average, and h is the number of samples in each response. An alternative expression for $H(z)$ is

$$H(z) = \frac{1}{N} \frac{1 - z^{Nh}}{1 - z^h} \qquad (2.25)$$

This is a moving average low-pass filter as discussed earlier, where the output is a function of the preceding value with a lag of h samples; in practice, the filter operates not on the time sequence but in the sweep sequence on corresponding samples.

The frequency response of the filter is shown in Figure 2.14 for different values of the parameter N. In this case, the sampling frequency f_s is the repetition frequency of the sweeps, and we may assume it to be 1 without loss of generality. The frequency response is characterized by a main lobe with the first zero corresponding to $f = 1/N$ and by successive secondary lobes separated by zeroes at intervals $1/N$. The width of each tooth decreases as well as the amplitude of the secondary lobes when increasing the number N of sweeps.

The desired signal is sweep-invariant, and it will be unaffected by the filter, while the broadband noise will be decreased. Some leakage of noise energy takes place in the center of the sidelobes and, of course, at zero frequency. Under the hypothesis of zero mean noise, the dc component has no effect, and the

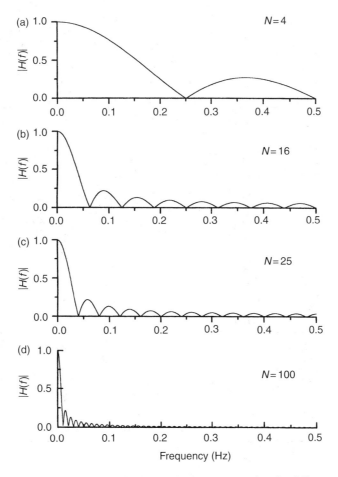

FIGURE 2.14 Equivalent frequency response for the signal-averaging procedure for different values of N (see text).

diminishing sidelobe amplitude implies the leakage to be not relevant for high frequencies. It is important to recall that the average filtering is based on the hypothesis of broadband distribution of the noise and lack of correlation between signal and noise. Unfortunately, these assumptions are not always verified in biologic signals. For example, the assumptions of independence of the background EEG and the evoked potential may be not completely realistic [Gevins and Remond, 1987]. In addition, much attention must be paid to the alignment of the sweeps; in fact, slight misalignments (fiducial point jitter) will lead to a low-pass filtering effect of the final result.

2.2.2.1 Example

As mentioned previously, one of the fields in which signal-averaging technique is employed extensively is in the evaluation of cerebral evoked response after a sensory stimulation. Figure 2.15a shows the EEG recorded from the scalp of a normal subject after a somatosensory stimulation released at time $t = 0$. The evoked potential ($N = 1$) is not visible because it is buried in the background EEG (upper panel). In the successive panels there is the same evoked potential after averaging different numbers of sweeps corresponding to the frequency responses shown in Figure 2.14. As N increases, the SNR is improved by a factor $\sqrt{N}$ (in rms value), and the morphology of the evoked potential becomes more recognizable while the EEG contribution is markedly diminished. In this way it is easy to evaluate the quantitative indices of clinical interest, such as the amplitude and the latency of the relevant waves.

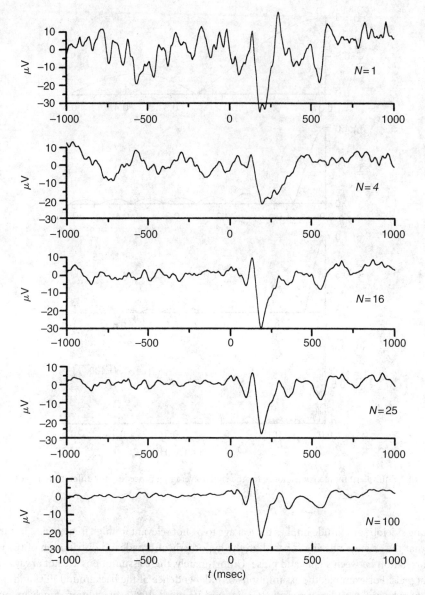

FIGURE 2.15 Enhancement of evoked potential (EP) by means of averaging technique. The EEG noise is progressively reduced, and the EP morphology becomes more recognizable as the number of averaged sweeps (N) is increased.

2.2.3 Spectral Analysis

The various methods to estimate the power spectrum density (PSD) of a signal may be classified as *nonparametric* and *parametric*.

2.2.3.1 Nonparametric Estimators of PSD

This is a traditional method of frequency analysis based on the Fourier transform that can be evaluated easily through the fast Fourier transform (FFT) algorithm [Marple, 1987]. The expression of the PSD as a function of the frequency $P(f)$ can be obtained directly from the time series $y(n)$ by using the periodogram expression

$$P(f) = \frac{1}{T_s} \left| T_s \sum_{k=0}^{N-1} y(k)e^{-j2\pi fkT_s} \right|^2 = \frac{1}{NT_s}|Y(f)|^2 \tag{2.26}$$

where T_s is the sampling period, N is the number of samples, and $Y(f)$ is the discrete time Fourier transform of $y(n)$.

On the basis of the Wiener–Khintchin theorem, PSD is also obtainable in two steps from the FFT of the autocorrelation function $\hat{R}_{yy}(k)$ of the signal, where $\hat{R}_{yy}(k)$ is estimated by means of the following expression:

$$\hat{R}_{yy}(k) = \frac{1}{N} \sum_{i=0}^{N-k-1} y(i)y^*(i+k) \tag{2.27}$$

where $*$ denotes the complex conjugate. Thus the PSD is expressed as

$$P(f) = T_s \cdot \sum_{k=-N}^{N} \hat{R}_{yy}(k)e^{-j2\pi fkT_s} \tag{2.28}$$

based on the available lag estimates $\hat{R}_{yy}(k)$, where $-(1/2T_s) \leq f \leq (1/2T_s)$.

FFT-based methods are widely diffused, for their easy applicability, computational speed, and direct interpretation of the results. Quantitative parameters are obtained by evaluating the power contribution at different frequency bands. This is achieved by dividing the frequency axis in ranges of interest and by integrating the PSD on such intervals. The area under this portion of the spectrum is the fraction of the total signal variance due to the specific frequencies. However, autocorrelation function and Fourier transform are theoretically defined on infinite data sequences. Thus errors are introduced by the need to operate on finite data records in order to obtain estimators of the true functions. In addition, for the finite data set it is necessary to make assumptions, sometimes not realistic, about the data outside the recording window; commonly they are considered to be zero. This implicit rectangular windowing of the data results in a special leakage in the PSD. Different windows that smoothly connect the side samples to zero are most often used in order to solve this problem, even if they may introduce a reduction in the frequency resolution [Harris, 1978]. Furthermore, the estimators of the signal PSD are not statistically consistent, and various techniques are needed to improve their statistical performances. Various methods are mentioned in the literature; the methods of Dariell [1946], Bartlett [1948], and Welch [1970] are the most diffused ones. Of course, all these procedures cause a further reduction in frequency resolution.

2.2.3.2 Parametric Estimators

Parametric approaches assume the time series under analysis to be the output of a given mathematical model, and no drastic assumptions are made about the data outside the recording window. The PSD is calculated as a function of the model parameters according to appropriate expressions. A critical point in this approach is the choice of an adequate model to represent the data sequence. The model is completely independent of the physiologic, anatomic, and physical characteristics of the biologic system but provides simply the input–output relationships of the process in the so-called black-box approach.

Among the numerous possibilities of modeling, linear models, characterized by a rational transfer function, are able to describe a wide number of different processes. In the most general case, they are represented by the following linear equation that relates the input-driving signal $w(k)$ and the output of an autoregressive moving average (ARMA) process:

$$y(k) = -\sum_{i=1}^{p} a_i y(k-i) + \sum_{j=1}^{q} b_j w(k-j) + w(k) \tag{2.29}$$

where $w(k)$ is the input white noise with zero mean value and variance λ^2, p and q are the orders of AR and MA parts, respectively, and a_i and b_j are the proper coefficients.

The ARMA model may be reformulated as an AR or an MA if the coefficients b_j or a_i are, respectively, set to zero. Since the estimation of the AR parameters results in liner equations, AR models are usually employed in place of ARMA or MA models, also on the basis of the Wold decomposition theorem [Marple, 1987] that establishes that any stationary ARMA or MA process of finite variance can be represented as a unique AR model of appropriate order, even infinite; likewise, any ARMA or AR process can be represented by an MA model of sufficiently high order.

The AR PPSD is then obtained from the following expression:

$$P(f) = \frac{\lambda^2 T_s}{|1 + \sum_{i=1}^{p} a_i z^{-i}|^2_{z=\exp(j2\pi f T_s)}} = \frac{\lambda^2 T_s}{\prod_{i=1}^{p} (z - z_l)|^2_{z=\exp(j2\pi f T_s)}} \tag{2.30}$$

The right side of the relation puts into evidence the poles of the transfer function that can be plotted in the z-transform plane. Figure 2.16b shows the PSD function of the HRV signal depicted in Figure 2.16a, while Figure 2.16c displays the corresponding pole diagram obtained according to the procedure described in the preceding section.

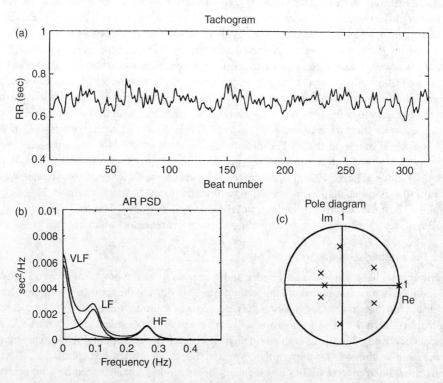

FIGURE 2.16 (a) Interval tachogram obtained from an ECG recording as the sequence of the RR time intervals expressed in seconds as a function of the beat number. (b) PSD of the signal (a) evaluated by means of an AR model (see text). (c) Pole diagram of the PSD shown in (b).

Parametric methods are methodologically and computationally more complex than the nonparametric ones, since they require an a priori choice of the structure and of the order of the model of the signal-generation mechanism. Some tests are required a posteriori to verify the whiteness of the prediction error, such as the Anderson test (autocorrelation test) [Box and Jenkins, 1976] in order to test the reliability of the estimation.

Postprocessing of the spectra can be performed as well as for nonparametric approaches by integrating the $P(f)$ function in predefined frequency ranges; however, the AR modeling has the advantage of allowing a spectral decomposition for a direct and automatic calculation of the power and frequency of each spectral component. In the z-transform domain, the autocorrelation function (ACF) $R(k)$ and the $P(z)$ of the signal are related by the following expression:

$$R(k) = \frac{1}{2\pi j} \int_{|z|=1} P(z)z^{k-1}\, dz \tag{2.31}$$

If the integral is calculated by means of the residual method, the ACF is decomposed into a sum of dumped sinusoids, each one related to a pair of complex conjugate poles, and of dumped exponential functions, related to the real poles [Zetterberg, 1969]. The Fourier transform of each one of these terms gives the expression of each spectral component that fits the component related to the relevant pole or pole pair. The argument of the pole gives the central frequency of the component, while the ith spectral component power is the residual γ_i in the case of real poles and $2\text{Re}(\gamma_i)$ in case of conjugate pole pairs. γ_i is computed from the following expression:

$$\gamma_i = z^{-1}(z - z_i)P(z)|_{z=z_i}$$

It is advisable to point out the basic characteristics of the two approaches that have been described above: the nonparametric and the parametric. The latter (parametric) has evident advantages with respect to the former, which can be summarized in the following:

- It has a more statistical consistency even on short segments of data; that is, under certain assumptions, a spectrum estimated through autoregressive modeling is a maximum entropy spectrum (MES).
- The spectrum is more easily interpretable with an "implicit" filtering of what is considered random noise.
- An easy and more reliable calculation of the spectral parameters (postprocessing of the spectrum), through the spectral decomposition procedure, is possible. Such parameters are directly interpretable from a physiologic point of view.
- There is no need to window the data in order to decrease the spectral leakage.
- The frequency resolution does not depend on the number of data.

On the other hand, the parametric approach

- Is more complex from a methodologic and computational point of view.
- Requires an a priori definition of the kind of model (AR, MA, ARMA, or other) to be fitted and mainly its complexity defined (i.e., the number of parameters).

Some figures of merit introduced in the literature may be of help in determining their value [Akaike, 1974]. Still, this procedure may be difficult in some cases.

2.2.3.3 Example

As an example, let us consider the frequency analysis of the heart rate variability (HRV) signal. In Figure 2.16a, the time sequence of the RR intervals obtained from an ECG recording is shown. The RR intervals are expressed in seconds as a function of the beat number in the so-called interval tachogram. It is worth noting that the RR series is not constant but is characterized by oscillations of up to the 10% of its mean value. These oscillations are not causal but are the effect of the action of the autonomic nervous system in controlling heart rate. In particular, the frequency analysis of such a signal (Figure 2.16b shows the PSD obtained by means of an AR model) has evidenced three principal contributions in the overall variability of the HRV signal. A very low frequency (VLF) component is due to the long-term regulation mechanisms that cannot be resolved by analyzing a few minutes of signal (3 to 5 min are generally studied in the traditional spectral analysis of the HRV signal). Other techniques are needed for a complete understanding of such mechanisms. The low-frequency (LF) component is centered around 0.1 Hz, in a range between 0.03 and 0.15 Hz. An increase in its power has always been observed in relation to sympathetic activations. Finally, the high-frequency (HF) component, in synchrony with the respiration rate, is due to the respiration activity mediated by the vagus nerve; thus it can be a marker of vagal activity. In particular, LF and HF power, both in absolute and in normalized units (i.e., as percentage value on the total power without the VLF contribution), and their ratio LF/HF are quantitative indices widely employed for the quantification of the sympathovagal balance in controlling heart rate [Malliani et al., 1991].

2.3   Conclusion

The basic aspects of signal acquisition and processing have been illustrated, intended as fundamental tools for the treatment of biologic signals. A few examples also were reported relative to the ECG signal, as well as EEG signals and EPs. Particular processing algorithms have been described that use digital filtering techniques, coherent averaging, and power spectrum analysis as reference examples on how traditional or innovative techniques of digital signal processing may impact the phase of informative parameter extraction from biologic signals. They may improve the knowledge of many physiologic systems as well as help clinicians in dealing with new quantitative parameters that could better discriminate between normal and pathologic cases.

Defining Terms

Aliasing: Phenomenon that takes place when, in A/D conversion, the sampling frequency f_s is lower than twice the frequency content f_b of the signal; frequency components above $f_s/2$ are folded back and are summed to the lower-frequency components, distorting the signal.

Averaging: Filtering technique based on the summation of N stationary waveforms buried in casual broadband noise. The SNR is improved by a factor of.

Frequency response: A complex quantity that, multiplied by a sinusoid input of a linear filter, gives the output sinusoid. It completely characterizes the filter and is the Fourier transform of the impulse response.

Impulse reaction: Output of a digital filter when the input is the impulse sequence $d(n)$. It completely characterizes linear filters and is used for evaluating the output corresponding to different kinds of inputs.

Notch filter: A stopband filter whose stopped band is very sharp and narrow.

Parametric methods: Spectral estimation methods based on the identification of a signal generating model. The power spectral density is a function of the model parameters.

Quantization error: Error added to the signal, during the A/D procedure, due to the fact that the analog signal is represented by a digital signal that can assume only a limited and predefined set of values.

Region of convergence: In the z-transform plane, the ensemble containing the z-complex points that makes a series converge to a finite value.

References

Akaike H. (1974). A new look at the statistical model identification. *IEEE Trans. Autom. Contr.* (AC-19): 716.

Antoniou A. (1979). *Digital Filters: Analysis and Design*. New York: McGraw-Hill.

Aunon J.L., McGillim C.D., and Childers D.G. (1981). Signal processing in evoked potential research: Averaging and modeling. *CRC Crit. Rev. Bioeng*. 5: 323.

Bartlett MS. (1948). Smoothing priodograms from time series with continuous spectra. *Nature* 61: 686.

Box G.E.P. and Jenkins G.M. (1976). *Time Series Analysis: Forecasting and Control*. San Francisco, Holden-Day.

Cappellini V., Constantinides A.G., and Emiliani P. (1978). *Digital Filters and Their Applications*. London, Academic Press.

Carassa F. (1983). *Comunicazioni Elettriche*. Torino, Boringhieri.

Cerutti S. (1983). *Filtri numerici per l'eleborazione di segnali biologici*. Milano, CLUP.

Challis R.E. and Kitney R.I. (1982). The design of digital filters for biomedical signal processing: 1. Basic concepts. *J. Biomed. Eng.* 5: 267.

Cobbold R.S.C. (1988). *Transducers for Biomedical Measurements*. New York, John Wiley & Sons.

Cohen A. (1983). *Biomedical Signal Processing: Time and Frequency Domains Analysis*. Boca Raton, FL, CRC Press.

Dariell P.J. (1946). On the theoretical specification and sampling properties of autocorrelated time-series (discussion). *J.R. Stat. Soc.* 8: 88.

Gardenhire L.W. (1964). Selecting sample rate. *ISA J.* 4: 59.

Gevins A.S. and Remond A. (Eds) (1987). *Handbook of Electrophysiology and Clinical Neurophysiology*. Amsterdam, Elsevier.

Glaser E.M. and Ruchkin D.S. (1976). *Principles of Neurophysiological Signal Processing*. New York, Academic Press.

Harris F.J. (1978). On the use of windows for harmonic analysis with the discrete Fourier transform. *Proc. IEEE* 64: 51.

Huta K. and Webster J.G. (1973). 60-Hz interference in electrocardiography. *IEEE Trans. Biomed. Eng.* 20: 91.

Jackson L.B. (1986). *Digital Signal Processing*. Hingham, Mas., Kluwer Academic.

Jaeger R.C. (1982). Tutorial: Analog data acquisition technology: II. Analog to digital conversion. *IEEE Micro.* 8: 46.

Malliani A., Pagani M., Lombardi F., and Cerutti S. (1991). Cardiovascular neural regulation explored in the frequency domain. *Circulation* 84: 482.

Marple S.L. (1987). *Digital Spectral Analysis with Applications*. Englewood Cliffs, NJ, Prentice-Hall.

Oppenheim A.V. and Schafer R.W. (1975). *Digital Signal Processing*. Englewood Cliffs, NJ, Prentice-Hall.

Rainer L.R., Cooley J.W., Helms H.D. et al. (1972). Terminology in digital signal processing. *IEEE Trans. Audio Electroac.* AU-20: 322.

Shannon C.E. (1949). Communication in presence of noise. *Proc IRE* 37: 10.

Simson M.B. (1981). Use of signals in the terminal QRS complex to identify patients with ventricular tachycardia after myocardial infarction. *Circulation* 64: 235.

Thakor N.V. (1987). Adaptive filtering of evoked potential. *IEEE Trans. Biomed. Eng.* 34: 1706.

Tompkins W.J. (Ed). (1993). *Biomedical Digital Signal Processing*. Englewood Cliffs, NJ, Prentice-Hall.

Tompkins W.J. and Webster J.G. (Eds) (1981). *Design of Microcomputer-Based Medical Instrumentation*. Englewood Cliffs, NJ, Prentice-Hall.

Webster J.G. (Ed) (1992). *Medical Instrumentation*, 2nd ed. Boston, Houghton-Mufflin.

Welch D.P. (1970). The use of fast Fourier transform for the estimation of power spectra: A method based on time averaging over short modified periodograms. *IEEE Trans. Acoust.* AU-15: 70.

Widrow B. (1956). A study of rough amplitude quantization by means of Nyquist sampling theory. *IRE Trans. Cric. Theory* 3: 266.

Widrow B., Glover J.R.J., Kaunitz J. et al. (1975). Adaptive noise cancelling: Principles and applications. *Proc IEEE* 63: 1692.

Zetterberg L.H. (1969). Estimation of parameters for a linear difference equation with application to EEG analysis. *Math. Biosci.* 5: 227.

Further Information

A book that provides a general overview of basic concepts in biomedical signal processing is *Digital Biosignal Processing*, by Rolf Weitkunat (Ed.) (Elsevier Science Publishers, Amsterdam, 1991). Contributions by different authors provide descriptions of several processing techniques and many applicative examples on biologic signal analysis. A deeper and more specific insight of actual knowledge and future perspectives on ECG analysis can be found in *Electrocardiography: Past and Future*, by Philippe Coumel and Oscar B. Garfein (Eds.) (Annals of the New York Academy Press, vol. 601, 1990). Advances in signal processing are monthly published in the journal *IEEE Transactions on Signal Processing*, while the *IEEE Transaction on Biomedical Engineering* provides examples of applications in biomedical engineering fields.

3

Compression of Digital Biomedical Signals

3.1   Introduction... 3-1
3.2   Time-Domain Coding of Biomedical Signals.......... 3-2
         Data Compression by DPCM • AZTEC ECG Compression
         Method • Turning Point ECG Compression Method • ECG
         Compression via Parameter Extraction
3.3   Frequency-Domain Data Compression Methods 3-4
3.4   Wavelet or Subband Coding 3-5
3.5   Hybrid Multichannel ECG Coding 3-6
         Preprocessor • Linear Transformer • Compression of the
         Transform Domain Signals • Subband Coder (SBC)
3.6   Conclusion 3-11
References 3-11
Further Information 3-12

A. Enis Çetin
Hayrettin Köymen
Bilkent University

3.1 Introduction

Computerized electrocardiogram (ECG), electroencephalogram (EEG), and magnetoencephalogram (MEG) processing systems have been widely used in clinical practice [1] and they are capable of recording and processing long records of biomedical signals. The use of such systems (1) enables the construction of large signal databases for subsequent evaluation and comparison, (2) makes the transmission of biomedical information feasible over telecommunication networks in real time or off line, and (3) increases the capabilities of ambulatory recording systems such as the Holter recorders for ECG signals. In spite of the great advances in VLSI memory technology, the amount of data generated by digital systems may become excessive quickly. For example, a Holter recorder needs more than 200 Mbits/day of memory space to store a dual-channel ECG signal sampled at a rate of 200 samples/sec with 10 bit/sample resolution. Since the recorded data samples are correlated with each other, there is an inherent redundancy in most biomedical signals. This can be exploited by the use of data compression techniques which have been successfully utilized in speech, image, and video signals [2] as well.

The aim of any biomedical signal compression scheme is to minimize the storage space without losing any clinically significant information, which can be achieved by eliminating redundancies in the signal, in a reasonable manner.

Data compression methods can be classified into two categories: (1) lossless and (2) lossy coding methods. In lossless data compression, the signal samples are considered to be realizations of a random variable or a random process and the entropy of the source signal determines the lowest compression ratio that can be achieved. In lossless coding the original signal can be perfectly reconstructed. For typical biomedical signals lossless (reversible) compression methods can only achieve Compression Ratios (CR) in the order of 2 to 1. On the other hand lossy (irreversible) techniques may produce CR results in the order of 10 to 1. In lossy methods, there is some kind of quantization of the input data which leads to higher CR results at the expense of reversibility. But this may be acceptable as long as no clinically significant degradation is introduced to the encoded signal. The CR levels of 2 to 1 are too low for most practical applications. Therefore, lossy coding methods which introduce small reconstruction errors are preferred in practice. In this section we review the lossy biomedical data compression methods.

3.2 Time-Domain Coding of Biomedical Signals

Biomedical signals can be compressed in time domain, frequency domain, or time–frequency domain. In this section the time domain techniques, which are the earlier approaches to biomedical signal compression, are reviewed.

3.2.1 Data Compression by DPCM

Differential pulse code modulation (DPCM) is a well-known data coding technique in which the main idea is to decorrelate the input signal samples by linear prediction. The current signal sample, $x(n)$, is estimated from the past samples by using either a fixed or adaptive linear predictor

$$\hat{x}(n) = \sum_{k=1}^{N} a_k x(n-k) \tag{3.1}$$

where $\hat{x}(n)$ is the estimate of $x(n)$ at discrete time instant n, and $\{a_k\}$ is the predictor weight. The samples of the estimation error sequence, $e(n) = x(n) - \hat{x}(n)$ are less correlated with each other compared to the original signal, $x(n)$ as the predictor removes the unnecessary information which is the predictable portion of the sample $x(n)$. In a typical DPCM encoder, the error sequence is quantized by using a nonuniform quantizer and quantizer outputs are entropy coded by assigning variable-length codewords to the quantized error sequence according to the frequency of occurrence. The variable-length codebook is constructed by Huffman coding which assigns shorter (longer) codewords to values occurring with higher (lower) probabilities. Huffman coding produces compression results that are arbitrarily close to the entropy of the quantized error sequence.

A CR of 7.8 was reported for an ECG signal recorded at a rate of 500 Hz with 8 bit/sample resolution [3]. This means that about 1 bit/sample is used to represent the ECG signal. The corresponding percent root mean square difference (PRD) was 3.5. The PRD is a measure of reconstruction error and it is defined as follows:

$$\text{PRD} = \sqrt{\frac{\sum_{n=0}^{N-1}[x(n) - x_{\text{rec}}(n)]^2}{\sum_{n=0}^{N-1} x^2(n)}} * 100 \tag{3.2}$$

where N is the total number of samples in the ECG signal, $x(n)$, and $x_{\text{rec}}(n)$ is the reconstructed ECG signal.

A typical DPCM encoder may become a lossless coder if the quantization step is skipped. In this case CR drops drastically to low values.

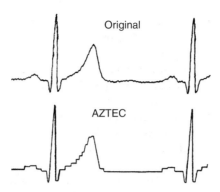

FIGURE 3.1 AZTEC representation of an ECG waveform.

3.2.2 AZTEC ECG Compression Method

The Amplitude Zone Time Epoch Coding (AZTEC) is one of the earliest ECG coding methods. It was developed by Cox et al. [4] as a preprocessing software for real-time monitoring of ECGs. It was observed to be useful for automatic analysis of ECGs such as QRS detection, but it is inadequate for visual presentation of the ECG signal as the reconstructed signal has a staircase appearance.

In this method the ECG signal is considered to consist of flat regions and "slopes." If the signal value stays within a predetermined constant for more than three consecutive samples then that region is assumed to be constant and stored by its duration (number of samples) and a fixed amplitude value. Otherwise the signal is assumed to have a slope. A slope is stored by its duration and the amplitude of the last sample point. Linear interpolation is used to reconstruct the ECG signal. As a result, the resulting signal has a discontinuous nature as shown in Figure 3.1.

Even through AZTEC produces a high compression ratio (CR = 10 to 1, for 500 Hz sampled data with 12 bit/sample resolution) the quality of the reconstructed signal is very low and it is not acceptable to cardiologists.

Various modified of AZTEC are proposed [5]. One notable example is the CORTES technique [6]. The CORTES technique is a hybrid of the AZTEC and the Turning Point method which is described in the next section.

3.2.3 Turning Point ECG Compression Method

The Turning Point data reduction method [7] is basically an adaptive downsampling method developed especially for ECGs. It reduces the sampling frequency of an ECG signal by a factor of two.

The method is based on the trends of the signal samples. Three input samples are processed at a time. Let $x(n)$ be the current sample at discrete-time instant n. Among the two consecutive input samples, $x(n + 1)$ and $x(n + 2)$, the one producing the highest slope (in magnitude) is retained and the other sample is dropped. In this way the overall sampling rate is reduced to one-half of the original sampling rate; no other coding is carried out. Therefore, the resulting CR is 2 to 1. A PRD of 5.3% is reported for an ECG signal sampled at 200 Hz with 12 bit/sample resolution [7]. In practice the CR value actually may be lower than two as the retained samples may not be equally spaced and some extra bits may be needed for timing determination.

3.2.4 ECG Compression via Parameter Extraction

In these methods, the signal is analyzed and some important features such as typical cycles, extreme locations, etc. are determined. These features are properly stored. Reconstruction is carried out by using appropriate interpolation schemes.

The location of the extrema or peaks in an ECG signal is important in diagnosis because they basically determine the shape of each ECG period. The ECG compression techniques described in Reference 8 take advantage of this feature and record only the maxima, minima, slope changes, zero-crossing intervals, etc. of the signal. During reconstruction various interpolation schemes such as polynomial fitting and spline functions are used. The performance of the extrema based methods is compared to the AZTEC method and it was reported that for a given CR the RMS error is half of that of AZTEC method [8].

Other parameter extraction methods include [9,10] where ECG signals are analyzed in a cycle-synchronous manner. An AR model is fitted to the MEG signal and parameters of the AR model are stored [11]. An ECG signal is modeled by splines and the data is compressed by storing the spline parameters [12].

Review of some other time-domain ECG data compression methods can be found in Reference 5.

3.3 Frequency-Domain Data Compression Methods

Transform Coding (TC) is the most important frequency-domain digital waveform compression method [2]. The key is to divide the signal into frequency components and judiciously allocate bits in the frequency domain.

In most TC methods, the input signal is first divided into blocks of data and each block is linearly transformed into the "frequency" domain. Let $x = [x_0, x_1, \ldots, x_{N-1}]^{\mathrm{T}}$ be a vector obtained from a block of N input samples. The transform domain coefficients, v_i, $i = 0, 1, \ldots, N - 1$, are given by

$$v = Ax \qquad (3.3)$$

where $v = [v_0 v_1 \ldots v_{N-1}]^{\mathrm{T}}$, and A is the $N \times N$ transform matrix representing the linear transform. A variety of transform matrices including the discrete Fourier transform matrix is used in digital waveform coding [2]. In this section discrete Karhunen–Loeve Transform (KLT) and Discrete Cosine Transform (DCT), which are the most used ones, are reviewed.

If the input signal is a wide sense stationary random process then the so-called optimum linear transform, KLT is well defined and it decorrelates the entries of the input vector. This is equivalent to removing all the unnecessary information contained in the vector x. Therefore, by coding the entries of the v vector, only the useful information is retained. The entries of the v vector are quantized and stored. Usually, different quantizers are used to quantize the entries of the v vector. In general, more bits are allocated to those entries which have high energies compared to the ones with low energies.

The KLT is constructed from the eigenvectors of the autocovariance matrix of the input vector x. In most practical waveforms the statistics of the input vector change from block to block. Thus for each block a new KLT matrix must be constructed. This is computationally very expensive (in some practical cases a fixed KLT matrix is estimated and it is assumed to be constant for a reasonable amount of duration). Furthermore, there is no fast algorithm similar to the Fast Fourier Transform (FFT) to compute the KLT.

The Discrete Cosine Transform (DCT) [2] was developed by Ahmed et al., to approximate KLT when there is high correlation among the input samples, which is the case in many digital waveforms including speech, music, and biomedical signals.

The DCT $v = [v_0, v_1, \ldots, v_{N-1}]^{\mathrm{T}}$ of the vector x is defined as follows:

$$v_0 = \frac{1}{\sqrt{N}} \sum_{n=0}^{N-1} x_n \qquad (3.4)$$

$$v_k = \sqrt{\frac{2}{N}} \sum_{n=0}^{N-1} x_n \cos \frac{(2n+1)k\pi}{2N} \qquad k = 1, 2, \ldots, (N-1) \qquad (3.5)$$

where v_k is the kth DCT coefficient. The inverse discrete cosine transform (IDCT) of v is given as follows:

$$x_n = \frac{1}{\sqrt{N}} v_0 + \sqrt{\frac{2}{N}} \sum_{k=1}^{N-1} v_k \cos \frac{(2n+1)k\pi}{2N} \qquad n = 0, 1, 2, \ldots, (N-1) \tag{3.6}$$

$$\left(\frac{k\pi}{4}, \frac{(k+1)\pi}{4} \right)_{k=0,1,2,3} \tag{3.6a}$$

There exist fast algorithms, Order ($N\log N$), to compute the DCT [2]. Thus, DCT can be implemented in a computationally efficient manner. Two recent image and video coding standards, JPEG and MPEG, use DCT as the main building block.

A CR of 3 to 1 for single channel ECG is reported by using DCT and KLT based coders [13]. For multi-lead systems, two-dimensional (2-D) transform based methods can be used. A CR of 12 to 1 was reported [14] for a three-lead system by using a 2-D KLT. Recently, Philips [15] developed a new transform by using time-warped polynomials and obtained a CR of 26 to 9. In this case a DCT based coding procedure produced a CR of 24 to 3.

Since signal recording conditions and noise levels vary from study to study, a thorough comparison of the coding methods is very difficult to make. But, frequency-domain coding methods produce higher coding results than time-domain coding methods.

3.4   Wavelet or Subband Coding

Wavelet Transform (WT) is a powerful time–frequency signal analysis tool and it is used in a wide variety of applications including signal and image coding [16]. WT and Subband Coding (SBC) are closely related to each other. In fact the fast implementation of WTs are carried out using Subband (SB) filter banks. Due to this reason WT based waveform coding methods are essentially similar to the SBC based methods.

In an SBC structure the basic building block is a digital filter bank which consists of a lowpass and a highpass filter. In the ideal case, the passband (stopband) of the lowpass filter is $[0, \pi/2]$ $[\pi/2, \pi]$. Let $H_l (e^{j\omega})$ $H_u (e^{j\omega})$ be the frequency response of the lowpass (highpass) filter. In SBC the input signal which is sampled at the rate of f_s is filtered by $H_l (e^{j\omega})$ and $H_u (e^{j\omega})$ and the filter outputs are downsampled by a factor of two (every other sample is dropped) in order to maintain the overall sampling rate to be equal to the original rate. In this way two subsignals, $x_i(n)$ and $x_u(n)$ which both have a sampling rate of $f_s/2$ are obtained. The block diagram of a two-level SBC structure is shown in Figure 3.1.

The subsignal, $x_i(n)$ [$x_u(n)$], contains the lowpass (highpass) frequency domain information of the original signal. The subsignals, $x_i(n)$ and $x_u(n)$, can be further divided into their frequency components in a similar manner. This SB division process can be repeated until the frequency domain is divided in a sufficient manner. In Reference 17, the two-level subband structure of Figure 3.2 which divides the frequency domain into four regions, is used to code a single channel ECG signal. The resulting subsignals can be encoded by various coding methods including DPCM, Entropy coding, and transform coding which should be designed to exploit the special nature of the subsignals to achieve the best possible CR for each band. Recently, very successful special encoders which take advantage of the tree structure of the decomposition were developed for compressing the subsignals [18]. The signal reconstruction from the coded subsignals is carried out by using a filter bank consisting of two filters, $G_l(e^{j\omega})$ and $G_u(e^{j\omega})$. In this case the subsignal, $x_i(n)$ [$x_u(n)$] is first upsampled by inserting a zero between every other sample and filtered by $G_l(e^{j\omega})$ [$G_u(e^{j\omega})$]. The reconstructed signal, $y(n)$, is the sum of the outputs of these two filters.

By properly selecting the filters, $H_l(z)$, $H_u(z)$, $G_l(z)$, and $G_u(z)$, perfect reconstruction is possible, that is,

$$y(n) = x(n - K) \tag{3.7}$$

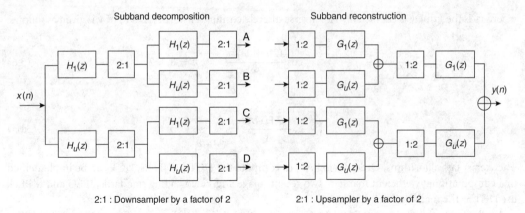

FIGURE 3.2 Two-level (four branch) subband coder structure. This structure divides the frequency domain into four regions.

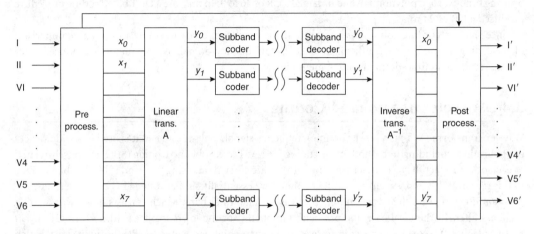

FIGURE 3.3 Block diagram of the multichannel ECG data compression scheme.

in the absence of quantization errors [16]. In other words, filtering and downsampling operations in the SB decomposition structure do not introduce any loss.

A CR 5.22 corresponding to a PRD of 5.94% is reported for an ECG signal sampled at 500 Hz with 12 bit/sample resolution [17].

Other WT based ECG coding methods include [16,19–21].

3.5 Hybrid Multichannel ECG Coding

In this section, a hybrid frequency domain multichannel compression method [22] for the so-called standard lead [23] ECG recording system is described. The block diagram of this system is shown in Figure 3.3. The main idea is to exploit not only the correlation between the consecutive ECG samples, but also the inherent correlation among the ECG channels.

The standard lead system has 12 ECG channels. In this method, the recorded digital signals are first passed through a preprocessor. The function of the preprocessor is to prepare raw ECG data for further processing. After preprocessing the input signals, the resulting discrete-time sequences are linearly transformed into another set of sequences. The aim of this linear transformation is to decorrelate the highly correlated ECG lead signals. In a way, this idea is similar to representing the RGB color components of an image in terms of luminance and chrominance components.

The transformation matrix, A, can be the matrix of the optimum transform, KLT, or the DCT matrix. Another approach is to use a nonlinear transform such as an Independent Component Analyzer (ICA) [24]. Lastly, to compress the transform domain signals, various coding schemes which exploit their special nature are utilized.

In the following sections, detailed descriptions of the sub-blocks of the multichannel ECG compression method are given.

3.5.1 Preprocessor

The standard lead ECG recording configuration consists of 12 ECG leads, I, II, III, AVR, AVL, AVF, V1, V2,...,V6. The leads, III, AVR, AVL, and AVF, are linearly related to I and II. Therefore, eight channels are enough to represent a standard 12-channel ECG recording system.

The preprocessor discards the redundant channels, III, AVR, AVL, and AVF, and rearranges the order of the ECG channels. The six precordial (chest) leads, V1,...,V6, represent variations of the electrical heart vector amplitude with respect to time from six different narrow angles. During a cardiac cycle it is natural to expect high correlation among precordial leads so the channels V1,...,V6 are selected as the first 6 signals, that is, $x_{i-1} = V_i, i = 1, 2, ..., 6$. The two horizontal lead waveforms (I and II) which have relatively less energy contents with respect to precordial ECG lead waveforms are chosen as seventh, $x_6 = $ I, and eighth channels, $x_7 = $ II. A typical set of standard ECG lead waveforms, $x_i, i = 0, 1, ..., 7$, are shown in Figure 3.4.

The aim of the reordering the ECG channels is to increase the efficiency of the linear transformation operation which is described in the next section.

3.5.2 Linear Transformer

The outputs of the preprocessor block, $x_i, i = 0, 1, ..., 7$, are fed to the linear transformer. In this block, the ECG channels are linearly transformed to another domain, and eight new transform domain signals y_i, $i = 0, 1, ..., 7$, are obtained which are significantly less correlated (ideally uncorrelated) than the ECG signal set, $x_i, i = 0, 1, ..., 7$. The transform domain samples at discrete-time instant m are given as follows:

$$Y_m = A \cdot X_m \tag{3.8}$$

where $Y_m = [y_0(m), ..., y_{N-1}(m)]T$, $X_m = [x_0(m), ..., x_{n-1}(m)]T$, and A is the $N \times N$ transform matrix.

The optimum linear transform, discrete KLT, can be properly defined for stationary random processes and the entries of the tranform matrix, A_{KLT} depending on the statistics of the random processes. For slowly varying, unstationary signals, an approximate KLT matrix can also be defined. Although ECG signals cannot be considered to be wide-sense stationary-random processes, a covariance matrix, $\hat{C}_x$, of the ECG channels is estimated as follows:

$$\hat{C}_x = \frac{1}{M} \sum_{i=0}^{M-1} \begin{bmatrix} x_0(i) \\ \vdots \\ x_{N-1}(i) \end{bmatrix} [x_0(i) \cdots x_{N-1}(i)] \tag{3.9}$$

where N is the number of the ECG channels and M is the number of ECG samples per channel used. The $N \times N$ ECG channel covariance matrix, $\hat{C}_x$, is used in the construction of an approximate KLT matrix. Rows of the approximate KLT matrix are the eigenvectors of $\hat{C}_x$. Typical approximate KLT matrices can be found in [22].

Although there is no fast algorithm to compute the KL transform, the computational burden is not high because $N = 8$. The DCT can also be used as a linear transformer because it approximates the KLT.

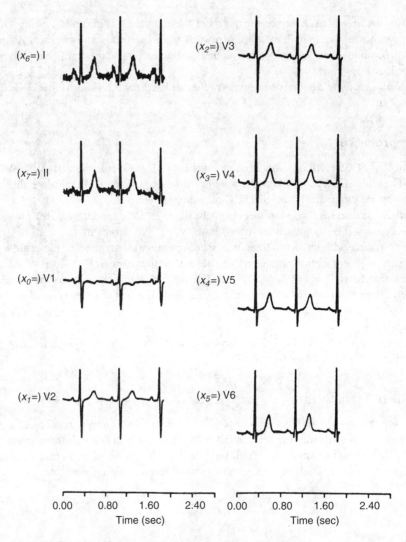

FIGURE 3.4   A typical set of standard ECG lead waveforms x_i, $i = 0, 1, \ldots, 7$.

3.5.3 Compression of the Transform Domain Signals

In this section the compression of the uncorrelated transform domain signals y_k, $k = 0, 1, \ldots, 7$, are described. In Figure 3.5 a typical set of uncorrelated signals, y_k, $k = 0, 1, \ldots, 7$, are shown. The signals in Figure 3.5 are obtained by KL transforming the ECG signals, x_k, $k = 0, 1, \ldots, 7$, shown in Figure 3.4.

Transform domain signals, y_k, $k = 0, 1, \ldots, 7$, are divided into two classes according to their energy contents. The first class of signals, $y_0, y_1, \ldots, y_4$, have higher energy than the second class of signals, y_5, y_6, and y_7. More bits are allocated to the high energy signals, $y_0, y_1, \ldots, y_4$, compared to the low energy signals, y_5, y_6, and y_7 in coding.

3.5.4 Subband Coder (SBC)

Higher energy signals, $y_0(n), y_1(n), \ldots, y_4(n)$, contain more information than the low energy signals, $y_5(n)$, $y_6(n)$, and $y_7(n)$. Therefore, the high energy signals, $y_0(n), \ldots, y_4(n)$ should be compressed very accurately. The signals, $y_0(n), \ldots, y_4(n)$, are compressed using the SBC [17] because this coding scheme does not introduce any visual degradation as pointed out in the previous section [9].

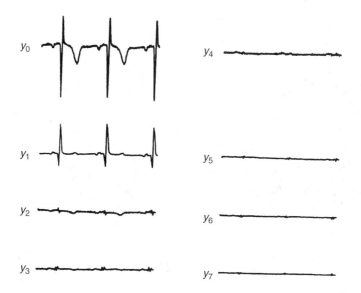

FIGURE 3.5 Uncorrelated signals y_i, $i = 0, 1, 2, \ldots, 7$, corresponding to the ECG signals shown in Figure 3.4.

Each signal y_i is decomposed into four subsignals by using a filter bank in a tree-structured manner. In this way the signal y_i is divided into four consecutive bands, $[l\pi/4, (l+1)\pi/4]$, $l = 0, 1, 2, 3$, in the frequency domain [2]. For example, y_{i00} (the subsignal at branch A of Figure 3.2) comes from the lowpass frequency band, $[0, \pi/4]$, of the signal y_i. In the coding of the subband signals, y_{ijk}, $j = 0, 1$; $k = 0, 1$, the advantage is taken of the nonuniform distribution of energy in the frequency domain to judiciously allocate the bits. The number of bits used to encode each frequency band can be different, so the encoding accuracy is always maintained at the required frequency bands [2].

It is observed that the energy of the signal y_i is mainly concentrated in the lowest frequency band $[0, \pi/4]$. Because of this, the lowband subsignal $y_{i,0,0}$ has to be carefully coded. High correlation among neighboring samples of $y_{i,0,0}$ makes this signal a good candidate for efficient predictive or transform coding. The subsignals $y_{i,0,0}$ are compressed using a DCT based scheme. After the application of DCT with a block size of 64 samples to the lowband subsignal, $y_{i,0,0}$, the transform domain coefficients, $g_{i,0,0}(k)$, $k = 0, 1, \ldots, 63$ are obtained and they are thresholded and quantized. The coefficients whose magnitudes are above a preselected threshold, b, are retained and the other coefficients are discarded. Thresholded DCT coefficients are quantized for bit level representation. Thresholded and quantized nonzero coefficients are variable-length coded by using an amplitude table and the zero values are runlength coded. The amplitude and runlength lookup tables are Huffman coding tables which are obtained according to the histograms of the DCT coefficients [22].

In practice, ECG recording levels do not change from one recording to another. If drastic variations occur, first scale the input by an appropriate factor, then apply DCT.

Bandpass and highpass subsignals, $y_{i,0,1}$, $y_{i,1,0}$, $y_{i,1,1}$ (branches B, C, and D), are coded using non-uniform quantizers. After quantization, a code assignment procedure is realized using variable length amplitude and runlength lookup tables for zero values. The look up tables are obtained according to the histograms of quantized subband signals.

The bit streams which are obtained from coding of four subband signals are multiplexed and stored. Appropriate decoders are assigned to each branch to convert the bit streams into time domain samples and the four-branch synthesis filter bank performs the reconstruction [17].

The low energy signals, $y_5(n)$, $y_6(n)$, $y_7(n)$, are also coded by using the SB coder previously explained. However, it is observed that all the subsignals except the subsignal at branch A of Figure 3.2 contain very little information when subband decomposition is applied to the signals $y_5(n)$, $y_6(n)$, $y_7(n)$. Due to this

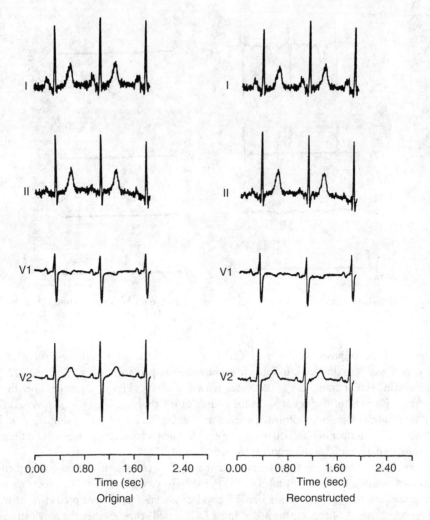

FIGURE 3.6   The original and reconstructed ECG lead signals I, II, V1, and V2 (CR = 6.17, APRD = 6).

fact, only the subsignals at branch A (lowband signals) are processed. The other branches which have very little energy are discarded.

Original and reconstructed ECG waveforms are shown in Figure 3.6 for CR = 6.17 (CR = 7.98) with PRD = 6.19% when DCT (KLT) is used as the Linear Transformer. Recorded ECG signals are sampled at 500 Hz with 12 bit/sample resolution. Also, the raw ECG signals are filtered to attenuate the high frequency noise with a 33-tap equiripple Parks–McClellan FIR filter whose cutoff frequency is equal to 125 Hz. In this case a CR = 9.41 is obtained for a PRD = 5.94%.

The effect of compressing the data on diagnostic computer analysis results is tested on Cardionics program, which is derived from the Mount Sinai program developed by Pordy et al., in conjunction with CRO-MED Bionics Company [25]. Morphological measurements include (1) intervals — PR, QRS, QT, (2) "width"s — Q, R, S, R′, S′, T, P, (3) amplitudes — P, Q, R, R′, S, S′, T, JJ, and (4) areas of QRS and QRST. There was no difference in the measurement results of both the compressed and the original data.

It is experimentally observed that the multichannel technique produces better compression results than single channel schemes. Also, the computational complexity of the multichannel scheme is comparable to single channel ECG coding schemes and the algorithm can be implemented by using digital signal processor for real-time applications, such as transmission of ECG signals over telephone lines.

3.6 Conclusion

In this section biomedical signal compression methods are reviewed. Most of the biomedical data compression methods have been developed for ECG signals. However, these methods can be applied to other biomedical signals with some modifications.

It is difficult to compare the efficiency of biomedical data compression schemes because coding results of various data compression schemes are obtained under different recording conditions such as (1) sampling frequency, (2) bandwidth, (3) sample precision, and (4) noise level, which may drastically affect the currently used performance measures.

References

[1] Willems, J. "Common standards for quantitative electrocardiography," *J. Med. Eng. Techn.*, 9, 209–217, 1985.

[2] Jayant, N.S. and Noll, P. *Digital Coding of Waveforms*, Englewood Cliffs, NJ, Prentice-Hall, 1984.

[3] Ruttiman, U.E. and Pipberger, H.V. "Compression of the ECG by prediction or interpolation and entropy coding," *IEEE Trans. Biomed. Eng.*, 26, 613–623, 1979.

[4] Cox J.R. et al., "AZTEC: a preprocessing program for real-time ecg rhythm analysis," *IEEE Trans. Biomed. Eng.*, 15, 128–129, 1968.

[5] Jalaleddine, S.M.S., Hutchens, C.G., Strattan, R.D., and Coberly, W.A. "ECG data compression techniques: a unified approach," *IEEE Trans. Biomed. Eng.*, BME-37, 329–343, 1990.

[6] Abenstein, J.P. and Tompkins, W.J. "New data reduction algorithm for real-time ECG analysis," *IEEE Trans. Biomed. Eng.*, 29, 43–48, 1982.

[7] Mueller, W.C. "Arrhythmia detection program for an ambulatory ECG monitor," *Biomed. Sci. Instrument*, 14, 81–85, 1978.

[8] Imai, H., Kimura, N., and Yoshida, Y. "An efficient encoding method for ECG using spline functions," *Syst. Comput, Jpn*, 16, 85–94, 1985.

[9] Jalaleddine, S.M.S., Hutchens, C.G., Strattan, R.D., and Coberly, W.A. "Compression of Holter ECG Data," *Biomed. Sci. Instrum.*, 24, 35–45, 1988.

[10] Hamilton, P.S. and Tompkins, W.J. "Compression of the ambulatory ECG by average beat subtraction and residual differencing," *IEEE Trans. Biomed. Eng.*, 38, 253–260, 1991.

[11] Angelidou, A. et al., "On AR modeling for MEG spectral estimation, data compression, and classification," *Comput. Biol Med.*, 22, 379–387, 1992.

[12] Karczewicz, M. and Gabbouj, M. "ECG data compression by spline approximation," *Signal Process.*, 59, 43–59, 1997.

[13] Ahmed, N., Milne, P.J., and Harris, S.G. "Electrocardiographic data compression via orthogonal transforms," *IEEE Trans. Biomed. Eng.*, 22, 484–487, 1975.

[14] Womble, M.E. et al. "Data compression for storing and transmitting ECGs/VCGs," *Proc. IEEE*, 65, 702–706, 1977.

[15] Philips, W. "ECG data compression with time-warped polynomials," *IEEE Trans. Biomed. Eng.*, 40, 1095–1101, 1993.

[16] Strang, G. and Nguyen, T. *Wavelets and Filter Banks*, Wellesley-Cambridge Press, MA, 1996.

[17] Aydin, M.C., Çetin, A.E., Köymen, H. "ECG data compression by sub-band coding," *Electron. Lett.*, 27, 359–360, 1991.

[18] Shapiro, J.M. "Embedded image coding using zerotrees of wavelet coefficients," *IEEE Trans.* SP, 41, 3445–3462, 1993.

[19] Crowe, J.A. et al., "Wavelet transform as a potential tool for ECG analysis and compression," *J. Biomed. Eng.*, 14, 268–272, 1992.

[20] Tai, S.C. "6-band subband coder on ECG waveforms," *Med. Biolog. Eng. Comput.*, 30, 187–192, 1992.

[21] Çetin, A.E., Tewfik, A.H. and Yardimci, Y. "ECG coding by wavelet transform extrema," *IEEE Symp. Time-Freq. and Time-Scale*, Philadelphia, 1994.

[22] Çetin, A.E., Köymen, H., and Aydn, M.C. "Multichannel ECG data compression by multirate signal processing and transform coding techniques," *IEEE Trans. Biomed. Eng.*, 40, 495–499, 1993.

[23] Wyngaarden, J.B. and Smith, L.H. *Textbook of Medicine*, W.B. Saunders, Toronto, 1985.

[24] Vigario, R. and Oja, E. "ICA fixed point algorithm in extraction of artifacts from EEG," NORSIG'96, Finland, pp. 383–386, 1996.

[25] Pordy, L., Jaffe, H., Chelsky, K., Freiedberg, C.K., Fullowes, L., and Bonner, R.E. "Computer diagnosis of electrodcardiograms: a computer program for contour analysis with classical results of rhythm and contour interpretation," *Comput. Biomed. Res.*, 1, 408–433, 1968.

[26] Bertrand, M., Guardo, R., Roberge, F.A., and Blondeau, P. "Microprocessor application for numerical ECG encoding and transmission," *Proc. IEEE*, 65, 714–722, 1977.

[27] Ider, Y.Z. and Köymen, H. "A new technique for line interference monitoring and reduction in biopotential amplifiers," *IEEE Trans. Biomed. Eng.*, 37, 624–631, 1990.

Further Information

Biomedical signal compression is a current research area and most of the research articles describing the advances in biomedical data compression appear in the following journals; IEEE Transactions on Biomedical Engineering and Signal Processing, Journal of Biomedical Engineering, and Medical and Biological Engineering and Computing.

4

Time-Frequency Signal Representations for Biomedical Signals

4.1   One-Dimensional Signal Representations   4-2
4.2   Desirable Properties of Time-Frequency
        Representations   4-2
4.3   TFR Classes...   4-3
        Cohen's Class of TFRs • Affine Class of TFRs • Hyperbolic
        Class of TFRs • *k*th Power Class
4.4   Common TFRs and Their Use in Biomedical
        Applications   4-17
        Wigner Distribution • Smoothed Wigner Distributions •
        Spectrogram • Choi–Williams Exponential and Reduced
        Interference Distributions • Scalogram or Wavelet
        Transform Squared Magnitude • Biomedical Applications
Acknowledgments..   4-20
References   4-20
Further Information   4-22

G. Faye
  Boudreaux-Bartels
Robin Murray
University of Rhode Island

The Fourier transform of a signal $x(t)$

$$X(f) = \int x(t) e^{-j2\pi ft} dt \tag{4.1}$$

is a useful tool for analyzing the spectral content of a stationary signal and for transforming difficult operations such as convolution, differentiation, and integration into very simple algebraic operations in the Fourier dual domain. The inverse Fourier transform equation

$$x(t) = \int X(f) e^{j2\pi ft} df \tag{4.2}$$

is a linear combination of complex sinusoids of infinite duration which implicitly assumes that each sinusoidal component is present at all times and, hence, that the spectral content of the signal does not change with time. However, many signals in bioengineering are produced by biologic systems whose spectral characteristics can change rapidly with time. To analyze these rapid spectral changes one needs a two-dimensional, mixed time-frequency signal representation (TFR) that is analogous to a musical score with time represented along one axis and frequency along the other, indicating which frequency components (notes) are present at each time instant.

The first purpose of this chapter is to review several TFRs defined in Table 4.1 and to describe many of the desirable properties listed in Table 4.2 that an ideal TFR should satisfy. TFRs will be grouped into classes satisfying similar properties to provide a more intuitive understanding of their similarities, advantages, and disadvantages. Further, each TFR within a given class is completely characterized by a unique set of kernels that provide valuable insight into whether or not a given TFR (1) satisfies other ideal TFR properties, (2) is easy to compute, and (3) reduces nonlinear cross-terms. The second goal of this chapter is to discuss applications of TFRs to signal analysis and detection problems in bioengineering. Unfortunately, none of the current TFRs is ideal; some give erroneous information when the signal's spectra are rapidly time-varying. Researchers often analyze several TFRs side by side, keeping in mind the relative strengths and weaknesses of each TFR before drawing any conclusions.

4.1 One-Dimensional Signal Representations

The instantaneous frequency and the group delay of a signal are one-dimensional representations that attempt to represent temporal and spectral signal characteristics simultaneously. The instantaneous frequency of the signal

$$f_x(t) = \frac{1}{2\pi} \frac{\mathrm{d}}{\mathrm{d}t} \arg\{x(t)\} \tag{4.3}$$

has been used in communication theory to characterize the time-varying frequency content of narrowband, frequency-modulated signals. It is a generalization of the fact that the frequency f_0 of a complex sinusoidal signal $x(t) = \exp(j2\pi f_0 t)$ is proportional to the derivative of the signal's phase. A dual concept used in filter analysis is the group delay

$$\tau_H(f) = -\frac{1}{2\pi} \frac{\mathrm{d}}{\mathrm{d}f} \arg\{H(f)\} \tag{4.4}$$

which can be interpreted as the time delay or distortion introduced by the filter's frequency response $H(f)$ at each frequency. Group delay is a generalization of the fact that time translations are coded in the derivative of the phase of the Fourier transform. Unfortunately, if the signal contains several signal components that overlap in time or frequency, then $f_x(t)$ or $\tau_H(f)$ only provides average spectral characteristics, which are not very useful.

4.2 Desirable Properties of Time-Frequency Representations

Mixed time-frequency representations (TFRs) map a one-dimensional signal into a two-dimensional function of time and frequency in order to analyze the time-varying spectral content of the signal. Before discussing any particular TFR in Table 4.1, it is helpful to first investigate what types of properties an "ideal" time-frequency representation should satisfy. The list of desirable TFR properties in Table 4.2 can be broken up conceptually into the following categories: covariance, statistical, signal analysis, localization, and inner products [Boashash, 1991; Claasen and Mecklenbräuker, 1980; Cohen, 1989; Flandrin, 1993; Hlawatsch and Boudreaux-Bartels, 1992]. The covariance properties P_1 to P_6 basically state that certain operations on the signal, such as translations, dilations, or convolution, should be preserved, that is, produce exactly the same operation on the signal's TFR. The second category of properties originates from the desire to generalize the concepts of the one-dimensional instantaneous signal energy $|x(t)|^2$ and power spectral density $|x(f)|^2$ into a two-dimensional statistical energy distribution $T_x(t_0, f_0)$ that provides a measure of the local signal energy or the probability that a signal contains a sinusoidal component of frequency f_0 at time t_0. Properties P_7 to P_{13} state that such an energy-distribution TFR should be real and nonnegative, have its marginal distributions equal to the signal's temporal and spectral energy densities $|x(t)|^2$ and $|X(f)|^2$, respectively, and preserve the signal energy, mean, variance, and other higher-order moments of the instantaneous signal energy and power spectral density. The next category of properties, P_{14} to P_{18}, arises from signal-processing considerations. A TFR should have the same duration and bandwidth as the signal under analysis. At any given time t, the average frequency should equal the instantaneous frequency of the signal, while the average or center of gravity in the time direction should equal the group delay of the signal. These two properties have been used to analyze the distortion of audio systems and the complex FM sonar signals used by bats and whales for echolocation. Property P_{18} is the TFR equivalent of the duality property of Fourier transforms. The group of properties P_{19} to P_{24} constitutes ideal TFR localization properties that are desirable for high resolution capabilities. Here, $d(a)$ is the Dirac function. These properties state that if a signal is perfectly concentrated in time or frequency, that is, an impulse or a sinusoid, then its TFR also should be perfectly concentrated at the same time or frequency. Properties P_{21} and P_{22} state that the TFRs of linear or hyperbolic spectral FM chirp signals should be perfectly concentrated along the chirp signal's group delay. Property P_{24} states that a signal modulated by a linear FM chirp should have a TFR whose instantaneous frequency has been sheared by an amount equal to the linear instantaneous frequency of the chirp. The last property, known as Moyal's formula or the unitarity property, states that TFRs should preserve the signal projections, inner products, and orthonormal signal basis functions that are used frequently in signal detection, synthesis, and approximation theory. Table 4.3 indicates which properties are satisfied by the TFRs listed in Table 4.1.

A TFR should be relatively easy to compute and interpret. Interpretation is greatly simplified if the TFR is linear, that is,

$$T_y(t,f) = \sum_{n=1}^{N} T_{x_n}(t,f) \qquad \text{for } y(t) = \sum_{n=1}^{N} x_n(t) \tag{4.5}$$

However, energy is a quadratic function of the signal, and hence so too are many of the TFRs in Table 4.1. The nonlinear nature of TFRs gives rise to troublesome cross-terms. If $y(t)$ contains N signal components or auto-terms $x_n(t)$ in Equation 4.5, then a quadratic TFR of $y(t)$ can have as many nonzero cross-terms as there are unique pairs of autoterms, that is, $N(N-1)/2$. For many TFRs, these cross-terms are oscillatory and overlap with autoterms, obscuring visual analysis of TFRs.

Two common methods used to reduce the number of cross-terms are to reduce any redundancy in the signal representation and to use local smoothing or averaging to reduce oscillating cross-terms. TFR analysis of real, bandpass signals should be carried out using the analytic signal representation, that is, the signal added to times its Hilbert transform, in order to remove cross-terms between the positive- and negative-frequency axis components of the signal's Fourier transform. As we will see in upcoming sections, cross-term reduction by smoothing is often achieved at the expense of significant autoterm distortion and loss of desirable TFR properties.

4.3 TFR Classes

This section will briefly review Cohen's class of shift covariant TFRs, the Affine class of affine covariant TFRs, the Hyperbolic class (developed for signals with hyperbolic group delay), and the Power class (which is useful for signals with polynomial group delay). Each class is formed by grouping TFRs that satisfy two properties. They provide very helpful insight as to which types of TFRs will work best in different situations. Within a class, each TFR is completely characterized by a unique set of TFR-dependent kernels which can

TABLE 4.1　List of Time–Frequency Representations (TFR) of a Signal $x(t)$ Whose Fourier Transform Is $X(f)$

Ackroyd distribution:
$$ACK_x(t,f) = \text{Re}\left\{x^*(t)X(f)e^{j2\pi ft}\right\}$$

Affine Wigner distribution
$$AWD_x(t,f;G,F) = \int G = \left(\frac{v}{f}\right)X\left(fF\left(\frac{v}{f}\right)+\frac{v}{2}\right)X^*\left(fF\left(\frac{v}{f}\right)-\frac{v}{2}\right)e^{j2\pi tv}\,dv$$

Altes-Marinovic distribution:
$$AM_x(t,f) = |f|\int X(fe^{u/2})X^*(fe^{-u/2})e^{j2\pi tfu}\,du = |f|\iint WAF_X(\tau,e^\beta)e^{j2\pi(tf\beta-f\tau)}\,d\tau\,d\beta$$

(Narrowband) ambiguity function:
$$AF_x(\tau,v) = \int x\left(t+\frac{\tau}{2}\right)x^*\left(t-\frac{\tau}{2}\right)e^{-j2\pi vt}\,dt = \int X\left(f+\frac{v}{2}\right)X^*\left(f-\frac{v}{2}\right)e^{j2\pi\tau f}\,df$$

Andrieux et al. distribution:
$$AND_x(t,f) = \iint \frac{1}{\sigma_{(t-t')}\sigma_{(f-f')}}\exp\left[-\left(\frac{(t-t')^2}{2\sigma_{(t-t')}^2}+\frac{\left(f-b_{(t-t')}(t-t')\right)^2}{2\sigma_{(f-f')}^2}\right)\right]$$
$$WD_x(t',f')\,dt'\,df'$$

where for $x(t) = e^{j2\pi\psi}$, then $b_t = \dfrac{d^2}{dt^2}\varphi(t)$, $\sigma_t = \left|\dfrac{d^3}{dt^3}\varphi(t)\right|^{-1/3}$, and $2\pi\sigma_t\sigma_f = \dfrac{1}{2}$

Autocorrelation function:

Temporal:
$$act_x(\tau) = \int x^*(t)x(t+\tau)\,dt = \int |X(f)|^2 e^{j2\pi\tau}\,df$$

Spectral:
$$ACF_X(v) = \int X^*(f)X(f+v)\,df = \int |x(t)|^2 e^{-j2\pi tv}\,dt$$

Bertramd P_k distribution:
$$BkD_x(t,f;\mu_k) = |f|\int X(f\lambda_k(u))X^*(f\lambda_k(-u))\mu_k(u)e^{j2\pi tf(\lambda k(u)-\lambda k(-u))}\,du \qquad k\neq 0,1,\ \mu_k(u)=\mu_k(-u)>0$$

with $\lambda_0(u)=\dfrac{u/2e^{u/2}}{\sinh(u/2)}$, $\lambda_1(u) = \exp\left[\dfrac{1+ue^{-u}}{e^{-u}-1}\right]$, $\lambda_k(u) = \left[k\dfrac{e^u-1}{e^{-ku}-1}\right]^{1/(k-1)}$

Born–Jordon distribution:
$$BJD_x(t,f) = \int \frac{1}{|\tau|}\left[\int_{t-|\tau|/2}^{t+|\tau|/2} x\left(t'+\frac{\tau}{2}\right)x^*\left(t'-\frac{\tau}{2}\right)dt'\right]e^{-j2\pi f\tau}\,d\tau$$

Butterworth distribution:
$$BUD_x(t,f) = \iint \left(1+\left(\frac{\tau}{\tau_0}\right)^{2M}\left(\frac{v}{v_0}\right)^{2N}\right)^{-1} AF_x(\tau,v)e^{j2\pi(tv-f\tau)}\,d\tau\,dv$$

Choi–Williams exponential distribution:
$$CWD_x(t,f) = \iint \sqrt{\frac{\sigma}{4\pi|\tau|^2}}\exp\left[-\frac{\sigma}{4}\left(\frac{t-t'}{\tau}\right)^2\right] x\left(t'+\frac{\tau}{2}\right)x^*\left(t'-\frac{\tau}{2}\right)e^{-j2\pi f\tau}\,dt'\,d\tau$$

Cohen's nonnegative distribution:

$$CND_x(t,f) = \frac{|x(t)|^2|X(f)|^2}{E_x}\left[1 + c\rho(\xi_x(t), \eta_x(f))\right]$$

with $\xi_x(t) = \dfrac{1}{E_x}\displaystyle\int_{-\infty}^{t}|x(\tau)|^2\,d\tau,\ \eta_x(f) = \dfrac{1}{E_x}\displaystyle\int_{-\infty}^{f}|X(f')|^2\,df',\ E_x = \displaystyle\int|x(t)|^2\,dt$

Cone–Kernel distribution:

$$CKD_x(t,f) = \int g(\tau)\left[\int_{t-|\tau|/2}^{t+|\tau|/2} x\left(t'+\frac{\tau}{2}\right)x^*\left(t'-\frac{\tau}{2}\right)dt'\right]e^{-j2\pi f\tau}\,d\tau$$

Cumulative attack spectrum:

$$CAS_x(t,f) = \left|\int_{-\infty}^{t} x(\tau)e^{-j2\pi f\tau}\,d\tau\right|^2$$

Cumulative decay spectrum:

$$CDS_x(t,f) = \left|\int_{t}^{\infty} x(\tau)e^{-j2\pi f\tau}\,d\tau\right|^2$$

Flandrin D-distribution:

$$FC_X(t,f) = |f|\int X\left(f\left[1+\frac{u^2}{4}\right]\right)X^*\left(f\left[1-\frac{u^2}{4}\right]\right)\left[1-\left(\frac{u}{4}\right)^2\right]e^{j2\pi fu}\,du$$

Gabor expansion, $Ge_x(n,k;g)$:

$$x(t) = \sum_n\sum_k Ge_x(nk;g)g(t - n\Delta T)e^{j2\pi(k\Delta F)t}$$

Generalized Altes distribution:

$$GAM_x(t,f;\alpha) = |f|\int e^{-\alpha u}X\left(fe^{((1/2)-\alpha)u}\right)X^*\left(fe^{-((1/2)+\alpha)u}\right)e^{j2\pi fu}\,du$$

Generalized exponential distribution:

$$GED_x(t,f) = \iint \exp\left[-\left(\frac{\tau}{\tau_0}\right)^{2M}\left(\frac{v}{v_0}\right)^{2N}\right]AF_x(\tau,v)e^{j2\pi(tv-f\tau)}\,d\tau\,dv$$

Generalized Wigner distribution:

$$GWD_x(t,f;\tilde{\alpha}) = \int_0^\infty x\left(t+\left(\frac{1}{2}+\tilde{\alpha}\right)\tau\right)x^*\left(t-\left(\frac{1}{2}-\tilde{\alpha}\right)\tau\right)e^{-j2\pi f\tau}\,d\tau$$

Hyperbolic ambiguity function:

$$HAF_X(\zeta,\beta) = \int_0^\infty X(fe^{\beta/2})X^*(fe^{-\beta/2})e^{j2\pi\zeta\ln(f/f_r)}\,df$$

Hyperbolic wavelet transform:

$$HWT_x(t,f;\Gamma) = \sqrt{\frac{f_r}{f}}\int_0^\infty X(\xi)\Gamma^*\left(\frac{f_r}{f}\xi\right)e^{j2\pi tf\ln(\xi f_r)}\,d\xi$$

Hyperbologram:

$$HYP_x(t,f;\Gamma) = \left|\sqrt{\frac{f_r}{f}}\int_0^\infty X(\xi)\Gamma^*\left(\frac{f_r}{f}\xi\right)e^{j2\pi tf\ln(\xi f_r)}\,d\xi\right|^2 = |HWT_x(t,f;\Gamma)|^2$$

Levin distribution:

$$LD_x(t,f) = -\frac{d}{dt}\left|\int_t^\infty x(\tau)e^{-j2\pi f\tau}\,d\tau\right|^2$$

Margineau–Hill distribution:

$$MH_x(t,f) = \text{Re}\left[x(t)X^*(f)e^{-j2\pi ft}\right]$$

Multiform, Tiltable distributions:

Let $\tilde{\mu}(\tilde{\tau},\tilde{v};\alpha,r,\beta,\gamma) = \left((\tilde{\tau})^2(\tilde{v})^2\right)^\alpha + \left((\tilde{\tau})^2\right)^\alpha(\tilde{v})^2 + 2r\left((\tilde{\tau}\tilde{v})^\beta\right)^\gamma$

Butterworth:

$$MTBD_x(t,f) = \iint\left[1-\tilde{\mu}^{2\lambda}\left(\frac{\tau}{\tau_0},\frac{v}{v_0};\alpha,r,\beta,\gamma\right)\right]^{-1}AF_x(\tau,v)e^{j2\pi(tv-f\tau)}\,d\tau\,dv$$

(Continued)

TABLE 4.1 (*Continued*) List of Time-Frequency Representations (TFR) of a Signal $x(t)$ Whose Fourier Transform Is $X(f)$

Exponential:

$$MTED_x(t,f) = \iint \exp\left\{-\pi\tilde{\mu}^{2\lambda}\left(\frac{\tau}{\tau_0},\frac{\nu}{\nu_0};\alpha,r,\beta,\gamma\right)\right\} AF_x(\tau,r)e^{j2\pi(t\nu-f\tau)}\,d\tau\,d\nu$$

(Inverse) Chebyshev:

$$MT(I)C_x(t,f) = \iint \left[1+\epsilon^2 C_\lambda^{\pm 2}\left(\tilde{\mu}\left(\frac{\tau}{\tau_0},\frac{\nu}{\nu_0};\alpha,r,\beta,\gamma\right)^{\pm 1}\right)\right]^{-1} AF_x(\tau,\nu)e^{j2\pi(t\nu-f\tau)}\,d\tau\,d\nu$$

where $C_\lambda(a)$ is a Chebyshev polynomial of order λ

Nutall–Griffin distribution:

$$ND_x(t,f) = \iint \exp\left\{-\pi\left[\left(\frac{\tau}{\tau_0}\right)^2+\left(\frac{\nu}{\nu_0}\right)^2+2r\left(\frac{\tau\nu}{\tau_0\nu_0}\right)\right]\right\} AF_x(\tau,\nu)e^{j2\pi(t\nu-f\tau)}\,d\tau\,d\nu$$

Page distribution:

kth power

$$PD_x(t,f) = \frac{d}{dt}\left|\int_{-\infty}^{t} x(\tau)e^{-j2\pi f\tau}\,d\tau\right|^2$$

Ambiguity function:

$$B_x^{(\kappa)}(\zeta,\beta) = AF_{W_\kappa x}\left(\frac{\zeta}{f_r},f_r\beta\right), (W_\kappa X)(f) = \frac{1}{\sqrt{f_r|\tau_\kappa(f_r\xi_\kappa^{-1}(f/f_r))|}} X\left(f_r\xi_\kappa^{-1}\left(\frac{f}{f_r}\right)\right)$$

Central member:

$$AM_X^{(\kappa)}(t,f) = WD_{W_\kappa x}\left(\frac{t}{f_r\tau_\kappa(f)},f_r\xi_\kappa\left(\frac{f}{f_r}\right)\right), \tau_\kappa(f) = \frac{d}{df}\xi_\kappa\left(\frac{f}{f_r}\right)$$

where $\xi_\kappa(b) = \begin{cases} \text{sgn}(b)|b|^\kappa, & b\in\mathcal{R} \text{ for } \kappa\neq 0 \\ \ln(b), & b>0 \text{ for } \kappa=0 \end{cases}$

and $\xi_\kappa^{-1}(b) = \begin{cases} \text{sgn}(b)|b|^{1/\kappa}, & b\in\mathcal{R}, \kappa\neq 0 \\ e^b, & b>0, \kappa\neq 0 \end{cases}$

Power spectral density:

$$PSD_x(f) = |X(f)|^2 = \int_0^\infty act_x(\tau)e^{-j2\pi f\tau}\,d\tau$$

Pseudo-Altes distribution:

$$PAD_X(t,f;\Gamma) = f_r \int_0^\infty AM_\Gamma\left(0,f_r,\frac{f}{f'}\right) AM_X\left(\frac{tf}{f'},f'\right)\frac{df'}{f'}$$

Pseudo-Wigner distribution:

$$PWD_x(t,f;\eta) = \int x\left(t+\frac{\tau}{2}\right) x^*\left(t-\frac{\tau}{2}\right) \eta\left(\frac{\tau}{2}\right) \eta^*\left(-\frac{\tau}{2}\right) e^{-j2\pi f\tau}\,d\tau$$

Radially adaptive Gaussian distribution:

$$RAGD_x(t,f) = \iint \exp\left[-\frac{(\tau/\tau_0)^2+\nu/\nu_0)^2}{2\sigma_x^2(\theta)}\right] AF_x(\tau,\nu)e^{j2\pi(t\nu-ft)}\,d\tau\,d\nu$$

where $\theta = \arctan\left[\frac{\nu/\nu_0}{\tau/\tau_0}\right]$

Real generalized Wigner distribution:
$$RGWD_x(t,f;\tilde{\alpha}) = \text{Re}\left\{\int x\left(t+\left(\frac{1}{2}-\tilde{\alpha}\right)\tau\right)x\left(t-\left(\frac{1}{2}-\tilde{\alpha}\right)\tau\right)e^{-j2\pi f\tau}\,d\tau\right\}$$

Reduced interference distribution:
$$RID_x(t,f;S_{RID}) = \iint \frac{1}{|\tau|}S_{RID}\left(\frac{t-t'}{\tau}\right)x\left(t'+\frac{\tau}{2}\right)x^*\left(t'-\frac{\tau}{2}\right)e^{-j2\pi f\tau}\,dt'\,d\tau$$

with $S_{RID}(\beta) \in \mathcal{R}$, $S_{RID}(0) = 1$, $\left\{\dfrac{d}{d\beta}S_{RID}(\beta)\bigg|_{\beta=0} = 0\right\}$, $\left\{S_{RID}(\alpha) = 0 \text{ for } |\alpha| > \dfrac{1}{2}\right\}$

Rihaczek distribution:
$$RD_x(t,f) = x(t)X^*(f)e^{-j2\pi tf}$$

Running spectrum, past and future:
$$RSP_x(t,f) = \int_{-\infty}^{t} x(u)e^{-j2\pi fu}\,du, \quad RSF_x(t,f) = \int_{t}^{\infty} x(u)e^{-j2\pi fu}\,du$$

Scalogram:
$$SCAL_x(t,f;\gamma) = \left|\int x(\tau)\sqrt{\left|\frac{f}{f_r}\right|}\gamma^*\left(\frac{f}{f_r}(\tau-t)\,d\tau\right)\right|^2 = |WT_x(t,f;\gamma)|^2$$

Short-time Fourier transform:
$$STFT_x(t,f;\gamma) = \int x(\tau)\gamma^*(\tau-t)e^{-j2\pi f\tau}\,d\tau = e^{-j2\pi tf}\int X(f')\Gamma^*(f'-f)e^{j2\pi tf'}\,df'$$

Smoothed Pseudo-Altes distribution:
$$SPAD_x(t,f;\Gamma,g) = \int g(tf-c)PAD_x\left(\frac{c}{f},f;\Gamma\right)\,dc$$

Smoothed Pseudo-Wigner distribution:
$$SPWD_x(t,f;\gamma,\eta) = \iint \gamma(t-t')\eta\left(\frac{\tau}{2}\right)\eta^*\left(-\frac{\tau}{2}\right)x\left(t'+\frac{\tau}{2}\right)x^*\left(t'-\frac{\tau}{2}\right)e^{-j2\pi f\tau}\,dt'\,d\tau$$

Spectrogram:
$$SPEC_x(t,f;\gamma) = \left|\int x(\tau)\gamma^*(\tau-t)e^{-j2\pi f\tau}\,d\tau\right|^2 = |STFT_x(t,f;\gamma)|^2$$

Unterberger active distribution:
$$UAD_x(t,f) = f\int_0^{\infty} X(fu)X^*(f/u)[1+u^{-2}]e^{j2\pi tf(u-1/u)}\,du$$

Unterberger passive distribution:
$$UPD_x(t,f) = 2f\int_0^{\infty} X(fu)X^*(f/u)[u^{-1}]e^{j2\pi tf(u-1/u)}\,du$$

Wavelet transform:
$$WT_x(t,f;\gamma) = \int x(\tau)\sqrt{\left|\frac{f}{f_r}\right|}\gamma^*\left(\frac{f}{f_r}(\tau-t)\right)\,d\tau = \int X(f')\sqrt{\left|\frac{f_r}{f}\right|}\Gamma^*\left(\frac{f_r}{f}f'\right)e^{j2\pi tf'}\,df'$$

Wideband ambiguity function:
$$WAF_x(\tau,\alpha) = \int_0^{\infty} X(f\sqrt{\alpha})X^*(f\sqrt{\alpha})e^{j2\pi\tau f}\,df$$

Wigner distribution:
$$WD_x(t,f) = \int x\left(t+\frac{\tau}{2}\right)x^*\left(t-\frac{\tau}{2}\right)e^{-j2\pi f\tau}\,d\tau = \int X\left(f+\frac{v}{2}\right)X^*\left(f-\frac{v}{2}\right)e^{j2\pi tv}\,dv$$

TABLE 4.2 List of Desirable Properties for Time–Frequency Representations and Their Corresponding Kernel Constraints

Property Name	TFR Property	Kernel Constraints for Cohen's Class	Kernel Constraints for Hyperbolic Class
P_1: Frequency-shift covariant	$T_y(t,f) = T_x(t, f - f_0)$ for $y(t) = x(t)e^{j2\pi f_0 t}$	Always satisfied	Always satisfied
P_2: Time-shift covariant	$T_y(t,f) = T_x(t - t_0, f)$ for $y(t) = x(t - t_0)$	Always satisfied	$\Psi_H(\zeta, \beta) = B_H(\beta)e^{-j2\pi\zeta \ln G(\beta)}$ with $G(\beta) = \dfrac{\beta/2}{\sinh(\beta/2)}$
P_3: Scale covariant	$T_y(t,f) = T_x(at, f/a)$ for $y(t) = \sqrt{|a|}x(at)$	$\Psi_C(\tau, \nu) = S_C(\tau\nu)$	Always satisfied
P_4: Hyperbolic time shift	$T_y(t,f) = T_x(t - c/f, f)$ if $Y(f) = \exp\left(-j2\pi c \ln\dfrac{f}{f_r}\right) X(f)$		Always satisfied
P_5: Convolution covariant	$T_y(t,f) = \int T_h(t - \tau, f)T_x(\tau, f)d\tau$ for $y(t) = \int h(t - \tau)x(\tau)d\tau$	$\Psi_C(\tau, \nu) = e^{\tau P_C(\nu)}$	$\Phi_H(b_1, \beta)\Phi_H(b_2, \beta) = e^{b_1}$ $\Phi_H(b_1, \beta)\delta(b_1 - b_2)$
P_6: Modulation covariant	$T_y(t,f) = \int T_h(t, f - f')T_x(t, f')df'$ for $y(t) = h(t)x(t)$	$\Psi_C(\tau, \nu) = e^{\nu P_C(\tau)}$	
P_7: Real-valued	$T_x^*(t,f) = T_x(t,f)$	$\Psi_C^*(-\tau, -\nu) = \Psi_C(\tau, \nu)$	$\Psi_H^*(-\zeta, -\beta) = \Psi_H(\zeta, \beta)$
P_8: Positivity	$T_x(t,f) \geq 0$	$\Psi_C(\tau, \nu) = AP_\gamma(-\tau, -\nu)$	$\Psi_H(\zeta, \beta) = HAF_T(-\zeta, -\beta)$
P_9: Time marginal	$\int T_x(t,f)df = |x(t)|^2$	$\Psi_C(0, \nu) = 1$	
P_{10}: Frequency marginal	$\int T_x(t,f)dt = |X(f)|^2$	$\Psi_C(\tau, 0) = 1$	$\Psi_H(\zeta, 0) = 1$
P_{11}: Energy distribution	$\iint T_x(t,f)dt\,df = \int |X(f)|^2 df$	$\Psi_C(0, 0) = 1$	$\Psi_H(0, 0) = 1$
P_{12}: Time moments	$\iint t^n T_x(t,f)dt\,df = \int t^n|x(t)|^2 dt$	$\Psi_C(0, \nu) = 1$	
P_{13}: Frequency moments	$\iint f^n T_x(t,f)dt\,df = \int f^n|X(f)|^2 df$	$\Psi_C(\tau, 0) = 1$	
P_{14}: Finite time support	$T_x(t,f) = 0$ for $t \notin (t_1, t_2)$ if $x(t) = 0$ for $t \notin (t_1, t_2)$	$\varphi_C(t, \tau) = 0, \left|\dfrac{t}{\tau}\right| > \dfrac{1}{2}$	

P_{15}: Finite frequency support	$T_x(t,f) = 0$ for $f \notin (f_1, f_2)$ if $X(f) = 0$ for $f \notin (f_1, f_2)$	$\Phi_C(f,\nu) = 0, \left\|\frac{f}{\nu}\right\| > \frac{1}{2}$	$\Phi_H(c,\zeta) = 0, \left\|\frac{c}{\zeta}\right\| > \frac{1}{2}$
P_{16}: Instantaneous frequency	$\dfrac{\int f T_x(t,f)\,df}{\int T_x(t,f)\,df} = \dfrac{1}{2\pi}\dfrac{d}{dt}\arg\{x(t)\}$	$\Psi_C(0,\nu) = 1$ and $\dfrac{\partial}{\partial\tau}\Psi_C(\tau,\nu)\,\|_{\tau=0} = 0$	
P_{17}: Group delay	$\dfrac{\int t T_x(t,f)\,dt}{\int T_x(t,f)\,dt} = -\dfrac{1}{2\pi}\dfrac{d}{df}\arg\{x(f)\}$	$\Psi_C(\tau,0) = 1$ and $\dfrac{\partial}{\partial\nu}\Psi_C(\tau,\nu)\|_{\nu=0} = 0$	$\Psi_H(\zeta,0) = 1$ and $\dfrac{\partial}{\partial\beta}\Psi_H(\zeta,\beta)\bigg\|_{\beta=0} = 0$
P_{18}: Fourier transform	$T_y(t,f) = T_x(-f,t)$ for $y(t) = X(t)$	$\Psi_C(-\nu,\tau) = \Psi_C(\tau,\nu)$	
P_{19}: Frequency localization	$T_x(t,f) = \delta(f - f_0)$ for $X(f) = \delta(f - f_0)$	$\Psi_C(\tau,0) = 1$	$\Psi_H(\zeta,0) = 1$
P_{20}: Time localization	$T_x(t,f) = \delta(t - t_0)$ for $x(t) = \delta(t - t_0)$	$\Psi_C(0,\nu) = 1$	
P_{21}: Linear chirp localization	$T_x(t,f) = \delta(t - cf)$ for $X(f) = e^{-j\pi cf^2}$	$\Psi_C(\tau,\nu) = 1$	
P_{22}: Hyperbolic localization	$T_x(t,f) = \dfrac{1}{f}\delta\left(t - \dfrac{c}{f}\right) f > 0$ if $X_c(f) = \dfrac{1}{\sqrt{f}}e^{-j2\pi c\ln(f/f_r)}, f > 0$		$\Psi_H(0,\beta) = 1$
P_{23}: Chirp convolution	$T_y(t,f) = T_x(t - f/c, f)$ for $y(t) = \int x(t-\tau)\sqrt{\|c\|}e^{j\pi c\tau^2}\,d\tau$	$\Psi_C\left(\tau - \dfrac{\nu}{c}, \nu\right) = \Psi_C(\tau,\nu)$	
P_{24}: Chirp multiplication	$T_y(t,f) = T_x(t, f - ct)$ for $y(t) = x(t)e^{j\pi ct^2}$	$\Psi_C(\tau, \nu - c\tau) = \Psi_C(\tau,\nu)$	
P_{25}: Moyal's formula	$\iint T_x(t,f)T_y^*(t,f)\,dt\,df = \left\|\int x(t)y^*(t)\,dt\right\|^2$	$\|\Psi_C(\tau,\nu)\| = 1$	$\|\Psi_H(\zeta,\beta)\| = 1$

TABLE 4.3 List of Desirable Properties Satisfied by Time–Frequency Representations

Class(es)	TFR c·a	ACK a·h	BOM	BJD a·c	BUD a·c	CWKD a·c	CAD c·a	CKAD a·c	CAD a·h	CCDS a·c	GED c·a	GAM	GEWD c·a	HYP a·h	LMDH c·a	MTED H·c	NPDD c·a	AMAK p·p	MAWD a·c	PWD	PWIRDD c·a	PRADL c·a	SCRAD H·c	SPAWDC a·h	SPEWDC c·a	SUAPDA a·a	UAPDA a·a	WWPDW c·a
Property																												
1 Frequency shift	✓	✓	✓	✓	✓	✓		✓	✓	✓	✓	✓	✓	✓	✓	✓			✓	✓	✓	✓		✓	✓	✓	✓	✓
2 Time shift	✓	✓	✓	✓	✓	✓	✓	✓	✓	✓	✓	✓	✓	✓	✓	✓			✓	✓	✓	✓	✓	✓	✓	✓	✓	✓
3 Scale covariance	✓	✓	✓¹	✓¹	✓			✓		✓¹	✓	✓	✓	✓	✓	✓			✓	✓	✓	✓	✓	✓	✓	✓	✓	✓
4 Hyperbolic time shift		✓									✓		✓⁹	✓	✓	✓		✓				✓			✓	✓		✓
5 Convolution						✓⁶					✓		✓¹⁰		✓	✓¹⁰			✓									✓
6 Modulation						✓⁷					✓		✓¹⁰		✓	✓¹⁰			✓									✓
7 Real-valued	✓	✓	✓	✓	✓⁴	✓		✓	✓	✓	✓		✓	✓	✓	✓			✓	✓	✓¹⁷	✓		✓	✓¹⁸	✓	✓	✓
8 Positivity	✓	✓									✓		✓															✓
9 Time marginal	✓	✓	✓	✓	✓	✓	✓	✓	✓	✓	✓	✓	✓¹¹	✓	✓	✓¹¹	✓	✓	✓¹³	✓	✓	✓		✓	✓			✓
10 Frequency marginal	✓	✓	✓	✓	✓	✓	✓	✓	✓	✓	✓	✓	✓¹¹	✓	✓	✓¹¹	✓	✓	✓¹³	✓	✓	✓		✓	✓			✓
11 Energy distribution	✓	✓	✓	✓	✓	✓	✓	✓	✓	✓	✓	✓	✓¹¹	✓⁸	✓	✓¹¹	✓	✓¹²	✓¹³	✓	✓	✓	✓¹⁶	✓	✓			✓
12 Time moments	✓					✓	✓			✓	✓		✓¹¹		✓	✓¹¹	✓		✓¹³	✓	✓	✓		✓	✓¹⁹			✓
13 Frequency moments	✓					✓					✓		✓¹¹		✓	✓¹¹	✓		✓	✓	✓	✓		✓		✓²⁰		✓
14 Finite time support		✓									✓		✓⁵		✓					✓	✓	✓		✓				✓
15 Finite frequency support	✓	✓									✓		✓⁵		✓				✓⁵	✓	✓	✓		✓				✓
16 Instantaneous frequency		✓	✓²	✓²		✓				✓	✓		✓¹¹		✓	✓¹¹				✓¹⁴	✓	✓						✓
17 Group delay	✓	✓	✓³	✓³		✓					✓		✓¹¹		✓	✓¹¹					✓	✓						✓
18 Fourier transform	✓	✓	✓¹	✓¹	✓	✓	✓	✓	✓	✓	✓	✓	✓⁹	✓	✓	✓⁹			✓		✓¹⁵	✓		✓		✓	✓	✓
19 Frequency localization	✓	✓	✓¹	✓¹	✓	✓		✓	✓	✓	✓		✓¹¹		✓	✓¹¹				✓¹³	✓	✓		✓		✓	✓	✓
20 Time localization	✓	✓	✓¹	✓¹	✓	✓	✓	✓	✓	✓	✓		✓¹¹		✓	✓¹¹				✓¹³	✓	✓		✓		✓	✓	✓
21 Linear chirp localization		✓								✓																		
22 Hyperbolic localization														✓				✓										✓
23 Chirp convolution		✓																										✓
24 Chirp multiplication		✓																										✓
25 Moyal's formula		✓								✓								✓										✓

A ✓ indicates that the TFR can be shown to satisfy the given property. A number following the ✓ indicates that additional constraints are needed to satisfy the property. The constraints are as follows: (1): $M = N$; (2): $M > 1/2$; (3): $N > 1/2$; (4): $g(\tau)$ even; (5): $|\alpha| < 1/2$; (6): $M = 1/2$; (7): $N = 1/2$; (8): $|\alpha| = 1$; (9): $\alpha = 1$; (10): $r = 0, \alpha = 1, \gamma = 1/4$; (11): $\alpha \neq 1$; (12): $|\rho_T(0)|^2 = (1/f_T)$; (13): $|\eta(0)| = 1$; (14): $\eta(0) = 1$; (15): $S_{RID}(\beta)$ even; (16): $\int |\Gamma(b)|^2 \, db/|b| = 1$; (17): $g(c) \in$ Real; (19): $|\Gamma(0)\eta(0)|^2 = 1$; (20): $\int |\nu(t)|^2 dt = 1$. In the second row, the letters c, a, h, and p indicate that the corresponding TFR is a member of the Cohen, Affine, Hyperbolic and κth Power class, respectively.

be compared against a class-dependent list of kernel constraints in Table 4.2 and Table 4.6 to quickly determine which properties the TFR satisfies.

4.3.1 Cohen's Class of TFRs

Cohen's class consists of all quadratic TFRs that satisfy the frequency-shift and time-shift covariance properties, that is, those TFRs with a check in the first two property rows in Table 4.3 [Claasen and Mecklenbräuker, 1980; Cohen, 1989; Flandrin, 1993; Hlawatsch and Boudreaux-Bartels, 1992]. Time- and frequency-shift covariances are very useful properties in the analysis of speech, narrowband Doppler systems, and multipath environments. Any TFR in Cohen's class can be written in one of the four equivalent "normal forms":

$$C_x(t, f; \Psi_C) = \iint \varphi_C(t - t', \tau) x \left(t' + \frac{\tau}{2} \right) x^* \left(t' - \frac{\tau}{2} \right) e^{-j2\pi f \tau} dt' d\tau \tag{4.6}$$

$$= \iint \Phi_C(f - f', \nu) X \left(f' + \frac{\nu}{2} \right) X^* \left(f' - \frac{\nu}{2} \right) e^{j2\pi t \nu} df' d\nu \tag{4.7}$$

$$= \iint \psi_C(t - t', f - f') WD_x(t', f') dt' df' \tag{4.8}$$

$$= \iint \Psi_C(\tau, \nu) AF_x(\tau, \nu) e^{j2\pi(t\nu - f\tau)} d\tau d\nu \tag{4.9}$$

Each normal form is characterized by one of the four kernels $\varphi_C(f, \tau)$, $\phi_C(f, \nu)$, $\psi_C(t, f)$, and $\Psi_C(\tau, \nu)$ which are interrelated by the following Fourier transforms:

$$\varphi_C(t, \tau) = \iint \Phi_C(f, \nu) e^{j2\pi(f\tau + \nu t)} df \, d\nu = \int \Psi_C(\tau, \nu) e^{j2\pi \nu t} d\nu \tag{4.10}$$

$$\psi_C(t, f) = \iint \Psi_C(\tau, \nu) e^{j2\pi(\nu t - ft)} d\tau \, d\nu = \int \Phi_C(f, \nu) e^{j2\pi \nu t} d\nu \tag{4.11}$$

The kernels for the TFRs in Cohen's class are given in Table 4.4.

The four normal forms offers various computational and analysis advantages. For example, the first two normal forms can be computed directly from the signal $x(t)$ or its Fourier transform $X(f)$ via a one-dimensional convolution with $\varphi_C(t, \tau)$ or $\Phi_C(f, \nu)$. If $\varphi_C(t, \tau)$ is of fairly short duration, then it may be possible to implement Equation 4.6 on a digital computer in real time using only a small number of signal samples. The third normal form indicates that any TFR in Cohen's shift covariant class can be computed by convolving the TFR-dependent kernel $\psi_C(t, f)$ with the Wigner distribution (WD) of the signal, defined in Table 4.1. Hence the WD is one of the key members of Cohen's class, and many TFRs correspond to smoothed WDs, as can be seen in the top of Table 4.5. Equation 4.11 and the fourth normal form in Equation 4.9 indicate that the two-dimensional convolution in Equation 4.8 transforms to multiplication of the Fourier transform of the kernel $\psi_C(t, f)$ with the Fourier transform of the WD, which is the ambiguity function (AF) in Table 4.1. This last normal form provides an intuitive interpretation that the "AF domain" kernel $\Psi_C(\tau, \nu)$ can be thought of as the frequency response of a two-dimensional filter.

The kernels in Equation 4.6 to Equation 4.11 are signal-independent and provide valuable insight into the performance of each Cohen class TFR, regardless of the input signal. For good cross-term reduction and little autoterm distortion, each TFR kernel $\Psi_C(\tau, \nu)$ given in Table 4.4 should be as close as possible to an ideal low-pass filter. If these kernels satisfy the constraints in the third column of Table 4.2, then the TFR properties in the first column are guaranteed to always hold [Claasen and Mecklenbräuker, 1980; Hlawatsch and Boudreaux-Bartels, 1992]. For example, the last row of Table 4.2 indicates that Moyal's

TABLE 4.4 Kernels of Cohen's Shift-Invariant Class of Time–Frequency Representations (TFR)

TFR	$\psi_C(t,f)$	$\Psi_C(\tau,\nu)$	$\varphi_C(t,\tau)$	$\Phi_C(f,\nu)$
ACK	$2\cos(4\pi t f)$	$\cos(\pi\tau\nu)$	$\dfrac{\delta(t+\tau/2)+\delta(t-\tau/2)}{2}$	$\dfrac{\delta(f-\nu/2)+\delta(f+\nu/2)}{2}$
BJD		$\dfrac{\sin(\pi\tau\nu)}{\pi\tau\nu}$	$\begin{cases}\dfrac{1}{|\tau|}, & |t/\tau|<1/2 \\ 0, & |t/\tau|>1/2\end{cases}$	$\begin{cases}\dfrac{1}{|\nu|}, & |f/\nu|<1/2 \\ 0, & |f/\nu|>1/2\end{cases}$
BUD		$\left(1+\left(\dfrac{\tau}{\tau_0}\right)^{2M}\left(\dfrac{\nu}{\nu_0}\right)^{2N}\right)^{-1}$		
CWD		$e^{-(2\pi\tau\nu)^2/\sigma}$	$\sqrt{\dfrac{\sigma}{4\pi}}\dfrac{1}{|\tau|}\exp\left[-\dfrac{\sigma}{4}\left(\dfrac{t}{\tau}\right)^2\right]$	$\sqrt{\dfrac{\sigma}{4\pi}}\dfrac{1}{|\nu|}\exp\left[-\dfrac{\sigma}{4}\left(\dfrac{f}{\nu}\right)^2\right]$
CKD		$g(\tau)|\tau|\dfrac{\sin(\pi\tau\nu)}{\pi\tau\nu}$	$\begin{cases}g(t), & |t/\tau|<1/2 \\ 0, & |t/\tau|>1/2\end{cases}$	
CAS		$\left[\dfrac{1}{2}\delta(\nu)+\dfrac{1}{j\nu}\right]e^{-j\pi|\tau|\nu}$		
CDS		$\left[\dfrac{1}{2}\delta(-\nu)+\dfrac{1}{j\nu}\right]e^{j\pi|\tau|\nu}$		
GED^2		$\exp\left[-\left(\dfrac{\tau}{\tau_0}\right)^{2M}\left(\dfrac{\nu}{\nu_0}\right)^{2N}\right]$	$\dfrac{\nu_0}{2\sqrt{\pi}}\left|\dfrac{\tau_0}{\tau}\right|^M\exp\left[\dfrac{-\nu_0^2\tau_0^{2M}t^2}{4\tau^{2M}}\right]$ $N=1$ only	$\dfrac{\tau_0}{2\sqrt{\pi}}\left|\dfrac{\nu_0}{\nu}\right|^N\exp\left[\dfrac{-\tau_0^2\nu_0^{2N}f^2}{4\nu^{2N}}\right]$ $M=1$ only
GRD		$\begin{cases}1, & \||\tau|^{MIN}|\nu|/\tau|<1 \\ 0, & \||\tau|^{MIN}|\nu|/\tau|>1\end{cases}$	$\dfrac{\sin(2\pi|\tau|t/|\tau|^{MIN})}{\pi\tau}$ $N=1$ only	
GWD	$\dfrac{1}{\tilde\alpha}e^{j2\pi tf/\tilde\alpha}$	$e^{j2\pi\tilde\alpha\tau\nu}$	$\delta(t+\tilde\alpha\tau)$	$\delta(f-\tilde\alpha\nu)$
LD		$e^{j\pi|\tau|\nu}$	$\delta(t+|\tau|/2)$	
MH		$\cos(\pi\tau\nu)$	$\dfrac{\delta(t+\tau/2)+\delta(t-\tau/2)}{2}$	$\dfrac{\delta(f-\nu/2)+\delta(f+\nu/2)}{2}$

MTBD	$\left[1 + \bar{\mu}^{-2\lambda}\left(\dfrac{\tau}{\tau_0}, \dfrac{\nu}{\nu_0}; \alpha, r, \beta, \gamma\right)\right]^{-1}$			
MTC	$\left[1 + \epsilon_p^2 C_\lambda^2\left(\bar{\mu}\left(\dfrac{\tau}{\tau_0}, \dfrac{\nu}{\nu_0}; \alpha, \rho, \beta, \gamma\right)\right)\right]^{-1}$			
MTED	$\exp\left[-\pi\bar{\mu}^{2\lambda}\left(\dfrac{\tau}{\tau_0}, \dfrac{\nu}{\nu_0}; \alpha, r, \beta, \gamma\right)\right]$			
MTIC	$\left[1 + \epsilon_s^2 C_\lambda^2\left(\bar{\mu}^{-1}\left(\dfrac{\tau}{\tau_0}, \dfrac{\nu}{\nu_0}; \alpha, r, \beta, \gamma\right)\right)\right]^{-1}$			
ND	$\exp\left[-\pi\bar{\mu}\left(\dfrac{\tau}{\tau_0}, \dfrac{\nu}{\nu_0}; 0, r, 1, 1\right)\right]$			
PD	$e^{-j\pi\tau|\nu}$		$\delta(t-|\tau|/2)$	
PWD	$\delta(t)WD_\eta(0,f)$	$\eta(\tau/2)\eta^*(-\tau/2)$	$\delta(t)\eta(\tau/2)\eta^*(-\tau/2)$	$WD_\eta(0,f)$
RGWD	$\dfrac{1}{|\bar{\alpha}|}\cos\left(2\pi t f/\bar{\alpha}\right)$	$\cos(2\pi\bar{\alpha}\tau\nu)$	$\dfrac{\delta(t+\bar{\alpha}\tau)+\delta(t-\bar{\alpha}\tau)}{2}$	$\dfrac{\delta(f-\bar{\alpha}\nu)+\delta(f+\bar{\alpha}\nu)}{2}$
RID	$\displaystyle\int \dfrac{1}{|\tau|}s_{RID}\left(\dfrac{t}{\tau}\right),$ $e^{-j2\pi ft}\,d\tau$	$s_{RID}(\tau\nu),$ $s_{RID}(\beta)\in \text{Real},\ s_{RID}(0)=1$	$\dfrac{1}{|\tau|}s_{RID}\left(\dfrac{t}{\tau}\right),$ $s_{RID}(\alpha)=0,\ |\alpha|>\tfrac{1}{2}$	$\dfrac{1}{|\nu|}s_{RID}\left(-\dfrac{f}{\nu}\right),$ $s_{RID}(\alpha)=0,\ |\alpha|>\tfrac{1}{2}$
RD	$2e^{-j4\pi tf}$	$e^{-j\pi\tau\nu}$	$\delta(t-\tau/2)$	$\delta(f+\nu/2)$
SPWD	$\gamma(t)WD_\eta(0,f)$	$\eta\left(\dfrac{\tau}{2}\right)\eta^*\left(-\dfrac{\tau}{2}\right)\Gamma(\nu)$	$\gamma\left(\dfrac{\tau}{2}\right)\eta^*\left(-\dfrac{\tau}{2}\right)$	$\Gamma(\nu)WD_\eta(0,f)$
SPEC	$WD_\gamma(-t,-f)$	$AF_\gamma(-\tau,\nu)$	$\gamma\left(-t-\dfrac{\tau}{2}\right)\gamma^*\left(-t+\dfrac{\tau}{2}\right)$	$\Gamma\left(f-\dfrac{\nu}{2}\right)\Gamma^*\left(-f+\dfrac{\nu}{2}\right)$
WD	$\delta(t)\delta(f)$	1	$\delta(t)$	$\delta(f)$

Here, $\bar{\mu}(\bar{\tau},\bar{\nu}; \alpha, r, \beta, \gamma) = ((\bar{\tau})^2(\bar{\nu})^2)^\alpha(\nu) + ((\bar{\tau})^2)^\alpha(\nu) + 2r((\bar{\tau}\bar{\nu})^\beta)\gamma^\gamma)$ and $C_\lambda(\alpha)$ is a Chebyshev polynomial of order λ. Functions with lowercase and uppercase letters, for example, $\gamma(t)$ and $\Gamma(f)$, indicate Fourier transform pairs.

TABLE 4.5 Many TFRs Are Equivalent to Smoothed or Warped Wigner Distributions

TFR Name	TFR formulation
Cohen's class TFR	$C_X(t,f;\psi_C) = \iint \psi_C(t-t',f-f')WD_x(t',f')dt'\,df'$
Pseudo-Wigner distribution	$PWD_x(t,f;\eta) = \int WD_\eta(0,f-f')WD_x(t,f')df'$
Scalogram	$SCAL_x(t,f;\gamma) = \iint WD_\gamma\left(\dfrac{f}{f_r}(t'-t),f_r\dfrac{f'}{f}\right)WD_x(t',f')dt'\,df'$
Smoothed Pseudo-Wigner distribution	$SPWD_x(t,f;\gamma,\eta) = \iint \gamma(t-t')WD_\eta(0,f-f')WD_x(t',f')dt'\,df'$
Spectogram	$SPEC_x(t,f;\gamma) = \iint WD_\gamma(t'-t,f'-f)WD_x(t',f')dt'\,df'$
Altes distribution	$AM_X(t,f) = WD_{WX}\left(\dfrac{tf}{f},f_r\ln\dfrac{f}{f_r}\right)$
κth Power Altes distribution	$AM_X^{(\kappa)}(t,f) = WD_{W_\kappa X}\left(\dfrac{t}{\kappa|f/f_r|^{\kappa-1}},f_r\mathrm{sgn}(f)|f/f_r|\kappa\right),\kappa\neq 0$
Hyperbologram	$HYP_X(t,f;\Gamma) = \displaystyle\int_{-\infty}^{\infty}\int_0^{\infty} WD_{W\Gamma}\left(t'-\dfrac{tf}{f_r},f'-f_r\ln\dfrac{f}{f_r}\right)WD_{WX}(t',f')dt'\,df'$
Pseudo-Altes distribution	$PAD_X(t,f;\Gamma) = f_r\displaystyle\int_0^{\infty} WD_{W\Gamma}\left(0,f_r\ln\dfrac{f}{f'}\right)WD_{WX}\left(\dfrac{tf}{f_r},f_r\ln\dfrac{f'}{f_r}\right)\dfrac{df'}{f'}$
Smoothed Pseudo-Altes distribution	$SPAD_X(t,f;\Gamma,g) = f_r\displaystyle\int_{-\infty}^{\infty}\int_0^{\infty} g(tf-c)WD_{W\Gamma}\left(0,f_r\ln\dfrac{f}{f'}\right)WD_{WX}\left(\dfrac{c}{f_r},f_r\ln\dfrac{f'}{f_r}\right)\dfrac{df'}{f'}dc$

where $f_r > 0$ is a positive reference frequency, $(\mathcal{W}H)(f) = \sqrt{e^{f/f_r}}H(f_re^{f/f_r}),(\mathcal{W}_\kappa H)(f) = |\kappa|f_r/f|^{(\kappa-1)/\kappa|-1/2}H(f_r\mathrm{sgn}(f)|f/f_r|^{1/\kappa}),\kappa\neq 0$, and $\mathrm{sgn}(f) = \begin{cases}1, & f>0 \\ -1, & f<0\end{cases}$ members of the affine class are the Bertrands' P_0 distribution, the scalogram, and the Unterberger distributions. All are defined in Table 4.1, and their kernel forms and TFR property constraints are listed in Table 4.6. Because of the scale covariance property, many TFRs in the Affine class exhibit constant-Q behavior, permitting multiresolution analysis.

formula is satisfied by any TFR whose AF domain kernel, listed in the third column of Table 4.4, has unit modulus, for example, the Rihaczek distribution. Since the AF domain kernel of the WD is equal to one, that is, $YWD(\tau,\nu) = 1$, then the WD automatically satisfies the kernel constraints in Table 4.2 for properties P_9 to P_{13} and P_{16} to P_{21} as well as Moyal's formula. However, it also acts as an all-pass filter, passing all cross-terms. The Choi-Williams Gaussian kernel in Table 4.4 was formulated to satisfy the marginal property constraints of having an AF domain kernel equal to one along the axes and to be a low-pass filter that reduces cross-terms.

4.3.2 Affine Class of TFRs

TFRs that are covariant to scale changes and time translations, that is, properties P_2 and P_3 in Tables 4.2 and 4.3, are members of the *Affine class* [Bertrand chapter in Boashash, 1991; Flandrin, 1993].

The scale covariance property P_3 is useful when analyzing wideband Doppler systems, signals with fractal structure, octave-band systems such as the cochlea of the inner ear, and detecting short-duration "transients." Any Affine class TFR can be written in four "normal form" equations similar to those of Cohen's class:

$$A_x(t,f;\Psi_A) = |f|\iint \varphi_A(f(t'-t),f\tau)x(t+\tau/2)x^*(t-\tau/2)dt'\,d\tau \tag{4.12}$$

$$= \frac{1}{|f|}\iint \Phi_A\left(\frac{f'}{f},\frac{\nu}{f}\right)X(f'+\nu/2)X^*(f'-\nu/2)e^{j2\pi t\nu}df'\,d\nu \tag{4.13}$$

$$= \iint \psi_A\left(f(t-t'),\frac{f'}{f}\right)WD_x(t',f')dt'\,df' \tag{4.14}$$

$$= \iint \Psi_A\left(f\tau,\frac{\nu}{f}\right)AF_x(\tau,\nu)e^{j2\pi t\nu}d\tau\,d\nu \tag{4.15}$$

TABLE 4.6 Affine Class Kernels and Constraints

TFR	$\psi_A(\zeta, \beta)$	$\Phi_A(b, \beta)$
BOD	$\dfrac{\beta/2}{\sinh \beta/2} e^{j2\pi\zeta\left[\frac{\beta}{2}\coth\frac{\beta}{2}\right]}$	$\dfrac{\beta/2}{\sinh \beta/2}\delta\left(b - \left[\frac{\beta}{2}\coth\frac{\beta}{2}\right]\right)$
FD	$\left[1 - \left(\dfrac{\beta}{4}\right)^2\right] e^{j2\pi\zeta\left[1+(\beta/4)^2\right]}$	$\left[1 - \left(\dfrac{\beta}{4}\right)^2\right]\delta\left(b - \left[1 + (\beta/4)^2\right]\right)$
GWD	$e^{-j2\pi\zeta[1-\xi\beta]}$	$\delta(b - [1 - \xi\beta])$
SCAL	$AF_\gamma(-\zeta/f_r, -f_r\beta)$	$f_r\Gamma(f_r(b - \beta/2))\Gamma^*(f_r(b + \beta/2))$
UAD	$e^{-j2\pi\zeta\sqrt{1+\beta^2/4}}$	$\delta\left(b = \sqrt{1 + \beta^2/4}\right)$
UPD	$\left[1 + \beta^2/4\right]^{-1/2} e^{-j2\pi\zeta 1+\beta^2/4}$	$\left[1 + \beta^2/4\right]^{-1/2}\delta\left(b - \sqrt{1 + \beta^2/4}\right)$
WD	$e^{-j2\pi\zeta}$	$\delta(b - 1)$

Property	Constraint on Kernel
P_1: Frequency shift	$\psi_A(\alpha_0 a, (b - 1)/\alpha_0 + 1) = \psi_A(a, b)$
P_2: Time shift	Always satisfied
P_3: Scale covariance	Always satisfied
P_4: Hyperbolic time shift	$\Phi_A(b, \beta) = G_A(\beta)\delta\left(b = \dfrac{\beta}{2}\coth\dfrac{\beta}{2}\right)$
P_5: Convolution	$\psi_A(\zeta, \beta) = e^{\xi P_A(\beta)}$
P_7: Real-valued	$\psi_A(\zeta, \beta) = \psi_A^*(-\zeta, -\beta)$
P_9: Time marginal	$\displaystyle\int \Phi_A(b, -2b)\dfrac{db}{|b|} = 1$
P_{10}: Frequency marginal	$\Phi_A(b, 0) = \delta(b - 1)$
P_{11}: Energy distribution	$\displaystyle\int \Phi_A(b, 0)\dfrac{db}{|b|} = 1$
P_{14}: Finite time support	$\varphi_A(a, \zeta) = 0, \left|\dfrac{a}{\zeta}\right| > \dfrac{1}{2}$
P_{15}: Finite frequency support	$\Phi_A(b, \beta) = 0, \left|\dfrac{b-1}{\beta}\right| > \dfrac{1}{2}$
P_{17}: Group delay	$\Phi_A(b, 0) = \delta(b - 1)$ and $\dfrac{\partial}{\partial\beta}\Phi_A(b, \beta)|_{\beta=0} = 0$
P_{19}: Frequency localization	$\Phi_A(b, 0) = \delta(b - 1)$
P_{25}: Moyal's formula	$\displaystyle\int \Phi_A^*(b\beta, \tilde\eta\beta)\Phi_A(\beta, \tilde\eta\beta)d\beta = \delta(b - 1), \forall\tilde\eta$

The Affine class kernels are interrelated by the same Fourier transforms given in Equation 4.10 and Equation 4.11. Note that the third normal form of the Affine class involves an Affine smoothing of the WD. Well-known members of the Affine class are the Bertrands' P_0 distribution, the scalogram, and the Unterberger distributions. All are defined in Table 4.1, and their kernel forms and TFR property constraints are listed in Table 4.6. Because of the scale covariance property, many TFRs in the Affine class exhibit constant-Q behavior, permitting multiresolution analysis.

4.3.3 Hyperbolic Class of TFRs

The Hyperbolic class of TFRs consists of all TFRs that are covariant to scale changes and hyperbolic time shifts, that is, properties P_3 and P_4 in Table 4.2 [Papandreou et al., 1993]. They can be analyzed using the

TABLE 4.7 Kernels of the Hyperbolic Class of Time–Frequency Representations

TFR	$\psi_H(c,b)$	$\psi_H(\zeta,\beta)$	$\varphi_H(c,\zeta)$	$\Phi_H(b,\beta)$
AM	$\delta(c)\delta(b)$	1	$\delta(c)$	$\delta(b)$
BOD	$\int \delta(b+\ln\lambda(\beta))e^{j2\pi c\beta}\,d\beta$	$e^{-j2x\zeta\ln\lambda(\beta)}$	$\int e^{j2\pi(c\beta-\zeta\ln\lambda(\beta))}\,d\beta$	$\delta(b+\ln\lambda(\beta))$
GAM	$\dfrac{1}{|\tilde{\alpha}|}e^{-j2\pi cb/\alpha}$	$e^{j2\pi\alpha\zeta\beta}$	$\delta(c+\tilde{\alpha}\zeta)$	$\delta(b-\tilde{\alpha}\beta)$
HYP	$AM_r\left(\dfrac{-c}{f_r e^{-b}},f_r e^{-b}\right)$	$HAF_r(-\zeta,-\beta)$	$\upsilon_r(-c,-\zeta)$	$V_r(-b,-\beta)$
PAD	$f_r\delta(c)AM_r(0,f_r e^b)$	$f_r\upsilon_r(0,\zeta)$	$f_r\delta(c)\upsilon_r(0,\zeta)$	$f_r AM_\Gamma(0,f_r e^b)$
SPAD	$f_r g(c)AM_r(0,f_r e^b)$	$f_r G(\beta)\upsilon_r(0,\zeta)$	$f_r g(c)\upsilon_r(0,\zeta)$	$f_r G(\beta)AM_\Gamma(0,f_r e^b)$

Here $\lambda(\beta)=(\beta/2/\sinh\beta/2)$, $V_\Gamma(b,\beta)=f_r e^b\Gamma(f_r e^{b+\beta/2})\Gamma^*(f_r e^{b-\beta/2})$, $u_\Gamma(c,\zeta)=\rho_\Gamma(c+\zeta/2)\rho_\Gamma(c-\zeta/2)$ and $\rho_\Gamma(c)=\int_0^\infty \Gamma(f)(f/f_r)^{j2\pi c}\dfrac{df}{\sqrt{f}}$.

following four normal forms:

$$H_X(t,f;\Psi_H)=\iint \varphi_H(tf-c,\zeta)\upsilon_X(c,\zeta)e^{-j2\pi|\ln(f/f_r)|\zeta}\,dc\,d\zeta \tag{4.16}$$

$$=\iint \Phi_H\left(\ln\frac{f}{f_r}-b,\beta\right)f_r e^b X(f_r e^{b+\beta/2})X^*(f_r e^{b-\beta/2})e^{j2\pi tf\beta}\,db\,d\beta \tag{4.17}$$

$$=\int_{-\infty}^\infty\int_0^\infty \psi_H\left(tf-t'f',\ln\frac{f}{f'}\right)AM_X(t',f')dt'\,df' \tag{4.18}$$

$$=\iint \Psi_H(\zeta,\beta)HAF_X(\zeta,\beta)e^{j2\pi(tf\beta-[\ln(f/f_r)\zeta])}\,d\zeta\,d\beta \tag{4.19}$$

where $AM_X(t,f)$ is the Altes distribution and $HAF_X(\zeta,\beta)$ is the hyperbolic ambiguity function defined in Table 4.1, $\upsilon_X(c,\zeta)$ is defined in Table 4.7, $(\mathcal{W}X)(f)=\sqrt{ef/f_r}X(f_r e^{f/f_r})$ is a unitary warping on the frequency axis of the signal, and the kernels are interrelated via the Fourier transforms in Equation 4.10 and Equation 4.11.

Table 4.3 reveals that the Altes-Marinovic, the Bertrands' P_0, and the hyperbologram distributions are members of the Hyperbolic class. Their kernels are given in Table 4.7, and kernel property constraints are given in Table 4.2. The hyperbolic TFRs give highly concentrated TFR representations for signals with hyperbolic group delay. Each Hyperbolic class TFR, kernel, and property corresponds to a warped version of a Cohen's class TFR, kernel, and property, respectively. For example, Table 4.5 shows that the Altes distribution is equal to the WD after both the signal and the time–frequency axes are warped appropriately. The WD's perfect location of linear FM chirps (P_{21}) corresponds to the Altes distribution's perfect localization for hyperbolic FM chirps (P_{22}). This one-to-one correspondence between the Cohen and Hyperbolic classes greatly facilitates their analysis and gives alternative methods for calculating various TFRs.

4.3.4 *k*th Power Class

The Power class of TFRs consists of all TFRs that are scale covariant and power time-shift covariant, that is,

$$PC_Y^{(\kappa)}(t,f)=PC_X^{(\kappa)}\left(t-c\frac{d}{df}\xi(f/f_r),f\right) \quad \text{for } Y(f)=e^{-j2\pi o\xi_\kappa(f/f_r)}X(f) \tag{4.20}$$

where $\zeta_\kappa(f)=\text{sgn}(f)|f|^\kappa$, for $\kappa\neq 0$ [Hlawatsch et al., 1993]. Consequently, the κth Power class perfectly represents group delay changes in the signal that are powers of frequency. When $\kappa=1$, the Power class is equivalent to the Affine class. The central member, $AM^{(\kappa)}$ in Table 4.1, is the Power class equivalent to the Altes-Marinovic distribution.

4.4 Common TFRs and Their Use in Biomedical Applications

This section will briefly review some of the TFRs commonly used in biomedical analysis and summarize their relative advantages and disadvantages.

4.4.1 Wigner Distribution

One of the oldest TFRs in Table 4.1 is the Wigner distribution (WD), which Wigner proposed in quantum mechanics as a two-dimensional statistical distribution relating the Fourier transform pairs of position and momentum of a particle. Table 4.3 reveals that the WD satisfies a large number of desirable TFR properties, P_1 to P_3, P_5 to P_7, P_9 to P_{21}, and P_{23} and P_{25}. It is a member of both the Cohen and the Affine classes. The WD is a high-resolution TFR for linear FM chirps, sinusoids, and impulses. Since the WD satisfies Moyal's formula, it has been used to design optimal signal-detection and synthesis algorithms. The drawbacks of the WD are that it can be negative, it requires the signal to be known for all time, and it is a quadratic TFR with no implicit smoothing to remove cross-terms.

4.4.2 Smoothed Wigner Distributions

Many TFRs are related to the WD by either smoothing or a warping, for example, see Equation 4.8 and Equation 4.18 and Table 4.5. An intuitive understanding of the effects of cross-terms on quadratic TFRs can be obtained by analyzing the WD of a multicomponent signal $y(t)$ in Equation 4.5 under the assumption that each signal component is a shifted version of a basic envelope, that is, $x_n(t) = x(t - t_n)$ $e^{j2\pi f_n t}$:

$$
\begin{aligned}
WD_y(t,f) = \sum_{n=1}^{N} WD_x(t - t_n, f - f_n) & \\
+ 2 \sum_{k=1}^{N-1} \sum_{q=k+1}^{N} WD_x(t - \bar{t}_{k,q}, f - \bar{f}_{k,q}) \cos(2\pi[\Delta f_{k,q}(t - \Delta t_{k,q}) & \\
- \Delta t_{k,q}(f - \Delta f_{k,q}) + \Delta f_{k,q}\Delta t_{k,q}]) &
\end{aligned}
\tag{4.21}
$$

where $\Delta f_{k,q} = f_k - f_q$ is the difference or "beat" frequency and $\bar{f}_{k,q} = (f_k + f_q)/2$ is the average frequency between the kth and qth signal components. Similarly, $\Delta t_{k,q}$ is the difference time and $\bar{t}_{k,q}$ is the average time. The auto-WD terms in the first summation properly reflect the fact that the WD is a member of Cohen's shift covariant class. Unfortunately, the cross-WD terms in the second summation occur midway in the time–frequency plane between each pair of signal components and oscillate with a spatial frequency proportional to the distance between them. The Pseudo-WD (PWD) and the smoothed PWD (SPWD) defined in Table 4.1 use low-pass smoothing windows $\eta(\tau)$ and $\gamma(t)$ to reduce oscillatory cross-components. However, Table 4.5 reveals that the Pseudo-WD performs smoothly only in the frequency direction. Short smoothing windows greatly reduce the limit of integration in the PWD and SPWD formulations and hence reduce computation time. However, Table 4.3 reveals that smoothing the WD reduces the number of desirable properties it satisfies from 18 to 7 for the PWD and to only 3 for the SPWD.

4.4.3 Spectrogram

One of the most commonly used TFRs for slowly time-varying or quasi-stationary signals is the spectrogram, defined in Table 4.1 and Table 4.5 [Rabiner and Schafer, 1978]. It is equal to the squared magnitude of the short-time Fourier transform, performing a local or "short-time" Fourier analysis by using a sliding analysis window $\gamma(t)$ to segment the signal into short sections centered near the output time t before computing a Fourier transformation. The spectrogram is easy to compute, using either FFTs or a parallel bank of filters, and it is often easy to interpret. The quadratic spectrogram smooths away all cross-terms except those which occur when two signal components overlap. This smoothing also distorts auto-terms. The spectrogram does a poor job representing rapidly changing spectral characteristics or resolving two closely spaced components because there is an inherent tradeoff between good time resolution, which requires a short analysis window, and good frequency resolution, which requires a long analysis window. The spectrogram satisfies only three TFR properties listed in Table 4.2 and Table 4.3; that is, it is a nonnegative number of Cohen's shift invariant class.

4.4.4 Choi–Williams Exponential and Reduced Interference Distributions

The Choi–Williams exponential distribution (CWD) and the reduced interference distribution (RID) in Table 4.1 are often used as a compromise between the high-resolution but cluttered WD versus the smeared but easy to interpret spectrogram [Jeong and Williams, 1992; Williams and Jeong, 1991]. Since they are members of both Cohen's class and the Affine class, their AF domain kernels in Table 4.4 have a very special form, that is, $\Psi_C(\tau, \nu) = S_C(\tau \nu)$, called a *product kernel*, which is a one-dimensional kernel evaluated at the product of its time–frequency variables [Hlawatsch and Boudreaux-Bartels, 1992]. The CWD uses a Gaussian product kernel in the AF plane to reduce cross-terms, while the RID typically uses a classic window function that is time-limited and normalized to automatically satisfy many desirable TFR properties (see Table 4.3). The CWD has one scaling factor σ that allows the user to select either good cross-term reduction or good auto-term preservation but, unfortunately, not always both. The generalized exponential distribution in Table 4.1 is an extension of the CWD that permits both [Hlawatsch and Boudreaux-Bartels, 1992]. Because the CWD and RID product kernels have hyperbolic isocontours in the AF plane, they always pass cross-terms between signal components that occur at either the same time or frequency, and they can distort auto-terms of linear FM chirp signals whose instantaneous frequency has a slope close to 1. The multiform tiltable exponential distribution (MTED) [Costa and Boudreaux-Bartels, 1994], another extension of the CWD, works well for any linear FM chirp.

4.4.5 Scalogram or Wavelet Transform Squared Magnitude

The scalogram [Flandrin, 1993], defined in Table 4.1 and Table 4.5, is the squared magnitude of the recently introduced wavelet transform (WT) [Daubechies, 1992; Meyer, 1993] and is a member of the Affine class. It uses a special sliding analysis window $\gamma(t)$, called the *mother wavelet*, to analyze local spectral information of the signal $x(t)$. The mother wavelet is either compressed or dilated to give a multiresolution signal representation. The scalogram can be thought of as the multiresolution output of a parallel bank of octave band-filters. High-frequency regions of the WT domain have very good time resolution, whereas low-frequency regions of the WT domain have very good spectral resolution. The WT has been used to model the middle- to high-frequency range operation of the cochlea, to track transients such as speech pitch and the onset of the QRS complex in ECG signals, and to analyze fractal and chaotic signals. One drawback of the scalogram is its poor temporal resolution at low-frequency regions of the time-frequency plane and poor spectral resolution at high frequencies. Moreover, many "classic" windows do not satisfy the conditions needed for a mother wavelet. The scalogram cannot remove cross-terms when signal components overlap. Further, many discrete WT implementations do not preserve the important time-shift covariance property.

4.4.6 Biomedical Applications

The electrocardiogram (ECG) signal is a recording of the time-varying electric rhythm of the heart. The short-duration QRS complex is the most predominant feature of the normal ECG signal. Abnormal heart rhythms can be identified on the ECG by detecting the QRS complex from one cycle to the next.

The transient detection capability of the wavelet transform (WT) has been exploited for detection of the QRS complex by Kadambe et al. [1992] and Li and Zheng [1993]. The WT exhibits local maxima which align across successive (dyadic) scales at the location of transient components, such as QRS complexes. The advantage of using the WT is that it is robust both to noise and to nonstationarities in the QRS complex.

Other pathologic features in the heart's electrical rhythm that appear only in high-resolution signal-averaged ECG signals are ventricular late potentials (VLPs). VLPs are small-amplitude, short-duration components that occur after the QRS complex and are precursors of dangerous, life-threatening cardiac arrhythmias. Tuteur [1989] used the peak of the WT at a fixed scale to identify simulated VLPs. More recently, Jones et al. [1992] compared different time-frequency techniques, such as the spectrogram, short-time spectral estimators, the smoothed WD, and the WT, in their ability to discriminate between normal patients and patients susceptible to dangerous arrhythmias. Morlet et al. [1993] used the transient detection capability of the WT to identify VLPs.

The WT has also been applied to the ECG signal in the context of ECG analysis and compression by Crowe et al. [1992]. Furthermore, Crowe et al. [1992] exploited the capability of the WT to analyze fractal-like signals to study heart rate variability (HRV) data, which have been described as having fractal-like properties.

The recording of heart sounds, or phonocardiogram (PCG) signal, has been analyzed using many time-frequency techniques. Bulgrin et al. [1993] compared the short-time Fourier transform and the WT for the analysis of abnormal PCGs. Picard et al. [1991] analyzed the sounds produced by different prosthetic valves using the spectrogram. The binomial RID, which is a fast approximation to the CWD, was used to analyze the short-time, narrow-bandwidth features of first heart sound in mongrel dogs by Wood et al. [1992].

TFRs have also been applied to nonstationary brain wave signals, including the electrocardiogram (EEG), the electrocorticogram (ECoG), and evoked potentials (EPs). Zaveri et al. [1992] used the spectrogram, the WD, and the CWD to characterize the nonstationary behavior of the ECoG of epileptic patients. Of the three techniques, the CWD exhibited superior results. The WT was used to identify the onset of epileptic seizures in the EEG by Schiff and Milton [1993], to extract a single EP by Bartnik et al. [1992], and to characterize changes in somatosensory EPs due to brain injury caused by oxygen deprivation by Thakor et al. [1993].

Crackles are lung sounds indicative of pathologic conditions. Verreault [1989] used AR models of slices of the WD to discriminate crackles from normal lung sounds.

The electrogastrogram (EGG) is a noninvasive measure of the time-varying electrical activity of the stomach. Promising results regarding abnormal EGG rhythms and the frequency of the EGG slow wave were obtained using the CWD by Lin and Chen [1994].

Widmalm et al. [1991] analyzed temporomandibular joint (TMI) clicking using the spectrogram, the WD, and the RID. The RID allowed for better time–frequency resolution of the TMJ sounds than the spectrogram while reducing the cross-terms associated with the WD. TMJ signals were also modeled using nonorthogonal Gabor logons by Brown et al. [1994]. The primary advantage of this technique, which optimizes the location and support of each Gabor log-on, is that only a few such logons were needed to represent the TMJ clicks.

Auditory applications of TFRs are intuitively appealing because the cochlea exhibits constant-bandwidth behavior at low frequencies and constant-Q behavior at middle to high frequencies. Applications include a wavelet-based model of the early stages of acoustic signal processing in the auditory system [Yang et al., 1992], a comparison of the WD and Rihaczek distribution on the response of auditory neurons to wideband noise stimulation [Eggermont and Smith, 1990], and spectrotemporal analysis of dorsal cochlear neurons in the guinea pig [Backoff and Clopton, 1992].

The importance of mammography, x-ray examination of the breast, lies in the early identification of tumors. Kaewlium and Longbotham [1993] used the spectrogram with a Gabor window as a texture discriminator to identify breast masses. Recently, a mammographic feature-enhancement technique using the WT was proposed by Laine et al. [1993]. The wavelet coefficients of the image are modified and then reconstructed to the desired resolution. This technique enhanced the visualization of mammographic features of interest without additional cost or radiation.

Magnetic resonance imaging (MRI) allows for the imaging of the soft tissues in the body. Weaver et al. [1992] reduced the long processing time of traditional phase encoding of MRI images by WT encoding. Moreover, unlike phase-encoded images, Gibb's ringing phenomena and motion artifacts are localized in WT encoded images.

The Doppler ultrasound signal is the reflection of an ultrasonic beam due to moving red blood cells and provides information regarding blood vessels and heart chambers. Doppler ultrasound signals in patients with narrowing of the aortic valve were analyzed using the spectrogram by Cloutier et al. [1991]. Guo and colleagues [1994] examined and compared the application of five different time–frequency representations (the spectrogram, short-time AR model, CWD, RID, and Bessel distributions) with simulated Doppler ultrasound signals of the femoral artery. Promising results were obtained from the Bessel distribution, the CWD, and the short-time AR model.

Another focus of bioengineering applications of TFRs has concerned the analysis of biologic signals of interest, including the sounds generated by marine mammals, such as dolphins and whales, and the sonar echolocation systems used by bats to locate and identify their prey. The RID was applied to sperm whale acoustic signals by Williams and Jeong [1991] and revealed an intricate time-frequency structure that was not apparent in the original time-series data. The complicated time-frequency characteristics of dolphin whistles were analyzed by Tyack et al. [1992] using the spectrogram, the WD, and the RID, with the RID giving the best results. Flandrin [1988] analyzed the time-frequency structure of the different signals emitted by bats during hunting, navigation, and identifying prey using the smoothed Pseudo-WD. In addition, the instantaneous frequency of the various signals was estimated using time-frequency representations. Saillant et al. [1993] proposed a model of the bat's echolocation system using the spectrogram. The most common application of the spectrogram is the analysis and modification of quasi-stationary speech signals [Rabiner and Schafer, 1978].

Acknowledgments

The authors would like to acknowledge the use of the personal notes of Franz Hlawatsch and Antonia Papandreou on TFR kernel constraints as well as the help given by Antonia Papandreou in critiquing the article and its tables.

References

Backoff P.M. and Clopton B.M. (1991). A spectrotemporal analysis of DCN single unit responses to wideband noise in guinea pig. *Hear. Res.* 53: 28.

Bartnik E.A., Blinowska K.J., and Durka P.J. (1992). Single evoked potential reconstruction by means of a wavelet transform. *Biol. Cybern.* 67: 175.

Boashash B. (ed). (1991). *Time–Frequency Signal Analysis — Methods and Applications.* Melbourne, Australia, Longman-Chesire.

Brown M.L., Williams W.J., and Hero A.O. (1994). Non-orthogonal Gabor representation for biological signals. In *Proc. Intl. Conf. ASSP*, Australia, pp. 305–308.

Bulgrin J.R., Rubal B.J., Thompson C.R., and Moody J.M. (1993). Comparison of short-time Fourier transform, wavelet and time-domain analyses of intracardiac sounds. *Biol. Sci. Instrum.* 29: 465.

Cloutier G., Lemire F., Durand L. et al. (1991). Change in amplitude distributions of Doppler spectrograms recorded below the aortic valve in patients with a valvular aortic stenosis. *IEEE Trans. Biomed. Eng.* 39: 502.

Cohen L. (1989). Time–frequency distributions — A review. *Proc. IEEE* 77: 941.

Claasen T.A.C.M. and Mecklenbräuker W.F.G. (1980). The Wigner distribution: a tool for time-frequency signal analysis, parts I–III. Philips *J. Res.* 35: 217, 35: 276, 35: 372.

Costa A. and Boudreaux-Bartels G.F. (1994). Design of time-frequency representations using multiform, tiltable kernels. In *Proc. IEEE-SP Intl. Symp. T-F and T-S Anal.* (Pacific Grove, CA).

Crowe J.A., Gibson N.M., Woolfson M.S., and Somekh M.G. (1992). Wavelet transform as a potential tool for ECG analysis and compression. *J. Biomed. Eng.* 14: 268.

Daubechies I. (1992). *Ten Lectures on Wavelets.* Montpelier, Vt, Capital City Press.

Eggermont J.J. and Smith G.M. (1990). Characterizing auditory neurons using the Wigner and Rihacek distributions: A comparison. *JASA* 87: 246.

Flandrin P. (1993). *Temps-Fréquence.* Hermes, Paris, France.

Flandrin P. (1988). Time-frequency processing of bat sonar signals. In Nachtigall P.E. and Moore P.W.B., (Eds.), *Animal Sonar: Processes and Performance,* pp. 797–802. New York, Plenum Press.

Guo Z., Durand L.G., and Lee H.C. (1994). Comparison of time-frequency distribution techniques for analysis of simulated Doppler ultrasound signals of the femoral artery. *IEEE Trans. Biomed. Eng.* 41: 332.

Hlawatsch F. and Boudreaux-Bartels G.F. (1992). Linear and quadratic time–frequency signal representations. *IEEE Sig. Proc. Mag.* March: 21.

Hlawatsch F., Papandreou A., and Boudreaux-Bartels G.F. (1993). Time-frequency representations: a generalization of the Affine and Hyperbolic classes. In *Proc. 26th Ann. Asil Conf. Sig. Syst. Comput.* (Pacific Grove, CA).

Jeong J. and Williams W.J. (1992). Kernel design for reduced interference distributions. *IEEE Trans. SP* 40: 402.

Jones D.L., Tovannas J.S., Lander P., and Albert D.E. (1992). Advanced time–frequency methods for signal averaged ECG analysis. *J. Electrocardiol.* 25: 188.

Kadambe S., Murray R., and Boudreaux-Bartels G.F. (1992). The dyadic wavelet transform based QRS detector. In *Proc. 26th Ann. Asil Conf. Sig. Syst. Comput.* (Pacific Grove, CA).

Kaewlium A. and Longbotham H. (1993). Application of Gabor transform as texture discriminator of masses in digital mammograms. *Biol. Sci. Instrum.* 29: 183.

Laine A., Schuler S., and Fan J. (1993). Mammographic feature enhancement by multiscale analysis. *IEEE Trans. Med. Imag.* (submitted).

Li C. and Zheng C. (1993). QRS detection by wavelet transform. In *Proc. Ann. Intl. Conf. IEEE EMBS,* pp. 330–331.

Lin Z.Y. and Chen J.D.Z. (1994). Time–frequency representation of the electrogastrogram: application of the exponential distribution. *IEEE Trans. Biomed. Eng.* 41: 267.

Morlet D., Peyrin F., Desseigne P. et al. (1993). Wavelet analysis of high resolution signal averaged ECGs in postinfarction patients. *J. Electrocardiol.* 26: 311.

Murray R. (1994). Summary of biomedical applications of time-frequency representations. Technical report no. 0195-0001, University of Rhode Island.

Papandreou A., Hlawatsch F., and Boudreaux-Bartels G.F. (1993). The Hyperbolic class of quadratic time–frequency representations: I. Constant-Q warping, the hyperbolic paradigm, properties, and members. *IEEE Trans. SP* 41: 3425.

Picard D., Charara J., Guidoin F. et al. (1991). Phonocardiogram spectral analysis simulator of mitral valve prostheses. *J. Med. Eng. Technol.* 15: 222.

Porat B. (1994). *Digital Processing of Random Signals: Theory and Methods.* Englewood Cliffs, NJ, Prentice-Hall.

Rabiner L.R. and Schafer R.W. (1978). *Digital Processing of Speech Signals.* Englewood Cliffs, NJ, Prentice-Hall.

Rioul O. and Vetterli M. (1991). Wavelets and signal processing. *IEEE Sig. Proc. Mag.* October 14.

Saillant P.A., Simmons J.A., and Dear S.P. (1993). A computational model of echo processing and acoustic imaging in frequency modulated echo-locating bats: the spectrogram correlation and transformation receiver. *JASA* 94: 2691.

Schiff S.J. and Milton J.G. (1993). Wavelet transforms for electroencephalographic spike and seizure detection. In *Proc. SPIE — Intl. Soc. Opt. Eng.,* pp. 50–56.

Tuteur F.B. (1989). Wavelet transformations in signal detection. In *Proc. Intl. Conf. ASSP*, pp. 1435–1438.

Tyack P.L., Williams W.J., and Cunningham G. (1992). Time-frequency fine structure of dolphin whistles. In *Proc. IEEE — SP Intl. Symp. T-F and T-S Anal.* (Victoria, BC, Canada), pp. 17–20.

Verreault E. (1989). Détection et Caractérisation des Rales Crépitants (French). PhD thesis, l'Université Laval, Faculte des Sciences et de Genie.

Weaver J.B., Xu Y., Healy D.M., and Driscoll J.R. (1992). Wavelet encoded MR imaging. *Magnet Reson. Med.* 24: 275.

Widmalm W.E., Williams W.J., and Zheng C. (1991). Reduced interference time–frequency distributions. In Boashash B. (Ed.), Time frequency distributions of TMJ sounds. *J. Oral. Rehabil.* 18: 403.

Williams W.J. and Jeong J. (1991). *Time–Frequency Signal Analysis — Methods and Applications*, pp. 878–881. Chesire, England, Longman.

Yang Z., Wang K., and Shamma S. (1992). Auditory representations of acoustic signals. *IEEE Trans. Info. Theory* 38: 824.

Zaveri H.P., Williams W.J., Iasemidis L.D., and Sackellares J.C. (1992). Time–frequency representations of electrocorticograms in temporal lobe epilepsy. *IEEE Trans. Biomed. Eng.* 39: 502.

Further Information

Several TFR tutorials exist on the Cohen class [Boashash, 1991; Cohen, 1989; Flandrin, 1993; Hlawatsch and Boudreaux-Bartels, 1992], Affine class [Bertrand chapter in Boashash, 1991; Flandrin, 1993], hyperbolic class [Papandreou et al., 1993], and power class [Hlawatsch et al., 1993]. Several special conferences or issues of IEEE journals devoted to TFRs and the WT include Proc. of the IEEE-SP Time Frequency and Time-Scale Workshop, 1992, *IEEE Sig. Proc. Soc.*; Special issue on wavelet transforms and multiresolution signal analysis, *IEEE Trans. Info. Theory*, 1992; and Special issue on wavelets and signal processing, *IEEE Trans. SP*, 1993. An extended list of references on the application of TFRs to problems in biomedical or bio-engineering can be found in Murray [1994].

5

Wavelet (Time-Scale) Analysis in Biomedical Signal Processing

5.1	Introduction..	**5-2**
5.2	The Wavelet Transform: Variable Time and Frequency Resolution............................	**5-2**
	Continuous Wavelet Transform • The Discrete Wavelet Transform	
5.3	A Multiresolution Theory: Decomposition of Signals	**5-7**
	Using Orthogonal Wavelets • Implementation of the Multiresolution Wavelet Transform: Analysis and Synthesis of Algorithms	
5.4	Further Developments of the Wavelet Transform	**5-10**
5.5	Applications	**5-11**
	Cardiac Signal Processing • Neurological Signal Processing • Other Applications	
5.6	Discussion and Conclusions	**5-23**
References		**5-23**

Nitish V. Thakor
Boris Gramatikov
David Sherman
Johns Hopkins School of Medicine

Signals recorded from the human body provide information pertaining to its organs. Their characteristic shape, or temporal and spectral properties, can be correlated with normal or pathological functions. In response to dynamical changes in the function of these organs, the signals may exhibit time-varying as well as nonstationary responses. Time–frequency and time-scale analysis techniques are well suited for such biological signals. Joint time-frequency signal analysis techniques include short-term Fourier transform and Wigner–Ville distribution, and related reduced interference distribution. Joint time-scale analysis includes continuous and discrete, orthonormal and non-orthonormal wavelets. These techniques find applications in the analysis of transient and time-varying events in biological signals. Examples of applications include cardiac signals (for detection of ischemia and reperfusion-related changes in QRS complex, and late potentials in ECG) and neurological signals (evoked potentials and seizure spikes).

5.1   Introduction

Digital signal processing uses sophisticated mathematical analysis and algorithms to extract information hidden in signals derived from sensors. In biomedical applications these sensors such as electrodes, accelerometers, optical imagers, etc., record signals from biological tissue with the goal of revealing their health and well-being in clinical and research settings. Refining those signal processing algorithms for biological applications requires building suitable signal models to capture signal features and components that are of diagnostic importance. As most signals of a biological origin are time-varying, there is a special need for capturing transient phenomena in both healthy and chronically ill states.

A critical feature of many biological signals is frequency domain parameters. Time localization of these changes is an issue for biomedical researchers who need to understand subtle frequency content changes over time. Certainly, signals marking the transition from severe normative to diseased states of an organism sometimes undergo severe changes which can easily be detected using methods such as the Short Time Fourier Transform (STFT) for deterministic signals and its companion, the spectrogram, for power signals. The basis function for the STFT is a complex sinusoid, e j2pft, which is suitable for stationary analyses of narrowband signals. For signals of a biological origin, the sinusoid may not be a suitable analysis signal. Biological signals are often spread out over wide areas of the frequency spectrum. Also as Rioul and Vetterli [1] point out, when the frequency content of a signal changes in a rapid fashion, the frequency content becomes smeared over the entire frequency spectrum as it does in the case of the onset of seizure spikes in epilepsy or a fibrillating heartbeat as revealed on an ECG. The use of a narrowband basis function does not accurately represent wideband signals. It is preferred that the basis functions be similar to the signal under study. In fact, for a compact representation using as few basis functions as possible, it is desirable to use basis functions that have a wider frequency spread as most biological signals do. Wavelet theory, which provides for wideband representation of signals [2–4], is therefore a natural choice for biomedical engineers involved in signal processing and currently under intense study [5–9].

5.2   The Wavelet Transform: Variable Time and Frequency Resolution

5.2.1   Continuous Wavelet Transform

A decomposition of a signal, based on a wider frequency mapping and consequently better time resolution is possible with the wavelet transform. The Continuous Wavelet Transform (CWT) [3] is defined thusly for a continuous signal, $x(t)$,

$$\text{CWT}_x(\tau, a) = \frac{1}{\sqrt{a}} \int x(at)g^* \left(\frac{t - \tau}{a} \right) dt \tag{5.1a}$$

or with change of variable as

$$\text{CWT}_x(\tau, a) = \sqrt{a} \int x(at)g^* \left(t - \frac{\tau}{a} \right) dt \tag{5.1b}$$

where $g(t)$ is the mother or basic wavelet, $*$ denotes a complex conjugate, a is the scale factor, and t is a time shift. Typically, $g(t)$ is a bandpass function centered around some center frequency, f_o. Scale a allows the compression or expansion of $g(t)$ [1,3,10]. A larger scale factor generates the same function compressed in time whereas a smaller scale factor generates the opposite. When the analyzing signal is contracted in time, similar signal features or changes that occur over a smaller time window can be studied. For the wavelet transform, the same basic wavelet is employed with only alterations in this signal arising from scale changes. Likewise, a smaller scale function enables larger time translations or delays in the basic signal.

The notion of scale is a critical feature of the wavelet transform because of time and frequency domain reciprocity. When the scale factor, a, is enlarged, the effect on frequency is compression as the analysis window in the frequency domain is contracted by the amount $1/a$ [10]. This equal and opposite frequency domain scaling effect can be put to advantageous use for frequency localization. Since we are using bandpass filter functions, a center frequency change at a given scale yields wider or narrower frequency response changes depending on the size of the center frequency. This is the same in the analog or digital filtering theories as "constant-Q or quality factor" analysis [1,10,11]. At a given Q or scale factor, frequency translates are accompanied by proportional bandwidth or resolution changes. In this regard, wavelet transforms are often written with the scale factor rendered as

$$a = \frac{f}{f_0} \tag{5.2}$$

or

$$\text{CWT}_x\left(\tau, a = \frac{f}{f_0}\right) = \frac{1}{\sqrt{f/f_0}} \int x(t) g^*\left(\frac{t-\tau}{f/f_0}\right) dt \tag{5.3}$$

This is the equivalent to logarithmic scaling of the filter bandwidth or octave scaling of the filter bandwidth for power-of-two growth in center frequencies. Larger center frequency entails a larger bandwidth and vice versa.

The analyzing wavelet, $g(t)$, should satisfy the following conditions:

1. Belong to L2 (R), that is, be square integrable (be of finite energy) [2]
2. Be analytic [$G(\omega) = 0$ for $\omega < 0$] and thus be complex-valued. In fact many wavelets are real-valued; however, analytic wavelets often provide valuable phase information [3], indicative of changes of state, particularly in acoustics, speech, and biomedical signal processing [8]
3. Be admissible. This condition was shown to enable invertibility of the transform [2,6,12]:

$$s(t) = \frac{1}{c_g} \int_{-\infty}^{\infty} \int_{a>0}^{\infty} W(\tau, a) \frac{1}{\sqrt{a}} g\left(\frac{t-\tau}{a}\right) \frac{1}{a^2} da d\tau \tag{5.3a}$$

where c_g is a constant that depends only on $g(t)$ and a is positive. For an analytic wavelet the constant should be positive and convergent:

$$c_g = \int_0^{\infty} \frac{|G(\omega)|^2}{\omega} d\omega < \infty \tag{5.3b}$$

which in turn imposes an admissibility condition on $g(t)$. For a real-valued wavelet, the integrals from both $-\infty$ to 0 and 0 to $+\infty$ should exist and be greater than zero.

The admissibility condition along with the issue of reversibility of the transformation is not so critical for applications where the emphasis is on signal analysis and feature extraction. Instead, it is often more important to use a fine sampling of both the translation and scale parameters. This introduces redundancy which is typical for the CWT, unlike for the discrete wavelet transform, which is used in its dyadic, orthogonal, and invertible form.

All admissible wavelets with g Œ L1(R) have no zero-frequency contribution. That is, they are of zero mean,

$$\int_{-\infty}^{+\infty} g(t) dt = 0 \tag{5.3c}$$

or equivalently $G(\omega) = 0$ for $\omega = 0$, meaning that $g(t)$ should not have nonzero DC [6,12]. This condition is often being applied also to nonadmissible wavelets.

The complex-valued Morlet's wavelet is often selected as the choice for signal analysis using the CWT. Morlet's wavelet [3] is defined as

$$g(t) = e^{j2\pi f_o t} e^{-(t^2/2)} \qquad (5.4a)$$

with its scaled version written as

$$g\left(\frac{t}{a}\right) = e^{j(2\pi f_o/a)t} e^{-(t^2/2a^2)} \qquad (5.4b)$$

Morlet's wavelet insures that the time-scale representation can be viewed as a time-frequency distribution as in Equation 5.3. This wavelet has the best representation in both time and frequency because it is based on the Gaussian window. The Gaussian function guarantees a minimum time-bandwidth product, providing for maximum concentration in both time and frequency domains [1]. This is the best compromise for a simultaneous localization in both time and frequency as the Gaussian function's Fourier transform is simply a scaled version of its time domain function. Also the Morlet wavelet is defined by an explicit function and leads to a quasi continuous discrete version [11]. A modified version of Morlet's wavelet leads to fixed center frequency, f_o, with width parameter, s,

$$g(\sigma, t) = e^{j2\pi f_o t} e^{-(t^2/2\sigma^2)} \qquad (5.4c)$$

Once again time–frequency (TF) reciprocity determines the degree of resolution available in time and frequency domains. Choosing a small window size, s, in the time domain, yields poor frequency resolution while offering excellent time resolution and vice versa [11,13]. To satisfy the requirement for admissibility and $G(0) = 0$, a correction term must be added. For $\omega > 5$, this correction term becomes negligibly small and can be omitted. The requirements for the wavelet to be analytic and of zero mean is best satisfied for $\omega 0 = 5.3$ [3].

Following the definition in Equation 5.1a and Equation 5.1b the discrete implementation of the CWT in the time-domain is a set of bandpass filters with complex-valued coefficients, derived by dilating the basic wavelet by the scale factor, a, for each analyzing frequency. The discrete form of the filters for each a is the convolution:

$$S(k, a) = \frac{1}{\sqrt{a}} \sum_{i=k-(\pi/2)}^{k+(\pi/2)} s(i) g_m * \left(\frac{i-k}{a}\right) = \frac{1}{\sqrt{a}} \sum_{i=-(\pi/2)}^{\pi/2} s(k-i) g_m * \left(\frac{i}{a}\right) \qquad (5.4d)$$

with $k = t/T_s$, where T_s is the sampling interval. The summation is over a number of terms, n. Because of the scaling factor a in the denominator of the argument of the wavelet, the wavelet has to be resampled at a sampling interval T_s/a for each scale a. Should the CWT cover a wide frequency range, a computational problem would arise. For example, if we wish to display the CWT over 10 octaves (a change by one octave corresponds to changing the frequency by a factor of 2), the computational complexity (size of the summation) increases by a factor of $2^{10} = 1024$. The algorithm by Holschneider et al. [14] solves this problem for certain classes of wavelets by replacing the need to resample the wavelet with a recursive application of an interpolating filter. Since scale is a multiplicative rather than an additive parameter, another way of reducing computational complexity would be by introducing levels between octaves (voices) [15]. Voices are defined to be the scale levels between successive octaves, uniformly distributed in a multiplicative sense [13,16]. Thus, the ratio between two successive voices is constant. For example, if one wishes to have ten voices per octave, then the ratio between successive voices is 21/10. The distance between two levels, ten voices apart is an octave.

The CWT can also be implemented in the frequency domain. Equation 5.1 may be formulated in the frequency domain as:

$$\text{CWT}(\tau, a) = \sqrt{a} \int S(\omega) G * (a\omega) e^{j\omega} d\omega \tag{5.5}$$

where $S(\omega)$ and $G(\omega)$ denote the Fourier transformed $s(t)$ and $g(t)$, and $j = (-1)1/2$. The analyzing wavelet $g(t)$ generally has the following Fourier transform:

$$G_{\tau,u}(\omega) = \sqrt{a} G(a\omega) e^{j\omega\tau} \tag{5.6a}$$

The Morlet wavelet [Equation 5.4a and Equation 5.4b] in frequency domain is a Gaussian function:

$$G_m(\omega) = \frac{1}{\sqrt{2\omega}} e^{-(\omega-\omega_0)^2/2} \tag{5.6b}$$

From Equation 5.6a and Equation 5.6b it can be seen that for low frequencies, ω, (larger scales a) the width, D/ω, of the Gaussian is smaller and vice versa. In fact, the ratio $D\omega/omega$ is constant [1], that is, Morlet wavelets may be considered filter banks of the constant-Q factor.

Based on Equation 5.5, Equation 5.6a, and Equation 5.6b the wavelet transform can be implemented in the frequency domain. At each scale, the Fourier image of the signal can be computed as

$$Y(\omega, a) = S(\omega) \bullet G_m(\omega, a) \tag{5.6c}$$

with $S(\omega)$ being the Fourier transform of the signal, $G_m(\omega, a)$ being the scaled Fourier image of the Morlet wavelet at scale a, and the operation c standing for element-by-element multiplication (windowing in frequency domain). The signal at each scale a will finally be obtained by applying the inverse Fourier transform:

$$\text{CWT}(\tau, a) = (\text{FFT})^{-1} Y(\omega, a) \tag{5.6d}$$

This approach has the advantage of avoiding computationally intensive convolution of time-domain signals by using multiplication in the frequency domain, as well as the need of resampling the mother wavelet in the time domain [17,18].

Note that the CWT is, in the general case, a complex-valued transformation. In addition to its magnitude, its phase often contains valuable information pertinent to the signal being analyzed, particularly in instants of transients [3]. Sometimes the TF distribution of the nonstationary signal is much more important. This may be obtained by means of real-valued wavelets. Alternatives to the complex-valued Morlet wavelet are simpler, real-valued wavelets that may be utilized for the purpose of the CWT. For example, the early Morlet wavelet, as used for seismic signal analysis [19], had the following real-valued form:

$$g(t) = \cos(5t) e^{-t^2/2} \tag{5.6e}$$

It had a few cycles of a sine wave tapered by a Gaussian envelope. Though computationally attractive, this idea contradicts the requirement for an analytic wavelet, that is, its Fourier transform $G(\omega) = 0$ for $\omega < 0$. An analytic function is generally complex-valued in the time domain and has its real and imaginary parts as Hilbert transforms of each other [2,20]. This guarantees only positive-frequency components of the analyzing signal.

A variety of analyzing wavelets have been proposed in recent years for time-scale analysis of the ECG. For example, Senhadji et al. [21] applied a pseudo-Morlet's wavelet to bandpass filtering to find out whether some abnormal ECG events like extrasystoles and ischemia are mapped on specific decomposition levels:

$$g(t) = C(1 + \cos(2\pi f_0 t))e^{-2i\pi k f_0 t} \qquad t \leq 1/2f_0 \quad \text{and} \quad k \text{ integer} \notin \{-1, 0, 1\} \qquad (5.6f)$$

with the product kf_0 defining the number of oscillations of the complex part, and C representing a normalizing constant such that $\|g\| = 1$. The above function is a modulated complex sine wave that would yield complex-valued CWT including phase information. However its envelope is a cosine, rather than a Gaussian, as in the case of the complex Morlet wavelet. It is well known that strictly the Gaussian function (both in time and frequency domain) guarantees the smallest possible time-bandwidth product which means maximum concentration in the time and frequency domains [22].

The STFT has the same time-frequency resolution regardless of frequency translations. The STFT can be written as

$$\text{STFT}(\tau, f) = \int_{-\infty}^{\infty} x(t)g * (t - \tau)e^{-2\pi j f t}\, dt \qquad (5.7)$$

where $g(t)$ is the time window that selects the time interval for analysis or otherwise known as the spectrum localized in time. Figure 5.1 shows comparative frequency resolution of both the STFT as well as the wavelet transform. The STFT is often thought to be analogous to a bank of bandpass filters, each shifted by a certain modulation frequency, f_0. In fact, the Fourier transform of a signal can be interpreted as passing the signal through multiple bandpass filters with impulse response, $g(t)e^{j2\pi ft}$, and then using complex demodulation to downshift the filter output. Ultimately, the STFT as a bandpass filter rendition simply translates the same low pass filter function through the operation of modulation. The characteristics of the filter stay the same though the frequency is shifted.

Unlike the STFT, the wavelet transform implementation is not frequency independent so that higher frequencies are studied with analysis filters with wider bandwidth. Scale changes are not equivalent to varying modulation frequencies that the STFT uses. The dilations and contractions of the basis function allow for variation of time and frequency resolution instead of uniform resolution of the Fourier transform [15].

Both the wavelet and Fourier transform are linear time–frequency representations (TFRs) for which the rules of superposition or linearity apply [10]. This is advantageous in cases of two or more separate signal constituents. Linearity means that cross-terms are not generated in applying either the linear TF or time-scale operations. Aside from linear TFRs, there are quadratic TF representations which are quite useful in displaying energy and correlation domain information. These techniques, also described elsewhere in this volume include the Wigner–Ville distribution (WVD), smoothed WVD, the reduced inference

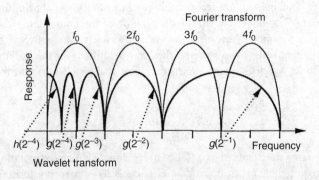

FIGURE 5.1 Comparative frequency resolution for STFT and WT. Note that frequency resolution of STFT is constant across frequency spectrum. The WT has a frequency resolution that is proportional to the center frequency of the bandpass filter.

distribution (RID), etc. One example of the smoothed Wigner-Ville distribution is

$$W(t,f) = \int s* \left(t - \frac{1}{2}\tau \right) e^{-j\tau 2\pi f} s* \left(t + \frac{1}{2}\tau \right) h \left(\frac{\tau}{2} \right) d\tau \tag{5.8a}$$

where $h(t)$, is a smoothing function. In this case the smoothing kernel for the generalized or Cohen's class of TFRs is

$$\phi(t,\tau) = h \left(\frac{\tau}{2} \right) \delta(t) \tag{5.8b}$$

These methods display joint TF information in such a fashion as to display rapid changes of energy over the entire frequency spectrum. They are not subject to variations due to window selection as in the case of the STFT. A problematic area for these cases is the elimination of those cross-terms that are the result of the embedded correlation.

It is to be noted that the scalogram or scaled energy representation for wavelets can be represented as a WVD as [1]

$$|CWT_x(\tau,a)|^2 = \iint W_x(u,n) W_g^* \left(\frac{u-t}{a}, an \right) du\,dn \tag{5.9a}$$

where

$$W_x(t,f) = \int x * \left(t - \frac{1}{2}\tau \right) e^{-j\tau 2\pi f} x * \left(t + \frac{1}{2}\tau \right) d\tau \tag{5.9b}$$

5.2.2 The Discrete Wavelet Transform

In the discrete TFRs both time and scale changes are discrete. Scaling for the discrete wavelet transform involves sampling rate changes. A larger scale corresponds to subsampling the signal. For a given number of samples a larger time swath is covered for a larger scale. This is the basis of signal compression schemes as well [23]. Typically, a dyadic or binary scaling system is employed so that given a discrete wavelet function, $y(x)$, is scaled by values that are binary. Thus

$$\psi_{2^j}(t) = 2^j \psi(2^j t) \tag{5.10a}$$

where j is the scaling index and $j = 0, -1, -2, \dots$. In a dyadic scheme, subsampling is always decimation-in-time by a power of 2. Translations in time will be proportionally larger as well as for a more sizable scale.

It is for discrete time signals that scale and resolution are related. When the scale is increased, resolution is lowered. Resolution is strongly related to frequency. Subsampling means lowered frequency content. Rioul and Vetterli [1] use the microscope analogy to point out that smaller scale (higher resolution) helps to explore fine details of a signal. This higher resolution is apparent with samples taken at smaller time intervals.

5.3 A Multiresolution Theory: Decomposition of Signals

5.3.1 Using Orthogonal Wavelets

One key result of the wavelet theory is that signals can be decomposed in a series of orthogonal wavelets. This is similar to the notion of decomposing a signal in terms of discrete Fourier transform components or Walsh or Haar functions. Orthogonality insures a unique and complete representation of the signal.

Likewise the orthogonal complement provides some measure of the error in the representation. The difference in terms of wavelets is that each of the orthogonal vector spaces offers component signals with varying levels of resolution and scale. This is why Mallat [24] named his algorithm the multiresolution signal decomposition. Each stage of the algorithm generates wavelets with sequentially finer representations of signal content. To achieve an orthogonal wavelet representation, a given wavelet function, $f(t)$, at a scaling index level equal to zero, is first dilated by the scale coefficient 2^j, then translating it by $2^{-j}n$ and normalizing by gives:

$$\sqrt{2^{-j}}\phi_{2j}(t - 2^{-j}n) \tag{5.10b}$$

The algorithm begins with an operator A_{2j} for discrete signals that takes the projections of a signal, $f(t)$ onto the orthonormal basis, V_{2j}:

$$A_{2j}f(t) = 2^{-j} \sum_{n=-\infty}^{\infty} \langle f(u), \phi_{2j}(u - 2^{-j}n)\rangle \phi_{2j}(t - 2^{-j}n) \tag{5.11}$$

where $2j$ defines the level of resolution. A_{2j} is defined as the multi-resolution operator that approximates a signal at a resolution $2j$. Signals at successively lower resolutions can be obtained by repeated application of the operator $A_{2j}(-J \leq j \leq -1)$, where J specifies the maximum resolution, such that $A_{2j}f(x)$ is the closest approximation of function $f(x)$ at resolution $2j$. Here we note that $\langle\rangle$ is simply a convolution defined thusly,

$$\langle f(u), \phi_{2j}(u - 2^{-j}n)\rangle = \int_{-\infty}^{\infty} f(u)\phi(u - 2^{-j}n)du \tag{5.12}$$

Here $f(x)$ is the impulse response of the scaling function. The Fourier transforms of these functions are lowpass filter functions with successively smaller halfband lowpass filters. This convolution synthesizes the coarse signal at a resolution/scaling level j:

$$C_j f = \langle f(t), \phi_{2j}(t - 2^{-j}n)\rangle \tag{5.13}$$

Each level j generates new basis functions of the particular orthonormal basis with a given discrete approximation. In this case, larger j provides for decreasing resolution and increasing the scale in proportional fashion for each level of the orthonormal basis. Likewise, each sequentially larger j provides for time shift in accordance with scale changes, as mentioned above, and the convolution or inner product operation generates the set of coefficients for the particular basis function. A set of scaling functions at decreasing levels of resolution, $j = 0, -1, -2, \ldots, -6$ is given in Reference 25.

The next step in the algorithm is the expression of basis function of one level of resolution, $f2^j$ by at a higher resolution, $f2^{j+1}$. In the same fashion as above, an orthogonal representation of the basis $V2^j$ in terms of $V2^{j+1}$ is possible, or

$$\phi_{2j}(t - 2^{-j}n) = 2^{-j-1} \sum_{k=-\infty}^{\infty} \langle \phi_{2j}(u - 2^{-j}n), \phi_{2j+1}(u - 2^{-j-1}k)\rangle \phi_{2j+1}(t - 2^{-j-1}k) \tag{5.14}$$

Here the coefficients are once again the inner products between the two basis functions. A means of translation is possible for converting the coefficients of one basis function to the coefficients of the basis function at a higher resolution:

$$C_{2^j} f = \langle f(u), \phi_{2^j}(t - 2^{-j} n) \rangle$$

$$= 2^{-j-1} \sum_{k=-\infty}^{\infty} \langle \phi_{2^j}(u - 2^{-j} n), \phi_{2^{j+1}}(u - 2^{-j-1} k) \rangle \langle f(u), \phi_{2^{j+1}}(t - 2^{-j-1} k) \rangle \tag{5.15}$$

Mallat [24] also conceives of the filter function, $h(n)$, whose impulse response provides this conversion, namely,

$$C_{2^j} f = \langle f(u), \phi_{2^j}(t - 2^{-j} n) \rangle = 2^{-j-1} \sum_{k=-\infty}^{\infty} \tilde{h}(2n - k) \langle f(u), \phi_{2^{j+1}}(t - 2^{-j-1} k) \rangle \tag{5.16}$$

where $h(n) = 2^{-j-1} \cdot f2^j(u - 2^{-j} n), f2^{j+1}(u - 2^{-j-1} k)Ò$ and $\tilde{h}(n) = h(-n)$ is the impulse response of the appropriate mirror filter.

Using the tools already described, Mallat [24] then proceeds to define the orthogonal complement, $O2^j$ to the vector space $V2^j$ at resolution level j. This orthogonal complement to $V2^j$ is the error in the approximation of the signal in $V2^{j+1}$ by use of basis function belonging to the orthogonal complement. The basis functions of the orthogonal complement are called orthogonal wavelets, $y(x)$, or simply wavelet functions. To analyze finer details of the signal, a wavelet function derived from the scaling function is selected. The Fourier transform of this wavelet function has the shape of a bandpass filter in frequency domain. A basic property of the function y is that it can be scaled according to

$$CWT_x(\tau, a) = \frac{1}{\sqrt{a}} \int x(at) g * \left(\frac{t - \tau}{a} \right) dt \tag{5.16a}$$

An orthonormal basis set of wavelet functions is formed by dilating the function $y(x)$ with a coefficient 2^j and then translating it by $2^{-j} n$, and normalizing by . They are formed by the operation of convolving the scale function with the quadrature mirror filter

$$\psi(\omega) = G\left(\frac{\omega}{2} \right) \phi\left(\frac{\omega}{2} \right) \tag{5.16b}$$

where $G(\omega) = e - j\omega—H(\omega + \pi)$ is the quadrature mirror filter transfer response and $g(n) = (-1)1 - nh(1 - n)$ is the corresponding impulse response function.

The set of scaling and wavelet functions presented here form a duality, together resolving the temporal signal into coarse and fine details, respectively. For a given level j then, this detail signal can once again be represented as a set of inner products:

$$D_{2^j} f = \langle f(t), \psi_{2^j}(x - 2^{-j} n) \rangle \tag{5.17}$$

For a specific signal, $f(x)$, we can employ the projection operator as before to generate the approximation to this signal on the orthogonal complement. As before, the detail signal can be decomposed using the higher resolution basis function:

$$D_{2^j} f = \langle f(u), \psi_{2^j}(t - 2^{-j} n) \rangle$$

$$= 2^{-j-1} \sum_{k=-\infty}^{\infty} \langle \psi_{2^j}(t - 2^{-j} n), \psi_{2^{j+1}}(u - 2^{-j-1} k) \rangle \langle f(u), \phi_{2^{j+1}}(t - 2^{-j-1} k) \rangle \acute{Y} \tag{5.18}$$

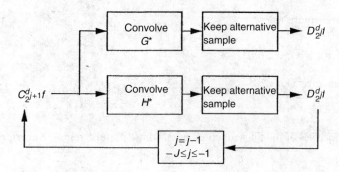

FIGURE 5.2   Flow chart of a multiresolution algorithm showing how successive coarse and detail components of resolution level, j, are generated from higher resolution level, $j + 1$.

or in terms of the synthesis filter response for the orthogonal wavelet

$$D_{2^j}f = \langle f(u), \psi_{2^j}(t - 2^{-j}n)\rangle = 2^{-j-1} \sum_{k=-\infty}^{\infty} \tilde{g}(2n - k)\langle f(u), \phi_{2^{j+1}}(t - 2^{-j-1}k)\rangle \qquad (5.19)$$

At this point, the necessary tools are here for a decomposition of a signal in terms of wavelet components, coarse and detail signals. Multiresolution wavelet description provides for the analysis of a signal into lowpass components at each level of resolution called coarse signals through the C operators. At the same time the detail components through the D operator provide information regarding bandpass components. With each decreasing resolution level, different signal approximations are made to capture unique signal features. Procedural details for realizing this algorithm follow.

5.3.2 Implementation of the Multiresolution Wavelet Transform: Analysis and Synthesis of Algorithms

A diagram of the algorithm for the multiresolution wavelet decomposition algorithm is shown in Figure 5.2. A step-by-step rendition of the analysis is as follows:

1. Start with N samples of the original signal, $x(t)$, at resolution level $j = 0$.
2. Convolve signal with original scaling function, $f(t)$, to find $C1 f$ as in Equation 5.13 with $j = 0$.
3. Find coarse signal at successive resolution levels, $j = -1, -2, \ldots, -J$ through Equation 5.16; keep every other sample of the output.
4. Find detail signals at successive resolution levels, $j = -1, -2, \ldots, -J$ through Equation 5.19; keep every other sample of the output.
5. Decrease j and repeat steps 3 through 5 until $j = -J$.

Signal reconstruction details are presented in References 24 and 26.

5.4   Further Developments of the Wavelet Transform

Of particular interest are Daubechies' orthonormal wavelets of compact support with the maximum number of vanishing moments [27,28]. In these works, wavelets of very short length are obtained (number of coefficients 4, 6, 8, etc.) thus allowing for very efficient data compression.

Another important development of the multiresolution decomposition is the wavelet packet approach [29]. Instead of the simple multiresolution three-stage filter bank (low-pass/high-pass/downsampling) described previously in this chapter, wavelet packets analyse all subsystems of coefficients at all scale levels, thus yielding the full binary tree for the orthogonal wavelet transform, resulting in a completely evenly spaced frequency resolution. The wavelet packet system gives a rich orthogonal structure that allows adaptation to particular signals or signal classes. An optimal basis may be found, minimizing some function on the signal sequences, on the manifold of orthonormal bases. Wavelet packets allow for a much more efficient adaptive data compression [30]. Karrakchou and Kunt report an interesting method of interference cancelling using a wavelet packet approach [8]. They apply "local" subband adaptive filtering by using a non-uniform filter bank, having a different filter for each subband (scale). Furthermore, the orthonormal basis has "optimally" been adapted to the spectral contents of the signal. This yields very efficient noise suppression without significantly changing signal morphology.

5.5   Applications

5.5.1   Cardiac Signal Processing

Signals from the heart, especially the ECG, are well suited for analysis by joint time-frequency and time-scale distributions. That is because the ECG signal has a very characteristic time-varying morphology, identified as the P-QRS-T complex. Throughout this complex, the signal frequencies are distributed (1) low frequency — P and T waves, (2) mid to high frequency — QRS complex [31,32]. Of particular diagnostic importance are changes in the depolarization (activation phase) of the myocardium, represented by the QRS complex. These changes cause alterations in the propagation of the depolarization wave detectable by time-frequency analysis of one-dimensional electrocardiographic signals recorded from the body surface. Two examples are presented below.

5.5.1.1   Analysis of the QRS Complex Under Myocardial Ischemia

Ischemia-related intra-QRS changes. When the heart muscle becomes ischemic or infarcted, characteristic changes are seen in the form of elevation or depression of the ST-segment. Detection of these changes requires an extension of the signal bandwidth to frequencies down to 0.05 Hz and less, making the measurements susceptible to motion artifact errors. Ischemia also causes changes in conduction velocity and action potential duration, which results in fragmentation in the depolarization front (Figure 5.3) and appearance of low-amplitude notches and slurs in the body surface ECG signals. These signal changes are detectable with various signal processing methods [33,34]. Depolarization abnormalities due to ischemia may also cause arrhythmogenic reentry [35], which is one more reason to detect intra-QRS changes precisely.

Identification of ischemia-related changes in the QRS complex is not as well known, and interpretation of the QRS complex would be less susceptible to artifactual errors, as compared to the ST analysis. Thus,

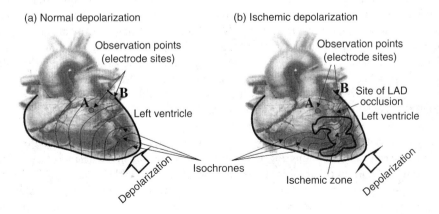

FIGURE 5.3   Idealized example of (a) normal propagation and (b) wavefront fragmentation due to an ischemic zone of slow conduction. The superimposed lines are isochrones, connecting points at which the depolarization arrives at the same time.

time-frequency or time-scale analysis would serve a useful function in localizing the ischemia-related changes within the QRS complex, but would be somewhat independent of the artifactual errors.

Experimental findings. In experimental animals, the response of the heart to coronary artery occlusion and then reperfusion was studied. The Left Anterior Descending (LAD) branch of the coronary artery was temporarily occluded for 20 min. Subsequent to that, the occlusion was removed, and resulting reperfusion more or less restored the ECG signal after 20 min. The coronary artery was occluded a second time for 60 min, and once again occlusion was removed and blood flow was restored. Single ECG cycles were analyzed using the continuous wavelet transform [33]. Figure 5.4 shows the time-scale plots for the ECG cycles for each of the five stages of this experiment. The three-dimensional plots give time in the P-QRS-T complex on one axis, the scale (or equivalent frequency) on another axis, and the normalized magnitude on the third axis. First occlusion results in a localized alteration around 100 ms and the midscale, which shows up as a bump in the three-dimensional plot or a broadening in the contour plot. Upon reperfusion, the time-scale plot returns to the pre-occlusion state. The second occlusion brings about a far more significant change in the time-scale plot, with increased response in the 0 to 200 msec and mid-scale ranges. This change is reversible. We were thus able to show, using time-scale technique, ischemia related changes in the QRS complex, and the effects of occlusion as well as reperfusion.

Potential role of ischemia-related intra-QRS changes in coronary angioplasty. The above results are also applicable to human ECGs and clinical cardiology. For example, a fairly common disorder is the occlusion of coronary vessels, causing cardiac ischemia and eventually infarction. An effective approach to the treatment of the occlusion injury is to open the coronary blood vessels using a procedure called coronary angioplasty (also known as percutaneous transluminal coronary angioplasty or PTCA). Vessels may be opened using a balloon-type or a laser-based catheter. When reperfusion occurs following the restoration of the blood flow, initially a reperfusion injury is known to occur (which sometimes leads to arrhythmias) [35]. The ST level changes as well, but its detection is not easy due to artifacts, common in a PTCA setting. In a clinical study, we analyzed ischemia and reperfusion changes before and after the PTCA procedure. Short-term occlusion and ischemia followed by reperfusion were carried out in a cardiac catheterization laboratory at the Johns Hopkins Hospital in connection with PTCA) [36]. Figure 5.5 shows time-scale plots of a patient derived from continuous wavelet transform. Characteristic midscale hump in the early stages of the QRS cycle is seen in the three-dimensional time-scale plot. Then, 60 min after angioplasty, the normal looking time-scale plot of the QRS complex is restored in this patient. This study suggests that time-scale analysis and resulting three-dimensional or contour plots may be usable in monitoring the effects of ischemia and reperfusion in experimental or clinical studies. In another study (4 patients, LAD) we monitored for intra-QRS changes during PTCA. Despite signal noise and availability of recordings only from limb leads, superimposed mid-frequency components during ischemic states of the heart were observed, which disappeared when perfusion was restored. There was at least one lead that responded to changes in coronary perfusion. Figure 5.6 shows five different stages of a PTCA procedure as time plots (lead I) and CWT TFDs (topo-plots). Despite the presence of noise, the WT was able to unveil elevation of intra-QRS time-frequency components around 20 Hz during balloon inflation (ischemia), and a drop in the same components with reperfusion after balloon deflation. Frequency components 20 to 25 Hz during inflation. No substantial ST changes can be observed in the time-domain plot. The arrows show the zones of change in TFDs with ischemia and reperfusion. Note the representation of power line interference (50 Hz) as "clouds" in (b) and (d) topo plots — far from the region of interest.

Another study analyzed ECG waveforms from patients undergoing the PTCA procedure by the multiresolution wavelet method, decomposing the whole P-QRS-T intervals into coarse and detail components [26,37], as can be seen from the analysis of one pre-angioplasty ECG cycle in Figure 5.7 [26]. The PTCA procedure results in significant morphological and spectral changes within the QRS complex. It was found that certain detail components are more sensitive than others: in this study, the detail components d6 and d5 corresponding to frequency band of 2.2 to 8.3 Hz are most sensitive to ECG changes following a successful PTCA procedure. From this study it was concluded that monitoring the energy of ECG signals at different detail levels may be useful in assessing the efficacy of angioplasty procedures [37]. A benefit of

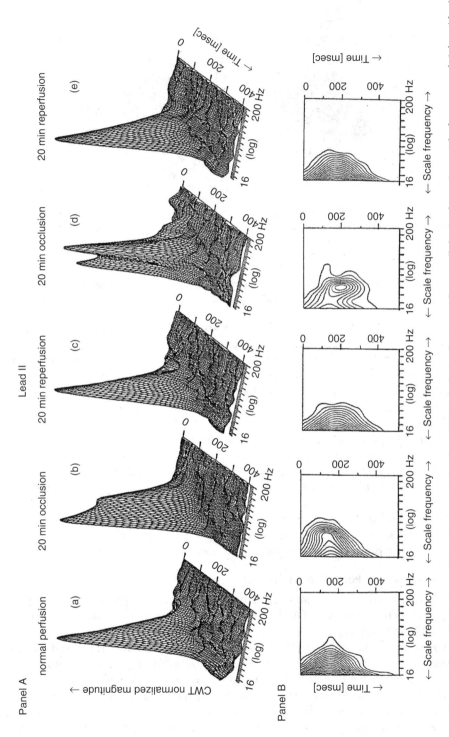

FIGURE 5.4 Time–frequency distributions of the vector magnitude of two ECG leads during five stages of a controlled animal experiment. The frequency scale is logarithmic, 16 to 200 Hz. The z-axis represents the modulus (normalized) of the complex wavelet-transformed signal.

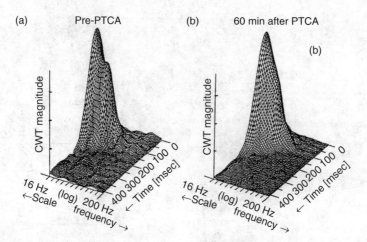

FIGURE 5.5 Time–frequency distributions of human ECG study using WT. Pre-angioplasty plot (a) shows a characteristic hump at about 35 Hz, which disappears as indicated by the second plot (b) taken 1 h after angioplasty treatment.

this approach is that a real-time monitoring instrument for the cardiac catheterization laboratory can be envisioned (whereas currently x-ray fluroscopy is needed).

Detection of reperfusion during thrombolytic therapy. Detecting reperfusion-related intra-QRS changes, along with ST changes, in the time–frequency domain would possibly find application in thrombolysis monitoring after myocardial infarction. At present, the ST elevation and its recovery are the main electrocardiographic indicators of acute coronary ischemia and reperfusion. Reports using continuous ST-segment monitoring have indicated that 25–50% of patients treated with intravenous thrombolytic therapy display unstable ST recovery [38], and additional reperfusion indicators are necessary. Signal averaged ECG and highest frequency ECG components (150–250 Hz) have been utilized as a reperfusion marker during thrombolysis and after angioplasty, but their utility is uncertain, since the degree of change of the energy values chosen does not appear to be satisfactory [39,40]. We have analyzed the QRS of the vector magnitude $V =$ of body surface orthogonal ECG leads X, Y and Z during thrombolytic therapy of two patients with myocardial infarction. Figure 5.8 shows how TFDs may be affected by reperfusion during thrombolysis. Two interesting trends may be observed on this figure: (1) a mid-frequency peak present during initial ischemia (a) disappears two hours after start of thrombolytic therapy (b) due to smoother depolarization front, and (2) high-frequency components appear with reestablished perfusion, possibly due to faster propagation velocity of the depolarization front.

5.5.1.2 Analysis of Late Potentials in the ECG

"Late potentials" are caused by fractionation of the depolarization front after myocardial infarction [35,41]. They have been shown to be predictive of life threatening reentrant arrhythmias. Late potentials occur in the terminal portion of the QRS complex and are characterized by small amplitude and higher frequencies than in the normal QRS complex. The presence of late potentials may indicate underlying dispersion of electrical activity of the cells in the heart, and therefore may provide a substrate for production of arrhythmias. The conventional Fourier transform does not readily localize these features in time and frequency [15,42]. STFT is more useful because the concentration of signal energy at various times in the cardiac cycle is more readily identified. The STFT techniques suffer from the problem of selecting a proper window function; for example, window width can affect whether high temporal or high spectral resolution is achieved [15]. Another approach sometimes considered is the Wigner-Ville distribution, which also produces a composite time-frequency distribution. However, the Wigner-Ville distribution suffers from the problem of interference from cross-terms. Comparative representations by smoothed

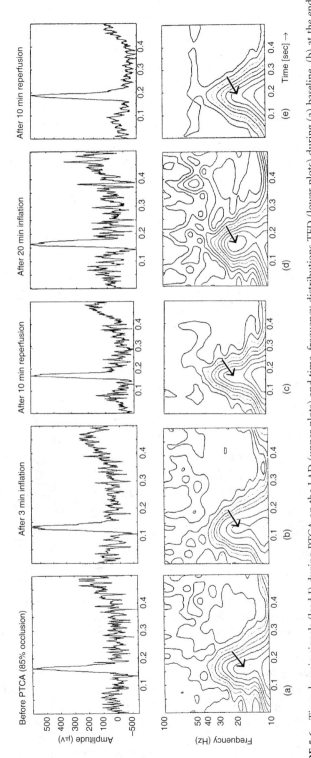

FIGURE 5.6 Time-domain signals (lead I) during PTCA on the LAD (upper plots) and time–frequency distributions TFD (lower plots) during (a) baseline, (b) at the end of a 3 min inflation (7 at), (c) 10 min after first inflation, reducing stenosis from 95 to 60%, (d) at the end of a 20 min inflation (6 at), (e) 10 min after first inflation, reducing stenosis from 95 to 60%. The arrows show the zones of change in TFDs with ischemia/reperfusion.

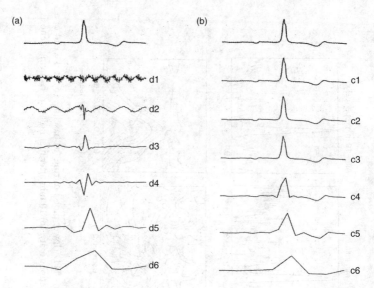

FIGURE 5.7 Detail and coarse components from one ECG cycle. The coarse components represent the low-pass filtered versions of the signal at successive scales. Detail components, d1 and d2, consist mainly of electrical interference.

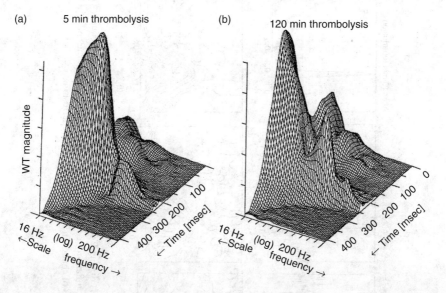

FIGURE 5.8 Change of the time–frequency distributions (QRS complex) of the vector magnitude of orthogonal leads X, Y, and Z during thrombolysis (a) 5 min after start, and (b) 2 h after initiation of therapy. A mid-frequency peak has disappeared due to smoother depolarization, and high-frequency components appear due to faster propagation.

Wigner-Ville, wavelet transform (scalogram), and traditional spectrogram are illustrated in Figure 5.9. This problem causes high levels of signal power to be seen at frequencies not representing the original signal; for example, signal energy contributed at certain frequencies by the QRS complex may mask the signal energy contributed by the late potentials. In this regard, wavelet analysis methods provide a more accurate picture of the localized time-scale features indicative of the late potentials [11,15,43–45]. Figure 5.10 shows that the signal energies at 60 Hz and beyond are localized in the late stage of the QRS and into the ST-segment. For comparison, the scalogram from a healthy person is illustrated in Figure 56.11. This spreading of the high frequencies into the late cycle stages of the QRS complex is a hallmark of the

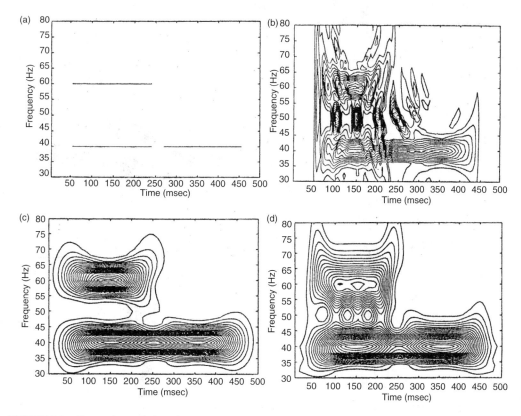

FIGURE 5.9 Comparison of time–frequency representations of sinusoids with specific on–off times (a) shows true time–frequency representation of 40 and 60 Hz sinusoids, (b) shows representation of smoothed Wigner-Ville transform, (c) spectrogram representation, (d) shows wavelet transform version of signal.

late potentials. Time-scale analysis of late potentials may therefore serve as a noninvasive diagnostic tool for predicting the likelihood of life threatening arrhythmias in the heart.

5.5.1.3 Role of Wavelets in Arrhythmia Analysis

Detection of altered QRS morphology. Further applications to the generalized field of arrhythmia classification can be envisaged [46]. When arrhythmias, such as premature ventricular contractions (PVCs) and tachycardia do occur, the P-QRS-T complex undergoes a significant morphological change. Abnormal beats, such as PVCs, have different time-scale signatures than normal beats. Often the QRS complex may widen and sometimes invert with PVCs. As the QRS complex widens, its power spectrum shows diminished contribution at higher frequencies and these are spread out over a wider body of the signal [47,48]. This empirical description of the time-domain features of the ECG signal lends itself particularly well to analysis by time–frequency and time-scale techniques. A more challenging problem is to distinguish multiform PVCs.

Use of the orthogonal wavelet decomposition to separate dynamical activities embedded in a time series. Another interesting application of the discrete wavelet transform to arrhythmia research is the dynamical analysis of the ECG before and during ventricular tachycardia and ventricular fibrillation. Earlier works on heart rate variability have shown that heart rhythm becomes rigidly constant prior to the onset of life threatening arrhythmias, whereas the correlation dimension as a measure of randomness increases to values above 1 during disorganized rhythms like fast ventricular tachycardia, ventricular flutter, and ventricular fibrillation. This fact was used to identify patients at risk, and is promising with regard to prediction of arrhythmic episodes. Encouraging results were recently obtained by combining

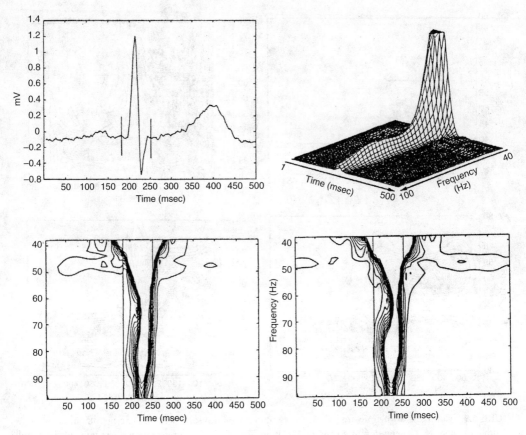

FIGURE 5.10 Healthy person (a) first recorded beat, (b) 3D representation of the modified WT for the first beat, (c) contour plot of the modified WT for the first beat, and (d) contour plot of the modified WT for the second beat.

multiresolution wavelet analysis and dynamical analysis, in an attempt to find a decorrelated scale best projecting changes in low-dimensional dynamics [49]. The authors used records 115 and 207 from the MIT Arrhythmia Database to study nonlinear dynamics preceding ventricular flutter. Distinct changes in the correlation dimension ($D2 \approx 3$) in frequency band 45 to 90 Hz were observed before the onset of arrythmia, indicating the presence of underlying low-dimensional activity.

5.5.2 Neurological Signal Processing

5.5.2.1 Evoked Potentials

Evoked potentials are the signals recorded from the brain in response to external stimulation. Evoked responses can be elicited by electrical stimulation (somatosensory evoked response), visual stimulation (visual evoked response), or auditory stimulation (brainstem auditory evoked response). Usually the signals are small, while the background noise, mostly the background EEG activity, is quite large. The low signal-to-noise ratio (SNR) necessitates use of ensemble averaging, sometimes signal averaging as many as a thousand responses [50]. After enhancing the SNR, one obtains a characteristic wave pattern that includes the stimulus artifact and an undulating pattern characterized by one or more peaks at specific latencies beyond the stimulus. Conventionally, the amplitude and the latency of the signal peaks is used in arriving at a clinical diagnosis. However, when the signals have a complex morphology, simple amplitude and latency analysis does not adequately describe all the complex changes that may occur as a result of

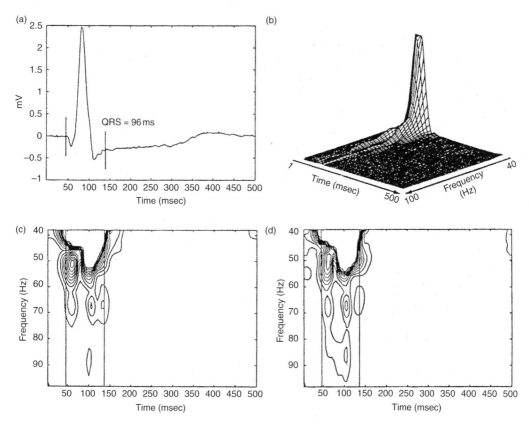

FIGURE 5.11 Patient with ventricular tachycardia diagnosis (a) first beat, (b) 3D representation of the modified WT for the first beat, (c) contour plot of the modified WT for the first beat, and (d) contour plot of the modified WT for the second beat.

brain injury or disease. Time-frequency and wavelet analysis have been shown to be useful in identifying the features localized within the waveform that are most indicative of the brain's response [51].

In one recent experimental study, we evaluated the somatosensory evoked response from experimental animals in whom injury was caused by oxygen deprivation. The evoked response signal was decomposed into its coarse and detail components with the aid of the multiresolution wavelet analysis technique (Figure 5.12) [25]. The magnitude of the detail components was observed to be sensitive to the cerebral hypoxia during its early stages. Figure 5.13a,b show a time trend of the magnitude of the detail components along with the trend of the amplitude and the latency of the primary peak of the somatosensory evoked response. The experimental animal was initially challenged by nitrous gas mixture with 100% oxygen (a non-injury causing event), and late by inspired air with 7 to 8% oxygen. As expected, the amplitude trend shows an initial rise because of the 100% oxygen, and later a gradual decline in response to hypoxia. The magnitude of the detail component shows a trend more responsive to injury: while there is not a significant change in response to the non-injury causing event, the magnitude of the detail component d4 drops quite rapidly when the brain becomes hypoxic. These data suggest that detail components of the evoked response may serve as indicators of early stages of brain injury. Evoked response monitoring can be useful in patient monitoring during surgery and in neurological critical care [52,53]. Other applications include study of cognitive or event-related potentials in human patients for normal cognitive function evaluation or for assessment of clinical situations, such as a response in Alzheimer's disease [54]. Proper characterization of evoked responses from multiple channel recordings facilitates localization of the source using the dipole localization theory [55].

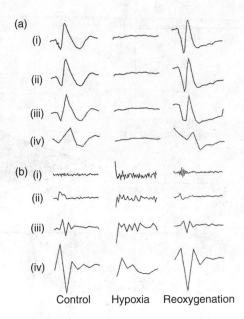

FIGURE 5.12   Coarse (a) and detail (b) components from somatosensory evoked potentials during normal, hypoxic, and reoxygenation phases of experiment.

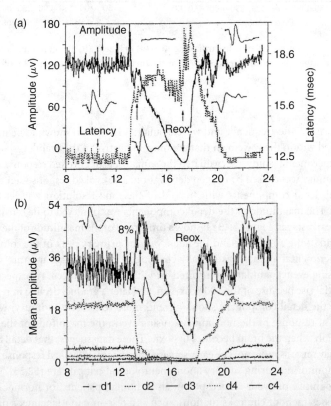

FIGURE 5.13   (a) Amplitude and latency of major evoked potential peak during control, hypoxic, and reoxygenation portions of experiment; (b) mean amplitude of respective detail components during phases of experiment.

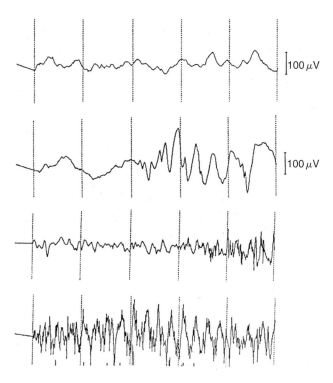

FIGURE 5.14   Example of epilepsy burst.

5.5.2.2 EEG and Seizures

Electroencephalographic signals are usually analyzed by spectrum analysis techniques, dividing the EEG signal into various arbitrary frequency bands (a, b, q, d). Conventional spectrum analysis is useful when these events are slowly unfolding, as when a person goes to sleep, the power in the EEG shifts from higher to lower frequency bands. However, when transient events such as epileptic seizures occur, there are often sharp spikes or a bursting series of events in the recorded waveform. This form of the signal, that is temporally well localized and has a spectrum that is distinctive from normal or ongoing events, lends itself to wavelet analysis. A patient's EEG recorded over an extended period, preceding and following the seizure, was recorded and analyzed. Figure 5.14 shows a short segment of the EEG signal with a seizure burst. The multiresolution wavelet analysis technique was employed to identify the initiation of the seizure burst. Figure 5.15 shows a sudden burst onset in the magnitude of the detail components when the seizure event starts. The bursting subsides at the end of the seizure, as seen by a significant drop in the magnitude of the detail components. Wavelet analysis, thus, may be employed for the detection of onset and termination of seizures. Further possibilities exist in the use of this technique for discriminating interictal spikes and classifying them [56]. Certain seizures, like the petit mal and the grand mal epilepsy seizures, have very characteristic morphologies (e.g., spike and dome pattern). These waveforms would be expected to lend themselves very well to wavelet analysis.

5.5.3 Other Applications

Wavelet, or time-scale analysis is applicable to problems in which signals have characteristic morphologies or equivalently differing spectral signature attributed to different parts of the waveform, and the events of diagnostic interest are well localized in time and scale. The examples of such situations and applications are many.

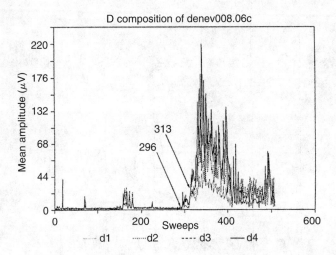

FIGURE 5.15   Localization of burst example with wavelet detail components.

In cardiac signal processing, there are several potential applications. Well localized features of ECG signals, such as the P-QRS-T lend themselves well to wavelet analysis [57]. The application of wavelet analysis to ischemic-reperfusion injury changes and the late potentials has been illustrated above. This idea has been extended to the study of body surface maps recorded using numerous electrodes placed on the chest. In a preliminary study [58], spatio-temporal maps can been constructed and interpreted using time-scale analysis techniques.

In many situations noise and artifact result in inaccurate detection of the QRS complex. Wavelet analysis may prove to be helpful in removal of electrical interference from ECG [59]. Wavelet techniques have successfully been used in removing the noise from functional MRI data [8]. A more challenging application would be in distinguishing artifact from signal. Since wavelet analysis naturally decomposes the signals at different scales at well localized times, the artifactual events can be localized and eliminated. Fast computational methods may prove to be useful in real-time monitoring of ECG signal at a bedside or in analysis of signals recorded by Holter monitors.

Other cardiovascular signals, such as heart sounds may be analyzed by time-frequency or time-scale analysis techniques. Characteristic responses to various normal and abnormal conditions along with sounds that are well localized in time and scale make these signals good candidates for wavelet analysis [60]. Normal patterns may be discriminated from pathological sound patterns, or sounds from various blood vessels can be identified [61]. Blood pressure waveform similarly has a characteristic pattern amenable to time-scale analysis. The dicrotic notch of the pressure waveform results from blood flow through the valves whose opening and closing affects the pressure signal pattern. The dicrotic notch can be detected by wavelet analysis [62]. Sounds from the chest, indicative of respiratory patterns are being investigated using wavelet techniques. Applications include analysis of respiratory patterns of infants [63] and respiration during sleep [64].

Two applications in neurological signal processing, evoked response and seizure detection, are described above. Other potential applications include detection and interpretation of signals from multiple neurons obtained using microelectrodes [65]. Since waveforms (called spikes) from individual neurons (called units) have different patterns because of their separation and orientation with respect to the recording microelectrode, multiunit spike analysis becomes a challenging problem. Time-scale analysis techniques may be employed to localize and analyze the responses of individual units and from that derive the overall activity and interrelation among these units so as to understand the behavior of neural networks. An analogous problem is that of detecting and discriminating signals from "motor units," that is, the muscle cells and fibers [66]. Signals from motor units are obtained by using small, micro or needle electrodes, and characteristic spike trains are obtained, which can be further analyzed by time-scale analysis techniques to discriminate normal and abnormal motor unit activity.

5.6 Discussion and Conclusions

Biological signals with their time-varying nature and characteristic morphologies and spectral signatures are particularly well suited for analysis and interpretation using time-frequency and time-scale analysis techniques. For example, the P-QRS-T complex of the ECG signal shows localized low frequencies in the P- and the ST-segments and high frequencies in the QRS complex. In time-scale frame, the ischemia related changes are seen in certain detail components of the QRS complex. The late segment of the QRS cycle exhibits the so-called late potentials more easily localized by means of time-scale analysis. Other cardiovascular signals, such as pressure waves, heart sounds, and blood flow are being analyzed by the newly developed wavelet analysis algorithms. Other examples of time-scale analysis include neurological signals with potential applications in the analysis of single and multiunit recordings from neurons, evoked response, EEG, and epileptic spikes and seizures.

The desirable requirements for a successful application of time-scale analysis to biomedical signals is that events are well localized in time and exhibit morphological and spectral variations within the localized events. Objectively viewing the signal at different scales should provide meaningful new information. For example, are there fine features of signal that are observable only at scales that pick out the detail components? Are there features of the signal that span a significant portion of the waveform so that they are best studied at a coarse scale. The signal analysis should be able to optimize the trade-off between time and scale, that is, distinguish short lasting events and long lasting events.

For these reasons, the signals described in this article have been found to be particularly useful models for data analysis. However, one needs to be cautious in using any newly developed tool or technology. Most important questions to be addressed before proceeding with a new application are: Is the signal well suited to the tool, and in applying the tool, are any errors inadvertently introduced? Does the analysis provide a new and more useful interpretation of the data and assist in the discovery of new diagnostic information?

Wavelet analysis techniques appear to have robust theoretical properties allowing novel interpretation of biomedical data. As new algorithms emerge, they are likely to find application in the analysis of more diverse biomedical signals. Analogously, the problems faced in the biomedical signal acquisition and processing world will hopefully stimulate development of new algorithms.

References

[1] Rioul, O. and Vetterli, M. Wavelets and signal processing, *IEEE Signal Proc. Mag.*, 14–38, 1991.

[2] Grossmann, A. and Morlet, J. Decomposition of Hardy functions into square integrable wavelets of constant shape, *SIAM J. Math. Anal.*, 15, 723–736, 1984.

[3] Kronland-Martinet, R., Morlet, J., and Grossmann, A. Analysis of sound patterns through wavelet transforms, *Intern. J. Pattern Rec. Artif. Intell.*, 1, 273–302, 1987.

[4] Daubechies, I. The wavelet transform, time–frequency localization, and signal analysis, *IEEE Trans. Info. Theory*, 36, 961–1005, 1990.

[5] Raghuveer, M., Samar, V., Swartz, K.P., Rosenberg, S., and Chaiyaboonthanit, T. Wavelet decomposition of event related potentials: toward the definition of biologically natural components. In: *Proc. Sixth SSAP Workshop on Statistical Signal and Array Processing*, Victoria, BC, CA, pp. 38–41, 1992.

[6] Holschneider, M. Wavelets. *An Analysis Tool*. Clarendon Press, Oxford, 1995.

[7] Strang, G. and Nguyen, T. *Wavelets and Filter Banks*. Wellesley-Cambridge Press, Wellesley, MA, 1996.

[8] Aldroubi, A. and Unser, M. *Wavelets in Medicine and Biology*. CRC Press, Boca Raton, FL, 1996.

[9] Ho, K.C. Fast CWT computation at integer scales by the generalized MRA structure, *IEEE Trans. Signal Process.*, 46, 501–506, 1998.

[10] Hlawatsch, F. and Bourdeaux-Bartels, G.F. Linear and quadratic time–frequency signal representations, *IEEE Signal Process. Mag.*, 21–67, 1992.

[11] Meste, O., Rix, H., Jane, P., Caminal, P., and Thakor, N.V. Detection of late potentials by means of wavelet transform, *IEEE Trans. Biomed. Eng.*, 41, 625–634, 1994.

[12] Chan, Y.T. *Wavelet Basics*. Kluwer Academic Publishers, Boston, 1995.

[13] Najmi, A.-H. and Sadowsky, J. The continuous wavelet transform and variable resolution time–frequency analysis, *The Johns Hopkins APL Tech. Dig.*, 18, 134–140, 1997.

[14] Holschneider, M., Kronland-Martinet, R., and Tchamitchian, P. A real-time algorithm for signal analysis with the help of the wavelet transform. In: *Wavelets: Time–Frequency Methods and Phase Space*, Combes, J., Grossmann, A., and Tchamitchian, P., Eds. Springer-Verlag, New York, pp. 286–297, 1989.

[15] Gramatikov, B. and Georgiev, I. Wavelets as an alternative to STFT in signal-averaged electrocardiography, *Med. Biolog. Eng. Comp.*, 33, 482–487, 1995.

[16] Sadowsky, J. The continuous wavelet transform: a tool for signal investigation and understanding, *Johns Hopkins APL Tech. Dig.*, 15, 306–318, 1994.

[17] Jones, D.L. and Baraniuk, R.G. Efficient approximation of continuous wavelet transforms, *Electron. Lett.*, 27, 748–750, 1991.

[18] Vetterli, M. and Kovacevic, J. *Wavelets and Subband Coding*. Prentice Hall, Englewood Cliffs, NJ, 1995.

[19] Goupillaud, P., Grossmann, A., and Morlet, J. Cycle-octave and related transforms in seismic signal analysis, *Geoexploration*, 23, 85–102, 1984.

[20] Oppenheim, A.V. and Schaffer, R.W. *Discrete-Time Signal Processing*. Prentice-Hall, Englewood Cliffs, NJ, 1989.

[21] Senhadji, L., Carrault, G., Bellanger, J.J., and Passariello, G. Some new applications of the wavelet transforms. In: *Proc. 14th Ann. Int. Conf. IEEE EMBS*, Paris, pp. 2592–2593, 1992.

[22] Tuteur, F.B. Wavelet transformation in signal detection, *Proc. IEEE Int. Conf. ASSP*, 1435–1438, 1988.

[23] Thakor, N.V., Sun, Y.C., Rix, H., and Caminal, P. Mulitwave: a wavelet-based ECG data compression algorithm, *IEICE Trans. Inf. Syst.*, E76-D, 1462–1469, 1993.

[24] Mallat, S. A theory for multiresolution signal decomposition: The wavelet representation, *IEEE Trans. Pattern Ana. Mach. Intell.*, 11, 674–693, 1989.

[25] Thakor, N.V., Xin-Rong, G., Yi-Chun, S., and Hanley, D.F. Multiresolution wavelet analysis of evoked potentials, *IEEE Trans. Biomed. Eng.*, 40, 1085–1094, 1993.

[26] Thakor, N.V., Gramatikov, B., and Mita, M. Multiresolution wavelet analysis of ecg during ischemia and reperfusion. In: *Proc. Comput. Cardiol.*, London, pp. 895–898, 1993.

[27] Daubechies, I. Orthogonal bases of compactly supported wavelets, *Commun. Pure Appl. Math.*, 41, 909–996, 1988.

[28] Daubechies, I. Orthonormal bases of compactly supported wavelets II. Variations on a theme, *SIAM J. Math. Anal.*, 24, 499–519, 1993.

[29] Burrus, C.S., Gopinath, R.A., and Guo, H. *Introduction to Wavelets and Wavelet Transforms*. Prentice Hall, Upper Saddle River, NJ, 1998.

[30] Hilton, M.L. Wavelet and wavelet packet compression of electrocardiograms, *IEEE Trans. Biomed. Eng.*, 44, 394–402, 1997.

[31] Thakor, N.V., Webster, J.G., and Tompkins, W.J. Estimation of QRS complex power spectra for design of QRS filter, *IEEE Trans. Biomed. Eng.*, 31, 702–706, 1984.

[32] Gramatikov, B. Digital filters for the detection of late potentials, *Med. Biol. Eng. Comp.*, 31, 416–420, 1993.

[33] Gramatikov, B. and Thakor, N. Wavelet analysis of coronary artery occlusion related changes in ECG. In: *Proc. 15th Ann. Int. Conf. IEEE Eng. Med. Biol. Soc.*, San Diego, p. 731, 1993.

[34] Pettersson, J., Warren, S., Mehta, N., Lander, P., Berbari, E.J., Gates, K., Sornmo, L., Pahlm, O., Selvester, R.H., and Wagner, G.S. Changes in high-frequency QRS components during prolonged coronary artery occlusion in humans, *J. Electrocardiol.*, 28 (Suppl), 225–227, 1995.

[35] Wit, A.L. and Janse, M.J. *The Ventricular Arrhythmias of Ischemia and Infarction: Electrophysiological Mechanisms.* Futura Publishing Company, New York, 1993.

[36] Thakor, N., Yi-Chun, S., Gramatikov, B., Rix, H., and Caminal, P. Multiresolution wavelet analysis of ECG: Detection of ischemia and reperfusion in angioplasty. In: *Proc. World Congress Med. Physics Biomed. Eng.*, Rio de Janeiro, p. 392, 1994.

[37] Gramatikov, B., Yi-Chun, S., Rix, H., Caminal, P., and Thakor, N. Multiresolution wavelet analysis of the body surface ECG before and after angioplasty, *Ann. Biomed. Eng.*, 23, 553–561, 1995.

[38] Kwon, K., Freedman, B., and Wilcox, I. The unstable ST segment early after thrombolysis for acute infarction and its usefulness as a marker of coronary occlusion, *Am. J. Cardiol.*, 67, 109, 1991.

[39] Abboud, S., Leor, J., and Eldar, M. High frequency ECG during reperfusion therapy of acute myocardial infarction. In: *Proc. Comput. Cardiol.*, pp. 351–353, 1990.

[40] Xue, Q., Reddy, S., and Aversano, T. Analysis of high-frequency signal-averaged ECG measurements, *J. Electrocardiol.*, 28 (Suppl), 239–245.

[41] Berbari, E.J. Critical review of late potential recordings, *J. Electrocardiol.*, 20, 125–127, 1987.

[42] Gramatikov, B. Detection of late potentials in the signal-averaged ECG — combining time and frequency domain analysis, *Med. Biol. Eng. Comp.*, 31, 333–339, 1993.

[43] Nikolov, Z., Georgiev, I., Gramatikov, B., and Daskalov, I. Use of the wavelet transform for time-frequency localization of late potentials. In: *Proc. Congress '93 of the German, Austrian and Swiss Society for Biomedical Engineering*, Graz, Austria, Biomedizinische Technik, Suppl. 38, pp. 87–89, 1993.

[44] Morlet, D., Peyrin, F., Desseigne, P., Touboul, P., and Roubel, P. Wavelet analysis of high-resolution signal-averaged ECGs in postinfarction patients, *J. Electrocardiol.*, 26, 311–320, 1993.

[45] Dickhaus, H., Khadral, L., and Brachmann, J. Quantification of ECG late potentials by wavelet transformation, *Comput. Meth. Programs Biomed.*, 43, 185–192, 1994.

[46] Jouney, I., Hamilton, P., and Kanapathipillai, M. Adaptive wavelet representation and classification of ECG signals. In: *Proc. IEEE Int.'l Conf. of the Eng. Med. Biol. Soc.*, Baltimore, MD, 1994.

[47] Thakor, N.V., Baykal, A., and Casaleggio, A. Fundamental analyses of ventricular fibrillation signals by parametric, nonparametric, and dynamical methods. In: Inbar IGaGF, ed., *Advances in Processing and Pattern Analysis of Biological Signals.* Plenum Press, New York, pp. 273–295, 1996.

[48] Baykal, A., Ranjan, R., and Thakor, N.V. Estimation of the ventricular fibrillation duration by autoregressive modeling, *IEEE Trans. Biomed. Eng.*, 44, 349–356, 1997.

[49] Casaleggio, A., Gramatikov, B., and Thakor, N.V. On the use of wavelets to separate dynamical activities embedded in a time series. In: *Proc. Computers in Cardiology*, Indianapolis, pp. 181–184, 1996.

[50] Aunon, J.I., McGillem, C.D., and Childers, D.G. Signal processing in evoked potential research: averaging, principal components, and modeling, *Crit. Rev. Biomed. Eng.*, 5, 323–367, 1981.

[51] Raz, J. Wavelet models of event-related potentials. In: *Proc. IEEE Int. Conf. Eng. Med. Biol. Soc.*, Baltimore, MD, 1994.

[52] Grundy, B.L., Heros, R.C., Tung, A.S., and Doyle, E. Intraoperative hypoxia detected by evoked potential monitoring, *Anesth. Analg.*, 60, 437–439, 1981.

[53] McPherson, R.W. Intraoperative monitoring of evoked potentials, *Prog. Neurol. Surg.*, 12, 146–163, 1987.

[54] Ademoglu, A., Micheli-Tzanakou, E., and Istefanopulos, Y. Analysis of pattern reversal visual evoked potentials (PRVEP) in Alzheimer's disease by spline wavelets. In: *Proc. IEEE Int. Conf. Eng. Med. Biol. Soc.*, 320–321, 1993.

[55] Sun, M., Tsui, F., and Sclabassi, R.J. Partially reconstructible wavelet decomposition of evoked potentials for dipole source localization. In: *Proc. IEEE Int. Conf. Eng. Med. Biol. Soc.*, pp. 332–333, 1993.

[56] Schiff, S.J. Wavelet transforms for epileptic spike and seizure detection. In: *Proc. IEEE Int. Conf. Eng. Med. Biol. Soc.*, Baltimore, MD, pp. 1214–1215, 1994.

[57] Li, C. and Zheng, C. QRS detection by wavelet transform. In: *Proc. IEEE Int. Conf. Eng. Med. Biol. Soc.*, pp. 330–331, 1993.

[58] Brooks, D.H., On, H., MacLeond, R.S., and Krim, H. Spatio-temporal wavelet analysis of body surface maps during PTCA-induced ischemia. In: *Proc. IEEE Int. Conf. Eng. Med. Biol. Soc.*, Baltimore, MD, 1994.

[59] Karrakchou, M. New structures for multirate adaptive filtering: application to intereference canceling in biomedical engineering. In: *Proc. IEEE Int. Conf. Eng. Med. Biol. Soc.*, Baltimore, MD, 1994.

[60] Bentley, P.M. and McDonnel, J.T.E. Analysis of heart sounds using the wavelet transform. In: *Proc. IEEE Int. Conf. Eng. Med. Biol. Soc.*, Baltimore, MD, 1994.

[61] Akay, M., Akay, Y.M., Welkowitz, W., and Lewkowicz, S. Investigating the effects of vasodilator drugs on the turbulent sound caused by femoral artery using short term Fourier and wavelet transform methods, *IEEE Trans. Biomed. Eng.*, 41, 921–928, 1994.

[62] Antonelli, L. Dicrotic notch detection using wavelet transform analysis. In: *Proc. IEEE Int. Conf. Eng. Med. Biol. Soc.*, Baltimore, MD, 1994.

[63] Ademovic, E., Charbonneau, G., and Pesquet, J.-C. Segmentation of infant respiratory sounds with Mallat's wavelets. In: *Proc. IEEE Int. Conf. Eng. Med. Biol. Soc.*, Baltimore, MD, 1994.

[64] Sartene, R., Wallet, J.C., Allione, P., Palka, S., Poupard, L., and Bernard, J.L. Using wavelet transform to analyse cardiorespiratory and electroencephalographic signals during sleep. In: *Proc. IEEE Int. Conf. Eng. Med. Biol. Soc.*, Baltimore, MD, 1994.

[65] Akay, Y.M. and Micheli-Tzanakou, E. Wavelet analysis of the multiple single unit recordings in the optic tectum of the frog. In: *Proc. IEEE Int. Conf. Eng. Med. Biol. Soc.*, pp. 334–335, 1993.

[66] Pattichis, M. and Pattichis, C.S. Fast wavelet transform in motor unit action potential analysis. In: *Proc. IEEE Int. Conf. Eng. Med. Biol. Soc.*, pp. 1225–1226, 1993.

6

Higher-Order Spectral Analysis

6.1 Introduction.. **6**-1
6.2 Definitions and Properties of HOS.................... **6**-2
6.3 HOS Computation from Real Data.................... **6**-4
Indirect Method • Direct Method
6.4 Linear Processes....................................... **6**-6
Nonparametric Methods • Parametric Methods
6.5 Nonlinear Processes **6**-8
6.6 HOS in Biomedical Signal Processing................. **6**-11
Acknowledgments... **6**-13
References **6**-14

Athina P. Petropulu
Drexel University

6.1 Introduction

The past 20 years witnessed an expansion of power spectrum estimation techniques, which have proved essential in many applications, such as communications, sonar, radar, speech/image processing, geophysics, and biomedical signal processing [1–3]. In power spectrum estimation, the process under consideration is treated as a superposition of statistically uncorrelated harmonic components. The distribution of power among these frequency components is the power spectrum. As such phase relations between frequency components are suppressed. The information in the power spectrum is essentially present in the autocorrelation sequence, which would suffice for the complete statistical description of a Gaussian process of known mean. However, there are applications where one would need to obtain information regarding deviations from the Gaussianity assumption and presence of nonlinearities. In these cases power spectrum is of little help, and a look beyond the power spectrum or autocorrelation domain is needed. Higher-order spectra (HOS) (of order greater than two), which are defined in terms of higher-order cumulants of the data, do contain such information [4]. The third order spectrum is commonly referred to as bispectrum and the fourth-order as trispectrum. The power spectrum is also a member of the higher-order spectral class; it is the second-order spectrum.

The HOS consist of higher-order moment spectra, which are defined for deterministic signals, and cumulant spectra, which are defined for random processes. In general there are three motivations behind the use of HOS in signal processing (1) to suppress Gaussian noise of unknown mean and variance, (2) to reconstruct the phase as well as the magnitude response of signals or systems, and (3) to detect and characterize nonlinearities in the data.

The first motivation stems from the property of Gaussian processes to have zero higher-order spectra of order greater than two. Due to this property, HOS are high signal-to-noise ratio domains in which one can perform detection, parameter estimation, or even signal reconstruction even if the time domain noise is spatially correlated. The same property of cumulant spectra can provide a means of detecting and characterizing deviations of the data from the Gaussian model.

The second motivation is based on the ability of cumulant spectra to preserve the Fourier phase of signals. In the modeling of time series, second-order statistics (autocorrelation) have been heavily used because they are the result of least-squares optimization criteria. However, an accurate phase reconstruction in the autocorrelation domain can be achieved only if the signal is at minimum phase. Nonminimum phase signal reconstruction can be achieved only in the HOS domain, due to the HOS ability to preserve the phase.

Being nonlinear functions of the data, HOS are quite natural tools in the analysis of nonlinear systems operating under a random input. General relations for stationary random data passing through an arbitrary linear system exist and have been studied extensively. Such expressions, however, are not available for nonlinear systems, where each type of nonlinearity must be studied separately. Higher-order correlations between input and output can detect and characterize certain nonlinearities [5], and for this purpose several higher-order spectra based methods have been developed.

This chapter is organized as follows. In Section 6.2 definitions and properties of cumulants and higher-order spectra are introduced. In Section 6.3 methods for estimation of HOS from finite length data are presented and the asymptotic statistics of the corresponding estimates are provided. In Section 6.4 methods for identification of a linear time-invariant system from HOS of the system output are outlined, while in Section 6.6, nonlinear system estimation is considered. Section 6.6 summarizes the research activity related to HOS as applied to biomedical signal analysis and provides details on a particular application, namely the improvement of resolution of medical ultrasound images via HOS is discussed.

6.2 Definitions and Properties of HOS

In this chapter only random one-dimensional processes are considered. The definitions can be easily extended to the two-dimensional case [6].

The joint moments of order r of the random variables $x_1, \ldots, x_n$ are given by [7]:

$$\mathrm{Mom}[x_1^{k_1}, \ldots, x_n^{k_n}] = E\{x_1^{k_1}, \ldots, x_n^{k_n}\}$$

$$= (-j)^r \left. \frac{\partial^r \Phi(\omega_1, \ldots, \omega_n)}{\partial \omega_1^{k_1} \ldots \partial \omega_n^{k_n}} \right|_{\omega_1 = \cdots = \omega_n = 0} \tag{6.1}$$

where $k_1 + \cdots + k_n = r$, and $\Phi(\cdot)$ is their joint characteristic function. The corresponding joint cumulants are defined as:

$$\mathrm{Cum}[x_1^{k_1}, \ldots, x_n^{k_n}] = (-j)^r \left. \frac{\partial^r \ln \Phi(\omega_1, \ldots, \omega_n)}{\partial \omega_1^{k_1} \ldots \partial \omega_n^{k_n}} \right\}_{\omega_1 = \cdots = \omega_n = 0} \tag{6.2}$$

For a stationary discrete time random process $x(k)$ (k denotes discrete time), the *moments* of order n are given by:

$$m_n^x(\tau_1, \tau_2, \ldots, \tau_{n-1}) = E\{x(k)x(k + \tau_1) \cdots x(k + \tau_{n-1})\} \tag{6.3}$$

where $E\{\cdot\}$ denotes expectation. The nth order cumulants are functions of the moments of order up to n, that is,

First-order cumulants:

$$c_1^x = m_1^x = E\{x(k)\} \quad \text{(mean)} \tag{6.4}$$

Second-order cumulants:

$$c_2^x(\tau_1) = m_2^x(\tau_1) - (m_1^x)^2 \quad \text{(covariance)} \tag{6.5}$$

Third-order cumulants:

$$c_3^x(\tau_1, \tau_2) = m_3^x(\tau_1, \tau_2) - (m_1^x)[m_2^x(\tau_1) + m_2^x(\tau_2) + m_2^x(\tau_2 - \tau_1)]2(m_1^x)^3 \tag{6.6}$$

Fourth-order cumulants:

$$
\begin{aligned}
c_4^x(\tau_1, \tau_2, \tau_3) = {}& m_4^x(\tau_1, \tau_2, \tau_3) - m_2^x(\tau_1)m_2^x(\tau_3 - \tau_2) - m_2^x(\tau_2)m_2^x(\tau_3 - \tau_1) - m_2^x(\tau_3)m_2^x(\tau_2 - \tau_1) \\
& - m_1^x[m_3^x(\tau_2 - \tau_1, \tau_3 - \tau_1) + m_3^x(\tau_2, \tau_3) + m_3^x(\tau_2, \tau_4) + m_3^x(\tau_1, \tau_2)] \\
& + (m_1^x)^2[m_2^x(\tau_1) + m_2^x(\tau_2) + m_2^x(\tau_3) + m_2^x(\tau_3 - \tau_1) + m_2^x(\tau_3 - \tau_2) \\
& + m_1^x(\tau_2 - \tau_1)] - 6(m_1^x)^4
\end{aligned}
\tag{6.7}
$$

The general relationship between cumulants and moments can be found in Reference 4.

Some important properties of moments and cumulants are summarized next.

[P1] If $x(k)$ is a jointly Gaussian process, then $c_n^x(\tau_1, \tau_2, \ldots, \tau_{n-1}) = 0$ for $n > 2$. In other words, all the information about a Gaussian process is contained in its first- and second-order cumulants. This property can be used to suppress Gaussian noise, or as a measure for non-Gaussianity in time series.

[P2] If $x(k)$ is symmetrically distributed, then $c_3^x(\tau_1, \tau_2) = 0$. Third-order cumulants suppress not only Gaussian processes, but also all symmetrically distributed processes, such as uniform, Laplace, and Bernoulli–Gaussian.

[P3] Additivity holds for cumulants. If $x(k) = s(k) + w(k)$, where $s(k)$, $w(k)$ are stationary and statistically independent random processes, then $c_n^x(\tau_1, \tau_2, \ldots, \tau_{n-1}) = c_n^s(\tau_1, \tau_2, \ldots, \tau_{n-1}) + c_n^w(\tau_1, \tau_2, \ldots, \tau_{n-1})$. It is important to note that additivity does not hold for moments.

If $w(k)$ is a Gaussian representing noise which corrupts the signal of interest, $s(k)$, then by means of (P2) and (P3), we conclude that $c_n^x(\tau_1, \tau_2, \ldots, \tau_{n-1}) = c_n^s(\tau_1, \tau_2, \ldots, \tau_{n-1})$, for $n > 2$. In other words, in higher-order cumulant domains the signal of interest propagates noise free. Property (P3) can also provide a measure of the statistical dependence of two processes.

[P4] if $x(k)$ has zero mean, then $c_n^x(\tau_1, \ldots, \tau_{n-1}) = m_n^x(\tau_1, \ldots, \tau_{n-1})$, for $n \leq 3$.

Higher-order spectra are defined in terms of either cumulants (e.g., cumulant spectra) or moments (e.g., moment spectra).

Assuming that the nth-order cumulant sequence is absolutely summable, the nth-order cumulant spectrum of $x(k)$, $C_n^x(\omega_1, \omega_2, \ldots, \omega_{n-1})$, exists, and is defined to be the $(n - 1)$-dimensional Fourier transform of the nth-order cumulant sequence. In general, $C_n^x(\omega_1, \omega_2, \ldots, \omega_{n-1})$ is complex, that is, it has magnitude and phase. In an analogous manner, moment spectrum is the multidimensional Fourier transform of the moment sequence.

If $v(k)$ is a stationary non-Gaussian process with zero mean and nth-order cumulant sequence

$$c_n^v(\tau_1, \ldots, \tau_{n-1}) = \gamma_n^v \delta(\tau_1, \ldots, \tau_{n-1}) \tag{6.8}$$

where $\delta(\cdot)$ is the delta function, $v(k)$ is said to be nth order white. Its nth order cumulant spectrum is then flat and equal to γ_n^x.

Cumulant spectra are more useful in processing random signals than moment spectra since they posses properties that the moment spectra do not share, that is, properties P1, P3, and flatness of spectra corresponding to higher-order white noise.

6.3 HOS Computation from Real Data

The definitions of cumulants presented in the previous section are based on expectation operations, and they assume infinite length data. In practice we always deal with data of finite length, therefore, the cumulants can only be estimated. Two methods for cumulants and spectra estimation are presented next for the third-order case.

6.3.1 Indirect Method

Let $x(k), k = 0, \ldots, N - 1$ be the available data.

1. Segment the data into K records of M samples each. Let $x^i(k), k = 0, \ldots, M - 1$, represent the ith record.
2. Subtract the mean of each record.
3. Estimate the moments of each segment $x^i(k)$ as follows:

$$l_1 = \max(0, -\tau_1, -\tau_2), l_2 = \min(M - 1 - \tau_1, M - 1 - \tau_2, M - 1), \ |\tau_1| < L, \ |\tau_2| < L,$$

$$i = 1, 2, \ldots, K. \tag{6.9}$$

Since each segment has zero mean, its third-order moments and cumulants are identical, that is, $c_3^{x_i}(\tau_1, \tau_2) = m_3^{x_i}(\tau_1, \tau_2)$.

4. Compute the average cumulants as:

$$\hat{c}_3^x(\tau_1, \tau_2) = \frac{1}{K} \sum_{i=1}^{K} m_3^{x_i}(\tau_1, \tau_2) \tag{6.10}$$

5. Obtain the third-order spectrum (bispectrum) estimate as the two-dimensional Discrete Fourier Transform of size $M \times M$ of the windowed $c_3^{x_i}(\tau_1, \tau_2)$, that is,

$$\hat{C}_3^x(k_1, k_2) = \sum_{\tau_1=-L}^{L} \sum_{\tau_2=-L}^{L} \hat{c}_3^x(\tau_1, \tau_2) e^{-j((2\pi/M)k_1\tau_1 + (2\pi/M)k_2\tau_2)} w(\tau_1, \tau_1), \quad k_1, k_2 = 0, \ldots, M - 1$$

$$\tag{6.11}$$

where $L < M - 1$, and $w(\tau_1, \tau_2)$ is a two-dimensional window of bounded support, introduced to smooth out edge effects. The bandwidth of the final bispectrum estimate is $\Delta = 1/L$.

A complete description of appropriate windows that can be used in Equation 6.11 and their properties can be found in Reference 4. A good choice of cumulant window is:

$$w(\tau_1, \tau_2) = d(\tau_1)d(\tau_2)d(\tau_1 - \tau_2) \tag{6.12}$$

where

$$
d(\tau) = \begin{cases} \dfrac{1}{\pi} \left| \sin \dfrac{\pi \tau}{L} \right| + \left(1 - \dfrac{|\tau|}{L} \right) \cos \dfrac{\pi \tau}{L} & |\tau| \leq L \\ 0 & |\tau| > L \end{cases} \tag{6.13}
$$

which is known as the minimum bispectrum bias supremum [8].

6.3.2 Direct Method

Let $x(k), k = 1, \ldots, N$ be the available data.

1. Segment the data into K records of M samples each. Let $x^i(k), k = 0, \ldots, M - 1$, represent the ith record.
2. Subtract the mean of each record.
3. Compute the Discrete Fourier Transform $X^i(k)$ of each segment, based on M points, that is,

$$
X^i(k) = \sum_{n=0}^{M-1} x^i(n) e^{-j(2\pi/M)nk}, \quad k = 0, 1, \ldots, M - 1, \ i = 1, 2, \ldots, K \tag{6.14}
$$

4. The third-order spectrum of each segment is obtained as

$$
C_3^{x_i}(k_1, k_2) = \frac{1}{M} X^i(k_1) X^i(k_2) X^{i*}(k_1 + k_2), \quad i = 1, \ldots, K \tag{6.15}
$$

   Due to the bispectrum symmetry properties, $C_3^{x_i}(k_1, k_2)$ needs to be computed only in the triangular region $0 \leq k_2 \leq k_1, k_1 + k_2 < M/2$.
5. In order to reduce the variance of the estimate, additional smoothing over a rectangular window of size $(M_3 \times M_3)$ can be performed around each frequency, assuming that the third-order spectrum is smooth enough, that is,

$$
\hat{C}_3^{x_i}(k_1, k_2) = \frac{1}{M_3^2} \sum_{n_1=-M_3/2}^{M_3/2-1} \sum_{n_2=-M_3/2}^{M_3/2-1} C_3^{x_i}(k_1 + n_1, k_2 + n_2) \tag{6.16}
$$

6. Finally, the third-order spectrum is given as the average over all third-order spectra, that is,

$$
\hat{C}_3^x(k_1, k_2) = \frac{1}{K} \sum_{i=1}^{K} \tilde{C}_3^{x_i}(k_1, k_2) \tag{6.17}
$$

The final bandwidth of this bispectrum estimate is $\Delta = M_3/M$, which is the spacing between frequency samples in the bispectrum domain.

   For large N, and as long as

$$
\Delta \to 0 \quad \text{and} \quad \Delta^2 N \to \infty \tag{6.18}
$$

both the direct and the indirect methods produce asymptotically unbiased and consistent bispectrum estimates, with real and imaginary part variances [9]:

$$\text{var}(\text{Re}[\hat{C}_3^x(k_1, k_2)]) = \text{var}(\text{Im}[\hat{C}_3^x(k_1, k_2)])$$

$$= \frac{1}{\Delta^2 N} C_2^x(k_1) C_2^x(k_2) C_2^x(k_1 + k_2) = \begin{cases} \dfrac{VL^2}{MK} C_2^x(k_1) C_2^x(k_2) C_2^x(k_1 + k_2) & \text{indirect} \\[2ex] \dfrac{M}{KM_3^2} C_2^x(k_1) C_2^x(k_2) C_2^x(k_1 + k_2) & \text{direct} \end{cases} \tag{6.19}$$

where V is the energy of the bispectrum window.

From the above expressions, it becomes apparent that the bispectrum estimate variance can be reduced by increasing the number of records, or reducing the size of the region of support of the window in the cumulant domain (L), or increasing the size of the frequency smoothing window (M_3), etc. The relation between the parameters M, K, L, M_3 should be such that 6.18 is satisfied.

6.4 Linear Processes

Let $x(k)$ be generated by exiting a linear, time-invariant (LTI), exponentially stable, mixed-phase system with frequency response $H(\omega)$ (or impulse response $h(k)$), with an nth order white, zero-mean, non-Gaussian stationary process $v(k)$, that is,

$$x(k) = v(k) * h(k) \tag{6.20}$$

where $*$ denotes convolution.

The output nth-order cumulant equals [10]:

$$c_n^x(\tau_1, \ldots, \tau_{n-1}) = \gamma_n^v \sum_{k=0}^{\infty} h(k) h(k + \tau_1) \cdots h(k + \tau_{n-1}), \quad n \geq 3 \tag{6.21}$$

where γ_n^v is a scalar constant and equals the nth-order spectrum of $v(k)$. The output nth-order cumulant spectrum is given by

$$C_n^x(\omega_1, \omega_2, \ldots, \omega_{n-1}) = \gamma_n^v H(\omega_1) \cdots H(\omega_{n-1}) H^*(\omega_1 + \cdots + \omega_{n-1}) \tag{6.22}$$

For a linear non-Gaussian random process $x(k)$, the nth-order spectrum can be factorized as in Equation 6.22 for every order n, while for a nonlinear process such a factorization might be valid for some orders only (it is always valid for $n = 2$).

It can be easily shown that the cumulant spectra of successive orders are related as follows:

$$C_n^x(\omega_1, \omega_2, \ldots, 0) - C_{n-1}^x(\omega_1, \omega_2, \ldots, \omega_{n-2}) H(0) \frac{\gamma_n^v}{\gamma_{n-1}^v} \tag{6.23}$$

For example, the power spectrum of a non-Gaussian linear process can be reconstructed from the bispectrum up to a scalar factor, that is,

$$C_3^x(\omega, 0) = C_2^x(\omega) \frac{\gamma_3^v}{\gamma_2^v} \tag{6.24}$$

While for $n = 2$, Equation 6.22 provides the magnitude only of $H(\omega)$, as a function of $C_n^x(\omega_1, \omega_2, \ldots, \omega_{n-1})$, for $n > 2$ both the magnitude and phase of $H(\omega)$ can be obtained. A significant amount of research has been devoted to estimating the system phase from the phase of the bispectrum or trispectrum [4,11–13].

Let

$$y(k) = x(k) + w(k) \tag{6.25}$$

where $x(k)$ was defined in Equation 6.20, and $w(k)$ is zero-mean Gaussian noise, uncorrelated to $x(k)$. Methods for reconstructing $h(k)$ from $y(k)$ can be divided into two main categories: nonparametric and parametric.

6.4.1 Nonparametric Methods

Nonparametric methods reconstruct the system by recovering its Fourier phase and magnitude. Some utilize the whole bispectrum (or polyspectrum) information [11,14–18], and others use fixed, one-dimensional polyspectrum slices [19,20]. In References 12 and 21, methods for system recovery from arbitrarily selected HOS slices have been proposed. A system method based on preselected polyspectrum slices, allows regions where polyspectrum estimates exhibit high variance, or regions where the ideal polyspectrum is expected to be zero, such as in the case of bandlimited systems to be avoided. Assuming that there existed a mechanism to select "good" slices, it can also lead to computational savings.

Let the bispectrum of $y(k)$ in Equation 6.25, that is, $C_3^x(\omega_1, \omega_2)$, be discretized on a square grid of size $2\pi/N \times 2\pi/N$, and let $\{C_3^y(m, l), m = 0, \ldots, N-1\}$, $\{C_3^y(m, l+r), m = 0, \ldots, N-1\}$ be two bispectral slices. In Reference 21 it was shown that unique identification of the system impulse response can be performed base on two horizontal slices of the discretized third-order spectrum of the system output, as long as the distance between slices, that is, r and N are co-prime numbers. Let

$$\hat{\mathbf{h}} = [\log H(1), \ldots, \log H(N-1)]^T ((N-1) \times 1) \tag{6.26}$$

where $H(k)$ is the Discrete Fourier Transform of $h(n)$. Then $\hat{\mathbf{h}}$ can be obtained as the solution of the system:

$$\mathbf{A}\hat{\mathbf{h}} = \mathbf{b} \tag{6.27}$$

where

$$b(k) = \log C_3^h(-k-r-l, l) - \log C_3^h(-k-r-l, l+r) + c_{l,r}$$

$$k = 0, \ldots, N-1$$

$$c_{l,r} = \frac{1}{N} \sum_{k=0}^{N-1} [\log C_3^y(k, l+r) - \log C_3^y(k, l)] \tag{6.28}$$

and A is a $[(N-1) \times (N-1)]$ sparse matrix; its first row contains a 1 at the rth column and 0s elsewhere. The kth row contains a -1 at column $(k-1) \, modulo N$, and a 1 at column $(k+r-1) \, modulo N$. Although $b(k)$ requires the computation of the logarithm of a complex quantity, it was shown in Reference 21, that the log-bispectrum can be computed based on the principal argument of the bispectral phase, thus bypassing the need for two-dimensional phase unwrapping. The bispectrum needed in this method can be substituted with a bispectral estimate, obtained with any of the methods outlined in Chapter 6.3. Reduction of the HOS estimate variance can be achieved via a low-rank approach [22–24].

The above described reconstruction method can be easily extended to any order spectrum [21]. Matlab code for this method can be found at http://www.ece.drexel.edu/CSPL.

6.4.2 Parametric Methods

These methods fit a parametric model to the data $x(k)$. For example, let us fit a real autoregressive moving average (ARMA) model to $x(k)$, that is,

$$\sum_{i=0}^{p} a(i)x(k-i) = \sum_{j=0}^{q} b(j)v(k-j) \tag{6.29}$$

where $v(k)$ is a stationary zero-mean nth order white non-Gaussian process, and $a(i)$ and $b(j)$ represent the AR and MA parameters. Let $y(k)$ be as defined in Equation 6.25. For estimation of the AR parameters from $y(k)$, equations analogous to the Yule-Walker equations can be derived based on third-order cumulants of $y(k)$, that is,

$$\sum_{i=0}^{p} a(i)c_3^y(\tau-i,j) = 0, \quad \tau > q \tag{6.30}$$

or

$$\sum_{i=1}^{p} a(i)c_3^y(\tau-i,j) = -c_3^y(\tau,j), \quad \tau > q \tag{6.31}$$

where it was assumed $a(0) = 1$. Concatenating Equation 6.31 for $\tau = q+1, \ldots, q+M, M \geq 0$, and $j = q - p, \ldots, q$, the matrix equation

$$Ca = c \tag{6.32}$$

can be formed, where C and c are a matrix and a vector, respectively, formed by third-order cumulants of the process according to Equation 6.31, and the vector a contains the AR parameters. If the AR order p is unknown and Equation 6.32 is formed based on an overestimate of p, the resulting matrix C always has rank p. In this case the AR parameters can be obtained using a low-rank approximation of C [25].

Using the estimated AR parameters, $\hat{a}(i)$, $i = 1, \ldots, p$, a, pth order filter with transfer function $\hat{A}(z) = 1 + \sum_{i=1}^{p} \hat{a}(i)z^{-i}$ can be constructed. Based on the filtered-through $\hat{A}(z)$ process $y(k)$, that is, $\tilde{y}(k)$, or otherwise known as the residual time series [25], the MA parameters can be estimated via any MA method [6], for example:

$$b(k) = \frac{c_3^{\tilde{y}}(q,k)}{c_3^{\tilde{y}}(q,0)}, \quad k = 0, 1, \ldots, q \tag{6.33}$$

known as the $c(q, k)$ formula [26].

Practical problems associated with the described approach are sensitivity to model order mismatch, and AR estimation errors that propagate in the estimation of the MA parameters. Additional parametric methods can be found in References 4, 6, and 27–31.

6.5 Nonlinear Processes

Despite the fact that progress has been established in developing the theoretical properties of nonlinear models, only a few statistical methods exist for detection and characterization of nonlinearities from a finite set of observations. In this chapter we will consider nonlinear Volterra systems excited by Gaussian

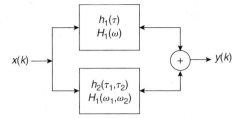

FIGURE 6.1   Second-order Volterra system. Linear and quadratic parts are connected in parallel.

stationary inputs. Let $y(k)$ be the response of a discrete time invariant, pth order, Volterra filter whose input is $x(k)$. Then,

$$y(k) = h_0 + \sum_i \sum_{\tau_1,\dots,\tau_i} h_i(\tau_1,\dots,\tau_i)x(k - \tau_1)\cdots x(k - \tau_i) \tag{6.34}$$

where $h_i(\tau_1,\dots,\tau_i)$ are the Volterra kernels of the system, which are symmetric functions of their arguments; for causal systems $h_i(\tau_1,\dots\tau_i) = 0$ for any $\tau_i < 0$.

The output of a second-order Volterra system when the input is zero-mean stationary is

$$y(k) = h_0 + \sum_{\tau_1} h_1(\tau_1)x(k - \tau_1) + \sum_{\tau_1}\sum_{\tau_2} h_2(\tau_1,\tau_2)x(k - \tau_1)x(k - \tau_2) \tag{6.35}$$

Equation 6.35 can be viewed as a parallel connection of a linear system $h_1(\tau_1)$ and a quadratic system $h_2(\tau_1,\tau_2)$ as illustrated in Figure 6.1. Let

$$c_2^{xy}(\tau) = E\{x(k + \tau)[y(k) - m_1^y]\} \tag{6.36}$$

be the cross-covariance of input and output, and

$$c_2^{xxy}(\tau_1,\tau_2) = E\{x(k + \tau_1)x(k + \tau_2)[y(k) - m_1^y]\} \tag{6.37}$$

be the third-order cross-cumulant sequence of input and output.

The system's linear part can be obtained by [32]

$$H_1(-\omega) = \frac{C_2^{xy}(\omega)}{C_2^x(\omega)} \tag{6.38}$$

and the quadratic part by

$$H_2(-\omega_1, -\omega_2) = \frac{C_3^{xxy}(\omega_1,\omega_2)}{2C_2^x(\omega_1)C_2^x(\omega_2)} \tag{6.39}$$

where $C_2^{xy}(\omega)$ and $C_3^{xxy}(\omega_1,\omega_2)$ are the Fourier transforms of $c_2^{xy}(t)$ and $c_2^{xxy}(\tau_1,\tau_2)$, respectively. It should be noted that the above equations are valid only for Gaussian input signals. More general results assuming non-Gaussian input have been obtained in References 33 and 34. Additional results on particular nonlinear systems have been reported in References 35 and 36.

An interesting phenomenon, caused by a second-order nonlinearity, is the quadratic-phase coupling. There are situations where nonlinear interaction between two harmonic components of a process contribute to the power of the sum and/or difference frequencies. The signal

$$x(k) = A\cos(\lambda_1 k + \theta_1) + B\cos(\lambda_2 k + \theta_2) \tag{6.40}$$

after passing through the quadratic system:

$$z(k) = x(k) + ex^2(k), \quad \epsilon \neq 0 \tag{6.41}$$

contains cosinusoidal terms in $(\lambda_1, \theta_1), (\lambda_2, \theta_2), (2\lambda_1, 2\theta_1), (2\lambda_2, 2\theta_2), (\lambda_1 + \lambda_2, \theta_1 + \theta_2), (\lambda_1 - \lambda_2, \theta_1 - \theta_2)$. Such a phenomenon that results in phase relations that are the same as the frequency relations is called quadratic phase coupling [37]. Quadratic phase coupling can arise only among harmonically related components. Three frequencies are harmonically related when one of them is the sum or difference of the other two. Sometimes it is important to find out if peaks at harmonically related positions in the power spectrum are in fact phase coupled. Due to phase suppression, the power spectrum is unable to provide an answer to this problem. As an example, consider the process [38]

$$x(k) = \sum_{i=1}^{6} \cos(\lambda_i k + \phi_i) \tag{6.42}$$

where $\lambda_1 > \lambda_2 > 0, \lambda_4 + \lambda_5 > 0, \lambda_3 = \lambda_1 + \lambda_2, \lambda_6 = \lambda_4 + \lambda_5, \phi_1, \ldots, \phi_5$ are all independent, uniformly distributed random variables over $(0, 2\pi)$, and $\phi_6 = \phi_4 + \phi_5$. Among the six frequencies $(\lambda_1, \lambda_2, \lambda_3)$ and $(\lambda_4, \lambda_5, \lambda_6)$ are harmonically related, however, only λ_6 is the result of phase coupling between λ_4 and λ_5. The power spectrum of this process consists of six impulses at $\lambda_i, i, \ldots, 6$ (Figure 6.2), offering no indication whether each frequency component is independent or a result of frequency coupling. On the other hand, the bispectrum of $x(k)$ (evaluated in its principal region) is zero everywhere, except at point

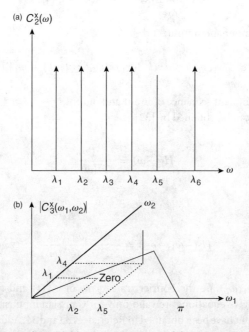

FIGURE 6.2 Quadratic phase coupling. (a) The power spectrum of the process described in Equation 6.42 cannot determine what frequencies are coupled. (b) The corresponding magnitude bispectrum is zero everywhere in the principle region, except at points corresponding to phase coupled frequencies.

(λ_4, λ_5) of the (ω_1, ω_2) plane, where it exhibits an impulse (Figure 6.2b). The peak indicates that only λ_4, λ_5 are phase coupled.

The biocoherence index, defined as

$$P_3^x(\omega_1, \omega_2) = \frac{C_3^x(\omega_1, \omega_2)}{\sqrt{C_2^x(\omega_1) C_2^x(\omega_2) C_2^x(\omega_1 + \omega_2)}} \tag{6.43}$$

has been extensively used in practical situations for the detection and quantification of quadratic phase coupling [37]. The value of the bicoherence index at each frequency pair indicates the degree of coupling among the frequencies of that pair. Almost all bispectral estimators can be used in Equation 6.43. However, estimates obtained based on parametric modeling of the bispectrum have been shown to yield resolution superior [38,39] to the ones obtained with conventional methods.

6.6 HOS in Biomedical Signal Processing

The applications of HOS on biomedical signals are clustered according to the HOS property they most rely on, that is, (1) the ability to describe non-Gaussian processes and preserve phase, (2) the Gaussian noise immunity, and (3) the ability to characterize nonlinearities.

In the first class are the works of References 40 to 42, where ultrasound imaging distortions are estimated from the ultrasound echo and subsequently compensated for, to improve the diagnostic quality of the image. HOS have been used in modeling the ultrasound radio-frequency (RF) echo [46], where schemes for estimation of resolvable periodicity as well as correlations among nonresolvable scatters have been proposed. The "tissue color," a quantity that describes the scatterer spatial correlations, and which can be obtained from the HOS of the RF echo, has been proposed [43] as a tissue characterization feature. The skewness and kurtosis of mammogram images have been proposed in Reference 44 as a tool for detecting microcalcifications in mammograms.

In the second class are methods that process multicomponent biomedical signals, treating one component as the signal of interest and the rest as noise. HOS have been used in Reference 45 to process lung sounds in order to suppress sound originating from the heart, and in Reference 46 to detect human afferent nerve signals, which are usually observed in very poor signal-to-noise ratio conditions.

Most of the HOS applications in the biomedical area belong to the third class, and usually investigate the formation and the nature of frequencies present in signals through the presence of quadratic phase coupling (QPC). The bispectrum has been applied in EEG signals of the rat during various vigilance states [47], where QPC between specific frequencies was observed. QPC changes in auditory evoked potentials of healthy subjects and subjects with Alzheimer's dementia has been reported [48]. Visual evoked potentials have been analyzed via the bispectrum in References 49 to 51. Bispectral analysis of interactions between electrocerebral activity resulting from stimulation of the left and right visual fields revealed nonlinear interactions between visual fields [52]. The bispectrum has been used in the analysis of electromyogram recruitment [53], and in defining the pattern of summation of muscle fiber twitches in the surface mechanomyogram generation [54]. QPC was also observed in the EEG of humans [55,56].

In the sequel, presented in some detail are the application of HOS on improving the resolution of ultrasound images, a topic that has recently attracted a lot of attention.

Ultrasonic imaging is a valuable tool in the diagnosis of tumors of soft tissues. Some of the distinctive features of ultrasound are its safe, nonionizing acoustic radiation, and its wide availability as a low cost, portable equipment. The major drawback that limits the use of ultrasound images in certain cases (e.g., breast imaging) is poor resolution. In B-Scan images, the resolution is compromised due to: (1) the finite bandwidth of the ultrasonic transducer, (2) the non-negligible beam width, and (3) phase aberrations and velocity variations arising from acoustic inhomogeneity of tissues themselves. The observed ultrasound image can be considered as a distorted version of the true tissue information. Along the axial direction the distortion is dominated by the pulse-echo wavelet of the imaging system, while along the lateral direction the distortion is mainly due to finite-width lateral beam profile. Provided that these distortions are known in advance, or non-invasively measurable, their effects can be compensated for in the observed image. With propagation in tissue, however, both axial and lateral distortions change due to the inhomogeneities of the media and the geometry of the imaging system. They also change among different tissue types and individuals. Distortions measure in a simplified setting, for example, in a water tank, are rarely applicable to clinical images, due to the effects of tissue-dependent components. Therefore, distortions must be estimated based on the backscattered RF data that lead to the B-mode image.

Assuming a narrow ultrasound beam, linear propagation and weak scattering, the ultrasonic RF echo, $y_i(n)$, corresponding to the ith axial line in the B-mode image is modeled as [40]:

$$y_i(n) = h_i(n) * f_i(n) + w_i(n), \quad i = 1, 2, \ldots \tag{6.44}$$

where n is the discrete time; $w_i(n)$ is observation noise; $f_i(n)$ represents the underlying tissue structure and is referred to as tissue response; and $h_i(n)$ represents the axial distortion kernel. Let us assume that: (A1) $y_i(n)$ is non-Gaussian; (A2) $f_i(n)$ is white, non-Gaussian random process; (A3) $w_i(n)$ is Gaussian noise uncorrelated with $f_i(n)$; and (A4) $y_i(n)$ is a short enough segment, so that the attenuation effects stay constant over its duration. (Long segments of data can be analyzed by breaking them into a sequence of short segments.) A similar model can be assumed to hold in the lateral direction of the RF image.

Even though the distortion kernels were known to be non-minimum phase [57], their estimation was mostly carried out using second-order statistics (SOS), such as autocorrelation or power spectrum, thereby neglecting Fourier phase information. Phase is important in preserving edges and boundaries in images. It is particularly important in medical ultrasound images where the nature of edges of a tumor provide important diagnostic information about the malignancy. Complex cepstrum-based operations that take phase information into account have been used [42] to estimate distortions. HOS retain phase and in addition, are not as sensitive to singularities as the cepstrum. HOS were used [40] for the first time to estimate imaging distortions from B-scan images. It was demonstrated that the HOS-based distortion estimation and subsequent image deconvolution significantly improved resolution. For the case of breast data, in was demonstrated [41] that deconvolution via SOS-based distortion estimates was not as good as its HOS counterpart.

In the following we present some results of distortion estimation followed by deconvolution of clinical B-scan images of human breast data. The data were obtained using a flat linear array transducer with a nominal center frequency of 7.5 MHz on a clinical imaging system UltraMark-9 Advanced Technology Laboratories. Data were sampled at a rate of 20 MHz. Figure 6.3a shows parts of the original image, where the the logarithm of the envelope has been used for display purposes. Axial and lateral distortion kernels were estimated from the RF data via the HOS-based non-parametric method outlined in Section 6.4 of this chapter [21], and also via an SOS power cepstrum based method [41]. Each kernel estimate was obtained from a rectangular block of RF data described by (x, y, N_x, N_y), where (x, y) are the co-ordinates of the upper left corner of the block, N_x is its lateral width, and N_y is the axial height. Note that y corresponds to the depth of the upper left corner of the image block from the surface of the transducer. In the following, all dimensions are specified in sample numbers. The size of the images used was 192×1024. Assuming that within the same block the axial distortion kernel does not significantly depend on the lateral location of the RF data, all axial RF data in the block can be concatenated to form a longer one-dimensional vector. In both HOS and SOS based axial kernel estimations, it was assumed that $N_x = 10, N_y = 128, N = 128$. Note that the $N_y = 128$ samples correspond to 5 mm in actual tissue space, as is reasonable to assume that attenuation over such a small distance may be assumed constant. Fifty kernels were estimated from the blocks $(x, 400, 10, 128)$, the x taking values in the range $1, \ldots, 50$. Lateral kernels were estimated from the same images with parameters $N_x = 192, N_y = 10$, and $N = 64$. All the kernels were estimated from the blocks $(1, y, 192, 10)$, the y taking values in the range $400, \ldots, 600$ increasing each time by 5. Data from all adjacent lateral image lines in the block were concatenated to

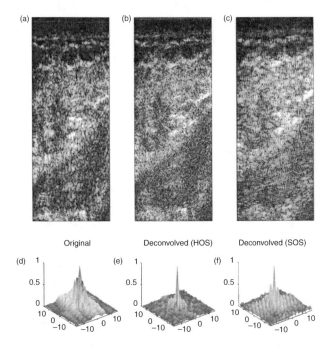

FIGURE 6.3   (a) Original image, (b) HOS-based deconvolution, (c) SOS-based deconvolution. In all cases the logarithm of the envelope is displayed. Autocovariance plots for (d) original, (e) HOS deconvolved, and (f) SOS deconvolved RF data.

make a long one-dimensional vector. Note that $N_y = 10$ corresponds to a very small depth, 0.4 mm in the real tissue space, hence he underlying assumption that the lateral distortion kernel does not vary much over this depth, should be reasonable.

Figure 6.3b,c show that the result of lateral followed by axial deconvolution of the image of Figure 6.3a, using respectively HOS- and SOS-based distortion kernel estimates. The deconvolution was performed via the constrained Wiener Filter technique [58]. According to Figure 6.3, the deconvolution in the RF-domain resulted in a significant reduction in speckle size. The speckle size appears smaller in the HOS-deconvolved image than in SOS-deconvolved ones, which is evidence of higher resolution. The resolution improvement can be quantified based on the width of the main lobe of the autocovariance of the image. The axial resolution gain for the HOS-based approach was 1.8 times that of the SOS-based approach. The lateral resolution gain for the HOS-based approach was 1.73 times as much. From a radiologist's point of view, overall, the HOS image appears to have better spatial resolution than the original as well as the SOS deconvolved images. Conversely, the SOS image seems to have incurred a loss of both axial and lateral resolution.

Acknowledgments

Parts of this chapter have been based on the book: Nikias, C.L. and Petropulu, A.P., Higher Order Spectra Analysis: A Nonlinear Signal Processing Framework, Prentice Hall, Englewood Cliffs, NJ, 1993.

Major support for this work came from the National Science Foundation under grant MIP-9553227, the Whitaker Foundation, the National Institute of Health under grant 2P01CA52823-07A1, Drexel University and the Laboratoire des Signaux et Systems, CNRS, Universite Paris Sud, Ecole Superieure d'Electric, France.

The author would like to thank Drs. F. Forsberg and E. Conant for providing the ultrasound image and for evaluating the processed image.

References

[1] Marple, Jr., S.L. *Digital Spectral Analysis with Applications*, Prentice-Hall, Inc., Englewood Cliffs, NJ, 1987.

[2] Kay, S.M. *Modern Spectral Estimation*, Prentice-Hall, Inc., Englewood Cliffs, NJ, 1988.

[3] Haykin, S. *Nonlinear Methods of Spectral Analysis*, 2nd ed., Springer-Verlag, Berlin, Germany, 1983.

[4] Nikias, C.L. and Petropulu, A.P. *Higher-Order Spectra Analysis: A Nonlinear Signal Processing Framework*, Prentice Hall Inc., Englewood Cliffs, NJ, 1993.

[5] Schetzen, M. *The Volterra and Wiener Theories on Nonlinear Systems*, updated edition, Krieger Publishing Company, Malabar, FL, 1989.

[6] Mendel, J.M. "Tutorial on Higher-Order Statistics (Spectra) in Signal Processing and System Theory: Theoretical Results and Some Applications," *IEEE Proc.*, 79: 278–305, 1991.

[7] Papoulis, A. *Probability Random Variables and Stochastic Processes*, McGraw-Hill, New York, 1984.

[8] Nikias, C.L. and Raghuveer, M.R. "Bispectrum Estimation: A Digital Signal Processing Framework," *Proc. IEEE*, 75: 869–891, 1987.

[9] Subba Rao, T. and Gabr, M.M. "An Introduction to Bispectral Analysis and Bilinear Time Series Models," *Lecture Notes in Statistics*, 24, New York: Springer-Verlag, 1984.

[10] Brillinger, D.R. and Rosenblatt, M. "Computation and Interpretation of kth-order Spectra," In: *Spectral Analysis of Time Series*, B Harris, Ed., John Wiley & Sons, New York, NY, pp. 189–232, 1967.

[11] Matsuoka, T. and Ulrych, T.J. "Phase Estimation Using Bispectrum," *Proc. IEEE*, 72: 1403–1411, October, 1984.

[12] Petropulu, A.P. and Abeyratne, U.R. "System Reconstruction from Higher-Order Spectra Slices," *IEEE Trans. Sig. Proc.*, 45: 2241–2251, 1997.

[13] Petropulu, A.P. and Pozidiz, H. "Phase Estimation from Bispectrum Slices," *IEEE Trans. Sig., Proc.*, 46: 527–531, 1998.

[14] Bartlet, H., Lohmann, A.W., and Wirnitzer, B. "Phase and Amplitude Recovery from Bispectra," *Applied Optics*, 23: 3121–3129, 1984.

[15] Petropulu, A.P. and Nikias, C.L. "Signal Reconstruction from the Phase of the Bispectrum," *IEEE Trans. Acoust., Speech, Signal Processing*, 40: 601–610, 1992.

[16] Rangoussi, M. and Giannakis, G.B. "FIR Modeling Using Log-Bispectra: Weighted Least-Squares Algorithms and Performance Analysis," *IEEE Trans. Circuits and Systems*, 38: 281–296, 1991.

[17] Pan, R. and Nikias, C.L. "The Complex Cepstrum of Higher-Order Cumulants and Nonminimum Phase System Identification," *IEEE Trans. Acoust., Speech, Signal Process.*, 36: 186–205, 1988.

[18] Le Roux, J. and Sole, P. "Least-Squared Error Reconstruction of a Deterministic Sampled Signal Fourier Transform Logarithm from its Nth Order Polyspectrum Logarithm," *Signal Process.*, 35: 75–81, 1994.

[19] Lii, K.S. and Rosenblatt, M. "Deconvolution and Estimation of Transfer Function Phase and Coefficients for Nongaussian Linear Processes," *Ann. Stat.*, 10: 1195–1208, 1982.

[20] Dianat, S.A. and Raghuveer, M.R. "Fast Algorithms for Phase and Magnitude Reconstruction from Bispectra," *Optical Engineering*, 29: 504–512, 1990.

[21] Pozidis, H. and Petropulu, A.P. "System Reconstruction from Selected Regions of the Discretized Higher-Order Spectrum," *IEEE Trans. Sig. Proc.*, 46: 3360–3377, 1998.

[22] Andre, T.F., Nowak, R.D., and Van Veen, B.D. "Low Rank Estimation of Higher Order Statistics," *IEEE Trans. Sig. Proc.*, 45: 673–685, March 1997.

[23] Bradaric, I. and Petropulu, A.P. "Low Rank Approach in System Identification Using Higher Order Statistics," *9th IEEE Sig. Processing Workshop on Statistical Signal and Array Processing — SSAP'98*, Portland, Oregon, September 1998.

[24] Bradaric, I. and Petropulu, A.P. "Subspace Design of Low Rank Estimators for Higher Order Statistics," *IEEE Trans. Sig. Proc.*, submitted in 1999.

[25] Giannakis, G.B. and Mendel, J.M. "Cumulant-Based Order Determination of Non-Gaussian ARMA Models," *IEEE Trans. Acous., Speech, and Sig. Proc.*, 38: 1411–1423, 1990.

[26] Giannakis, G.B. "Cumulants: A Powerful Tool in Signal Processing," *Proc. IEEE*, 75, 1987.

[27] Alshbelli, S.A., Venetsanopoulos, A.N., and Cetin, A.E. "Cumulant Based Identification Approaches for Nonminimum Phase Systems," *IEEE Trans. Sig. Proc.*, 41: 1576–1588, 1993.

[28] Fonollosa, J.A.R. and Vidal, J. "System Identification Using a Linear Combination of Cumulant Slices," *IEEE Trans. Sig. Process.*, 41: 2405–2411, 1993.

[29] Petropulu, A.P. "Noncausal Nonminimum Phase ARMA Modeling of Non-Gaussian Processes," *IEEE Trans. Sig. Process.*, 43: 1946–1954, 1995.

[30] Tugnait, J. "Fitting Non-Causal AR Signal Plus Noise Models to Noisy Non-Gaussian Linear Processes," *IEEE Trans. Automat. Control*, 32: 547–552, 1987.

[31] Tugnait, J. "Identification of Linear Stochastic Systems via Second- and Fourth-Order Cumulant Matching," *IEEE Trans. Inform. Theory*, 33: 393–407, 1987.

[32] Tick, L.J. "The Estimation of Transfer Functions of Quadratic Systems," *Technometrics*, 3: 562–567, 1961.

[33] Hinich, M.J. "Identification of the Coefficients in a Nonlinear Time Series of the Quadratic Type," *J. Econom.*, 30: 269–288, 1985.

[34] Powers, E.J., Ritz, C.K., et al. "Applications of Digital Polyspectral Analysis to Nonlinear Systems Modeling and Nonlinear Wave Phenomena," *Workshop on Higher-Order Spectral Analysis*, pp. 73–77, Vail, CO, 1989.

[35] Brillinger, D.R. "The Identification of a Particular Nonlinear Time Series System," *Biometrika*, 64: 509–515, 1977.

[36] Rozzario, N. and Papoulis, A. "The Identification of Certain Nonlinear Systems by Only Observing the Output," *Workshop on Higher-Order Spectral Analysis*, pp. 73–77, Vail, CO, 1989.

[37] Kim, Y.C. and Powers, E.J. "Digital Bispectral Analysis of Self-Excited Fluctuation Spectra," *Phys. Fluids*, 21: 1452–1453, 1978.

[38] Raghuveer, M.R. and Nikias, C.L. "Bispectrum Estimation: A Parametric Approach," *IEEE Trans. Acous., Speech, and Sig. Proc.*, ASSP, 33: 1213–1230, 1985.

[39] Raghuveer, M.R. and Nikias, C.L. "Bispectrum Estimation via AR Modeling," *Sig. Proc.*, 10: 35–45, 1986.

[40] Abeyratne, U., Petropulu, A.P., and Reid, J.M. "Higher-Order Spectra Based Deconvolution of Ultrasound Images," *IEEE Trans. Ultrason. Ferroelec., Freq. Con.*, 42: 1064–1075, 1995.

[41] Abeyratne, U.R., Petropulu, A.P., Golas, T., Reid, J.M., Forsberg, F., and Consant, E. "Blind Deconvolution of Ultrasound Breast Images: A Comparative Study of Autocorrelation Based Versus Higher-Order Statistics Based Methods," *IEEE Trans. Ultrason. Ferroelec., Freq. Con.*, 44: 1409–1416, 1997.

[42] Taxt, T. "Comparison of Cepstrum-Based Methods for Radial Blind Deconvolution of Ultrasound Images," *IEEE Trans. Ultrason., Ferroelec., and Freq. Con.*, 44, 1997.

[43] Abeyratne, U.R., Petropulu, A.P., and Reid, J.M. "On Modeling the Tissue Response from Ultrasound Images," *IEEE Trans. Med. Imag.*, 14: 479–490, 1996.

[44] Gurcan, M.N., Yardimci, Y., Cetin, A.E., and Ansari, R. "Detection of Microcalcifications in Mammograms Using Higher-Order Statistics," *IEEE Sig. Proc. Lett.*, 4, 1997.

[45] Hadjileontiadis, L. and Panas, S.M. "Adaptive Reduction of Heart Sounds from Lung Sounds Using Fourth-Order Statistics," *IEEE Trans. Biomed. Eng.*, 44, 1997.

[46] Upshaw, B. "SVD and Higher-Order Statistical Processing of Human Nerve Signals," *Proc. International Conference of the IEEE Engineering in Medicine and Biology*, 1996.

[47] Ning, T. and Bronzino, J.D. "Bispectral Analysis of the EEG During Various Vigilance States," *IEEE Trans. Biomed. Eng.*, 36: 497–499, 1989.

[48] Samar, V.J., Swartz, K.P., et al. "Quadratic Phase Coupling in Auditory Evoked Potentials from Healthy Old Subjects and Subjects with Alzheimer's Dementia," *IEEE Signal Processing Workshop on Higher-Order Statistics*, pp. 361–365, Tahoe, CA, 1993.

[49] Tang, Y. and Norcia, A.M. "Coherent Bispectral Analysis of the Steady-State VEP," *Proc. International Conference of the IEEE Engineering in Medicine and Biology*, 1995.

[50] Husar, P. and Henning, G. "Bispectrum Analysis of Visually Evoked Potentials," *IEEE Eng. Med. Biol.*, 16, 1997.

[51] Henning, G. and Husar, P. "Statistical Detection of Visually Evoked Potentials," *IEEE Eng. Med. Biol.*, 14: 386–390, 1995.

[52] "Bispectral Analysis of Visual Field Interactions," *Proc. International Conference of the IEEE Engineering in Medicine and Biology*, vol. 3, Amsterdam, Netherlands, 1996.

[53] Yana, K., Mizuta, H., and Kajiyama, R. "Surface Electromyogram Recruitment Analysis Using Higher-Order Spectrum," *Proc. International Conference of the IEEE Engineering in Medicine and Biology*, 1995.

[54] Orizio, C., Liberati, D., Locatelli, C., De Grandis, D., Veicsteinas, A., "Surface Mechanomyogram Reflects Muscle Fibres Twitches Summation," *J. Biomech.*, 29, 1996.

[55] Barnett, T.P., Johnson, L.C., et al., "Bispectrum Analysis of Electroencephalogram Signals During Waking and Sleeping," *Science*, 172: 401–402, 1971.

[56] Husar, P.J., Leiner, B., et al., "Statistical Methods for Investigating Phase Relations in Stochastic Processes," *IEEE Trans. Audio and Electroacoust.*, 19: 78–86, 1971.

[57] Jensen, J.A. and Leeman, S. "Nonparametric Estimation of Ultrasound Pulses," *IEEE Trans. Biomed. Eng.*, 41: 929–936, 1994.

[58] Treitel, S. and Lines, L.R. "Linear Inverse Theory and Deconvolution," *Geophysics*, 47: 1153–1159, 1982.

[59] Cohen, F.N. "Modeling of Ultrasound Speckle with Applications in Flaw Detection in Metals," *IEEE Trans. Sig. Proc.*, 40: 624–632, 1992.

[60] Giannakis, G.B. and Swami, A. "On Estimating Noncausal Nonminimum Phase ARMA Models of Non-Gaussian Processes," *IEEE Tran. Acous., Speech, Sig. Process.*, 38: 478–495, 1990.

[61] Jensen, J.A. "Deconvolution of Ultrasound Images," *Ultrasonic Imaging*, 14: 1–15, 1992.

[62] Le Roux, J, Coroyer, C., and Rossille, D. "Illustration of the Effects of Sampling on Higher-Order Spectra," *Sig. Process.*, 36: 375–390, 1994.

[63] Ning, T. and Bronzino, J.D. "Autogressive and Bispectral Analysis Techniques: EEG Applications," *IEEE Engineering in Medicine and Biology*, March 1990.

[64] Oppenheim, A.V. and Schafer, R.W. *Discrete-Time Signal Processing*, Prentice-Hall, Englewood Cliffs, NJ, 1989.

[65] Petropulu, A.P. "Higher-Order Spectra in Signal Processing," *Signal Processing Handbook*, CRC Press, Boca Raton, FL, 1998.

[66] Swami, A. and Mendel, J.M. "ARMA Parameter Estimation Using Only Output Cumulants," *IEEE Trans. Acoust., Speech and Sig. Process.*, 38: 1257–1265, 1990.

7

Neural Networks in Biomedical Signal Processing

7.1 Neural Networks in Sensory Waveform Analysis 7-2
     Multineuronal Activity Analysis • Visual Evoked Potentials
7.2 Neural Networks in Speech Recognition 7-5
7.3 Neural Networks in Cardiology 7-7
7.4 Neural Networks in Neurology 7-11
7.5 Discussion 7-11
References 7-11

Evangelia
Micheli-Tzanakou
Rutgers University

Computing with neural networks (NNs) is one of the faster growing fields in the history of artificial intelligence (AI), largely because NNs can be trained to identify nonlinear patterns between input and output values and can solve complex problems much faster than digital computers. Owing to their wide range of applicability and their ability to learn complex and nonlinear relationships — including noisy or less precise information — NNs are very well suited to solving problems in biomedical engineering and, in particular, in analyzing biomedical signals.

Neural networks have made strong advances in continuous speech recognition and synthesis, pattern recognition, classification of noisy data, nonlinear feature detection, and other fields. By their nature, NNs are capable of high-speed parallel signal processing in real time. They have an advantage over conventional technologies because they can solve problems that are too complex — problems that do not have an algorithmic solution or for which an algorithmic solution is too complex to be found. NNs are trained by example instead of rules and are automated. When used in medical diagnosis, they are not affected by factors such as human fatigue, emotional states, and habituation. They are capable of rapid identification, analysis of conditions, and diagnosis in real time.

The most widely used architecture of an NN is that of a multilayer perceptron (MLP) trained by an algorithm called backpropagation (BP). Backpropagation is a gradient-descent algorithm that tries to minimize the average squared error of the network. In real applications, the network is not a simple one-dimensional system, and the error curve is not a smooth, bowl-shaped curve. Instead, it is a highly complex, multidimensional curve with hills and valleys (for a mathematical description of the algorithm).

BP was first developed by Werbos in 1974 [1], rediscovered by Parker in 1982 [2], and popularized later by Rummelhart et al. in 1986 [3]. There exist many variations of this algorithm, especially trying to improve its speed and performance in avoiding getting stuck into local minima — one of its main drawbacks.

In my work, I use the ALOPEX algorithm developed by my colleagues and myself (see Chapter 182) [4–10], and my colleagues and I have applied it in a variety of world problems of considerable complexity. This chapter will examine several applications of NNs in biomedical signal processing. One- and two-dimensional signals are examined.

7.1 Neural Networks in Sensory Waveform Analysis

Mathematical analysis of the equations describing the processes in NNs can establish any dependencies between quantitative network characteristics, the information capacity of the network, and the probabilities of recognition and retention of information. It has been proposed that electromyographic (EMG) patterns can be analyzed and classified by NNs [11] where the standard BP algorithm is used for decomposing surface EMG signals into their constituent action potentials (APs) and their firing patterns [12]. A system such as this may help a physician in diagnosing time-behavior changes in the EMG.

The need for a knowledge-based system using NNs for evoked potential recognition was described by Bruha and Madhavan [13]. In this chapter, the authors used syntax pattern-recognition algorithms as a first step, while a second step included a two-layer perceptron to process the list of numerical features produced by the first step.

Myoelectric signals (MES) also have been analyzed by NNs [14]. A discrete Hopfield network was used to calculate the time-series parameters for a moving-average MES. It was demonstrated that this network was capable of producing the same time-series parameters as those produced by a conventional sequential least-squares algorithm. In the same paper, a second implementation of a two-layered perceptron was used for comparison. The features used were a time-series parameter and the signal power in order to train the perceptron on four separate arm functions, and again, the network performed well.

Moving averages have been simulated for nonlinear processes by the use of NNs [15]. The results obtained were comparable with those of linear adaptive techniques.

Moody et al. [16] used an adaptive approach in analyzing visual evoked potentials. This method is based on spectral analysis that results in spectral peaks of uniform width in the frequency domain. Tunable data windows were used. Specifically, the modified Bessel functions $I_o - \sin h$, the gaussian, and the cosine-taper windows are compared. The modified Bessel function window proved to be superior in classifying normal and abnormal populations.

Pulse-transmission NNs — networks that consist of neurons that communicates with other neurons via pulses rather than numbers — also have been modeled [7,17]. This kind of network is much more realistic, since, in biological systems, action potentials are the means of neuronal communication. Dayhoff [18] has developed a pulse-transmission network that can temporally integrate arriving signals and also display some resistance to temporal noise.

Another method is optimal filtering, which is a variation of the traditional matched filter in noise [19]. This has the advantage of separating even overlapping waveforms. It also carries the disadvantage that the needed knowledge of the noise power spectral density and the Fourier transform of the spikes might not be always available.

Principal-components analysis also has been used. Here the incoming spike waveforms are represented by templates given by eigenvectors from their average autocorrelation functions [20]. The authors found that two or three eigenvectors are enough to account for 90% of the total energy of the signal. This way each spike can be represented by the coordinates of its projection onto the eigenvector space. These coordinates are the only information needed for spike classification, which is further done by clustering techniques.

7.1.1 Multineuronal Activity Analysis

When dealing with single- or multineuron activities, the practice is to determine how many neurons (or units) are involved in the "spike train" evoked by some sensory stimulation. Each spike in a spike train represents an action potential elicited by a neuron in close proximity to the recording electrode. These action potentials have different amplitudes, latencies, and shape configurations and, when superimposed on each other, create a complex waveform — a composite spike. The dilemma that many scientists face is how to decompose these composite potentials into their constituents and how to assess the question of how many neurons their electrode is recording from. One of the most widely used methods is window discrimination, in which different thresholds are set, above which the activity of any given neuron is assigned, according to amplitude. Peak detection techniques also have been used [21]. These methods perform well if the number of neurons is very small and the spikes are well separated. Statistical methods of different complexity also have been used [22–24] involving the time intervals between spikes. Each spike is assigned a unique instant of time so that a spike train can be described by a process of time points corresponding to the times where the action potential had occurred. Processes such as these are called point processes, since they are characterized by only one number. Given this, a spike train can be treated as a stochastic point process that may or may not be stationary. In the former case, its statistics do not vary in the time of observation [25]. In the second case, when nonstationarity is assumed, any kind of statistical analysis becomes formidable.

Correlations between spike trains of neurons can be found because of many factors, but mostly because of excitatory or inhibitory interactions between them or due to a common input to both. Simulations on each possibility have been conducted in the past [26]. In our research, when recording from the optic tectum of the frog, the problem is the reversed situation of the one given above. That is, we have the recorded signal with noise superimposed, and we have to decompose it to its constituents so that we can make inferences on the neuronal circuitry involved. What one might do would be to set the minimal requirements on a neural network, which could behave the same way as the vast number of neurons that could have resulted in a neural spike train similar to the one recorded.

This is a very difficult problem to attack with no unique solution. A method that has attracted attention is the one developed by Gerstein et al. [22,27]. This technique detects various functional groups in the recorded data by the use of the so-called gravitational clustering method. Although promising, the analysis becomes cumbersome due to the many possible subgroups of neurons firing in synchrony. Temporal patterns of neuronal activity also have been studied with great interest. Some computational methods have been developed for the detection of favored temporal patterns [28–31]. My group also has been involved in the analysis of complex waveforms by the development of a novel method, the ST-scan method [32]. This method is based on well-known tomographic techniques, statistical analysis, and template matching. The method proved to be very sensitive to even small variations of the waveforms due to the fact that many orientations of them are considered, as it is done in tomographic imaging. Each histogram represents the number of times a stroke vector at a specific orientation is cutting the composite waveform positioned at the center of the window. These histograms were then fed to a NN for categorization. The histograms are statistical representations of individual action potentials. The NN therefore must be able to learn to recognize histograms by categorizing them with the action potential waveform that they represent. The NN also must be able to recognize any histogram as belonging to one of the "learned" patterns or not belonging to any of them [33]. In analyzing the ST-histograms, the NN must act as an "adaptive demultiplexer." That is, given a set of inputs, the network must determine the correspondingly correct output. This is a categorization procedure performed by a perceptron, originally described by Rosenblatt [34]. In analyzing the ST-histograms, the preprocessing is done by a perceptron, and the error is found either by an LMS algorithm [35] or by an ALOPEX algorithm [36–38].

7.1.2 Visual Evoked Potentials

Visual evoked potentials (VEPs) have been used in the clinical environment as a diagnostic tool for many decades. Stochastic analysis of experimental recordings of VEPs may yield useful information that is not well understood in its original form. Such information may provide a good diagnostic criterion in differentiating normal subjects from subjects with neurological diseases as well as provide an index of the progress of diseases.

These potentials are embedded in noise. Averaging is then used in order to improve the signal-to-noise (S/N) ratio. When analyzing these potentials, several methods have been used, such as spectral analysis of their properties [39], adaptive filtering techniques [40,41], and some signal enhancers, again based on adaptive processes [42]. In this latter method, no a priori knowledge of the signal is needed. The adaptive signal enhancer consists of a bank of adaptive filters, the output of which is shown to be a minimum mean-square error estimate of the signal.

If we assume that the VEP represents a composite of many action potentials and that each one of these action potentials propagates to the point of the VEP recording, the only differences between the various action potentials are their amplitudes and time delays. The conformational changes observed in the VEP waveforms of normal individuals and defected subjects can then be attributed to an asynchrony in the arrival of these action potentials at a focal point (integration site) in the visual cortex [36]. One can simulate this process by simulating action potentials and trying to fit them to normal and abnormal VEPs with NNs.

Action potentials were simulated using methods similar to those of Moore and Ramon [43] and Bell and Cook [44]. Briefly, preprocessing of the VEP waveforms is done first by smoothing a five-point filter that performs a weighted averaging over its neighboring points

$$S(n) = [F(n-2) + 2F(n-1) + 3F(n) + 2F(n+1) + F(n+2)]/9 \qquad (7.1)$$

The individual signals v_j are modulated so that at the VEP recording site each v_j has been changed in amplitude $am(j)$ and in phase $ph(j)$. The amplitude change represents the propagation decay, and the phases represent the propagation delays of signals according to the equation

$$v_j(i) = am(j) \cdot AP[i - ph(j)] \qquad (7.2)$$

For a specific choice of $am(j)$ and $ph(j), j = 1, 2, \ldots, N$, the simulated VEP can be found by

$$VEP = b + k \sum_{j=1}^{N} v_j^{\alpha} \qquad (7.3)$$

where k is a scaling factor, b is a d.c. component, and α is a constant [37,38].

The ALOPEX process was used again in order to adjust the parameters (amplitude and phase) so that the cost function reaches a minimum and therefore the calculated waveform coincides with the experimental one.

The modified ALOPEX equation is given by

$$p_i(n) = p_i(n-1) + \gamma \Delta p_i(n) \Delta R(n) + \mu r_i(n) \qquad (7.4)$$

where $p_i(n)$ are the parameters at iteration n, and γ and μ are scaling factors of the deterministic and random components, respectively, which are adjusted so that at the beginning γ is small and μ is large. As the number of iterations increases, γ increases while μ decreases. The cost function R is monitored until convergence has been achieved at least 80% or until a preset number of iterations has been covered.

The results obtained show a good separation between normal and abnormal VEPs. This separation is based on an index λ, which is defined as the ratio of two summations, namely, the summation of amplitudes whose $ph(i)$ is less than 256 msec and the summation of amplitudes whose $ph(i)$ is greater than 256 msec. A large value of l indicates an abnormal VEP, while a small l indicates a normal VEP.

The convergences of the process for a normal and an abnormal VEP are shown in Figure 7.1 and Figure 7.2, respectively, at different iteration numbers. The main assumption here is that in normal individuals, the action potentials all arrive at a focal point in the cortex in resonance, while in abnormal subjects there exists as asynchrony of the arrival times. Maier and colleagues [45] noted the importance of

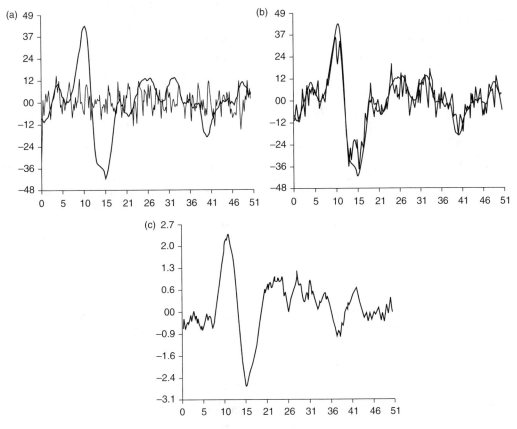

FIGURE 7.1 Normal VEP. (a) The fitting at the beginning of the process, (b) after 500 iterations, and (c) after 1000 iterations. Only one action potential is repeated 1000 times. The x-axis is $\times 10$ msec; the y-axis is in millivolts.

source localization of VEPs in humans in studying the perceptual behavior in humans. The optimization procedure used in this section can help that task, since individual neuronal responses are optimally isolated. One of the interesting points is that signals (action potentials) with different delay times result in composite signals of different forms. Thus the reverse solution of this problem, that is, extracting individual signals from a composite measurement, can help resolve the problem of signal source localization. The multiunit recordings presented in the early sections of this paper fall in the same category with that of decomposing VEPs. This analysis might provide insight as to how neurons communicate.

7.2 Neural Networks in Speech Recognition

Another place where NNs find wide application is in speech recognition. Tebelski et al. [46] have studied the performance of linked predictive NNs (LPNNs) for large-vocabulary, continuous-speech recognition. The authors used a six-state phoneme topology, and without any other optimization, the LPNN achieved an average of 90, 58, and 39% accuracy on tasks with perplexity of 5, 11, and 402, respectively, which is better than the performance of several other simpler NNs tested. These results show that the main advantages of predictive networks are mainly that they produce nonbinary distortion measures in a simple way and that they can model dynamic properties such as those found in speech. Their weakness is that they show poor discrimination, which may be corrected by corrective training and function work modeling.

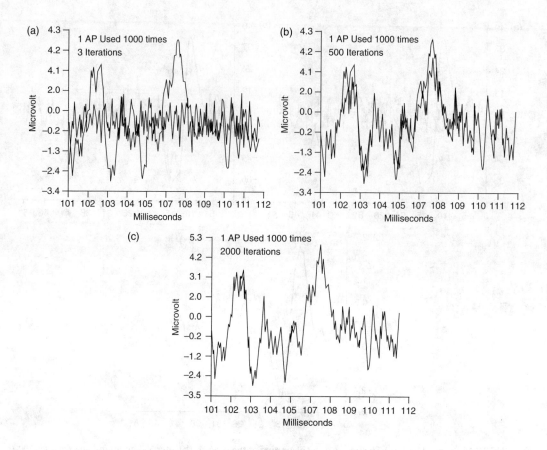

FIGURE 7.2 Abnormal VEP. (a) Fitting at $t = 3$ iterations, (b) after 500 iterations, and (c) after 2000 iterations. One action potential was used 1000 times.

Allen and Kanam [47] designed in NN architecture that locates word boundaries and identifies words from phoneme sequences. They tested the model in three different regimes with a highly redundant corpus and a restricted vocabulary, and the NN was trained with a limited number of phonemic variations for the words in the corpus. These tests yielded a very low error rate. In a second experiment, the network was trained to identify words from expert transcriptions of speech. The error rate for correct simultaneous identification of words and word boundaries was 18%. Finally, they tested the use of the output of a phoneme classifier as the input to the word and word boundary identification network. The error rate increased almost exponentially to 49%.

The best discrimination came from hybrid systems such as the use of an MLP and a hidden Markov model (HMM). These systems incorporate multiple sources of evidence such as features and temporal context without any restrictive assumptions of distributions or statistical independence. Bourland et al. [48] used MLPs as linear predictions for autoregressive HMMs. This approach, although more compatible with the HMM formalism, still suffers from several limitations. Although these authors generalized their approach to take into account time correlations between successive observations without any restrictive assumptions about the driving noise, the reputed results show that many of the tricks used to improve standard HMMs are also valid for this hybrid approach.

In another study, Intrator [49] used an unsupervised NN for dimensionality reduction that seeks directions emphasizing multimodality and derived a new statistical insight to the synaptic modification equations learning as in the Bienenstock, Cooper, and Munro (BCM) neurons [50]. The speech data consisted of 20 consecutive time windows of 32 msec with 30-msec overlap aligned at the beginning of the time. For each window, a set of 22 energy levels was computed corresponding to the Zwicker critical-band filters [51]. The classification results were compared with those of a backpropagation network. These results showed that the backpropagation network does well in finding structures useful for classification of the trained data, but these structures are more sensitive to voicing. Classification results using a BCM network, on the other hand, suggest that for the specified task, structures that are more sensitive to voicing can be extracted, even though voicing imposes several effects on the speech signal. These features are more speaker-invariant.

Phan et al. [52] have attempted to solve the "cocktail party effect," which describes phenomena in which humans can selectively focus attention on one sound source among competing sound sources. This is an ability that is hampered for the hearing-impaired. A system was developed that successfully identifies a speaker in the presence of competing speakers for short utterances. Features used for identification are monaural, whose feature space represent a 90% data reduction from the original data. This system is presently used off-line and also has been applied successfully to intraspeaker speech recognition. The features used in the preprocessing were obtained by wavelet analysis. This multiresolution analysis decomposes a signal into a hierarchical system of subspaces that are one-dimensional and are square integrable. Each subspace is spanned by basis functions that have scaling characteristics of either dilation or compression depending on the resolution. The implementation of these basis functions is incorporated in a recursive pyramidal algorithm in which the discrete approximation of a current resolution is convolved with quadrature mirror filters in the subsequent resolution [53]. After preprocessing, speech waveform is analyzed by the wavelet transform. Analysis is limited to four octaves. For pattern-recognition input configuration, the wavelet coefficients are mapped to a vector and used as inputs to a neural network trained by the ALOPEX algorithm. White noise was superimposed on the features as well in order to establish a threshold of robustness of the algorithm.

7.3 Neural Networks in Cardiology

Two-dimensional echocardiography is an important noninvasive clinical tool for cardiac imaging. The endocardial and epicardial boundaries of the left ventricle (LV) are very useful quantitative measures of various functions of the heart. Cardiac structures detection in ECG images is very important in recognizing the image parts.

A lot of research in the last couple of years has taken place around these issues and the application of neural networks in solving them. Hunter et al. [54] have used NNs in detecting echocardiographic LV boundaries and the center of the LV cavity. The points detected are then linked by a "snake" energy-minimizing function to give the epicardial and endocardial boundaries. A snake is an energy-minimizing deformable curve [55] fined by an internal energy that is the controller of the differential properties in terms of its curvature and its metrics. The most robust results were obtained by a 9×9 square input vector with a resolution reduction of $32 : 1$. Energy minimization is carried out by simulated annealing. The minimum energy solution was obtained after 1000 iterations over the entire snake. The use of NNs as edge detectors allows the classification of points to be done by their probability of being edges rather than by their edge strength, a very important factor for echocardiographic images due to their wide variations in edge strength.

A complex area in electrocardiography is the differentiation of wide QRS tachycardias in ventricular (VT) and supraventricular tachycardia (SVT). A set of criteria for this differentiation has been proposed recently by Brugada et al. [56]. One important aspect of applying NNs in interpreting ECGs is to use parameters that not only make sense but are also meaningful for diagnosis. Dassen et al. [57] developed an induction algorithm that further improved the criteria set by Brugada et al., also using NNs.

Nadal and deBossan [58] used principal-components analysis (PCA) and the relative R-wave to R-wave intervals of P-QRS complexes to evaluate arrhythmias. Arrhythmias are one of the risks of sudden cardiac arrest in coronary care units. In this study, the authors used the first 10 PCA coefficients (PCCs) to reduce the data of each P-QRS complex and a feedforward NN classifier that splits the vector space generated by the PCCs into regions that separate the different classes of beats in an efficient way. They obtained better classification than using other methods, with correct classification of 98.5% for normal beats, 98.5% for ventricular premature beats, and 93.5% for fusion beats, using only the first two PCCs. When four PCCs were used, these classifications improved to 99.2, 99.1, and 94.1%, respectively. These results are better than those obtained by logistic regression when the input space is composed of more than two classes of beats. The difficulties encountered include the elimination of redundant data in order not to overestimate the importance of normal beat detection by the classifier.

In another work, Silipo et al. [59] used an NN as an autoassociator. In previous work they had proved that NNs had better performances than the traditional clustering and statistical methods. They considered beat features derived from both morphologic and prematurity information. Their classification is adequate for ventricular ectopic beats, but the criteria used were not reliable enough to characterize the supraventricular ectopic beat.

A lot of studies also have used NNs for characterization of myocardial infarction (MI). Myocardial infarction is one of the leading causes of death in the United States. The currently available techniques for diagnosis are accurate enough, but they suffer from certain drawbacks, such as accurate quantitative measure of severity, extent, and precise location of the infarction. Since the acoustic properties in the involved region are mostly changing, one can study them by the use of ultrasound.

Baxt [60] used an NN to identify MI in patients presented to an emergency department with anterior chest pain. An NN was trained on clinical pattern sets retrospectively derived from patients hospitalized with a high likelihood of having MI, and the ability of the NN was compared with that of physicians caring for the same patients. The network performed with a sensitivity of 92% and a specificity of 96%. These figures were better than the physicians, with a sensitivity of 88% and a specificity of 71%, or any other computer technology (88% sensitivity, 74% specificity) [61].

Diagnosis of inferior MI with NNs was studied by Hedén et al. [62] with sensitivity of 84% and a specificity of 97%, findings that are similar to those of Pahlm et al. [63].

Yi et al. [64] used intensity changes in an echocardiogram to detect MI. Once an echocardiogram is obtained, it is digitized and saved in a file as a gray-scale image (512 × 400) (Figure 7.3). A window of the region of interest is then selected between the systole and diastole of the cardiac cycle and saved in a different file. The window can be either of a constant size or it can be adaptive (varying) in size. This new file can be enlarged (zoom) for examination of finer details in the image. All image artifacts are filtered out, and contrast enhancement is performed. This new image is then saved and serves as input to the NN. A traditional three-layer NN with 300 input nodes (one node for each pixel intensity in the input file), a varying number of hidden nodes, and two output nodes were used. The output node indicates the status of the patient under testing. A "one" indicates normal and a "zero" an abnormal case.

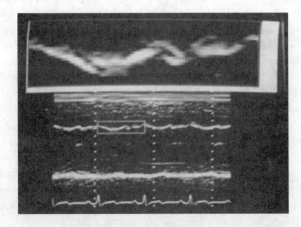

FIGURE 7.3 Selection of region of interest. The intensity pattern in the box is used as input to the NN.

The weights of the connections were calculated using the optimization algorithms of ALOPEX. One sub-ALOPEX was used for the weights between hidden nodes and input nodes, and a second sub-ALOPEX was used for those from the output to the hidden layer.

The network was trained with a population of 256 patients, some with scars and some normal. These patients were used to obtain "templates" for each category. These templates were then used for comparison with the test images. None of these testing images was included in the training set. The cost function used for the process was the least-squares rule, which, although slow, produces reliable results.

A similar process is used for the output layer. The noise was made adaptable. The intensities of the images are normalized before being submitted to the NN. A cutoff of 0.2 was used. Therefore, anything above 0.8 is normal, below 0.2 is scar, and all the in-between values are classified as unknown. Due to the fact that the scar training set was very small compared with the normals, a better classification of normals than scars was observed. A study was also made as to how the number of hidden nodes influences the results for the same standard deviation of noise.

In another study, Kostis et al. [65] used NNs in estimating the prognosis of acute MI. Patients who survive the acute phase of an MI have an increased risk of mortality persisting up to 10 years or more. Estimation of the probability of being alive at a given time in the future is important to the patients and their physicians and is usually ascertained by the use of statistical methods. The purpose of the investigation was to use an NN to estimate future mortality of patients with acute MI. The existence of a large database (Myocardial Infarction Data Acquisition Systems, or MIDAS) that includes MI occurring in the state of New Jersey and has long-term follow-up allows the development and testing of such a computer algorithm. Since the information included in the database does not allow the exact prediction of vital status (dead or alive) in all patients with 100% accuracy, the NN should be able to categorize patients according to the probability of dying within a given period of time.

Since information included in the database is not sufficient to allow the exact prediction of vital status (dead or alive) in all patients with 100% accuracy, we developed an NN able to categorize patients according to the probability of dying within a given period of time rather than predicting categorically whether a patient will be dead or alive at a given time in the future. It was observed that there were many instances where two or more patients had identical input characteristics while some were dead and some alive at the end of the study period. For this reason, it is difficult to train a standard NN. Since there is no unique output value for all input cases, the network had difficulty converging to a unique set of solutions. To alleviate this problem, a conflict-resolution algorithm was developed. The algorithm takes templates with identical input vectors and averages each of their input characteristics to produce a single case. Their output values of vital status are averaged, producing, in effect, a percentage probability of mortality for the particular set of input characteristics. As each new subject template is read into the program, its input characteristics are compared with those of all previous templates. If no match is found, its input values and corresponding output value are accepted. If a match is found, the output value is brought together with the stored output value (percentage probability of mortality and the number of templates on which it is based), and a new output value is calculated, representing the percentage average mortality of the entire characteristic group. Since each member of the group is an identical input case, no input characteristic averaging is necessary, thus preserving the statistical significance of the average mortality with respect to that exact case.

This new algorithm, using the two-hidden-layer perceptron optimized by ALOPEX, has converged to greater than 98% using several thousand input cases. In addition, 10 output nodes were used in the final layer, each corresponding to a range of percent chance or mortality (e.g., node 1: 0 to 10%; node 2: 10 to 20%; etc.). The outputs of the network are designed to maximize one of the 10 potential output "binds," each corresponding to a decile of mortality between 0 and 100%. The output node containing the correct probability value was set to a value of 1.0; the others to 0.0. In this manner, the network should be able to provide percentage probability of mortality and also to resolve input-case conflicts. An SAS program was written to present the predicted probability of mortality separately in patients who are dead or alive at the end of the follow-up period. The NNs constructed as described above were able to be trained and evaluated according to several definitions of network response: matching the output value at every output

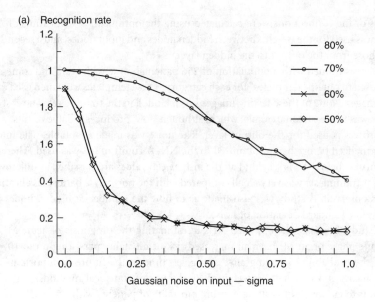

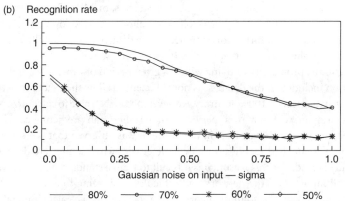

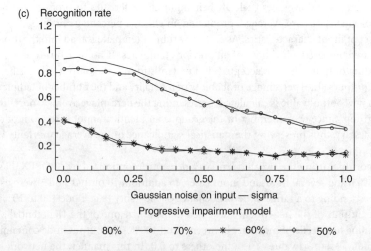

FIGURE 7.4 Recognition rate versus standardization of noise added to the inputs. Different curves correspond to various learning levels with damaged weights. (a) Noise added only to the inputs. (b) Noise added to the weights to mimic "brain damage," $s = 0.05$. (c) Noise on the weights with $s = 0.1$. Notice how much more robust the "brain" is to noise with higher levels of education.

node, identifying the correct location of which node was to contain the peak output value, and matching the output value at the peak output location.

The network was tested on known and then on unknown cases. A correspondence of the observed to the predicted probability of being alive at a given time was observed. The categorical classifications (dead or alive) yielded an overall accuracy of 74%. A reciprocal relationship between sensitivity and specificity of the rules for determination of vital status was observed.

7.4 Neural Networks in Neurology

Neural networks found applications in neurology as well and, in particular, in characterizing memory defects, as are apparent in diseases such as Parkinson's and Alzheimer's. Both diseases exhibit devastating effects and disrupt the lives of those affected.

For several decades, in an attempt to further understand brain functions, computational neuroscientists have addressed the issue by modeling biologic neural network structure with computer simulations. A recent article by Stern et al. [66] reports on an important relationship of Alzheimer's disease expression and levels of education. A similar inverse relationship was earlier reported by Zhang et al. [67] in a Chinese population. This inverse relationship was attributed to a protective role of the brain reserve capacity [68]. Such a capacity becomes important, since in an educated person's brain more synapses exist, which might protect the individual in the expression of symptoms of the disease. It is not argued, however, that the disease will not be acquired; rather, that it will be delayed. Zahner et al. [69] have employed a three-layer feedforward NN trained with ALOPEX to simulate the effects of education in dementia, age-related changes, and in general, brain damage. Our results show that the higher the level of training of the NN, 50, 60, 70, 80%, etc., the slower is the damage on the "brain." Damage was simulated by systematically adding noise on the weights of the network. Noise had a gaussian distribution with varying standard deviations and mean of zero. Figure 7.4 shows the results of these simulations as recognition rate versus standard deviation of noise added to the inputs for increasingly damaged weights at various levels of training. Each point corresponds to an average of 100 samples. Notice how much slower the drop in recognition is for the 70 and 80% curves as compared with the 50 and 60% training. Also notice the distances of the starting points of the curves as we follow the progress of dementia at different stages (Figure 7.4, a vs. b vs. c). All curves demonstrate impairment with damage, but they also show some threshold in the training level, after which the system becomes more robust.

7.5 Discussion

Neural networks provide a powerful tool for analysis of biosignals. This chapter has reviewed applications of NNs in cardiology, neurology, speech processing, and brain waveforms. The literature is vast, and this chapter is by no means exhaustive. In the last 10 years, NNs have been used more and more extensively in a variety of fields, and biomedical engineering is not short of it. Besides the applications, a lot of research is still going on in order to find optimal algorithms and optimal values for the parameters used in these algorithms. In industry, an explosion of VLSI chip designs on NNs has been observed. The parallel character of NNs makes them very desirable solutions to computational bottlenecks.

References

[1] Werbos P. 1974. Beyond regression: New tools for prediction and analysis in the behavioral sciences. Ph.D. thesis, Harvard University, Cambridge, Mass.

[2] Parker D.B. 1985. *Learning logic*, S-81-64, file 1, Office of Technology Licensing, Stanford University, Stanford, Calif.

[3] Rumelhart D.E., Hinton G.E., and Williams R.J. 1986. Learning internal representations by error propagation. In Rumelhart, D.E. and McClelland J.L. (Eds.), *Parallel Distributed Processing*, Vol. 2: Foundations. Cambridge, Mass, MIT Press.

[4] Harth E. and Tzanakou E. 1974. A stochastic method for determining visual receptive fields. *Vision Res.* 14: 1475.

[5] Tzanakou E., Michalak R., and Harth E. 1984. The ALOPEX process: Visual receptive fields with response feedback. *Biol. Cybernet.* 51: 53.

[6] Micheli-Tzanakou E. 1984. Nonlinear characteristics in the frog's visual system. *Biol. Cybernet.* 51: 53.

[7] Deutsch S. and Micheli-Tzanakou E. 1987. *Neuroelectric Systems*. New York, NYU Press.

[8] Marsic I. and Micheli-Tzanakou E. 1990. Distributed optimization with the ALOPEX algorithms. *Proceedings of the 12th Annual International Conference of the IEEE/EMBS* 12: 1415.

[9] Dasey T.J. and Micheli-Tzanakou E. 1989. A pattern recognition application of the ALOPEX process with hexagonal arrays. *International Joint Conference on Neural Networks* 12: 119.

[10] Xiao L.-T., Micheli-Tzanakou E., and Dasey T.J. 1990. Analysis of composite neuronal waveforms into their constituents. *Proceedings of the 12th Annual International Conference of the IEEE/EMBS* 12: 1433.

[11] Hiraiwa A., Shimohara K., and Tokunaga Y. 1989. EMG pattern analysis and classification by Neural Networks. In *IEEE International Conference on Systems, Man and Cybernetics*, part 3, pp. 1113–1115.

[12] Huang Q., Graupe D., Huang Y.-F., and Liu R.W. 1989. Identification of firing patterns of neuronal signals. In *Proceedings of the 28th IEEE Conference on Decision and Control*, Vol. 1, pp. 266–271.

[13] Bruha I. and Madhavan G.P. 1989. Need for a knowledge-based subsystem in evoked potential neural-net recognition system. In *Proceedings of the 11th Annual International Conference of the IEEE/EMBS*, Vol. 11, part 6, pp. 2042–2043.

[14] Kelly M.F., Parker P.A., and Scott R.N. 1990. Applications of neural networks to myoelectric signal analysis: A preliminary study. *IEEE Trans. Biomed. Eng.* 37: 221.

[15] Ramamoorthy P.A., Govid G., and Iyer V.K. 1988. Signal modeling and prediction using neural networks. *Neural Networks* 1: 461.

[16] Moody E.B. Jr, Micheli-Tzanakou E., and Chokroverty S. 1989. An adaptive approach to spectral analysis of pattern-reversal visual evoked potentials. *IEEE Trans. Biomed. Eng.* 36: 439.

[17] Dayhoff J.E. 1990. Regularity properties in pulse transmission networks. *Proc. IJCNN* 3: 621.

[18] Dayhoff J.E. 1990. A pulse transmission (PT) neural network architecture that recognizes patterns and temporally integrates. *Proc. IJCNN* 2: A-979.

[19] Roberts W.M. and Hartile D.K. 1975. Separation of multi-unit nerve impulse trains by the multichannel linear filter algorithm. *Brain Res.* 94: 141.

[20] Abeles M. and Goldstein M.H. 1977. Multiple spike train analysis. *Proc. IEEE* 65: 762.

[21] Wiemer W., Kaack D., and Kezdi P. 1975. Comparative evaluation of methods for quantification of neural activity. *Med. Biol. Eng.* 358.

[22] Perkel D.H., Gerstein G.L., and Moore G.P. 1967. Neuronal spike trains and stochastic point processes: I. The single spike train. *Biophys. J.* 7: 391.

[23] Perkel D.H., Gerstein G.L., and Moore G.P. 1967. Neuronal spike trains and stochastic point processes: II. Simultaneous spike trains. *Biophys. J.* 7: 419.

[24] Gerstein G.L., Perkel D.H., and Subramanian K.N. 1978. Identification of functionally related neuronal assemblies. *Brain Res.* 140: 43.

[25] Papoulis A. 1984. *Probability, Random Variables and Stochastic Processes*, 2nd ed. New York, McGraw-Hill.

[26] Moore G.P., Segundo J.P., Perkel D.H., and Levitan H. 1970. Statistical signs of synaptic interactions in neurons. *Biophys. J.* 10: 876.

[27] Gerstein G.L., Perkel D.H., and Dayhoff J.E. 1985. Cooperative firing activity in simultaneously recorded populations of neurons: detection and measurement. *J. Neurosci.* 5: 881.

[28] Dayhoff J.E. and Gerstein G.L. 1983. Favored patterns in nerve spike trains: I. Detection. *J. Neurophysiol.* 49: 1334.

[29] Dayhoff J.E. and Gerstein G.L. 1983. Favored patterns in nerve spike trains: II. Application. *J. Neurophysiol.* 49: 1349.

[30] Abeles M. and Gerstein G.L. 1988. Detecting spatiotemporal firing patterns among simultaneously recorded single neurons. *J. Neurophysiol.* 60: 909.

[31] Frostig R.D. and Gerstein G.L. 1990. Recurring discharge patterns in multispike trains. *Biol. Cybernet.* 62: 487.

[32] Micheli-Tzanakou E. and Iezzi R. 1985. Spike recognition by stroke density function calculation. In *Proceedings of the 11th Northeast Bioengineering Conference*, pp. 309–312.

[33] Iezzi R. and Micheli-Tzanakou E. 1990. Neural network analysis of neuronal spike-trains. *Annual International Conference of the IEEE/EMBS*, 12: 1435–1436.

[34] Rosenblatt F. 1962. *Principles of Neurodynamics*. Washington, Spartan Books.

[35] Davilla C.E., Welch A.J., and Rylander H.G. 1986. Adaptive estimation of single evoked potentials. In *Proceedings of the 8th IEEE EMBS Annual Conference*, pp. 406–409.

[36] Wang J.-Z. and Micheli-Tzanakou E. 1990. The use of the ALOPEX process in extracting normal and abnormal visual evoked potentials. *IEEE/EMBS Mag.* 9: 44.

[37] Micheli-Tzanakou E. and O'Malley K.G. 1985. Harmonic context of patterns and their correlations to VEP waveforms. In *Proceedings of IEEE, 9th Annual Conference EMBS*, pp. 426–430.

[38] Micheli-Tzanakou E. 1990. A neural network approach of decomposing brain waveforms to their constituents. In *Proceedings of the IASTED International Symposium on Computers and Advanced Technology in Medicine, Healthcare and Bioengineering*, pp. 56–60.

[39] Nahamura M., Nishida S., and Shibasaki H. 1989. Spectral properties of signal averaging and a novel technique for improving the signal to noise ration. *J. Biomed. Eng.* 2: 72.

[40] Orfanidis S., Aafif F., and Micheli-Tzanakou E. 1987. Visual evoked potentials extraction by adaptive filtering. In *Proceedings of the IEEE/EMBS International Conference*, Vol. 2, pp. 968–969.

[41] Doncarli C. and Goerig I. 1988. Adaptive smoothing of evoked potentials: A new approach. In *Proceedings of the Annual International Conference on the IEEE/EMBS*, part 3 (of 4), pp. 1152–1153.

[42] Davilla E., Welch A.J., and Rylander H.G. 1986. Adaptive estimation of single evoked potentials. In *Proceedings of the 8th IEEE/EMBS Annual International Conference*, pp. 406–409.

[43] Moore J. and Ramon F. 1974. On numerical integration of the Hodgkin and Huxley equations for a membrane action potential. *J. Theor. Biol.* 45: 249.

[44] Bell J. and Cook L.P. 1979. A model of the nerve action potential. *Math. Biosci.* 46: 11.

[45] Maier J., Dagnelie G., Spekreijse H., and Van Duk W. 1987. Principal component analysis for source localization of VEPs in man. *Vis. Res.* 27: 165.

[46] Tebelski J., Waibel A., Bojan P., and Schmidbauer O. 1991. Continuous speech recognition by linked predictive neural networks. In Lippman P.R., Moody J.E., and Touretzky D.S. (Eds.), *Advances in Neural Information Processing Systems 3*, pp. 199–205. San Mateo, Calif, Morgan Kauffman.

[47] Allen R.B. and Kanam C.A. 1991. A recurrent neural network for word identification from continuous phonemena strings. In Lippman P.R., Moody J.E., and Touretzky D.S. (Eds.), *Advances in Neural Information Processing Systems 3*, pp. 206–212. San Mateo, Calif, Morgan Kauffman.

[48] Bourland H., Morgan N., and Wooters C. 1991. Connectionist approaches to the use of Markov models speech recognition. In Lippman P.R., Moody J.E., and Touretzky D.S. (Eds.), *Advances in Neural Information Processing systems 3*, pp. 213–219. San Mateo, Calif, Morgan Kauffman.

[49] Intrator N. 1991. Exploratory feature extraction in speech signals. In Lippman P.R., Moody J.E., and Touretzky D.S. (Eds.), *Advances in Neural Information Processing Systems 3*, pp. 241–247. San Mateo, Calif, Morgan Kauffman.

[50] Bienenstock E.L., Cooper L.N., and Munro P.W. 1992. Theory for the development of neuron selectivity: orientation specificity and binocular interaction in visual cortex. *J. Neurosci.* 2: 32.

[51] Zwicker E. 1961. Subdivision of the audible frequency range into critical bands (frequenagruppen). *J. Acoust. Soc. Am.* 33: 248.

[52] Phan F., Zahner D., Micheli-Tzanakou E., and Sideman S. 1994. Speaker identification through wavelet multiresolution decomposition and Alopex. In *Proceedings of the 1994 Long Island Conference on Artificial Intelligence and Computer Graphics*, pp. 53–68.

[53] Mallat S.G. 1989. A theory of multiresolution signal decomposition: the wavelet representation. *IEEE Trans. Pattern Anal. Mach. Int.* 11: 674.

[54] Hunter I.A., Soraghan J.J., Christie J., and Durani T.S. 1993. Detection of echocardiographic left ventricle boundaries using neural networks. *Comput. Cardiol.* 201.

[55] Cohen L.D. 1991. On active contour models and balloons. *CVGIP Image Understanding* 53: 211.

[56] Brugada P., Brugada T., Mont L. et al. 1991. A new approach to the differential diagnosis of a regular tachycardia with a wide QRS complex. *Circulation* 83: 1649.

[57] Dassen W.R.M., Mulleneers R.G.A., Den Dulk K. et al. 1993. Further improvement of classical criteria for differentiation of wide-QRS tachycardia in SUT and VT using artificial neural network techniques. *Comput. Cardiol.* 337.

[58] Nadal J. and deBossan M.C. 1993. Classification of cardiac arrhythmias based on principal components analysis and feedforward neural networks. *Comput. Cardiol.* 341.

[59] Silipo R., Gori M., and Marchesi C. 1993. Autoassociator structured neural network for rhythm classification of long-term electrocardiogram. *Comput. Cardiol.* 349.

[60] Baxt W.B. 1991. Use of an artificial neural network for the diagnosis of myocardial infarction. *Ann. Intern. Med.* 115: 843.

[61] Goldman L., Cook S.F., Brand D.A., et al. 1988. A computer protocol to predict myocardial infarction in emergency department patients with chest pain. *N. Engl. J. Med.* 18: 797.

[62] Hedén B., Edenbrandt L., Haisty W.K. Jr, and Pahlm O. 1993. Neural networks for ECG diagnosis of inferior myocardial infarction. *Comput. Cardiol.* 345.

[63] Pahlm O., Case D., Howard G. et al. 1990. Decision rules for the ECK diagnosis of inferior myocardial infarction. *Comput. Biomed. Res.* 23: 332.

[64] Yi C., Micheli-Tzanakou E., Shindler D., and Kostis J.B. 1993. A new neural network algorithm to study myocardial ultrasound for tissue characterization. In *Proceedings of the 19th Northeastern Bioengineering Conference*, NJIT, pp. 109–110.

[65] Kostis W.J., Yi C., and Micheli-Tzanakou E. 1993. Estimation of long-term mortality of myocardial infarction using a neural network based on the ALOPEX algorithm. In Cohen M.E. and Hudson D.L. (Eds.), *Comparative Approaches in Medical Reasoning*.

[66] Stern Y., Gurland B., Tatemichi T.K. et al. 1994. Influence of education and occupation on the incidence of Alzheimer's disease. *JAMA* 271: 1004.

[67] Zhang M., Katzman R., Salmon D. et al. 1990. The prevalence of dementia and Alzheimer's disease in Shanghai, China: impact of age, gender and education. *Ann. Neurol.* 27: 428.

[68] Satz P. 1993. Brain reserve capacity on symptom onset after brain injury: a formulation and review of evidence for threshold theory. *Neurophysiology* 7: 723.

[69] Zahner D.A., Micheli-Tzanakou E., Powell A. et al. 1994. Protective effects of learning on a progressively impaired neural network model of memory. In *Proceedings of the 16th IEEE/EMBS Annual International Conference*, Baltimore, MD. Vol. 2, pp. 1065–1066.

8

Complexity, Scaling, and Fractals in Biomedical Signals

8.1   Complex Dynamics 8-2
       Overcoming the Limits of Newtonian Mathematics • Critical
       Phenomena: Phase Transitions • An Illustration of Critical
       Phenomena: Magnetism • A Model for Phase Transitions:
       Percolation • Self-Organized Criticality • Dynamics at the
       Edge of Chaos
8.2   Introduction to Scaling Theories 8-6
       Fractal Preliminaries • Mathematical and Natural Fractals •
       Fractal Measures • Power Law and 1/f Processes •
       Distributed Relaxation Processes • Multifractals
8.3   An Example of the Use of Complexity Theory in the
       Development of a Model of the Central Nervous
       System 8-9
Defining Terms 8-10
References 8-10

Banu Onaral
Drexel University

Joseph P. Cammarota
Naval Air Warfare Center

Complexity, a contemporary theme embraced by physical as well as social sciences, is concerned with the collective behavior observed in composite systems in which long-range order is induced by short-range interactions of the constituent parts. Complex forms and functions abound in nature. Particularly in biology and physiology, branched, nested, granular, or otherwise richly packed, irregular, or disordered objects are the rule rather than the exception. Similarly ubiquitous are distributed, broad-band phenomena that appear to fluctuate randomly. The rising science of complexity holds the promise to lead to powerful tools to analyze, model, process, and control the global behavior of complex biomedical systems.

The basic tenets of the complexity theory rest on the revelation that large classes of complex systems (composed of a multitude of richly interacting components) are reducible to simple rules. In particular, the structure and dynamics of complex systems invariably exist or evolve over a multitude of spatial and temporal scales. Moreover, they exhibit a systematic relationship between scales. From the biomedical engineering standpoint, the worthwhile outcome is the ability to characterize these intricate objects and processes in terms of straightforward **scaling** and **fractal** concepts and measures that often can be translated into simple iterative rules. In this sense, the set of concepts and tools, emerging under the rubric of complexity, complements the prediction made by the **chaos** theory that simple (low-order deterministic) systems may generate complex behavior.

In their many incarnations, the concepts of complexity and scaling are playing a refreshingly unifying role among diverse scientific pursuits; therein lie compelling opportunities for scientific discoveries and technical innovations. Since these advances span a host of disciplines, hence different scientific languages, cultures, and dissemination media, finding one's path has become confusing. One of the aims of this presentation is to serve as a resource for key literature. We hope to guide the reader toward substantial contributions and away from figments of fascination in the popular press that have tended to stretch emerging concepts ahead of the rigorous examination of evidence and the scientific verification of facts.

This chapter is organized in three mains parts. The first part is intended to serve as a primer for the fundamental aspects of the complexity theory. An overview of the attendant notions of scaling theories constitutes the core of the second part. In the third part, we illustrate the potential of the complexity approach by presenting an application to predict acceleration-induced loss of consciousness in pilots.

8.1 Complex Dynamics

There exists a class of systems in which very complex spatial and temporal behavior is produced through the rich interactions among a large number of local subsystems. Complexity theory is concerned with systems that have many degrees of freedom (composite systems), are spatially extended (systems with both spatial and temporal degrees of freedom), and are dissipative as well as nonlinear due to the interplay among local components (agents). In general, such systems exhibit **emergent global behavior**. This means that macroscopic characteristics cannot be deduced from the microscopic characteristics of the elementary components considered in isolation. The global behavior emerges from the interactions of the local dynamics.

Complexity theories draw their power from recognition that the behavior of a complex dynamic system does not, in general, depend on the physical particulars of the local elements but rather on how they interact to collectively (cooperatively or competitively) produce the globally observable behavior. The local agents of a complex dynamic system interact with their neighbors through a set of usually (very) simple rules.

The emergent global organization that occurs through the interplay of the local agents arises without the intervention of a central controller. That is, there is **self-organization**, a spontaneous emergence of global order. Long-range correlations between local elements are not explicitly defined in such models, but they are induced through local interactions. The global organization also may exert a top-down influence on the local elements, providing feedback between the macroscopic and microscopic structures [Forrest, 1990] (Figure 8.1).

8.1.1 Overcoming the Limits of Newtonian Mathematics

Linearity, as well as the inherent predictive ability, was an important factor in the success of Newtonian mechanics. If a linear system is perturbed by a small amount, then the system response will change by a proportionally small amount. In nonlinear systems, however, if the system is perturbed by a small amount, the response could be no change, a small change, a large change, oscillations (limit cycle), or chaotic behavior. The response depends on the state of the system at the time it was perturbed. Since most of nature is nonlinear, the key to success in understanding nature lies in embracing this nonlinearity.

Another feature found in linear systems is the property of superposition. Superposition means that the whole is equal to the sum of the parts. All the properties of a linear system can be understood through the analysis of each of its parts. This is not the case for complex systems, where the interaction among simple local elements can produce complex emergent global behavior.

Complexity theory stands in stark contrast to a purely reductionist approach that would seek to explain global behavior by breaking down the system into its most elementary components. The reductionist approach is not guaranteed to generate knowledge about the behavior of a complex system, since it is likely that the information about the local interactions (which determine the global behavior) will not be revealed in such an analysis. For example, knowing everything there is to know about a single ant will

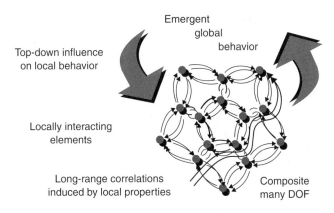

FIGURE 8.1 A complex dynamic system.

reveal nothing about why an ant colony is capable of such complex behaviors as waging war, farming, husbandry, and the ability to quickly adapt to changing environmental conditions. The approach that complexity theory proposes is to look at the system as a whole and not merely as a collection of irreducible parts.

Complexity research depends on digital computers for simulation of interactions. **Cellular automata** (one of the principal tools of complexity) have been constructed to model sand piles, earthquakes, traffic patterns, satellite communication networks, evolution, molecular autocatalysis, forest fires, and species interactions (among others) [Toffoli and Margoulis, 1987]. We note here that complexity is building on, and in some cases unifying, developments made in the fields of chaotic dynamics [Devaney, 1992], critical phenomena, **phase transitions**, **renormalization** [Wilson, 1983], **percolation** [Stauffer and Aharony, 1992], neural networks [Harvey, 1994; Simpson, 1990], genetic algorithms [Goldberg, 1989] and artificial life [Langton, 1989; Langton et al., 1992].

8.1.2 Critical Phenomena: Phase Transitions

For the purpose of this discussion, a phase transition can be defined as any abrupt change between the physical and/or dynamic states of a system. The most familiar examples of phase transitions are between the fundamental stages of matter: solid, liquid, gas, and plasma. Phase transitions are also used to define other changes in matter, such as changes in the crystalline structure or state of magnetism. There are also phase transitions in the dynamics of systems from ordered (fixed-point and limit-cycle stability) to disordered (chaos). Determining the state of matter is not always straightforward. Sometimes the apparent state of matter changes when the scale of the observation (macroscopic versus microscopic) is changed. A critical point is a special case of phase transitions where order and disorder are intermixed at all scales [Wilson, 1983]. At **criticality**, all spatial and temporal features become scale invariant or self-similar. Magnetism is a good example of this phenomenon.

8.1.3 An Illustration of Critical Phenomena: Magnetism

The atoms of a ferromagnetic substance have more electrons with spins in one direction than in the other, resulting in a net magnetic field for the atom as a whole. The individual magnetic fields of the atoms tend to line up in one direction, with the result that there is a measurable level of magnetism in the material. At a temperature of absolute zero, all the atomic dipoles are perfectly aligned. At normal room temperature, however, some of the atoms are not aligned to the global magnetic field due to thermal fluctuations. This creates small regions that are nonmagnetic, although the substance is still magnetic. Spatial renormalization, or coarse graining, is the process of averaging the microscopic properties of the substance over a specified range in order to replace the multiple elements with a single equivalent element.

If measurements of the magnetic property were taken at a very fine resolution (without renormaliz-ation), there would be some measurements that detect small pockets of nonmagnetism, although most measurements would indicate that the substance was magnetic. As the scale of the measurements is increased, that is, spatially renormalized, the small pockets of nonmagnetism would be averaged out and would not be measurable. Therefore, measurements at the larger scale would indicate that the substance is magnetic, thereby decreasing its apparent temperature and making the apparent magnetic state depend-ent on the resolution of the measurements. The situation is similar (but reversed) at high temperatures. That is, spatial renormalization results in apparently higher temperatures, since microscopic islands of magnetism are missed because of the large areas of disorder in the material.

At the Curie temperature there is long-range correlation in both the magnetic and nonmagnetic regions. The distribution of magnetic and nonmagnetic regions is invariant under the spatial renormalization transform. These results are independent of the scale at which the measure is taken, and the apparent temperature does not change under the renormalization transform. This scale invariance (**self-similarity**) occurs at only three temperatures: absolute zero, infinity, and the Curie temperature. The Curie temper-ature represents a critical point (criticality) in the tuning parameter (temperature) that governs the phase transition from a magnetic to a nonmagnetic state [Pietgen and Richter, 1986].

8.1.4 A Model for Phase Transitions: Percolation

A percolation model is created by using a simple regular geometric framework and by establishing simple interaction rules among the elements on the grid. Yet these models give rise to very complex structures and relationships that can be described by using scaling concepts such as fractals and power laws. A percolation model can be constructed on any regular infinite n-dimensional lattice [Stauffer and Aharony, 1992]. For simplicity, the example discussed here will use a two-dimensional finite square grid. In site percolation, each node in the grid has only two states, occupied or vacant. The nodes in the lattice are populated-based on a uniform probability distribution, independent of the sate of any other node. The probability of a node being occupied is p (and thus the probability of a node being vacant is $1 - p$). Nodes that are neighbors on the grid link together to form clusters (Figure 8.2).

Clusters represent connections between nodes in the lattice. Anything associated with the cluster can therefore travel (flow) to any node that belongs to the cluster. Percolation can describe the ability of water to flow through a porous medium such as igneous rock, oil fields, or finely ground Colombian coffee. As the occupation probability increases, the clusters of the percolation network grow from local connectedness to global connectedness [Feder, 1988]. At the critical occupation probability, a cluster that spans the entire lattice emerges. It is easy to see how percolation could be used to describe such phenomena as phase transitions by viewing occupied nodes as ordered matter, with vacant nodes representing disordered matter. Percolation networks have been used to model magnetism, forest fires, and the permeability of ion channels in cell membranes.

8.1.5 Self-Organized Criticality

The concept of self-organized criticality has been introduced as a possible underlying principle of com-plexity [Bak et al., 1988; Bak and Chen, 1991]. The class of self-organized critical systems is spatially extended, composite, and dissipative with many locally interacting degrees of freedom. These systems have the capability to naturally evolve (i.e., there is no explicit tuning parameter such as temperature or pressure) toward a critical state.

Self-organized criticality is best illustrated by a sand pile. Start with a flat plate. Begin to add sand one grain at a time. The mound will continue to grow until criticality is reached. This criticality is dependent only on the local interactions among the grains of sand. The local slope determines what will happen if another grain of sand is added. If the local slope is below the criticality (i.e., flat) the new grain of sand will stay put and increase the local slope. If the local slope is at the criticality, then adding the new grain of sand will increase the slope beyond the criticality, causing it to collapse. The collapsing grains of sand spread

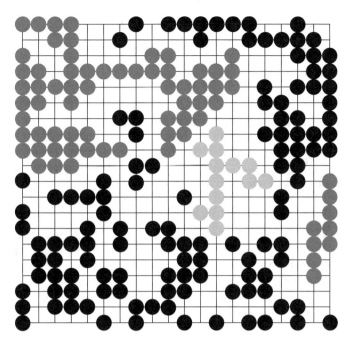

FIGURE 8.2 A percolation network.

to adjoining areas. If those areas are at the criticality, then the avalanche will continue until local areas with slopes below the criticality are reached. Long-range correlations (up to the length of the sand pile) may emerge from the interactions of the local elements. Small avalanches are very common, while large avalanches are rare. The size (and duration) of the avalanche plotted against the frequency of occurrence of the avalanche can be described by a power law [Bak et al., 1988]. The sand pile seeks the criticality on its own. The slope in the sand pile will remain constant regardless of even the largest avalanches. These same power laws are observed in traffic patterns, earthquakes, and many other complex phenomena.

8.1.6 Dynamics at the Edge of Chaos

The dynamics of systems can be divided into several categories. Dynamic systems that exhibit a fixed-point stability will return to their initial state after being perturbed. A periodic evolution of states will result from a system that exhibits a limit-cycle stability. Either of these systems may display a transient evolution of states before the stable regions are reached. Dynamic systems also may exhibit chaotic behavior. The evolution of states associated with chaotic behavior is aperiodic, well-bounded, and very sensitive to initial conditions and resembles noise but is completely deterministic [Tsonis and Tsonis, 1989].

The criticality that lies between highly ordered and highly disordered dynamics has been referred to as the edge of chaos [Langton, 1990] and is analogous to a phase transition between states of matter, where the highly ordered system can be thought of as a solid and the highly disordered system a liquid.

The edge of chaos is the critical boundary between order and chaos. If the system dynamics are stagnant (fixed-point stability, highly ordered system), then there is no mechanism for change. The system cannot adapt and evolve because new states cannot be encoded into the system. If the system dynamics are chaotic (highly disordered), then the system is in a constant state of flux, and there is no memory, no learning, and no adaptation (some of the main qualities associated with life). Systems may exhibit transients in the evolution of states before settling down into either fixed-point or limit-cycle behavior. As the dynamics of a complex system enter the edge of chaos region, the length of these transients quickly grows. The chaotic region is where the length of the "transient" is infinite. At the edge of chaos (the dynamic phase transition) there is no characteristic scale due to the emergence of arbitrarily long correlation lengths in space and time [Langton, 1990]. The self-organized criticality in the sand piles of Per Bak is an example of a system that exists at the edge of chaos. It is in this region that there is no characteristic space or time scale. A single grain of sand added to the pile could cause an avalanche that consists of two grains of sand, or it could cause an avalanche that spreads over the entire surface of the sand pile.

8.2   Introduction to Scaling Theories

Prior to the rise of complexity theories, the existence of a systematic relationship between scales eluded the mainstream sciences. As a consequence, natural structures and dynamics have been commonly dismissed as too irregular and complex and often rejected as monstrous formations, intractable noise, or artifacts. The advent of scaling concepts [Mandelbrot, 1983] has uncovered a remarkable hierarchical order that persists over a significant number of spatial or temporal scales.

Scaling theories capitalize on scale-invariant symmetries exhibited by many natural broadband (i.e., multiscale) phenomena. According to the theory of self-organized criticality (see Section 8.1), this scaling order is a manifestation of dilation (compression) symmetries that define the organization inherent to complex systems which naturally evolve toward a critical state while dissipating energies on broad ranges of space and time scales. Long overlooked, this symmetry is now added to the repertoire of mathematical modeling concepts, which had included approaches based largely on displacement invariances under translation and/or rotation.

Many natural forms and functions maintain some form of exact or statistical invariance under transformations of scale and thus belong in the scaling category. Objects and processes that remain invariant under ordinary geometric similarity constitute the self-similar subset in this class.

Methods to capture scaling information in the form of simple rules that relate features on different scales are actively developed in many scientific fields [Barnsley, 1993]. Engineers are coping with scaling nature of forms and functions by investigating multiscale system theory [Basseville et al., 1992], multiresolution and multirate signal processing [Akansu and Hadad, 1992; Vaidyanathan, 1993], subband coding, wavelets, and filter banks [Meyer, 1993], and fractal compression [Barnsley and Hurd, 1993].

These emerging tools empower engineers to reexamine old data and to re-formulate the question at the root of many unresolved inverse problems — What can small patterns say about large patterns, and vice versa? They also offer the possibility to establish cause–effect relationships between a given physical (spatial) medium and the monitored dynamic (temporal) behavior that constitutes the primary preoccupation of diagnostic scientists.

8.2.1   Fractal Preliminaries

In the broadest sense, the noun or adjective fractal refers to physical objects or dynamic processes that reveal new details on space or time magnification. A staple of a truly fractal object or process is therefore the lack of characteristic scale in time or space. Most structures in nature are broadband over a finite range, covering at least a number of frequency decades in space or time. Scaling fractals often consist of a hierarchy or heterarchy of spatial or temporal structures in cascade and are often accomplished through recursive replication of patterns at finer scales. If the replication rule preserves scale invariance throughout the entity, such fractals are recognized as self-similar in either an exact or a statistical sense.

A prominent feature of fractals is their ability to pack structure with economy of resources, whether energy, space, or whatever other real estate. Fitting nearly infinite networks into finite spaces is just one such achievement. These types of fractals are pervasive in physiology, that is, the branching patterns of the bronchi, the cardiovascular tree, and the nervous tissue [West and Goldberger, 1987], which have the additional feature of being "fault tolerant" [West, 1990].

Despite expectations heightened by the colorful publicity campaign mounted by promoters of fractal concepts, it is advisable to view fractals only as a starting approximation in analyzing scaling shapes and fluctuations in nature. Fractal concepts are usually descriptive at a phenomenologic level without pretense to reveal the exact nature of the underlying elementary processes. They do not offer, for that matter, conclusive evidence of whatever particular collective, coupled, or isolated repetitive mechanism that created the fractal object.

In many situations, the power of invoking fractal concepts resides in the fact that they bring the logic of constraints, whether in the form of asymmetry of motion caused by defects, traps, energy barriers, residual memories, irreversibility, or any other appropriate interaction or coupling mechanisms that hinder free random behavior. As discussed earlier, the spontaneous or forced organization and the ensuing divergence in correlations and coherences that emerges out of random behavior are presumably responsible for the irregular structures pervasive throughout the physical world.

More important, the versatility of fractal concepts as a magnifying tool is rooted in the facility to account for scale hierarchies and/or scale invariances in an exact or statistical sense. In the role of a scale microscope, they suggest a fresh look, with due respect to all scales of significance, at many structural and dynamic problems deemed thus far anomalous or insoluble.

8.2.2 Mathematical and Natural Fractals

The history of mathematics is rife with "pathologic" constructions of the iterated kind which defy the euclidian dimension concepts. The collection once included an assortment of anomalous dust sets, lines, surfaces, volumes, and other mathematical miscellenia mostly born out of the continuous yet nondifferentiable category of functions such as the Weierstrass series.

The feature unifying these mathematical creations with natural fractals is the fractional or integer dimensions distinct from the euclidian definition. Simply stated, a fractional dimension positions an object in between two integer dimensions in the euclidian sense, best articulated by the critical dimension in the Hausdorff-Besicovith derivation [Feder, 1988]. When this notion of dimension is pursued to the extreme and the dimension reaches an integer value, one is confronted with the counterintuitive reality of space-filling curves, volume-filling planes, etc. These objects can be seen readily to share intrinsic scaling properties with the nearly infinite networks accomplished by the branching patterns of bronchi and blood vessels and the intricate folding of the cortex.

A rewarding outcome afforded by the advent of scaling concepts is the ability to characterize such structures in terms of straightforward "scaling" or "dimension" measures. From these, simple iterative rules may be deduced to yield models with maximum economy (or minimum number) or parameters [Barnsley, 1993]. This principle is suspected to underlie the succinct, coding adopted by nature in order to store extensive information needed to create complex shapes and forms.

8.2.3 Fractal Measures

The measure most often used in the diagnosis of a fractal is the basic fractal dimension, which, in the true spirit of fractals, has eluded a rigorous definition embracing the entire family of fractal objects. The guiding factor in the choice of the appropriate measures is the recognition that most fractal objects scale self-similarly; in other words, they can be characterized by a measure expressed in the form of a power factor, or scaling exponent ∂, that links the change in the observed dependent quantity V to the independent variable x as $V(x) \approx x\partial$ [Falconer, 1990: 36]. Clearly, ∂ is proportional to the ratio of the logarithm of $V(x)$ and x, that is, $\partial = \log V(x)/\log x$. In the case of fractal objects, ∂ is the scaling exponent in the fractal sense and may have a fractional value. In the final analysis, most scaling relationships can be cast into some form of a logarithmic dependence on the independent variable with respect to which a scaling property is analyzed, the latter also expressed on the logarithmic scale. A number of dimension formulas have been developed based on this observation, and comprehensive compilations are now available [Falconer, 1990; Feder, 1988].

One approach to formalize the concept of scale invariance utilizes the homogeneity or the renormalization principle given by $f(m) = f(am)/b$, where a and b are constants and m is the independent variable [West and Goldberger, 1987]. The function f that satisfies this relationship is referred as a scaling function.

The power-law function $f(m) \approx m b$ is a prominent example in this category provided $b = \log b / \log a$. The usefulness of this particular scaling function has been proven many times over in many areas of science, including the thermodynamics of phase transitions and the threshold behavior of percolation networks [Schroeder, 1991; Stauffer and Aharony, 1992; Wilson, 1983].

8.2.4 Power Law and 1/f Processes

The revived interest in power-law behavior largely stems from the recognition that a large class of noisy signals exhibits spectra that attenuate with a fractional power dependence on frequency [West and Shlesinger, 1989; Wornell, 1993]. Such behavior is often viewed as a manifestation of the interplay of a multitude of local processes evolving on a spectrum of time scales that collectively give rise to the so-called 1/f b or, more generally, the 1/f-type behavior. As in the case of spatial fractals that lack a characteristic length scale, **1/f processes** such as the **fractional brownian motion** cannot be described adequately within the confines of a "characteristic" time scale and hence exhibit the "fractal time" property [Mandelbrot, 1967].

8.2.5 Distributed Relaxation Processes

Since the later part of the nineteenth century, the fractional power function dependence of the frequency spectrum also has been recognized as a macroscopic dynamic property manifested by strongly interacting dielectric, viscoelastic, and magnetic materials and interfaces between different conducting materials [Daniel, 1967]. More recently, the 1/f-type dynamic behavior has been observed in percolating networks composed of random mixtures of conductors and insulators and layered wave propagation in heterogeneous media [Orbach, 1986]. In immittance (impedance or admittance) studies, this frequency dispersion has been analyzed conventionally to distinguish a broad class of the so-called anomalous, that is, nonexponential, relaxation/dispersion systems from those which can be described by the "ideal" single exponential form due to Debye [Daniel, 1967].

The fractal time or the multiplicity of times scales prevalent in distributed relaxation systems necessarily translates into fractional constitutive models amenable to analysis by fractional calculus [Ross, 1977] and fractional state-space methods [Bagley and Calico, 1991]. This corresponds to logarithmic distribution functions ranging in symmetry from the log-normal with even center symmetry at one extreme to single-sided hyperbolic distributions with diverging moments at the other. The realization that systems that do not possess a characteristic time can be described in terms of distributions renewed the interest in the field of dispersion/relaxation analysis. Logarithmic distribution functions have been used conventionally as means to characterize such complexity [West, 1994].

8.2.6 Multifractals

Fractal objects and processes in nature are rarely strictly homogeneous in their scaling properties and often display a distribution of scaling exponents that echos the structural heterogeneities occurring at a myriad of length or time scales. In systems with spectra that attenuate following a pure power law over extended frequency scales, as in the case of Davidson–Cole dispersion [Daniel, 1967], the corresponding distribution of relaxation times is logarithmic and single-tailed. In many natural relaxation systems, however, the spectral dimension exhibits a gradual dependence on frequency, as in phenomena conventionally modeled by the Cole–Cole type dispersion. The equivalent distribution functions exhibit double-sided symmetries on the logarithmic relaxation time scale ranging from the even symmetry of the log-normal through intermediate symmetries down to strictly one-sided functions.

The concept that a fractal structure can be composed of fractal subsets with uniform scaling property within the subset has gained popularity in recent years [Feder, 1988]. From this perspective, one may view a complicated fractal object, say, the strange attractor of a chaotic process, as a superposition of simple fractal subsystems. The idea has been formalized under the term multifractal. It follows that each individual member contributes to the overall scaling behavior according to a spectrum of scaling exponents or dimensions. The latter function is called the multifractal spectrum and summarizes the global scaling information of the complete set.

8.3   An Example of the Use of Complexity Theory in the Development of a Model of the Central Nervous System

Consciousness can be viewed as an emergent behavior arising from the interactions among a very large number of local agents, which, in this case, range from electrons through neurons and glial cells to networks of neurons. The hierarchical organization of the brain [Churchland and Sejnowski, 1992; Newell, 1990], which exists and evolves on a multitude of spatial and temporal scales, is a good example of the scaling characteristics found in many complex dynamic systems. There is no master controller for this emergent behavior, which results from the intricate interactions among a very large number of local agents.

A model that duplicates the global dynamics of the induction of unconsciousness in humans due to cerebral ischemia produced by linear acceleration stress (G-LOC) was constructed using some of the tenets of complexity [Cammarota, 1994]. It was an attempt to provide a theory that could both replicate historical human acceleration tolerance data and present a possible underlying mechanism. The model coupled the realization that an abrupt loss of consciousness could be thought of as a phase transition from consciousness to unconsciousness with the proposed neurophysiologic theory of G-LOC [Whinnery, 1989]. This phase transition was modeled using a percolation network to evaluate the connectivity of neural pathways within the central nervous system.

In order to construct the model, several hypotheses had to be formulated to account for the unobservable interplay among the local elements of the central nervous system. The inspiration for the characteristics of the locally interacting elements (the nodes of the percolation lattice) was provided by the physiologic mechanism of arousal (the all-or-nothing aspect of consciousness), the utilization of oxygen in neural tissue during ischemia, and the response of neural cells to metabolic threats. The neurophysiologic theory of acceleration tolerance views unconsciousness as an active protective mechanism that is triggered by a metabolic threat which in this case is acceleration-induced ischemia. The interplay among the local systems is determined by using a percolation network that models the connectivity of the arousal mechanism (the reticular activating system). When normal neuronal function is suppressed due to local cerebral ischemia, the corresponding node is removed from the percolation network. The configuration of the percolation network varies as a function of time. When the network is no longer able to support arousal, unconsciousness results.

The model simulated a wide range of human data with a high degree of fidelity. It duplicated the population response (measured as the time it took to lose consciousness) over a range of stresses that varied from a simulation of the acute arrest of cerebral circulation to a gradual application of acceleration stress. Moreover, the model was able to offer a possible unified explanation for apparently contradictory historical data. An analysis of the parameters responsible for the determination of the time of LOC indicated that there is a phase transition in the dynamics that was not explicitly incorporated into the construction of the model. The model spontaneously captured an interplay of the cardiovascular and neurologic systems that could not have been predicted based on existing data.

The keys to the model's success are the reasonable assumptions that were made about the characteristics and interaction of the local dynamic subsystems through the integration of a wide range of human and animal physiologic data in the design of the model. None of the local parameters was explicitly tuned to produce the global (input–output) behavior. By successfully duplicating the observed global behavior of humans under acceleration stress, however, this model provided insight into some (currently) unobservable inner dynamics of the central nervous system. Furthermore, the model suggests new experimental protocols specifically aimed at exploring further the microscopic interplay responsible for the macroscopic (observable) behavior.

Defining Terms

1/f process: Signals or systems that exhibit spectra which attenuate following a fractional power dependence on frequency.

Cellular automata: Composite discrete-time and discrete space dynamic systems defined on a regular lattice. Neighborhood rules determine the state transitions of the individual local elements (cells).

Chaos: A state the produces a signal that resembles noise and is aperiodic, well-bounded, and very sensitive to initial conditions but is governed by a low-order deterministic differential or difference equation.

Complexity: Complexity theory is concerned with systems that have many degrees of freedom (composite systems), are spatially extended (systems with both spatial and temporal degrees of freedom), and are dissipative as well as nonlinear due to the rich interactions among the local components (agents). Some of the terms associated with such systems are emergent global behavior, collective behavior, cooperative behavior, self-organization, critical phenomena, and scale invariance.

Criticality: A state of a system where spatial and/or temporal characteristics are scale invariant.

Emergent global behavior: The observable behavior of a system that cannot be deduced from the properties of constituent components considered in isolation and results from the collective (cooperative or competitive) evolution of local events.

Fractal: Refers to physical objects or dynamic processes that reveal new details on space or time magnification. Fractals lack a characteristic scale.

Fractional brownian motion: A generalization of the random function created by the record of the motion of a "brownian particle" executing random walk. Brownian motion is commonly used to model diffusion in constraint-free media. Fractional brownian motion is often used to model diffusion of particles in constrained environments or anomalous diffusion.

Percolation: A simple mathematical construct commonly used to measure the extent of connectedness in a partially occupied (site percolation) or connected (bond percolation) lattice structure.

Phase transition: Any abrupt change between the physical and/or the dynamic states of a system, usually between ordered and disordered organization or behavior.

Renormalization: Changing the characteristic scale of a measurement though a process of systematic averaging applied to the microscopic elements of a system (also referred to as coarse graining).

Scaling: Structures or dynamics that maintain some form of exact or statistical invariance under transformations of scale.

Self-organization: The spontaneous emergence of order. This occurs without the direction of a global controller.

Self-similarity: A subset of objects and processes in the scaling category that remain invariant under ordinary geometric similarity.

References

Akansu A.N. and Haddad R.A. 1992. *Multiresolution Signal Decomposition: Transforms, Subbands, and Wavelets.* New York, Academic Press.

Bagley R. and Calico R. 1991. Fractional order state equations for the control of viscoelastic damped structures. *J. Guid.* 14: 304.

Bak P., Tang C., and Wiesenfeld K. 1988. Self-organized criticality. *Phys. Rev. A.* 38: 364.

Bak P. and Chen K. 1991. Self-organized. *Sci. Am. J.*: 45.

Barnsley M.F. 1993. *Fractals Everywhere*, 2nd ed. New York, Academic Press.

Barnsley M.F. and Hurd L.P. 1993. *Fractal Image Compression.* Wellesley, AK Peters.

Basseville M., Benveniste A., Chou K.C. et al. 1992. Modeling and estimation of multiresolution stochastic processes. *IEEE Trans. Inf. Theor.* 38: 766.

Cammarota J.P. 1994. A Dynamic Percolation Model of the Central Nervous System under Acceleration (+Gz) Induced/Hypoxic Stress. Ph.D. thesis, Drexel University, Philadelphia.

Churchland P.S. and Sejnowski T.J. 1992. *The Computational Brain.* Cambridge, Mass., MIT Press.

Daniel V. 1967. *Dielectric Relaxation.* New York, Academic Press.

Devaney R.L. 1992. *A First Course in Chaotic Dynamical Systems: Theory and Experiment.* Reading, Mass., Addison-Wesley.

Falconer K. 1990. *Fractal Geometry: Mathematical Foundations and Applications.* New York, John Wiley & Sons.

Feder J. 1988. *Fractals.* New York, Plenum Press.

Forrest S. 1990. Emergent computation: self-organization, collective, and cooperative phenomena in natural and artificial computing networks. *Physica D* 42: 1.

Goldberg D.E. 1989. *Genetic Algorithms in Search, Optimization, and Machine Learning.* Reading, Mass., Addison-Wesley.

Harvey R.L. 1994. *Neural Network Principles.* Englewood Cliffs, NJ, Prentice-Hall.

Langton C.G. 1989. *Artificial Life: Proceedings of an Interdisciplinary Workshop on the Synthesis and Simulation of Living Systems,* September 1987, Los Alamos, New Mexico, Redwood City, Calif, Addison-Wesley.

Langton C.G. 1990. Computation at the edge of the chaos: Phase transitions and emergent computation. *Physica D* 42: 12.

Langton C.G., Taylor C., Farmer J.D., and Rasmussen S. 1992. *Artificial Life II: Proceedings of the Workshop on Artificial Life,* February 1990, Sante Fe, New Mexico. Redwood City, Calif, Addison-Wesley.

Mandelbrot B. 1967. Some noises with $1/f$ spectrum, a bridge between direct current and white noise. *IEEE Trans. Inf. Theor.* IT-13: 289.

Mandelbrot B. 1983. *The Fractal Geometry of Nature.* New York, WH Freeman.

Meyer Y. 1993. *Wavelets: Algorithms and Applications.* Philadelphia, SIAM.

Newell A. 1990. *Unified Theories of Cognition.* Cambridge, Mass., Harvard University Press.

Orbach R. 1986. Dynamics of fractal networks. *Science* 231: 814.

Peitgen H.O. and Richter P.H. 1986. *The Beauty of Fractals.* New York, Springer-Verlag.

Ross B. 1977. Fractional calculus. *Math. Mag.* 50: 115.

Shroeder M. 1990. *Fractals, Chaos, Power Laws.* New York, WH Freeman.

Simpson P.K. 1990. *Artificial Neural Systems: Foundations, Paradigms, Applications, and Implementations.* New York, Pergamon Press.

Stauffer D. and Aharony A. 1992. *Introduction to Percolation.* 2nd ed. London, Taylor & Francis.

Toffoli T. and Margolus N. 1987. *Cellular Automata Machines: A New Environment for Modeling.* Cambridge, Mass., MIT Press.

Tsonis P.A. and Tsonis A.A. 1989. Chaos: Principles and implications in biology. *Comput. Appl. Biosci.* 5: 27.

Vaidyanathan P.P. 1993. *Multi-Rate Systems and Filter Banks.* Englewood Cliffs, NJ, Prentice-Hall.

West B.J. 1990. Physiology in fractal dimensions: error tolerance. *Ann. Biomed. Eng.* 18: 135.

West B.J. 1994. Scaling statistics in biomedical phenomena. In *Proceedings of the IFAC Conference on Modeling and Control in Biomedical Systems,* Galveston, Texas.

West B.J. and Goldberger A. 1987. Physiology in fractal dimensions. *Am. Scientist* 75: 354.

West B.J. and Shlesinger M. 1989. On the ubiquity of $1/f$ noise. *Int J. Mod. Phys.* 3: 795.

Whinnery J.E. 1989. Observations on the neurophysiologic theory of acceleration (+Gz) induced loss of consciousness. *Aviat. Space Environ. Med.* 60: 589.

Wilson K.G. 1983. The renormalization group and critical phenomena. *Rev. Mod. Phys.* 55: 583.

Wornell G.W. 1993. Wavelet-based representations for the $1/f$ family of fractal processes. *IEEE Proc.* 81: 1428.

9

Future Directions: Biomedical Signal Processing and Networked Multimedia Communications

Banu Onaral
Drexel University

9.1   Public Switched Network and Asynchronous Transfer
       Mode.. **9**-2
9.2   Wireless Communication **9**-2
9.3   Photonics **9**-3
9.4   Virtual Reality **9**-3
Acknowledgment.. **9**-3
Defining Terms **9**-3
References **9**-4

The long anticipated "information age" is taking shape at the cross-section of **multimedia** signal processing and telecommunications-based networking. By defying the traditional concepts of space and time, these emerging technologies promise to affect all facets of our lives in a pervasive and profound manner [Mayo, 1992]. The physical constraints of location have naturally led, over the centuries, to the creation of the conventional patient care services and facilities. As the "information superhighway" is laid down with branches spanning the nation, and eventually the world via wired and wireless communication channels, we will come closer to a bold new era in health care delivery, namely, the era of remote monitoring, diagnosis, and intervention.

Forward-looking medical industries are engaging in research and development efforts to capitalize on the emerging technologies. Medical institutions in particular recognize the transforming power of the impending revolution. A number of hospitals are undertaking pilot projects to experiment with the potentials of the new communication and interaction media that will constitute the foundations of futuristic health care systems. There is consensus among health care administrators that the agility and effectiveness with which an institution positions itself to fully embrace the new medical lifestyle will decide its viability in the next millennium.

Although multimedia communications is yet in its infancy, recent developments foretell a bright future. Many agree that multimedia networking is becoming a reality thanks to advances in digital signal-processing research and development. Trends toward implementation of algorithms by fewer components are leading to decreasing hardware complexity while increasing processing functionality [Andrews, 1994]. The vast and vibrant industry producing multimedia hardware and software ranging from application-specific digital signal processors and video chip sets to videophones and multimedia terminals heavily relies on digital signal processing know-how.

As in the case of generic digital signal processing, biomedical signal processing is expected to play a key role in mainstreaming patient care at a distance. Earlier in this section, emerging methods in biomedical signal analysis that promise major enhancements in our ability to extract information from vital signals were introduced. This chapter provides a glimpse of the future — when biomedical signals will be integrated with other patient information and transmitted via networked multimedia — by examining trends in key communications technologies, namely, public switched-network protocols, wireless communications, **photonics**, and **virtual reality**.

9.1 Public Switched Network and Asynchronous Transfer Mode

The public switched network already can accommodate a wide array of networked multimedia communications. The introduction of new standards such as the **asynchronous transfer mode (ATM)** is a strong sign that the network will evolve to handle an array of novel communication services.

ATM is a technology based on a switched network that uses dedicated media connections [ATM Networking, 1994]. Each connection between users is physically established by setting up a path or virtual channel through a series of integrated circuits in the switch. In conventional shared media networks, connections are made by breaking the information into packets labeled with their destination; these packets then share bandwidth until they reach their destination. In switched networks, instead of sharing bandwidth, connections can be run in parallel, since each connection has its own pathway. This approach prevents degradation of the response time despite an increased number of users who are running intensive applications on the network, such as videoconferencing. Therefore, ATM offers consistently high performance to all users on the network, particularly in real-time networked multimedia applications which often encounter severe response time degradation on shared media networks. Also, the ATM standards for both local area networks (LANs) and wide area networks (WANs) are the same; this allows for seamless integration of LANs and WANs.

Small-scale experiments based on ATM-based multimedia communications have already been launched in a number of medical centers. Early examples involve departments where doctors and staff can remotely work on chest x-rays, **CT** exams, and **MRI** images around the hospital over an ATM switched network. Since ATM integrates LANs and WANs, collaborating institutions will be able to access the same information in the future. Similar patient multimedia information-sharing efforts are underway which integrate all vital information including physiologic signals and sounds, images, and video and patient data and make them available remotely. In some recent experiments, the access is accomplished in real time such that medical conferencing, and hence remote diagnosis, becomes a possibility.

9.2 Wireless Communication

Wireless communication is the fastest growing sector of the telecommunications industry [Wittman, 1994]. **Wireless networking** technology is rapidly coming of age with the recent passage of initial standards, widespread performance improvements, and the introduction of personal communications networks (PCNs). Pocket-sized portable "smart" terminals are combined with wireless communication to free users from the constraints of wired connection to networks. The progress in this direction is closely monitored by the health care community because the technology holds the potential to liberate ambulatory patients who require long-term monitoring and processing of biomedical signals for timely intervention. Wireless and interactive access by medical personnel to physiologic multimedia information will no doubt be a staple of the future distributed health care delivery systems.

9.3 Photonics

Photonics, or lightwave, is an evolving technology with the capacity to support a wide range of high-bandwidth multimedia applications. In current practice, photonics plays a complementary role to electronics in the hybrid technology referred to as electro-optics. Optical fibers are widely used for transmission of signals, from long-distance links to undersea cables to local loops linking customers with the central switching office. The trend in photonics is to move beyond functions limited to transmission toward logic operations. Recent advances in photonic logic devices suggest that optical computers may present characteristics more desirable than electronics in many biomedical processing applications requiring parallel tasks. A case in point is online pattern recognition, which may bring a new dimension to remote diagnosis.

9.4 Virtual Reality

Virtual reality — the ultimate networked multimedia service — is a simulated environment that enables one to remotely experience an event or a place in all dimensions. Virtual reality makes telepresence possible. The nascent technology builds on the capabilities of interactive telecommunications and is expected to become a consumer reality early in the next century. Applications in the field of endoscopic surgery are being developed. Demonstration projects in remote surgery are underway, paving the way for remote medical intervention.

Acknowledgment

Contributions by Prabhakar R. Chitrapu, Dialogic Corporation, to material on networked multimedia communications in this chapter are gratefully acknowledged.

Defining Terms

ATM (asynchronous transfer mode): Technology based on a switched network that uses dedicated media connections.

CT: Computer tomography.

MRI: Magnetic resonance imaging.

Multimedia: Technology to integrate sights, sounds, and data. The media may include audio signals such as speech, music, biomedical sounds, images, animation, and video signals, as well as text, graphics, and fax. One key feature is the common linkage, synchronization, and control of the various media that contribute to the overall multimedia signal. In general, multimedia services and products are interactive, hence real-time, as in the case of collaborative computing and videoconferencing.

Photonics: Switching, computing, and communications technologies based on lightwave.

Virtual reality: Technology that creates a simulated environment enabling one to remotely experience an event or a place in all dimensions.

Wireless network: Technology based on communication between nodes such as stationary desktops, laptops, or personal digital assistants (PDAs) and the LAN hub or access point using a wireless adapter with radio circuitry and an antenna. The LAN hub has a LAN attachment on one interface and one or more antennas on another.

References

Andrews, D. 1994. Digital signal processing: the engine to make multimedia mainstream. *Byte* 22.

ATM Networking: increasing performance on the network. *HEPC Syllabus* 3: 12, 1994.

Mayo, J.S. 1992. The promise of networked multimedia communications. *Bear Stearns Sixth Annual Media and Communications Conference*, Coronado, CA.

Wittmann, A. 1994. Will wireless win the war? *Network Computing* 58.

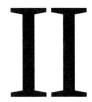

Imaging

Warren S. Grundfest
David Geffen School of Medicine

10 X-Ray
Robert E. Shroy, Jr., Michael S. Van Lysel, Martin J. Yaffe 10-1

11 Computed Tomography
Ian A. Cunningham, Philip F. Judy 11-1

12 Magnetic Resonance Imaging
Steven Conolly, Albert Macovski, John Pauly, John Schenck, Kenneth K. Kwong,
David A. Chesler, Xiaoping Hu, Wei Chen, Maqbool Patel, Kamil Ugurbil 12-1

13 Nuclear Medicine
Barbara Y. Croft, Benjamin M.W. Tsui 13-1

14 Ultrasound
Richard L. Goldberg, Stephen W. Smith, Jack G. Mottley, K. Whittaker Ferrara 14-1

15 Magnetic Resonance Microscopy
Xiaohong Zhou, G. Allan Johnson 15-1

16 Positron-Emission Tomography (PET)
Thomas F. Budinger, Henry F. VanBrocklin 16-1

17 Electrical Impedance Tomography
D.C. Barber 17-1

18 Medical Applications of Virtual Reality Technology
Walter Greenleaf, Tom Piantanida 18-1

I MAGING HAS BECOME AN INTEGRAL PART of medical care. The ability to obtain information about the anatomic and physiologic status of the body without the need for direct visualization has dramatically altered the practice of medicine.

X-rays provided the first technical capability to image inside the body. X-rays provide a two-dimensional image of a three-dimensional space. Their contrast mechanism is primarily dependent upon the absorption of high-energy photons by water and calcium salts within the body. X-rays are therefore very effective at imaging bony structures but less sensitive to soft tissue defects. The use of contrast materials based on x-ray absorbing substances such as barium and iodine allow visualization of the gastrointestinal tract, urinary tract, and cardiovascular system. X-ray techniques initially required a large x-ray generator and a film holder to obtain an image. More recently all-digital systems have been introduced reducing or eliminating the need for film.

Digital mammography has found widespread acceptance. Detectors used in digital mammography demonstrate significantly improved detective quantum efficiency curves compared with screen film mammography systems [1]. This improves the ability to detect fine, low-contrast detail at the same radiation dose or reduced dose to maintain the same level of image quality. A variety of digital mammography systems based on charge-couple devices, amorphous silicon technology, and amorphous selenium technology are on the market. Digital systems allow optimization of each stage in the imaging chain. Further image improvement is achieved through image processing techniques and the use of high-resolution displays. New imaging reconstruction techniques are currently being explored. However, x-ray imaging still requires the patient, the clinician, and the technicians to be exposed to radiation. The need for shielding and the desire for continuous imaging without the need for radiation stimulated the search for alternative imaging techniques.

Optical imaging techniques beyond direct physical observation were made feasible by the development of fiber optics and optical relay systems. Endoscopy, the use of optical imaging systems to look inside the body, makes use of the body's channels to gain access to hollow organs. Laparoscopy, arthroscopy, thoracoscopy, and other similar techniques distend potential spaces within the body, such as the abdominal cavity, joint cavities, and pleural spaces, to allow placement of a rigid telescope that brings light into the space and relays images out to the clinician. The development of small TV cameras which could be attached directly to the endoscope eliminated the need for the clinician to have his/her eye at the end of the endoscope. The creation of video endoscopy greatly facilitated the use of endoscopic techniques for both diagnostic and therapeutic purposes. As the endoscopes became more sophisticated the ability to guide procedures with these devices grew rapidly. In 1987 there were no laparoscopic cholecystectomies in the United States. The technique, which uses a rigid endoscope and a series of tools to operate within the peritoneal cavity, permits minimally invasive surgical removal of the gallbladder. By 1995 more than 550,000 laparoscopic cholecystectomies were performed yearly in the United States. Hospital stay decreased from 5–7 days to 1–2 days per patient with a concomitant reduction in need for pain medication and a dramatic decrease in overall costs of the procedure.

Flexible endoscopy has had a similar impact on the diagnosis and treatment of colonic polyps, esophageal stricture, and pulmonary biopsy procedures. Rigid endoscopy has been effectively applied to orthopedics, where it is used to inspect large and small joints and permits surgeons to perform repairs without opening the joint. As with other imaging modalities, the ability to observe and define pathology becomes the basis for the development of new therapeutic techniques. More than 10 million endoscopic procedures are performed annually in the United States. Optical techniques cannot see inside solid organs, and the ability to apply optical imaging is limited to those procedures that can be accomplished under direct visualization.

Ultrasound technologies can generate images of solid organs with mobile systems that do not require exposure to radiation. Ultrasound is particularly effective at imaging the heart, kidneys, liver, and other solid organs. Unfortunately, ultrasound does not effectively penetrate bone or air–water interfaces. Therefore imaging of the brain and lungs is rarely possible with ultrasonic techniques. Ultrasound can provide information on the flow of blood through arteries and veins, and Doppler techniques can identify the direction of flow. Fetal ultrasound is responsible for dramatic advances in the development of neonatal medicine and the treatment of congenital defects in utero. Recent developments in ultrasonic imaging include dramatic reductions in the size of the instruments, the ability to generate three-dimensional data sets, and the use of ultrasound to guide procedures such as breast and liver biopsies. As techniques have improved sensitivity has increased, and the ability to identify and localize pathologic tissue has increased. The development of all these techniques has, in general, shortened hospital stay and allowed for earlier and more accurate diagnosis of disease and development of more effective treatment plans.

Naqvi reported extensive use of three-dimensional ultrasound for cardiac procedures [2]. This technology provides the clinician with an effective presentation of cardiac structure, which allows bedside diagnosis. Echocardiography is the predominant imaging modality for assessing patients with congenital heart disease [3]. It is simple to use, provides high-resolution images with real-time feedback, and now allows characterization of myocardial strain rate. These data provide the clinician with a clear indication of cardiac function. Ultrasonography also provides precise anatomic information in the study of vascular occlusive disease, particularly in the analysis of carotid stenosis [4]. The development of contrast media for ultrasound is improving the ability of ultrasound to identify specific tissues and localize organs [5]. Miniaturized ultrasound transducers have extended high-resolution ultrasonic imaging to the vascular tree and the digestive tract. These new imaging formats provide a wealth of three-dimensional data on the structure of these anatomic systems.

Computed tomography (CT) scanning provided the first high-resolution, three-dimensional imaging capability. Two-dimensional slices were obtained and reassembled to form a three-dimensional reconstruction of solid organs. In the 1970s true three-dimensional images obtained in live patients became a reality. Over the last 35 years CT scanning has evolved and now employs helical and electron beam technologies to produce faster, more accurate scans. Advances in CT computer programs permit virtual endoscopic representations of the gastrointestinal tract, pulmonary tree, and cardiovascular tree. The ability to perform organ segmentation and generate three-dimensional reconstructions from two-dimensional slices is driving the development of both CT and MR colonography and CT bronchography, cystography, and arthrography. The American Gastroenterological Association studied the current status of CT colonography [6]. They concluded that it was an attractive imaging modality with a significant potential impact on the practice of gastroenterology. The report details the broad variability seen in the literature on the current effectiveness of this technology. Cotton et al. [7] concluded that the technology held promise but was not yet ready for widespread clinical application. As the technology improves these imaging technologies are likely to alter the current practice of medicine.

As the ability to image anatomic structures improved, clinicians desired techniques to monitor function of specific organs. Radiopharmaceuticals provided a means of obtaining images that were based on the physiologic function of an organ. The ability to define the functional status of multiple organs including the heart, the liver, the kidneys, the gallbladder, etc. allowed clinicians to correlate physiology with disease states. As radiopharmaceutical chemistry improved, the ability to make imaging agents for specific organs required the development of unique radionuclides. When linked to the right carrier molecule, radionuclides provide imaging agents for cardiac ischemia, breast cancer imaging, kidney function, and prostate cancer imaging. The principal limitation of these techniques is the inability to precisely define the location of the problem in a three-dimensional system.

Positron emission tomography (PET) was developed in part to address the limitations of standard radionuclide imaging. As detailed in the chapter by Budinger and VanBrocklin, PET scanning can generate two-dimensional images from a one-dimensional projection seen at different angles. These two-dimensional constructs can be assembled into a three-dimensional map.

The successes of x-ray, ultrasound, and radionuclide imaging demonstrated the value of these techniques in patient care, but the limitations of these techniques stimulated scientists to explore new methods of imaging. Magnetic resonance imaging (MRI) uses radiofrequency energy and oscillating electromagnetic fields to determine the chemical structure of materials within a magnetic field. This information is then processed to generate a three-dimensional reconstruction based on the signals obtained from excitation of the hydrogen nuclei, as detailed in Chapter 63. Like x-ray systems, MRI can be enhanced by the use of unique dyes. Under the proper conditions MRI imaging can give true three-dimensional data regarding a particular area within the body or provide data on the functional status of a particular tissue.

Functional magnetic resonance imaging (FMRI) uses blood oxygenation levels as a contrast medium. This technique has been applied to investigation of the brain. Recent studies have expanded the use of bold fMRI with the use of high-field (3.0 T or greater) magnets [8]. High-field magnetic resonance spectroscopy allows greater accuracy in quantitative measurements and decrease in voxel size. Improvements in MR spectroscopy improve our understanding of the organization of the brain. Diffusion tensor imaging allows MR imaging of actual fiber tracts within the brain. At high-field strength DTI techniques reveal the complexity of neuronal interconnections [9]. High-field MRI is gaining acceptance across a broad range of applications. Investigations have noted some unpleasant transient phenomena but no long-term sequelae from these intense magnetic fields. The increases in signal-to-noise lead to dramatic improvements in image quality. MRI angiography improves as vessels appear brighter and smaller vessels become visible. At 3 T the combination of improved background suppression and increased signal-to-noise extends the capability of MRA to the smaller vessels. Orthopedic and cardiac imaging are significantly improved as well. In higher magnetic fields it is possible to use phosphorus, carbon, sodium, and fluorine as the basis for imaging. Studies exploring the use of these nuclei are now feasible at higher fields [10].

Cardiac MRI is rapidly becoming the imaging modality of choice for studying cardiac structure, function, perfusion, and viability at the same time. In many situations it is superior to other modalities. Cardiac magnetic resonance has been applied to the diagnosis of aortic aneurismal disease, valvular heart disease, congenital heart disease, and ischemic heart disease. Cardiac MRI perfusion techniques are now competing with nuclear medicine techniques. Comprehensive assessment of the coronary arteries and functional status of the underlying ventricle has been shown to be feasible but is not yet routinely performed. Interventional techniques based on magnetic resonance fluoroscopy are of great interest to the cardiovascular community, but several significant hurdles, including the cost of the instrumentation, the need for nonmagnetic guidewires and stents, and the difficulty in defining small vessels, are only now being addressed [11].

Positron emission tomography (PET) allows for collection of functionally based images using 18F-FDG as a radiotracer. 18F-FDG permits detection of small tumors but is difficult to precisely locate. The challenge has been to fuse imaging techniques while retaining the advantages of each modality. PET scans are now routinely combined with CT scans. Recent articles by Goerres [12], Townsend [13], Gaa [14], Buscombe [15], Wahl [16], and Kim [17] demonstrate the trend of combining PET with CT or MRI. In each of these papers PET identifies an area of potential malignancy and the CT or MRI scan provides the anatomic details. Registration algorithms allow for precise localization of the PET data into the three-dimensional anatomic image constructed from the CT or MR data. PET/CT and PET/MRI improves the diagnostic accuracy compared to PET alone. The ability to integrate information is becoming critical to the patient care process [5]. Images are now moved through picture archiving and communications systems (PACS) via networks and work stations. The availability of fused data allows for greater precision in planning surgical procedures and radiation therapy.

Advances in digital or filmless systems and the use of flat panel displays has changed the design and improved the flexibility of the radiology suite. As digital radiography becomes more prominent archiving the information in digital form will become more commonplace. Systems that allow for long-range consulting, teleradiology, are being developed. Thus an individual with great skill, such as a pediatric orthopedic radiologist, can receive information from hundreds to thousands of miles away, interpret an image, and provide feedback to an emergency room physician.

The following chapters provide a concise review of the techniques, instrumentation, and applications involved in imaging systems: Chapter 10: x-ray equipment; Chapter 11: computed tomography (CT); Chapter 12: magnetic resonance imaging (MRI); Chapter 13: nuclear medicine; Chapter 14: ultrasound techniques; Chapter 15: magnetic resonance microscopy (MRM); Chapter 16: positron emission tomography (PET); Chapter 17: electrical impedance tomography (EIT).

Chapter 18 discusses medical applications of virtual reality (VR) technology, an area that is taking advantage of rapid advances in computer processing power and improved display techniques. VR applications including virtual colonoscopy, preoperative planning, surgical simulations, and training systems are the subject of detailed investigation to identify their role in healthcare. While still in their infancy these technologies will drive development of less invasive technologies and improve the outcome of surgical procedures.

References

[1] James J.J. The current status of digital mammography. *Clin. Radiol.* 2004, 59: 1–10.

[2] Naqvi T.Z. Recent advances in echocardiography. *Expert. Rev. Cardiovasc. Ther.* 2004, 2: 89–96.

[3] Pignatelli R.H., McMahon C.J., Chung T., and Vick G.W. III. Role of echocardiography versus MRI for the diagnosis of congenital heart disease. *Curr. Opin. Cardiol.* 2003, 18: 357–365.

[4] Nederkoorn P.J., van der Graaf Y., and Hunink M.G. Duplex ultrasound and magnetic resonance angiography compared with subtraction angiography in carotid artery stenosis: a systematic review. *Stroke*, 2003, 34: 1324–1332. Epub 2003 Apr 10.

[5] Margulis A.R. and Sunshine J.H. Radiology at the Turn of the Millennium. *Radiology* 2000, 214: 15–23.

[6] van Dam J., Cotton P., Johnson C.D., McFarland B. et al. American Gastroenterological Association. AGA future trends report: CT colonography. *Gastroenterology* 2004, 127.

[7] Cotton P.B., Durkalski V.L., Pineau B.C. et al. Computed tomographic colonography (virtual colonoscopy): a multicenter comparison with standard colonoscopy for detection of colorectal neoplasia. *JAMA* 2004, 291.

[8] Kim D.S. and Garwood M. High-field magnetic resonance techniques for brain research. *Curr. Opin. Neurobiol.* 2003, 13, 612–619.

[9] Takahashi M., Uematsu H., and Hatabu H. MR imaging at high magnetic fields. *Eur. J. Radiol.* 2003, 46: 45–52.

[10] Hu X. and Norris D.G. Advances in high-field magnetic resonance imaging. *Ann. Rev. Biomed. Eng.* 2004, 6: 157–184.

[11] Constantine G., Shan K., Flamm S.D., and Sivananthan M.U. Role of MRI in clinical cardiology. *Lancet* 2004, 363: 2162–2171.

[12] Goerres G.W., von Schulthess G.K., and Steinert H.C. Why Most PET of lung and head-and-neck cancer will be PET/CT. *J. Nuc. Med.* 2004, 45: 66S–71S.

[13] Townsend D.W., Carney J.P.J., Yap J.T., and Hall N.C. PET/CT today and tomorrow. *J. Nuclear Med.* 2004, 45: 4S–14S.

[14] Gaa J., Rummeny E.J., and Seemann M.D. Whole-body imaging with PET/MRI. *Eur. J. Med. Res.* 2004, 9: 309–312.

[15] Buscombe J.R., Holloway B., Roche N., and Bombardieri E. Position of nuclear medicine modalities in the diagnostic work-up of breast cancer. *Quant. J. Nuclear Med. Mol. Imaging.* 2004, 48: 109–118.

[16] Wahl R.L. Why nearly all pet of abdominal and pelvic cancers will be performed as PET/CT. *J. Nuclear Med.* 2004, 45: 82S–95S.

[17] Kim E.E. Whole-body positron emission tomography and positron emission tomography/computed tomography in gynecologic oncology. *Int. J. Gyn. Cancer* 2004, 14: 12.

10

X-Ray

10.1	X-Ray Equipment	10-1
	Production of X-Rays • Image Detection: Screen Film Combinations • Image Detection: X-Ray Image Intensifiers with Televisions • Image Detection: Digital Systems	
	Defining Terms	10-7
	References	10-7
	Further Information	10-8
10.2	X-Ray Projection Angiography	10-8
	X-Ray Generation • Image Formation • Digital Angiography • Summary	
	Defining Terms	10-18
	References	10-18
	Further Information	10-19
10.3	Mammography	10-19
	Principles of Mammography • Physics of Image Formation • Equipment • Quality Control • Stereotactic Biopsy Devices • Digital Mammography • Summary	
	Defining Terms	10-34
	References	10-34
	Further Information	10-35

Robert E. Shroy, Jr.
Picker International

Michael S. Van Lysel
University of Wisconsin

Martin J. Yaffe
University of Toronto

10.1 X-Ray Equipment

Robert E. Shroy, Jr.

Conventional x-ray radiography produces images of anatomy that are shadowgrams based on x-ray absorption. The x-rays are produced in a region that is nearly a point source and then are directed on the anatomy to be imaged. The x-rays emerging from the anatomy are detected to form a two-dimensional image, where each point in the image has a brightness related to the intensity of the x-rays at that point. Image production relies on the fact that significant numbers of x-rays penetrate through the anatomy and that different parts of the anatomy absorb different amounts of x-rays. In cases where the anatomy of interest does not absorb x-rays differently from surrounding regions, contrast may be increased by introducing strong x-ray absorbers. For example, barium is often used to image the gastrointestinal tract.

X-rays are electromagnetic waves (like light) having an energy in the general range of approximately one to several hundred kiloelectronvolts (**keV**). In medical x-ray imaging, the x-ray energy typically lies between 5 and 150 keV, with the energy adjusted to the anatomic thickness and the type of study being performed.

X-rays striking an object may either pass through unaffected or may undergo an interaction. These interactions usually involve either the photoelectric effect (where the x-ray is absorbed) or scattering (where the x-ray is deflected to the side with a loss of some energy). X-rays that have been scattered may undergo deflection through a small angle and still reach the image detector; in this case they reduce image contrast and thus degrade the image. This degradation can be reduced by the use of an air gap between the anatomy and the image receptor or by use of an **antiscatter grid**.

Because of health effects, the doses in radiography are kept as low as possible. However, x-ray quantum noise becomes more apparent in the image as the dose is lowered. This noise is due to the fact that there is an unavoidable random variation in the number of x-rays reaching a point on an image detector. The quantum noise depends on the average number of x-rays striking the image detector and is a fundamental limit to radiographic image quality.

The equipment of conventional x-ray radiography mostly deals with the creation of a desirable beam of x-rays and with the detection of a high-quality image of the transmitted x-rays. These are discussed in the following sections.

10.1.1 Production of X-Rays

10.1.1.1 X-Ray Tube

The standard device for production of x-rays is the rotating anode x-ray tube, as illustrated in Figure 10.1. The x-rays are produced from electrons that have been accelerated in vacuum from the cathode to the anode. The electrons are emitted from a filament mounted within a groove in the cathode. Emission occurs when the filament is heated by passing a current through it. When the filament is hot enough, some electrons obtain a thermal energy sufficient to overcome the energy binding the electron to the metal of the filament. Once the electrons have "boiled off" from the filament, they are accelerated by a voltage difference applied from the cathode to the anode. This voltage is supplied by a generator (see Section 10.1.1.2).

After the electrons have been accelerated to the anode, they will be stopped in a short distance. Most of the electrons' energy is converted into heating of the anode, but a small percentage is converted to x-rays by two main methods. One method of x-ray production relies on the fact that deceleration of a charged particle results in emission of electromagnetic radiation, called bremmstrahlung radiation. These x-rays will have a wide, continuous distribution of energies, with the maximum being the total energy

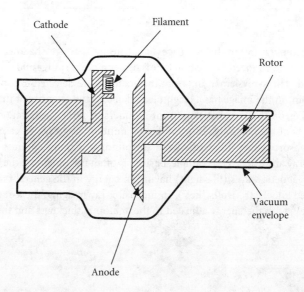

FIGURE 10.1   X-ray tube.

the electron had when reaching the anode. The number of x-rays is relatively small at higher energies and increases for lower energies.

A second method of x-ray production occurs when an accelerated electron strikes an atom in the anode and removes an inner electron from this atom. The vacant electron orbital will be filled by a neighboring electron, and an x-ray may be emitted whose energy matches the energy change of the electron. The result is production of large numbers of x-rays at a few discrete energies. Since the energy of these characteristic x-rays depends on the material on the surface of the anode, materials are chosen partially to produce x-rays with desired energies. For example, molybdenum is frequently used in anodes of mammography x-ray tubes because of its 20-keV characteristic x-rays.

Low-energy x-rays are undesirable because they increase dose to the patient but do not contribute to the final image because they are almost totally absorbed. Therefore, the number of low-energy x-rays is usually reduced by use of a layer of absorber that preferentially absorbs them. The extent to which low-energy x-rays have been removed can be quantified by the **half-value layer** of the x-ray beam.

It is ideal to create x-rays from a point source because any increase in source size will result in blurring of the final image. Quantitatively, the effects of the blurring are described by the **focal spot**'s contribution to the system **modulation transfer function (MTF)**. The blurring has its main effect on edges and small objects, which correspond to the higher frequencies. The effect of this blurring depends on the geometry of the imaging and is worse for larger distances between the object and the image receptor (which corresponds to larger geometric magnifications).

To avoid this blurring, the electrons must be focused to strike a small spot of the anode. The focusing is achieved by electric fields determined by the exact shape of the cathode. However, there is a limit to the size of this focal spot because the anode material will melt if too much power is deposited into too small an area. This limit is improved by use of a rotating anode, where the anode target material is rotated about a central axis and new (cooler) anode material is constantly being rotated into place at the focal spot. To further increase the power limit, the anode is made with an angle surface. This allows the heat to be deposited in a relatively large spot while the apparent spot size at the detector will be smaller by a factor of the sine of the anode angle. Unfortunately, this angle cannot be made too small because it limits the area that can be covered with x-rays. In practice, tubes are usually supplied with two (or more) focal spots of differing sizes, allowing choice of a smaller (sharper, lower-power) spot or a larger (more blurry, higher-power) spot.

The x-ray tube also limits the total number of x-rays that can be used in an exposure because the anode will melt if too much total energy is deposited in it. This limit can be increased by using a more massive anode.

10.1.1.2 Generator

The voltages and currents in an x-ray tube are supplied by an x-ray generator. This controls the cathode-anode voltage, which partially defines the number of x-rays made because the number of x-rays produced increases with voltage. The voltage is also chosen to produce x-rays with desired energies: higher voltages makes x-rays that generally are more penetrating but give a lower contrast image. The generator also determines the number of x-rays created by controlling the amount of current flowing from the cathode to anode and by controlling the length of time this current flows. This points out the two major parameters that describe an x-ray exposure: the peak kilovolts (peak kilovolts from the anode to the cathode during the exposure) and the milliampere-seconds (the product of the current in milliamperes and the exposure time in seconds).

The peak kilovolts and milliampere-seconds for an exposure may be set manually by an operator based on estimates of the anatomy. Some generators use manual entry of kilovolts and milliamperes but determine the exposure time automatically. This involves sampling the radiation either before or after the image sensor and is referred to as phototiming.

The anode–cathode voltage (often 15 to 150 kV) can be produced by a transformer that converts 120 or 220 V ac to higher voltages. This output is then rectified and filtered. Use of three-phase transformers gives voltages that are nearly constant versus those from single-phase transformers, thus avoiding low kilovoltages that produce undesired low-energy x-rays. In a variation of this method, the transformer output can be controlled at a constant voltage by electron tubes. This gives practically constant voltages and, further, allows the voltage to be turned on and off so quickly that millisecond exposure times can be achieved. In a third approach, an ac input can be rectified and filtered to produce a nearly dc voltage, which is then sent to a solid-state inverter that can turn on and off thousands of times a second. This higher-frequency ac voltage can be converted more easily to a high voltage by a transformer. Equipment operating on this principle is referred to as midfrequency or high-frequency generators.

10.1.2 Image Detection: Screen Film Combinations

Special properties are needed for image detection in radiographic applications, where a few high-quality images are made in a study. Because decisions are not immediately made from the images, it is not necessary to display them instantly (although it may be desirable).

The most commonly used method of detecting such a radiographic x-ray image uses light-sensitive negative film as a medium. Because high-quality film has a poor response to x-rays, it must be used together with x-ray-sensitive screens. Such screens are usually made with $CaWo_2$ or phosphors using rare earth elements such as doped Gd_2O_2S or LaOBr. The film is enclosed in a light-tight cassette in contact with an x-ray screen or in between two x-ray screens. When a x-ray image strikes the cassette, the x-rays are absorbed by the screens with high efficiency, and their energy is converted to visible light. The light then exposes a negative image on the film, which is in close contact with the screen.

Several properties have been found to be important in describing the relative performance of different films. One critical property is the contrast, which describes the amount of additional darkening caused by an additional amount of light when working near the center of a film's exposure range. Another property, the latitude of a film, describes the film's ability to create a usable image with a wide range in input light levels. Generally, latitude and contrast are competing properties, and a film with a large latitude will have a low contrast. Additionally, the modulation transfer function (MTF) of a film is an important property. MTF is most degraded at higher frequencies; this high-frequency MTF is also described by the film's resolution, its ability to image small objects.

X-ray screens also have several key performance parameters. It is essential that screens detect and use a large percentage of the x-rays striking them, which is measured as the screen's **quantum detection efficiency**. Currently used screens may detect 30% of x-rays for images at higher peak kilovolts and as much 60% for lower peak kilovolt images. Such efficiencies lead to the use of two screens (one on each side of the film) for improved x-ray utilization. As with films, a good high-frequency MTF is needed to give good visibility of small structures and edges. Some MTF degradation is associated with blurring that occurs when light spreads as it travels through the screen and to the film. This leads to a compromise on thickness; screens must be thick enough for good quantum detection efficiency but thin enough to avoid excess blurring.

For a film/screen system, a certain amount of radiation will be required to produce a usable amount of film darkening. The ability of the film/screen system to make an image with a small amount of radiation is referred to as its speed. The speed depends on a number of parameters: the quantum detection efficiency of the screen, the efficiency with which the screen converts x-ray energy to light, the match between the color emitted by the screen and the colors to which the film is sensitive, and the amount of film darkening for a given amount of light. The number of x-rays used in producing a radiographic image will be chosen to give a viewable amount of exposure to the film. Therefore, patient dose will be reduced by the use of a high-speed screen/film system. However, high-speed film/screen combinations gives a "noisier" image because of the smaller number of x-rays detected in its creation.

10.1.3 Image Detection: X-Ray Image Intensifiers with Televisions

Although screen-film systems are excellent for radiography, they are not usable for fluoroscopy, where lower x-ray levels are produced continuously and many images must be presented almost immediately.

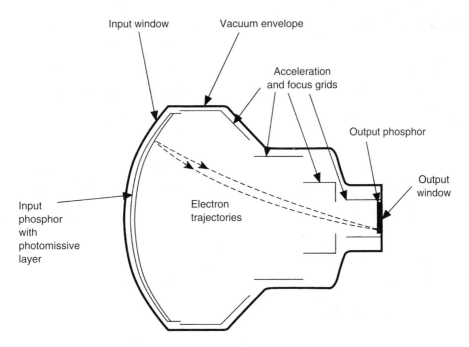

Input window

Vacuum envelope

Acceleration
and focus grids

Output phosphor

Output
window

Input
phosphor
with
photomissive
layer

Electron
trajectories

FIGURE 10.2 X-ray image intensifier.

Fluoroscopic images are not used for diagnosis but rather as an aid in performing tasks such as placement of catheters in blood vessels during angiography. For fluoroscopy, x-ray image intensifiers are used in conjunction with television cameras. An x-ray image intensifier detects the x-ray image and converts it to a small, bright image of visible light. This visible image is then transferred by lenses to a television camera for final display on a monitor.

The basic structure of an x-ray image intensifier is shown in Figure 10.2. The components are held in a vacuum by an enclosure made of glass and/or metal. The x-rays enter through a low-absorption window and then strike an input phosphor usually made of doped Cesium iodide (CsI). As in the x-ray screens described above, the x-rays are converted to light in the CsI. On top of the CsI layer is a photoemitter, which absorbs the light and emits a number of low-energy electrons that initially spread in various directions. The photoelectrons are accelerated and steered by a set of grids that have voltages applied to them. The electrons strike an output phosphor structure that converts their energy to the final output image made of light. This light then travels through an output window to a lens system. The grid voltages serve to add energy to the electrons so that the output image is brighter. Grid voltages and shapes are also chosen so that the x-ray image is converted to a light image with minimal distortion. Further, the grids must be designed to take photoelectrons that are spreading from a point on the photoemitter and focus them back together at a point on the output phosphor.

It is possible to adjust grid voltages on an image intensifier so that it has different fields of coverage. Either the whole input area can be imaged on the output phosphor, or smaller parts of the input can be imaged on the whole output. Use of smaller parts of the input is advantageous when only smaller parts of anatomy need to be imaged with maximum resolution and a large display. For example, an image intensifier that could cover a 12-in.-diameter input also might be operated so that a 9-in.-diameter or 6-in.-diameter input covers all the output phosphor.

X-ray image intensifiers can be described by a set of performance parameters not unlike those of screen/film combinations. It is important that x-rays be detected and used with a high efficiency; current image intensifiers have quantum detection efficiencies of 60 to 70% for 59-keV x-rays. As with film/screens, a good high-frequency MTF is needed to image small objects and sharp edges without blurring. However, low-frequency MTF also must be controlled carefully in image intensifiers, since it can be degraded by internal scattering of x-rays, photoelectrons, and light over relatively large distances. The amount of intensification depends on brightness and size of the output image for a given x-ray input. This is described either by the gain (specified relative to a standard x-ray screen) or by conversion efficiency (a light output per radiation input measured in $(cd/m^2)/(mR/min)$). Note that producing a smaller output image is as important as making a light image with more photons because the small image can be handled more efficiently by the lenses that follow. Especially when imaging the full input area, image intensifiers introduce a pincushion distortion into the output image. Thus a square object placed off-center will produce an image that is stretched in the direction away from the center.

Although an image intensifier output could be viewed directly with a lens system, there is more flexibility when the image intensifier is viewed with a television camera and the output is displayed on a monitor. Televisions are currently used with pickup tubes and with CCD sensors.

When a television tube is used, the image is focused on a charged photoconducting material at the tube's input. A number of materials are used, including SbS_3, PbO, and $SeTeAs$. The light image discharges regions of the photoconductor, converting the image to a charge distribution on the back of the photoconducting layer. Next, the charge distribution is read by scanning a small beam of electrons across the surface, which recharges the photoconductor. The recharging current is proportional to the light intensity at the point being scanned; this current is amplified and then used to produce an image on a monitor. The tube target is generally scanned in an interlaced mode in order to be consistent with broadcast television and allow use of standard equipment.

In fluoroscopy, it is desirable to use the same detected dose for all studies so that the image noise is approximately constant. This is usually achieved by monitoring the image brightness in a central part of the image intensifier's output, since brightness generally increases with dose. The brightness may be monitored by a photomultiplier tube that samples it directly or by analyzing signal levels in the television. However, maintaining a constant detected dose would lead to high patient doses in the case of very absorptive anatomy. To avoid problems here, systems are generally required by federal regulations to have a limit on the maximum patient dose. In those cases where the dose limit prevents the image intensifier from receiving the usual dose, the output image becomes darker. To compensate for this, television systems are often operated with automatic gain control that gives an image on the monitor of a constant brightness no matter what the brightness from the image intensifier.

10.1.4 Image Detection: Digital Systems

In both radiography and fluoroscopy, there are advantages to the use of digital images. This allows image processing for better displayed images, use of lower doses in some cases, and opens the possibility for digital storage with a PACS system or remote image viewing via teleradiology. Additionally, some digital systems provide better image quality because of fewer processing steps, lack of distortion, or improved uniformity.

A common method of digitizing medical x-ray images uses the voltage output from an image-intensifier/TV system. This voltage can be digitized by an analog-to-digital converter at rates fast enough to be used with fluoroscopy as well as radiography.

Another technology for obtaining digital radiographs involves use of photostimulable phosphors. Here the x-rays strike an enclosed sheet of phosphor that stores the x-ray energy. This phorphor can then be taken to a read-out unit, where the phosphor surface is scanned by a small light beam of proper wavelength. As a point on the surface is read, the stored energy is emitted as visible light, which is then detected, amplified, and digitized. Such systems have the advantage that they can be used with existing systems designed for screen-film detection because the phosphor sheet package is the same size as that for screen films.

A new method for digital detection involves use of active-matrix thin-film-transistor technology, in which an array of small sensors is grown in hydrogenated amorphous silicon. Each sensor element includes an electrode for storing charge that is proportional to its x-ray signal. Each electrode is coupled to a transistor that either isolates it during acquisition or couples it to digitization circuitry during read-out. There are two common methods for introducing the charge signal on each electrode. In one method, a layer of x-ray absorber (typically selenium) is deposited on the array of sensors; when this layer is biased and x-rays are absorbed there, their energy is converted to electron-hole pairs and the resulting charge is collected on the electrode. In the second method, each electrode is part of the photodiode that makes electron-hole pairs when exposed to light; the light is produced from x-rays by a layer of scintillator (such as CsI) that is deposited on the array.

Use of a digital system provides several advantages in fluoroscopy. The digital image can be processed in real time with edge enhancement, smoothing, or application of a median filter. Also, frame-to-frame averaging can be used to decrease image noise, at the expense of blurring the image of moving objects. Further, digital fluoroscopy with TV system allows the TV tube to be scanned in formats that are optimized for read-out; the image can still be shown in a different format that is optimized for display. Another advantage is that the displayed image is not allowed to go blank when x-ray exposure is ended, but a repeated display of the last image is shown. This last-image-hold significantly reduces doses in those cases where the radiologist needs to see an image for evaluation, but does not necessarily need a continuously updated image.

The processing of some digital systems also allows the use of pulsed fluoroscopy, where the x-rays are produced in a short, intense burst instead of continuously. In this method the pulses of x-rays are made either by biasing the x-ray tube filament or by quickly turning on and off the anode–cathode voltage. This has the advantage of making sharper images of objects that are moving. Often one x-ray pulse is produced for every display frame, but there is also the ability to obtain dose reduction by leaving the x-rays off for some frames. With such a reduced exposure rate, doses can be reduced by a factor of two or four by only making x-rays every second or fourth frame. For those frames with no x-ray pulse, the system repeats a display of the last frame with x-rays.

Defining Terms

Antiscatter grid: A thin structure made of alternating strips of lead and material transmissive to x-rays. Strips are oriented so that most scattered x-rays go through lead sections and are preferentially absorbed, while unscattered x-rays go through transmissive sections.

Focal spot: The small area on the anode of an x-ray tube from where x-rays are emitted. It is the place where the accelerated electron beam is focused.

Half-value layer (HVL): The thickness of a material (often aluminum) needed to absorb half the x-ray in a beam.

keV: A unit of energy useful with x-rays. It is equal to the energy supplied to an electron when accelerated through 1 kV.

Modulation transfer function (MTF): The ratio of the contrast in the output image of a system to the contrast in the object, specified for sine waves of various frequencies. Describes blurring (loss of contrast) in an imaging system for different-sized objects.

Quantum detection efficiency: The percentage of incident x-rays effectively used to create an image.

References

Bushberg, J.T., Seibert, J.A., Leidholdt, E.M., and Boone, J.M. 1994. The *Essential Physics of Medical Imaging*. Baltimore, Williams and Wilksins.

Curry, T.S., Dowdey, J.E., and Murry, R.C. 1984. *Christensen's Introduction to the Physics of Diagnostic Radiology*. Philadelphia, Lea and Febiger.

Hendee, W.R. and Ritenour, R. 1992. *Medical Imaging Physics*. St. Louis, Mosby-Year Book.

Ter-Pogossian, M.M. 1969. *The Physical Aspects of Diagnostic Radiology*. New York, Harper and Row.

Further Information

Medical Physics is a monthly scientific and informational journal published for the American Association of Physicists in Medicine. Papers here generally cover evaluation of existing medical equipment and development of new systems. For more information, contact the American Association of Physicists in Medicine, One Physics Ellipse, College Park, MD 20740-3846.

The Society of Photo-Optical Instrumentation Engineers (SPIE) sponsors numerous conferences and publishes their proceedings. Especially relevant is the *annual conference on Medical Imaging*. Contact SPIE, P.O. Box 10, Bellham, WA 98277-0010.

Several corporations active in medical imaging work together under the National Electrical Manufacturers Association to develop definitions and testing standards for equipment used in the field. Information can be obtained from NEMA, 2101 L Street, N.W., Washington, DC 20037.

Critical aspects of medical x-ray imaging are covered by rules of the Food and Drug Administration, part of the Department of Health and Human Services. These are listed in the *Code of Federal Regulations*, Title 21. Copies are for sale by the Superintendent of Documents, U.S. Government Printing Office, Washington, DC 20402.

10.2   X-Ray Projection Angiography

Michael S. Van Lysel

Angiography is a diagnostic and, increasingly, therapeutic modality concerned with diseases of the circulatory system. While many imaging modalities (ultrasound, computed tomography, magnetic resonance imaging, angioscopy) are now available, either clinically or for research, to study vascular structures, this section will focus on projection radiography. In this method, the vessel of interest is opacified by injection of a radiopaque contrast agent. Serial radiographs of the contrast material flowing through the vessel are then acquired. This examination is performed in an angiographic suite, a special procedures laboratory, or a cardiac catheterization laboratory.

Contrast material is needed to opacify vascular structures because the radiographic contrast of blood is essentially the same as that of soft tissue. Contrast material consists of an iodine-containing ($Z = 53$) compound, with maximum iodine concentrations of about 350 mg/cm^3. Contrast material is injected through a catheter ranging in diameter roughly from 1 to 3 mm, depending on the injection flow rate to be used. Radiographic images of the contrast-filled vessels are recorded using either film or video.

Digital imaging technology has become instrumental in the acquisition and storage of angiographic images. The most important application of digital imaging is **digital subtraction angiography (DSA)**. **Temporal subtraction** is a DSA model in which a preinjection image (the mask) is acquired, the injection of contrast agent is then performed, and the sequential images of the opacified vessel(s) are acquired and subtracted from the mask. The result, ideally, is that the fixed anatomy is canceled, allowing contrast enhancement (similar to computed tomographic windowing and leveling) to provide increased contrast sensitivity.

An increasingly important facet of the angiographic procedure is the use of transluminal interventional techniques to effect a therapeutic result. These techniques, including angioplasty, atherectomy, laser ablation, and intraluminal stents, rely on digital angiographic imaging technology to facilitate the precise catheter manipulations necessary for a successful result. In fact, digital enhancement, storage, and retrieval of fluoroscopic images have become mandatory capabilities for digital angiographic systems.

Figure 10.3 is a schematic representation of an angiographic imaging system. The basic components include an x-ray tube and generator, image intensifier, video camera, cine camera (optional for cardiac imaging), and digital image processor.

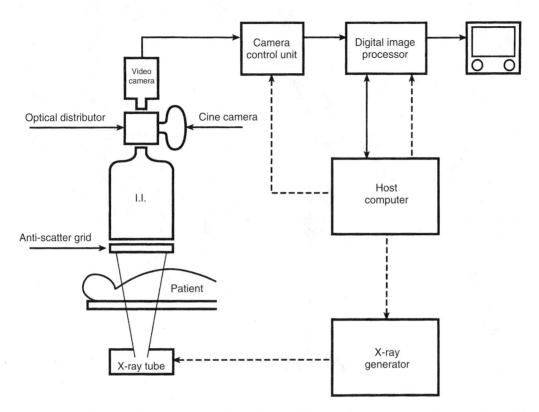

FIGURE 10.3 Schematic diagram of an image intensifier-based digital angiographic and cine imaging system. Solid arrows indicate image signals, and dotted arrows indicate control signals.

10.2.1 X-Ray Generation

Angiographic systems require a high-power, sophisticated x-ray generation system in order to produce the short, intense x-ray pulses needed to produce clear images of moving vessels. Required exposure times range from 100 to 200 msec for cerebral studies to 1 to 10 msec for cardiac studies. Angiographic systems use either a constant potential generator, or, increasingly, a medium/high-frequency inverter generator. Power ratings for angiographic generators are generally greater than or equal to 80 kW at 100 kW and must be capable of producing reasonably square x-ray pulses. In most cases (pediatric cardiology being an exception), pulse widths of 5 msec or greater are necessary to keep the x-ray tube potential in the desirable, high-contrast range of 70 to 90 kVp.

The x-ray tube is of the rotating-anode variety. Serial runs of high-intensity x-ray pulses result in high heat loads. Anode heat storage capacities of 1 mega-heat units (MHU) or greater are required, especially in the case of cine angiography. Electronic "heat computers," which calculate and display the current heat load of the x-ray tube, are very useful in preventing damage to the x-ray tube. In a high-throughput angiographic suite, forced liquid cooling of the x-ray tube housing is essential. Angiographic x-ray tubes are of multifocal design, with the focal spot sizes tailored for the intended use. A 0.6-mm (50-kW loading), 1.2-mm (100-kW loading) bifocal insert is common. The specified heat loads for a given focal spot are for single exposures. When serial angiographic exposures are performed, the focal spot load limit must be derated (reduced) to account for the accumulation of heat in the focal spot target during the run. Larger focal spots (e.g., 1.8 mm) can be obtained for high-load procedures. A smaller focal spot (e.g., 0.3 and 0.1 mm [bias]) is needed for magnification studies. Small focal spots have become increasingly desirable for high-resolution fluoroscopic interventional studies performed with 1000-line video systems.

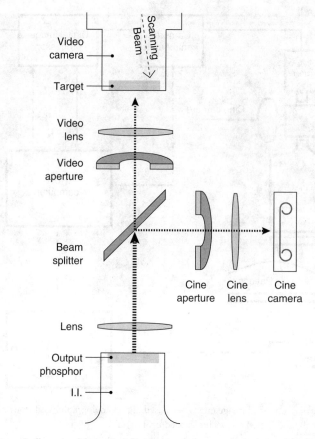

FIGURE 10.4 Schematic diagram of the optical distributor used to couple the image intensifier (I.I.) output phosphor to a video and cine camera. (From Van Lysel, M.S. In S. Baum (ed.), *Abrams' Angiography*, 4th ed. Boston, Little, Brown. With permission.)

10.2.2 Image Formation

10.2.2.1 Film

From the 1950s to 1980s, the dominant detector system used for recording the angiographic procedure was film/screen angiography using a rapid film changer [Amplatz, 1997]. However, digital angiography, described below, has almost completely replaced this technology. Film provides a higher spatial resolution than digital. However, as the spatial resolution of digital continues to improve, the overwhelming advantages of ease of use and image processing algorithms have prevailed. While film changers can still be found in use, few new film/screen systems are being purchased.

One application where film use is still common is cardiac imaging. Cine angiography is performed with a 35-mm motion picture camera optically coupled to the image intensifier output phosphor (Figure 10.4). The primary clinical application is coronary angiography and ventriculography. During cine angiography, x-ray pulses are synchronized both with the cine camera shutter and the vertical retrace of the system video camera. To limit motion blurring, it is desirable to keep the x-ray pulses as short as possible, but no longer than 10 msec.

Imaging runs generally last from 5 to 10 sec in duration at a frame rate of 30 to 60 frames/sec (fps). Sixty fps is generally used for pediatric studies, where higher heart rates are encountered, while 30 fps is more typical for adult studies ("digital cine," discussed below, generally is performed at 15 fps). Some cine angiographic installations provide biplane imaging in which two independent imaging chains can acquire orthogonal images of the injection sequence. The eccentricity of coronary lesions and the asymmetric nature of cardiac contraction abnormalities require that multiple x-ray projections be acquired. Biplane systems allow this to be done with a smaller patient contrast load. For this reason, biplane systems are considered a requirement for pediatric cath labs. They are relatively uncommon for adult cath labs, however, where the less complicated positioning of a single plane system is often valued over the reduced number of injections possible with a biplane system. The AP and lateral planes of a biplane system are energized out of phase, which results in the potential for image degradation due to detection of the radiation scattered from the opposite plane. Image intensifier blanking, which shuts down the accelerating voltage of the nonimaging plane, is used to eliminate this problem.

While film remains in common use for cardiac imaging, here too the medium is being replaced by digital. Digital angiographic systems (described below) were integrated into the cardiac catheterization imaging system beginning in the 1980s, to provide short term image storage and replay. However, the high resolution and frame rate required for cardiac imaging precluded the use of digital hardware for long-term (greater than one day) storage. Film and cine are acquired simultaneously using the beam splitting mirror in the optical distributor (Figure 10.4). This situation is rapidly changing, as high-speed video servers and the recordable compact disc (CD-R) now provide acceptable performance for this application. Most new cardiac imaging systems are purchased without a cine film camera.

10.2.2.2   Image Intensifier/Video Camera

The image intensifier (II) is fundamental to the modern angiographic procedure. The purpose of the image intensifier is (1) to produce a light image with sufficient brightness to allow the use of video and film cameras and (2) to produce an output image of small enough size to allow convenient coupling to video and film cameras. The image intensifier provides both real-time imaging capability (fluoroscopy), which allows patient positioning and catheter manipulation, and recording of the angiographic injection (digital angiography, analog video recording, photospot, cine).

Image intensifier output phosphors are approximately 25 mm in diameter, although large (e.g., 50 to 60 mm) output phosphor image intensifiers have been developed to increase spatial resolution. The modulation transfer function (MTF) of the image intensifier is determined primarily by the input and output phosphor stages, so mapping a given input image to a larger output phosphor will improve the MTF of the system. The input phosphor of a modern image intensifier is cesium iodide (CsI). The largest currently available image intensifier input phosphors are approximately 16 in. The effective input phosphor diameter is selectable by the user. For example, an image intensifier designated 9/7/5 allows the user to select input phosphor diameters of 9, 7, or 5 in. These selections are referred to as image intensifier modes. The purpose of providing an adjustable input phosphor is to allow the user to trade off between spatial resolution and field of view. A smaller mode provides higher spatial resolution both because the MTF of the image intensifier improves and because it maps a smaller field of view to the fixed size of the video camera target. Generally speaking, angiographic suites designed exclusively for cardiac catheterization use 9-in. image intensifiers, neuroangiography suites use 12-in. intensifiers, while suites that must handle pulmonary, renal, or peripheral angiography require the larger (i.e., 14 to 16 in.) intensifiers.

The brightness gain of the image intensifier derives from two sources (1) the increase in electron energy produced by the accelerating potential (the flux gain) and (2) the decrease in size of the image as it is transferred from the input to the output phosphor (the minification gain). The product of these two factors can exceed 5000. However, since the minification gain is a function of the area of the input phosphor exposed to the radiation beam (i.e., the image intensifier mode), the brightness gain drops as smaller image intensifier modes are selected. This is compensated for by a combination of increasing x-ray exposure to maintain the image intensifier light output and opening the video camera aperture. Image intensifier brightness gain declines with age and must be monitored to allow timely replacement. The specification used for this purpose is the image intensifier conversion factor, defined as the light output of the image intensifier per unit x-ray exposure input. Modern image intensifiers have a conversion factor of 100 cd/m^2/mR/sec or more for the 9-in. mode.

With the increasing emergence of digital angiography as the primary angiographic imaging modality, image intensifier performance has become increasingly important. In the field, the high-spatial-frequency of an image intensifier is assessed by determining the limiting resolution [in the neighborhood of 4 to 5 line-pairs/mm (lp/mm) in the 9-in. mode], while the low-spatial-frequency response is assessed using the contrast ratio (in the neighborhood of 15 : 1 to 30 : 1). The National Electrical Manufacturers Association (NEMA) has defined test procedures for measuring the contrast ratio [NEMA, 1992]. The detective quantum efficiency (DQE), which is a measure of the efficiency with which the image intensifier utilizes the x-ray energy incident on it, is in the neighborhood of 65% (400 μm phosphor thickness, 60 keV). A tabulation of the specifications of several commercially available image intensifiers has been published by Siedband [1994].

10.2.2.3 Optical Distributor

The image present at the image intensifier output phosphor is coupled to the video camera, and any film camera present (e.g., cine), by the optical distributor. The components of the distributor are shown in Figure 10.4. There is an aperture for each camera to allow the light intensity presented to each camera to be adjusted independently. The video camera aperture is usually a motor-driven variable iris, while the film camera aperture is usually fixed. It is important to realize that while the aperture does ensure that the proper light level is presented to the camera, more fundamentally, the aperture determines the x-ray exposure input to the image intensifier. As a result, both the patient exposure and the level of quantum noise in the image are set by the aperture. The noise amplitude in a fluoroscopic or digital angiographic image is inversely proportional to the f-number of the optical system. Because the quantum sink of a properly adjusted fluorographic system is at the input of the image intensifier, the aperture diameter is set, for a given type of examination, to provide the desired level of quantum mottle present in the image. The x-ray exposure factors are then adjusted for each patient, by an automatic exposure control (AEC) system, to produce the proper postaperture light level. However, some video systems do provide for increasing the video camera aperture during fluoroscopy when the maximum entrance exposure does not provide adequate light levels on a large patient.

The beam-splitting mirror was originally meant to provide a moderate-quality video image simultaneous with cine recording in order to monitor the contrast injection during cardiac studies. More recently, as the importance of digital angiography has mushroomed, precision-quality mirrors with higher transmission have been used in order to provide simultaneous diagnostic-quality cine and video. The latest development has been the introduction of *cine-less* digital cardiac systems, in which the video image is the sole recording means. The introduction of these systems has sometimes been accompanied by the claim that a *cine-less* system requires less patient exposure due to the fact that light does not have to be provided to the cine camera. However, a conventional cine system operates with an excess of light (i.e., the cine camera aperture is stopped down). Because the image intensifier input is the quantum sink of the system, exposure is determined by the need to limit quantum mottle, not to maintain a given light level at the image intensifier output. Therefore, the validity of this claim is dubious. It should be noted, however, that because of the difference in spatial resolution capabilities of cine and video, the noise power spectrum of images acquired with equal exposure will be different. It is possible that observers accept a lower exposure in a video image than in the higher-resolution film image.

10.2.2.4 Video System

The video system in an angiographic suite consists of several components, including the camera head, camera control unit (CCU), video monitors, and video recording devices. In addition, a digital image processor is integrated with the video system.

The video camera is responsible for signal generation. Traditionally, pickup-tube based cameras (discussed below) have been used. Recently, high resolution (1024^2), high frame rate (30 frame/sec) charge-coupled device (CCD) video cameras have become available and are replacing tube-based cameras in some angiographic installations. This trend will probably continue. The image quality ramifications are a matter of current research [Blume, 1998]. The advantages of CCD cameras include low-voltage operation, reliability, little required setup tuning, and freedom from geometric distortions. Frame-charge transfer is the preferred CCD read-out scheme, due to the higher optical fill factor of this configuration.

Video camera pickup tubes used for angiography are of the photoconductive *vidicon-style* of construction. This type of tube uses a low-velocity scanning beam and generates a signal from the recharge of the target by the scanning electron beam. There are several types of vidicon-style tubes in use (Plumbicon, Primicon, Saticon, Newvicon) which differ from each other in the material and configuration used for target construction. There is an unfortunate confusion in terminology because the original vidicon-style tube is referred to simply as a vidicon. The original vidicon has an antimony trisulfide target (Sb_2S_3) and exhibits such a high degree of lag (image retention) that it is not useful for angiographic work. Even with *low-lag* angiographic cameras, the residual lag can result in artifacts in subtraction images. Light bias is often used to further reduce lag by ensuring that the target surface is not driven to a negative potential by energetic electrons in the scanning beam [Sandrik, 1984].

Image noise in a well-designed system is due to x-ray quantum fluctuations and noise related to signal generation in the video camera. When used for digital angiographic purposes, it is important that the video camera exhibit a high signal-to-noise ratio (at least 60 dB) so that video camera noise does not dominate the low-signal (dark) portions of the image. In order to achieve this, the pickup tube must be run at high beam currents (2 to 3 μA). Because long-term operation of the tube at these beam currents can result in damage to the target, beam current is usually either blanked when imaging is not being performed, or the current is held at a low level (e.g., 400 nA) and boosted only when high-quality angiographic images are required. All pickup tubes currently in use for angiographic imaging exhibit a linear response to light input (i.e., $\gamma = 1$, where the relationship between signal current I and image brightness B is described by a relationship of the form $I/I_o = (B/B_o)\gamma$). This has the disadvantage that the range in image brightness presented to the camera often exceeds the camera's dynamic range when a highly transmissive portion of the patient's anatomy (e.g., lung) or unattenuated radiation is included in the image field, either saturating the highlights, forcing the rest of the image to a low signal level, or both. To deal with this problem, it is desirable for the operator to mechanically **bolus** the bright area with metal filters, saline bags, etc. Specially constructed filters are available for commonly encountered problems, such as the transmissive region between the patient's legs during runoff studies of the legs, and most vendors provide a controllable metal filter in the x-ray collimator that the operator can position over bright spots with a joystick.

In addition to mechanical bolusing performed by the laboratory staff, most system vendors have incorporated some form of *gamma curve modification* into the systems. Usually performed using analog processing in the CCU, the technique applies a nonlinear transfer curve to the originally linear data. There are two advantages to this technique. First, the CRT of the display monitor has reduced gain at low signal, so imposing a transfer function with $\gamma \approx 0.5$ via gamma-curve modification provides a better match between the video signal and the display monitor. Second, if the modification is performed prior to digitization, a $\gamma < 1$ results in a more constant ratio between the ADC step size and the image noise amplitude across the full range of the video signal. This results in less contouring in the dark portions of the digital image, especially in images that have been spatially filtered. It is important to note, however, that gamma-curve modification does not eliminate the desirable effects of mechanically bolusing the image field prior to image acquisition. This is so because bolusing allows more photon flux to be selectively applied to the more attenuating regions of the patient, which decreases both quantum and video noise in those regions. Bolusing is especially important for subtraction imaging.

The video system characteristic most apparent to the user is the method employed in scanning the image. Prior to the advent of the digital angiography, EIA RS-170 video (525-line, 30 Hz frames, 2:1 interlace) was the predominant standard used for fluoroscopic systems in the United States. However, this method of scanning has definite disadvantages for angiography, including low resolution and image artifacts related to the interlaced format. The inclusion of a digital image processor in the imaging chain, functioning as an image buffer, allows the scanning mode to be tailored to the angiographic procedure. Many of the important video scanning modes used for angiographic work are dependent on the ability of image processors to perform scan conversion operations. Two typical *scan conversion* operations are progressive-to-interlaced conversion and **upscanning**. Progressive-to-interlaced scan conversion allows **progressive**

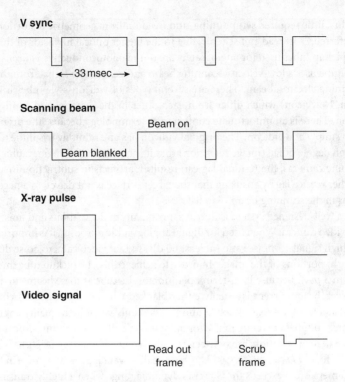

FIGURE 10.5 Timing diagram for image acquisition using the pulsed-progressive mode. (From Van Lysel M.S. In, S. Baum (Ed.), *Abrams' Angiography*, 4th ed. Boston, Little, Brown. With permission.)

scanning (also referred to as *sequential scanning*) to be used for image acquisition and interlaced scanning for image display. Progressive scanning is a noninterlaced scan mode in which all the lines are read out in a single vertical scan. Progressive scanning is especially necessary when imaging moving arteries, such as during coronary angiography [Seibert et al., 1984]. In noncardiac work, progressive scan acquisition is usually combined with beam blanking. Beam blanking refers to the condition in which the pickup tube beam current is blanked (turned off) for one or more integer number of frames. This mode is used in order to allow the image to integrate on the camera target prior to readout (Figure 10.5). In this way, x-ray pulses shorter than one frame period can be acquired without scanning artifacts, and x-ray pulses longer than one frame period can be used in order to increase the x-ray quantum statistics of an image. Upscanning refers to the acquisition of data at a low line rate (e.g., 525 lines) and the display of that data at a higher line rate (e.g., 1023 lines) [Holmes et al., 1989]. The extra lines are produced by either replication of the actual data or, more commonly, by interpolation (either linear or spline). Upscanning also can be performed in the horizontal direction as well, but this is less typical. Upscanning is used to decrease the demands on the video camera, system bandwidth, and digital storage requirements while improving display contrast and decreasing interfield flicker.

The image buffering capability of a digital system can provide several operations aimed at reducing patient exposure. If fluoroscopy is performed with pulsed rather than continuous x-rays, then the operator has the freedom to choose the frame rate. During **pulsed-progressive fluoroscopy**, the digital system provides for display refresh without flicker. Frame rates of less than 30 fps can result in lower patient exposure, though; because of the phenomenon of eye integration, the x-ray exposure per pulse must be increased as the frame rate drops in order to maintain low contrast detectability [Aufrichtig et al., 1994]. *Last image hold*, which stores and displays the last acquired fluoroscopic frame, also can result in an exposure reduction. Combining last image hold with graphic overlays allows collimator shutters and bolus filters to be positioned with the x-rays turned off.

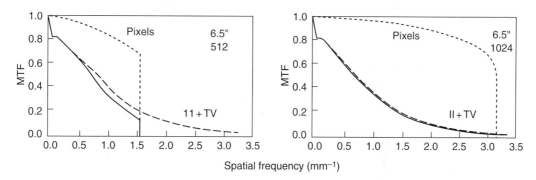

FIGURE 10.6 Detector modulation transfer function, including limits due to the image intensifier (II), video camera (TV), and sampling, including the antialiasing filter (pixels). Figures are for the 6.5-in. image intensifier mode for 512- and 1024-pixel matrices. In both cases, the total detector MTF is given by the solid line. Data used for this figure from Verhoeven [1985].

10.2.3 Digital Angiography

Digital imaging technology has quickly replaced film-based recording for most angiographic procedures. Digital image processing provides the ability to manipulate the contrast and spatial-frequency characteristics of the angiographic image, as well as providing immediate access to the image data during the procedure.

The rapid application of digital imaging technology to the angiographic procedure was facilitated by the fact that the image intensifier and video camera imaging chain was already in use when digital imaging appeared. It is a relatively simple matter to digitize the video camera output. Theoretically, additional noise is added to the image due to quantitization errors associated with the digitization process. This additional noise can be kept insignificantly small by using a sufficient number of digital levels so that the amplitude of one digital level is approximately equal to the amplitude of the standard deviation in image values associated with the noise (x-ray quantum and electronic noise) in the image prior to digitization [Kruger et al., 1981]. To meet this condition, most digital angiographic systems employ a 10-bit (1024-level) analog-to-digital convertor (ADC). Those systems which are designed to digitize high-noise (i.e., low x-ray exposure) images exclusively can employ an 8-bit (256-level) ADC. Such systems include those designed for cardiac and fluoroscopic applications.

The spatial resolution of a digital angiographic image is determined by several factors, including the size of the x-ray tube focal spot, the modulation transfer function of the image intensifier-video camera chain, and the size of the pixel matrix. The typical image matrix dimensions for non-cardiac digital angiographic images is 1024×1024. Cardiac systems use 512×512, $1024(H) \times 512(V)$, or 1024×1024. Sampling rates required to digitize 512^2 and 1024^2 matrices in the 33-msec frame period of conventional video are 10 and 40 MHz, respectively. Figure 10.6 shows an example of the detector MTF of a digital angiographic system. The product of the image intensifier and video system MTF constitute the presampling MTF [Fujita et al., 1985]. It is seen that the effect of sampling with a 512-pixel matrix is to truncate the high-frequency tail of the presampling MTF, while a 1024-pixel matrix imposes few additional limitations beyond that associated with the analog components (especially for small image intensifier modes) [Verhoeven, 1985]. However, because of blurring associated with the x-ray tube focal spot, the full advantage of the higher density pixel matrix can rarely be realized, clinically (Figure 10.7).

10.2.3.1 Digital Image Processor

The digital image processor found in a modern angiographic suite is a dedicated device designed specially to meet the demands of the angiographic procedure. Hardware is structured as a pipeline processor to perform real-time processing at video rates. Image-subtraction, integration, spatial-filtration, and temporal-filtration algorithms are hardwired to meet this requirement. Lookup tables (LUTs) are used to

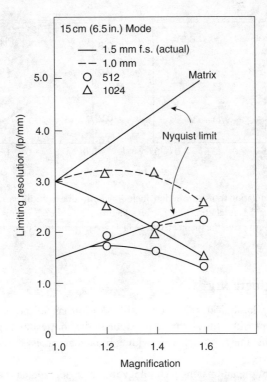

FIGURE 10.7 Experimental determination of the limiting resolution (high-contrast object and high x-ray exposure) for 512- and 1024-pixel matrices, focal spots of actual dimensions 1.0 and 1.5 mm, and a 6.5-in. image intensifier mode, as a function of geometric magnification. (From Mistretta, C.A. and Peppler, W.W. 1988. *Am. J. Card. Imag.* 2: 26. With permission.)

perform intensity transformations (e.g., contrast enhancement and logarithmic transformation). A more general-purpose host computer is used to control the pipeline processor and x-ray generator, respond to user input, and perform nonreal-time image manipulations.

The most clinically important image-processing algorithm is temporal subtraction (DSA). Subtraction imaging is used for most vascular studies. Subtraction allows approximately a factor of 2 reduction in the amount of injected contrast material. As a result, DSA studies can be performed with less contrast load and with smaller catheters than film/screen angiography. The primary limitation of DSA is a susceptibility to misregistration artifacts resulting from patient motion. Some procedures that are particularly susceptible to motion artifacts are routinely performed in a nonsubtracted mode. Unsubtracted digital angiographic studies are usually performed with the same amount of contrast material as film/screen studies. Cardiac angiography is one procedure that is generally performed without subtraction, although in any particular study, if patient and respiratory motion are absent, it is possible to obtain high-quality time subtractions using phase-matched mask subtractions in which the preinjection mask and postinjection contrast images are matched with respect to cardiac phase. In order to do this efficiently, it is necessary to digitize the ECG signal along with the image data.

Additional examples of unsubtracted digital angiographic studies are those in uncooperative patients (e.g., trauma) and digital runoff studies of the vessels in the leg. In a digital runoff study it is necessary to follow the bolus down the legs by moving the patient (or the image gantry). This motion causes difficulties with both mask registration and uniform exposure intensities between the mask and contrast images. The high contrast sensitivity of DSA is valuable for runoff studies, however, because the small vessels and slow flow in the lower extremities can make vessel visualization difficult. Recently, making use of programmed table (or gantry) motion and pixel-shifting strategies, x-ray vendors have begun to offer a viable digital subtraction runoff mode.

In addition to subtraction angiography, two filtration algorithms have become clinically important. The first is high-pass spatial filtration for the purposes of providing edge enhancement. Real-time edge enhancement of fluoroscopy is especially important for interventional procedures, such as angioplasty, where the task requires visualization of high-frequency objects such as vessel edges and guidewires. Because increasing the degree of edge enhancement also increases image noise, operator control of the degree of enhancement (accomplished by adjusting the size and weighing of the convolution kernel) is an important feature.

The second filtration algorithm often available from a digital angiographic system is low-pass temporal filtration (recursive filtering) [Rowlands, 1992]. Temporal filtration is used to reduce quantum noise levels in fluoroscopic images without increasing patient exposure. Recursive filtering is a more desirable method than simple image integration because it requires only two memory planes and because it is a simple matter to turn the filtering algorithm off, on a pixel-by-pixel basis, when motion is detected. Motion-detection circuits monitor the frame-to-frame change in pixel values and assume that an object has moved into or out of the pixel if the change exceeds a preset threshold.

10.2.3.2 Image Storage

Storage needs during the angiographic procedure are easily met by modern hard drives. These often are configured to provide real-time (i.e., video rate) storage. The immediate access to images provided by real-time disk technology is one of the major advantages of digital angiography over film. Not only is it unnecessary to wait for film to be developed, but review of the image data after the patient's procedure is completed is facilitated by directories and specialized review software. For example, a popular image menu feature is the presentation to users of a low-resolution collage of available images from which they may select a single image or entire run for full-resolution display.

While online storage of recent studies is a strength of digital angiography, long-term (archival) storage is a weakness. Archival devices provided by vendors are generally proprietary devices that make use of various recording media. There is an established communications protocol (ACR-NEMA) [NEMA, 1993] for network transfer of images. For the time being, while large institutions and teaching hospitals are investing in sophisticated digital **picture archiving and communications systems (PACS)**, archival needs at most institutions are met by storage of hardcopy films generated from the digital images. Hardcopy devices include multiformat cameras (laser or video) and video thermal printers. Laser cameras, using either an analog or a digital interface to the digital angiographic unit, can provide diagnostic-quality, large-format, high-contrast, high-resolution films. Multiformat video cameras, which expose the film with a CRT, are a less expensive method of generating diagnostic-quality images but are also more susceptible to drift and geometric distortions. Thermal printer images are generally used as convenient method to generate temporary hardcopy images.

Cardiac angiography labs have long employed a similar method, referred to as **parallel cine**, in which both digital and cine images are recorded simultaneously by use of the semitransparent mirror in the image intensifier optical distributor. Immediate diagnosis would be performed off the digital monitor while the 35-mm film would provide archival storage and the ability to share the image data with other institutions. However, due to the promulgation of an image transfer standard using the recordable CD (CD-R), many laboratories are abandoning cine film. While CD-R cannot replay images at full real-time rates, the read-rate (>1 MB/sec) is sufficient to load old data quickly from CD-R to a workstation hard drive for review. Low volume laboratories can use CD-R as an archival storage method. Higher volume labs are installing networked video file servers to provide online or near-line access to archived patient studies.

10.2.4 Summary

For decades, x-ray projection film/screen angiography was the only invasive modality available for the diagnosis of vascular disease. Now several imaging modalities are available to study the cardiovascular system, most of which are less invasive than x-ray projection angiography. However, conventional angiography also has changed dramatically during the last decade. Digital angiography has replaced film/screen angiography in most applications. In addition, the use and capabilities of transluminal interventional techniques have mushroomed, and digital angiographic processor modes have expanded significantly in support of these interventional procedures. As a consequence, while less invasive technologies, such as MR angiography, make inroads into conventional angiography's diagnostic applications, it is likely that x-ray projection angiography will remain an important clinical modality for many years to come.

Defining Terms

Bolus: This term has two, independent definition (1) material placed in a portion of the x-ray beam to reduce the sense dynamic range and (2) the injection contrast material.

Digital subtraction angiography (DSA):   Methodology in which digitized angiographic images are subtracted in order to provide contrast enhancement of the opacified vasculature. Clinically, temporal subtraction is the algorithm used, though energy subtraction methods also fall under the generic term DSA.

Parallel cine: The simultaneous recording of digital and cine-film images during cardiac angiography. In this mode, digital image acquisition provides diagnostic-quality images.

Picture archiving and communications systems (PACS):   Digital system or network for the electronic storage and retrieval of patient images and data.

Progressive scanning: Video raster scan method in which all horizontal lines are read out in a single vertical scan of the video camera target.

Pulsed-progressive fluoroscopy: Method of acquiring fluoroscopic images in which x-rays are produced in discrete pulses coincident with the vertical retrace period of the video camera. The video camera is then read out using progressive scanning. This compares with the older fluoroscopic method of producing x-rays continuously, coupled with interlaced video camera scanning.

Temporal subtraction: Also known as time subtraction or mask-mode subtraction. A subtraction mode in which an unopacified image (the mask, usually acquired prior to injection) is subtracted from an opacified image.

Upscanning: Scan conversion method in which the number of pixels or video lines displayed is higher (usually by a factor of 2) than those actually acquired from the video camera. Extra display data are produced by either replication or interpolation of the acquired data.

References

Amplatz, K. 1997. Rapid film changers. In S. Baum (Ed.), *Abrams' Angiography*, Chapter 6. Boston, Little, Brown and Company.

Aufrichtig, R., Xue, P., Thomas, C.W. et al. 1994. Perceptual comparison of pulsed and continuous fluoroscopy. *Med. Phys.* 21: 245.

Blume, H. 1998. The imaging chain. In Nickoloff, E.L. and Strauss, K.J. (Eds.) *Categorical Course in Diagnostic Radiology Physics: Cardiac Catheterization Imaging*, pp. 83–103. Oak Brook, IL, Radiological Society of North America.

Fujita, H., Doi, K., and Lissak Giger, M. 1985. Investigation of basic imaging properties in digital radiography: 6. MTFs of II-TV digital imaging systems. *Med. Phys.* 12: 713.

Holmes, D.R. Jr, Wondrow, M.A., Reeder, G.S. et al. 1989. Optimal display of the coronary arterial tree with an upscan 1023-line video display system. *Cathet. Cardiovasc. Diagn.* 18: 175.

Kruger, R.A., Mistretta, C.A., and Riederer, S.J. 1981. Physical and technical considerations of computerized fluoroscopy difference imaging. *IEEE Trans. Nucl. Sci.* 28: 205.

National Electrical Manufacturers Association. 1992. Test Standard for the Determination of the System Contrast Ratio and System Veiling Glare Index of an X-Ray Image Intensifier System, NEMA Standards Publication No. XR 16. Washington, National Electrical Manufacturers Association.

National Electric Manufacturers Association. 1993. Digital Imaging and Communications in Medicine (DICOM), NEMA Standards Publication PS3.0. Washington, National Electrical Manufacturers Association.

Rowlands, J.A. 1992. Real-time digital processing of video image sequences for videofluoroscopy. *SPIE Proc.* 1652: 294.

Sandrik, J.M. 1984. The video camera for medical imaging. In G.D. Fullerton, W.R. Hendee, J.C. Lasher et al. (Eds.), *Electronic Imaging in Medicine*, pp. 145–183. New York, American Institute of Physics.

Seibert, J.A., Barr, D.H., Borger, D.J. et al. 1984. Interlaced versus progressive readout of television cameras for digital radiographic acquisitions. *Med. Phys.* 11: 703.

Siedband, M.P. 1994. Image intensification and television. In J.M. Taveras and J.T. Ferrucci (Eds.), *Radiology: Diagnosis-Imaging-Intervention*, Chapter 10. Philadelphia, JB Lippincott.

Verhoeven, L.A.J. 1985. DSA imaging: Some physical and technical aspects. *Medicamundi* 30: 46.

Further Information

Balter, S. and Shope, T.B. (Eds.). 1995. *A Categorical Course in Physics: Physical and Technical Aspects of Angiography and Interventional Radiology.* Oak Brook, IL, Radiological Society of North America.

Baum S. (Ed.). 1997. *Abrams' Angiography*, 4th ed. Boston Little, Brown and Company.

Kennedy, T.E., Nissen, S.E., Simon, R., Thomas, J.D., and Tilkemeier, P.L. 1997. *Digital Cardiac Imaging in the 21st Century: A Primer.* Bethesda, MD, The Cardiac and Vascular Information Working Group (American College of Cardiology).

Moore, R.J. 1990. *Imaging Principles of Cardiac Angiography.* Rockville, MD, Aspen Publishers.

Nickoloff, E.L. and Strauss, K.J. (Eds.). 1998. *Categorical Course in Diagnostic Radiology Physics: Cardiac Catheterization Imaging.* Oak Brook, IL, Radiological Society of North America.

Seibert, J.A., Barnes, G.T., and Gould, R.G. (Eds.). 1994. Medical Physics Monograph No. 20: *Specification, Acceptance Testing and Quality Control of Diagnostic X-Ray Imaging Equipment.* Woodbury, NY, American Institute of Physics.

10.3   Mammography

Martin J. Yaffe

Mammography is an x-ray imaging procedure for examination of the breast. It is used primarily for the detection and diagnosis of breast cancer, but also for pre-surgical localization of suspicious areas and in the guidance of needle biopsies.

Breast cancer is a major killer of women. Approximately 179,000 women were diagnosed with breast cancer in the United States in 1998 and 43,500 women died of this disease [Landis, 1998]. Its cause is not currently known; however, it has been demonstrated that **survival** is greatly improved if disease is detected at an early stage [Tabar, 1993; Smart, 1993]. Mammography is at present the most effective means of detecting early stage breast cancer. It is used both for investigating symptomatic patients (diagnostic mammography) and for **screening** of asymptomatic women in selected age groups.

Breast cancer is detected on the basis of four types of signs on the mammogram:

1. The characteristic morphology of a tumor mass
2. Certain presentations of mineral deposits as specks called microcalcifications
3. Architectural distortion of normal tissue patterns caused by the disease
4. Asymmetry between corresponding regions of images of the left and right breast

10.3.1 Principles of Mammography

The mammogram is an x-ray shadowgram formed when x-rays from a quasi-point source irradiate the breast and the transmitted x-rays are recorded by an **image receptor**. Because of the spreading of the x-rays from the source, structures are magnified as they are projected onto the image receptor. The signal is a result of differential attenuation of x-rays along paths passing through the structures of the breast.

The essential features of image quality are summarized in Figure 10.8. This is a one-dimensional profile of x-ray transmission through a simplified computer model of the breast [Fahrig, 1992], illustrated in Figure 10.9. A region of reduced transmission corresponding to a structure of interest such as a tumor, a calcification, or normal *fibroglandular* tissue is shown. The imaging system must have sufficient *spatial resolution* to delineate the edges of fine structures in the breast. Structural detail as small as 50 μm must be adequately resolved. Variation in x-ray attenuation among tissue structures in the breast gives rise to contrast. The detectability of structures providing subtle contrast is impaired, however, by an overall random fluctuation in the profile, referred to as mottle or noise. Because the breast is sensitive to ionizing radiation, which at least for high doses is known to cause breast cancer, it is desirable to use the lowest radiation dose compatible with excellent image quality. The components of the imaging system will be described and their design will be related to the imaging performance factors discussed in this section.

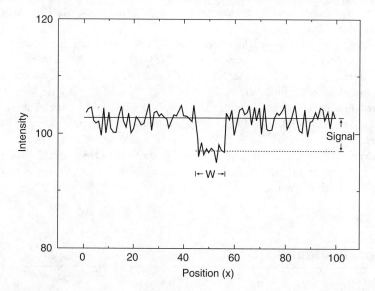

FIGURE 10.8   Profile of a simple x-ray projection image illustrating the role of contrast, spatial resolution, and noise in mammographic image quality.

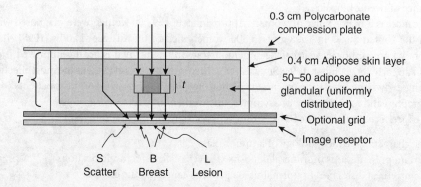

FIGURE 10.9   Simplified computer model of the mammographic image acquisition process.

10.3.2 Physics of Image Formation

In the model of Figure 10.9, an "average" breast composed of 50% adipose tissue and 50% **fibroglandular tissue** is considered. For the simplified case of monoenergetic x-rays of energy, E, the number of x-rays recorded in a fixed area of the image is proportional to

$$N_B = N_0(E)e^{-\mu T} \tag{10.1}$$

in the "background" and

$$N_L = N_0(E)e^{-[\mu(T-t)+\mu' t]} \tag{10.2}$$

in the shadow of the lesion or other structure of interest. In Equation 61.1 and Equation 61.2, $N_0(E)$ is the number of x-rays that would be recorded in the absence of tissue in the beam, μ and μ' are the attenuation coefficients of the breast tissue and the lesion, respectively, T is the thickness of the breast, and t is the thickness of the lesion.

The difference in x-ray transmission gives rise to subject contrast which can be defined as:

$$C_0 = \frac{N_B - N_L}{N_B + N_L} \tag{10.3}$$

For the case of monoenergetic x-rays and temporarily ignoring scattered radiation,

$$\frac{1 - e^{-[\mu'-\mu t]}}{1 + e^{-[\mu'-\mu t]}} \tag{10.4}$$

that is, contrast would depend only on the thickness of the lesion and the difference between its attenuation coefficient and that of the background material. These are not valid assumptions and in actuality contrast also depends on μ and T.

Shown in Figure 10.10 are x-ray attenuation coefficients measured vs. energy on samples of three types of materials found in the breast: adipose tissue, normal fibroglandular breast tissue, and infiltrating ductal carcinoma (one type of breast tumor) [Johns, 1987]. Both the attenuation coefficients themselves and their difference $(\mu' - \mu)$ decrease with increasing E. As shown in Figure 10.11, which is based on Equation 10.4, this causes C_s to fall as x-ray energy increases. Note that the subject contrast of even small calcifications in the breast is greater than that for a tumor because of the greater difference in attenuation coefficient between calcium and breast tissue.

For a given image recording system (image receptor), a proper exposure requires a specific value of x-ray energy transmitted by the breast and incident on the receptor, that is, a specific value of NB. The breast entrance skin exposure[1] (ESE) required to produce an image is, therefore, proportional to

$$N_0 = N_B(E)e^{+\mu T} \tag{10.5}$$

Because μ decreases with energy, the required exposure for constant signal at the image receptor, N_B, will increase if E is reduced to improve image contrast. A better measure of the risk of radiation-induced breast cancer than ESE is the mean glandular dose (MGD) [BEIR V, 1990]. MGD is calculated as the product of the ESE and a factor, obtained experimentally or by Monte Carlo radiation transport calculations, which converts from incident exposure to dose [Wu, 1991, 1994]. The conversion factor increases with E so that MGD does not fall as quickly with energy as does entrance exposure. The trade-off between image contrast and radiation dose necessitates important compromises in establishing mammographic operating conditions.

---

[1] Exposure is expressed in Roentgers (R) (which is not an SI unit) or in Coulombs of ionization collected per kilogram of air.

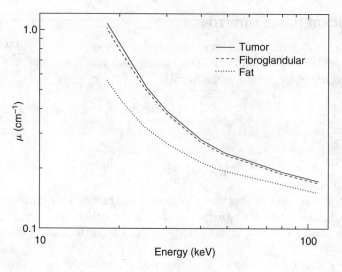

FIGURE 10.10 Measured x-ray linear attenuation coefficients of breast fibroglandular tissue, breast fat, and infiltrating ductal carcinoma plotted vs. x-ray energy.

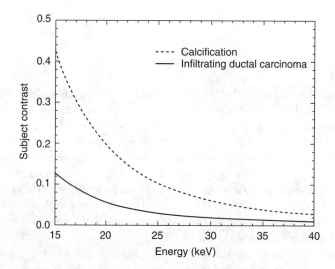

FIGURE 10.11 Dependence of mammographic subject contrast on x-ray energy.

10.3.3 Equipment

The mammography unit consists of an x-ray tube and an image receptor mounted on opposite sides of a mechanical assembly or gantry. Because the breast must be imaged from different aspects and to accommodate patients of different height, the assembly can be adjusted in a vertical axis and rotated about a horizontal axis as shown in Figure 10.12.

Most general radiography equipment is designed such that the image field is centered below the x-ray source. In mammography, the system's geometry is arranged as in Figure 10.13a where a vertical line from the x-ray source grazes the chest wall of the patient and intersects orthogonally with the edge of the image receptor closest to the patient. If the x-ray beam were centered over the breast as in Figure 10.13b, some of the tissue near the chest wall would be projected inside of the patient where it could not be recorded.

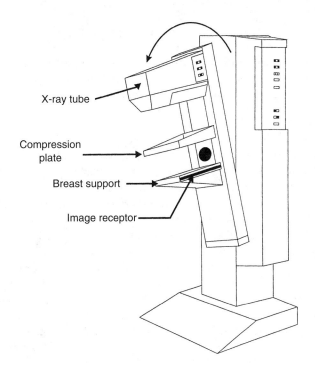

FIGURE 10.12 Schematic diagram of a dedicated mammography machine.

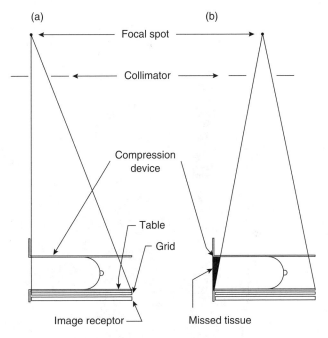

FIGURE 10.13 Geometric arrangement of system components in mammography. (a) Correct alignment provides good tissue coverage, (b) incorrect alignment causes tissue near the chest wall not to be imaged.

Radiation leaving the x-ray tube passes through a metallic spectral-shaping filter, a beam-defining aperture, and a plate which compresses the breast. Those rays transmitted through the breast are incident on an antiscatter "**grid**" and then strike the image receptor where they interact and deposit most of their energy locally. A fraction of the x-rays pass through the receptor without interaction and impinge upon a sensor which is used to activate the automatic exposure control mechanism of the unit.

10.3.3.1 X-Ray Source

Practical monoenergetic x-ray sources are not available and the x-rays used in mammography arise from bombardment of a metal target by electrons in a hot-cathode vacuum tube. The x-rays are emitted from the target over a spectrum of energies, ranging up to the peak kilovoltage applied to the x-ray tube. Typically, the x-ray tube employs a rotating anode design in which electrons from the cathode strike the anode target material at a small angle (0 to 16°) from normal incidence (Figure 10.14). Over 99% of the energy from the electrons is dissipated as heat in the anode. The angled surface and the distribution of the electron bombardment along the circumference of the rotating anode disk allows the energy to be spread over a larger area of target material while presenting a much smaller effective **focal spot** as viewed from the imaging plane. On modern equipment, the typical "nominal" focal spot size for normal contact mammography is 0.3 mm, while the smaller spot used primarily for magnification is 0.1 mm. The specifications for x-ray focal spot size tolerance, established by NEMA (National Electrical Manufacturers Association) or the IEC (International Electrotechnical Commission) allow the effective focal spot size to be considerably larger than these nominal sizes. For example, the NEMA specification allows the effective focal spot size to be 0.45 mm in width and 0.65 mm in length for a nominal 0.3 mm spot and 0.15 mm in each dimension for a nominal 0.1 mm spot.

The nominal focal spot size is defined relative to the effective spot size at a "reference axis." As shown in Figure 10.14, this reference axis, which may vary from manufacturer to manufacturer, is normally specified at some mid-point in the image. The effective size of the focal spot will monotonically increase from the anode side to the cathode side of the imaging field. Normally, x-ray tubes are arranged such that the cathode side of the tube is adjacent to the patient's chest wall, since the highest intensity of x-rays is available at the cathode side, and the attenuation of x-rays by the patient is generally greater near the chest wall of the image.

The spatial resolution capability of the imaging system is partially determined by the effective size of the focal spot and by the degree of magnification of the anatomy at any plane in the breast. This is illustrated

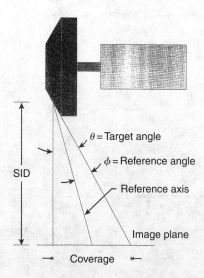

FIGURE 10.14 Angled-target x-ray source provides improved heat loading but causes effective focal spot size to vary across the image.

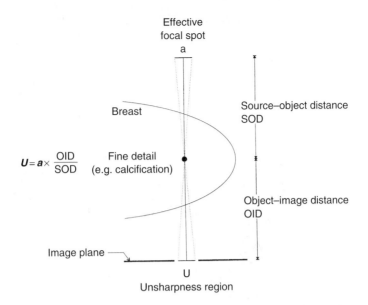

FIGURE 10.15 Dependence of focal spot unsharpness on focal spot size and magnification factor.

in Figure 10.15 where, by similar triangles, the unsharpness region due to the finite size of the focal spot is linearly related to the effective size of the spot and to the ratio of OID to SOD, where SOD is the source-object distance and OID is the object–image receptor distance. Because the breast is a three-dimensional structure, this ratio and, therefore, the unsharpness will vary for different planes within the breast.

The size of the focal spot determines the heat loading capability of the x-ray tube target. For smaller focal spots, the current through the x-ray tube must be reduced, necessitating increased exposure times and the possibility of loss of resolution due to motion of anatomical structures. Loss of geometric resolution can be controlled in part by minimizing OID/SOD, that is, by designing the equipment with greater source-breast distances, by minimizing space between the breast and the image receptor, and by compressing the breast to reduce its overall thickness.

Magnification is often used intentionally to improve the signal-to-noise ratio of the image. This is accomplished by elevating the breast above the image receptor, in effect reducing SOD and increasing OID. Under these conditions, resolution is invariably limited by focal spot size and use of a small spot for magnification imaging (typically a nominal size of 0.1 mm) is critical.

Since monoenergetic x-rays are not available, one attempts to define a spectrum providing energies which give a reasonable compromise between radiation dose and image contrast. The spectral shape can be controlled by adjustment of the kilovoltage, choice of the target material, and the type and thickness of metallic filter placed between the x-ray tube and the breast.

Based on models of the imaging problem in mammography, it has been suggested that the optimum energy for imaging lies between 18 and 23 keV, depending on the thickness and composition of the breast [Beaman, 1982]. It has been found that for the breast of typical thickness and composition, the characteristic x-rays from molybdenum at 17.4 and 19.6 keV provide good imaging performance. For this reason, molybdenum target x-ray tubes are used on the vast majority of mammography machines.

Most mammography tubes use beryllium exit windows between the evacuated tube and the outside world since glass or other metals used in general purpose tubes would provide excessive attenuation of the useful energies for mammography. Figure 10.16 compares tungsten target and molybdenum target spectra for beryllium window x-ray tubes. Under some conditions, tungsten may provide appropriate image quality for mammography; however, it is essential that the intense emission of L radiation from tungsten be filtered from the beam before it is incident upon the breast, since extremely high doses to the skin would result from this radiation without useful contribution to the mammogram.

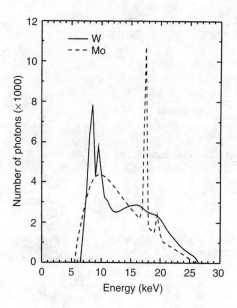

FIGURE 10.16 Comparison of tungsten and molybdenum target x-ray spectra.

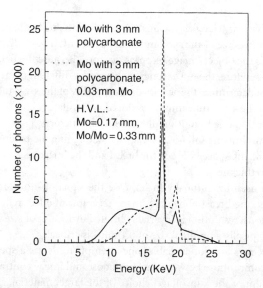

FIGURE 10.17 Molybdenum target spectrum filtered by 0.03 mm Mo foil.

10.3.3.2 Filtration of the X-Ray Beam

In conventional radiology, filters made of aluminum or copper are used to provide selective removal of low x-ray energies from the beam before it is incident upon the patient. In mammography, particularly when a molybdenum anode x-ray tube is employed, a molybdenum filter 20–35 μm thick is generally used. This filter attenuates x-rays both at low energies and those above its own K-absorption edge allowing the molybdenum characteristic x-rays from the target to pass through the filter with relatively high efficiency. As illustrated in Figure 10.17, this K edge filtration results in a spectrum enriched with x-ray energies in the range of 17–20 keV.

Although this spectrum is relatively well suited for imaging the breast of average attenuation, slightly higher energies are desirable for imaging dense thicker breasts. Because the molybdenum target spectrum is so heavily influenced by the characteristic x-rays, an increase in the kilovoltage alone does not substantially change the shape of the spectrum. The beam can be "hardened," however, by employing filters of higher atomic number than molybdenum. For example, rhodium (atomic no. 45) has a K absorption edge at 23 keV, providing strong attenuation both for x-rays above this energy and for those at substantially lower energies. Used with a molybdenum target x-ray tube and slightly increased kilovolt, it provides a spectrum with increased penetration (reduced dose) compared to the Mo/Mo combination.

It is possible to go further in optimizing imaging performance, by "tuning" the effective spectral energy by using other target materials in combination with appropriate K-edge filters [Jennings, 1993]. One manufacturer employs an x-ray tube incorporating both molybdenum and rhodium targets, where the electron beam can be directed toward one or the other of these materials [Heidsieck, 1991]. With this system, the filter material (rhodium, molybdenum, etc.) can be varied to suit the target that has been selected. Similarly, work has been reported on K-edge filtration of tungsten spectra [Desponds, 1991], where the lack of pronounced K characteristic peaks provides more flexibility in spectral shaping with filters.

10.3.3.3 Compression Device

There are several reasons for applying firm (but not necessarily painful) compression to the breast during the examination. Compression causes the different tissues to be spread out, minimizing superposition from different planes and thereby improving a conspicuity of structures. As will be discussed later, scattered radiation can degrade contrast in the mammogram. The use of compression decreases the ratio of scattered to directly transmitted radiation reaching the image receptor. Compression also decreases the distance from any plane within the breast to the image receptor (i.e., OID) and in this way reduces geometric unsharpness. The compressed breast provides lower overall attenuation to the incident x-ray beam, allowing the radiation dose to be reduced. The compressed breast also provides more uniform attenuation over the image. This reduces the exposure range which must be recorded by the imaging system, allowing more flexibility in choice of films to be used. Finally, compression provides a clamping action which reduces anatomical motion during the exposure reducing this source of image unsharpness.

It is important that the compression plate allows the breast to be compressed parallel to the image receptor, and that the edge of the plate at the chest wall be straight and aligned with both the focal spot and image receptor to maximize the amount of breast tissue which is included in the image (see Figure 10.13).

10.3.3.4 Antiscatter Grid

Lower x-ray energies are used for mammography than for other radiological examinations. At these energies, the probability of photoelectric interactions within the breast is significant. Nevertheless, the probability of Compton scattering of x-rays within the breast is still quite high. Scattered radiation recorded by the image receptor has the effect of creating a quasi-uniform haze on the image and causes the subject contrast to be reduced to

$$C_s = \frac{C_c}{1 + \text{SPR}} \tag{10.6}$$

where C_0 is the contrast in the absence of scattered radiation, given by Equation 10.4 and SPR is the scatter-to-primary (directly transmitted) x-ray ratio at the location of interest in the image. In the absence of an anti-scatter device, 37 to 50% of the total radiation incident on the image receptor would have experienced a scattering interaction within the breast, that is, the scatter-to-primary ratio would be $0.6 : 1.0$. In addition to contrast reduction, the recording of scattered radiation uses up part of the dynamic range of the image receptor and adds statistical noise to the image.

Antiscatter *grids* have been designed for mammography. These are composed of linear lead (Pb) septa separated by a rigid interspace material. Generally, the grid septa are not strictly parallel but focused (toward the x-ray source). Because the primary x-rays all travel along direct lines from the x-ray source to the image receptor, while the scatter diverges from points within the breast, the grid presents a smaller acceptance aperture to scattered radiation than to primary radiation and thereby discriminates against scattered radiation. Grids are characterized by their *grid ratio* (ratio of the path length through the interspace material to the interseptal width) which typically ranges from 3.5:1 to 5:1. When a grid is used, the SPR is reduced typically by a factor of about 5, leading in most cases to a substantial improvement in image contrast [Wagner, 1991].

On modern mammography equipment, the grid is an integral part of the system, and during x-ray exposure is moved to blur the image of the grid septa to avoid a distracting pattern in the mammogram. It is important that this motion be uniform and of sufficient amplitude to avoid nonuniformities in the image, particularly for short exposures that occur when the breast is relatively lucent.

Because of absorption of primary radiation by the septa and by the interspace material, part of the primary radiation transmitted by the patient does not arrive at the image receptor. In addition, by removing some of the scattered radiation, the grid causes the overall radiation fluence to be reduced from that which would be obtained in its absence. To obtain a radiograph of proper optical density, the entrance exposure to the patient must be increased by a factor known as the Bucky factor to compensate for these losses. Typical Bucky factors are in the range of 2 to 3.

A linear grid does not provide scatter rejection for those quanta traveling in planes parallel to the septa. Recently a crossed grid that consists of septa that run in orthogonal directions has been introduced for this purpose. The improved scatter rejection is accomplished at doses comparable to those required with a linear grid, because the interspace material of the crossed grid is air rather than solid. To avoid artifacts, the grid is moved in a very precise way during the exposure to ensure a uniform blurring of the image of the grid itself.

10.3.3.5 Image Receptor

10.3.3.5.1 Fluorescent Screens

When first introduced, mammography was carried out using direct exposure radiographic film in order to obtain the high spatial resolution required. Since the mid-1970s, high resolution fluorescent screens have been used to convert the x-ray pattern from the breast into an optical image. These screens are used in conjunction with single-coated radiographic film, and the configuration is shown in Figure 10.18. With this arrangement, the x-rays pass through the cover of a light-tight cassette and the film to impinge upon the screen. Absorption is exponential, so that a large fraction of the x-rays are absorbed near the entrance surface of the screen. The phosphor crystals which absorb the energy produce light in an isotropic distribution. Because the film emulsion is pressed tightly against the entrance surface of the screen, the

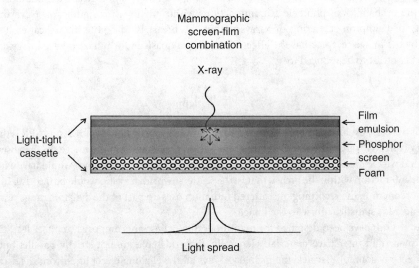

FIGURE 10.18 Design of a screen-film image receptor for mammography.

majority of the light quanta have only a short distance to travel to reach the film. Light quanta traveling longer distances have an opportunity to spread laterally (see Figure 10.18), and in this way degrade the spatial resolution. To discriminate against light quanta which travel along these longer oblique paths, the phosphor material of the screen is generally treated with a dye which absorbs much of this light, giving rise to a sharper image. A typical phosphor used for mammography is gadolinium oxysulphide (Gd_2O_2S). Although the K-absorption edge of gadolinium occurs at too high an energy to be useful in mammography, the phosphor material is dense (7.44 g/cm^3) so that the **quantum efficiency** (the fraction of incident x-rays which interact with the screen), is good (about 60%). Also, the **conversion efficiency** of this phosphor (fraction of the absorbed x-ray energy converted to light) is relatively high. The light emitted from the fluorescent screen is essentially linearly dependent upon the total amount of energy deposited by x-rays within the screen.

10.3.3.5.2 Film

The photographic film emulsion for mammography is designed with a characteristic curve such as that shown in Figure 10.19, which is a plot of the optical density (blackness) provided by the processed film vs. the logarithm of the x-ray exposure to the screen. Film provides nonlinear input–output transfer characteristics. The local gradient of this curve controls the display contrast presented to the radiologist. Where the curve is of shallow gradient, a given increment of radiation exposure provides little change in optical density, rendering structures imaged in this part of the curve difficult to visualize. Where the curve is steep, the film provides excellent image contrast. The range of exposures over which contrast is appreciable is referred to as the latitude of the film. Because the film is constrained between two optical density values — the *base + fog* density of the film, where no intentional x-ray exposure has resulted, and the maximum density provided by the emulsion — there is a compromise between maximum gradient of the film and the latitude that it provides. For this reason, some regions of the mammogram will generally be underexposed or overexposed, that is, rendered with sub-optimal contrast.

10.3.3.5.3 Film Processing

Mammography film is processed in an automatic processor similar to that used for general radiographic films. It is important that the development temperature, time, and rate of replenishment of the developer

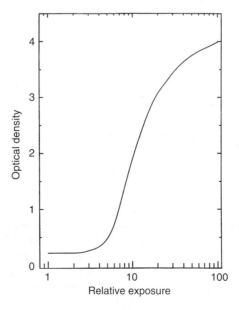

FIGURE 10.19   Characteristic curve of a mammographic screen-film image receptor.

chemistry be compatible with the type of film emulsion used and be designed to maintain good contrast of the film.

10.3.3.6   Noise and Dose

Noise in mammography results primarily from two sources — the random absorption of x-rays in the detector and the granularity associated with the screen and the film emulsion. The first, commonly known as quantum noise, is governed by Poisson statistics so that for a given area of image the standard deviation in the number of x-rays recorded is equal to the square root of the mean number recorded. In other words, the noise in the image is dependent on both the amount of radiation which strikes the imaging system per unit area, and the quantum efficiency of the imaging system. The quantum efficiency is related to the attenuation coefficient of the phosphor material and the thickness of the screen. In order to maintain high spatial resolution, the screen must be made relatively thin to avoid lateral diffusion of light. The desirability of maintaining a relatively low quantum noise level in the image mandates that the conversion efficiency of the screen material and the sensitivity of the film not be excessively high. With very high conversion efficiency, the image could be produced at low dose but with an inadequate number of quanta contributing to the image. Similarly, film granularity increases as more sensitive films are used, so that again film speed must be limited to maintain high image quality. For current high quality mammographic imaging employing an anti-scatter grid, with films exposed to a mean optical density of at least 1.6, the mean glandular dose to a 5-cm thick compressed breast consisting of 50% fibroglandular and 50% adipose tissue is in the range of 1 to 2 mGy [Conway, 1992].

10.3.3.7   Automatic Exposure Control

It is difficult for the technologist to estimate the attenuation of the breast by inspection and, therefore, modern mammography units are equipped with automatic exposure control (AEC). The AEC radiation sensors are located behind the image receptor so that they do not cast a shadow on the image. The sensors measure the x-ray fluence transmitted through both the breast and the receptor and provide a signal which can be used to discontinue the exposure when a certain preset amount of radiation has been received by the image receptor. The location of the sensor must be adjustable so that it can be placed behind the appropriate region of the breast in order to obtain proper image density. AEC devices must be calibrated so that constant image optical density results are independent of variations in breast attenuation, kilovoltage setting, or field size. With modern equipment, automatic exposure control is generally microprocessor-based so that relatively sophisticated corrections can be made during the exposure for the above effects and for *reciprocity law* failure of the film.

10.3.3.7.1   Automatic Kilovoltage Control

Many modern mammography units also incorporate automatic control of the kilovoltage or target/filter/kilovoltage combination. Penetration through the breast depends on both breast thickness and composition. For a breast that is dense, it is possible that a very long exposure time would be required to achieve adequate film blackening. This results in high dose to the breast and possibly blur due to anatomical motion. It is possible to sense the compressed breast thickness and the transmitted exposure rate and to employ an algorithm to automatically choose the x-ray target and/or beam filter as well as the kilovoltage.

10.3.4   Quality Control

Mammography is one of the most technically demanding radiographic procedures, and in order to obtain optimal results, all components of the system must be operating properly. Recognizing this, the American College of Radiology implemented and administers a Mammography Accreditation Program [McClelland, 1991], which evaluates both technical and personnel-related factors in facilities applying for accreditation.

In order to verify proper operation, a rigorous quality control program should be in effect. In fact, the U.S. Mammography Quality Standards Act stipulates that a quality control program must be in place in all facilities performing mammography. A program of tests (summarized in Table 10.1) and methods

TABLE 10.1 Mammographic Quality Control Minimum Test Frequencies

Test	Performed By	Minimum Frequency
Darkroom cleanliness	Radiologic technologist	Daily
Processor quality control		Daily
Screen cleanliness		Weekly
Viewboxes and viewing conditions		Weekly
Phantom images		Weekly
Visual check list		Monthly
Repeat analysis		Quarterly
Analysis of fixer retention in film		Quarterly
Darkroom fog		Semi-annually
Screen-film contact		Semi-annually
Compression		Semi-annually
Mammographic unit assembly evaluation	Medical physicist	Annually
Collimation assessment		Annually
Focal spot size performance		Annually
kVp accuracy/reproducibility		Annually
Beam quality assessment (half-value-layer)		Annually
Automatic exposure control (AEC) system performance assessment		Annually
Uniformity of screen speed		Annually
Breast entrance exposure and mean glandular dose		Annually
Image quality — Phantom evaluation		Annually
Artifact assessment		Annually
Radiation output rate		Annually
Viewbox luminance and room illuminance		Annually
Compression release mechanism		Annually

Source: Hendrick, R.E. et al., 1999. *Mammography Quality Control Manuals* (radiologist, radiologic technologist, medical physicist). American College of Radiology, Reston, VA.

for performing them are contained in the quality control manuals for mammography published by the American College of Radiology [Hendrick, 1999].

10.3.5 Stereotactic Biopsy Devices

Stereoscopic x-ray imaging techniques are currently used for the guidance of needle "core" biopsies. These procedures can be used to investigate suspicious mammographic or clinical findings without the need for surgical excisional biopsies, resulting in reduced patient risk, discomfort, and cost. In these stereotactic biopsies, the gantry of a mammography machine is modified to allow angulated views of the breast (typically ±15° from normal incidence) to be achieved. From measurements obtained from these images, the three-dimensional location of a suspicious lesion is determined and a needle equipped with a spring-loaded cutting device can be accurately placed in the breast to obtain tissue samples. While this procedure can be performed on an upright mammography unit, special dedicated systems have recently been introduced to allow its performance with the patient lying prone on a table. The accuracy of sampling the appropriate tissue depends critically on the alignment of the system components and the quality of the images produced. A thorough review of stereotactic imaging, including recommended quality control procedures is given by Hendrick and Parker [1994].

10.3.6 Digital Mammography

There are several technical factors associated with screen-film mammography which limit the ability to display the finest or most subtle details, and produce images with the most efficient use of radiation dose to the patient. In screen-film mammography, the film must act as an image acquisition detector as well as

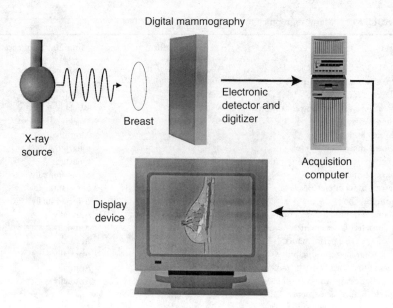

FIGURE 10.20 Schematic representation of a digital mammography system.

a storage and display device. Because of its sigmoidal shape, the range of x-ray exposures over which the film display gradient is significant, that is, the image latitude, is limited. If a tumor is located in either a relatively lucent or more opaque region of the breast, then the contrast displayed to the radiologist may be inadequate because of the limited gradient of the film. This is particularly a concern in patients whose breasts contain large amounts of fibroglandular tissue, the so-called dense breast.

Another limitation of film mammography is the effect of structural noise due to the granularity of the film emulsion used to record the image. This impairs the detectibility of microcalcifications and other fine structures within the breast. While Poisson quantum noise is unavoidable, it should be possible to virtually eliminate structural noise by technical improvements. Existing screen-film mammography also suffers because of the inefficiency of grids in removing the effects of scattered radiation and with compromises in spatial resolution vs. quantum efficiency inherent in the screen-film image receptor.

Many of the limitations of conventional mammography can be effectively overcome with a digital *mammography* imaging system (Figure 10.20), in which image acquisition, display, and storage are performed independently, allowing optimization of each. For example, acquisition can be performed with low noise, highly linear x-ray detectors, while since the image is stored digitally, it can be displayed with contrast independent of the detector properties and defined by the needs of the radiologist. Whatever image processing techniques are found useful, ranging from simple contrast enhancement to histogram modification and spatial frequency filtering, could conveniently be applied.

The challenges in creating a digital mammography system with improved performance are mainly related to the x-ray detector and the display device. There is active development of high resolution display monitors and hard copy devices to meet the demanding requirements (number of pixels, luminance, speed, multi-image capacity) of displaying digital mammography images, and suitable systems for this purpose should be available in the near future. The detector should have the following characteristics:

1. Efficient absorption of the incident radiation beam
2. Linear response over a wide range of incident radiation intensity
3. Low intrinsic noise
4. Spatial resolution on the order of 10 cycles/mm (50 μm sampling)
5. Can accommodate at least an 18 × 24 cm and preferably a 24 × 30 cm field size
6. Acceptable imaging time and heat loading of the x-ray tube

Two main approaches have been taken in detector development — area detectors and slot detectors. In the former, the entire image is acquired simultaneously, while in the latter only a portion of the image is acquired at one time and the full image is obtained by scanning the x-ray beam and detector across the breast. Area detectors offer convenient fast image acquisition and could be used with conventional x-ray machines, but may still require a grid, while slot systems are slower and require a scanning x-ray beam, but use relatively simple detectors and have excellent intrinsic efficiency at scatter rejection.

At the time of writing, small-format (5 × 5 cm) digital systems for guidance of stereotactic breast biopsy procedures are in widespread use. These use a lens or a fiberoptic taper to couple a phosphor to a CCD whose format is approximately square and typically provides 1 × 1 K images with 50 μm pixels (Figure 10.21a). Adjustment of display contrast enhances the localization of the lesion while the immediate display of images (no film processing is required) greatly accelerates the clinical procedure.

Four designs of full breast digital mammography systems are undergoing clinical evaluation. Various detector technologies are being developed and evaluated for use in digital mammography. In three of the systems, x-rays are absorbed by a cesium iodide (CsI) phosphor layer and produce light. In one system, the phosphor is deposited directly on a matrix of about 2000^2 photodiodes with thin film transistor switches fabricated on a large area amorphous silicon plate. The electronic signal is read out on a series of data lines as the switches in each row of the array are activated. In another system, the light is coupled through demagnifying fiberoptic tapers to a CCD readout. A mosaic of 3 × 4 detector modules is formed (Figure 10.21b) to obtain a detector large enough to cover the breast [Cheung, 1998]. A third system also uses fiberoptic coupling of CsI to CCDs; however, the detector is in a slot configuration and is scanned beneath the breast in synchrony with a fan beam of x-rays to acquire the transmitted signal (Figure 10.21c). The fourth system employs a plate formed of a photostimulable phosphor material. When exposed to x-rays, traps in the phosphor are filled with electrons, the number being related to x-ray intensity. The plate is placed in a reader device and scanned with a red HeNe laser beam which stimulates the traps to release the electrons. The transition of these electrons through energy levels in the phosphor crystal result in the formation of blue light, which is measured as a function of the laser position on the plate to form the image signal.

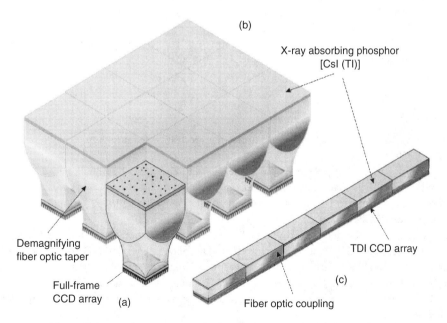

FIGURE 10.21 (a) Small-format detector system for biopsy imaging, (b) full-breast detector incorporating 12 detector modules, (c) slot detector for a full-breast scanning digital mammography system.

Other materials in which x-ray energy is directly converted to charge are under development for digital mammography. These materials include lead iodide, amorphous selenium, zinc cadmium telluride, and thallium bromide. A review of the current status of digital mammography is given in [Yaffe, 1994; Pisano, 1998] and of detectors for digital x-ray imaging in Yaffe [1997].

10.3.7 Summary

Mammography is a technically demanding imaging procedure which can help reduce mortality from breast cancer. To be successful at this purpose, both the technology and technique used for imaging must be optimized. This requires careful system design and attention to quality control procedures. Imaging systems for mammography are still evolving and, in the future, are likely to make greater use of digital acquisition and display methods.

Defining Terms

Conversion efficiency: The efficiency of converting the energy from x-rays absorbed in a phosphor material into that of emitted light quanta.

Fibroglandular tissue: A mixture of tissues within the breast composed of the functional glandular tissue and the fibrous supporting structures.

Focal spot: The area of the anode of an x-ray tube from which the useful beam of x-rays is emitted. Also known as the target.

Grid: A device consisting of evenly spaced lead strips which functions like a venetian blind in preferentially allowing x-rays traveling directly from the focal spot without interaction in the patient to pass through, while those whose direction has been diverted by scattering in the patient strike the slats of the grid and are rejected. Grids improve the contrast of radiographic images at the price of increased dose to the patient.

Image receptor: A device that records the distribution of x-rays to form an image. In mammography, the image receptor is generally composed of a light-tight cassette containing a fluorescent screen, which absorbs x-rays and produces light, coupled to a sheet of photographic film.

Quantum efficiency: The fraction of incident x-rays which interact with a detector or image receptor.

Screening: Examination of asymptomatic individuals to detect disease.

Survival: An epidemiological term giving the fraction of individuals diagnosed with a given disease alive at a specified time after diagnosis, for example, "10-year survival".

References

Beaman, S.A. and Lillicrap, S.C. 1982. Optimum x-ray spectra for mammography. *Phys. Med. Biol.* 27: 1209–1220.

Cheung, L., Bird, R., Ashish, C., Rego, A., Rodriguez, C., and Yuen, J. 1998. Initial operating and clinical results of a full-field mammography system.

Health Effects of Exposure to Low Levels of Ionizing Radiation (BEIR V) 1990. National Academy Press, Washington, D.C. 163–170.

Landis, S.H., Murray, T., Bolden, S., and Wingo, P. 1998. Cancer Statistics, *CA: Cancer J. Clin.* 48, 6–29.

Conway, B.J., Suleiman, O.H., Rueter, F.G., Antonsen, R.G., Slayton, R.J., and McCrohan, J.L. 1992. Does credentialing make a difference in mammography? *Radiology* 185: 250.

Desponds, L., Depeursinge, C., Grecescu, M., Hessler, C., Samiri, A. and Valley, J.F. 1991. Image of anode and filter material on image quality and glandular dose for screen-film mammography. *Phys. Med. Biol.* 36: 1165–1182.

Fahrig, R., Maidment, A.D.A., and Yaffe, M.J. 1992. Optimization of peak kilovoltage and spectral shape for digital mammography. *Proc. SPIE* 1651: 74–83.

Heidsieck, R., Laurencin, G., Ponchin, A., Gabbay, E., and Klausz, R. 1991. Dual target x-ray tubes for mammographic examinations: dose reduction with image quality equivalent to that with standard mammographic tubes. *Radiology* 181: 311.

Hendrick, R.E. et al. 1994. *Mammography Quality Control Manuals (Radiologist, Radiologic Technologist, Medical Physicist)*. American College of Radiology, Reston, VA.

Hendrick, R.E. and Parker, S.H. 1994. Stereotaxic imaging. In *A Categorical Course in Physics: Technical Aspects of Breast Imaging*, 3rd ed. Haus, A.G. and Yaffe, M.J. (Eds.), RSNA Publications, Oak Brook, IL, pp. 263–274.

Jennings, R.J., Quinn, P.W., Gagne, R.M., and Fewell, T.R. 1993. Evaluation of x-ray sources for mammography. *Proc. SPIE* 1896: 259–268.

Johns, P.C. and Yaffe, M.J. 1987. X-ray characterization of normal and neoplastic breast tissues. *Phys. Med. Biol.* 32: 675–695.

Karellas, A., Harris, L.J. and D'Orsi, C.J. 1990. Small field digital mammography with a 2048 × 2048 pixel charge-coupled device. *Radiology* 177: 288.

McClelland, R., Hendrick, R.E., Zinninger, M.D., and Wilcox, P.W. 1991. The American College of Radiology Mammographic Accreditation Program. *Am. J. Roentgenol.* 157: 473–479.

Nishikawa, R.M. and Yaffe, M.J. 1985. Signal-to-noise properties of mammography film-screen systems. *Med. Phys.* 12: 32–39.

Pisano, E.D. and Yaffe, M.J. 1998. Digital mammography. *Contemp. Diagn. Radiol.* 21: 1–6.

Smart, C.R., Hartmann, W.H., Beahrs, O.H. et al. 1993. Insights into breast cancer screening of younger women: evidence from the 14-year follow-up of the breast cancer detection demonstration project. *Cancer* 72: 1449–1456.

Tabar, L., Duffy, S.W., and Burhenne, L.W. 1993. New Swedish breast cancer detection results for women aged 40–49. *Cancer* (Suppl.) 72: 1437–1448.

Wagner, A.J. 1991. Contrast and grid performance in mammography. In *Screen Film Mammography: Imaging Considerations and Medical Physics Responsibilities*. Barnes, G.T. and Frey, G.D. (Eds.) Medical Physics Publishing, Madison, WI, pp. 115–134.

Wu, X., Barnes, G.T., and Tucker, D.M. 1991. Spectral dependence of glandular tissue dose in screen-film mammography. *Radiology* 179: 143–148.

Wu, X., Gingold, E.L., Barnes, G.T., and Tucker, D.M. 1994. Normalized average glandular dose in molybdenum target-rhodium filter and rhodium target-rhodium filter mammography. *Radiology* 193: 83–89.

Yaffe, M.J. 1994. Digital mammography. In *A Categorical Course in Physics: Technical Aspects of Breast Imaging*, 3rd ed. Haus, A.G. and Yaffe, M.J. (Eds.), RSNA Publications, Oak Brook, IL, pp. 275–286.

Yaffe, M.J. and Rowlands, J.A. 1997. X-ray detectors for digital radiography. *Phys. Med. Biol.* 42: 1–39.

Further Information

Yaffe, M.J. et al. 1993. *Recommended Specifications for New Mammography Equipment*: ACR-CDC Cooperative Agreement for Quality Assurance Activities in Mammography, ACR Publications, Reston, VA.

Haus, A.G. and Yaffe, M.J. 1994. *A Categorical Course in Physics: Technical Aspects of Breast Imaging*. RSNA Publications, Oak Brook, IL. In this syllabus to a course presented at the Radiological Society of North America all technical aspects of mammography are addressed by experts and a clinical overview is presented in language understandable by the physicist or biomedical engineer.

Screen Film Mammography: Imaging Considerations and Medical Physics Responsibilities. G.T. Barnes and Frey, G.D. (Eds.). Medical Physics Publishing, Madison, WI. Considerable practical information related to obtaining and maintaining high quality mammography is provided here.

Film Processing in Medical Imaging. Haus, A.G. (Ed.), Medical Physics Publishing. Madison, WI. This book deals with all aspects of medical film processing with particular emphasis on mammography.

11

Computed Tomography

11.1	Instrumentation	11-1
	Data-Acquisition Geometries • X-Ray System • Patient Dose Considerations • Summary	
	Defining Terms	11-10
	References	11-12
	Further Information	11-12
11.2	Reconstruction Principles	11-13
	Image Processing: Artifact and Reconstruction Error • Projection Data to Image: Calibrations • Projection Data to Image: Reconstruction	
	References	11-16

Ian A. Cunningham
Victoria Hospital
The John P. Roberts
Research Institute
The University of Western Ontario

Philip F. Judy
Brigham and Women's Hospital
Harvard Medical School

11.1 Instrumentation

Ian A. Cunningham

The development of **computed tomography (CT)** in the early 1970s revolutionized medical radiology. For the first time, physicians were able to obtain high-quality tomographic (cross-sectional) images of internal structures of the body. Over the next ten years, 18 manufacturers competed for the exploding world CT market. Technical sophistication increased dramatically, and even today, CT continues to mature, with new capabilities being researched and developed.

Computed tomographic images are reconstructed from a large number of measurements of **x-ray transmission** through the patient (called **projection data**). The resulting images are tomographic "maps" of the x-ray linear **attenuation** coefficient. The mathematical methods used to **reconstruct** CT images from projection data are discussed in the next section. In this section, the hardware and instrumentation in a modern scanner are described.

The first practical CT instrument was developed in 1971 by **Dr. G.N. Hounsfield** in England and was used to image the brain [Hounsfield, 1980]. The projection data were acquired in approximately 5 min, and the tomographic image was reconstructed in approximately 20 min. Since then, CT technology has developed dramatically, and CT has become a standard imaging procedure for virtually all parts of the body in thousands of facilities throughout the world. Projection data are typically acquired in approximately 1 sec, and the image is reconstructed in 3 to 5 sec. One special-purpose scanner described below acquires the projection data for one tomographic image in 50 msec. A typical modern CT scanner is shown in Figure 11.1, and typical CT images are shown in Figure 11.2.

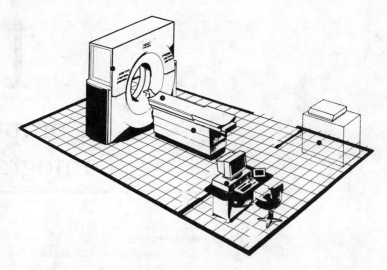

FIGURE 11.1 Schematic drawing of a typical CT scanner installation, consisting of (1) control console, (2) gantry stand, (3) patient table, (4) head holder, and (5) laser imager. (Courtesy of Picker International, Inc.)

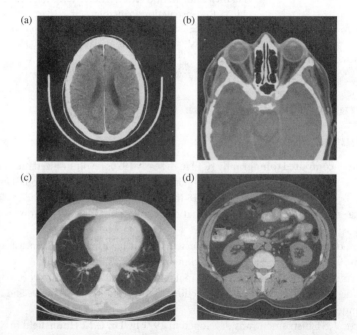

FIGURE 11.2 Typical CT images of (a) brain, (b) head showing orbits, (c) chest showing lungs, and (d) abdomen.

The fundamental task of CT systems is to make an extremely large number (approximately 500,000) of highly accurate measurements of x-ray transmission through the patient in a precisely controlled geometry. A basic system generally consists of a **gantry**, a patient table, a **control console**, and a computer. The gantry contains the **x-ray source**, **x-ray detectors**, and the **data-acquisition system (DAS)**.

11.1.1 Data-Acquisition Geometries

Projection data may be acquired in one of several possible geometries described below, based on the scanning configuration, scanning motions, and detector arrangement. The evolution of these geometries

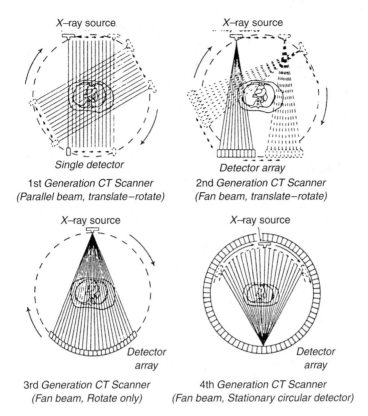

FIGURE 11.3 Four generations of CT scanners illustrating the parallel- and fan-beam geometries. (Taken from Robb R.A. 1982, CRC *Crit. Rev. Biomed. Eng.* 7: 265.)

is descried in terms of "generations," as illustrated in Figure 11.3, and reflects the historical development [Newton and Potts, 1981; Seeram, 1994]. Current CT scanners use either third-, fourth-, or fifth-generation geometries, each having their own pros and cons.

11.1.1.1 First Generation: Parallel-Beam Geometry

Parallel-beam geometry is the simplest technically and the easiest with which to understand the important CT principles. Multiple measurements of x-ray transmission are obtained using a single highly collimated x-ray **pencil beam** and detector. The beam is translated in a linear motion across the patient to obtain a projection profile. The source and detector are then rotated about the patient isocenter by approximately 1 degree, and another projection profile is obtained. This translate-rotate scanning motion is repeated until the source and detector have been rotated by 180 degrees. The highly collimated beam provides excellent rejection of radiation scattered in the patient; however, the complex scanning motion results in long (approximately 5-min) **scan times**. This geometry was used by Hounsfield in his original experiments [Hounsfield, 1980] but is not used in modern scanners.

11.1.1.2 Second Generation: Fan Beam, Multiple Detectors

Scan times were reduced to approximately 30 sec with the use of a **fan beam** of x-rays and a linear **detector array**. A translate-rotate scanning motion was still employed; however, a larger rotate increment could be used, which resulted in shorter scan times. The reconstruction algorithms are slightly more complicated than those for first-generation algorithms because they must handle fan-beam projection data.

11.1.1.3 Third Generation: Fan Beam, Rotating Detectors

Third-generation scanners were introduced in 1976. A fan beam of x-rays is rotated 360 degrees around the isocenter. No translation motion is used; however, the fan beam must be wide enough to completely contain the patient. A curved detector array consisting of several hundred independent detectors is mechanically coupled to the x-ray source, and both rotate together. As a result, these rotate-only motions acquire projection data for a single image in as little as 1 sec. Third-generation designs have the advantage that thin tungsten septa can be placed between each detector in the array and focused on the x-ray source to reject **scattered radiation**.

11.1.1.4 Fourth Generation: Fan Beam, Fixed Detectors

In a fourth-generation scanner, the x-ray source and fan beam rotate about the isocenter, while the detector array remains stationary. The detector array consists of 600 to 4800 (depending on the manufacturer) independent detectors in a circle that completely surrounds the patient. Scan times are similar to those of third-generation scanners. The detectors are no longer coupled to the x-ray source and hence cannot make use of **focused septa** to reject scattered radiation. However, detectors are calibrated twice during each rotation of the x-ray source, providing a self-calibrating system. Third-generation systems are calibrated only once every few hours.

Two detector geometries are currently used for fourth-generation systems (1) a rotating x-ray source inside a fixed detector array and (2) a rotating x-ray source outside a nutating detector array. Figure 11.4 shows the major components in the gantry of a typical fourth-generation system using a fixed-detector array. Both third- and fourth-generation systems are commercially available, and both have been highly successful clinically. Neither can be considered an overall superior design.

11.1.1.5 Fifth Generation: Scanning Electron Beam

Fifth-generation scanners are unique in that the x-ray source becomes an integral part of the system design. The detector array remains stationary, while a high-energy electron beams is electronically swept along a semicircular tungsten strip **anode**, as illustrated in Figure 11.5. X-rays are produced at the point where the electron beam hits the anode, resulting in a source of x-rays that rotates about the patient with no moving parts [Boyd et al., 1979]. Projection data can be acquired in approximately 50 msec, which is fast enough to image the beating heart without significant motion artifacts [Boyd and Lipton, 1983].

An alternative fifth-generation design, called the dynamic spatial reconstructor (DSR) scanner, is in use at the Mayo Clinic [Ritman, 1980, 1990]. This machine is a research prototype and is not available commercially. It consists of 14 x-ray tubes, scintillation screens, and video cameras. **Volume CT** images can be produced in as little as 10 msec.

11.1.1.6 Spiral/Helical Scanning

The requirement for faster scan times, and in particular for fast multiple scans for **three-dimensional imaging**, has resulted in the development of spiral (**helical**) scanning systems [Kalendar et al., 1990]. Both third- and fourth-generation systems achieve this using self-lubricating slip-ring technology (Figure 11.6) to make the electrical connections with rotating components. This removes the need for power and signal cables which would otherwise have to be rewound between scans and allows for a continuous rotating motion of the x-ray fan beam. Multiple images are acquired while the patient is translated through the gantry in a smooth continuous motion rather than stopping for each image. Projection data for multiple images covering a volume of the patient can be acquired in a single breath hold at rates of approximately one **slice** per second. The reconstruction algorithms are more sophisticated because they must accommodate the spiral or helical path traced by the x-ray source around the patient, as illustrated in Figure 11.7.

11.1.2 X-Ray System

The x-ray system consists of the x-ray source, detectors, and a data-acquisition system.

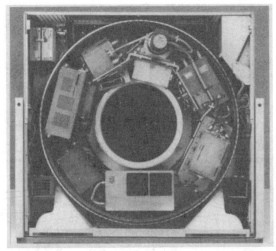

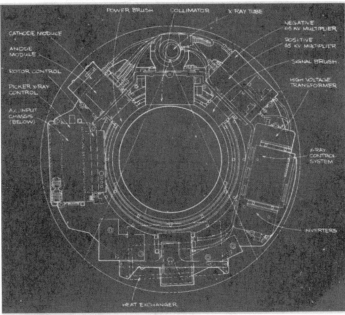

FIGURE 11.4   The major internal components of a fourth-generation CT gantry are shown in a photograph with the gantry cover removed (upper) and identified in the line drawing (lower). (Courtesy of Picker International, Inc.)

11.1.2.1   X-Ray Source

With the exception of one fifth-generation system described above, all CT scanners use bremsstrahlung x-ray tubes as the source of radiation. These tubes are typical of those used in diagnostic imaging and produce x-rays by accelerating a beam of electrons onto a target anode. The anode area from which x-rays are emitted, projected along the direction of the beam, is called the **focal spot**. Most systems have two possible focal spot sizes, approximately 0.5×1.5 mm and 1.0×2.5 mm. A collimator assembly is used to control the width of the fan beam between 1.0 and 10 mm, which in turn controls the width of the imaged slice.

The power requirements of these tubes are typically 120 kV at 200 to 500 mA, producing x-rays with an energy spectrum ranging between approximately 30 and 120 keV. All modern systems use high-frequency generators, typically operating between 5 and 50 kHz [Brunnett et al., 1990]. Some spiral systems use a

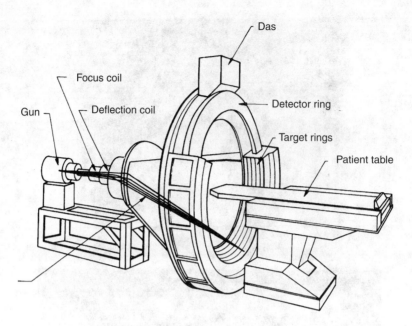

FIGURE 11.5   Schematic illustration of a fifth-generation ultrafast CT system. Image data are acquired in as little as 50 msec, as an electron beam is swept over the strip anode electronically. (Courtesy of Imatron, Inc.)

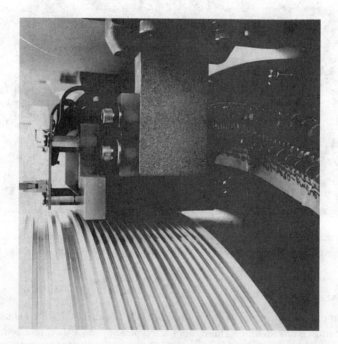

FIGURE 11.6   Photograph of the slip rings used to pass power and control signals to the rotating gantry. (Courtesy of Picker International, Inc.)

stationary generator in the gantry, requiring high-voltage (120-kV) slip rings, while others use a rotating generator with lower-voltage (480-V) slip rings. Production of x-rays in bremsstrahlung tubes is an inefficient process, and hence most of the power delivered to the tubes results in heating of the anode. A heat exchanger on the rotating gantry is used to cool the tube. **Spiral scanning**, in particular, places heavy demands on the heat-storage capacity and cooling rate of the x-ray tube.

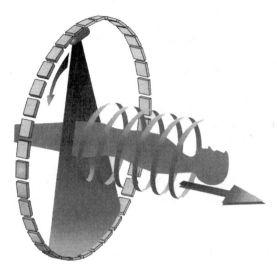

FIGURE 11.7   Spiral scanning causes the focal spot to follow a spiral path around the patient as indicated. (Courtesy of Picker International, Inc.)

The intensity of the x-ray beam is attenuated by **absorption** and scattering processes as it passes through the patient. The degree of attenuation depends on the energy spectrum of the x-rays as well as on the average atomic number and mass density of the patient tissues. The transmitted intensity is given by

$$I_t = I_o e^{-\int_0^L \mu(x)dx} \tag{11.1}$$

where I_o and I_t are the incident and transmitted beam intensities, respectively; L is the length of the x-ray path; and $m(x)$ is the **x-ray linear attenuation coefficient**, which varies with tissue type and hence is a function of the distance x through the patient. The integral of the attenuation coefficient is therefore given by

$$\int_0^L \mu(x)dx = -\frac{1}{L}\ln(I_t/I_o) \tag{11.2}$$

The reconstruction algorithm requires measurements of this integral along many paths in the fan beam at each of many angles about the isocenter. The value of L is known, and I_o is determined by a system calibration. Hence values of the integral along each path can be determined from measurements of I_t.

11.1.2.2   X-Ray Detectors

X-ray detectors used in CT systems must (a) have a high overall efficiency to minimize the patient radiation dose, have a large dynamic range, (b) be very stable with time, and (c) be insensitive to temperature variations within the gantry. Three important factors contributing to the detector efficiency are geometric efficiency, quantum (also called capture) efficiency, and conversion efficiency [Villafanaet et al., 1987]. Geometric efficiency refers to the area of the detectors sensitive to radiation as a fraction of the total exposed area. Thin septa between detector elements to remove scattered radiation, or other insensitive regions, will degrade this value. Quantum efficiency refers to the fraction of incident x-rays on the detector that are absorbed and contribute to the measured signal. Conversion efficiency refers to the ability to accurately convert the absorbed x-ray signal into an electrical signal (but is not the same as the energy conversion efficiency). Overall efficiency is the product of the three, and it generally lies between 0.45 and 0.85. A value of less than 1 indicates a nonideal detector system and results in a required increase in patient radiation

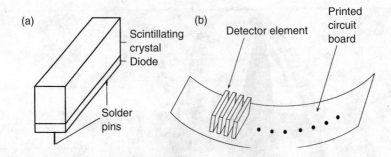

FIGURE 11.8 (a) A solid-state detector consists of a scintillating crystal and photodiode combination. (b) Many such detectors are placed side by side to form a detector array that may contain up to 4800 detectors.

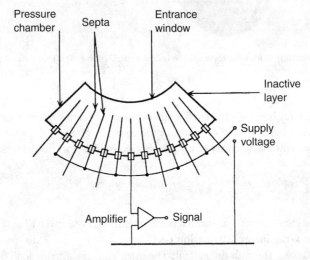

FIGURE 11.9 Gas ionization detector arrays consist of high-pressure gas in multiple chambers separated by thin septa. A voltage is applied between alternating septa. The septa also act as electrodes and collect the ions created by the radiation, converting them into an electrical signal.

dose if image quality is to be maintained. The term dose efficiency sometimes has been used to indicate overall efficiency.

Modern commercial systems use one of two detector types: solid-state or gas ionization detectors.

Solid-State Detectors. Solid-state detectors consist of an array of scintillating crystals and photodiodes, as illustrated in Figure 11.8. The scintillators generally are either cadmium tungstate (CdWO4) or a ceramic material made of rare earth oxides, although previous scanners have used bismuth germanate crystals with photomultiplier tubes. Solid-state detectors generally have very high quantum and conversion efficiencies and a large dynamic range.

Gas Ionization Detectors. Gas ionization detectors, as illustrated in Figure 11.9, consist of an array of chambers containing compressed gas (usually xenon at up to 30 atm pressure). A high voltage is applied to tungsten septa between chambers to collect ions produced by the radiation. These detectors have excellent stability and a large dynamic range; however, they generally have a lower quantum efficiency than solid-state detectors.

11.1.2.3 Data-Acquisition System

The transmitted fraction I_t/I_o in Equation 11.2 through an obese patient can be less than 10 to 4. Thus it is the task of the data-acquisition system (DAS) to accurately measure I_t over a dynamic

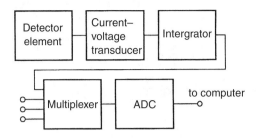

FIGURE 11.10 The data-acquisition system converts the electrical signal produced by each detector to a digital value for the computer.

range of more than 104, encode the results into digital values, and transmit the values to the system computer for reconstruction. Some manufacturers use the approach illustrated in Figure 11.10, consisting of precision preamplifiers, current-to-voltage converters, analog integrators, multiplexers, and analog-to-digital converters. Alternatively, some manufacturers use the preamplifier to control a synchronous voltage-to-frequency converter (SVFC), replacing the need for the integrators, multiplexers, and analog-to-digital converters [Brunnett et al., 1990]. The logarithmic conversion required in Equation 11.2 is performed with either an analog logarithmic amplifier or a digital lookup table, depending on the manufacturer.

Sustained data transfer rates to the computer are as high as 10 Mbytes/sec for some scanners. This can be accomplished with a direct connection for systems having a fixed detector array. However, third-generation slip-ring systems must use more sophisticated techniques. At least one manufacturer uses optical transmitters on the rotating gantry to send data to fixed optical receivers [Siemens, 1989].

11.1.2.4 Computer System

Various computer systems are used by manufacturers to control system hardware, acquire the projection data, and reconstruct, display, and manipulate the tomographic images. A typical system is illustrated in Figure 11.11, which uses 12 independent processors connected by a 40-Mbyte/sec multibus. Multiple custom array processors are used to achieve a combined computational speed of 200 MFLOPS (million floating-point operations per second) and a reconstruction time of approximately 5 sec to produce an image on a 1024 × 1024 pixel display. A simplified UNIX operating system is used to provide a multitasking, multiuser environment to coordinate tasks.

11.1.3 Patient Dose Considerations

The patient dose resulting from CT examinations is generally specified in terms of the CT dose index (CTDI) [Felmlee et al., 1989; Rothenberg and Pentlow, 1992], which includes the dose contribution from radiation scattered from nearby slices. A summary of CTDI values, as specified by four manufacturers, is given in Table 11.1.

11.1.4 Summary

Computed tomography revolutionized medical radiology in the early 1970s. Since that time, CT technology has developed dramatically, taking advantage of developments in computer hardware and detector technology. Modern systems acquire the projection data required for one tomographic image in approximately 1 sec and present the reconstructed image on a 1024 × 1024 matrix display within a few seconds. The images are high-quality tomographic "maps" of the x-ray linear attenuation coefficient of the patient tissues.

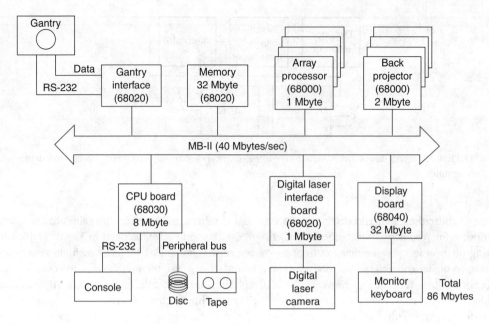

FIGURE 11.11 The computer system controls the gantry motions, acquires the x-ray transmission measurements, and reconstructs the final image. The system shown here uses 1,268,000-family CPUs. (Courtesy of Picker International, Inc.)

TABLE 11.1   Summary of the CT Dose Index (CTDI) Values at Two Positions (Center of the Patient and Near the Skin) as Specified by Four CT Manufacturers for Standard Head and Body Scans

Manufacturer	Detector	kVp	mA	Scan time (sec)	CTDI, center (mGy)	CTDI, skin (mGy)
A, head	Xenon	120	170	2	50	48
A, body	Xenon	120	170	2	14	25
A, head	Solid state	120	170	2	40	40
A, body	Solid state	120	170	2	11	20
B, head	Solid state	130	80	2	37	41
B, body	Solid state	130	80	2	15	34
C, head	Solid state	120	500	2	39	50
C, body	Solid state	120	290	1	12	28
D, head	Solid state	120	200	2	78	78
D, body	Solid state	120	200	2	9	16

Defining Terms

Absorption: Some of the incident x-ray energy is absorbed in patient tissues and hence does not contribute to the transmitted beam.

Anode: A tungsten bombarded by a beam of electrons to produce x-rays. In all but one fifth-generation system, the anode rotates to distribute the resulting heat around the perimeter. The anode heat-storage capacity and maximum cooling rate often limit the maximum scanning rates of CT systems.

Attenuation: The total decrease in the intensity of the primary x-ray beam as it passes through the patient, resulting from both scatter and absorption processes. It is characterized by the linear attenuation coefficient.

Computed tomography (CT): A computerized method of producing x-ray tomographic images. Previous names for the same thing include computerized tomographic imaging, computerized axial tomography (CAT), computer-assisted tomography (CAT), and reconstructive tomography (RT).

Control console: The control console is used by the CT operator to control the scanning operations, image reconstruction, and image display.

Cormack, Dr. Allan MacLeod: A physicist who developed mathematical techniques required in the reconstruction of tomographic images. Dr. Cormack shared the Nobel Prize in Medicine and Physiology with Dr. G.N. Hounsfield in 1979 [Cormack, 1980].

Data-acquisition system (DAS): Interfaces the x-ray detectors to the system computer and may consist of a preamplifier, integrator, multiplexer, logarithmic amplifier, and analog-to-digital converter.

Detector array: An array of individual detector elements. The number of detector elements varies between a few hundred and 4800, depending on the acquisition geometry and manufacturer. Each detector element functions independently of the others.

Fan beam: The x-ray beam is generated at the focal spot and so diverges as it passes through the patient to the detector array. The thickness of the beam is generally selectable between 1.0 and 10 mm and defines the slice thickness.

Focal spot: The region of the anode where x-rays are generated.

Focused septa: Thin metal plates between detector elements which are aligned with the focal spot so that the primary beam passes unattenuated to the detector elements, while scattered x-rays which normally travel in an altered direction are blocked.

Gantry: The largest component of the CT installation, containing the x-ray tube, collimators, detector array, DAS, other control electronics, and the mechanical components required for the scanning motions.

Helical scanning: The scanning motions in which the x-ray tube rotates continuously around the patient while the patient is continuously translated through the fan beam. The focal spot therefore traces a helix around the patient. Projection data are obtained which allow the reconstruction of multiple contiguous images. This operation is sometimes called spiral, volume, or three-dimensional CT scanning.

Hounsfield, Dr. Godfrey Newbold: An engineer who developed the first practical CT instrument in 1971. Dr. Hounsfield received the McRobert Award in 1972 and shared the Nobel Prize in Medicine and Physiology with Dr. A.M. Cormack in 1979 for this invention [Hounsfield, 1980].

Image plane: The plane through the patient that is imaged. In practice, this plane (also called a slice) has a selectable thickness between 1.0 and 10 mm centered on the image plane.

Pencil beam: A narrow, well-collimated beam of x-rays.

Projection data: The set of transmission measurements used to reconstruct the image.

Reconstruct: The mathematical operation of generating the tomographic image from the projection data.

Scan time: The time required to acquire the projection data for one image, typically 1.0 sec.

Scattered radiation: Radiation that is removed from the primary beam by a scattering process. This radiation is not absorbed but continues along a path in an altered direction.

Slice: See Image plane.

Spiral scanning: See Helical scanning.

Three-dimensional imaging: See Helical scanning.

Tomography: A technique of imaging a cross-sectional slice.

Volume CT: See Helical scanning.

X-ray detector: A device that absorbs radiation and converts some or all of the absorbed energy into a small electrical signal.

X-ray linear attenuation coefficient m: Expresses the relative rate of attenuation of a radiation beam as it passes through a material. The value of m depends on the density and atomic number of the material and on the x-ray energy. The units of m are cm^{-1}.

X-ray source: The device that generates the x-ray beam. All CT scanners are rotating-anode bremsstrahlung x-ray tubes except one-fifth generation system, which uses a unique scanned electron beam and a strip anode.

X-ray transmission: The fraction of the x-ray beam intensity that is transmitted through the patient without being scattered or absorbed. It is equal to I_t/I_o in Equation 11.2, can be determined by measuring the beam intensity both with (I_t) and without (I_o) the patient present, and is expressed as a fraction. As a rule of thumb, n^2 independent transmission measurements are required to reconstruct an image with an $n \times n$ sized pixel matrix.

References

Body D.P. et al. 1979. A proposed dynamic cardiac 3D densitometer for early detection and evaluation of heart disease. *IEEE Trans. Nucl. Sci.* 2724.

Boyd D.P. and Lipton M.J. 1983. Cardiac computed tomography. *Proc. IEEE* 198.

Brunnett C.J., Heuscher D.J., Mattson R.A., and Vrettos C.J. 1990. CT Design Considerations and Specifications. Picker International, CT Engineering Department, Ohio.

Cormack A.M. 1980. Nobel award address: early two-dimensional reconstruction and recent topics stemming from it. *Med. Phys.* 7(4): 277.

Felmlee J.P., Gray J.E., Leetzow M.L., and Price J.C. 1989. Estimated fetal radiation dose from multislice CT studies. *Am. Roent. Ray. Soc.* 154: 185.

Hounsfield G.N. 1980. Nobel award address: computed medical imaging. *Med. Phys.* 7(4): 283.

Kalendar W.A., Seissler W., Klotz E. et al. 1990. Spiral volumetric CT with single-breath-hold technique, continuous transport, and continuous scanner rotation. *Radiology* 176: 181.

Newton T.H. and Potts D.G. (eds). 1981. *Radiology of the Skull and Brain: Technical Aspects of Computed Tomography.* St. Louis, Mosby.

Picker. 1990. *Computed Dose Index PQ2000 CT Scanner.* Ohio, Picker International.

Ritman E.L. 1980. Physical and technical considerations in the design of the DSR, and high temporal resolution volume scanner. *AJR* 134: 369.

Ritman E.L. 1990. Fast computed tomography for quantitative cardiac analysis —state of the art and future perspectives. *Mayo Clin. Proc.* 65: 1336.

Robb R.A. 1982. X-ray computed tomography: an engineering synthesis of multiscientific principles. *CRC Crit. Rev. Biomed. Eng.* 7: 265.

Rothenberg L.N. and Pentlow K.S. 1992. Radiation dose in CT. *RadioGraphics* 12: 1225.

Seeram E. 1994. *Computed Tomography: Physical Principles, Clinical Applications and Quality Control.* Philadelphia, Saunders.

Siemens. 1989. *The Technology and Performance of the Somatom Plus.* Erlangen, Germany, Siemens Aktiengesellschaft, Medical Engineering Group.

Villafana T., Lee S.H., and Rao K.C.V.G. (eds). 1987. *Cranial Computed Tomography.* New York, McGraw-Hill.

Further Information

A recent summary of CT instrumentation and concepts is given by E. Seeram in *Computed Tomography: Physical Principles, Clinical Applications and Quality Control.* The author summarizes CT from the perspective of the nonmedical, nonspecialist user. A summary of average CT patient doses is described by Rothenberg and Pentlow [1992] in *Radiation Dose in CT.* Research papers on both fundamental and practical aspects of CT physics and instrumentation are published in numerous journals, including *Medical Physics, Physics in Medicine and Biology, Journal of Computer Assisted Tomography, Radiology, British Journal of Radiology,* and the IEEE Press. A comparison of technical specifications of CT systems provided by the manufacturers is available from ECRI to help orient the new purchaser in a selection process.

Their Product Comparison System includes a table of basic specifications for all the major international manufactures.

11.2   Reconstruction Principles

Philip F. Judy

Computed tomography (CT) is a two-step process (1) the transmission of an x-ray beam is measured through all possible straight-line paths as in a plane of an object, and (2) the attenuation of an x-ray beam is estimated at points in the object. Initially, the transmission measurements will be assumed to be the results of an experiment performed with a narrow monoenergetic beam of x-rays that are confined to a plane. The designs of devices that attempt to realize these measurements are described in the preceding section. One formal consequence of these assumptions is that the logarithmic transformation of the measured x-ray intensity is proportional to the line integral of attenuation coefficients. In order to satisfy this assumption, computer processing procedures on the measurements of x-ray intensity are necessary even before image reconstruction is performed. These linearization procedures will reviewed after background.

Both analytical and iterative estimations of linear x-ray attenuation have been used for transmission CT reconstruction. Iterative procedures are of historic interest because an iterative reconstruction procedure was used in the first commercially successful CT scanner [EMI, Mark I, Hounsfield, 1973]. They also permit easy incorporation of physical processes that cause deviations from the linearity. Their practical usefulness is limited. The first EMI scanner required 20 min to finish its reconstruction. Using the identical hardware and employing an analytical calculation, the estimation of attenuation values was performed during the 4.5-min data acquisition and was made on a 160×160 matrix. The original iterative procedure reconstructed the attenuation values on an 80×80 matrix and consequently failed to exploit all the spatial information inherent in transmission data.

Analytical estimation, or direct reconstruction, uses a numerical approximation of the inverse Radon transform [Radon, 1917]. The direct reconstruction technique (convolution-backprojection) presently used in x-ray CT was initially applied in other areas such as radio astronomy [Bracewell and Riddle, 1967] and electron microscopy [Crowther et al., 1970; Ramachandran and Lakshminarayana, 1971]. These investigations demonstrated that the reconstructions from the discrete spatial sampling of band-limited data led to full recovery of the cross-sectional attenuation. The random variation (noise) in x-ray transmission measurements may not be bandlimited. Subsequent investigators [Herman and Rowland, 1973; Shepp and Logan, 1974; Chesler and Riederer, 1975] have suggested various bandlimiting windows that reduce the propagation and amplification of noise by the reconstruction. These issues have been investigated by simulation, and investigators continue to pursue these issues using a computer phantom [e.g., Guedon and Bizais, 1994, and references therein] described by Shepp and Logan. The subsequent investigations of the details of choice of reconstruction parameters has had limited practical impact because real variation of transmission data is bandlimited by the finite size of the focal spot and radiation detector, a straightforward design question, and because random variation of the transmission tends to be uncorrelated. Consequently, the classic precedures suffice.

11.2.1   Image Processing: Artifact and Reconstruction Error

An artifact is a reconstruction defect that is obviously visible in the image. The classification of an image feature as an artifact involves some visual criterion. The effect must produce an image feature that is greater than the random variation in image caused by the intrinsic variation in transmission measurements. An artifact not recognized by the physician observer as an artifact may be reported as a lesion. Such false-positive reports could lead to an unnecessary medical procedure, for example, surgery to remove an imaginary tumor. A reconstruction error is a deviation of the reconstruction value from its expected value. Reconstruction errors are significant if the application involves a quantitative measurement, not a common medical application. The reconstruction errors are characterized by identical material at different points in the object leading to different reconstructed attenuation values in the image which are not visible in the medical image.

Investigators have used computer simulation to investigate artifact [Herman, 1980] because image noise limits the visibility of their visibility. One important issue investigated was required spatial sampling of transmission slice plane [Crawford and Kak, 1979; Parker et al., 1982]. These simulations provided a useful guideline in design. In practice, these aliasing artifacts are overwhelmed by random noise, and designers tend to oversample in the slice plane. A second issue that was understood by computer simulation was the partial volume artifact [Glover and Pelc, 1980]. This artifact would occur even for mononergetic beams and finite beam size, particularly in the axial dimension. The axial dimension of the beams tend to be greater (about 10 mm) than their dimensions in the slice plane (about 1 mm). The artifact is created when the variation of transmission within the beam varies considerably, and the exponential variation within the beam is summed by the radiation detector. The logarithm transformation of the detected signal produces a nonlinear effect that is propagated throughout the image by the reconstruction process. Simulation was useful in demonstrating that isolated features in the same cross-section act together to produce streak artifacts. Simulations have been useful to illustrate the effects of patient motion during the data-acquisition streaks off high-contrast objects.

11.2.2 Projection Data to Image: Calibrations

Processing of transmission data is necessary to obtain high-quality images. In general, optimization of the projection data will optimize the reconstructed image. Reconstruction is a process that removes the spatial correlation of attenuation effects in the transmitted image by taking advantage of completely sampling the possible transmissions. Two distinct calibrations are required: registration of beams with the reconstruction matrix and linearization of the measured signal.

Without loss of generalization, a projection will be considered a set of transmissions made along parallel lines in the slice plane of the CT scanner. Without loss of generalization means that essential aspects of all calibration and reconstruction procedures required for fan-beam geometries are captured by the calibration and reconstruction procedures described for parallel projections. One line of each projection is assumed to pass through the center of rotation of data collection. Shepp et al. [1979] showed that errors in the assignment of that center-of-rotation point in the projections could lead to considerable distinctive artifacts and that small errors (0.05 mm) would produce these effects. The consequences of these errors have been generalized to fan-beam collection schemes, and images reconstructed from 180-degree projection sets were compared with images reconstructed from 360-degree data sets [Kijewski and Judy, 1983]. A simple misregistration of the center of rotation was found to produce blurring of image without the artifact. These differences may explain the empirical observation that most commercial CT scanners collect a full 360-degree data set even though 180 degree of data will suffice.

The data-acquisition scheme that was designed to overcome the limited sampling inherent in third-generation fan-beam systems by shifting detectors a quarter sampling distance while opposite 180-degree projection is measured, has particularly stringent registration requirements. Also, the fourth-generation scanner does not link the motion of the x-ray tube and the detector; consequently, the center of rotation is determined as part of a calibration procedure, and unsystematic effects lead to artifacts that mimic noise besides blurring the image.

Misregistration artifacts also can be mitigated by feathering. This procedure requires collection of redundant projection data at the end of the scan. A single data set is produced by linearly weighting the redundant data at the beginning and end of the data collection [Parker et al., 1982]. These procedures have be useful in reducing artifacts from gated data collections [Moore et al., 1987].

The other processing necessary before reconstruction of project data is linearization. The formal requirement for reconstruction is that the line integrals of some variable be available; this is the variable that ultimately is reconstructed. The logarithm of x-ray transmission approximates this requirement. There are physical effects in real x-ray transmissions that cause deviations from this assumption. X-ray beams of sufficient intensity are composed of photons of different energies. Some photons in the beam interact with objects and are scattered rather than absorbed. The spectrum of x-ray photons of different attenuation coefficients means the logarithm of the transmission measurement will not be proportional to the line integral of the attenuation coefficient along that path, because an attenuation coefficient cannot even be defined. An effective attenuation coefficient can only be defined uniquely for a spectrum for a small mass of material that alters that intensity. It has to be small enough not to alter the spectrum [McCullough, 1979].

A straightforward approach to this nonunique attenuation coefficient error, called hardening, is to assume that the energy dependence of the attenuation coefficient is constant and that differences in attenuation are related to a generalized density factor that multiplies the spectral dependence of attenuation. The transmission of an x-ray beam then can be estimated for a standard material, typically water, as a function of thickness. This assumption is that attenuations of materials in the object, the human body, differ because specific gravities of the materials differ. Direct measurements of the transmission of an actual x-ray beam may provide initial estimates that can be parameterized. The inverse of this function provides the projection variable that is reconstructed. The parameters of the function are usually modified as part of a calibration to make the CT image of a uniform water phantom flat.

Such a calibration procedure does not deal completely with the hardening effects. The spectral dependence of bone differs considerably from that of water. This is particularly critical in imaging of the brain, which is contained within the skull. Without additional correction, the attenuation values of brain are lower in the center than near the skull.

The detection of scattered energy means that the reconstructed attenuation coefficient will differ from the attenuation coefficient estimated with careful narrow-beam measurements. The x-rays appear more penetrating because scattered x-rays are detected. The zero-ordered scatter, a decrease in the attenuation coefficient by some constant amount, is dealt with automatically by the calibration that treats hardening. First-order scattering leads to a widening of the x-ray beam and can be dealt with by a modification of the reconstruction kernel.

11.2.3 Projection Data to Image: Reconstruction

The impact of CT created considerable interest in the formal aspects of reconstruction. There are many detailed descriptions of direct reconstruction procedures. Some are presented in textbooks used in graduate courses for medical imaging [Barrett and Swindell, 1981; Cho et al., 1993]. Herman [1980] published a textbook that was based on a two-semester course that dealt exclusively with reconstruction principles, demonstrating the reconstruction principles with simulation.

The standard reconstruction method is called convolution-backprojection. The first step in the procedure is to convolve the projection, a set of transmissions made along parallel lines in the slice plane, with a reconstruction kernel derived from the inverse Radon transform. The choice of kernel is dictated by bandlimiting issues [Herman and Rowland, 1973; Shepp and Logan, 1974; Chesler and Riederer, 1975]. It can be modified to deal with the physical aperture of the CT system [Bracewell, 1977], which might include the effects of scatter. The convolved projection is then backprojected onto a two-dimensional image matrix. Backprojection is the opposite of projection; the value of the projection is added to each point along the line of the projection. This procedure makes sense in the continuous description, but in the discrete world of the computer, the summation is done over the image matrix.

Consider a point of the image matrix; very few, possibly no lines of the discrete projection data intersect the point. Consequently, to estimate the projection value to be added to that point, the procedure must interpolate between two values of sampled convolve projection. The linear interpolation scheme is a significant improvement over nearest project nearest to the point. More complex schemes get confounded with choices of reconstruction kernel, which are designed to accomplish standard image processing in the image, for example, edge enhancement.

Scanners have been developed to acquire a three-dimensional set of projection data [Kalender et al., 1990]. The motion of the source defines a spiral motion relative to the patient. The spiral motion defines an axis. Consequently, only one projection is available for reconstruction of the attenuation values in the plane. This is the back-projection problem just discussed; no correct projection value is available from the discrete projection data set. The solution is identical: a projection value is interpolated from the existing projection values to estimate the necessary projections for each plane to be reconstructed. This procedure has the advantage that overlapping slices can be reconstructed without additional exposure, and this eliminates the risk that a small lesion will be missed because it straddles adjacent slices. This data-collection scheme is possible because systems that continuously rotate have been developed. The spiral scan motion is realized by moving the patient through the gantry. Spiral CT scanners have made possible the acquisition of an entire data set in a single breath hold.

References

Barrett H.H. and Swindell W. 1981. *Radiological Imaging: The Theory and Image Formation, Detection, and Processing*, Vol. 2. New York, Academic Press.

Bracewell R.N. and Riddle A.C. 1967. Inversion of fan-beam scans in radio astronomy. *The Astrophys. J.* 150: 427–434.

Chesler D.A. and Riederer S.J. 1975. Ripple suppression during reconstruction in transverse tomography. *Phys. Med. Biol.* 20(4): 632–636.

Cho Z., Jones J.P. and Singh M. 1993. *Foundations of Medical Imaging.* New York, Wiley & Sons, Inc.

Crawford C.R. and Kak A.C. 1979. Aliasing artifacts in computerized tomography. *Appl. Opt.* 18: 3704–3711.

Glover G.H. and Pelc N.J. 1980. Nonlinear partial volume artifacts in x-ray computed tomography. *Med. Phys.* 7: 238–248.

Guedon J.-P. and Bizais. 1994. Bandlimited and harr filtered back-projection reconstruction. *IEEE Trans. Med. Imag.* 13(3): 430–440.

Herman G.T. and Rowland S.W. 1973. Three methods for reconstruction objects for x-rays — a comparative study. *Comp. Graph. Imag. Process.* 2: 151–178.

Herman G.T. 1980. *Image Reconstruction from Projection: The Fundamentals of Computerized Tomography.* New York, Academic Press.

Hounsfield, G.N. 1973. Computerized transverse axial scanning (tomography): Part I. *Brit. J. Radiol.* 46: 1016–1022.

Kalender W.A., Weissler, Klotz E. et al. 1990. Spiral volumetric CT with single-breath-hold technique, continuous transport, and continuous scanner rotation. *Radiology* 176: 181–183.

Kijewski M.F. and Judy P.F. 1983. The effect of misregistration of the projections on spatial resolution of CT scanners. *Med. Phys.* 10: 169–175.

McCullough E.C. 1979. Specifying and evaluating the performance of computed tomographic (CT) scanners. *Med. Phys.* 7: 291–296.

Moore S.C., Judy P.F., Garnic J.D. et al. 1983. The effect of misregistration of the projections on spatial resolution of CT scanners. *Med. Phys.* 10: 169–175.

12

Magnetic Resonance Imaging

Steven Conolly
Albert Macovski
John Pauly
Stanford University

John Schenck
General Electric Corporate Research and Development Center

Kenneth K. Kwong
David A. Chesler
Massachusetts General Hospital Harvard University Medical School

Xiaoping Hu
Wei Chen
Maqbool Patel
Kamil Ugurbil
Center for Magnetic Resonance Research
The University of Minnesota Medical School

12.1 Acquisition and Processing............................ **12**-1
　　Fundamentals of MRI • Contrast Mechanisms
Defining Terms.. **12**-8
References **12**-9
12.2 Hardware/Instrumentation **12**-9
　　Fundamentals of MRI Instrumentation • Static Field Magnets • Gradient Coils • Radiofrequency Coils • Digital Data Processing • Current Trends in MRI
Defining Terms.. **12**-19
References **12**-21
Further Information **12**-21
12.3 Functional MRI **12**-22
　　Advances in Functional Brain Mapping • Mechanism • Problem and Artifacts in fMRI: The Brain–Vein Problem? The Brain-Inflow Problem? • Techniques to Reduce the Large Vessel Problems
References **12**-29
12.4 Chemical-Shift Imaging: An Introduction to Its Theory and Practice **12**-31
　　General Methodology • Practical Examples • Summary
Acknowledgments.. **12**-38
References **12**-38

12.1 Acquisition and Processing

Steven Conolly, Albert Macovski, and John Pauly

Magnetic resonance imaging (MRI) is a clinically important medical imaging modality due to its exceptional soft-tissue contrast. MRI was invented in the early 1970s [1]. The first commercial scanners appeared about 10 years later. Noninvasive MRI studies are now supplanting many conventional invasive procedures. A 1990 study [2] found that the principal applications for MRI are examinations of the head (40%), spine (33%), bone and joints (17%), and the body (10%). The percentage of bone and joint studies was growing in 1990.

Although typical imaging studies range from 1 to 10 min, new fast imaging techniques acquire images in less than 50 msec. MRI research involves fundamental tradeoffs between resolution, imaging time, and signal-to-noise ratio (SNR). It also depends heavily on both gradient and receiver coil hardware innovations.

In this section we provide a brief synopsis of basic nuclear magnetic resonance (NMR) physics. We then derive the *k*-**space** analysis of MRI, which interprets the received signal as a scan of the Fourier transform of the image. This powerful formalism is used to analyze the most important imaging sequences. Finally, we discuss the fundamental contrast mechanisms for MRI.

12.1.1 Fundamentals of MRI

Magnetic resonance imaging exploits the existence of induced nuclear magnetism in the patient. Materials with an odd number of protons or neutrons possess a weak but observable nuclear magnetic moment. Most commonly protons (^{1}H) are imaged, although carbon (^{13}C), phosphorous (^{31}P), sodium (^{23}Na), and fluorine (^{19}F) are also of significant interest. The nuclear moments are normally randomly oriented, but they align when placed in a strong magnetic field. Typical field strengths for imaging range between 0.2 and 1.5 T, although spectroscopic and functional imaging work is often performed with higher field strengths. The nuclear **magnetization** is very weak; the ratio of the induced magnetization to the applied fields is only 4×10^{-9}. The collection of nuclear moments is often referred to as magnetization or **spins**.

The static nuclear moment is far too weak to be measured when it is aligned with the strong static magnetic field. Physicists in the 1940s developed resonance techniques that permit this weak moment to be measured. The key idea is to measure the moment while it oscillates in a plane perpendicular to the static field [3,4]. First one must tip the moment away from the static field. When perpendicular to the static field, the moment feels a torque proportional to the strength of the static magnetic field. The torque always points perpendicular to the magnetization and causes the spins to oscillate or precess in a plane perpendicular to the static field. The frequency of the rotation ω_0 is proportional to the field:

$$\omega_0 = -\gamma B_0$$

where γ, the **gyromagnetic ratio**, is a constant specific to the nucleus, and B_0 is the magnetic field strength. The direction of B_0 defines the z-axis. The **precession** frequency is called the **Larmor frequency**. The negative sign indicates the direction of the precession.

Since the precessing moments constitute a time-varying flax, they produce a measurable voltage in a loop antenna arranged to receive the x and y components of induction. It is remarkable that in MRI we are able to directly measure induction from the precessing nuclear moments of water protons.

Recall that to observe this precession, we first need to tip the magnetization away from the static field. This is accomplished with a weak rotating radiofrequency (RF) field. It can be shown that a rotating RF field introduces a fictitious field in the z direction of strength ω/γ. By tuning the frequency of the RF field to ω_0, we effectively delete the B_0 field. The RF slowly nutates the magnetization away from the z-axis. The Larmor relation still holds in this "rotating frame," so the frequency of the nutation is γB_1, where B_1 is the amplitude of the RF field. Since the coils receive x and y (transverse) components of induction, the signal is maximized by tipping the spins completely into the transverse plane. This is accomplished by a $\pi/2$ RF pulse, which requires $\gamma B_1 \tau = \pi/2$, where τ is the duration of the RF pulse. Another useful RF pulse rotates spins by π radians. This can be used to invert spins. It also can be used to refocus transverse spins that have dephased due to B_0 field inhomogeneity. This is called a **spin echo** and is widely used in imaging.

NMR has been used for decades in chemistry. A complex molecule is placed in a strong, highly uniform magnetic field. Electronic shielding produces microscopic field variations within the molecule so that geometrically isolated nuclei rotate about distinct fields. Each distinct magnetic environment produces a peak in the spectra of the received signal. The relative size of the spectral peaks gives the ratio of nuclei in each magnetic environment. Hence the NMR spectrum is extremely useful for elucidating molecular structure.

The NMR signal from a human is due predominantly to water protons. Since these protons exist in identical magnetic environments, they all resonate at the same frequency. Hence the NMR signal is simply proportional to the volume of the water. They key innovation for MRI is to impose spatial variations on the magnetic field to distinguish spins by their location. Applying a magnetic field gradient causes each region of the volume to oscillate at a distinct frequency. The most effective nonuniform field is a linear gradient where the field and the resulting frequencies vary linearly with distance along the object being studied. Fourier analysis of the signal obtains a map of the spatial distribution of spins. This argument is formalized below, where we derive the powerful k-space analysis of MRI [5,6].

12.1.1.1 k-Space Analysis of Data Acquisition

In MRI, we receive a volume integral from an array of oscillators. By ensuring that the phase, "signature" of each oscillator is unique, one can assign a unique location to each spin and thereby reconstruct an image. During signal reception, the applied magnetic field points in the z direction. Spins precess in the xy plane at the Larmor frequency. Hence a spin at position $\mathbf{r} = (x, y, z)$ has a unique phase θ that describes its angle relative to the y axis in the xy plane:

$$s(t) \propto \frac{d}{dt} \int_V M(\mathbf{r})\, e^{-i\theta(\mathbf{r},t)/} \, dr \tag{12.1}$$

where $B_z(\mathbf{r}, t)$ is the z component of the instantaneous, local magnetic flux density. This formula assumes there are no x and y field components.

A coil large enough to receive a time-varying flux uniformly from the entire volume produces an EMF proportional to

$$\theta(\mathbf{r}, t) = -\gamma \int_0^t B_z(\mathbf{r}, \tau)d\tau \tag{12.2}$$

where $M(\mathbf{r})$ represents the equilibrium moment density at each point $\mathbf{r}$.

The key idea for imaging is to superimpose a linear field gradient on the static field B_0. This field points in the direction z, and its magnitude varies linearly with a coordinate direction. For example, an x gradient points in the z direction and varies along the coordinate x. This is described by the vector field $xG_x\hat{\mathbf{z}}$, where $\hat{\mathbf{z}}$ is the unit vector in the z direction. In general, the gradient is $(xG_x + yG_y + zG_z)\hat{\mathbf{z}}$, which can be written compactly as the dot product $\mathbf{G} \cdot \mathbf{r}\hat{\mathbf{z}}$. These gradient field components can vary with time, so the total z field is

$$B_z(\mathbf{r}, t) = B_0 + \mathbf{G}(t) \cdot \mathbf{r} \tag{12.3}$$

In the presence of this general time-varying gradient, the received signal is

$$s(t) \propto \frac{d}{dt} \int_V e^{i\gamma B_0 t} M(\mathbf{r}) e^{-i\gamma \int_0^t \mathbf{G}(\tau)\cdot\mathbf{r}\, d\tau} \, dr \tag{12.4}$$

The center frequency γB_0 is always much larger than the bandwidth of the signal. Hence the derivative operation is approximately equivalent to multiplication by $-i\omega_0$. The signal is demodulated by the waveform $e^{i\gamma B_0 t}$ to obtain the "baseband" signal:

$$s(t) \propto -i\omega_0 \int_V M(\mathbf{r}) e^{-i\gamma \int_0^t \mathbf{G}(\tau)\cdot\mathbf{r}\, d\tau} \, dr \tag{12.5}$$

It will be helpful to define the term $\mathbf{k}(t)$:

$$\mathbf{k}(t) = \gamma \int_0^t \mathbf{G}(\tau)\, d\tau \tag{12.6}$$

Then we can rewrite the received baseband signal as

$$S(t) \propto \int_V M(\mathbf{r})e^{-i\mathbf{k}(t)\cdot\mathbf{r}}\, dr \tag{12.7}$$

which we can now identify as the spatial Fourier transform of $M(\mathbf{r})$ evaluated at $\mathbf{k}(t)$. That is, $S(t)$ scans the spatial frequencies of the function $M(\mathbf{r})$. This can be written explicitly as

$$S(t) \propto \mathcal{M}(\mathbf{k}(t)) \tag{12.8}$$

where $\mathcal{M}(\mathbf{k})$ is the three-dimensional Fourier transform of the object distribution $M(\mathbf{r})$. Thus we can view MRI with linear gradients as a "scan" of k-space or the spatial Fourier transform of the image. After the desired portion of k-space is scanned, the image $M(\mathbf{r})$ is reconstructed using an inverse Fourier transform.

12.1.1.1.1 2D Imaging

Many different gradient waveforms can be used to scan k-space and to obtain a desired image. The most common approach, called *two-dimensional Fourier transform imaging* (**2D FT**), is to scan through k-space along several horizontal lines covering a rectilinear grid in 2D k-space. See Figure 12.1 for a schematic of the k-space traversal. The horizontal grid lines are acquired using 128 to 256 excitations separated by a time TR, which is determined by the desired contrast, RF flip angle, and the T_1 of the desired components of the image. The horizontal-line scans through k-space are offset in k_y by a variable area y-gradient pulse, which happens before data acquisition starts. These variable offsets in k_y are called *phase encodes* because they affect the phase of the signal rather than the frequency. Then for each k_y phase encode, signal is acquired while scanning horizontally with a constant x gradient.

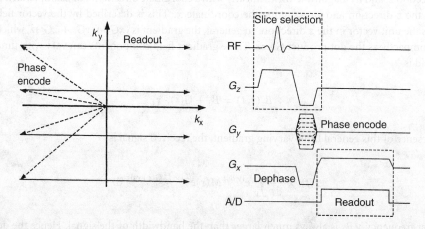

FIGURE 12.1 The drawing on the left illustrates the scanning pattern of the 2D Fourier transform imaging sequence. On the right is a plot of the gradient and RF waveforms that produce this pattern. Only four of the N_y horizontal k-space lines are shown. The phase-encode period initiates each acquisition at a different k_y and at $-k_x$(max). Data are collected during the horizontal traversals. After all N_y k-space lines have been acquired, a 2D FFT reconstructs the image. Usually 128 or 256 k_y lines are collected, each with 256 samples along k_x. The RF pulse and the z gradient waveform together restrict the image to a particular slice through the subject.

12.1.1.1.2 Resolution and Field of View

The fundamental image characteristics of resolution and field of view (FOV) are completely determined by the characteristics of the k-space scan. The extent of the coverage of k-space determines the resolution of the reconstructed image. The resolution is inversely proportional to the highest spatial frequency acquired:

$$\frac{1}{\Delta x} = \frac{k_x(\max)}{\pi} = \frac{\gamma G_x T}{2\pi} \tag{12.9}$$

$$\frac{1}{\Delta y} = \frac{k_y(\max)}{\pi} = \frac{\gamma G_y T_{\text{phase}}}{\pi} \tag{12.10}$$

where G_x is the readout gradient amplitude and T is the readout duration. The time T_{phase} is the duration of the phase-encode gradient G_y. For proton imaging on a 1.5-T imaging system, a typical gradient strength is $G_x = 1$ G/cm. The signal is usually read for about 8 msec. For water protons, $\gamma = 26,751$ rad/sec/G, so the maximum excursion in k_x is about 21 rad/mm. Hence we cannot resolve an object smaller than 0.3 mm in width. From this one might be tempted to improve the resolution dramatically using very strong gradients or very long readouts. But there are severe practical obstacles, since higher resolution increases the scan time and also degrades the image SNR.

In the phase-encode direction, the k-space data are sampled discretely. This discrete sampling in k-space introduces replication in the image domain [7]. If the sampling in k-space is finer than 1/FOV, then the image of the object will not fold back on itself. When the k-space sampling is coarser than 1/FOV, the image of the object does fold back over itself. This is termed *aliasing*. Aliasing is prevented in the readout direction by the sampling filter.

12.1.1.1.3 Perspective

For most imaging systems, diffraction limits the resolution. That is, the resolution is limited to the wavelength divided by the angle subtended by the receiver aperture, which means that the ultimate resolution is approximately the wavelength itself. This is true for imaging systems based on optics, ultrasound, and x-rays (although there are other important factors, such as quantum noise, in x-ray).

MRI is the only imaging system for which the resolution is independent of the wavelength. In MRI, the wavelength is often many meters, yet submillimeter resolution is routinely achieved. The basic reason is that no attempt is made to focus the radiation pattern to the individual pixel or voxel (volume element), as is done in all other imaging modalities. Instead, the gradients create spatially varying magnetic fields so that individual pixels emit unique waveform signatures. These signals are decoded and assigned to unique positions. An analogous problem is isolating the signals from two transmitting antenna towers separated by much less than a wavelength. Directive antenna arrays would fail because of diffraction spreading. However, we can distinguish the two signals if we use the a priori knowledge that the two antennas transmit at different frequencies. We can receive both signals with a wide-angle antenna and then distinguish the signals through frequency-selective filtering.

12.1.1.1.4 SNR Considerations

The signal strength is determined by the EMF induced from each voxel due to the processing moments. The magnetic moment density is proportional to the polarizing field B_0. Recall that the EMF is proportional to the rate of change of the coil flux. The derivative operation multiples the signal by the Larmor frequency, which is proportional to B_0, so the received signal is proportional to B_0^2 times the volume of the voxel V_v.

In a well-designed MRI system, the dominant noise source is due to thermally generated currents within the conductive tissues of the body. These currents create a time-varying flux which induces noise voltages in the receiver coil. Other noise sources include the thermal noise from the antenna and from the first amplifier. These subsystems are designed so that the noise is negligible compared with the noise from the patient. The noise received is determined by the total volume seen by the antenna pattern V_n and the effective resistivity and temperature of the conductive tissue. One can show [8] that the standard deviation of the noise from conductive tissue varies linearly with B_0. The noise is filtered by an integration over the total acquisition time T_{acq}, which effectively attenuates the noise standard deviation by $\sqrt{T_{acq}}$. Therefore, the SNR varies as

$$\text{SNR} \propto \frac{B_0^2 V_v}{B_0 V_n / \sqrt{T_{acq}}} = B_0 \sqrt{T_{acq}}(V_v / V_n) \tag{12.11}$$

The noise volume V_n is the effective volume based on the distribution of thermally generated currents. For example, when imaging a spherical object of radius r, the noise standard deviation varies as $r^{5/2}$ [9]. The effective resistance depends strongly on the radius because currents near the outer radius contribute more to the noise flux seen by the receiver coil.

To significantly improve the SNR, most systems use *surface coils*, which are simply small coils that are just big enough to see the desired region of the body. Such a coil effectively maximizes the voxel-volume to noise-volume ratio. The noise is significantly reduced because these coils are sensitive to currents from a smaller part of the body. However, the field of view is somewhat limited, so "phased arrays" of small coils are now being offered by the major manufacturers [10]. In the phased array, each coil sees a small noise volume, while the combined responses provide the wide coverage at a greatly improved SNR.

12.1.1.1.5 Fast Imaging

The 2D FT scan of k-space has the disadvantage that the scan time is proportional to the number of phase encodes. It is often advantageous to trade off SNR for a shorter scan time. This is especially true when motion artifacts dominate thermal noise. To allow for a flexible tradeoff of SNR for imaging time, more than a single line in k-space must be covered in a single excitation. The most popular approach, called echo-planar imaging (EPI), traverses k-space back and forth on a single excitation pulse. The k-space trajectory is drawn in Figure 12.2.

It is important that the tradeoff be flexible so that you can maximize the imaging time given the motion constraints. For example, patients can hold their breath for about 12 sec. So a scan of 12 sec duration gives the best SNR given the breath-hold constraint. The EPI trajectory can be interleaved to take full advantage of the breath-hold interval. If each acquisition takes about a second, 12 interleaves can be collected. Each interleaf acquires every twelfth line in k-space.

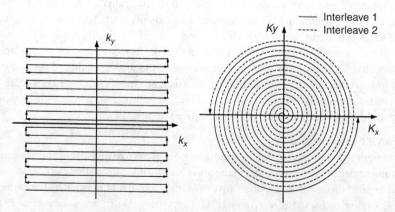

FIGURE 12.2 Alternative methods for the rapid traversal of k-space. On the left is the echo planar trajectory. Data are collected during the horizontal traversals. When all N_y horizontal lines in k-space have been acquired, the data are sent to a 2D FFT to reconstruct the image. On the right is an interleaved spiral trajectory. The data are interpolated to a 2D rectilinear grid and then Fourier transformed to reconstruct the image. These scanning techniques allow for imaging within a breathhold.

Another trajectory that allows for a flexible tradeoff between scan time and SNR is the spiral trajectory. Here the trajectory starts at the origin in k-space and spirals outward. Interleaving is accomplished by rotating the spirals. Figure 12.2 shows two interleaves in a spiral format. Interleaving is very helpful for reducing the hardware requirements (peak amplitude, peak slew rate, average dissipation, etc.) for the gradients amplifiers. For reconstruction, the data are interpolated to a 2D rectilinear grid and then Fourier-transformed. Our group has found spiral imaging to be very useful for imaging coronary arteries within a breath-hold scan [11]. The spiral trajectory is relatively immune to artifacts due to the motion of blood.

12.1.2 Contrast Mechanisms

The tremendous clinical utility of MRI is due to the great variety of mechanisms that can be exploited to create image contrast. If magnetic resonance images were restricted to water density, MRI would be considerably less useful, since most tissues would appear identical. Fortunately, many different MRI contrast mechanisms can be employed to distinguish different tissues and disease processes.

The primary contrast mechanisms exploit *relaxation* of the magnetization. The two types of relaxations are termed **spin–lattice relaxation**, characterized by a relaxation time T_1, and **spin–spin relaxation**, characterized by a relaxation time T_2.

Spin–lattice relaxation describes the rate of recovery of the z component of magnetization toward equilibrium after it has been disturbed by RF pulses. The recovery is given by

$$M_z(t) = M_0(1 - e^{-t/T_1}) + M_z(0)e^{-t/T_1} \tag{12.12}$$

where M_0 is the equilibrium magnetization. Differences in the T_1 time constant can be used to produce image contrast by exciting all magnetization and then imaging before full recovery has been achieved. This is illustrated on the left in Figure 12.3. An initial $\pi/2$ RF pulse destroys all the longitudinal magnetization. The plots show the recovery of two different T_1 components. The short T_1 component recovers faster and produces more signal. This gives a T_1-weighted image.

Spin–spin relaxation describes the rate at which the NMR signal decays after it has been created. The signal is proportional to the transverse magnetization and is given by

$$M_{xy}(t) = M_{xy}(0)e^{-t/T_2} \tag{12.13}$$

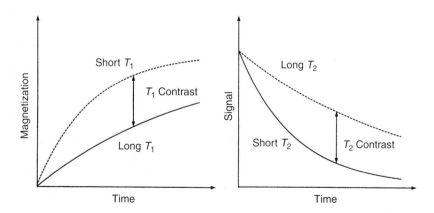

FIGURE 12.3   The two primary MRI contrast mechanisms, T_1 and T_2. T_1, illustrated on the left, describes the rate at which the equilibrium M_{zk} magnetization is restored after it has been disturbed. T_1 contrast is produced by imaging before full recovery has been obtained. T_2, illustrated on the right, describes the rate at which the MRI signal decays after it has been created. T_2 contrast is produced by delaying data acquisition, so shorter T_2 components produce less signal.

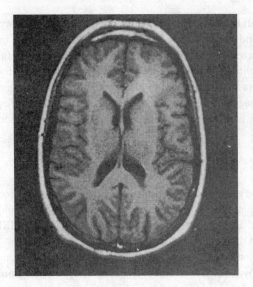 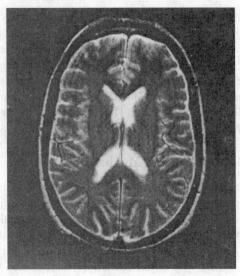

FIGURE 12.4 Example images of a normal volunteer demonstrating T_1 contrast on the left and T_2 contrast on the right.

Image contrast is produced by delaying the data acquisition. The decay of two different T_2 species is plotted on the right in Figure 12.3. The signal from the shorter T_2 component decays more rapidly, while that of the longer T_2 component persists. At the time of data collection, the longer T_2 component produces more signal. This produces a T_2-weighted image.

Figure 12.4 shows examples of these two basic types of contrast. These images are of identical axial sections through the brain of a normal volunteer. The image of the left was acquired with an imaging method that produces T_1 contrast. The very bright ring of subcutaneous fat is due to its relatively short T_1. White matter has a shorter T_1 than gray matter, so it shows up brighter in this image. The image on the right was acquired with an imaging method that produces T_2 contrast. Here the cerebrospinal fluid in the ventricles is bright due to its long T_2. White matter has a shorter T_2 than gray matter, so it is darker in this image.

There are many other contrast mechanisms that are important in MRI. Different chemical species have slightly different resonant frequencies, and this can be used to image one particular component. It is possible to design RF and gradient waveforms so that the image shows only moving spins. This is of great utility in MR angiography, allowing the noninvasive depiction of the vascular system. Another contrast mechanism is called T_2. This relaxation parameter is useful for functional imaging. It occurs when there is a significant spread of Larmor frequencies within a voxel. The superposition signal is attenuated faster than T_2 due to destructive interference between the different frequencies.

In addition to the intrinsic tissue contrast, artificial MRI contrast agents also can be introduced. These are usually administered intravenously or orally. Many different contrast mechanisms can be exploited, but the most popular agents decrease both T_1 and T_2. One agent approved for clinical use is gadolinium DPTA. Decreasing T_1 causes faster signal recovery and a higher signal on a T_1-weighted image. The contrast-enhanced regions then show up bright relative to the rest of the image.

Defining Terms

Gyromagnetic ratio γ: An intrinsic property of a nucleus. It determines the Larmor frequency through the relation $\omega_0 = -\gamma B_0$.

k-**space**: The reciprocal of object space, k-space describes MRI data acquisition in the spatial Fourier transform coordinate system.

Larmor frequency ω_0:   The frequency of precession of the spins. It depends on the product of the applied flux density B_0 and on the gyromagnetic ratio γ. The Larmor frequency is $\omega_0 = -\gamma B_0$.

Magnetization M: The macroscopic ensemble of nuclear moments. The moments are induced by an applied magnetic field. At body temperatures, the amount of magnetization is linearly proportional ($M_0 = 4 \times 10^{-9} H_0$) to the applied magnetic field.

Precession: The term used to describe the motion of the magnetization about an applied magnetic field. The vector locus traverses a cone. The precession frequency is the frequency of the magnetization components perpendicular to the applied field. The precession frequency is also called the *Larmor frequency* ω_0.

Spin echo: The transverse magnetization response to a π RF pulse. The effects of field inhomogeneity are refocused at the middle of the spin echo.

Spin–lattice relaxation T_1:   The exponential rate constant describing the decay of the z component of magnetization toward the equilibrium magnetization. Typical values in the body are between 300 and 3000 msec.

Spin–spin relaxation T_2:   The exponential rate constant describing the decay of the transverse components of magnetization (M_x and M_y).

Spins M: Another name for magnetization.

2D FT: A rectilinear trajectory through k-space. This popular acquisition scheme requires several (usually 128 to 256) excitations separated by a time TR, which is determined by the desired contrast, RF flip angle, and the T_1 of the desired components of the image.

References

[1] Lauterbur P.C. 1973. *Nature* 242: 190.
[2] Evens R.G. and Evens J.R.G. 1991. *AJR* 157: 603.
[3] Bloch F., Hansen W.W., and Packard M.E. 1946. *Phys. Rev.* 70: 474.
[4] Bloch F. 1946. *Phys. Rev.* 70: 460.
[5] Twieg D.B. 1983. *Med. Phys.* 10: 610.
[6] Ljunggren S. 1983. *J. Magn. Reson.* 54: 338.
[7] Bracewell R.N. 1978. *The Fourier Transform and Its Applications.* New York, McGraw-Hill.
[8] Hoult D.I. and Lauterbur P.C. 1979. *J. Magn. Reson.* 34: 425.
[9] Chen C.N. and Hoult D. 1989. *Biomedical Magnetic Resonance Technology.* New York, Adam Hilger.
[10] Roemer P.B., Edelstein W.A., Hayes C.E. *et al.* 1990. *Magn. Reson. Med.* 16: 192.
[11] Meyer C.H., Hu B.S., Nishimura D.G., and Macovski A. 1992. *Magn. Reson. Med.* 28: 202.

12.2   Hardware/Instrumentation

John Schenck

This section describes the basic components and the operating principles of MRI scanners. Although scanners capable of making diagnostic images of the human internal anatomy through the use of **magnetic resonance imaging** (MRI) are now ubiquitous devices in the radiology departments of hospitals in the United States and around the world, as recently as 1980 such scanners were available only in a handful of research institutions. Whole-body superconducting magnets became available in the early 1980s and greatly increased the clinical acceptance of this new imaging modality. Market research data indicate that between 1980 and 1996 more than 100 million clinical MRI scans were performed worldwide. By 1996 more than 20 million MRI scans were being performed each year.

MRI scanners use the technique of **nuclear magnetic resonance (NMR)** to induce and detect a very weak radio frequency signal that is a manifestation of **nuclear magnetism**. The term *nuclear magnetism* refers to weak magnetic properties that are exhibited by some materials as a consequence of the nuclear

spin that is associated with their atomic nuclei. In particular, the proton, which is the nucleus of the hydrogen atom, possesses a nonzero nuclear spin and is an excellent source of NMR signals. The human body contains enormous numbers of hydrogen atoms — especially in water (H_2O) and lipid molecules. Although biologically significant NMR signals can be obtained from other chemical elements in the body, such as phosphorous and sodium, the great majority of clinical MRI studies utilize signals originating from protons that are present in the lipid and water molecules within the patient's body.

The patient to be imaged must be placed in an environment in which several different magnetic fields can be simultaneously or sequentially applied to elicit the desired NMR signal. Every MRI scanner utilizes a strong static field magnet in conjunction with a sophisticated set of **gradient coil**s and radiofrequency coils. The gradients and the radiofrequency components are switched on and off in a precisely timed pattern, or **pulse sequence**. Different pulse sequences are used to extract different types of data from the patient. MR images are characterized by excellent contrast between the various forms of soft tissues within the body. For patients who have no ferromagnetic foreign bodies within them, MRI scanning appears to be perfectly safe and can be repeated as often as necessary without danger [Shellock and Kanal, 1998]. This provides one of the major advantages of MRI over conventional x-ray and computed tomographic (CT) scanners. The NMR signal is not blocked at all by regions of air or bone within the body, which provides a significant advantage over ultrasound imaging. Also, unlike the case of nuclear medicine scanning, it is not necessary to add radioactive tracer materials to the patient.

12.2.1 Fundamentals of MRI Instrumentation

Three types of magnetic fields — main fields or static fields (B_2), gradient fields, an radiofrequency (RF) fields (B_1) — are required in MRI scanners. In practice, it is also usually necessary to use coils or magnets that produce shimming fields to enhance the spatial uniformity of the static field B_0. Most MRI hardware engineering is concerned with producing and controlling these various forms of magnetic fields. The ability to construct NMR instruments capable of examining test tube-sized samples has been available since shortly after World War II. The special challenge associated with the design and construction of medical scanners was to develop a practical means of scaling these devices up to sizes capable of safely and comfortably accommodating an entire human patient. Instruments capable of human scanning first became available in the late 1970s. The successful implementation of MRI requires a two-way flow of information between analog and digital formats (Figure 12.5). The main magnet, the gradient and RF coils, and the gradient and RF power supplies operate in the analog domain. The digital domain is centered on a general-purpose computer (Figure 12.6) that is used to provide control information (signal timing and amplitude) to the gradient and RF amplifiers, to process time-domain MRI signal data returning from

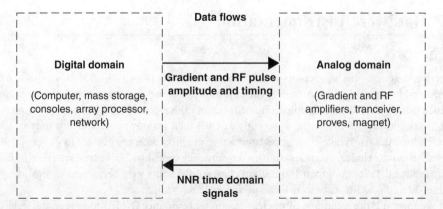

FIGURE 12.5   Digital and analog domains for MRI imaging. MRI involves the flow of data and system commands between these two domains (Courtesy of WM Leue. Reprinted with permission from Schenck and Leue, 1991).

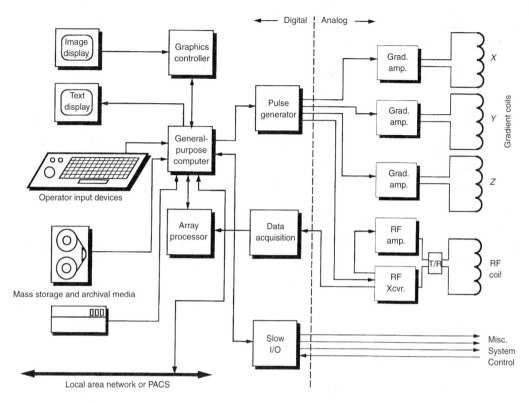

FIGURE 12.6   Block diagram for an MRI scanner. A general-purpose computer is used to generate the commands that control the pulse sequence and to process data during MR scanning. (Courtesy of WM Leue. Reprinted with permission from Schenck and Leue, 1991.)

the receiver, and to drive image display and storage systems. The computer also provides miscellaneous control functions, such as permitting the operator to control the position of the patient table.

12.2.2 Static Field Magnets

The main field magnet [Thomas, 1993] is required to produce an intense and highly uniform, **static magnetic field** over the entire region to be imaged. To be useful for imaging purposes, this field must be extremely uniform in space and constant in time. In practice, the spatial variation of the main field of a whole-body scanner must be less than about 1 to 10 parts per million (ppm) over a region approximately 40 cm in diameter. To achieve these high levels of homogeneity requires careful attention to magnet design and to manufacturing tolerances. The temporal drift of the field strength is normally required to be less than 0.1 ppm/h.

Two units of magnetic field strength are now in common use. The gauss (G) has a long historical usage and is firmly embedded in the older scientific literature. The tesla (T) is a more recently adopted unit, but is a part of the SI system of units and, for this reason, is generally preferred. The tesla is a much larger unit than the gauss — 1 T corresponds to 10,000 G. The magnitude of the earth's magnetic field is about 0.05 mT (5000 G). The static magnetic fields of modern MRI scanners arc most commonly in the range of 0.5 to 1.5 T; useful scanners, however, have been built using the entire range from 0.02 to 8 T. The signal-to-noise ration (SNR) is the ratio of the NMR signal voltage to the ever-present noise voltages that arise within the patient and within the electronic components of the receiving system. The SNR is one of the key parameters that determine the performance capabilities of a scanner. The maximum available

SNR increases linearly with field strength. The improvement in SNR as the field strength is increased is the major reason that so much effort has gone into producing high-field magnets for MRI systems.

Magnetic fields can be produced by using either electric currents or permanently magnetized materials as sources. In either case, the field strength falls off rapidly away from the source, and it is not possible to create a highly uniform magnetic field on the outside of a set of sources. Consequently, to produce the highly uniform field required for MRI, it is necessary to more or less surround the patient with a magnet. The main field magnet must be large enough, therefore, to effectively surround the patient; in addition, it must meet other stringent performance requirements. For these reasons, the main field magnet is the most important determinant of the cost, performance, and appearance of an MRI scanner. Four different classes of main magnets — (1) permanent magnets, (2) electromagnets, (3) resistive magnets, and (4) superconducting magnets — have been used in MRI scanners.

12.2.2.1 Permanent Magnets and Electromagnets

Both these magnet types use magnetized materials to produce the field that is applied to the patient. In a permanent magnet, the patient is placed in the gap between a pair of permanently magnetized pole faces. Electromagnets use a similar configuration, but the pole faces are made of soft magnetic materials, which become magnetized only when subjected to the influence of electric current coils that are wound around them. Electromagnets, but not permanent magnets, require the use of an external power supply. For both types of magnets, the magnetic circuit is completed by use of a soft iron yoke connecting the pole faces to one another (Figure 12.7). The gap between the pole faces must be large enough to contain the patient as well as the gradient and RF coils. The permanent magnet materials available for use in MRI scanners include high-carbon iron, alloys such as Alnico, ceramics such as barium ferrite, and rare earth alloys such as samarium cobalt.

Permanent magnet scanners have some advantages: they produce a relatively small fringing field and do not require power supplies. However, they tend to be very heavy (up to 100 T) can produce only relatively low fields — on the order of 0.3 T or less. They are also subject to temporal field drift caused by temperature changes. If the pole faces are made from an electrically conducting material, eddy currents induced in the pole faces by the pulsed gradient fields can limit performance as well. A recently introduced

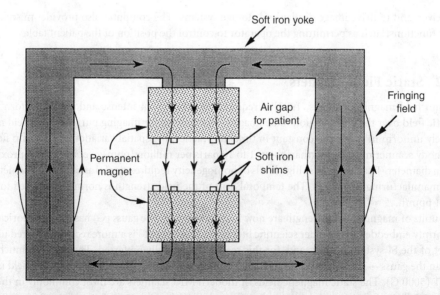

FIGURE 12.7 Permanent magnet. The figure shows a schematic cross-section of a typical permanent magnet configuration. Electromagnets have a similar construction but are energized by current-carrying coils wound around the iron yoke. Soft magnetic shims are used to enhance the homogeneity of the field. (Reprinted with permission from Schenck and Leue, 1991.)

alloy of neodymium, boron, and iron (usually referred to as *neodymium iron*) has been used to make lighter-weight permanent magnet scanners.

12.2.2.2 Resistive Magnets

The first whole-body scanners, manufactured in the late 1970s and early 1980s, used four to six large coils of copper or aluminum wire surrounding the patient. These coils are energized by powerful (40–100 kW) direct-current (dc) power supplies. The electrical resistance of the coils leads to substantial joule heating, and the use of cooling water flowing through the coils is necessary to prevent overheating. The heat dissipation increases rapidly with field strength, and it is not feasible to build resistive magnets operating at fields much higher than 0.15–0.3 T. At present, resistive magnets are seldom used except for very low field strength (0.02–0.06 T) applications.

12.2.2.3 Superconducting Magnets

Since the early 1980s, the use of cryogenically cooled superconducting magnets [Wilson, 1983] has been the most satisfactory solution to the problem of producing the static magnet field for MRI scanners. The property of exhibiting absolutely no electrical resistance near absolute zero has been known as an exotic property of some materials since 1911. Unfortunately, the most common of these materials, such as lead, tin, and mercury, exhibit a phase change back to the normal state at relatively low magnetic field strengths and cannot be used to produce powerful magnetic fields. In the 1950s, a new class of materials (type II superconductors) was discovered. These materials retain the ability to carry loss-free electric currents in very high fields. One such material, an alloy of niobium and titanium, has been used in most of the thousands of superconducting whole-body magnets that have been constructed for use in MRI scanners (Figure 12.8). The widely publicized discovery in 1986 of another class of materials which remain superconducting at much higher temperatures than any previously known material has not yet lead to any material capable of carrying sufficient current to be useful in MRI scanners.

Figure 12.9 illustrates the construction of a typical superconducting whole-body magnet. In this case, six coils of superconducting wire are connected in a series and carry an intense current — on the order of 200 A — to produce the 1.5-T magnetic field at the magnet's center. The diameter of the coils is about 1.3 m, and the total length of wire is about 65 km (40 miles). The entire length of this wire must be

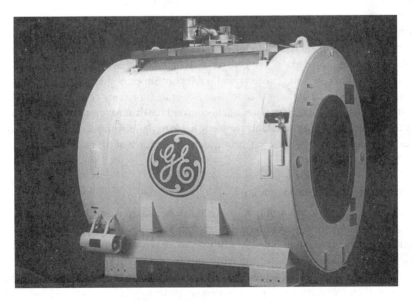

FIGURE 12.8   Superconducting magnet. This figure shows a 1.5-T whole-body superconducting magnet. The nominal warm bore diameter is 1 m. The patient to be imaged, as well as the RF and gradient coils, are located within this bore. (Courtesy of General Electric Medical Systems. Reprinted with permission from Schenck and Leue, 1991.)

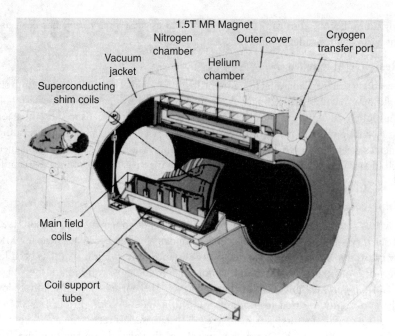

FIGURE 12.9 Schematic drawing of a superconducting magnet. The main magnet coils and the superconducting shim coils are maintained at liquid helium temperature. A computer-controlled table is used to advance the patient into the region of imaging. (Reprinted with permission from Schenck and Leue, 1991.)

without any flaws — such as imperfect welds — that would interrupt the superconducting properties. If the magnet wire has no such flaws, the magnet can be operated in the persistent mode — that is, once the current is established, the terminals may be connected together, and a constant persistent current flow indefinitely so long as the temperature of the coils is maintained below the superconducting transition temperature. This temperature is about 10 K for niobium–titanium wire. The coils are kept at this low temperature by encasing them in a double-walled cryostat (analogous to a Thermos bottle) that permits them to be immersed in liquid helium at a temperature of 4.2 K. The gradual boiling of liquid helium caused by inevitable heat leaks into the cryostat requires that the helium be replaced on a regular schedule. Many magnets now make use of cryogenic refrigerators that reduce or eliminate the need for refilling the liquid helium reservoir. The temporal stability of superconducting magnets operating in the persistent mode is truly remarkable — magnets have operated for years completely disconnected from power supplies and maintained their magnetic field constant to within a few parts per million. Because of their ability to achieve very strong and stable magnetic field strengths without undue power consumption, superconducting magnets have become the most widely used source of the main magnetic fields for MRI scanners.

12.2.2.4 Magnetic Field Homogeneity

The necessary degree of spatial uniformity of the field can be achieved only by carefully placing the coils at specific spatial locations. It is well known that a single loop of wire will produce, on its axis, a field that is directed along the coil axis and that can be expressed as a sum of spherical harmonic fields. The first term in this sum is constant in space and represents the desired field that is completely independent of position. The higher-order terms represent contaminating field inhomogeneities that spoil the field uniformity. More than a century ago, a two-coil magnet system — known as the *Helmholtz pair* — was developed which produced a much more homogeneous field at its center than is produced by a single current loop. This design is based on the mathematical finding that when two coaxial coils of the same radius are separated by a distance equal to their radius, the first nonzero contaminating term in the harmonic expansion is of the fourth order. This results in an increased region of the field homogeneity, which, although it is useful in many applications, is far too small to be useful in MRI scanners. However, the principle of eliminating low-order harmonic fields can be extended by using additional coils. This is the method now used to increase the volume of field homogeneity to values that are useful for MRI. For example, in the commonly used six-coil system, it is possible to eliminate all the error fields through the twelfth order.

In practice, manufacturing tolerances and field perturbations caused b extraneous magnetic field sources — such as steel girders in the building surrounding the magnet — produce additional inhomogeneity in the imaging region. These field imperfections are reduced by the use of shimming fields. One approach — *active shimming* — uses additional coils (either resistive coils, superconducting coils, or some of each) which are designed to produce a magnetic field corresponding to a particular term in the spherical harmonic expansion. When the magnet is installed, the magnetic field is carefully mapped, and the currents in the shim coils are adjusted to cancel out the terms in the harmonic expansion to some prescribed high order. The alternative approach — *passive shimming* — utilizes small permanent magnets that are placed at the proper locations along the inner walls of the magnet bore to cancel out contaminating fields. If a large object containing magnetic materials — such as a power supply — is moved in the vicinity of superconducting magnets, it may be necessary to reset the shimming currents or magnet locations to account for the changed pattern of field inhomogeneity.

12.2.2.5 Fringing Fields

A large, powerful magnet produces a strong magnetic field in the region surrounding it as well as in its interior. This fringing field can produce undesirable effects such as erasing magnetic tapes (and credit cards). It is also a potential hazard to people with implanted medical devices such as cardiac pacemakers. For safety purposes, it is general practice to limit access to the region where the fringing field becomes intense. A conventional boundary for this region is the "5-gaussline," which is about 10 to 12 m from the center of an unshielded 1.5-T magnet. Magnetic shielding — in the form of iron plates (passive shielding) or external coils carrying current in the direction opposite to the main coil current (active shielding) — is frequently used to restrict the region in which the fringing field is significant.

12.2.3 Gradient Coils

Three gradient fields, one each for the x, y, and z directions of a Cartesian coordinate system, are used to code position information into the MRI signal and to permit the imaging of thin anatomic slices [Thomas, 1993]. Along with their larger size, it is the use of these gradient coils that distinguishes MRI scanners from the conventional NMR systems such as those used in analytical chemistry. The direction of the static field, along the axis of the scanner, is conventionally taken as the z direction, and it is only the Cartesian component of the gradient field in this direction that produces a significant contribution to the resonant behavior of the nuclei. Thus, the three relevant gradient fields are $B_z = G_x X$, $B_z = G_y Y$, and $B_z = G_z Z$. MRI scans are carried out by subjecting the spin system to a sequence of pulsed gradient and RF fields. Therefore, it is necessary to have three separate coils — one for each of the relevant gradient fields — each with its own power supply and under independent computer control. Ordinarily, the most practical method for constructing the gradient coils is to wind them on a cylindrical coil form that surrounds the patient and is located inside the warm bore of the magnet. The z gradient field can be produced by sets of circular coils wound around the cylinder with the current direction reversed for coils on the opposite sides of the magnet center ($z = 0$). To reduce deviations from a perfectly linear B_z gradient field, a spiral winding can be used with the direction of the turns reversed at $z = 0$ and the spacing between windings decreasing away from the coil center (Figure 12.10). A more complex current pattern is required to produce the transverse (x and y) gradients. As indicated in Figure 12.11, transverse gradient fields are produced by windings which utilize a four-quadrant current pattern.

The generation of MR images requires that a rapid sequence of time-dependent gradient fields (on all three axes) be applied to the patient. For example, the commonly used technique of **spin-warp imaging**

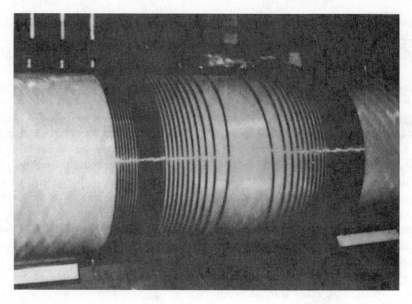

FIGURE 12.10 *Z*-gradient coil. The photograph shows a spiral coil wound on a cylindrical surface with an overwiding near the end of the coil. (Courtesy of R.J. Dobberstein, General Electric Medical Systems. Reprinted with permission from Schenck and Leue, 1991.)

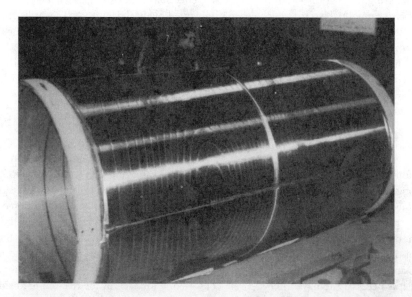

FIGURE 12.11 Transverse gradient coil. The photograph shows the outer coil pattern of an actively shielded transverse gradient coil. (Courtesy of R.J. Dobberstien, General Electric Medical Systems. Reprinted with permission from Schenck and Leue, 1991.)

[Edelstein et al., 1980] utilizes a slice-selection gradient pulse to select the spins in a thin (3–10 mm) slice of the patient and then applies readout and phase-encoding gradients in the two orthogonal directions to encode two-dimensional spatial information into the NMR signal. This, in turn, requires that the currents in the three gradient coils be rapidly switched by computer-controlled power supplies. The rate at which gradient currents can be switched is an important determinant of the imaging capabilities of a scanner. In typical scanners, the gradient coils have an electrical resistance of about 1 Ω and an inductance of about 1 mH, and the gradient field can be switched from 0 to 10 mT/m (1 G/cm) in about 0.5 msec. The current must be switched from 0 to about 100 A in this interval, and the instantaneous voltage on the coils, $L\,di/dt$, is on the order of 200 V. The power dissipation during the switching interval is about 20 kW. In more demanding applications, such as are met in cardiac MRI, the gradient field may be as high as 4–5 mT/m and switched in 0.2 msec or less. In this case, the voltage required during gradient switching is more than 1 kV. In many pulse sequences, the switching duty cycle is relatively low, and coil heating is not significant. However, fast-scanning protocols use very rapidly switched gradients at a high duty cycle. This places very strong demands on the power supplies, and it is often necessary to use water cooling to prevent overheating the gradient coils.

12.2.4 Radiofrequency Coils

Radiofrequency (RF) coils are components of every scanner and are used for two essential purposes — transmitting and receiving signals at the resonant frequency of the protons within the patient [Schenck, 1993]. The precession occurs at the **Larmor frequency** of the protons, which is proportional to the static magnetic field. At 1T this frequency is 42.58 MHz. Thus in the range of field strengths currently used in whole-body scanners, 0.02 to 4 T, the operating frequency ranges from 0.85 to 170.3 MHz. For the commonly used 1.5-T scanners, the operating frequency is 63.86 MHz. The frequency of MRI scanners overlaps the spectral region used for radio and television broadcasting. As an example, the frequency of a 1.5-T scanner is within the frequency hand 60 to 66 MHz, which is allocated to television channel 3. Therefore, it is not surprising that the electronic components in MRI transmitter and receiver chains closely resemble corresponding components in radio and television circuitry. An important difference between MRI scanners and broadcasting systems is that the transmitting and receiving antennas of broadcast systems operate in the far field of the electromagnetic wave. These antennas are separated by many wavelengths. On the other hand, MRI systems operate in the near field, and the spatial separation of the sources and receivers is much less than a wavelength. In far-field systems, the electromagnetic energy is shared equally between the electric and magnetic components of the wave. However, in the near field of magnetic dipole sources, the field energy is almost entirely in the magnetic component of the electromagnetic wave. This difference accounts for the differing geometries that are most cost effective for broadcast and MRI antenna structures.

Ideally, the RF field is perpendicular to the static field, which is in the z direction. Therefore, the RF field can be linearly polarized in either the x or y direction. However, the most efficient RF field results from quadrature excitation, which requires a coil that is capable of producing simultaneous x and y fields with a 90-degree phase shift between them. Three classes of RF coils — body coils, head coils, and surface coils — are commonly used in MRI scanners. These coils are located in the space between the patient and the gradient coils. Conducting shields just inside the gradient coils are used to prevent electromagnetic coupling between the RF coils and the rest of the scanner. Head and body coils are large enough to surround the legion being imaged and are designed to produce an RF magnetic field that is uniform across the region to be imaged. Body coils are usually constructed on cylindrical coil forms and have a large enough diameter (50 to 60 cm) to entirely surround the patient's body. Coils are designed only for head imaging (Figure 12.12) have a smaller diameter (typically 28 cm). Surface coils are smaller coils designed to image a restricted region of the patient's anatomy. They come in a wide variety of shapes and sizes. Because they can be closely applied to the region of interest, surface coils can provide SNR advantages over head and body coils for localized regions, but because of their asymmetric design, they do not have uniform sensitivity.

A common practice is to use separate coils for the transmitter and receiver functions. This permits the use of a large coil — such as the body coil — with a uniform excitation pattern as the transmitter and a small surface coil optimized to the anatomic region — such as the spine — being imaged. When this two-coil approach is used, it is important to provide for electronically decoupling of the two coils because they are tuned at the same frequency and will tend to have harmful mutual interactions.

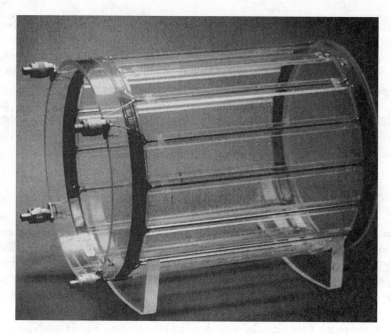

FIGURE 12.12   Birdcage resonator. This is a head coil designed to operate in a 4-T scanner at 170 MHz. Quadrature excitation and receiver performance are achieved by using two adjacent ports with a 90-degree phase shift between them. (Reprinted with permission from Schenck and Leue, 1991.)

12.2.5   Digital Data Processing

A typical scan protocol calls for a sequence of tailored RF and gradient pulses with duration controlled in steps of 0.1 msec. To achieve sufficient dynamic range in control of pulse amplitudes, 12- to 16-bit digital-to-analog converters are used. The RF signal at the Larmor frequency (usually in the range from 1 to 200 MHz) is mixed with a local oscillator to produce a baseband signal which typically has a **bandwidth** of 16–32 kHz. The data-acquisition system must digitize the baseband signal at the Nyquist rate, which requires sampling the detected RF signal at a rate one digital data point every 5–20 msec. Again, it is necessary to provide sufficient dynamic range. Analog-to-digital converters with 16–18 bits are used to produce the desired digitized signal data. During the data acquisition, information is acquired at a rate on the order of 800 kilobytes per second, and each image can contain up to a megabyte of digital data. The array processor (AP) is a specialized computer that is designed for the rapid performance of specific algorithms, such as the **fast Fourier transform (FFT)**, which are used to convert the digitized time-domain data to image data. Two-dimensional images are typically displayed as 256 × 128, 256 × 256, or 512 × 512 **pixel** arrays. The images can be made available for viewing within about 1 sec after data acquisition. Three-dimensional imagining data, however, require more computer processing, and this results in longer delays between acquisition and display.

A brightness number, typically containing 16 bits of gray-scale information, is calculated for each pixel element of the image, and this corresponds to the signal intensity originating in each **voxel** of the object. To make the most effective use of the imaging information, sophisticated display techniques, such as multi-image displays, rapid sequential displays (cine loop), and three-dimensional renderings of anatomic surfaces, are frequently used. These techniques are often computationally intensive and require the use of specialized computer hardware. Interfaces to microprocessor-based workstations are frequently used to provide such additional display and analysis capabilities. MRI images are available as digital data; therefore, there is considerable utilization of local area networks (LANs) to distribute information throughout the hospital, and long-distance digital transmission of the images can be used for purposes of teleradiology.

12.2.6 Current Trends in MRI

At present, there is a substantial effort directed at enhancing the capabilities and cost-effectiveness of MR imagers. The activities include efforts to reduce the cost of these scanners, improve image quality, reduce scan times, and increase the number of useful clinical applications. Examples of these efforts include the development of high-field scanners, the advent of MRI-guided therapy, and the development of niche scanners that are designed for specific anatomical and clinical applications. Scanners have been developed that are dedicated to low-field imaging of the breast and other designs are dedicated to orthopedic applications such as the knees, wrists, and elbows. Perhaps the most promising incipient application of MRI is to cardiology. Scanners are now being developed to permit studies of cardiac wall motion, cardiac perfusion, and the coronary arteries in conjunction with cardiac stress testing. These scanners emphasize short magnet configurations to permit close monitoring and interaction with the patient, and high strength rapidly switched gradient fields.

Conventional spin-warp images typically require several minutes to acquire. The fast spin echo (FSE) technique can reduce this to the order of 20 sec, and gradient-echo techniques can reduce this time to a few seconds. The echo-planar technique (EPI) [Wehrli, 1990; Cohen and Weisskoff, 1991] requires substantially increased gradient power and receiver bandwidth but can produce images in 40 to 60 msec. Scanners with improved gradient hardware that are capable of handling higher data-acquisition rates are now available.

For most of the 1980s and 1990s, the highest field strength commonly used in MRI scanners was 1.5 T. To achieve better SNRs, higher-field scanners, operating at fields up to 4 T, were studied experimentally. The need for very high-field scanners has been enhanced by the development of functional brain MRI. This technique utilizes magnetization differences between oxygenated and deoxygenated hemoglobin, and this difference is enhanced at higher field strengths. It has now become possible to construct 3- and 4-T and even 8-T [Robitaille et al., 1998], whole-body scanners of essentially the same physical size (or footprint) as conventional 1.5-T systems. Along with the rapidly increasing clinical interest in functional MRI, this is resulting in a considerable increase in the use of high-field systems.

For the first decade or so after their introduction, MRI scanners were used almost entirely to provide diagnostic information. However, there is now considerable interest in systems capable of performing image-guided, invasive surgical procedures. Because MRI is capable of providing excellent soft-tissue contrast and has the potential for providing excellent positional information with submillimeter accuracy, it can be used for guiding biopsies and stereotactic surgery. The full capabilities of MRI-guided procedures can only be achieved if it is possible to provide surgical access to the patient simultaneously with the MRI scanning. This has lead to the development of new system designs, including the introduction of a scanner with a radically modified superconducting magnet system that permits the surgeon to operate at the patient's side within the scanner (Figure 12.13) [Schenck et al., 1995; Black et al., 1997]. These systems have lead to the introduction of magnetic field-compatible surgical instruments, anesthesia stations, and patient monitoring equipment [Schenck, 1996].

Defining Terms

Bandwidth: The narrow frequency range, approximately 32 kHz, over which the MRI signal is transmitted. The bandwidth is proportional to the strength of the readout gradient field.

Echo-planar imaging (EPI): A pulse sequence used to produce very fast MRI scans. EPI times can be as short as 50 msec.

Fast Fourier transform (FFT): A mathematical technique used to convert data sampled from the MRI signal into image data. This version of the Fourier transform can be performed with particular efficiency on modern array processors.

Gradient coil: A coil designed to produce a magnetic field for which the field component B: varies linearly with position. Three gradient coils, one each for the x, y, and z directions, are required MRI. These coils are used to permit slice selection and to encode position information into the MRI signal.

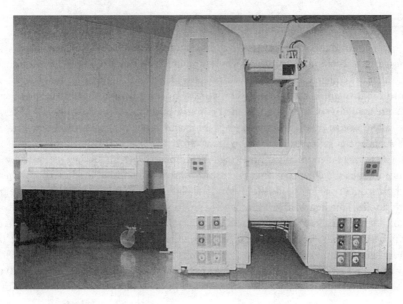

FIGURE 12.13   Open magnet for MEI-guided therapy. This open-geometry superconducting magnet provides a surgeon with direct patient access and the ability to interactively control the MRI scanner. This permits imaging to be performed simultaneously with surgical interventions.

Larmor frequency: The rate at which the magnetic dipole moment of a particle precesses in an applied magnetic field. It is proportional to the field strength and is 42.58 MHz for protons in a 1-T magnetic field.

Magnetic resonance imaging (MRI):   A technique for obtaining images of the internal anatomy based on the use of nuclear magnetic resonance signals. During the 1980s, it became a major modality for medical diagnostic imaging.

Nuclear magnetic resonance (NMR):   A technique for observing and studying nuclear magnetism. It is based on partially aligning the nuclear spins by use of a strong, static magnetic field, stimulating these spins with a radiofrequency field oscillating at the Larmor frequency, and detecting the signal that is induced at this frequency.

Nuclear magnetism: The magnetic properties arising from the small magnetic dipole moments possessed by the atomic nuclei of some materials. This form of magnetism is much weaker than the more familiar form that originates from the magnetic dipole moments of the atomic electrons.

Pixel: A single element or a two-dimensional array of image data.

Pulse sequence: A series of gradient and radiofrequency pulses used to organize the nuclear spins into a pattern that encodes desired imaging information into the NMR signal.

Quadrature excitation and detection: The use of circularly polarized, rather than linearly polarized, radio frequency fields to excite an detect the NMR signal. It provides a means of reducing the required excitation power by 1/2 and increasing the signal-to-noise ratio by 2.

Radiofrequency (RF) coil: A coil designed to excite and/or detect NMR signals. These coils can usually be tuned to resonate at the Larmor frequency of the nucleus being studied.

Spin: The property of a particle, such as an electron or nucleus, that leads to the presence of an intrinsic angular momentum and magnetic moment.

Spin-warp imagining: The pulse sequence used in the most common method of MRI imaging. It uses a sequence of gradient field pulses to encode position information into the NMR signal and applies Fourier transform mathematics to this signal to calculate the image intensity value for each pixel.

Static magnetic field: The field of the main magnet that is used to magnetize the spins and to drive their Larmor precession.

Voxel: The volume element associated with a pixel. The voxel volume is equal to the pixel area multiplied by the slice thickness.

References

Black P.Mc.L., Moriarty T., Alexander E. III. *et al.* 1997. Development and implementation of intraoperative magnetic resonance imaging and its neurosurgical applications. *Neurosurgery* 41: 831.

Cohen M.S. and Weisskoff R.M. 1991. Ultra-fast imaging. *Magn. Reson. Imag.* 9: 1.

Edelstein W.A., Hutchinson J.M.S., Johnson G., and Redpath T.W. 1980. Spin-warp NMR imaging and applications to human whole-body imaging. *Phys. Med. Biol.* 25: 751.

Robitaille P.-M.L., Abdujalil A.M., Kangarlu A. *et al.* 1998. Human magnetic resonance imaging at 8 T. *NMR Biomed.* 11: 263.

Schenck JF. 1993. Radiofrequency coils: types and characteristics. In M.I. Bronskill and P. Sprawls (Eds.), *The Physics of MRI, Medical Physics Monograph No. 21*, pp. 98–134. Woodbury, NY, American Institute of Physics.

Schenck J.F. 1996. The role of magnetic susceptibility in magnetic resonance imaging: magnetic field compatibility of the first and second kinds. *Med. Phys.* 23: 815.

Schenck J.F. and Leue W.M. 1996. Instrumentation: magnets coils and hardware. In S.W. Atlas (Ed.), *Magnetic Resonance Imaging of the Brain and Spine*, 2nd ed., pp. 1–27. Philadelphia, Lippincott-Raven.

Schenck J.F., Jolesz A., Roemer P.B. *et al.* 1995. Superconducting open-configuration MR imaging system for image-guided therapy. *Radiology* 195: 805.

Shellock F.G. and Kanal E. 1998. *Magnetic Resonance: Bioeffects, Safety and Patient Management*, 2nd ed. Philadelphia, Saunders.

Thomas S.R. 1993. Magnet and gradient coils: types and characteristics. In M.J. Bronskill and P. Sprawls (Eds.), *The Physics of MRI, Medical Physics Monograph No. 21*, pp. 56–97. Woodbury, NY, American Institute of Physics.

Wehrli F.W. 1990. Fast scan magnetic resonance: principles and applications. *Magn. Reson. Q.* 6: 165.

Wilson M.N. 1983. *Superconducting Magnets*. Oxford, Clarendon Press.

Further Information

There are several journals devoted entirely to MR imaging. These include *Magnetic Resonance in Medicine*, *JMRI — Journal of Magnetic Resonance Imaging*, and *NMR in Biomedicine*, all three of which are published by Wiley-Liss, 605 Third Avenue, New York, NY 10158. Another journal dedicated to this field is *Magnetic Resonance Imaging* (Elsevier Publishing, 655 Avenue of the Americas, New York, NY 10010). The clinical aspects of MRI are covered extensively in *Radiology* (Radiological Society of North America, 2021 Spring Road, Suite 600, Oak Brook, IL 60521), *The American Journal of Radiology* (American Roentgen Ray Society, 1891 Preston White Drive, Reston, VA 20191), as well as in several other journals devoted to the practice of radiology. There is a professional society, now known as the International Society for Magnetic Resonance in Medicine (ISMRM), devoted to the medical aspects of magnetic resonance. The main offices of this society are at 2118 Milvia, *Suite* 201, Berkeley, CA 94704. This society holds an annual meeting that includes displays of equipment and the presentation of approximately 2800 technical papers on new developments in the field. The annual *Book of Abstracts* of this meeting provides an excellent summary of current activities in the field. Similarly, the annual meeting of the Radiological Society of North America (RSNA) provides extensive coverage of MRI that is particularly strong on the clinical applications. The RSNA is located at 2021 Spring Road, Suite 600, Oak Brook, IL 60521.

Several book-length accounts of MRI instrumentation and techniques are available. *Biomedical Magnetic Resonance Technology* [Adam Higler, Bristol, 1989] by Chen and D.I. Hoult, *The Physics of MRI* (Medical Physics Monograph 21, American Institute of Physics, Woodbury, NY, 1993), edited by

M.J. Bronskill and P. Sprawls, and *Electromagnetic Analysis and Design in Magnetic Resonance Imaging* (CRC Press, Boca Raton, FL, 1998) by J.M. Jin each contain thorough accounts of instrumentation and the physical aspects of MRI. There are many books that cover the clinical aspects of MRI. Of particular interest are *Magnetic Resonance Imaging*, 3rd edition [Mosby, St. Louis, 1999], edited by D.D. Stark and W.G. Bradley, Jr., and *Magnetic Resonance Imaging of the Brain and Spine*, 2nd ed. (Lipincott-Raven, Philadelphia, 1996), edited by S.W. Atlas.

12.3 Functional MRI

Kenneth K. Kwong and David A. Chesler

Functional magnetic resonance imaging (fMRI), a technique that images intrinsic blood signal change with magnetic resonance (MR) imagers, has in the last 3 years become one of the most successful tools used to study blood flow and perfusion in the brain. Since changes in neuronal activity are accompanied by focal changes in cerebral blood flow (CBF), blood volume (CBV), blood oxygenation, and metabolism, these physiologic changes can be used to produce functional maps of mental operations.

There are two basic but completely different techniques used in fMRI to measure CBF. The first one is a classic steady-state perfusion technique first proposed by Detre et al. [1], who suggested the use of saturation or inversion of incoming blood signal to quantify absolute blood flow [1–5]. By focusing on blood flow *change* and not just steady-state blood flow, Kwong et al. [6] were successful in imaging brain visual functions associated with quantitative perfusion change. There are many advantages in studying blood flow change because many common baseline artifacts associated with MRI absolute flow techniques can be subtracted out when we are interested only in changes. And one obtains adequate information in most functional neuroimaging studies with information of flow change alone.

The second technique also looks at change of a blood parameter — blood oxygenation *change* during neuronal activity. The utility of the change of blood oxygenation characteristics was strongly evident in Turner's work [7] with cats with induced hypoxia. Turner et al. found that with hypoxia, the MRI signal from the cats' brains went down as the level of deoxyhemoglobin rose, a result that was an extension of an earlier study by Ogawa et al. [8,9] of the effect of deoxyhemoglobin on MRI signals in animals' veins. Turner's new observation was that when oxygen was restored, the cats' brain signals climbed up and went *above* their baseline levels. This was the suggestion that the vascular system overcompensated by bringing more oxygen, and with more oxygen in the blood, the MRI signal would rise beyond the baseline.

Based on Turner's observation and the perfusion method suggested by Detre et al., movies of human visual cortex activation utilizing both the perfusion and blood oxygenation techniques were successfully acquired in May of 1991 (Figure 12.14) at the Massachusetts General Hospital with a specially equipped superfast 1.5-T system known as an *echo-planar imaging* (EPI) MRI system [10]. fMRI results using intrinsic blood contrast were first presented in public at the Tenth Annual Meeting of the Society of Magnetic Resonance in Medicine in August of 1991 [6,11]. The visual cortex activation work was carried out with flickering goggles, a photic stimulation protocol employed by Belliveau et al. [12] earlier to acquire the MRI functional imaging of the visual cortex with the injection of the contrast agent gadolinium-DTPA. The use of an external contrast agent allows the study of change in blood volume. The intrinsic blood contrast technique, sensitive to blood flow and blood oxygenation, uses no external contrast material. Early model calculation showed that signal due to blood perfusion change would only be around 1% above baseline, and the signal due to blood oxygenation change also was quite small. It was quite a pleasant surprise that fMRI results turned out to be so robust and easily detectable.

The blood oxygenation–sensitive MRI signal change, coined *blood oxygenation level dependent* (BOLD) by Ogawa et al. [8,9,13], is in general much larger than the MRI perfusion signal change during brain activation. Also, while the first intrinsic blood contrast fMRI technique was demonstrated with a superfast EPI MRI system, most centers doing fMRI today are only equipped with conventional MRI systems, which are really not capable of applying Detre's perfusion method. Instead, the explosive growth of MR functional

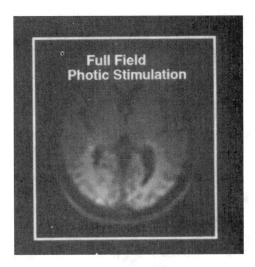

FIGURE 12.14 Functional MR image demonstrating activation of the primary visual cortex (V1). Image acquired on May 9, 1991 with a blood oxygenation–sensitive MRI gradient-echo (GE) technique.

neuroimaging [14–33] in the last three years relies mainly on the measurement of blood oxygenation change, utilizing a MR parameter called T_2. Both high speed echo planar (EPI) and conventional MR have now been successfully employed for functional imaging in MRI systems with magnet field strength ranging from 1.5 to 4.0 T.

12.3.1 Advances in Functional Brain Mapping

The popularity of fMRI is based on many factors. It is safe and totally noninvasive. It can be acquired in single subjects for a scanning duration of several minutes, and it can be repeated on the same subjects as many times as necessary. The implementation of the blood oxygenation sensitive MR technique is universally available. Early neuroimaging, work focused on time-resolved MR topographic mapping of human primary visual (VI) (Figure 12.15 and Figure 12.16), motor (MI), somatosensory (S1), and auditory (A1) cortices during task activation. Today, with BOLD technique combined with EPI, one can acquire 20 or more contiguous brain slices covering the whole head (3×3 mm in plane and 5 mm slice thickness) every 3 sec for a total duration of several minutes. Conventional scanners can only acquire a couple of slices at a time. The benefits of whole-head imaging are many. Not only can researchers identify and test their hypotheses on known brain activation centers, they can also search for previous unknown or unsuspected sites. High resolution work done with EPI has a resolution of 1.5×1.5 mm in plane and a slice thickness of 3 mm. Higher spatial resolution has been reported in conventional 1.5-T MR systems [34].

Of note with Figure 12.16 is that with blood oxygenation–sensitive MR technique, one observers an undershoot [6,15,35] in signal in V1 when the light stimulus is turned off. The physiologic mechanism underlying the undershoot is still not well understood.

The data collected in the last 3 years have demonstrated that fMRI maps of the visual cortex correlate well with known retinotopic organization [24,36]. Higher visual regions such as V5/MT [37] and motor-cortex organization [6,14,27,38] have been explored successfully. Preoperative planning work (Figure 12.17) using motor stimulation [21,39,40] has helped neurosurgeons who attempt to preserve primary areas from tumors to be resected. For higher cognitive functions, several fMRI language studies have already demonstrated known language-associated regions [25,26,41,42] (Figure 12.18). There is more detailed modeling work on the mechanism of functional brain mapping by blood-oxygenation change [43–46]. Postprocessing techniques that would help to alleviate the serious problem of motion/displacement artifacts are available [47].

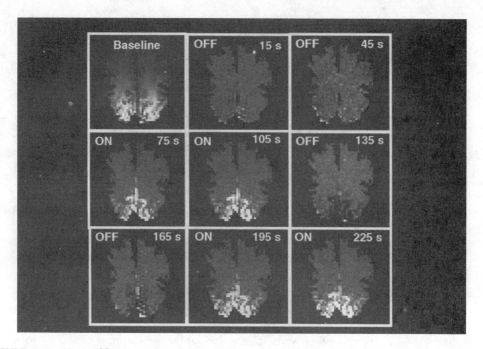

FIGURE 12.15   Movie of fMRI mapping of primary visual cortex (V1) activation during visual stimulation. Images are obliquely aligned along the calcarie fissures with the occipital pole at the bottom. Images were acquired at 3-sec intervals using a blood oxygenation–sensitive MRI sequence (80 images total). A baseline image acquired during darkness (*upper left*) was subtracted from subsequent images. Eight of these subtraction images are displayed, chosen when the image intensities reached a steady-state signal level during darkness (OFF) and during 8-Hz photic stimulation (ON). During stimulation, local increases in signal intensity are detected in the posteromedial regions of the occipital lobes along the calcarine fissures.

12.3.2   Mechanism

Flow-sensitive images show increased perfusion with stimulation, while blood oxygenation–sensitive images show changes consistent with an increase in venous blood oxygenation. Although the precise biophysical mechanisms responsible for the signal changes have yet to be determined, good hypotheses exist to account for our observations.

Two fundamental MRI relaxation rates, T_1 and T_2, are used to describe the fMRI signal. T_1 is the rate at which the nuclei approach thermal equilibrium, and perfusion change can be considered as an additional T_1 change. T_2 represents the rate of the decay of MRI signal due to magnetic field inhomogeneities, and the change of T_2 is used to measure blood-oxygenation change.

T_2 changes reflect the interplay between changes in cerebral blood flow, volume, and oxygenation. As hemoglobin becomes deoxygenated, it becomes more paramagnetic than the surrounding tissue [48] and thus creates a magnetically inhomogeneous environment. The observed *increased* signal on T_2-weighted images during activation reflects a decrease in deoxyhemoglobin content, that is, an increase in venous blood oxygenation. Oxygen delivery, cerebral blood flow, and cerebral blood volume all increase with neuronal activation. Because CBF (and hence oxygen-delivery) changes exceed CBV changes by 2 to 4 times [49], while blood–oxygen extraction increases only slightly [50,51], the total paramagnetic blood deoxyhemoglobin content within brain tissue voxels will decrease with brain activation. The resulting decrease in the tissue-blood magnetic susceptibility difference leads to less intravoxel dephasing within brain tissue voxels and hence *increased* signal on T_2-weighted images [6,14,15,17]. These results independently confirm PET observations that activation-induced changes in blood flow and volume are accompanied by little or no increases in tissue oxygen consumption [50–52].

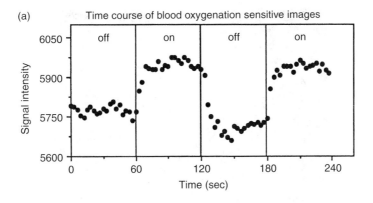

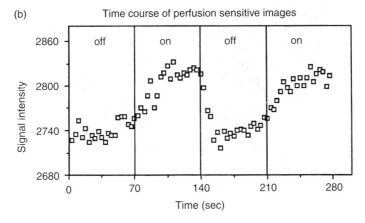

FIGURE 12.16 Signal intensity changes for a region of interest ($\sim$60 mm^2) within the visual cortex during darkness and during 8-Hz photic stimulation. Results using oxygenation-sensitive (*top graph*) and flow-sensitive (*bottom graph*) techniques are shown. The flow-sensitive data were collected once every 3.5 sec, and the oxygenation-sensitive data were collected once every 3 sec. Upon termination of photic stimulation, an undershoot in the oxygenation-sensitive signal intensity is observed.

Since the effect of volume susceptibility difference $\Delta\chi$ is more pronounced at high field strength [53], higher-field imaging magnets [17] will increase the observed T_2 changes.

Signal changes can also be observed on T_1-weighted MR images. The relationship between T_1 and regional blood flow was characterized by Detre et al. [1]:

$$\frac{dM}{dt} = \frac{M_0 - M}{T_1} + fM_b - \frac{f}{\lambda}M \tag{12.14}$$

where M is tissue magnetization and M_b is incoming blood signal. M_0 is proton density, f is the flow in ml/gm/unit time, and λ is the brain–blood partition coefficient of water ($\sim$0.95 ml/g). From this equation, the brain tissue magnetization M relaxes with an apparent T_1 time constant $T_{1\,\text{app}}$ given by

$$\frac{f}{\lambda} = \frac{1}{T_{1\,\text{app}}} - \frac{1}{T_1} \tag{12.15}$$

where the $T_{1\,\text{app}}$ is the observed (apparent) longitudinal relaxation time with flow effects included. T_1 is the true tissue longitudinal relaxation time in the absence of flow. If we assume that the true tissue T_1

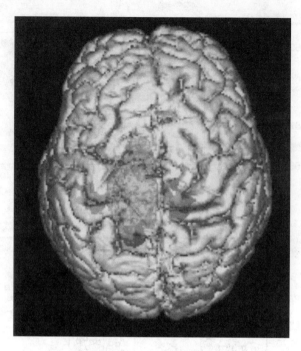

FIGURE 12.17 Functional MRI mapping of motor cortex for preoperative planning. This three-dimensional rendering of the brain represents fusion of functional and structural anatomy. Brain is viewed from the top. A tumor is shown in the left hemisphere, near the midline. The other areas depict sites of functional activation during movement of the right hand, right foot, and left foot. The right foot cortical representation is displaced by tumor mass effect from its usual location. (Courtesy of Dr. Brad Buchbinder.)

remains constant with stimulation, a change in blood flow Δf will lead to a change in the observed $T_{1\,app}$:

$$\Delta \frac{1}{T_{1\,app}} = \Delta \frac{f}{\lambda} \qquad (12.16)$$

Thus the MRI signal change can be used to estimate the change in blood flow.

From Equation 12.14, if the magnetization of blood and tissue always undergoes a similar T_1 relaxation, the flow effect would be minimized. This is a condition that can be approximated by using a flow-nonsensitive T_1 technique inverting *all* the blood coming into the imaged slice of interest. This flow-nonsensitive sequence can be subtracted from a flow-sensitive T_1 technique to provide an index of CBF without the need of external stimulation [54,55] (Figure 12.19). Initial results with tumor patients show that such flow-mapping techniques are useful for mapping out blood flow of tumor regions [55].

Other flow techniques under investigation include the continuous inversion of incoming blood at the carotid level [1] or the use of a single inversion pulse at the carotid level (EPIstar) inverting the incoming blood [56,57]. Compared with the flow-nonsensitive and flow-sensitive methods, the blood-tagging techniques at the carotid level are basically similar concepts except that the MRI signal of tagged blood is expected to be smaller by a factor that depends on the time it takes blood to travel from the tagged site to the imaged slice of interest [55]. The continuous-inversion technique also has a significant problem of magnetization transfer [1] that contaminates the flow signal with a magnetization transfer signal that is several times larger. On the other hand, the advantage of the continuous inversion is that it can under optimal conditions provide a flow contrast larger than all the other methods by a factor of e [55].

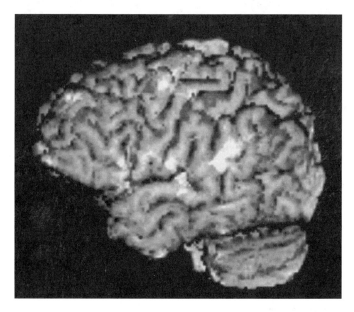

FIGURE 12.18 Left hemisphere surface rendering of functional data (EPI, gradient-echo, ten oblique coronal slices extending to posterior sylvian fissure) and high-resolution anatomic image obtained on a subject (age 33 years) during performance of a same-different (visual matching) task of pairs of words or nonwords (false font strings). Foci of greatest activation for this study are located in dominant perisylvian cortex, that is, inferior frontal gyrus (Broca's area), superior temporal gyrus (Wernicke's area), and inferior parietal lobule (angular gyrus). Also active in this task are sensorimotor cortex and prefrontal cortex. The perisylvian sites of activation are known to be key nodes in a left hemisphere language network. Prefrontal cortex probably plays a more general, modulatory role in attentional aspects of the task. Sensorimotor activation is observed in most language studies despite the absence of overt vocalization. (Courtesy of Dr. Randall Benson.)

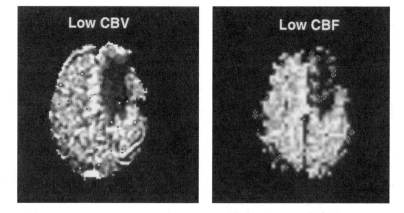

FIGURE 12.19 Functional MRI cerebral blood flow (CBF) index (*right*) of a low-flow brain tumor (dark region right of the midline) generated by the subtraction of a flow-nonsensitive image from a flow-sensitive image. This low-flow region matches well with a cerebral blood volume (CBV) map (*left*) of the tumor region generated by the injection of a bolus of MRI contrast agent Gd-DTPA, a completely different and established method to measure hemodynamics with MRI.

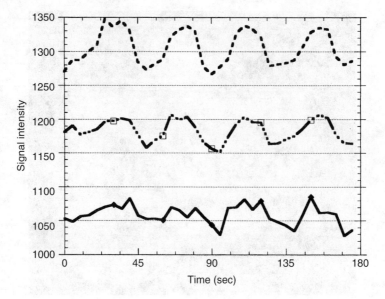

FIGURE 12.20 The curves represent time courses of MRI response to photic stimulation (off-on-off-on ...) with different levels of velocity-dephasing gradients turned on to remove MRI signals coming from the flowing blood of large vessels. The top curve had no velocity-dephasing gradients turned on. The bottom curve was obtained with such strong velocity-dephasing gradients turned on that all large vessel signals were supposed to have been eliminated. The middle curve represents a moderate amount of velocity-dephasing gradients, a tradeoff between removing large vessel signals and retaining a reasonable amount of MRI signal to noise.

12.3.3 Problem and Artifacts in fMRI: The Brain–Vein Problem? The Brain-Inflow Problem?

The artifacts arising from large vessels pose serious problems to the interpretation of oxygenation sensitive fMRI data. It is generally believed that microvascular changes are specific to the underlying region of neuronal activation. However, MRI gradient echo (GE) is sensitive to vessels of all dimensions [46,58], and there is concern that macrovascular changes distal to the site of neuronal activity can be induced [20]. This has been known as the *brain–vein problem*. For laboratories not equipped with EPI, gradient echo (GE) sensitive to variations in T_2 and magnetic susceptibility are the only realistic sequences available for fMRI acquisition, so the problem is particularly acute.

In addition, there is a non-deoxyhemoglobin-related problem, especially acute in conventional MRI. This is the inflow problem of fresh blood that can be time-locked to stimulation [28,29,59]. Such nonparenchymal and macrovascular responses can introduce error in the estimate of activated volumes.

12.3.4 Techniques to Reduce the Large Vessel Problems

In dealing with the inflow problems, EPI has special advantages over conventional scanners. The use of long repetition times (2 to 3 sec) in EPI significantly reduces the brain-inflow problem. Small-flip-angle methods in conventional MRI scanners can be used to reduce inflow effect [59]. Based on inflow modeling, one observes that at an angle smaller than the Ernst angle [60], the inflow effect drops much faster than the tissue signal response to activation. Thus one can effectively remove the inflow artifacts with small-flip-angle techniques.

A new exciting possibility is to add small additional velocity-dephasing gradients to suppress slow in-plane vessel flow [60,61]. Basically, moving spins lose signals, while stationary spins are unaffected. The addition of these velocity-dephasing gradients drops the overall MRI signal (Figure 12.20). The hypothesis that large vessel signals are suppressed while tissue signals remain intact is a subject of ongoing research.

Another advantage with EPI is that another oxygenation-sensitive method such as the EPI T_2-weighted spin-echo (T2SE) is also available. T2SE methods are sensitive to the MRI parameter T_2, which is affected by microscopic susceptibility and hence blood oxygenation. Theoretically, T2SE methods are far less sensitive to large vessel signals [1,6,46,58]. For conventional scanners, T2SE methods take too long to perform and therefore are not practical options.

The flow model [1] based on T_1-weighted sequences and independent of deoxyhemoglobin is also not so prone to large vessel artifacts, since the T_1 model is a model of perfusion at the tissue level.

Based on the study of volunteers, the average T_2-weighted GE signal percentage change at V1 was $2.5 \pm 0.8\%$. The average oxygenation-weighted T2SE signal percentage change was $0.7 \pm 0.3\%$. The average perfusion-weighted and T_1-weighted MRI signal percentage change was $1.5 \pm 0.5\%$. These results demonstrate that T2SE and T_1 methods, despite their ability to suppress large vessels, are not competitive with T_2 effect at 1.5 T. However, since the microscopic effect detected by T2SE scales up with field strength [62], we expect the T2SE to be a useful sequence at high field strength such as 3 or 4 T. Advancing field strength also should benefit T_1 studies due to better signal-to-noise and to the fact that T_1 gets longer at higher field strength.

While gradient-echo sequence has a certain ambiguity when it comes to tissue versus vessels, its sensitivity at current clinical field strength makes it an extremely attractive technique to identify activation sites. By using careful paradigms that rule out possible links between the primary activation site and secondary sites, one can circumvent many of the worries of "signal from the primary site draining down to secondary sites." A good example is as follows: photic stimulation activates both the primary visual cortex and the extrastriates. To show that the extrastriates are not just a drainage from the primary cortex, one can utilize paradigms that activate the primary visual cortex but not the extrastriate, and vice versa. There are many permutations of this [37]. This allows us to study the higher-order functions umambiguously even if we are using gradient-echo sequences.

The continuous advance of MRI mapping techniques utilizing intrinsic blood-tissue contrast promises the development of a functional human neuroanatomy of unprecedented spatial and temporal resolution.

References

[1] Detre J., Leigh J., Williams D., and Koretsky A. 1992. *Magn. Reson. Med.* 23: 37.

[2] Williams D.S., Detre J.A., Leigh J.S., and Koretsky A.P. 1992. *Proc. Natl Acad. Sci. USA* 89: 212.

[3] Zhang W., Williams D.S., and Detre J.A. 1992. *Magn. Reson. Med.* 25: 362.

[4] Zhang W., Williams D.S., and Koretsky A.P. 1993. *Magn. Reson. Med.* 29: 416.

[5] Dixon W.T., Du L.N., Faul D. *et al.* 1986. *Magn. Reson. Med.* 3: 454.

[6] Kwong K.K., Belliveau J.W., Chesler D.A. *et al.* 1992. *Proc. Natl Acad. Sci. USA* 89: 5675.

[7] Turner R., Le Bihan D., Moonen C.T. *et al.* 1991. *Magn. Reson. Med.* 22: 159.

[8] Ogawa S., Lee T.M., Kay A.R., and Tank D.W. 1990. *Proc. Natl Acad. Sci. USA* 87: 9868.

[9] Ogawa S. and Lee T.M. 1990. *Magn. Reson. Med.* 16: 9.

[10] Cohen M.S. and Weisskoff R.M. 1991. *Magn. Reson. Imag.* 9: 1.

[11] Brady T.J. 1991. *Society of Magnetic Resonance in Medicine*, San Francisco, CA Vol. 2.

[12] Belliveau J.W., Kennedy D.N. Jr, McKinstry R.C. *et al.* 1991. *Science* 254: 716.

[13] Ogawa S., Lee T.M., Nayak A.S., and Glynn P. 1990. *Magn. Reson. Med.* 14: 68.

[14] Bandettini P.A., Wong E.C., Hinks R.S. *et al.* 1992. *Magn. Reson. Med.* 25: 390.

[15] Ogawa S., Tank D.W., Menon R. *et al.* 1992. *Proc. Natl Acad. Sci. USA* 89: 5951.

[16] Frahm J., Bruhn H., Merboldt K., and Hanicke W. 1992. *J. Magn. Reson. Imag.* 2: 501.

[17] Turner R., Jezzard P., Wen H. *et al.* 1992. *Society of Magnetic Resonance in Medicine Eleventh Annual Meeting*, Berlin.

[18] Blamire A., Ogawa S., Ugurbil K. *et al.* 1992. *Proc. Natl Acad. Sci. USA* 89: 11069.

[19] Menon R., Ogawa S., Tank D., and Ugurbil K. 1993. *Magn. Reson. Med.* 30: 380.

[20] Lai S., Hopkins A., Haacke E. *et al.* 1993. *Magn. Reson. Med.* 30: 387.

[21] Cao Y., Towle V.L., Levin D.N. *et al.* 1993. *Society of Magnetic Resonance in Medicine Meeting.*

[22] Connelly A., Jackson G.D., Frackowiak R.S.J. *et al.* 1993. *Radiology* 125.

[23] Kim S.G., Ashe J., Georgopouplos A.P. *et al.* 1993. *J. Neurophys.* 69: 297.

[24] Schneider W., Noll D.C., and Cohen J.D. 1993. *Nature* 365: 150.

[25] Hinke R.M., Hu X., Stillman A.E. *et al.* 1993. *Neurol. Rep.* 4: 675.

[26] Binder J.R., Rao S.M., Hammeke T.A. *et al.* 1993. *Neurology* (suppl. 2): 189.

[27] Rao S.M., Binder J.R., Bandettini P.A. *et al.* 1993. *Neurology* 43: 2311.

[28] Gomiscek G., Beisteiner R., Hittmair K. *et al.* 1993. *MAGMA* 1: 109.

[29] Duyn J., Moonen C., de Boer R. *et al.* 1993. *Society of Magnetic Resonance in Medicine, 12th Annual Meeting*, New York.

[30] Hajnal J.V., Collins A.G., White S.J. *et al.* 1993. *Magn. Reson. Med.* 30: 650.

[31] Hennig J., Ernst T., Speck O. *et al.* 1994. *Magn. Reson. Med.* 31: 85.

[32] Constable R.T., Kennan R.P., Puce A. *et al.* 1994. *Magn. Reson. Med.* 31: 686.

[33] Binder J.R., Rao S.M., Hammeke T.A. *et al.* 1994. *Ann. Neurol.* 35: 662.

[34] Frahm J., Merboldt K., and Hänicke W. 1993. *Magn. Reson. Med.* 29: 139.

[35] Stern C.E., Kwong K.K., Belliveau J.W. *et al.* 1992. *Society of Magnetic Resonance in Medicine Annual Meeting*, Berlin, Germany.

[36] Belliveau J.W., Kwong K.K., Baker J.R. *et al.* 1992. *Society of Magnetic Resonance in Medicine Annual Meeting*, Berlin, Germany.

[37] Tootell R.B.H., Kwong K.K., Belliveau J.W. *et al.* 1993. *Investigative Ophthalmology and Visual Science*, p. 813.

[38] Kim S.-G., Ashe J., Hendrich K. *et al.* 1993. *Science* 261: 615.

[39] Buchbinder B.R., Jiang H.J., Cosgrove G.R. *et al.* 1994. *ASNR* 162.

[40] Jack C.R., Thompson R.M., Butts R.K. *et al.* 1994. *Radiology* 190: 85.

[41] Benson R.R., Kwong K.K., Belliveau J.W. *et al.* 1993. *Soc. Neurosci.*

[42] Benson R.R., Kwong K.K., Buchbinder B.R. *et al.* 1994. *Society of Magnetic Resonance*, San Francisco.

[43] Ogawa S., Menon R., Tank D. *et al.* 1993. *Biophys. J.* 64: 803.

[44] Ogawa S., Lee T.M., and Barrere B. 1993. *Magn. Reson. Med.* 29: 205.

[45] Kennan R.P., Zhong J., and Gore J.C. 1994. *Magn. Reson. Med.* 31: 9.

[46] Weisskoff R.M., Zuo C.S., Boxerman J.L., and Rosen B.R. 1994. *Magn. Reson. Med.* 31: 601.

[47] Bandettini P.A., Jesmanowicz A., Wong E.C., and Hyde J.S. 1993. *Magn. Reson. Med.* 30: 161.

[48] Thulborn K.R., Waterton J.C., Matthews P.M., and Radda G.K. 1982. *Biochim. Biophys. Acta* 714: 265.

[49] Grubb R.L., Raichle M.E., Eichling J.O., and Ter-Pogossian M.M. 1974. *Stroke* 5: 630.

[50] Fox P.T. and Raichle M.E. 1986. *Proc. Natl Acad. Sci. USA* 83: 1140.

[51] Fox P.T., Raichle M.E., Mintun M.A., and Dence C. 1988. *Science* 241: 462.

[52] Prichard J., Rothman D., Novotny E. *et al.* 1991. *Proc. Natl Acad. Sci. USA* 88: 5829.

[53] Brooks R.A. and Di Chiro G. 1987. *Med. Phys.* 14: 903.

[54] Kwong K., Chesler D., Zuo C. *et al.* 1993. *Society of Magnetic Resonance in Medicine, 12th Annual Meeting*, New York, p. 172.

[55] Kwong K.K., Chesler D.A., Weisskoff R.M., and Rosen B.R. 1994. *Society of Magnetic Resonance*, San Francisco.

[56] Edelman R., Sievert B., Wielopolski P. *et al.* 1994. *JMRI* 4.

[57] Warach S., Sievert B., Darby D. *et al.* 1994. *JMRI* 4: S8.

[58] Fisel C.R., Ackerman J.L., Buxton R.B. *et al.* 1991. *Magn. Reson. Med.* 17: 336.

[59] Frahm J., Merboldt K., and Hanicke W. 1993. *Society of Magnetic Resonance in Medicine, 12th Annual Meeting*, New York, p. 1427.

[60] Kwong K.K., Chesler D.A., Boxerman J.L. *et al.* 1994. *Society of Magnetic Resonance*, San Francisco.

[61] Song W., Bandettini P., Wong E., and Hyde J. 1994. Personal communication.

[62] Zuo C., Boxerman J., and Weisskoff R. 1992. *Society of Magnetic Resonance in Medicine, 11th Annual Meeting*, Berlin, p. 866.

12.4 Chemical-Shift Imaging: An Introduction to Its Theory and Practice

Xiaoping Hu, Wei Chen, Maqbool Patel, and Kamil Ugurbil

Over the past two decades, there has been a great deal of development in the application of nuclear magnetic resonance (NMR) to biomedical research and clinical medicine. Along with the development of magnetic resonance imaging [1], *in vivo* magnetic resonance spectroscopy (MRS) is becoming a research tool for biochemical studies of humans as well as a potentially more specific diagnostic tool, since it provides specific information on individual chemical species in living systems. Experimental studies in animals and humans have demonstrated that MRS can be used to study the biochemical basis of disease and to follow the treatment of disease.

Since biologic subjects (e.g., humans) are heterogeneous, it is necessary to spatially localize the spectroscopic signals to a well-defined volume or region of interest (VOI or ROI, respectively) in the intact body. Toward this goal, various localization techniques have been developed (see Reference 2 for a recent review). Among these techniques, chemical-shift imaging (CSI) or spectroscopic imaging [3–6] is an attractive technique, since it is capable of producing images reflecting the spatial distribution of various chemical species of interest. Since the initial development of CSI in 1982 [3], further developments have been made to provide better spatial localization and sensitivity, and the technique has been applied to numerous biomedical problems.

In this section we will first present a qualitative description of the basic principles of chemical-shift imaging and subsequently present some practical examples to illustrate the technique. Finally, a summary is provided in the last subsection.

12.4.1 General Methodology

In an NMR experiment, the subject is placed in a static magnetic field B_0. Under the equilibrium condition, nuclear spins with nonzero magnetic moment are aligned along B_0, giving rise to an induced bulk magnetization. To observe the bulk magnetization, it is tipped to a direction perpendicular to B_0 (transverse plane) with a radiofrequency (RF) pulse that has a frequency corresponding to the resonance frequency of the nuclei. The resonance frequency is determined by the product of the gyromagnetic ratio of the nucleus γ and the strength of the static field, that is, γB_0, and is called the *Larmor frequency*. The Larmor frequency also depends on the chemical environment of the nuclei, and this dependency gives rise to chemical shifts that allow one to identify different chemical species in an NMR spectrum. Upon excitation, the magnetization in the transverse plane (perpendicular to the main B_0 field direction) oscillates with the Larmor frequencies of all the different chemical species and induces a signal in a receiving RF coil; the signal is also termed the *free induction decay (FID)*. The FID can be Fourier transformed with respect to time to produce a spectrum in frequency domain.

In order to localize an NMR signal from an intact subject, spatially selective excitation and/or spatial encoding are usually utilized. Selective excitation is achieved as follows: in the excitation, an RF pulse with a finite bandwidth is applied in the presence of a linear static magnetic field gradient. With the application of the gradient, the Larmor frequency of spins depends linearly on the spatial location along the direction of the gradient. Consequently, only the spins in a slice whose resonance frequency falls into the bandwidth of the RF pulse are excited.

The RF excitation rotates all or a portion of the magnetization to the transverse plane, which can be detected by a receiving RF coil. Without spatial encoding, the signal detected is the integral of the signals over the entire excited volume. In CSI based on Fourier imaging, spatial discrimination is achieved by phase encoding. Phase encoding is accomplished by applying a gradient pulse after the excitation and before the data acquisition. During the gradient pulse, spins precess at Larmor frequencies that vary linearly along the direction of the gradient and accrue a phase proportional to the position along the phase-encoding gradient as well as the strength and the duration of the gradient pulse. This acquired spatially encoded phase is typically expressed as $\vec{k} \cdot \vec{r} = \int \gamma \vec{g}(t) \cdot \vec{r} dt$, where γ is the gyromagnetic ratio; $\vec{r}$ is the vector designating spatial location; $\vec{g}(t)$ defines the magnitude, the direction, and the time dependence of the magnetic field gradient applied during the phase-encoding; and the integration is performed over time when the phase-encoding gradient is on. Thus, in one-dimensional phase encoding, if the phase encoding is along, for example, the y axis, the phase acquired becomes $k \times y = \int \gamma g_y(t) \times y \, dt$. The acquired signal $S(t)$ is the integral of the spatially distributed signals modulated by a spatially dependent phase, given by the equation

$$S(t) = \int \rho(\vec{r}, t) e^{(i\vec{k} \cdot \vec{r})} d^3 r \tag{12.17}$$

where ρ is a function that describes the spatial density and the time evolution of the transverse magnetization of all the chemical species in the sample. This signal mathematically corresponds to a sample of the Fourier transform along the direction of the gradient. The excitation and detection process is repeated with various phase-encoding gradients to obtain many phase-encoded signals that can be inversely Fourier-transformed to resolve an equal number of pixels along this direction. Taking the example of one-dimensional phase-encoding along the y axis to obtain a one-dimensional image along this direction of n pixels, the phase encoding gradient is incremented n times so that n FIDs are acquired, each of which is described as

$$S(t, n) = \int \rho^*(y, t) e^{(ink_0 y)} dy \tag{12.18}$$

where ρ^* is already integrated over the x and z directions, and k_0 is the phase-encoding increment; the latter is decided on using the criteria that the full field of view undergo a 360-degree phase difference when $n = 1$, as dictated by the sampling theorem. The time required for each repetition (TR), which is dictated by the longitudinal relaxation time, is usually on the order of seconds.

In CSI, phase encoding is applied in one, two, or three dimensions to provide spatial localization. Meanwhile, selective excitation also can be utilized in one or more dimensions to restrict the volume to be resolved with the phase encodings. For example, with selective excitation in two dimensions, CSI in one spatial dimension can resolve voxels within the selected column. In multidimensional CSI, all the phase-encoding steps along one dimension need to be repeated for all the steps along the others. Thus, for three dimensions with M, N, and L number of phase encoding steps, one must acquire $M \times N \times L$ number of FIDS:

$$S(t, m, n, l) = \int \rho(\vec{r}, t) e^{i(mkx_0 x + nky_0 y + lkz_0 z)} d^3 \vec{r} \tag{12.19}$$

where m, n, and l must step through M, N, and L in integer steps, respectively. As a result, the time needed for acquiring a chemical-shift image is proportional to the number of pixels desired and may be very long. In practice, due to the time limitation as well as the signal-to-noise ratio (SNR) limitation, chemical-shift imaging is usually performed with relatively few spatial encoding steps, such as 16×16 or 32×32 in a two-dimensional experiment.

The data acquired with the CSI sequence need to be properly processed before the metabolite information can be visualized and quantitated. The processing consists of spatial reconstruction and spectral processing. Spatial reconstruction is achieved by performing discrete inverse Fourier transformation, for each of the spatial dimensions, with respect to the phase-encoding steps. The spatial Fourier transform is applied for all the points of the acquired FID. For example, for a data set from a CSI in two spatial dimensions with 32×32 phase-encoding steps and 1024 sampled data points for each FID, a 32×32 two-dimensional inverse Fourier transform is applied to each of the 1024 data points. Although the nominal spatial resolution achieved by the spatial reconstruction is determined by the number of phase-encoding steps and the field of view (FOV), it is important to note that due to the limited number of phase-encoding steps used in most CSI experiments, the spatial resolution is severely degraded by the truncation artifacts, which results in signal "bleeding" between pixels. Various methods have been developed to reduce this problem [7–14].

The localized FIDs derived from the spatial reconstruction are to be further processed by spectral analysis. Standard procedures include Fourier transformation, filtering, zero-filling, and phasing. The localized spectra can be subsequently presented for visualization or further processed to produce quantitative metabolite information. The presentation of the localized spectra in CSI is not a straightforward task because there can be thousands of spectra. In one-dimensional experiments, localized spectra are usually presented in a stack plot. In two-dimensional experiments, localized spectra are plotted in small boxes representing the extent of the pixels, and the plots can be overlaid on corresponding anatomic image for reference. Spectra from three-dimensional CSI experiments are usually presented slice by slice, each displaying the spectra as in the two-dimensional case.

To derive metabolite maps, peaks corresponding to the metabolites of interest need to be quantified. In principle, the peaks can be quantified using the standard methods developed for spectral quantification [15–17]. The most straightforward technique is to calculate the peak areas by integrating the spectra over the peak of interest if it does not overlap with other peaks significantly. In integrating all the localized spectra, spectral shift due to B_0 inhomogeneity should be taken into account. A more robust approach is to apply spectral fitting programs to each spectrum to obtain various parameters of each peak. The fitted area for the peak of interest can then be used to represent the metabolite signal. The peak areas are then used to generate metabolite maps, which are images with intensities proportional to the localized peak area. The metabolite map can be displayed by itself as a gray-scale image or color-coded image or overlaid on a reference anatomic image.

12.4.2 Practical Examples

To illustrate the practical utility of CSI, we present two representative CSI studies in this section. The sequence for the first study is shown in Figure 12.21. This is a three-dimensional sequence in which phase encoding is applied in all three directions and no slice selection is used. Such a sequence is usually used with a surface RF coil whose spatial extent of sensitivity defines the field of view. In this sequence, the FID is acquired immediately after the application of the phase-encoding gradient to minimize the decay of the transverse magnetization, and the sequence is suitable for imaging metabolites with short transverse relaxation time (e.g., ATP).

With the sequence shown in Figure 12.21, a phosphorus-31 CSI study of the human brain was conducted using a quadrature surface coil. A nonselective RF pulse with an Ernest angle (40 degrees) optimized for the repetition time was used for the excitation. Phase-encoding gradients were applied for a duration of 500 μsec; the phase-encoding gradients were incremented according to a FOV of 25 × 25 × 20 cm^3. Phase-encoded FIDs were acquired with 1024 complex data points over a sampling window of 204.8 msec; the corresponding spectral width was 5000 Hz. To reduce intervoxel signal contamination, a technique that utilizes variable data averaging to introduce spatial filtering during the data acquisition for optimal signal-to-noise ratio is employed [7–10], resulting in spherical voxels with diameter of 3 cm (15 cc volume). The data were acquired with a *TR* of 1 sec, and the total acquisition time was approximately 28 min.

The acquired data were processed to generate three-dimensional voxels, each containing a localized phosphorus spectrum, in a 17 × 13 × 17 matrix. In Figure 12.22a–c, spectra in three slices of the three-dimensional CSI are presented; these spectra are overlaid on the corresponding anatomic images obtained with a T_1-weighted imaging sequence. One representative spectrum of the brain is illustrated in Figure 12.22d, where the peaks corresponding to various metabolites are labeled. It is evident that the localized phosphorus spectra contain a wealth of information about several metabolites of interest, including adenosine triphosphate (ATP), phosphocreatine (PCr), phosphomonoester (PME), inorganic phosphate (P$_i$), and phosphodiester (PDE). In pathologic cases, focal abnormalities

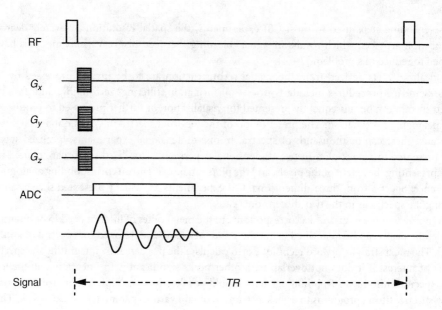

FIGURE 12.21 Sequence diagram for a three-dimensional chemical shift imaging sequence using a nonselective RF pulse.

in phosphorus metabolites have been detected in patients with tumor, epilepsy, and other diseases [18–25].

The second study described below is performed with the sequence depicted in Figure 12.23. This is a two-dimensional spin-echo sequence in which a slice is selectively excited by a 90-degree excitation pulse. The 180-degree refocusing pulse is selective with a slightly broader slice profile. Here the phase-encoding gradients are applied before the refocusing pulse; they also can be placed after the 180-degree pulse or split to both sides of the 180-degree pulse. This sequence was used for a proton CSI experiment. In proton CSI, a major problem arises from the strong water signal that overwhelms that of the metabolites. In order to suppress the water signal, many techniques have been devised [26–29]. In this study, a three-pulse CHESS [26] technique was applied before the application of the excitation pulse as shown in Figure 12.23. The CSI experiment was performed on a 1.4-cm slice with 32×32 phase encodings over a 22×22 cm^2 FOV. The second half of the spin-echo was acquired with 512 complex data points over a sampling window of 256 msec, corresponding to a spectral width of 2000 Hz. Each phase-encoding FID was acquired twice for data averaging. The repetition time (*TR*) and the echo time (*TE*) used were 1.2 sec and 136 msec, respectively. The total acquisition time was approximately 40 min.

Another major problem in proton CSI study of the brain is that the signal from the subcutaneous lipid usually is much stronger than those of the metabolites, and this strong signal leaks into pixels within the brain due to truncation artifacts. To avoid lipid signal contamination, many proton CSI studies of the brain are performed within a selected region of interest excluding the subcutaneous fat [30–34]. Recently, several techniques have been proposed to suppress the lipid signal and consequently suppress the lipid signal contamination. These include the use of WEFT [27] and the use of outer-volume signal suppression [34]. In the example described below, we used a technique that utilizes the spatial location of the lipid to extrapolate data in the *k*-space to reduce the signal contamination due to truncation [35].

In Figure 12.24, the results from the proton CSI study are presented. In panel (a), the localized spectra are displayed. Note that the spectra in the subcutaneous lipid are ignored because they are all off the scale. The nominal spatial resolution is approximately 0.66 cc. A spectrum from an individual pixel in this study is presented in Figure 12.24b with metabolite peaks indicated. Several metabolite peaks, such as those corresponding to the *N*-acetyl aspartate (NAA), creatine/phosphocreatine (Cr/PCr), and choline (Cho), are readily identified. In addition, there is still a noticeable amount of residual lipid signal contamination despite the use of the data extrapolation technique. Without the lipid suppression technique, the brain spectra would be severely contaminated by the lipid signal, making the detection of the metabolite peaks formidable. The peak of NAA in these spectra is fitted to generate the metabolite map shown in panel (c). Although the metabolite map is not corrected for coil sensitivity and other factors and only provides a relative measure of the metabolite concentration in the brain, it is a reasonable measure of the NAA distribution in the brain slice. The spatial resolution of the CSI study can be appreciated from the brain structure present in the map. In biomedical research, proton CSI is potentially the most promising technique, since it provides best sensitivity and spatial resolution. Various *in vivo* applications of proton spectroscopy can be found in the literature [36].

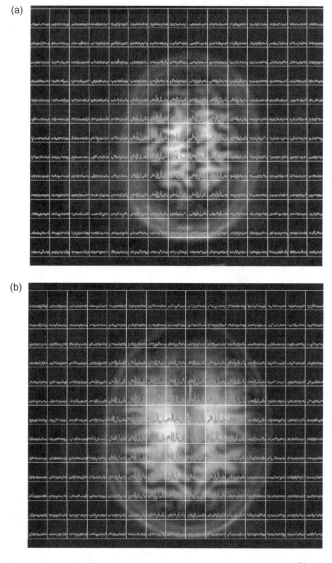

(a)

(b)

FIGURE 12.22 (a)–(c) Boxed plot of spectra in three slices from the three-dimensional ^{31}P CSI experiment overlaid on corresponding anatomic images. The spectral extent displayed is from 10 to 20 ppm. A 20-Hz line broadening is applied to all the spectra.

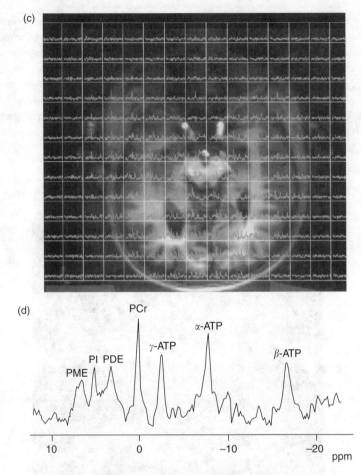

FIGURE 12.22   (d) Representative spectrum from the three-dimensional ^{31}P CSI shown in (b). Metabolite peaks are labeled.

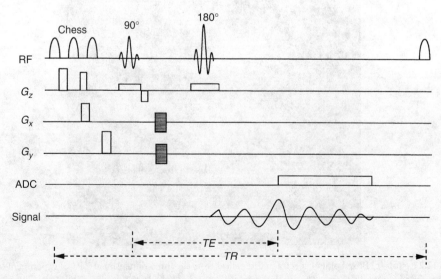

FIGURE 12.23   A two-dimensional spin-echo CSI sequence with chemical selective water suppression (CHESS) for proton study.

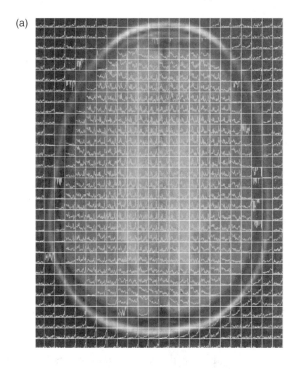

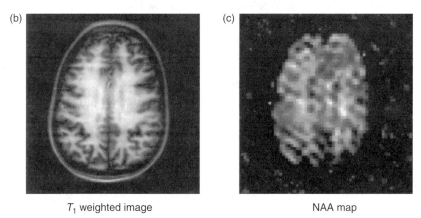

T_1 weighted image   NAA map

FIGURE 12.24   (a) Boxed plot of spectra for the two-dimensional proton study overlaid on the anatomic image. A spectral range of 1.7 to 3.5 ppm is used in the plot to show Cho, PCr/Cr, and NAA. A 5-Hz line broadening is applied in the spectral processing. (b) A representative spectrum from the two-dimensional CSI in panel (a). Peaks corresponding to Cho, PCr/Cr, and NAA are indicated. (c) A map of the area under the NAA peak obtained by spectral fitting. The anatomic image is presented along with the metabolite map for reference. The spatial resolution of the metabolite image can be appreciated from the similarities between the two images. The lipid suppression technique has successfully eliminated the signal contamination from the lipid in the skull.

12.4.3   Summary

CSI is a technique for generating localized spectra that provide a wealth of biochemical information that can be used to study the metabolic activity of living system and to detect disease associated biochemical changes. This section provides an introduction to the technique and illustrates it by two representative examples. More specific topics concerning various aspects of CSI can be found in the literature.

Acknowledgments

The authors would like to thank Dr. Xiao-Hong Zhu for assisting data acquisition and Mr. Gregory Adriany for hardware support. The studies presented here are supported by the National Institute of Health (RR08079).

References

[1] Lauterbur P.C. 1973. Image formation by induced local interactions: examples employing nuclear magnetic resonance. *Nature* 242: 190.

[2] Alger J.R. 1994. Spatial localization for *in vivo* magnetic resonance spectroscopy: concepts and commentary. In R.J. Gillies (ed.), *NMR in Physiology and Biomedicine*, pp. 151–168. San Diego, CA, Academic Press.

[3] Brown T.R., Kincaid M.B., and Ugurbil K. 1982. NMR chemical shift imaging in three dimensions. *Proc. Natl Acad. Sci. USA* 79: 3523.

[4] Maudsley A.A., Hilal S.K., Simon H.E., and Perman W.H. 1983. Spatially resolved high resolution spectroscopy by "four dimensional" NMR. *J. Magn. Reson.* 51: 147.

[5] Haselgrove J.C., Subramanian V.H., Leigh J.S. Jr. *et al.* 1983. *In vivo* one-dimensional imaging of phosphorous metabolites by phosphorus-31 nuclear magnetic resonance. *Science* 220: 1170.

[6] Maudsley A.A., Hilal S.K., Simon H.E., and Wittekoek S. 1984. *In vivo* MR spectroscopic imaging with P-31. *Radiology* 153: 745.

[7] Garwood M., Schleich T., Ross B.D. *et al.* 1985. A modified rotating frame experiment based on a Fourier window function: application to *in vivo* spatially localized NMR spectroscopy. *J. Magn. Reson.* 65: 239.

[8] Garwood M., Robitalle P.M., and Ugurbil K. 1987. Fourier series windows on and off resonance using multiple coils and longitudinal modulation. *J. Magn. Reson.* 75: 244.

[9] Mareci T.H. and Brooker H.R. 1984. High-resolution magnetic resonance spectra from a sensitive region defined with pulsed gradients. *J. Magn. Reson.* 57: 157.

[10] Brooker H.R., Mareci T.H., and Mao J.T. 1987. Selective Fourier transform localization. *Magn. Reson.* Med. 5: 417.

[11] Hu X., Levin D.N., Lauterbur P.C., and Spraggins T.A. 1988. SLIM: spectral localization by imaging. *Magn. Reson. Med.* 8: 314.

[12] Liang Z.P. and Lauterbur P.C. 1991. A generalized series approach to MR spectroscopic imaging. *IEEE Trans. Med. Imag.* MI-10: 132.

[13] Hu X. and Stillman A.E. 1991. Technique for reduction of truncation artifact in chemical shift images. *IEEE Trans. Med. Imag.* MI-10 3: 290.

[14] Hu X., Patel M.S., and Ugurbil K. 1993. A new strategy for chemical shift imaging. *J. Magn. Reson.* B103: 30.

[15] van den Boogaart A., Ala-Korpela M., Jokisaari J., and Griffiths J.R. 1994. Time and frequency domain analysis of NMR data compared: an application to 1D 1H spectra of lipoproteins. *Magn. Reson. Med.* 31: 347.

[16] Ernst T., Kreis R., and Ross B. 1993. Absolute quantification of water and metabolites in human brain: I. Compartments and water. *J. Magn. Reson.* 102: 1.

[17] Kreis R., Ernst T., and Ross B. 1993. Absolute quantification of water and metabolites in human brain. II. Metabolite concentration. *J. Magn. Reson.* 102: 9.

[18] Lenkinski R.E., Holland G.A., Allman T. *et al.* 1988. Integrated MR imaging and spectroscopy with chemical shift imaging of P-31 at 1.5 T: Initial clinical experience. *Radiology* 169: 201.

[19] Hugg J.W., Matson G.B., Twieg D.B. *et al.* ^{31}P MR spectroscopic imaging of normal and pathological human brains. *Magn. Reson. Imag.* 10: 227.

[20] Vigneron D.B., Nelson S.J., Murphy-Boesch J. *et al.* 1990. Chemical shift imaging of human brain: axial, sagittal, and coronal ^{31}P metabolite images. *Radiology* 177: 643.

[21] Hugg J.W., Laxer K.D., Matson G.B. *et al.* 1992. Lateralization of human focal epilepsy by ^{31}P magnetic resonance spectroscopic imaging. *Neurology* 42: 2011.

[22] Meyerhoff D.J., Maudsley A.A., Schafer S., and Weiner M.W. 1992. Phosphorous-31 magnetic resonance metabolite imaging in the human body. *Magn. Reson. Imag.* 10: 245.

[23] Bottomley P.A., Hardy C., and Boemer P. 1990. Phosphate metabolite imaging and concentration measurements in human heart by nuclear magnetic resonance. *J. Magn. Reson. Med.* 14: 425.

[24] Robitaille P.M., Lew B., Merkle H. *et al.* 1990. Transmural high energy phosphate distribution and response to alterations in workload in the normal canine myocardium as studied with spatially localized ^{31}P NMR spectroscopy. *Magn. Reson. Med.* 16: 91.

[25] Ugurbil K., Garwood M., Merkle H. *et al.* 1989. Metabolic consequences of coronary stenosis: transmurally heterogeneous myocardial ischemia studied by spatially localized ^{31}P NMR spectroscopy. *NMR Biomed.* 2: 317.

[26] Hasse A., Frahm J., Hanicker H., and Mataei D. 1985. ^{1}H NMR chemical shift selective (CHESS) imaging. *Phys. Med. Biol.* 30: 341.

[27] Patt S.L. and Sykes B.D. 1972. T_1 water eliminated Fourier transform NMR spectroscopy. *Chem. Phys.* 56: 3182.

[28] Moonen C.T.W. and van Zijl P.C.M. 1990. Highly effective water suppression for *in vivo* proton NMR spectroscopy (DRYSTEAM). *J. Magn. Reson.* 88: 28.

[29] Ogg R., Kingsley P., and Taylor J.S. 1994. WET: A T_1 and B_1 insensitive water suppression method for *in vivo* localized ^{1}H *NMR Spectroscopy*, B104: 1.

[30] Lampman D.A., Murdoch J.B., and Paley M. 1991. *In vivo* proton metabolite maps using MESA 3D technique. *Magn. Reson. Med.* 18: 169.

[31] Luyten P.R., Marien A.J.H., Heindel W. *et al.* 1990. Metabolic imaging of patients with intracranial tumors: [1]H MR spectroscopic imaging and PET. *Radiology* 176: 791.

[32] Arnold D.L., Matthews P.M., Francis G.F. *et al.* 1992. Proton magnetic resonance spectroscopic imaging for metabolite characterization of demyelinating plaque. *Ann. Neurol.* 31: 319.

[33] Duijin J.H., Matson G.B., Maudsley A.A. *et al.* 1992. Human brain infarction: proton MR spectroscopy. *Radiology* 183: 711.

[34] Duyn J.H., Gillen J., Sobering G. *et al.* 1993. Multisection proton MR spectroscopic imaging of the brain. *Radiology* 188: 277.

[35] Patel M.S. and Hu X. 1994. Selective data extrapolation for chemical shift imaging. *Soc. Magn. Reson. Abstr.* 3: 1168.

[36] Rothman D.L. 1994. ^{1}H NMR studies of human brain metabolism and physiology. In R.J. Gillies (ed.), *NMR in Physiology and Biomedicine*, pp. 353–372. San Diego, CA, Academic Press.

13

Nuclear Medicine

13.1 Instrumentation **13**-1
  Parameters for Choices in Nuclear Medicine • Detection of
  Photon Radiation • Various Detector Configurations •
  Ancillary Electronic Equipment for Detection • Place of
  Planar Imaging in Nuclear Medicine Today:
  Applications and Economics

Defining Terms **13**-9
Further Information **13**-9

13.2 SPECT (Single-Photon Emission Computed
  Tomography).. **13**-10
  Basic Principles of SPECT • SPECT Instrumentation •
  Reconstruction Methods • Sample SPECT Images •
  Discussion

References **13**-27

Barbara Y. Croft
National Institutes of Health

Benjamin M.W. Tsui
University of North Carolina

13.1 Instrumentation

Barbara Y. Croft

Nuclear medicine can be defined as the practice of making patients radioactive for diagnostic and therapeutic purposes. The radioactivity is injected intravenously, rebreathed, or ingested. It is the internal circulation of radioactive material that distinguishes nuclear medicine from diagnostic radiology and radiation oncology in most of its forms. This section will examine only the diagnostic use and will concentrate on methods for detecting the radioactivity from outside the body without trauma to the patient. Diagnostic nuclear medicine is successful for two main reasons (1) It can rely on the use of very small amounts of materials (picomolar concentrations in chemical terms) thus usually not having any effect on the processes being studied, and (2) the radionuclides being used can penetrate tissue and be detected outside the patient. Thus the materials can trace processes or "opacify" organs without affecting their function.

13.1.1 Parameters for Choices in Nuclear Medicine

Of the various kinds of emanations from radioactive materials, photons alone have a range in tissue great enough to escape so that they can be detected externally. Electrons or beta-minus particles of high energy can create bremsstrahlung in interactions with tissue, but the radiation emanates from the site of the interaction, not the site of the beta ray's production. Positrons or beta-plus particles annihilate with electrons to create gamma rays so that they can be detected (see Chapter 16). For certain radionuclides, the emanation being detected is x-rays, in the 50- to 100-keV energy range.

TABLE 13.1   Gamma Ray Detection

Type of sample	Activity (μCi)	Energy (keV)	Type of instrument
Patient samples, for example, blood, urine	0.001	0–5000	Gamma counter with annular NaI(TI) detector, 1 or 2 PMTs, external Pb shielding
Small organ function <30 cm field of view at 60 cm distance	5–200	20–1500	2–4-in. NaI(TI) detector with flared Pb collimator
Static image of body part, for example, liver, lung	0.2–30	50–650	Rectilinear scanner with focused Pb collimator
Dynamic image of body part, for example, xenon in airways	2–30	80–300	Anger camera and parallel-hole Pb collimator
Static tomographic image of body part	See Section 13.1		

The half-lives of materials in use in nuclear medicine range from a few minutes to weeks. The half-life must be chosen with two major points in mind: the time course of the process being studied and the radiation dose to the target organ, that is, that organ with the highest concentration over the longest time (the cumulated activity or area underneath the activity versus time curve). In general, it is desired to stay under 5 **rad** to the target organ.

The choice of the best energy range to use is also based on two major criteria: the energy that will penetrate tissue but can be channeled by heavy metal shielding and collimation and that which will interact in the detector to produce a pulse. Thus the ideal energy is dependent on the detector being used and the kind of examination being performed. Table 13.1 describes the kinds of gamma-ray detection, the activity and energy ranges, and an example of the kind of information to be gained. The lesser amounts of activity are used in situations of lesser spatial resolution and of greater sensitivity. Positron imaging is omitted because it is treated elsewhere.

Radiation dose is affected by all the emanations of a radionuclide, not just the desirable ones, thus constricting the choice of nuclide further. There can be no alpha radiation used in diagnosis; the use of materials with primary beta radiation should be avoided because the beta radiation confers a radiation dose without adding to the information being gained. For imaging, in addition, even if there is a primary gamma ray in the correct energy window for the detector, there should be no large amount of radiation, either of primary radiation of higher energy, because it interferes with the image collimation, or of secondary radiation of a very similar energy, because it interferes with the perception of the primary radiation emanating from the site of interest.

For imaging using heavy-metal collimation, the energy range is constrained to be that which will emanate from the human body and which the collimation can contain, or about 50 to 500 keV.

Detectors must be made from materials that exhibit some detectable change when ionizing radiation is absorbed and that are of a high enough atomic number and density to make possible stopping large percentages of those gamma rays emanating (high sensitivity). In addition, because the primary gamma rays are not the only rays emanating from the source — a human body and therefore a distributed source accompanied by an absorber — there must be energy discrimination in the instrument to prevent the formation of an image of the scattered radiation. To achieve pulse size proportional to energy, and therefore to achieve identification of the energy and source of the energy, the detector must be a proportional detector. This means that Geiger-Muller detection, operating in an all-or-none fashion, is not acceptable.

Gaseous detectors are not practical because their density is not great enough. Liquid detectors (in which any component is liquid) are not practical because the liquid can spill when the detector is positioned; this problem can be compensated for if absolutely necessary, but it is better to consider it from the outset. Another property of a good detector is its ability to detect large numbers of gamma rays per time unit. With detection capabilities to separate 100,000 counts per second or a dead time of 2 msec, the system is still only detecting perhaps 1,000 counts per square centimeter per second over a 10 × 10 cm area. The precision of the information is governed by **Poisson statistics**, so the imprecision in information collected

TABLE 13.2 Ways of Imaging Using Lead Collimation

Moving probe; rectilinear scanner
Array of multiple crystals; autofluoroscope, "fly-eye" camera
Two moving probes: dual-head rectilinear scanner
Large single-crystal system: Anger camera
Two crystals on opposite sides of patient for two views using Anger logic
Large multiple-crystal systems using Anger logic SPECT
Other possibilities

for 1 sec in a square centimeter is ±3% at the 1 standard deviation level. Since we would hope for better spatial resolution than 1 cm^2, the precision is obviously worse than this. This points to the need for fast detectors, in addition to the aforementioned sensitivity. The more detector that surrounds the patient, the more sensitive the system will be. Table 13.2 lists in order from least sensitive to most sensitive some of the geometries used for imaging in nuclear medicine. This generally is also a listing from the older methods to the more recent.

For the purposes of this section, we shall consider that the problems of counting patient and other samples and of detecting the time course of activity changes in extended areas with probes are not our topic and confine ourselves to the attempts made to image distributions of gamma-emitting radionuclides in patients and research subjects. The previous section treats the three-dimensional imaging of these distributions; this section will treat detection of the distribution in a planar fashion or the image of the projection of the distribution onto a planar detector.

13.1.2 Detection of Photon Radiation

Gamma rays are detected when atoms in a detector are ionized and the ions are collected either directly as in gaseous or semiconductor systems or by first conversion of the ionized electrons to light and subsequent conversion of the light to electrons in a photomultiplier tube (P-M tube or PMT). In all cases there is a voltage applied across some distance that causes a pulse to be created when a photon is absorbed.

The gamma rays are emitted according to Poisson statistics because each decaying nucleus is independent of the others and has an equal probability of decaying per unit time. Because the uncertainty in the production of gamma rays is therefore on the order of magnitude of the square root of the number of gamma rays, the more gamma rays that are detected, the less the proportional uncertainty will be. Thus sensitivity is a very important issue for the creation of images, since the rays will be detected by area. To get better resolution, one must have the numbers of counts and the apparatus to resolve them spatially. Having the large numbers of counts also means the apparatus must resolve them temporally.

The need for **energy resolution** carries its own burden. Depending on the detector, the energy resolution may be easily achieved or not (Table 13.3). In any case, the attenuation and scattering inside the body means that there will be a range of gamma rays emitted, and it will be difficult to tell those scattered through very small angles from those not scattered at all. This affects the spatial resolution of the instrument.

The current practice of nuclear medicine has defined the limits of the amount of activity that can be administered to a patient by the amount of radiation dose. Since planar imaging with one detector allows only 2 pi detection at best and generally a view of somewhat less because the source is in the patient and the lead collimation means that only rays that are directed from the decay toward the crystal will be detected, it is of utmost importance to detect every ray possible. To the extent that no one is ever satisfied with the resolution of any system and always wishes for better, there is the need to be able to get spatial resolution better than the intrinsic 2 mm currently achievable. Some better collimation system, such as envisioned in a coincidence detection system like that used in PET, might make it possible to avoid stopping so many of the rays with the collimator.

We have now seen that energy resolution, sensitivity and resolving time of the detector are all bound up together to produce the spatial resolution of the instrument as well as the more obvious temporal

TABLE 13.3 Detector Substances and Size Considerations, Atomic Number of the Attenuator, Energy Resolution Capability

---

PMT connected
  NaI(TI): up to 50 cm across; 63; 5–10%
  Plastic scintillators: unlimited; 6; only Compton absorption for gamma rays used in imaging
  CsI(TI): <3 × 3 cm; 53, 55; poorer than NaI(TI)
  BiGermanate: <3 × 3 cm; 83; poorer than NaI(TI)
Semiconductors: Liquid nitrogen operation and liquid nitrogen storage
  GeLi: <3 × 3 cm; 32; <1%
  SiLi: <3 × 3 cm; 14; <1%

TABLE 13.4 Calculation of Number of Counts Achieved with Anger Camera

	cpm	cps
Activity	0.001	
mCi/cm^3		
counts/sec		3.7×10^7
counts/min	2.22×10^9	
2π geometry	1.11×10^9	1.85×10^7
Attenuated by tissue of 0.12/cm attenuation and 3 cm thick	7.44×10^8	1.29×10^7
X Camera efficiency of 0.0006	4.64×10^5	7744
Good uptake in liver = 5 mCi/1000 g = 0.005 mCi/g	2.32×106	3.8×10^4
Thyroid uptake of Tc-99m = (2 mCi/37 g)*	4.6×10^5	7.7×10^3
2% = 0.001 mCi/G		

resolution. The need to collimate to create an image rather than a blush greatly decreases the numbers of counts and makes Poisson statistics a major determinant of the appearance of nuclear medical images.

Table 13.4 shows a calculation for the NaI(TI)-based Anger camera showing 0.06% efficiency for the detection system. Thus the number of counts per second is not high and so is well within the temporal resolving capabilities of the detector system. The problem is the 0.06% efficiency, which is the effect of both the crystal thickness being optimized for imaging rather than for stopping all the gamma rays, and the lead collimation. Improvements in nuclear medicine imaging resolution can only come if both these factors are addressed.

13.1.3 Various Detector Configurations

The detectors in clinical nuclear medicine are NaI(TI) crystals. In research applications, other substances are employed, but the engineering considerations for the use of other detectors are more complex and have been less thoroughly explored (Table 13.3).

The possibilities for configuring the detectors have been increasing, although the older methods tend to be discarded as the new ones are exploited (see Table 13.2). This is in part because each laboratory cannot afford to have one of every kind of instrument, although there are tasks for which each one is ideally suited.

The first instruments possible for plane-projection imaging consisted of a moving single crystal probe, called a rectilinear scanner. The probe consisted of a detector (beginning with NaI(TI) but later incorporating small semiconductors) that was collimated by a focused lead collimator of appreciable thickness (often 2 in. of lead or more) with hole sizes and thicknesses of septa consonant with the intended energy and organ size and depth to be imaged. The collimated detector was caused to move across the patient at a constant speed; the pulses from the detector were converted to visible signals either by virtue of markings on a sheet or of light flashes exposing a film. This detector could see only one spot at a time, so only slow

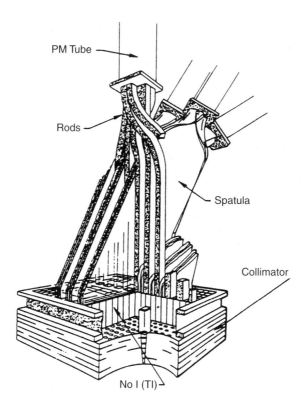

FIGURE 13.1   The Bender–Blau autofluoroscope is a multicrystal imager with a rectangular array of crystals connected to PMTs by plastic light guides. There is a PMT for each row of crystals and a PMT for each column of crystals, so an N by M array would have $(N + M)$ PMTs.

temporal changes in activity could be appreciated. A small organ such as the thyroid could be imaged in this fashion very satisfactorily. Bone imaging also could be done with the later versions of this instrument.

To enlarge the size of the detector, several probes, each with its own photomultiplier tube and collimator, could be used. Versions of this idea were used to create dual-probe instruments to image both sides of the patient simultaneously, bars of probes to sweep down the patient and create a combined image, etc.

To go further with the multiple crystals to create yet larger fields of view, the autofluoroscope (Figure 13.1) combined crystals in a rectangular array. For each to have its own photomultiplier tube required too many PMTs, so the instrument was designed with a light pipe to connect each crystal with a PMT to indicate its row and a second one to indicate its column. The crystals are separated by lead septa to prevent scattered photons from one crystal affecting the next. Because of the large number of crystals and PMTs, the instrument is very fast, but because of the size of the crystals, the resolution is coarse. To improve the resolution, the collimator is often jittered so that each crystal is made to see more than one field of view to create a better resolved image. For those dynamic examinations in which temporal resolution is more important than spatial resolution, the system has a clear advantage. It has not been very popular for general use, however. In its commercial realization, the field of view was not large enough to image either lungs or livers or bones in any single image fashion.

As large NaI(TI) crystals became a reality, new ways to use them were conceived. The Anger camera (Figure 13.2) is one of the older of these methods. The idea is to use a single crystal of diameter large enough to image a significant part of the human body and to back the crystal by an array of photomultiplier tubes to give positional sensitivity. Each PMT is assigned coordinates (Figure 13.3). When a photon is absorbed by the crystal, a number of PMTs receive light and therefore emit signals. The X and Y signal values for the emanation are determined by the strength of the signal from each of the tubes and its x and

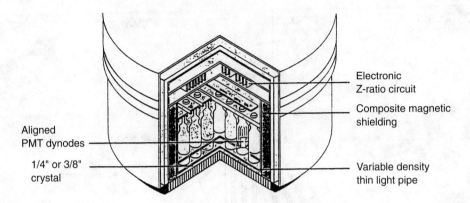

FIGURE 13.2 Anger camera detector design. This figure shows a cross section through the camera head. The active surface is pointed down. Shielding surrounds the assembly on the sides and top.

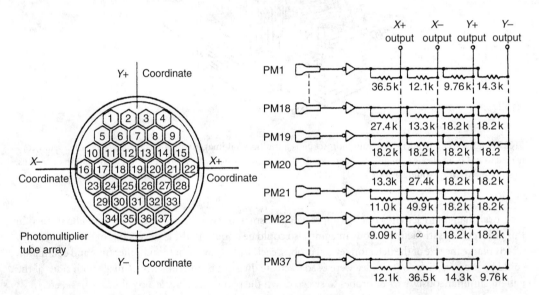

FIGURE 13.3 An array of PMTs in the Anger camera showing the geometric connection between the PMTs and the X and Y output.

y position, and the energy of the emanation (which determines if it will be used to create the image) is the sum of all the signals (the Z pulse). If the discriminator passes the Z pulse, then the X and Y signals are sent to whatever device is recording the image, be it an oscilloscope and film recording system or the analog-to-digital (A/D) converters of a computer system. More recently, the A/D conversion is done earlier in the system so that the X and Y signals are themselves digital. The Anger camera is the major instrument in use in nuclear medicine today. It has been optimized for use with the 140-keV radiation from Tc-99m, although collimators have been designed for lower and higher energies, as well as optimized for higher sensitivity and higher resolution. The early systems used circular crystals, while the current configuration is likely to be rectangular or square.

A combination of the Anger positional logic and the focused collimator in a scanner produced the PhoCon instrument, which, because of the design of its collimators, had planar tomographic capabilities (the instrument could partially resolve activity in different planes, parallel to the direction of movement of the detector).

13.1.4   Ancillary Electronic Equipment for Detection

The detectors used in nuclear medicine are attached to preamplifiers, amplifiers, and pulse shapers to form a signal that can be examined for information about the energy of the detected photon (Figure 13.4). The energy discriminator has lower and upper windows that are set with reference radionuclides so that typically the particular nuclide in use can be dialed in along with the width of the energy window. A photon with an energy that falls in the selected range will cause the creation of a pulse of a voltage that falls in between the levels; all other photon energies will cause voltages either too high or too low. If only gross features are being recorded, any of the instruments may be used as probe detectors and the results recorded on strip-chart recordings of activity vs. time.

The PMT "multiplies" photons (Figure 13.5) because it has a quartz entrance window which is coated to release electrons when it absorbs a light photon and there is a voltage drop; the number of electrons

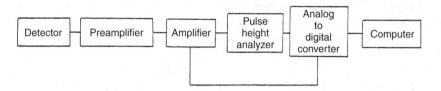

FIGURE 13.4   Schematic drawing of a generalized detector system. There would be a high-voltage power supply for the detector in an NaI(TI)-PMT detector system.

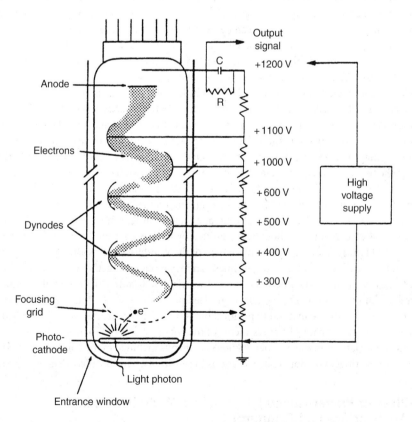

FIGURE 13.5   Schematic drawing of a photomultiplier tube (PMT). Each of the dynodes and the anode is connected to a separate pin in the tube socket. The inside of the tube is evacuated of all gas. Dynodes are typically copper with a special oxidized coating for electron multiplication.

released is proportional to the amount of light that hits the coating. The electrons are guided through a hole and caused to hit the first dynode, which is coated with a special substance to allow it to release electrons when it is hit by an electron. There are a series of dynodes each with a voltage that pulls the electrons from the last dynodes toward it. The surface coating not only releases electrons but also multiplies the electron shower. In a cascade through 10–12 dynodes, there is a multiplication of approximately 106, so that pulses of a few electrons become currents of the order of 10–12 A. The PMTs must be protected from other influences, such as stray radioactivity or strong magnetic fields, which might cause extraneous electron formation or curves in the electron path. Without the voltage drop from one dynode to the next, there is no cascade of electrons and no counting.

For imaging, the x and y positions of those photons in the correct energy range will be recorded in the image because they have a Z pulse. Once the pulse has been accepted and the position determined, that position may be recorded to make an image either in analog or digital fashion; a spot may be made on an oscilloscope screen and recorded on film or paper, or the position may be digitized and stored in a computer file for later imaging on an oscilloscope screen and/or for photography. In general, the computers required are very similar to those used for other imaging modalities, except for the hardware that allows the acceptance of the pulse. The software is usually specifically created for nuclear medicine because of the unique needs for determination of function.

The calibration of the systems follows a similar pattern, no matter how simple or complex the instrument. Most probe detectors must be "peaked," which means that the energy of the radioactivity must be connected with some setting of the instrument, often meant to read in kiloelectronvolts. This is accomplished by counting a sample with the instrument, using a reasonably narrow energy window, while varying the high voltage until the count rate reading is a maximum. The window is then widened for counting samples to encompass all the energy peak being counted. The detector is said to be liner if it can be set with one energy and another energy can be found where it should be on the kiloelectronvolt scale.

To ensure that the images of the radioactivity accurately depict the distribution in the object being imaged, the system must be initialized correctly and tested at intervals. The several properties that must be calibrated and corrected are sensitivity, uniformity, energy pulse shape, and linearity.

These issues are addressed in several ways. The first is that all the PMTs used in an imaging system must be chosen to have matched sensitivities and energy spectra. Next, during manufacture, and at intervals during maintenance, the PMTs' response to voltage is matched so that the voltage from the power supply causes all the tubes to have maximum counts at the same voltage. The sensitivities of all the tubes are also matched during periodic maintenance. Prior to operation, usually at the start of each working day, the user will check the radioactive peak and then present the instrument with a source of activity to give an even exposure over the whole crystal. This uniform "flood" is recorded. The image may be used by the instrument for calibration; recalibration is usually performed at weekly intervals. The number of counts needed depends on the use the instrument is to be put to, but generally the instrument must be tested and calibrated with numbers of counts at least equal to those being emitted by the patients and other objects being imaged.

Because the PMT placement means that placement of the x and y locations is not perfect over the face of the crystal but has the effect of creating wiggly lines that may be closer together over the center of the PMT and farther apart at the interstices between tubes, the image may suffer from spatial nonlinearity. This can be corrected for by presenting the system with a lead pattern in straight-line bars or holes in rows and using a hard-wired or software method to position the X and Y signals correctly. This is called a linearity correction. In addition, there may be adjustments of the energy spectra of each tube to make them match each other so that variations in the number of kiloelectronvolts included in the window (created by varying the discriminator settings) will not create variations in sensitivity. This is called an energy correction.

13.1.5 Place of Planar Imaging in Nuclear Medicine Today: Applications and Economics

There are various ways of thinking about diagnostic imaging and nuclear medicine. If the reason for imaging the patient is to determine the presence of disease, then there are at least two possible strategies. One is to do the most complicated examination that will give a complete set of results on all patients. The other is to start with a simple examination and hope to categorize patients, perhaps into certain abnormals and all others, or even into abnormals, indeterminates, and normals. Then a subsequent, more complex examination is used to determine if there are more abnormals, or perhaps how abnormal they are. If the reason for imaging the patient is to collect a set of data that will be compared with results from that patient at a later time and with a range of normal results from all patients, then the least complex method possible for collecting the information should be used in a regular and routine fashion so that the comparison are possible.

In the former setting, where the complexity of the examination may have to be changed after the initial results are seen, in order to take full advantage of the dose of radioactive material that has been given to the patient, it is sensible to have the equipment available that will be able to perform the more complex examination and not to confine the equipment available to that capable of doing only the simple first examination. For this reason and because for some organs, such as the brain, the first examination is a SPECT examination, the new Anger cameras being sold today are mostly capable of doing rotating SPECT. The added necessities that SPECT brings to the instrument specifications are of degree: better stability, uniformity, and resolution. Thus they do not obviate the use of the equipment for planar imaging but rather enhance it. In the setting of performing only the examination necessary to define the disease, the Anger SPECT camera can be used for plane projection imaging and afterward for SPECT to further refine the examination. There are settings in which a planar camera will be purchased because of the simplicity of all the examinations (as in a very large laboratory that can have specialized instruments, a thyroid practice, or in the developing countries), but in the small- to medium-sized nuclear medicine practice, the new cameras being purchased are all SPECT-capable.

Nuclear medicine studies are generally less expensive than x-ray computed tomography or magnetic resonance imaging and more so than planar x-ray or ultrasound imaging. The general conduct of a nuclear medicine laboratory is more complex than these others because of the radioactive materials and the accompanying regulations. The specialty is practice both in clinics and in hospitals, but again, the complication imposed by the presence of the radioactive materials tips the balance of the practices toward the hospital. In that setting the practitioners may be imagers with a broad range of studies offered or cardiologists with a concentration on cardiac studies. Thus the setting also will determine what kind of instrument is most suitable.

Defining Terms

Energy resolution: Full width at half maximum of graph of detected counts vs. energy, expressed as a
        percentage of the energy.

Poisson statistics: Expresses probability in situations of equal probability for an event per unit of time,
        such as radioactive decay or cosmic-ray appearance. The standard deviation of a mean number
        of counts is the square root of the mean number of counts, which is a decreasing fraction of the
        number of counts when expressed as a fraction of the number of counts.

rad: The unit of radiation energy absorption (dose) in matter, defined as the absorption of 100 ergs
        per gram of irradiated material. The unit is being replaced by the gray, an SI unit, where 1 gray
        (Gy) = 100 rad.

Further Information

A good introduction to nuclear medicine, written as a text for technologists, is *Nuclear Medicine Technology and Techniques*, edited by D.R. Bernier, J.K. Langan, and L.D. Wells. A treatment of many of the nuclear medicine physics issues is given in L.E. Williams' *Nuclear Medicine Physics*, published in three volumes. Journals that publish nuclear medicine articles include the monthly *Journal of Nuclear Medicine, the European Journal of Nuclear Medicine, Clinical Nuclear Medicine, IEEE Transactions in Nuclear Science, IEEE Transactions in Medical Imaging, and Medical Physics*. Quarterly and annual publications include *Seminars in Nuclear Medicine, Yearbook of Nuclear Medicine, and Nuclear Medicine Annual*.

The Society of Nuclear Medicine holds an annual scientific meeting that includes scientific papers, continuing education which could give the novice a broad introduction, poster sessions, and a large equipment exhibition. Another large meeting, devoted to many radiologic specialties is the Radiologic Society of North America's annual meeting, held just after Thanksgiving.

13.2 SPECT (Single-Photon Emission Computed Tomography)

Benjamin M.W. Tsui

During the last three decades, there has been much excitement in the development of diagnostic radiology. The development is fueled by inventions and advances made in a number of exciting new medical imaging modalities, including ultrasound (US), x-ray CT (computed tomography), PET (positron emission tomography), SPECT (single-photon emission computed tomography), and MRI (magnetic resonance imaging). These new imaging modalities have revolutionized the practice of diagnostic radiology, resulting in substantial improvement in patient care.

Single-photon emission computed tomography (SPECT) is a medical imaging modality that combines conventional nuclear medicine (NM) imaging techniques and CT methods. Different from x-ray CT, SPECT uses radioactive-labeled pharmaceuticals, that is, radiopharmaceuticals, that distribute in different internal tissues or organs instead of an external x-ray source. The spatial and uptake distributions of the radiopharmaceuticals depend on the biokinetic properties of the pharmaceuticals and the normal or abnormal state of the patient. The gamma photons emitted from the radioactive source are detected by radiation detectors similar to those used in conventional nuclear medicine. The CT method requires projection (or planar) image data to be acquired from different views around the patient. These projection data are subsequently reconstructed using image reconstruction methods that generate cross-sectional images of the internally distributed radiopharmaceuticals. The SPECT images provide much improved contrast and detailed information about the radiopharmaceutical distribution as compared with the planar images obtained from conventional nuclear medicine methods.

As an emission computed tomographic (ECT) method, SPECT differs from PET in the types of radionuclides used. PET uses radionuclides such as C-11, N-13, O-15, and F-18 that emit positrons with subsequent emission of two coincident 511 keV annihilation photons. These radionuclides allow studies of biophysiologic functions that cannot be obtained from other means. However, they have very short half-lives, often requiring an on-site cyclotron for their production. Also, detection of the annihilation photons requires expensive imaging systems. SPECT uses standard radionuclides normally found in nuclear medicine clinics and which emit individual gamma-ray photons with energies that are much lower than 511 keV. Typical examples are the 140-keV photons from Tc-99m and the ~70-keV photons from TI-201. Subsequently, the costs of SPECT instrumentation and of performing SPECT are substantially less than PET.

Furthermore, substantial advances have been made in the development of new radiopharmaceuticals, instrumentation, and image processing and reconstruction methods for SPECT. The results are much improved quality and quantitative accuracy of SPECT images. These advances, combined with the relatively lower costs, have propelled SPECT to become an increasingly more important diagnostic tool in nuclear medicine clinics.

This section will present the basic principles of SPECT and the instrumentation and image processing and reconstruction methods that are necessary to reconstruct SPECT images. Finally, recent advances and future development that will continue to improve the diagnostic capability of SPECT will be discussed.

13.2.1 Basic Principles of SPECT

Single-photon emission computed tomography (SPECT) is a medical imaging technique that is based on the conventional nuclear medicine imaging technique and tomographic reconstruction methods. General review of the basic principles, instrumentation, and reconstruction technique for SPECT can be found in

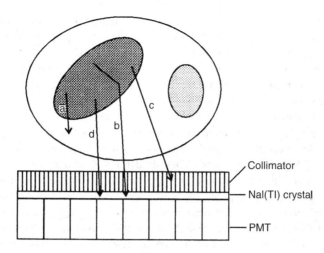

FIGURE 13.6 The conventional nuclear medicine imaging process. Gamma-ray photons emitted from the internally distributed radioactivity may experience photoelectric (a) or scatter (b) interactions. Photons that are not traveling in the direction within the acceptance analog of the collimator (c) will be intercepted by the lead collimator. Photons that experience no interaction and travel within the acceptance angle of the collimator will be detected (d).

a few review articles [Jaszczak et al., 1980; Jaszczak and Coleman, 1985a; Barrett, 1986; Jaszczak and Tsui, 1994].

13.2.1.1 The SPECT Imaging Process

The imaging process of SPECT can be simply depicted as in Figure 13.6. Gamma-ray photons emitted from the internal distributed radiopharmaceutical penetrate through the patient's body and are detected by a single or a set of collimated radiation detectors. The emitted photons experience interactions with the intervening tissues through basic interactions of radiation with matter [Evans, 1955]. The photoelectric effect absorbs all the energy of the photons and stops their emergence from the patient's body. The other major interaction is Compton interaction, which transfers part of the photon energy to free electrons. The original photon is scattered into a new direction with reduced energy that is dependent on the scatter angle. Photons that escape from the patient's body include those that have not experienced any interactions and those which have experienced Compton scattering. For the primary photons from the commonly used radionuclides in SPECT, for example, 140-keV of TC-99m and ~70-keV of TI-201, the probability of pair production is zero.

Most of the radiation detectors used in current SPECT systems are based on a single or multiple NaI(TI) scintillation detectors. The most significant development in nuclear medicine is the scintillation camera (or Anger camera) that is based on a large-area (typically 40 cm in diameter) NaI(TI) crystal [Anger, 1958, 1964]. An array of photomultiplier tubes (PMTs) is placed at the back of the scintillation crystal. When a photon hits and interacts with the crystal, the scintillation generated will be detected by the array of PMTs. An electronic circuitry evaluates the relative signals from the PMTs and determines the location of interaction of the incident photon in the scintillation crystal. In addition, the scintillation cameras have built-in energy discrimination electronic circuitry with finite energy resolution that provides selection of the photons that have not been scattered or been scattered within a small scattered angle. The scintillation cameras are commonly used in commercial SPECT systems.

Analogous to the lens in an optical imaging system, a scintillation camera system consists of a collimator placed in front of the NaI(TI) crystal for the imaging purpose. The commonly used collimator is made of a large number of parallel holes separated by lead septa [Anger, 1964; Keller, 1968; Tsui, 1988]. The geometric dimensions, that is, length, size, and shape of the collimator apertures, determine the directions of photons that will be detected by the scintillation crystals or the geometric response of the collimator.

The width of the geometric response function increases (or the spatial resolution worsens) as the source distance from the collimator increases. Photons that do not pass through the collimator holes properly will be intercepted and absorbed by the lead septal walls of the collimator. In general, the detection efficiency is approximately proportional to the square of the width of the geometric response function of the collimator. This tradeoff between detection efficiency and spatial resolution is a fundamental property of a typical SPECT system using conventional collimators.

The amount of radioactivity that is used in SPECT is restricted by the allowable radiation dose to the patient. Combined with photon attenuation within the patient, the practical limit on imaging time, and the tradeoff between detection efficiency and spatial resolution of the collimator, the number of photons that are collected by a SPECT system is limited. These limitations resulted in SPECT images with relatively poor spatial resolution and high statistical noise fluctuations as compared with other medical imaging modalities. For example, currently a typical brain SPECT image has a total of about 500K counts per image slice and a spatial resolution in the order of approximately 8 mm. A typical myocardial SPECT study using TI-201 has about 150K total count per image slice and a spatial resolution of approximately 15 mm.

In SPECT, projection data are acquired from different views around the patient. Similar to x-ray CT, image processing and reconstruction methods are used to obtain transaxial or cross-sectional images from the multiple projection data. These methods consist of preprocessing and calibration procedures before further processing, mathematical algorithms for reconstruction from projections, and compensation methods for image degradation due to photon attenuation, scatter, and detector response.

The biokinetics of the radiopharmaceutical used, anatomy of the patient, instrumentation for data acquisition, preprocessing methods, image reconstruction techniques, and compensation methods have important effects on the quality and quantitative accuracy of the final SPECT images. A full understanding of SPECT cannot be accomplished without clear understanding of these factors. The biokinetics of radiopharmaceuticals and conventional radiation detectors have been described in the previous section on conventional nuclear medicine. The following subsections will present the major physical factors that affect SPECT and a summary review of the instrumentation, image reconstruction techniques, and compensation methods that are important technological and engineering aspects in the practice of SPECT.

13.2.1.2 Physical and Instrumentation Factors that Affect SPECT Images

There are several important physical and instrumentation factors that affect the measured data and subsequently the SPECT images. The characteristics and effects of these factors can be found in a few review articles [Jaszczak et al., 1981; Jaszczak and Tsui, 1994; Tsui et al., 1994a, 1994b]. As described earlier, gamma-ray photons that emit from an internal source may experience photoelectric absorption within the patient without contributing to the acquired data, Compton scattering with change in direction and loss of energy, or no interaction before exiting the patient's body. The exiting photons will be further selected by the geometric response of the collimator–detector. The photoelectric and Compton interactions and the characteristics of the collimator–detector have significant effects on both the quality and quantitative accuracy of SPECT image.

Photon attenuation is defined as the effect due to photoelectric and Compton interactions resulting in a reduced number of photons that would have been detected without them. The degree of attenuation is determined by the linear attenuation coefficient, which is a function of photon energy and the amount and types of materials contained in the attenuating medium. For example, the attenuation coefficient for the 140-keV photon emitted from the commonly used Tc-99m in water or soft tissue is 0.15 cm^{-1}. This gives rise to a half-valued-layer, the thickness of material that attenuates half the incident photons, or 4.5 cm H_2O for the 140-keV photon. Attenuation is the most important factor that affects the quantitative accuracy of SPECT images.

Attenuation effect is complicated by the fact that within the patient the attenuation coefficient can be quite different in various organs. The effect is most prominent in the thorax, where the attenuation coefficients range from as low as 0.05 cm^{-1} in the lung to as high as 0.18 cm^{-1} in the compact bone for the 140-keV photons. In x-ray CT, the attenuation coefficient distribution is the target for image reconstruction. In SPECT, however, the wide range of attenuation coefficient values and the variations of attenuation coefficient distributions among patients are major difficulties in obtaining quantitative accurate SPECT images. Therefore, compensation for attenuation is important to ensure good image quality and quantitatively high accuracy in SPECT. Review of different attenuation methods that have been used in SPECT is a subject of discussion later in this chapter.

Photons that have been scattered before reaching the radiation detector provide misplaced spatial information about the origin of the radioactive source. The results are inaccurate quantitative information and poor contrast in the SPECT images. For radiation detectors with perfect energy discrimination, scattered photons can be completely rejected. In a typical scintillation camera system, however, the energy resolution is in the order of 10% at 140 keV. With this energy resolution, the ratio of scattered to scattered total photons detected by a typical scintillation detector is about 20–30% in brain and about 30–40% in cardiac and body SPECT studies for 140-keV photons. Furthermore, the effect of scatter depends on the distribution of the radiopharmaceutical, the proximity of the source organ to the target organ, and the energy window used in addition to the photon energy and the energy resolution of the scintillation detector. The compensation of scatter is another important aspect of SPECT to ensure good image quality and quantitative accuracy.

The advances in SPECT can be attributed to simultaneous development of new radiopharmaceuticals, instrumentation, reconstruction methods, and clinical applications. Most radiopharmaceuticals that are developed for conventional nuclear medicine can readily be used in SPECT, and review of these developments is beyond the scope of this chapter. Recent advances include new agents that are labeled with iodine and technetium for blood perfusion for brain and cardiac studies. Also, the use of receptor agents and labeled antibiotics is being investigated. These developments have resulted in radiopharmaceuticals with improved uptake distribution, biokinetics properties, and potentially new clinical applications. The following subsections will concentrate on the development of instrumentation and image reconstruction methods that have made substantial impact on SPECT.

13.2.2 SPECT Instrumentation

Review of the advances in SPECT instrumentation can be found in several recent articles [Jaszczak et al., 1980; Rogers and Ackermann, 1992; Jaszczak and Tsui, 1994]. A typical SPECT system consists of a single or multiple units of radiation detectors arranged in a specific geometric configuration and a mechanism for moving the radiation detector(s) or specially designed collimators to acquire data from different projection views. In general, SPECT instrumentation can be divided into three general categories (1) arrays of multiple scintillation detectors, (2) one or more scintillation cameras, and (3) hybrid scintillation detectors combining the first two approaches. In addition, special collimator designs have been proposed for SPECT for specific purposes and clinical applications. The following is a brief review of these SPECT systems and special collimators.

13.2.2.1 Multidetector SPECT System

The first fully functional SPECT imaging acquisition system was designed and constructed by Kuhl and Edwards [Kuhl and Edwards, 1963, 1964, 1968] in the 1960s, well before the conception of x-ray CT. As shown in Figure 13.7a, the MARK IV brain SPECT system consisted of four linear arrays of eight discrete NaI(TI) scintillation detectors assembled in a square arrangement. Projection data were obtained by rotating the square detector array around the patient's head. Although images from the pioneer MARK IV SPECT system were unimpressive without the use of proper reconstruction methods that were developed in later years, the multidetector design has been the theme of several other SPECT systems that were developed. An example is the Gammatom-1 developed by Cho et al. [1982]. The design concept also was used in a dynamic SPECT system [Stokely et al., 1980] and commercial multidetector SPECT systems marketed by Medimatic, A/S (Tomomatic-32). Recently, the system design was extended to a multislice SPECT system with the Tomomatic-896, consisting of eight layers of 96 scintillation detectors. Also, the system allows both body and brain SPECT imaging by varying the aperture size.

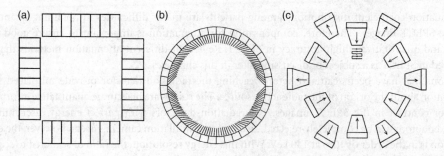

FIGURE 13.7 Examples of multidetector-based SPECT systems. (a) The MARK IV system consists of four arrays of eight individual NaI(TI) detectors arranged in a square configuration. (b) The Headtome-II system consists of a circular ring of detectors. A set of collimator vanes that swings in front of the discrete detector is used to collect projection data from different views. (c) A unique Cleon brain SPECT system consists of 12 detectors that scan both radially and tangentially.

Variations of the multiple-detectors arrangement have been proposed for SPECT system designs. Figure 13.7b shows the Headtome-II system by Shimadzu Corporation [Hirose et al., 1982], which consists of a stationary array of scintillation detectors arranged in a circular ring. Projection data are obtained by a set of collimator vanes that swings in front of the discrete detectors. A unique Cleon brain SPECT system (see Figure 13.7c), originally developed by Union Carbide Corporation in the 1970s, consists of 12 detectors that scan both radially and tangentially [Stoddart and Stoddart, 1979]. Images from the original system were unimpressive due to inadequate sampling, poor axial resolution, and a reconstruction algorithm that did not take full advantage of the unique system design and data acquisition strategy. A much improved version of the system with a new reconstruction method [Moore et al., 1984] is currently marketed by Strichman Corporation.

The advantages of multidetector SPECT systems are their high sensitivity per image slice and high counting rate capability resulting from the array of multidetectors fully surrounding the patient. However, disadvantages of multidetector SPECT systems include their ability to provide only one or a few noncontiguous cross-sectional image slices. Also, these systems are relatively more expensive compared with camera-based SPECT systems described in the next section. With the advance of multicamera SPECT systems, the disadvantages of multidetector SPECT systems outweigh their advantages. As a result, they are less often found in nuclear medicine clinics.

13.2.2.2 Camera-Based SPECT Systems

The most popular SPECT systems are based on single or multiple scintillation cameras mounted on a rotating gantry. The successful design was developed almost simultaneously by three separate groups [Budinger and Gullberg, 1977; Jaszczak et al., 1977; Keyes et al., 1977]. In 1981, General Electric Medical Systems offered the first commercial SPECT system based on a single rotating camera and brought SPECT to clinical use. Today, there are over ten manufacturers (e.g., ADAC, Elscint, General Electric, Hitachi, Picker, Siemens, Sopha, Toshiba, Trionix) offering an array of commercial SPECT systems in the marketplace.

An advantage of camera-based SPECT systems is their use of off-the-shelf scintillation cameras that have been widely used in conventional nuclear medicine. These systems usually can be used in both conventional planar and SPECT imaging. Also, camera-based SPECT systems allow truly three-dimensional (3D) imaging by providing a large set of contiguous transaxial images that cover the entire organ of interest. They are easily adaptable for SPECT imaging of the brain or body by simply changing the radius of rotation of the camera.

A disadvantage of a camera-based SPECT system is its relatively low counting rate capability. The dead time of a typical state-of-the-art scintillation camera gives rise to a loss of 20% of its true counts at about 80K counts per second. A few special high-count-rate systems give the same count rate loss at about 150K

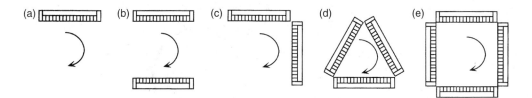

FIGURE 13.8   Examples of camera-based SPECT systems. (a) Single-camera system. (b) Dual-camera system with the two cameras placed at opposing sides of patient during rotation. (c) Dual-camera system with the two cameras placed at right angles. (d) Triple-camera system. (e) Quadruple-camera system.

counts per second. For SPECT systems using a single scintillation camera, the sensitivity per image slice is relative low compared with a typical multidetector SPECT system.

Recently, SPECT systems based on multiple cameras became increasingly more popular. Systems with two [Jaszczak et al., 1979a], three [Lim et al., 1980, 1985], and four cameras provide increased sensitivity per image slice that is proportional to the number of cameras. Figure 13.8 shows the system configurations of these camera-based SPECT systems. The dual-camera systems with two opposing cameras (Figure 13.8b) can be used for both whole-body scanning and SPECT, and those with two right-angled cameras (Figure 13.8c) are especially useful for 180-degree acquisition in cardiac SPECT. The use of multicameras has virtually eliminated the disadvantages of camera-based SPECT systems as compared with multidetector SPECT systems. The detection efficiency of camera-based SPECT systems can be further increased by using converging-hole collimators such as fan, cone, and astigmatic collimators at the cost of a smaller field of view. The use of converging-hole collimators in SPECT will be described in a later section.

13.2.2.3 Novel SPECT System Designs

There are several special SPECT systems designs that do not fit into the preceding two general categories. The commercially available CERESPECT (formerly known as ASPECT) [Genna and Smith, 1988] is a dedicated brain SPECT system. As shown in Figure 13.9a, it consists of a single fixed-annular NaI(TI) crystal that completely surrounds the patient's head. Similar to a scintillation camera, an array of PMTs and electronics circuitry are placed behind the crystal to provide positional and energy information about photons that interact with the crystal. Projection data are obtained by rotating a segmented annular collimator with parallel holes that fits inside the stationary detector. A similar system is also being developed by Larsson et al. [1991] in Sweden.

Several unique SPECT systems are currently being developed in research laboratories. They consist of modules of small scintillation cameras that surround the patient. The hybrid designs combine the advantage of multidetector and camera-based SPECT systems with added flexibility in system configuration. An example is the SPRINT II brain SPECT system developed at the University of Michigan [Rogers et al., 1988]. As shown in Figure 13.9b, the system consists of 11 detector modules arranged in a circular ring around the patient's head. Each detector module consists of 44 one-dimensional (1D) bar NaI(TI) scintillation cameras. Projection data are required through a series of narrow slit openings on a rotating lead ring that fits inside the circular detector assemblies. A similar system was developed at the University of Iowa [Chang et al., 1990] with 22 detector modules, each consisting of four bar detectors. A set of rotating focused collimators is used to acquire projection data necessary for image reconstruction. At the University of Arizona, a novel SPECT system is being developed that consists of 20 small modular scintillation cameras [Milster et al., 1990] arranged in a hemispherical shell surrounding the patient's head [Rowe et al., 1992]. Projection data are acquired through a stationary hemispherical array of pinholes that are fitted inside the camera array. Without moving parts, the system allows acquisition of dynamic 3D SPECT data.

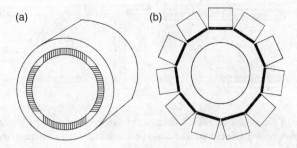

FIGURE 13.9   Examples of novel SPECT system designs. (a) The CERESPECT brain SPECT system consists of a single fixed annular NaI(TI) crystal and a rotating segmented annular collimator. (b) The SPRINT II brain SPECT system consists of 11 detector modules and a rotating lead ring with slit opening.

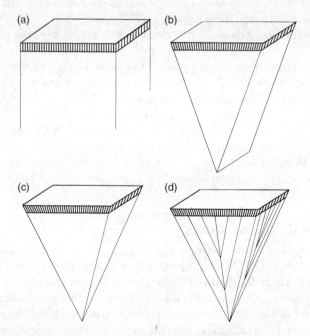

FIGURE 13.10   Collimator designs used in camera-based SPECT systems. (a) The commonly used parallel-hole collimator. (b) The fan-beam collimator, where the collimator holes are converged to a line that is parallel to the axis of rotation. (c) The cone-beam collimator, where the collimator holes are converged to a point. (d) A varifocal collimator, where the collimator holes are converged to various focal points.

13.2.2.4   Special Collimator Designs for SPECT Systems

Similar to conventional nuclear medicine imaging, parallel-hole collimators (Figure 13.10a) are commonly used in camera-based SPECT systems. As described earlier, the tradeoff between detection efficiency and spatial resolution of parallel-hole collimator is a limiting factor for SPECT. A means to improve SPECT system performance is to improve the tradeoff imposed by the parallel-hole collimation.

To achieve this goal, converging-hole collimator designs that increase the angle of acceptance of incoming photons without sacrificing spatial resolution have been developed. Examples are fan-beam [Jaszczak et al., 1979b; Tsui et al., 1986], cone-beam [Jaszczak et al., 1987], astigmatic [Hawman and Hsieh, 1986], and more recently varifocal collimators. As shown in Figure 13.10b, the collimator holes converge to a line that is oriented parallel to the axis of rotation for a fan-beam collimator, to a point for a cone-beam collimator, and to various points for a varifocal collimator, respectively. The gain in detection efficiency of a typical fan-beam and cone-beam collimator is about 1.5 and 2 times of that of a parallel-hole collimator with the same spatial resolution. The anticipated gain in detection efficiency and corresponding decrease in image noise are the main reasons for the interest in applying converging-hole collimators in SPECT.

Despite the advantage of increased detection efficiency, the use of converging-hole collimators in SPECT poses special problems. The tradeoff for increase in detection efficiency as compared with parallel-hole collimators is a decrease in field of view (see Figure 13.10). Consequently, converging-hole collimators are restricted to imaging small organs or body parts such as the head [Jaszczak et al., 1979b; Tsui et al., 1986] and heart [Gullberg et al., 1991]. In addition, the use of converging-hole collimators requires special data-acquisition strategies and image reconstruction algorithms. For example, for cone-beam tomography using a conventional single planar orbit, the acquired projection data become increasingly insufficient for reconstructing transaxial image sections that are further away from the central plane of the cone-beam geometry. Active research is underway to study special rotational orbits for sufficient projection data acquisition and 3D image reconstruction methods specific for cone-beam SPECT.

13.2.3   Reconstruction Methods

As discussed earlier, SPECT combines conventional nuclear medicine image techniques and methods for image reconstruction from projections. Aside from radiopharmaceuticals and instrumentation, image reconstruction methods are another important engineering and technological aspect of the SPECT imaging technique.

In x-ray CT, accurate transaxial images can be obtained through the use of standard algorithms for image reconstruction from projections. The results are images of attenuation coefficient distribution of various organs within the patient's body. In SPECT, the goal of image reconstruction is to determine the distribution of administered radiopharmaceutical in the patient. However, the presence of photon attenuation affects the measured projection data. If conventional reconstruction algorithms are used without proper compensation for the attenuation effects, inaccurate reconstructed images will be obtained. Effects of scatter and the finite collimator–detector response impose additional difficulties on image reconstruction in SPECT.

In order to achieve quantitatively accurate images, special reconstruction methods are required for SPECT. Quantitatively accurate image reconstruction methods for SPECT consist of two major components. They are the standard algorithms for image reconstruction from projections and methods that compensate for the image-degrading effects described earlier. Often, image reconstruction algorithms are inseparable from the compensation methods, resulting in a new breed of reconstruction method not found in other tomographic medical imaging modalities. The following ssssssections will present the reconstruction problem and a brief review of conventional algorithms for image reconstruction from projections. Then quantitative SPECT reconstruction methods that include additional compensation methods will be described.

13.2.3.1   Image Reconstruction Problem

Figure 13.11 shows a schematic diagram of the two-dimensional (2D) image reconstruction problem. Let $f(x, y)$ represent a 2D object distribution that is to be determined. A 1D detector array is oriented at an angle q with respect to the x-axis of the laboratory coordinates system (x, y). The data collected into each detector element at location t, called the projection data $p(t, q)$, is equal to the sum of $f(x, y)$ along a ray that is perpendicular to the detector array and intersects the detector at position t; that is,

$$p(t, \theta) = c \int_{-\alpha}^{\alpha} f(x, y) \, ds \qquad (13.1)$$

where (s, t) represents a coordinate system with s along the direction of the ray sum and t parallel to the 1D detector array, and c is the gain factor of the detection system. The angle between the s and x-axes is θ. The relationship between the source position (x, y), the projection angle θ, and the position of detection

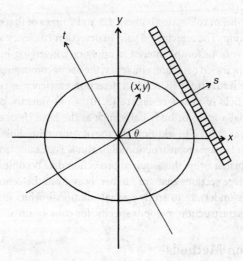

FIGURE 13.11 Schematic diagram of the two-dimensional image reconstruction problem. The projection data are line integrals of the object distribution along rays that are perpendicular to the detector. A source point (x, y) is projected onto a point $p(t, \theta)$, where t is a position along the projection and θ is the projection angle.

on the 1D detector array is given by

$$t = y \cos \theta - x \sin \theta \tag{13.2}$$

In 2D tomographic imaging, the 1D detector array rotates around the object distribution $f(x, y)$ and collects projection data from various projection data from various projection angles θ. The integral transform of the object distribution to its projections given by Equation 13.1 is called the Radon transform [Radon, 1917]. The goal of image reconstruction is to solve the inverse Radon transform. The solution is the reconstructed image estimate $\hat{f}(x, y)$ of the object distribution $f(x, y)$.

In x-ray CT, the measured projection data is given by

$$p'(t, \theta) = c_t I_0 \exp\left[-\int_{-\alpha}^{+\alpha} \mu(x, y) \, ds\right] \tag{13.3}$$

where I_0 is the intensity of the incident x-ray, $\mu(x, y)$ is the 2D attenuation coefficient, and c_t is the gain factor which transforms x-ray intensity to detected signals. The reconstruction problem can be rewritten as

$$p(t, \theta) = \ln\left[\frac{I_0}{p'(t, \theta)}\right] = \int_{-\alpha}^{+\alpha} \mu(x, y) \, ds \tag{13.4}$$

with the goal to solve for the attenuation coefficient distribution $\mu(x, y)$. Also, in x-ray CT, if parallel rays are used, the projection data at opposing views are the same, that is, $p(t, \theta) = p(\theta + p)$, and projection data acquired over 180 degrees will be sufficient for reconstruction. The number of linear samples along the 1D projection array and angular samples, that is, the number of projection views, over 180 degrees must be chosen carefully to avoid aliasing error and resolution loss in the reconstructed images.

In SPECT, if the effects of attenuation, scatter, and collimator–detector response are ignored, the measured projection data can be written as the integral of radioactivity along the projection rays; that is,

$$p(t, \theta) = c_e \int_{-\alpha}^{+\alpha} \rho(x, y) \, ds \tag{13.5}$$

where $\rho(x, y)$ is the radioactivity concentration distribution of the object, and c_e is the gain factor which transforms radioactivity concentration to detected signals. Equation 13.5 fits in the form of the Radon transform, and similar to x-ray CT, the radioactivity distribution can be obtained by solving the inverse Radon transform problem.

If attenuation is taken into consideration, the attenuated Radon transform [Gullberg, 1979] can be written as

$$p(t, \theta_i) = c_e \int_{-\alpha}^{+\alpha} \rho(x, y) \exp\left[-\int_{(x,y)}^{+\alpha} \mu(u, v)\, ds' \right] ds \tag{13.6}$$

where $\mu(u, v)$ is the 2D attenuation coefficient distribution, and $\int_{x,y}^{+\alpha} \mu(u, v)\, ds$ is the attenuation factor for photons that originate from (x, y), travel along the direction perpendicular to the detector array, and are detected by the collimator–detector. A major difficulty in SPECT image reconstruction lies in the attenuation factor, which makes the inverse problem given by Equation 13.6 difficult to solve analytically. However, the solution is important in cardiac SPECT, where the widely different attenuation coefficients are found in various organs within the thorax. Also, due to the attenuation factor, the projection views at opposing angles are different. Hence full 360-degree projection data are usually necessary for image reconstruction in SPECT.

Different from x-ray CT, small differences in attenuation coefficient are not as important in SPECT. When the attenuation coefficient in the body region can be considered constant, the attenuated Radon transform given by Equation 13.6 can be written as [Tretiak and Metz, 1980]

$$p(t, \theta) = c_e \int_{-\alpha}^{+\alpha} \rho(x, y) \exp[-\mu l(x, y)]\, ds \tag{13.7}$$

where μ is the constant attenuation coefficient in the body region, and $l(x, y)$ is the path length between the point (x, y) and the edge of the attenuator (or patient's body) along the direction of the projection ray. The solution of the inverse problem with constant attenuator has been a subject of several investigations. It forms the basis for analytical methods for compensation of uniform attenuation described later in this chapter.

When scatter and collimator–detector response are taken into consideration, the assumption that the projection data can be represented by line integrals given by Equation 13.1 to Equation 13.7 will no longer be exactly correct. Instead, the integration will have to include a wider region covering the field of view of the collimator–detector (or the collimator–detector response function). The image reconstruction problem is further complicated by the nonstationary properties of the collimator–detector and scatter response functions and their dependence on the size and composition of the patient's body.

13.2.3.2 Algorithms for Image Reconstruction from Projections

The application of methods for image reconstruction from projections was a major component in the development of x-ray CT in the 1970s. The goal was to solve for the inverse Radon transform problem given in Equation 13.1. There is an extensive literature on these reconstruction algorithms. Reviews of the applications of these algorithms to SPECT can be found in several articles [Budinger and Gullberg, 1974; Brooks and Di Chiro, 1975, 1976; Barrett, 1986].

Simple backprojection: An intuitive image reconstruction method is simple backprojection. Here, the reconstructed image is formed simply by spreading the values of the measured projection data uniformly along the projection ray into the reconstructed image array. By backprojecting the measured projection data from all projection views, an estimate of the object distribution can be obtained. Mathematically, the simple backproject operation is given by

$$\hat{f}(x,y) = \sum_{j=1}^{m} p(y\cos\theta_j - x\sin\theta_j, \theta_j)\Delta\theta \tag{13.8}$$

where θ_j is the jth projection angle, m is the number of projection views, and $\Delta\theta$ is the angular spacing between adjacent projections. The simple backprojected image $\hat{f}(x,y)$ is a poor approximation of the true object distribution $f(x,y)$. It is equivalent to the true object distribution blurred by a blurring function in the form of $1/r$.

There are two approaches for accurate image reconstruction, and both have been applied to SPECT. The first approach is based on direct analytical methods and is widely used in commercial SPECT systems. The second approach is based on statistical criteria and iterative algorithms. They have been found useful in reconstruction methods that include compensation for the image-degrading effects.

Analytical reconstruction algorithms: filtered backprojection: The most widely used analytical image-reconstruction algorithm is the filtered backprojection (FBP) method, which involves backprojecting the filtered projections [Bracewell and Riddle, 1967; Ramachandran and Lakshminarayanan, 1971]. The algorithm consists of two major steps:

1. Filter the measured projection data at different projection angles with a special function
2. Backproject the filtered projection data to form the reconstructed image

The first step of the filtered backprojection method can be implemented in two different ways. In the spatial domain, the filter operation is equivalent to convolving the measured projection data using a special convolving function $h(t)$; that is,

$$p'(t,\theta) = p(t,\theta) * h(t) \tag{13.8a}$$

where $*$ is the convolution operation. With the advance of FFT methods, the convolution operation can be replaced by a more efficient multiplication in the spatial frequency domain. The equivalent operation consists of three steps:

1. Fourier-transform the measured projection data into spatial frequency domain using the FFT method, that is, $P(v,\theta) = \text{FT}\{p(t,\theta)\}$, where FT is the Fourier transform operation.
2. Multiply the Fourier-transformed projection data with a special function that is equal to the Fourier transform of the special function used in the convolution operation described above, that is, $P'(v,\theta) = P(v,\theta) \cdot H(v)$, where $H(v) = \text{FT}\{h(x)\}$ is the Fourier transform of $h(x)$.
3. Inverse Fourier transform the product $P'(v,\theta)$ into spatial domain.

Again, the filtered projections from different projection angles are backprojected to form the reconstructed images.

The solution of the inverse Radon transform given in Equation 13.1 specifies the form of the special function. In the spatial domain, the special function h(x) used in the convolution operation in Equation 13.8 is given by

$$h(x) = \frac{1}{2(\Delta x)^2}\left\{\text{sinc}\left[\frac{x}{(\Delta x)}\right]\right\} - \frac{1}{4(\Delta x)^2}\left\{\text{sinc}^2\left[\frac{x}{2(\Delta x)}\right]\right\} \tag{13.9}$$

where Δx is the linear sampling interval, and $\text{sinc}(z) = [\sin(z)]/z$. The function $h(x)$ consists of a narrow central peak with high magnitude and small negative side lobes. It removes the blurring from the $1/r$ function found in the simple backprojected images.

In the frequency domain, the special function $H(v)$ is equivalent to the Fourier transform of $h(x)$ and is a truncated ramp function given by

$$H(v) = |v| \cdot \text{rect}(v) \qquad (13.10)$$

where $|v|$ is the ramp function, and

$$\text{rect}(v) = \begin{cases} 1, & |v| \le 0.5 \\ 0, & v < 0.5 \end{cases} \qquad (13.11)$$

that is, the rectangular function $\text{rect}(v)$ has a value of 1 when the absolute value of v is less than the Nyquist frequency at 0.5 cycles per pixel.

For noisy projection data, the ramp function tends to amplify the high-frequency noise. In these situations, an additional smoothing filter is often applied to smoothly roll off the high-frequency response of the ramp function. Examples are Hann and Butterworth filters [Huesman et al., 1977]. Also, deconvolution filters have been used to provide partial compensation of spatial resolution loss due to the collimator-detection response and noise smoothing. Examples are the Metz and Wiener filters (see later).

Iterative reconstruction algorithms: Another approach to image reconstruction is based on statistical criteria and iterative algorithms. They were investigated for application in SPECT before the development of analytical image reconstruction methods [Kuhl and Edwards, 1968; Gordon et al., 1970; Gilbert, 1972; Goitein, 1972]. The major drawbacks of iterative reconstruction algorithms are the extensive computations and long processing time required. For these reasons, the analytical reconstruction methods have gained widespread acceptance in clinical SPECT systems. In recent years, there has been renewed interest in the use of iterative reconstruction algorithms in SPECT to achieve accurate quantitation by compensating for the image-degrading effects.

A typical iterative reconstruction algorithm starts with an initial estimate of the object source distribution. A set of projection data is estimated from the initial estimate using a projector that models the imaging process. The estimated projection data are compared with the measured projection data at the same projection angles, and their differences are calculated. Using an algorithm derived from specific statistical criteria, the differences are used to update the initial image estimate. The updated image estimate is then used to recalculate a new set of estimated projection data that are again compared with the measured projection data. The procedure is repeated until the difference between the estimated and measured projection data are smaller than a preselected small value. Statistical criteria that have been used in formulating iterative reconstruction algorithms include the minimum mean squares error (MMSE) [Budinger and Gullberg, 1977], weighted least squares (WLS) [Huesman et al., 1977], maximum entropy (ME) [Minerbo, 1979], maximum likelihood (ML) [Shepp and Vardi, 1982], and maximum a posteriori approaches [Geman and McClure, 1985; Barrett, 1986; Levitan and Herman, 1987; Liang and Hart, 1987; Johnson et al., 1991]. Iterative algorithms that have been used in estimating the reconstructed images include the conjugate gradient (CG) [Huesman et al., 1977] and expectation maximization (EM) [Lange and Carson, 1984].

Recently, interest in the application of iterative reconstruction algorithms in SPECT has been revitalized. The interest is sparked by the need to compensate for the spatially variant and/or nonstationary image-degrading factors in the SPECT imaging process. The compensation can be achieved by modeling the imaging process that includes the image-degrading factors in the projection and backprojection operations of the iterative steps. The development is aided by advances made in computer technology and custom-dedicated processors. The drawback of long processing time in using these algorithms is substantially reduced. Discussion of the application of iterative reconstruction algorithms in SPECT will be presented in a later section.

13.2.3.3 Compensation Methods

For a typical SPECT system, the measured projection data are severely affected by attenuation, scatter, and collimator–detector response. Direct reconstruction of the measured projection data without compensation of these effects produces images with artifacts, distortions, and inaccurate quantitation. In recent years, substantial efforts have been made to develop compensation methods for these image-degrading effects. This development has produced much improved quality and quantitatively accurate reconstructed images. The following sections will present a brief review of some of these compensation methods.

Compensation for attenuation: Methods for attenuation compensation can be grouped into two categories (1) methods that assume the attenuation coefficient is uniform over the body region, and (2) methods that address situations of nonuniform attenuation coefficient distribution. The assumption of uniform attenuation can be applied to SPECT imaging of the head and abdomen regions. The compensation methods seek to solve for the inverse of the attenuated Radon transform given in Equation 13.7. For cardiac and lung SPECT imaging, nonuniform attenuation compensation methods must be used due to the very different attenuation coefficient values in various organs in the thorax. Here, the goal is to solve the more complicated problem of the inverse of the attenuated Radon transform in Equation 13.6.

There are several approximate methods for compensating uniform attenuation. They include methods that preprocess the projection data or postprocess the reconstructed image. The typical preprocess methods are those which use the geometric or arithmetic mean [Sorenson, 1974] of projections from opposing views. These compensation methods are easy to implement and work well with a single, isolated source. However, they are relatively inaccurate for more complicated source configurations. Another method achieves uniform attenuation compensation by processing the Fourier transform of the sinogram [Bellini et al., 1979]. The method provides accurate compensation even for complicated source configurations.

A popular compensation method for uniform attenuation is that proposed by Chang [1978]. The method requires knowledge of the body contour. The information is used in calculating the average attenuation factor at each image point from all projection views. The array of attenuation factors is used to multiply the reconstructed image obtained without attenuation compensation. The result is the attenuation-compensated image. An iterative scheme also can be implemented for improved accuracy. In general, the Chang method performs well for uniform attenuation situations. However, the noise level in the reconstructed images increases with iteration number. Also, certain image features tend to fluctuate as a function of iteration. For these reasons, no more than one or two iterations are recommended.

Another class of methods for uniform attenuation compensation is based on analytical solution of the inverse of the attenuation Radon transform given in Equation 13.7 for a convex-shaped medium [Tretiak and Metz, 1980; Gullberg and Budinger, 1981]. The resultant compensation method involves multiplying the projection data by an exponential function. Then the FBP algorithm is used in the image reconstruction except that the ramp filter is modified such that its value is zero in the frequency range between 0 and $\mu/2\pi$, where μ is the constant attenuation coefficient. The compensation method is easy to implement and provides good quantitative accuracy. However, it tends to amplify noise in the resulting image, and smoothing is required to obtain acceptable image quality [Gullberg and Budinger, 1981].

An analytical solution for the more complicated inverse attenuated Radon transform with nonuniform attenuation distribution (Equation 13.6) has been found difficult [Gullberg, 1979]. Instead, iterative approaches have been used to estimate a solution of the problem. The application is especially important in cardiac and lung SPECT studies. The iterative methods model the attenuation distribution in the projection and backprojection operations [Manglos et al., 1987; Tsui et al., 1989]. The ML criterion with the EM algorithm [Lange and Carson, 1984] has been used with success [Tsui et al., 1989]. The compensation method requires information about the attenuation distribution of the region to be imaged. Recently, transmission CT methods are being developed using existing SPECT systems to obtain attenuation distribution from the patient. The accurate attenuation compensation of cardiac SPECT promises to provide much improved quality and quantitative accuracy in cardiac SPECT images [Tsui et al., 1989, 1994a].

Compensation for scatter: As described earlier in this chapter, scattered photons carry misplaced positional information about the source distribution resulting in lower image contrast and inaccurate quantitation in SPECT images. Compensation for scatter will improve image contrast for better image quality and images that will more accurately represent the true object distribution. Much research has been devoted to develop scatter compensation methods that can be grouped into two general approaches. In the first approach, various methods have been developed to estimate the scatter contribution in the measured data. The scatter component is then subtracted from the measured data or from the reconstructed images to obtain scatter-free reconstructed images. The compensation method based on this approach tends to increase noise level in the compensated images.

One method estimates the scatter contribution as a convolution of the measured projection data with an empirically derived function [Axelsson et al., 1984]. Another method models the scatter component as the convolution of the primary (or unscattered) component of the projection data with an exponential function [Floyd et al., 1985]. The convolution method is extended to 3D by estimating the 2D scatter component [Yanch et al., 1988]. These convolution methods assume that the scatter response function is stationary, which is only an approximation.

The scatter component also has been estimated using two energy windows acquisition methods. One method estimates the scatter component in the primary energy window from the measured data obtained from a lower and adjacent energy window [Jaszczak et al., 1984, 1985b]. In a dual photopeak window (DPW) method, two nonoverlapping windows spanning the primary photopeak window are used [King et al., 1992]. This method provides more accurate estimation of the scatter response function.

Multiple energy windows also have been used to estimate the scatter component. One method uses two satellite energy windows that are placed directly above and below the photopeak window to estimate the scatter component in the center window [Ogawa et al., 1991]. In another method, the energy spectrum detected at each image pixel is used to predict the scatter contribution [Koral et al., 1988]. An energy-weighted acquisition (EWA) technique acquires data from multiple energy windows. The images reconstructed from these data are weighted with energy-dependent factors to minimize scatter contribution to the weighted image [DeVito et al., 1989; DeVito and Hamill, 1991]. Finally, the holospectral imaging method [Gagnon et al., 1989] estimates the scatter contribution from a series of eigenimages derived from images reconstructed from data obtained from a series of multiple energy windows.

In the second approach, the scatter photons are utilized in estimating the true object distribution. Without subtracting the scatter component, the compensated images are less noisy than those obtained from the first approach. In one method, an average scatter response function can be combined with the geometric response of the collimator–detector to form the total response of the imaging system [Gilland et al., 1988; Tsui et al., 1994a]. The total response function is then used to generate a restoration filter for an approximate geometric and scatter response compensation (see later).

Another class of methods, characterizes the exact scatter response function and incorporates it into iterative reconstruction algorithms for accurate compensation for scatter [Floyd et al., 1985; Frey and Tsui, 1992]. Since the exact scatter response functions are nonstationary and are asymmetric in shape, implementation of the methods requires extensive computations. However, efforts are being made to parameterize the scatter response function and to optimize the algorithm for substantial reduction in processing time [Frey and Tsui, 1991; Frey et al., 1993].

Compensation for collimator–detector response: As described earlier, for a typical collimator–detector, the response function broadens as the distance from the collimator face increases. The effect of the collimator–detector response is loss of spatial resolution and blurring of fine detail in SPECT images. Also, the spatially variant detector response function will cause nonisotropic point response in SPECT images [Knesaurek et al., 1989; Maniawski et al., 1991]. The spatially variant collimator–detector response is a major difficulty in its exact compensation.

By assuming an average and stationary collimator–detector response function, restoration filters can be used to provide partial and approximate compensation for the effects of the collimator–detector. Examples are the Metz [King et al., 1984, 1986] and Wiener [Penney et al., 1990] filters, where the inverse of the average collimator–detector response function is used in the design of the restoration filters. Two-dimensional compensation is achieved by applying the 1D restoration filters to the 1D projection data, and 3D compensation by applying the 2D filters to the 2D projection images [Tsui et al., 1994b].

Analytical methods have been developed for compensation of the spatially variant detector response. A spatially variant filtering method has been proposed which is based on the frequency distance principle (FDP) [Edholm et al., 1986; Lewitt et al., 1989]. The method has been shown to provide an isotropic point response function in phantom SPECT images [Glick et al., 1993].

Iterative reconstruction methods also have been used to accurately compensate for both nonuniform attenuation and collimator–detector response by modeling the attenuation distribution and spatially variant detector response function in the projection and backprojection steps. The compensation methods have been applied in 2D reconstruction [Tsui et al., 1988; Formiconi et al., 1990], and more recently in 3D reconstruction [Zeng et al., 1991; Tsui et al., 1994b]. It has been found that the iterative reconstruction methods provide better image quality and more accurate quantitation when compared with the conventional restoration filtering techniques. Furthermore, 3D compensation outperforms 2D compensation at the expense of more extensive computations [Tsui et al., 1994b].

13.2.4 Sample SPECT Images

This section presents sample SPECT images to demonstrate the performance of various reconstruction and compensation methods. Two data sets were used. The first set was acquired from a 3D physical phantom that mimics a human brain perfusion study. The phantom study provided knowledge of the true radioactivity distribution for evaluation purposes. The second data set was obtained from a patient myocardial SPECT study using thallium-201.

Figure 13.12a shows the radioactivity distribution from a selected slice of a 3D brain phantom manufactured by the Data Spectrum Corporation. The phantom design was based on PET images from a normal patient to simulate cerebral blood flow [Hoffman et al., 1990]. The phantom was filled with water containing 74 mBq of Tc-99m. A single-camera-based GE 400AC/T SPECT system fitted with a high-resolution collimator was used for data collection. The projection data were acquired into 128×128 matrices at 128 views over 360 degrees. Figure 13.12b shows the reconstructed image obtained from the FBP algorithm without any compensation. The poor image quality is due to statistical noise fluctuations, effects of attenuation (especially at the central portion of the image), loss of spatial resolution due to the collimator–detector response, and loss of contrast due to scatter.

Figure 13.12c shows the reconstructed image obtained with the application of a noise-smoothing filter and compensation for the uniform attenuation and scatter. The resulting image has lower noise level, reduced attenuation effect, and higher contrast as compared with the image shown in Figure 13.12b. Figure 13.12d is similar to Figure 13.12c except for an additional application of a Metz filter to partially compensate for the collimator–detector blurring. Figure 13.12e shows the reconstructed image obtained from the iterative ML-EM algorithm that accurately modeled the attenuation and spatially variant detector response. The much superior image quality is apparent.

Figure 13.13a shows a selected FBP reconstructed transaxial image slice from a typical patient myocardial SPECT study using thallium-201. Figure 13.13b shows the reconstructed image obtained from the Chang algorithm for approximate nonuniform attenuation compensation and 2D processing using a Metz filter for approximate compensation for collimator–detector response. Figure 13.13c shows the reconstructed image obtained from the iterative ML-EM algorithm using a measured transmission CT image for accurate attenuation compensation and a 2D model of the collimator–detector response for accurate collimator–detector response compensation. The reconstructed image in Figure 13.13d is similar to that in Figure 13.13b except that the Metz filter was implemented in 3D. Finally, the reconstructed image in Figure 13.13e is similar to that in Figure 13.13c except that a 3D model of the collimator–detector response is used. The superior image quality obtained from using an accurate 3D model of the imaging process is evident.

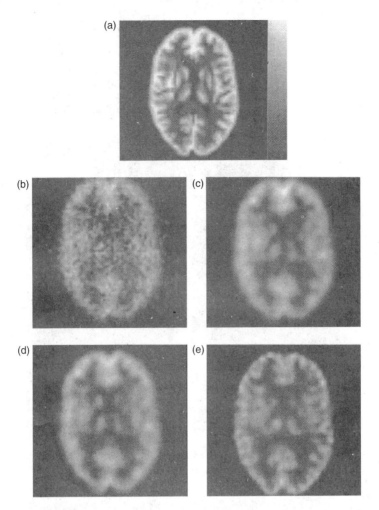

FIGURE 13.12   Sample images from a phantom SPECT study. (a) Radioactivity distribution from a selected slice of a 3D brain phantom. (b) Reconstructed image obtained from the FBP algorithm without any compensation. (c) Reconstructed image obtained with the application of noise-smoothing filter and compensation for uniform attenuation and scatter. (d) Similar to (c) except for an additional application of a Metz filter to partially compensate for the collimator–detector blurring. (e) Reconstructed image similar to that obtained from the iterative ML-EM algorithm that accurately models the attenuation and spatially variant detector response. (From Tsui BMW, Frey EC, Zhao X-D, et al. 1994. *Phys. Med. Biol.* 39: 509. Reprinted with permission.)

13.2.5   Discussion

The development of SPECT has been a combination of advances in radiopharmaceuticals, instrumentation, image processing and reconstruction methods, and clinical applications. Although substantial progress has been made during the last decade, there are many opportunities for contributions from biomedical engineering in the future.

The future SPECT instrumentation will consist of more detector area to fully surround the patient for high detection efficiency and multiple contiguous transaxial slice capability. Multicamera SPECT systems will continue to dominate the commercial market. The use of new radiation detector materials and detector systems with high spatial resolution will receive increased attention. Continued research is needed to investigate special converging-hole collimator design geometries, fully 3D reconstruction algorithms, and their clinical applications.

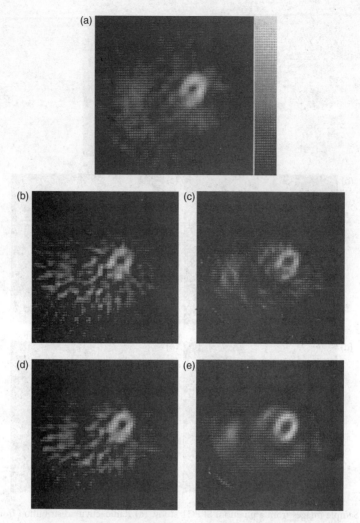

FIGURE 13.13 Sample images from a patient myocardial SPECT study using TI-201. (a) A selected transaxial image slice from a typical patient myocardial SPECT study using TI-201. The reconstructed image was obtained with the FBP algorithm without any compensation. (b) Reconstructed image obtained from the Chang algorithm for approximate nonuniform attenuation compensation and 2D processing using a Metz filter for approximate compensation for collimator–detector response. (c) Reconstructed image obtained from the iterative ML-EM algorithm using a measured transmission CT image for accurate attenuation compensation and 2D model of the collimator–detector response for accurate collimator–detector response compensation. (d) Similar to (b) except that the Metz filter was implemented in 3D. (e) Similar to (c) except that a 3D model of the collimator–detector response is used.

To improve image quality and to achieve quantitatively accurate SPECT images will continue to be the goals of image processing and image reconstruction methods for SPECT. An important direction of research in analytical reconstruction methods will involve solving the inverse Radon transform, which includes the effects of attenuation, the spatially variant collimator–detector response function, and scatter. The development of iterative reconstruction methods will require more accurate models of the complex SPECT imaging process, faster and more stable iterative algorithms, and more powerful computers and special computational hardware.

These improvements in SPECT instrumentation and image reconstruction methods, combined with newly developed radiopharmaceuticals, will bring SPECT images with increasingly higher quality and more accurate quantitation to nuclear medicine clinics for improved diagnosis and patient care.

References

Anger H.O. (1958). Scintillation camera. *Rev. Sci. Instrum.* 29: 27.

Anger H.O. (1964). Scintillation camera with multichannel collimators. *J. Nucl. Med.* 5: 515.

Axelsson B., Msaki P., and Israelsson A. (1984). Subtraction of Compton-scattered photons in single-photon emission computed tomography. *J. Nucl. Med.* 25: 490.

Barrett H.H. (1986). Perspectives on SPECT. *Proc. SPIE* 671: 178.

Bellini S., Piacentini M., Cafforio C. et al. (1979). Compensation of tissue absorption in emission tomography. *IEEE Trans. Acoust. Speech Signal Process.* ASSP 27: 213.

Bracewell R.N. and Riddle A.C. (1967). Inversion of fan-beam scans in radio astronomy. *Astrophys. J.* 150: 427.

Brooks R.A. and Di Chiro G. (1975). Theory of image reconstruction in computed tomography. *Radiology* 117: 561.

Brooks R.A. and Di Chiro G. (1976). Principles of computer assisted tomography (CAT) in radiographic and radioisotopic imaging. *Phys. Med. Biol.* 21: 689.

Budinger T.F. and Gullberg G.T. (1974). Three-dimensional reconstruction in nuclear medicine emission imaging. *IEEE Trans. Nucl. Sci. NS* 21: 2.

Budinger T.F. and Gullberg G.T. (1977). Transverse section reconstruction of gamma-ray emitting radionuclides in patients. In M.M. Ter-Pogossian, M.E. Phelps, G.L. Brownell et al. (Eds), *Reconstruction Tomography in Diagnostic Radiology and Nuclear Medicine*. Baltimore, University Park Press.

Chang L.T. (1978). A method for attenuation correction in radionuclide computed tomography. *IEEE Trans. Nucl. Sci. NS* 25: 638.

Chang W., Huang G., and Wang L. (1990). A multi-detector cylindrical SPECT system for phantom imaging. In *Conference Record of the 1990 Nuclear Science Symposium*, Vol. 2, pp. 1208–1211. Piscataway, NJ, IEEE.

Cho Z.H., Yi W., Jung K.J. et al. (1982). Performance of single photon tomography system-Gamma-tom-1. *IEEE Trans. Nucl. Sci. NS* 29: 484.

DeVito R.P. and Hamill J.J. (1991). Determination of weighting functions for energy-weighted acquisition. *J. Nucl. Med.* 32: 343.

DeVito R.P., Hamill J.J., Treffert J.D., and Stoub E.W. (1989). Energy-weighted acquisition of scintigraphic images using finite spatial filters. *J. Nucl. Med.* 30: 2029.

Edholm P.R., Lewitt R.M., and Lindholm B. (1986). Novel properties of the Fourier decomposition of the sinogram. *Proc. SPIE* 671: 8.

Evans R.D. (1955). *The Atomic Nucleus*. Malabar, FL, Robert E. Krieger.

Floyd C.E., Jaszczak R.J., Greer K.L., and Coleman R.E. (1985). Deconvolution of Compton scatter in SPECT. *J. Nucl. Med.* 26: 403.

Formiconi A.R., Pupi A., and Passeri A. (1990). Compensation of spatial system response in SPECT with conjugate gradient reconstruction technique. *Phys. Med. Biol.* 34: 69.

Frey E.C., Ju Z.-W., and Tsui B.M.W. (1993). A fast projector-backprojector pair modeling the asymmetric, spatially varying scatter response function for scatter compensation in SPECT imaging. *IEEE Trans. Nucl. Sci. NS* 40: 1192.

Frey E.C. and Tsui B.M.W. (1991). Spatial properties of the scatter response function in SPECT. *IEEE Trans. Nucl. Sci. NS* 38: 789.

Frey E.C. and Tsui B.M.W. (1992). A comparison of scatter compensation methods in SPECT: subtraction-based techniques versus iterative reconstruction with an accurate scatter model. In *Conference Record of the 1992 Nuclear Science Symposium and the Medical Imaging Conference*, October 27–31, Orlando, FL, pp. 1035–1037.

Gagnon D., Todd-Pokropek A., Arsenault A., and Dupros G. (1989). Introduction to holospectral imaging in nuclear medicine for scatter subtraction. *IEEE Trans. Med. Imag.* 8: 245.

Geman S. and McClure D.E. (1985). Bayesian image analysis: an application to single photon emission tomography. In *Proceedings of the Statistical Computing Section*. Washington, American Statistical Association.

Genna S. and Smith A. (1988). The development of ASPECT, an annular single crystal brain camera for high efficiency SPECT. *IEEE Trans. Nucl. Sci.* NS 35: 654.

Gilland D.R., Tsui B.M.W., Perry J.R. et al. (1988). Optimum filter function for SPECT imaging. *J. Nucl. Med.* 29: 643.

Gilbert P. (1972). Iterative methods for the three-dimensional reconstruction of an object from projections. *J. Theor. Biol.* 36: 105.

Glick S.J., Penney B.C., King M.A., and Byrne C.L. (1993). Non-iterative compensation for the distance-dependent detector response and photon attenuation in SPECT imaging. *IEEE Trans. Med. Imag.* 13: 363.

Goitein M. (1972). Three-dimensional density reconstruction from a series of two-dimensional projections. *Nucl. Instrum. Meth.* 101: 509.

Gordon R. (1974). A tutorial on ART (Algebraic reconstruction techniques). *IEEE Trans. Nucl. Sci.* 21: 78.

Gordon R., Bender R., and Herman G.T. (1970). Algebraic reconstruction techniques (ART) for three-dimensional electron microscopy and x-ray photography. *J. Theor. Biol.* 29: 471.

Gullberg G.T. (1979). The attenuated Radon transform: theory and application in medicine and biology. Ph.D. dissertation, University of California at Berkeley.

Gullberg G.T. and Budinger T.F. (1981). The use of filtering methods to compensate for constant attenuation in single-photon emission computed tomography. *IEEE Trans. Biomed. Eng.* BME 28: 142.

Gullberg G.T., Christian P.E., Zeng G.L. et al. (1991). Cone beam tomography of the heart using single-photon emission-computed tomography. *Invest. Radiol.* 26: 681.

Hawman E.G. and Hsieh J. (1986). An astigmatic collimator for high sensitivity SPECT of the brain. *J. Nucl. Med.* 27: 930.

Hirose Y., Ikeda Y., Higashi Y. et al. (1982). A hybrid emission CT-HEADTOME II. *IEEE Trans. Nucl. Sci.* NS 29: 520.

Hoffman E.J., Cutler P.D., Kigby W.M., and Mazziotta J.C. (1990). 3-D phantom to simulate cerebral blood flow and metabolic images for PET. *IEEE Trans. Nucl. Sci.* NS 37: 616.

Huesman R.H., Gullberg G.T., Greenberg W.L., and Budinger T.F. (1977). *RECLBL Library Users Manual, Donner Algorithms for Reconstruction Tomography*. Lawrence Berkeley Laboratory, University of California.

Jaszczak R.J., Chang L.T., and Murphy P.H. (1979). Single photon emission computed tomography using multi-slice fan beam collimators. *IEEE Trans. Nucl. Sci.* NS 26: 610.

Jaszczak R.J., Chang L.T., Stein N.A., and Moore F.E. (1979). Whole-body single-photon emission computed tomography using dual, large-field-of-view scintillation cameras. *Phys. Med. Biol.* 24: 1123.

Jaszczak R.J. and Coleman R.E. (1985). Single photon emission computed tomography (SPECT) principles and instrumentation. *Invest. Radiol.* 20: 897.

Jaszczak R.J., Coleman R.E., and Lim C.B. (1980). SPECT: single photon emission computed tomography. *IEEE Trans. Nucl. Sci.* NS 27: 1137.

Jaszczak R.J., Coleman R.E., and Whitehead F.R. (1981). Physical factors affecting quantitative measurements using camera-based single photon emission computed tomography (SPECT). *IEEE Trans. Nucl. Sci.* NS 28: 69.

Jaszczak R.J., Floyd C.E., and Coleman R.E. (1985). Scatter compensation techniques for SPECT. *IEEE Trans. Nucl. Sci.* NS 32: 786.

Jaszczak R.J., Floyd C.E., Manglos S.M. et al. (1987). Cone beam collimation for single photon emission computed tomography: Analysis, simulation, and image reconstruction using filtered backprojection. *Med. Phys.* 13: 484.

Jaszczak R.J., Greer K.L., Floyd C.E. et al. (1984). Improved SPECT quantification using compensation for scattered photons. *J. Nucl. Med.* 25: 893.

Jaszczak R.J., Murphy P.H., Huard D., and Burdine J.A. (1977). Radionuclide emission computed tomography of the head with 99 mTc and a scintillation camera. *J. Nucl. Med.* 18: 373.

Jaszczak R.J. and Tsui B.M.W. (1994). Single photon emission computed tomography. In H.N. Wagner and Z. Szabo (Eds), Principles of Nuclear Medicine, 2nd ed. Philadelphia, Saunders.

Johnson V.E., Wong W.H., Hu X., and Chen C.T. (1991). Image restoration using Gibbs priors: boundary modeling, treatment of blurring and selection of hyperparameters. *IEEE Trans. Pat.* 13: 413.

Keller E.L. (1968). Optimum dimensions of parallel-hole, multiaperture collimators for gamma-ray camera. *J. Nucl. Med.* 9: 233.

Keyes J.W., Jr, Orlandea N., Heetderks W.J. et al. (1977). The humogotron — a scintillation-camera transaxial tomography. *J. Nucl. Med.* 18: 381.

King M.A., Hademenos G., and Glick S.J. (1992). A dual photopeak window method for scatter correction. *J. Nucl. Med.* 33: 605.

King M.A., Schwinger R.B., Doherty P.W., and Penney B.C. (1984). Two-dimensional filtering of SPECT images using the Metz and Wiener filters. *J. Nucl. Med.* 25: 1234.

King M.A., Schwinger R.B., and Penney B.C. (1986). Variation of the count-dependent Metz filter with imaging system modulation transfer function. *Med. Phys.* 25: 139.

Knesaurek K., King M.A., Glick S.J. et al. (1989). Investigation of causes of geometric distortion in 180 degree and 360 degree angular sampling in SPECT. *J. Nucl. Med.* 30: 1666.

Koral K.F., Wang X., Rogers W.L., and Clinthorne N.H. (1988). SPECT Compton-scattering correction by analysis of energy spectra. *J. Nucl. Med.* 29: 195.

Kuhl D.E. and Edwards R.Q. (1963). Image separation radioisotope scanning. *Radiology* 80: 653.

Kuhl D.E. and Edwards R.Q. (1964). Cylindrical and section radioisotope scanning of the liver and brain. *Radiology* 83: 926.

Kuhl D.E. and Edwards R.Q. (1968). Reorganizing data from transverse section scans of the brain using digital processing. *Radiology* 91: 975.

Lange K. and Carson R. (1984). EM reconstruction algorithms for emission and transmission tomography. *J. Comput. Assist. Tomogr.* 8: 306.

Levitan E. and Herman G.T. (1987). A maximum a posteriori probability expectation maximization algorithm for image reconstruction in emission tomography. *IEEE Trans. Med. Imag. MI* 6: 185.

Liang Z. and Hart H. (1987). Bayesian image processing of data from constrained source distribution: I. Nonvalued, uncorrelated and correlated constraints. *Bull. Math. Biol.* 49: 51.

Larsson S.A., Hohm C., Carnebrink T. et al. (1991). A new cylindrical SPECT Anger camera with a decentralized transputer based data acquisition system. *IEEE Trans. Nucl. Sci. NS* 38: 654.

Lassen N.A., Sveinsdottir E., Kanno I. et al. (1978). A fast moving single photon emission tomograph for regional cerebral blood flow studies in man. *J. Comput. Assist. Tomogr.* 2: 661.

Lewitt R.M., Edholm P.R., and Xia W. (1989). Fourier method for correction of depth dependent collimator blurring. *Proc. SPIE* 1092: 232.

Lim C.B., Chang J.T., and Jaszczak R.J. (1980). Performance analysis of three camera configurations for single photon emission computed tomography. *IEEE Trans. Nucl. Sci. NS* 27: 559.

Lim C.B., Gottschalk S., Walker R. et al. (1985). Tri-angular SPECT system for 3-D total organ volume imaging: design concept and preliminary imaging results. *IEEE Trans. Nucl. Sci. NS* 32: 741.

Manglos S.H., Jaszczak R.J., Floyd C.E. et al. (1987). Nonisotropic attenuation in SPECT: phantom test of quantitative effects and compensation techniques. *J. Nucl. Med.* 28: 1584.

Maniawski P.J., Morgan H.T., and Wackers F.J.T. (1991). Orbit-related variations in spatial resolution as a source of artifactual defects in thallium-201 SPECT. *J. Nucl. Med.* 32: 871.

Milster T.D., Aarsvold J.N., Barrett H.H. et al. (1990). A full-field modular gamma camera. *J. Nucl. Med.* 31: 632.

Minerbo G. (1979). Maximum entropy reconstruction from cone-beam projection data. *Comput. Biol. Med.* 9: 29.

Moore S.C., Doherty M.D., Zimmerman R.E., and Holman B.L. (1984). Improved performance from modifications to the multidetector SPECT brain scanner. *J. Nucl. Med.* 25: 688.

Ogawa K., Harata Y., Ichihara T. et al. (1991). A practical method for position-dependent Compton scatter correction in SPECT. *IEEE Trans. Med. Imag.* 10: 408.

Penney B.C., Glick S.J., and King M.A. (1990). Relative importance of the errors sources in Wiener restoration of scintigrams. *IEEE Trans. Med. Imag.* 9: 60.

Radon J. (1917). Uber die bestimmung von funktionen durch ihre integral-werte langs gewisser mannigfaltigkeiten. *Ber. Verh. Sachs. Akad. Wiss.* 67: 26.

Ramachandran G.N. and Lakshminarayanan A.V. (1971). Three-dimensional reconstruction from radiographs and electron micrographs: application of convolutions instead of Fourier transforms. *Proc. Natl Acad. Sci. USA* 68: 2236.

Roger W.L. and Ackermann R.J. (1992). SPECT instrumentation. *Am. J. Physiol. Imag.* 314: 105.

Rogers W.L., Clinthorne N.H., Shao L. et al. (1988). SPRINT II: a second-generation single photon ring tomograph. *IEEE Trans. Med. Imag.* 7: 291.

Rowe R.K., Aarsvold J.N., Barrett H.H. et al. (1992). A stationary, hemispherical SPECT imager for 3D brain imaging. *J. Nucl. Med.* 34: 474.

Sorenson J.A. (1974). Quantitative measurement of radiation *in vivo* by whole body counting. In G.H. Hine and J.A. Sorenson (Eds), Instrumentation in Nuclear Medicine, Vol. 2, pp. 311–348. New York, Academic Press.

Shepp L.A. and Vardi Y. (1982). Maximum likelihood reconstruction for emission tomography. *IEEE Trans. Med. Imag. MI* 1: 113.

Stoddart H.F. and Stoddart H.A. (1979). A new development in single gamma transaxial tomography Union Carbide focused collimator scanner. *IEEE Trans. Nucl. Sci. NS* 26: 2710.

Stokely E.M., Sveinsdottir E., Lassen N.A., and Rommer P. (1980). A single photon dynamic computer assisted tomography (DCAT) for imaging brain function in multiple cross-sections. *J. Comput. Assist. Tomogr.* 4: 230.

Tretiak O.J. and Metz C.E. (1980). The exponential Radon transform. *SIAM J. Appl. Math.* 39: 341.

Tsui B.M.W. (1988). Collimator design, properties and characteristics. Chapter 2. In G.H. Simmons (Ed.), *The Scintillation Camera*, pp. 17–45. New York, The Society of Nuclear Medicine.

Tsui B.M.W., Frey E.C., Zhao X.-D. et al. (1994). The importance and implementation of accurate 3D compensation methods for quantitative SPECT. *Phys. Med. Biol.* 39: 509.

Tsui B.M.W., Gullberg G.T., Edgerton E.R. et al. (1986). The design and clinical utility of a fan beam collimator for a SPECT system. *J. Nucl. Med.* 247: 810.

Tsui B.M.W., Gullberg G.T., Edgerton E.R. et al. (1989). Correction of nonuniform attenuation in cardiac SPECT imaging. *J. Nucl. Med.* 30: 497.

Tsui B.M.W., Hu H.B., Gilland D.R., and Gullberg G.T. (1988). Implementation of simultaneous attenuation and detector response correction in SPECT. *IEEE Trans. Nucl. Sci. NS* 35: 778.

Tsui B.M.W., Zhao X.-D., Frey E.C., and McCartney W.H. (1994). Quantitative single-photon emission computed tomography: basics and clinical considerations. *Semin. Nucl. Med.* 24: 38.

Yanch J.C., Flower M.A., and Webb S. (1988). Comparison of deconvolution and windowed subtraction techniques for scatter compensation in SPECT. *IEEE Trans. Med. Imag.* 7: 13.

Zeng G.L., Gullberg G.T., Tsui B.M.W., and Terry J.A. (1991). Three-dimensional iterative reconstruction algorithms with attenuation and geometric point response correction. *IEEE Trans. Nucl. Sci. NS* 38: 693.

14

Ultrasound

14.1 Transducers... **14-1**
   Transducer Materials • Scanning with Array Transducers •
   Linear-Array Transducer Performance • Designing a
   Phased-Array Transducer • Summary
Defining Terms **14-14**
References **14-15**
Further Information **14-16**
14.2 Ultrasonic Imaging **14-16**
   Fundamentals • Applications and Example Calculations •
   Economics
Defining Terms **14-21**
Reference **14-22**
Further Information **14-22**
14.3 Blood Flow Measurement Using Ultrasound **14-22**
   Fundamental Concepts • Velocity Estimation Techniques •
   New Directions
Defining Terms **14-38**
References **14-38**
Further Information **14-40**

Richard L. Goldberg
University of North Carolina

Stephen W. Smith
Duke University

Jack G. Mottley
University of Rochester

K. Whittaker Ferrara
Riverside Research Institute

14.1 Transducers

Richard L. Goldberg and Stephen W. Smith

An ultrasound transducer generates acoustic waves by converting magnetic, thermal, and electrical energy into mechanical energy. The most efficient technique for medical ultrasound uses the piezoelectric effect, which was first demonstrated in 1880 by Jacques and Pierre Curie [Curie and Curie, 1880]. They applied a stress to a quartz crystal and detected an electrical potential across opposite faces of the material. The Curies also discovered the inverse piezoelectric effect by applying an electric field across the crystal to induce a mechanical deformation. In this manner, a piezoelectric transducer converts an oscillating electric signal into an acoustic wave, and vice versa.

Many significant advances in ultrasound imaging have resulted from innovation in transducer technology. One such instance was the development of linear-array transducers. Previously, ultrasound systems had made an image by manually moving the transducer across the region of interest. Even the faster scanners had required several seconds to generate an ultrasound image, and as a result, only static targets could be scanned. On the other hand, if the acoustic beam could be scanned rapidly, clinicians could visualize moving targets such as a beating heart. In addition, real-time imaging would provide instantaneous feedback to the clinician of the transducer position and system settings.

To implement real-time imaging, researchers developed new types of transducers that rapidly steer the acoustic beam. Piston-shaped transducers were designed to wobble or rotate about a fixed axis to mechanically steer the beam through a sector-shaped region. Linear sequential arrays were designed to electronically focus the beam in a rectangular image region. Linear phased-array transducers were designed to electronically steer and focus the beam at high speed in a sector image format.

This section describes the application of piezoelectric ceramics to transducer arrays for medical ultrasound. Background is presented on transducer materials and beam steering with phased arrays. Array performance is described, and the design of an idealized array is presented.

14.1.1　Transducer Materials

Ferroelectric materials strongly exhibit the piezoelectric effect, and they are ideal materials for medical ultrasound. For many years, the ferroelectric ceramic lead–zirconate–titanate (PZT) has been the standard transducer material for medical ultrasound, in part because of its high electromechanical conversion efficiency and low intrinsic losses. The properties of PZT can be adjusted by modifying the ratio of zirconium to titanium and introducing small amounts of other substances, such as lanthanum [Berlincourt, 1971]. Table 14.1 shows the material properties of linear-array elements made from PZT-5H.

PZT has a high dielectric constant compared with many piezoelectric materials, resulting is favorable electrical characteristics. The ceramic is mechanically strong, and it can be machined to various shapes and sizes. PZT can operate at temperatures up to $100°C$ or higher, and it is stable over long periods of time.

The disadvantages of PZT include its high **acoustic impedance** ($Z = 30$ MRayls) compared with body tissue ($Z = 1.5$ MRayls) and the presence of **lateral modes** in array elements. One or more acoustic matching layers can largely compensate for the acoustic impedance mismatch. The effect of lateral modes can be diminished by choosing the appropriate element dimensions or by subdicing the elements.

Other piezoelectric materials are used for various applications. Composites are made from PZT interspersed in an epoxy matrix [Smith, 1992]. Lateral modes are reduced in a composite because of its inhomogeneous structure. By combining the PZT and epoxy in different ratios and spatial distributions, one can tailor the composite's properties for different applications. Polyvinylidene difluoride (PVDF) is a ferroelectric polymer that has been used effectively in high-frequency transducers [Sherar and Foster, 1989]. The copolymer of PVDF with trifluoroethylene has an improved electromechanical conversion efficiency. Relaxor ferroelectric materials, such as lead–magnesium–niobate (PMN), become piezoelectric when a large direct-current (dc) bias voltage is applied [Takeuchi et al., 1990]. They have a very large dielectric constant ($\varepsilon > 20,000\varepsilon_0$), resulting in higher transducer capacitance and a lower electrical impedance.

14.1.2　Scanning with Array Transducers

Array transducers use the same principles as acoustic lenses to focus an acoustic beam. In both cases, variable delays are applied across the transducer aperture. With a sequential or phased array, however,

TABLE 14.1　Material Properties of Linear-Array Elements
Made of PZT-5H

Parameter	Symbol	Value	Units
Density	ρ	7500	kg/m^3
Speed of sound	c	3970	m/sec
Acoustic impedance	Z	29.75	MRayls
Relative dielectric constant	ϵ/ϵ_0	1475	None
Electromechanical coupling coefficient	k	0.698	None
Mechanical loss tangent	$\tan \delta_m$	0.015	None
Electrical loss tangent	$\tan \delta_e$	0.02	None

the delays are electronically controlled and can be changed instantaneously to focus the beam in different regions. Linear arrays were first developed for radar, sonar, and radio astronomy [Allen, 1964; Bobber, 1970], and they were implemented in a medical ultrasound system by Somer in 1968 [Somer, 1968].

Linear-array transducers have increased versatility over piston transducers. Electronic scanning involves no moving parts, and the focal point can be changed dynamically to any location in the scanning plane. The system can generate a wide variety of scan formats, and it can process the received echoes for other applications, such as dynamic receive focusing [von Ramm and Thurstone, 1976], correction for phase aberrations [Flax and O'Donnell, 1988; Trahey et al., 1990], and synthetic aperture imaging [Nock and Trahey, 1992].

The disadvantages of linear arrays are due to the increased complexity and higher cost of the transducers and scanners. For high-quality ultrasound images, many identical array elements are required (currently 128 and rising). The array elements are typically less than a millimeter on one side, and each has a separate connection to its own transmitter and receiver electronics.

The widespread use of array transducers for many applications indicates that the advantages often outweigh the disadvantages. In addition, improvement in transducer fabrication techniques and integrated circuit technology have led to more advanced array transducers and scanners.

14.1.2.1 Focusing and Steering with Phased Arrays

This section describes how a phased-array transducer can focus and steer an acoustic beam along a specific direction. An ultrasound image is formed by repeating this process over 100 times to interrogate a two- (2D) or three-dimensional (3D) region of the medium.

Figure 14.1a illustrates a simple example of a six-element linear array focusing the transmitted beam. One can assume that each array element is a point source that radiates a spherically shaped wavefront into the medium. Since the top element is farthest from the focus in this example, it is excited first. The remaining elements are excited at the appropriate time intervals so that the acoustic signals from all

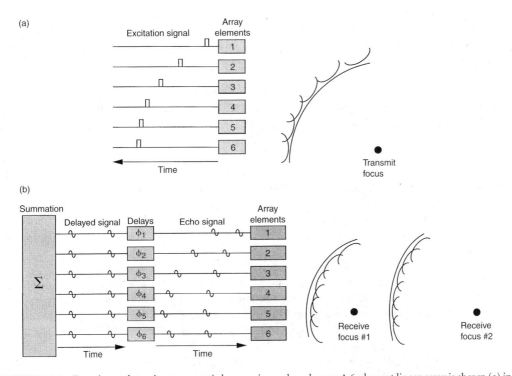

FIGURE 14.1   Focusing and steering an acoustic beam using a phased array. A 6-element linear array is shown (a) in the transmit mode and (b) in the receive mode. Dynamic focusing in receive allows the scanner focus to track the range of returning echoes.

the elements reach the focal point at the same time. According to Huygens' principle, the net acoustic signal is the sum of the signals that have arrived from each source. At the focal point, the contributions from every element add in phase to produce a peak in the acoustic signal. Elsewhere, at least some of the contributions add out of phase, reducing the signal relative to the peak.

For receiving an ultrasound echo, the phased array works in reverse. Figure 14.1b shows an echo originating from focus 1. The echo is incident on each array element at a different time interval. The received signals are electronically delayed so that the delayed signals add in phase for an echo originating at the focal point. For echoes originating elsewhere, at least some of the delayed signals will add out of phase, reducing the receive signal relative to the peak at the focus.

In the receive mode, the focal point can be dynamically adjusted so that it coincides with the range of returning echoes. After transmission of an acoustic pulse, the initial echoes return from targets near the transducer. Therefore, the scanner focuses the phased array on these targets, located at focus 1 in Figure 14.1b. As echoes return from more distant targets, the scanner focuses at a greater depth (focus 2 in the figure). Focal zones are established with adequate depth of field so that the targets are always in focus in receive. This process is called dynamic receive focusing and was first implemented by von Ramm and Thurstone in 1976 [von Ramm and Thurstone, 1976].

14.1.2.2 Array-Element Configurations

An ultrasound image is formed by repeating the preceding process many times to scan a 2D or 3D region of tissue. For a 2D image, the scanning plane is the *azimuth dimension*; the *elevation dimension* is perpendicular to the azimuth scanning plane. The shape of the region scanned is determined by the array-element configuration, described in the paragraph below.

Linear Sequential Arrays: Sequential linear arrays have as many as 512 elements in current commercial scanners. A subaperture of up to 128 elements is selected to operate at a given time. As shown in Figure 14.2a, the scanning lines are directed perpendicular to the face of the transducer; the acoustic beam is focused but not steered. The advantage of this scheme is that the array elements have high sensitivity when the beam is directed straight ahead. The disadvantage is that the field of view is limited to the rectangular region directly in front of the transducer. Linear-array transducers have a large footprint to obtain an adequate field of view.

Curvilinear Arrays: Curvilinear or convex arrays have a different shape than sequential linear arrays, but they operate in the same manner. In both cases, the scan lines are directed perpendicular to the transducer face. A curvilinear array, however, scans a wider field of view because of its convex shape, as shown in Figure 14.2b.

Linear Phased Arrays: The more advanced linear phased arrays have 128 elements. All the elements are used to transmit and receive each line of data. As shown in Figure 14.2c, the scanner steers the ultrasound beam through a sector-shaped region in the azimuth plane. Phased arrays scan a region that is significantly wider than the footprint of the transducer, making them suitable for scanning through restricted acoustic windows. As a result, these transducers are ideal for cardiac imaging, where the transducer must scan through a small window to avoid the obstructions of the ribs (bone) and lungs (air).

1.5D Arrays: The so-called 1.5D array is similar to a 2D array in construction but a 1D array in operation. The 1.5D array contains elements along both the azimuth and **elevation dimensions**. Features such dynamic focusing and phase correction can be implemented in both dimensions to improve image quality. Since a 1.5D array contains a limited number of elements in elevation (e.g., 3 to 9 elements), steering is not possible in that direction. Figure 14.2d illustrates a B-scan made with a 1.5D phased array. Linear sequential scanning is also possible with 1.5D arrays.

2D Phased Arrays: A 2D phased-array has a large number of elements in both the azimuth and elevation dimensions. Therefore, 2D arrays can focus and steer the acoustic beam in both dimensions. Using parallel receive processing [Shattuck et al., 1984], a 2D array can scan a pyramidal region in real time to produce a volumetric image, as shown in Figure 14.2e [von Ramm and Smith, 1990].

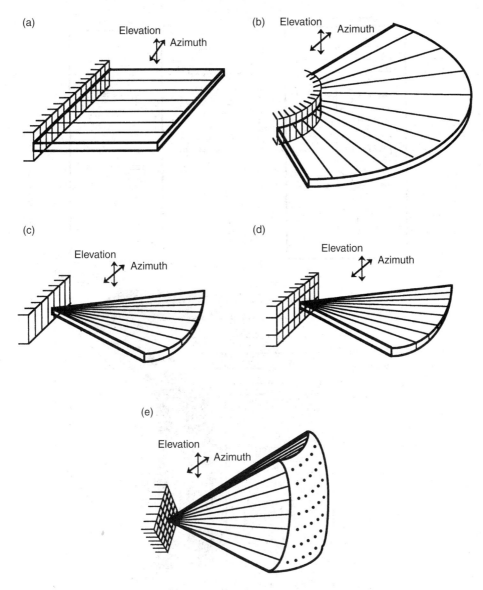

FIGURE 14.2 Array-element configurations and the region scanned by the acoustic beam. (a) A sequential linear array scans a rectangular region; (b) a curvilinear array scans a sector-shaped region; (c) a linear phased array scans a sector-shaped region; (d) a 1.5D array scans a sector-shaped region; and (e) a 2D array scans a pyramidal-shaped region.

14.1.3 Linear-Array Transducer Performance

Designing an ultrasound transducer array involves many compromises. Ideally, a transducer has high sensitivity or SNR, good spatial resolution, and no artifacts. The individual array elements should have wide **angular response** in the steering dimensions, low cross-coupling, and an electrical impedance matched to the transmitter.

Figure 14.3a illustrates the connections to the transducer assembly. The transmitter and receiver circuits are located in the ultrasound scanner and are connected to the array elements through 1 to 2 m of coaxial cable. **Electrical matching networks** can be added to tune out the capacitance of the coaxial cable and/or the transducer element and increase the signal-to-noise ratio (SNR).

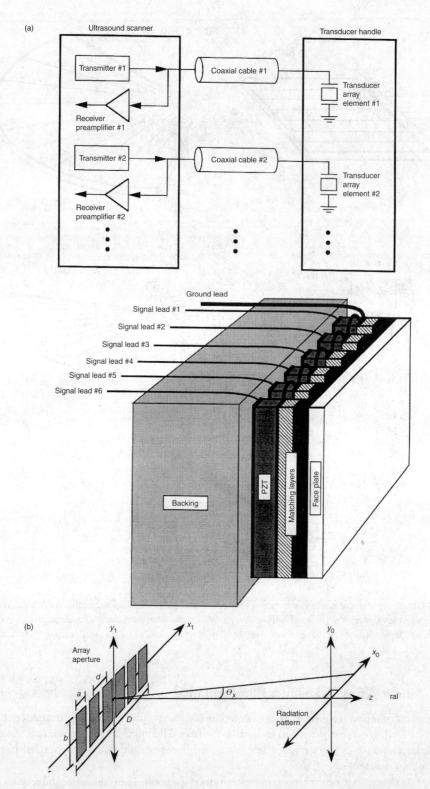

FIGURE 14.3 (a) The connections between the ultrasound scanner and the transducer assembly for two elements of an array. (b) A more detailed picture of the transducer assembly for six elements of an array. (c) Coordinate system and labeling used to describe an array transducer.

A more detailed picture of six-transducer elements is shown in Figure 14.3b. Electrical leads connect to the ground and signal electrodes of the piezoelectric material. Acoustically, the array elements are loaded on the front side by one or two **quarter-wave matching layers** and the tissue medium. The matching layers may be made from glass or epoxy. A backing material, such as epoxy, loads the back side of the array elements. The faceplate protects the transducer assembly and also may act as an acoustic lens. Faceplates are often made from silicone or polyurethane.

The following sections describe several important characteristics of an array transducer. Figure 14.3c shows a six-element array and its dimensions. The element thickness, width, and length are labeled as t, a, and b, respectively. The interelement spacing is d, and the total aperture size is D in azimuth. The acoustic wavelength in the load medium, usually human tissue, is designated as l, while the wavelength in the transducer material is λ_t.

Examples are given below for a 128-element linear array operating at 5 MHz. The array is made of PZT-5H with element dimensions of $0.1 \times 5 \times 0.3$ mm^3. The interelement spacing is $d = 0.15$ mm in azimuth, and the total aperture is $D = 128 \times 0.15$ mm $= 19.3$ mm (see Table 14.1 for the piezoelectric material characteristics). The elements have an epoxy backing of $Z = 3.25$ MRayls. For simplicity, the example array does not contain a $\lambda/4$ matching layer.

14.1.3.1 Axial Resolution

Axial resolution determines the ability to distinguish between targets aligned in the axial direction (the direction of acoustic propagation). In pulse-echo imaging, the echoes off of two targets separated by $r/2$ have a path length difference of r. If the acoustic pulse length is r, then echoes off the two targets are just distinguishable. As a result, the **axial resolution** is often defined as one-half the pulse length [Christensen, 1988]. A transducer with a high resonant frequency and a broad bandwidth has a short acoustic pulse and good axial resolution.

14.1.3.2 Radiation Pattern

The radiation pattern of a transducer determines the insonified region of tissue. For good **lateral resolution** and sensitivity, the acoustic energy should be concentrated in a small region. The radiation pattern for a narrow-band or continuous-wave (CW) transducer is described by the Rayleigh–Sommerfeld diffraction formula [Goodman, 1986]. For a pulse-echo imaging system, this diffraction formula is not exact due to the broadband acoustic waves used. Nevertheless, the Rayleigh–Sommerfeld formula is a reasonable first-order approximation to the actual radiation pattern.

The following analysis considers only the azimuth scanning dimension. Near the focal point or in the far field, the Fraunhofer approximation reduces the diffraction formula to a Fourier transform formula. For a circular or rectangular aperture, the far field is at a range of

$$z > \frac{D^2}{4\lambda} \tag{14.1}$$

Figure 14.3c shows the coordinate system used to label the array aperture and its radiation pattern. The array aperture is described by

$$\text{Array}\,(x_1) = \text{rect}\left(\frac{x_1}{a}\right) * \text{comb}\left(\frac{x_1}{d}\right) \cdot \text{rect}\left(\frac{x_1}{D}\right) \tag{14.2}$$

where the rect(x) function is a rectangular pulse of width x, and the comb(x) function is a delta function repeated at intervals of x. The diffraction pattern is evaluated in the x_0 plane at a distance z from the transducer, and θ_x is the angle of the point x_0 from the normal axis. With the Fraunhofer approximation, the normalized diffraction pattern is given by

$$P_x(\theta_x) = \text{sinc}\left(\frac{a\sin\theta_x}{\lambda}\right) \cdot \text{comb}\left(\frac{d\sin\theta_x}{\lambda}\right) * \text{sinc}\left(\frac{D\sin\theta_x}{\lambda}\right) \tag{14.3}$$

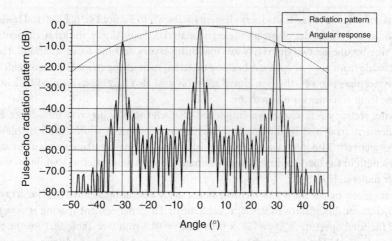

FIGURE 14.4   Radiation pattern of Equation 14.3 for a 16-element array with $a = \lambda$, $d = 2\lambda$, and $D = 32\lambda$. The angular response, the first term of Equation 14.3, is also shown as a dashed line.

in azimuth, where the Fourier transform of Equation 14.2 has been evaluated at the spatial frequency

$$f_x = \frac{x_0}{\lambda z} = \frac{\sin\theta_x}{\lambda} \tag{14.4}$$

Figure 14.4 shows a graph of Equation 14.3 for a 16-element array with $a = \lambda$, $d = 2\lambda$, and $D = 32\lambda$. In the graph, the significance of each term is easily distinguished. The first term determines the angular response weighting, the second term determines the location of **grating lobes** off-axis, and the third term determines the shape of the main lobe and the grating lobes. The significance of *lateral resolution*, angular response, and grating lobes is seen from the CW diffraction pattern.

Lateral resolution determines the ability to distinguish between targets in the azimuth and elevation dimensions. According to the Rayleigh criterion [Goodman, 1986], the lateral resolution can be defined by the first null in the main lobe, which is determined from the third term of Equation 14.3.

$$\theta_x = \sin^{-1}\frac{\lambda}{D} \tag{14.5}$$

in the **azimuth dimension**. A larger aperture results in a more narrow main lobe and better resolution.

A broad angular response is desired to maintain sensitivity while steering off-axis. The first term of Equation 14.3 determines the one-way angular response. The element is usually surrounded by a soft baffle, such as air, resulting in an additional cosine factor in the radiation pattern [Selfridge et al., 1980]. Assuming transmit/receive reciprocity, the pulse-echo angular response for a single element is

$$P_x(\theta_x) = \frac{\sin^2(\pi a/\lambda \cdot \sin\theta_x)}{(\pi a/\lambda \cdot \sin\theta_x)} \cdot \cos^2\theta_x \tag{14.6}$$

in the azimuth dimension. As the aperture size becomes smaller, the element more closely resembles a point source, and the angular response becomes more broad. Another useful indicator is the −6-dB angular response, defined as the full-width at half-maximum of the angular response graph.

Grating lobes are produced at a location where the path length difference to adjacent array elements is a multiple of a wavelength (the main lobe is located where the path length difference is zero). The acoustic contributions from the elements constructively interfere, producing off-axis peaks. The term grating lobe was originally used to describe the optical peaks produced by a diffraction grating. In ultrasound, grating

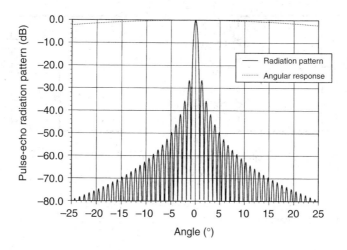

FIGURE 14.5 Radiation pattern of the example array element with $a = 0.1$ mm, $d = 0.15$ mm, $D = 19.2$ mm, and $\lambda = 0.3$ mm. The angular response of Equation 14.6 was substituted into Equation 14.3 for this graph.

lobes are undesirable because they represent acoustic energy steered away from the main lobe. From the comb function in Equation 14.3, the grating lobes are located at

$$\theta_x = \sin^{-1}\frac{i\lambda}{d} \quad i = 1, 2, 3, \ldots \tag{14.7}$$

in azimuth.

If d is a wavelength, then grating lobes are centered at ± 90 degrees from the steering direction in that dimension. Grating lobes at such large angles are less significant because the array elements have poor angular response in those regions. If the main lobe is steered at a large angle, however, the grating lobes are brought toward the front of the array. In this case, the angular response weighting produces a relatively weak main lobe and a relatively strong grating lobe. To eliminate grating lobes at all steering angles, the interelement spacing is set to $\lambda/2$ or less [Steinberg, 1967].

Figure 14.5 shows the theoretical radiation pattern of the 128-element example. For this graph, the angular response weighting of Equation 14.6 was substituted into Equation 14.3. The lateral resolution, as defined by Equation 14.7, $\theta_x = 0.9$ degrees at the focal point. The -6-dB angular response is ± 40 degrees from Equation 14.6.

14.1.3.3 Electrical Impedance

The electric impedance of an element relative to the electrical loads has a significant impact on transducer signal-to-noise ratio (SNR). At frequencies away from resonance, the transducer has electrical characteristics of a capacitor. The construction of the transducer is a parallel-plate capacitor with clamped capacitance of

$$C_0 = \varepsilon^s \frac{ab}{t} \tag{14.8}$$

where ε^s is the clamped dielectric constant.

Near resonance, equivalent circuits help to explain the impedance behavior of a transducer. The simplified circuit of Figure 14.6a is valid for transducers operating at series resonance without losses and with low acoustic impedance loads [Kino, 1987]. The mechanical resistance R_m represents the acoustic

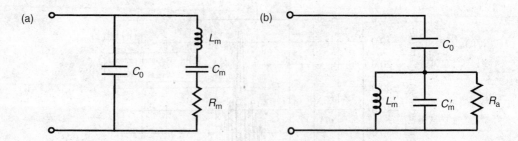

FIGURE 14.6 Simplified equivalent circuits for a piezoelectric transducer (a) near-series resonance and (b) near-parallel resonance.

loads as seen from the electrical terminals:

$$R_m = \frac{\pi}{4k^2 \omega C_0} \cdot \frac{Z_1 + Z_2}{Z_C} \tag{14.9}$$

where k is the electromechanical coupling coefficient of the piezoelectric material, Z_C is the acoustic impedance of the piezoelectric material, Z_1 is the acoustic impedance of the transducer backing, and Z_2 is the acoustic impedance of the load medium (body tissue). The power dissipated through R_m corresponds to the acoustic output power from the transducer.

The mechanical inductance L_m and mechanical capacitance C_m are analogous to the inductance and capacitance of a mass-spring system. At the series resonant frequency of

$$f_s = \frac{1}{2\pi \sqrt{L_m C_m}} \tag{14.10}$$

the impedances of these components add to zero, resulting in a local impedance minimum.

The equivalent circuit of Figure 14.6a can be redrawn in the form shown in Figure 14.6b. In this circuit, C_0 is the same as before, but the mechanical impedances have values of L'_m, C'_m, and R_a. The resistive component R_a is

$$R_a = \frac{4k^2}{\pi \omega C_0} \cdot \frac{Z_C}{Z_1 - Z_2} \tag{14.11}$$

The inductor and capacitor combine to form an open circuit at the parallel resonant frequency of

$$f_p = \frac{1}{2\pi \sqrt{L'_m C'_m}} \tag{14.12}$$

The parallel resonance, which is at a slightly higher frequency than the series resonance, is indicated by a local impedance maximum.

Figure 14.7 shows a simulated plot of magnitude and phase versus frequency for the example array element described at the beginning of this subsection. The series resonance frequency is immediately identified at 5.0 MHz with an impedance minimum of $|Z| = 350\ \Omega$. Parallel resonance occurs at 6.7 MHz with an impedance maximum of $|Z| = 4000\ \Omega$. Note the capacitive behavior (approximately -90-degree phase) at frequencies far from resonance.

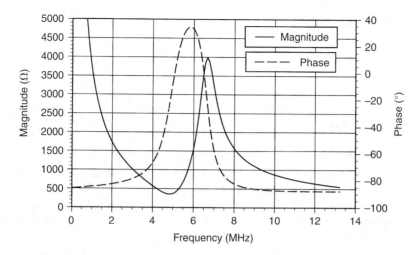

FIGURE 14.7   Complex electrical impedance of the example array element. Series resonance is located at 5.0 MHz, and parallel resonance is located at 6.7 MHz.

14.1.4   Designing a Phased-Array Transducer

In this section the design of an idealized phased-array transducer is considered in terms of the performance characteristics described above. Criteria are described for selecting array dimensions, acoustic backing and matching layers, and electrical matching networks.

14.1.4.1   Choosing Array Dimensions

The array element thickness is determined by the parallel resonant frequency. For $\lambda/2$ resonance, the thickness is

$$t = \frac{\lambda_t}{2}\,\frac{c_t}{2f_p} \tag{14.13}$$

where c_t is the longitudinal speed of sound in the transducer material.

There are three constraints for choosing the element width and length (1) a nearly square cross-section should be avoided so that lateral vibrations are not coupled to the thickness vibration; as a rule of thumb [Kino and DeSilets, 1979],

$$a/t \leq 0.6 \quad \text{or} \quad a/t \geq 10 \tag{14.14}$$

(2) a small width and length are also desirable for a wide angular response weighting function; and (3) an interelement spacing of $\lambda/2$ or less is necessary to eliminate grating lobes.

Fortunately, these requirements are consistent for PZT array elements. For all forms of PZT, $c_t > 2c$, where c is the speed of sound in body tissue (an average of 1540 m/sec). At a given frequency, then $\lambda_t > 2\lambda$. Also, Equation 14.13 states that $\lambda_t = 2t$ at a frequency of f_p. By combining these equations, $t > \lambda$ for PZT array elements operating at a frequency of f_p. If $d = \lambda/2$, then $a < \lambda/2$ because of the finite kerf width that separates the elements. Given this observation, then $a < t/2$. This is consistent with Equation 14.14 to reduce lateral modes.

An element having $d = \lambda/2$ also has adequate angular response. For illustrative purposes, one can assume a zero kerf width so that $a = \lambda/2$. In this case, the -6-dB angular response is $\theta_x = \pm 35$ degrees according to Equation 14.6.

The array dimensions determine the transducer's lateral resolution. In the azimuth dimension, if $d = \lambda/2$, then the transducer aperture is $D = n\lambda/2$, where n is the number of elements in a fully sampled array. From Equation 14.5, the lateral resolution in azimuth is

$$\theta_x = \sin^{-1}\frac{2}{n} \tag{14.15}$$

Therefore, the lateral resolution is independent of frequency in a fully sampled array with $d = \lambda/2$. For this configuration, the lateral resolution is improved by increasing the number of elements.

14.1.4.2 Acoustic Backing and Matching Layers

The backing and matching layers affect the transducer bandwidth and sensitivity. While a lossy, matched backing improves bandwidth, it also dissipates acoustic energy that could otherwise be transmitted into the tissue medium. Therefore, a low-impedance acoustic backing is preferred because it reflects the acoustic pulses toward the front side of the transducer. In this case, adequate bandwidth is maintained by acoustically matching the transducer to the tissue medium using matching layers.

Matching layers are designed with a thickness of $\lambda/4$ at the center frequency and an acoustic impedance between those of the transducer Z_T and the load medium Z_L. The ideal acoustic impedances can be determined from several different models [Hunt et al., 1983]. Using the KLM equivalent circuit model [Desilets et al., 1978], the ideal acoustic impedance is

$$Z_1 = \sqrt[3]{Z_T Z_L^2} \tag{14.16}$$

for a single matching layer. For matching PZT-5H array elements ($Z_T = 30$ MRayls) to a water load ($Z_L = 1.5$ MRayls), a matching layer of $Z_1 = 4.1$ MRayls should be chosen. If two matching layers are used, they should have acoustic impedances of

$$Z_1 \sqrt[7]{Z_T^4 Z_L^3} \tag{14.17a}$$

$$Z_2 \sqrt[7]{Z_T Z_L^6} \tag{14.17b}$$

In this case, $Z_1 = 8.3$ MRayls and $Z_2 = 2.3$ MRayls for matching PZT-5H to a water load.

When constructing a transducer, a practical matching layer material is not always available, with the ideal acoustic impedance (Equation 14.16 or Equation 14.17). Adequate bandwidth is obtained by using materials that have an impedance close to the ideal value. With a single matching layer, for example, conductive epoxy can be used with $Z = 5.1$ MRayls.

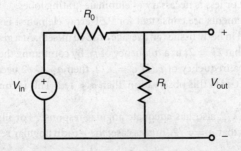

FIGURE 14.8 A transducer of real impedance R_t being excited by a transmitter with source impedance R_0 and source voltage V_{in}.

14.1.4.3 Electrical Impedance Matching

Signal-to-noise ratio and bandwidth are also improved when electrical impedance of an array element is matched to that of the transmit circuitry. Consider the simplified circuit in Figure 14.8 with a transmitter of impedance R_0 and a transducer of real impedance R_t. The power output is proportional to the power dissipated in R_t, as expressed as

$$P_{out} = \frac{V_{out}^2}{R_t} \text{ where } V_{out} = \frac{R_t}{R_0 + R_t} V_{in} \tag{14.18}$$

The power available from the transmitter is

$$P_{in} = \frac{(V_{in}/2)^2}{R_0} \tag{14.19}$$

into a matched load. From the two previous equations, the power efficiency is

$$\frac{P_{out}}{P_{in}} = \frac{4R_0 R_t}{(R_0 + R_t)^2} \tag{14.20}$$

For a fixed-source impedance, the maximum efficiency is obtained by taking the derivative of Equation 14.20 with respect to R_t and setting it to zero. Maximum efficiency occurs when the source impedance is matched to the transducer impedance, $R_0 = R_t$.

In practice, the transducer has a complex impedance of R_m in parallel with C_0 (see Figure 14.6), which is excited by a transmitter with a real impedance of 50 Ω. The transducer has a maximum efficiency when the imaginary component is tuned out and the real component is 50 Ω. This can be accomplished with electrical matching networks.

The capacitance C_0 is tuned out in the frequency range near Ω_0 using an inductor of

$$L_0 = \frac{1}{\omega_0^2 C_0} \tag{14.21}$$

for an inductor in shunt, or

$$L_1 \frac{1}{\omega_0^2 C_0 + 1/R_m^2 C_0} \tag{14.22}$$

for an inductor in series. The example array elements described in the preceding subsection have $C_0 = 22$ pF and $R_m = 340\ \Omega$ at series resonance of 5.0 MHz. Therefore, tuning inductors of $L_0 = 46$ mH or $L_1 = 2.4$ mH should be used.

A shunt inductor also raises the impedance of the transducer, as seen from the scanner, while a series inductor lowers the terminal impedance [Hunt et al., 1983]. For more significant changes in terminal impedance, transformers are used.

A transformer of turns ratio 1 : N multiplies the terminal impedance by $1/N^2$. In the transmit mode, N can be adjusted so that the terminal impedance matches the transmitter impedance. In the receive mode, the open-circuit sensitivity varies as $1/N$ because of the step-down transformer. The lower terminal impedance of the array element, however, provides increased ability to drive an electrical load.

More complicated circuits can be used for better electrical matching across a wide bandwidth [Hunt et al., 1983]. These circuits can be either passive, as above, or active. Inductors also can be used in the scanner to tune out the capacitance of the coaxial cable that loads the transducer on receive.

Another alternative for electrical matching is to use multilayer piezoelectric ceramics [Goldberg and Smith, 1994]. Figure 14.9 shows an example of a single layer and a five-layer array element with the same overall dimensions of a, b, and t. Since the layers are connected electrically in parallel, the clamped

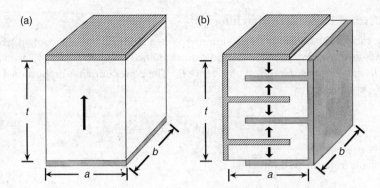

FIGURE 14.9 (a) Conventional single-layer ceramic; (b) five-layer ceramic of the same overall dimensions. The layers are electrically in parallel and acoustically in series. The arrows indicate the piezoelectric poling directions of each layer.

capacitance of a multilayer ceramic (MLC) element is

$$C_0 = N \cdot \varepsilon^S \cdot \frac{ab}{t/N} = N^2 \cdot C_{\text{single}} \qquad (14.23)$$

where C_{single} is the capacitance of the single-layer element (Equation 14.8). As a result, the MLC impedance is reduced by a factor of N^2. Acoustically, the layers of the MLC are in series so the $\lambda/2$ resonant thickness is t, the stack thickness.

To a first order, an N-layer ceramic has identical performance compared with a 1:N transformer, but the impedance is transformed within the ceramic. MLCs also can be fabricated in large quantities more easily than hand-wound transformers. While MLCs do not tune out the reactive impedance, they make it easier to tune a low capacitance array element. By lowering the terminal impedance of an array element, MLCs significantly improve transducer SNR.

14.1.5 Summary

The piezoelectric transducer is an important component in the ultrasound imaging system. The transducer often consists of a liner array that can electronically focus an acoustic beam. Depending on the configuration of array elements, the region scanned may be sector shaped or rectangular in two dimensions or pyramidal shaped in three dimensions.

The transducer performance large determines the resolution and the signal-to-noise ratio of the resulting ultrasound image. The design of an array involves many compromises in choosing operating frequency and array-element dimensions. Electrical matching networks and quarter-wave matching layers may be added to improve transducer performance.

Further improvements in transducer performance may result from several areas of research. Newer materials, such as composites, are gaining widespread use in medical ultrasound. In addition, 1.5D arrays or 2D arrays may be employed to control the acoustic beam in both azimuth and elevation. Problems in fabrication and electrical impedance matching must be overcome to implement these arrays in an ultrasound system.

Defining Terms

Acoustic impedance: In an analogy to transmission line impedance, the acoustic impedance is the ratio of pressure to particle velocity in a medium; more commonly, it is defined as $Z = \rho c$, where ρ = density and c = speed of sound in a medium [the units are kg/(m^2 sec) or Rayls].

Angular response: The radiation pattern versus angle for a single element of an array.

Axial resolution: The ability to distinguish between targets aligned in the axial direction (the direction of acoustic propagation).

Azimuth dimension: The lateral dimension that is along the scanning plane for an array transducer.

Electrical matching networks: Active or passive networks designed to tune out reactive components of the transducer and match the transducer impedance to the source and receiver impedance.

Elevation dimension: The lateral dimension that is perpendicular to the scanning plane for an array transducer.

Grating lobes: Undesirable artifacts in the radiation pattern of a transducer; they are produced at a location where the path length difference to adjacent array elements is a multiple of a wavelength.

Lateral modes: Transducer vibrations that occur in the lateral dimensions when the transducer is excited in the thickness dimension.

Lateral resolution: The ability to distinguish between targets in the azimuth and elevation dimensions (perpendicular to the axial dimension).

Quarter-wave matching layers: One or more layers of material placed between the transducer and the load medium (water or human tissue); they effectively match the acoustic impedance of the transducer to the load medium to improve the transducer bandwidth and signal-to-noise ratio.

References

Allen J.L. 1964. Array antennas: new applications for an old technique. *IEEE Spect.* 1: 115.

Berlincourt D. 1971. Piezoelectric crystals and ceramics. In O.E. Mattiat (Ed.), *Ultrasonic Transducer Materials.* New York, Plenum Press.

Bobber R.J. 1970. *Underwater Electroacoustic Measurements.* Washington, Naval Research Laboratory.

Christensen D.A. 1988. *Ultrasonic Bioinstrumentation.* New York, Wiley.

Curie P. and Curie J. 1980. Development par pression de l'electricite polaire dans les cristaux hemiedres a faces enclinees. *Comp. Rend.* 91: 383.

Desilets C.S., Fraser J.D., and Kino G.S. 1978. The design of efficient broad-band piezoelectric transducers. *IEEE Trans. Son. Ultrason.* SU-25: 115.

Flax S.W. and O'Donnell M. 1988. Phase aberration correction using signals from point reflectors and diffuse scatters: basic principles. *IEEE Trans. Ultrason. Ferroelec. Freq. Contr.* 35: 758.

Goldberg R.L. and Smith S.W. 1994. Multi-layer piezoelectric ceramics for two-dimensional array transducers. *IEEE Trans. Ultrason. Ferroelec. Freq. Contr.*

Goodman W. 1986. *Introduction to Fourier Optics.* New York, McGraw-Hill.

Hunt J.W., Arditi M., and Foster F.S. 1983. Ultrasound transducers for pulse-echo medical imaging. *IEEE Trans. Biomed. Eng.* 30: 453.

Kino G.S. 1987. *Acoustic Waves.* Englewood Cliffs, NJ, Prentice-Hall.

Kino G.S. and DeSilets C.S. 1979. Design of slotted transducer arrays with matched backings. *Ultrason. Imag.* 1: 189.

Nock L.F. and Trahey G.E. 1992. Synthetic receive aperture imaging with phase correction for motion and for tissue inhomogeneities: I. Basic principles. *IEEE Trans. Ultrason. Ferroelec. Freq. Contr.* 39: 489.

Selfridge A.R., Kino G.S., and Khuri-Yahub B.T. 1980. A theory for the radiation pattern of a narrow strip acoustic transducer. *Appl. Phys. Lett.* 37: 35.

Shattuck D.P., Weinshenker M.D., Smith S.W., and von Ramm O.T. 1984. Explososcan: a parallel processing technique for high speed ultrasound imaging with linear phased arrays. *J. Acoust. Soc. Am.* 75: 1273.

Sherar M.D. and Foster F.S. 1989. The design and fabrication of high frequency poly(vinylidene fluoride) transducers. *Ultrason. Imag.* 11: 75.

Smith W.A. 1992. New opportunities in ultrasonic transducers emerging from innovations in piezoelectric materials. In F.L. Lizzi (Ed.), *New Developments in Ultrasonic Transducers and Transducer Systems,* pp. 3–26. New York, SPIE.

Somer J.C. 1968. Electronic sector scanning for ultrasonic diagnosis. *Ultrasonics* 153.

Steinberg B.D. 1976. *Principles of Aperture and Array System Design*. New York, Wiley.

Takeuchi H., Masuzawa H., Nakaya C., and Ito Y. 1990. Relaxor ferroelectric transducers. *Proceedings of IEEE Ultrasonics Symposium*, IEEE cat no 90CH2938-9, pp. 697–705.

Trahey G.E., Zhao D., Miglin J.A., and Smith S.W. 1990. Experimental results with a real-time adaptive ultrasonic imaging system for viewing through distorting media. *IEEE Trans. Ultrason. Ferroelec. Freq. Contr.* 37: 418.

von Ramm O.T. and Smith S.W. 1990. Real time volumetric ultrasound imaging system. In *SPIE Medical Imaging IV: Image Formation*, Vol. 1231, pp. 15–22. New York, SPIE.

von Ramm O.T. and Thurstone F.L. 1976. Cardiac imaging using a phased array ultrasound system: I. System design. *Circulation* 53: 258.

Further Information

A good overview of linear array design and performance is contained in von O.T. Ramm and S.W. Smith [1983], Beam steering with linear arrays, *IEEE Trans. Biomed. Eng.* 30: 438. The same issue contains a more general article on transducer design and performance: J.W. Hunt, M.'Arditi, and F.S. Foster [1983], Ultrasound transducers for pulse-echo medical imaging, *IEEE Trans. Biomed. Eng.* 30: 453.

The journal *IEEE Transactions on Ultrasonics, Ferroelectrics, and Frequency Control* frequently contains articles on medical ultrasound transducers. For subscription information, contact IEEE Service Center, 445 Hoes Lane, P.O. Box 1331, Piscataway, NJ 08855-1331, phone (800) 678-IEEE.

Another good source is the proceedings of the IEEE Ultrasonics Symposium, published each year. Also, the proceedings from *New Developments in Ultrasonics Transducers and Transducer Systems*, edited by F.L. Lizzi, was published by SPIE, Vol. 1733, in 1992.

14.2 Ultrasonic Imaging

Jack G. Mottley

It was recognized long ago that the tissues of the body are inhomogeneous and that signals sent into them, like pulses of high-frequency sound, are reflected and scattered by those tissues. **Scattering**, or redirection of some of an incident energy signal to other directions by small particles, is why we see the beam of a spotlight in fog or smoke. That part of the scattered energy that returns to the transmitter is called the **backscatter**.

Ultrasonic imaging of the soft tissues of the body really began in the early 1970s. At that time, the technologies began to become available to capture and display the echoes backscattered by structures within the body as images, at first as static **compound images** and later as real-time moving images. The development followed much the same sequence (and borrowed much of the terminology) as did radar and sonar, from initial crude single-line-of-sight displays (**A-mode**) to recording these side by side to build up recordings over time to show motion (**M-mode**), to finally sweeping the transducer either mechanically or electronically over many directions and building up two-dimensional views (**B-mode or 2D**).

Since this technology was intended for civilian use, applications had to wait for the development of inexpensive data handling, storage, and display technologies. A-mode was usually shown on oscilloscopes, M-modes were printed onto specially treated light-sensitive thermal paper, and B-mode was initially built up as a static image in analog scan converters and shown on television monitors. Now all modes are produced in real time in proprietary scan converters, shown on television monitors, and recorded either on commercially available videotape recorders (for organs or studies in which motion is a part of the diagnostic information) or as still frames on photographic film (for those cases in which organ dimensions and appearance are useful, but motion is not important).

Using commercial videotape reduces expenses and greatly simplifies the review of cases for quality control and training, since review stations can be set up in offices or conference rooms with commonly

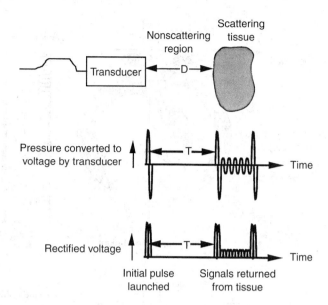

FIGURE 14.10   Schematic representation of the signal received from along a single line of sight in a tissue. The rectified voltage signals are displayed for A-mode.

available monitors and videocassette recorders, and tapes from any imaging system can be played back. Also, the tapes are immediately available and do not have to be chemically processed.

Since the earliest systems were mostly capable of showing motion, the first applications were in studying the heart, which must move to carry out its function. A-mode and M-mode displays (see Figures 14.10–14.12) were able to demonstrate the motion of valves, thickening of heart chamber walls, relationships between heart motion and pressure, and other parameters that enabled diagnoses of heart problems that had been difficult or impossible before. For some valvular diseases, the preferred display format for diagnosis is still the M-mode, on which the speed of valve motions can be measured and the relations of valve motions to the electrocardiogram (ECG) are easily seen.

Later, as 2D displays became available, ultrasound was applied more and more to imaging of the soft abdominal organs and in obstetrics (Figure 14.13). In this format, organ dimensions and structural relations are seen more easily, and since the images are now made in real time, motions of organs such as the heart are still well appreciated. These images are used in a wide variety of areas from obstetrics and gynecology to ophthalmology to measure the dimensions of organs or tissue masses and have been widely accepted as a safe and convenient imaging modality.

14.2.1   Fundamentals

Strictly speaking, ultrasound is simply any sound wave whose frequency is above the limit of human hearing, which is usually taken to be 20 kHz. In the context of imaging of the human body, since frequency and wavelength (and therefore resolution) are inversely related, the lowest frequency of sound commonly used is around 1 MHz, with a constant trend toward higher frequencies in order to obtain better resolution. Axial resolution is approximately one wavelength, and at 1 MHz, the wavelength is 1.5 mm in most soft tissues, so one must go to 1.5 MHz to achieve 1-mm resolution.

Attenuation of ultrasonic signals increases with frequency in soft tissues, and so a tradeoff must be made between the depth of penetration that must be achieved for a particular application and the highest frequency that can be used. Applications that require deep penetration (e.g., cardiology, abdominal, obstetrics) typically use frequencies in the 2- to 5-MHz range, while those applications which only require shallow penetration but high resolution (e.g., ophthalmology, peripheral vascular, testicular) use

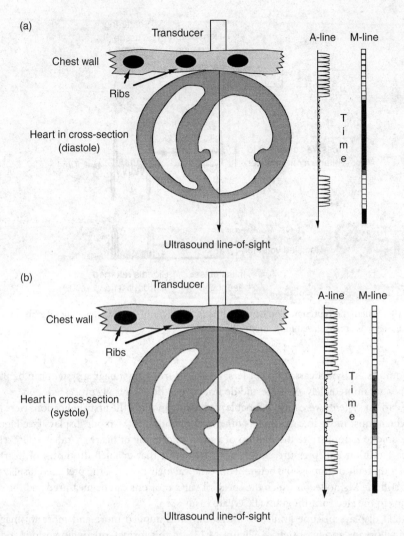

FIGURE 14.11 Example of M-mode imaging of a heart at two points during the cardiac cycle. (a) Upper panel shows heart during diastole (relaxation) with a line of sight through it and the corresponding A-line converted to an M-line. (b) The lower panel shows the same heart during systole (contraction) and the A- and M-lines. Note the thicker walls and smaller ventricular cross-section during systole.

frequencies up to around 20 MHz. Intra-arterial imaging systems, requiring submillimeter resolution, use even higher frequencies of 20 to 50 MHz, and laboratory applications of ultrasonic microscopy use frequencies up to 100 or even 200 MHz to examine structures within individual cells.

There are two basic equations used in ultrasonic imaging. One relates the (one-way) distance d of an object that caused an echo from the transducer to the (round-trip) time delay t and speed of sound in the medium c:

$$d = \frac{1}{2} tc \tag{14.24}$$

The speed of sound in soft body tissues lies in a fairly narrow range from 1450 to 1520 m/sec. For rough estimates of time of flight, one often uses 1500 m/sec, which can be converted to 1.5 mm/μsec, a more convenient set of units. This leads to delay times for the longest-range measurements (20 cm) of 270 μsec.

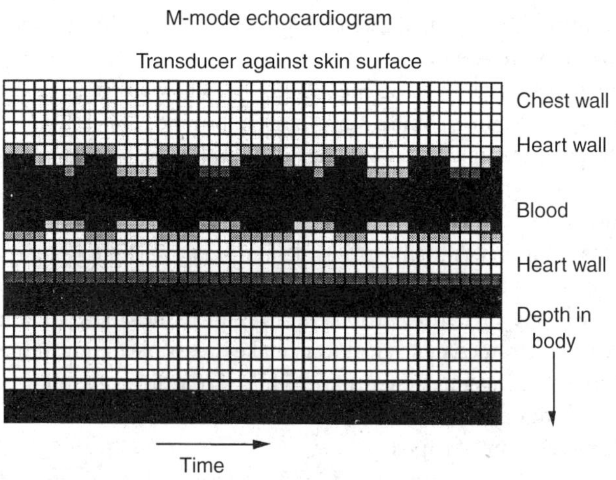

M-mode echocardiogram

Transducer against skin surface

Chest wall

Heart wall

Blood

Heart wall

Depth in body

Time

FIGURE 14.12 Completed M-mode display obtained by showing the M-lines of Figure 14.11 side by side. The motion of the heart walls and their thickening and thinning are well appreciated. Often the ECG or heart sounds are also shown in order to coordinate the motions of the heart with other physiologic markers.

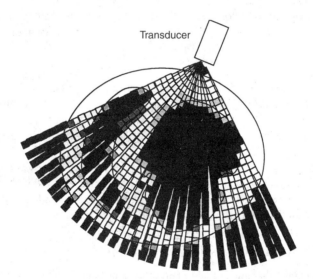

Transducer

FIGURE 14.13 Schematic representation of a heart and how a 2D image is constructed by scanning the transducer.

To allow echoes and reverberations to die out, one needs to wait several of these periods before launching the next interrogating pulse, so pulse repetition frequencies of about a kilohertz are possible.

The other equation relates the received signal strength $S(t)$ to the transmitted signal $T(t)$, the transducer's properties $B(t)$, the attenuation of the signal path to and from the scatterer $A(t)$, and the strength of the scatterer $h(t)$:

$$S(t) = T(t) \otimes B(t) \otimes A(t) \otimes \eta(t) \tag{14.25}$$

where $\otimes$ denotes time-domain convolution. Using the property of Fourier transforms that a convolution in the time domain is a multiplication in the frequency domain, this is more often written in the frequency domain as

$$S(f) = T(f)B(f)A(f)\eta(f) \tag{14.26}$$

where each term is the Fourier transform of the corresponding term in the time-domain expression 14.25 and is written as a function of frequency f.

The goal of most imaging applications is to measure and produce an image based on the local values of the scattering strength, which requires some assumptions to be made concerning each of the other terms. The amplitude of the transmitted signal $T(f)$ is a user-adjustable parameter that simply adds a scale factor to the image values, unless it increases the returned signal to the point of saturating the receiver amplifier. Increasing the transmit power increases the strength of return from distant or faint echoes simply by increasing the power that illuminates them, like using a more powerful flashlight lets you see farther at night. Some care must be taken to not turn the transmit power up too high, since very high power levels are capable of causing acoustic cavitation or local heating of tissues, both of which can cause cellular damage. Advances in both electronics and transducers make it possible to transmit more and more power. For this reason, new ultrasonic imaging systems are required to display an index value that indicates the transmitted power. If the index exceeds established thresholds, it is possible that damage may occur, and the examiner should limit the time of exposure.

Most imaging systems are fairly narrow band, so the transducer properties $B(f)$ are constant and produce only a scale factor to the image values. On phased-array systems it is possible to change the depth of focus on both transmit and receive. This improves image quality and detection of lesions by matching the focusing characteristics of the transducer to best image the object in question, like focusing a pair of binoculars on a particular object.

As the ultrasonic energy travels along the path from transmitter to scatterer and back, attenuation causes the signal to decrease with distance. This builds up as a line integral from time 0 to time t as

$$A(f, t) = e^{-\int_0^t \alpha(f)c\,dt'}$$

An average value of attenuation can be corrected for electronically by increasing the gain of the imaging system as a function of time (variously called time gain compensation [TGC] or depth gain compensation [DGC]). In addition, some systems allow for lateral portions of the image region to have different attenuation by adding a lateral gain compensation in which the gain is increased to either side of the center region of the image.

Time gain compensation is usually set to give a uniform gray level to the scattering along the center of the image. Most operators develop a "usual" setting on each machine, and if it becomes necessary to change those settings to obtain acceptable images on a patient, then that indicates that the patient has a higher attenuation or that there is a problem with the electronics, transducer, or acoustic coupling.

14.2.2 Applications and Example Calculations

As an example of calculating the time of flight of an ultrasonic image, consider the following.

Example 1. A tissue has a speed of sound $c = 1460$ m/sec, and a given feature is 10 cm deep within. Calculate the time it will take an ultrasonic signal to travel from the surface to the feature and back.

Answer: $t = 2 \times (10 \text{ cm})/(1460 \text{ m/sec}) = 137 \ \mu\text{sec}$, where the factor of 2 is to account for the round trip the signal has to make (i.e., go in and back out).

Example 2. Typical soft tissues attenuate ultrasonic signals at a rate of 0.5 dB/cm/MHz. How much attenuation would be suffered by a 3-MHz signal going through 5 cm of tissue and returning?
Answer: $a = 3 \text{ MHz} \times (0.5 \text{ dB/cm/MHz})/(8.686 \text{ dB/neper}) = 0.173 \text{ neper/cm}$, $A(3 \text{ MHz}, 5 \text{ cm}) = e^{(-0.173 \text{ neper/cm}) \times (5 \text{ cm}) \times 2} = 0.177$.

14.2.3 Economics

Ultrasonic imaging has many economic advantages over other imaging modalities. The imaging systems are typically much less expensive than those used for other modalities and do not require special preparations of facilities such as shielding for x-rays or uniformity of magnetic field for MRI. Most ultrasonic imaging systems can be rolled easily from one location to another, so one system can be shared among technicians or examining rooms or even taken to patients' rooms for critically ill patients.

There are minimal expendables used in ultrasonic examinations, mostly the coupling gel used to couple the transducer to the skin and videotape or film for recording. Transducers are reusable and amortized over many examinations. These low costs make ultrasonic imaging one of the least expensive modalities, far preferred over others when indicated. The low cost also means these systems can be a part of private practices and used only occasionally.

As an indication of the interest in ultrasonic imaging as an alternative to other modalities, in 1993, the *Wall Street Journal* reported that spending in the United States on MRI units was approximately $520 million, on CT units $800 million, and on ultrasonic imaging systems $1000 million, and that sales of ultrasound systems was growing at 15% annually [1].

Defining Terms

A-mode: The original display of ultrasound measurements, in which the amplitude of the returned echoes along a single line is displayed on an oscilloscope.

Attenuation: The reduction is signal amplitude that occurs per unit distance traveled. Some attenuation occurs in homogeneous media such as water due to viscous heating and other phenomena, but that is very small and is usually taken to be negligible over the 10- to 20-cm distances typical of imaging systems. In inhomogeneous media such as soft tissues, the attenuation is much higher and increases with frequency. The values reported for most soft tissues lie around 0.5 dB/cm/MHz.

Backscatter: That part of a scattered signal that goes back toward the transmitter of the energy.

B-mode or 2D: The current display mode of choice. This is produced by sweeping the transducer from side to side and displaying the strength of the returned echoes as bright spots in their geometrically correct direction and distance.

Compound images: Images built up by adding, or compounding, data obtained from a single transducer or multiple transducers swept through arcs. Often these transducers were not fixed to a single point of rotation but could be swept over a surface of the body like the abdomen in order to build up a picture of the underlying organs such as the liver. This required an elaborate position-sensing apparatus attached to the patient's bed or the scanner and that the organ in question be held very still throughout the scanning process, or else the image was blurred.

M-mode: Followed A-mode by recording the strength of the echoes as dark spots on moving light-sensitive paper. Objects that move, such as the heart, caused standard patterns of motion to be displayed, and a lot of diagnostic information such as valve closure rates, whether valves opened or closed completely, and wall thickness could be obtained from M-mode recordings.

Real-time images: Images currently made on ultrasound imaging systems by rapidly sweeping the transducer through an arc either mechanically or electronically. Typical images might have 120 scan lines in each image, each 20 cm long. Since each line has a time of flight of 267 μsec, a single frame takes 120×267 μsec $= 32$ msec. It is therefore possible to produce images at standard video frame rates (30 frames/sec, or 33.3 msec/frame).

Reflection: Occurs at interfaces between large regions (much larger than a wavelength) of media with differing acoustic properties such as density or compressibility. This is similar to the reflection of light at interfaces and can be either total, like a mirror, or partial, like a half-silvered mirror or the ghostlike reflection seen in a sheet of glass.

Scattering: Occurs when there are irregularities or inhomogeneities in the acoustic properties of a medium over distances comparable with or smaller than the wavelength of the sound. Scattering from objects much smaller than a wavelength typically increases with frequency (the blue-sky law in optics), while that from an object comparable to a wavelength is constant with frequency (why clouds appear white).

Reference

[1] Naj A.K. 1993. Industry focus: big medical equipment makers try ultrasound market; cost-cutting pressures prompt shift away from more expensive devices. *Wall Street J.*, November 30, B-4.

Further Information

There are many textbooks that contain good introduction to ultrasonic imaging. *Physical Principles of Ultrasonic Diagnosis*, by P. N. Wells, is a classic, and there is a new edition of another classic, *Diagnostic Ultrasound*: *Principles, Instruments and Exercises*, 4th ed., by Frederick Kremkau. Books on medical imaging that contain introductions to ultrasonic imaging include *Medical Imaging Systems*, by Albert Macovski; *Principles of Medical Imaging*, by Kirk Shung, Michael Smith, and Benjamin Tsui; and *Foundations of Medical Imaging*, by Zang-Hee Cho, Joie P. Jones, and Manbir Singh.

The monthly journals *IEEE Transactions on Ultrasonics, Ferroelectrics, and Frequency Control* and *IEEE Transactions on Biomedical Engineering* often contain information and research reports on ultrasonic imaging. For subscription information, contact IEEE Service Center, 445 Hoes Lane, P.O. Box 1331, Piscataway, NJ 08855-1331, phone (800) 678-4333. Another journal that often contains articles on ultrasonic imaging is the *Journal of the Acoustical Society of America*. For subscription information, contact AIP Circulation and Fulfillment Division, 500 Sunnyside Blvd., Woodbury, NY 11797-2999, phone (800) 344-6908; e-mail: elecprod\@pinet.aip.org.

There are many journals that deal with medical ultrasonic imaging exclusively. These include *Ultrasonic Imaging, the Journal of Ultrasound in Medicine*, American Institute of Ultrasound of Medicine (AIUM), 14750 Sweitzer Lane, Suite 100, Laurel, MD 20707-5906, and the Journal of Ultrasound in Medicine and Biology, Elsevier Science, Inc., 660 White Plains Road, Tarrytown, NY 10591-5153, e-mail: esuk.usa@elsevier.com.

There are also specialty journals for particular medical areas, e.g., the *Journal of the American Society of Echocardiography*, that are available through medical libraries and are indexed in Index Medicus, Current Contents, Science Citation Index, and other databases.

14.3   Blood Flow Measurement Using Ultrasound

K. Whittaker Ferrara

In order to introduce the fundamental challenges of blood velocity estimation, a brief description of the unique operating environment produced by the ultrasonic system, intervening tissue, and the scattering of ultrasound by blood is provided. In providing an overview of the parameters that differentiate this problem from radar and sonar target estimation problems, an introduction to the fluid dynamics of the cardiovascular system is presented, and the requirements of specific clinical applications are summarized. An overview of blood flow estimation systems and their performance limitations is then presented. Next, an overview of the theory of moving target estimation, with its roots in radar and sonar signal processing, is provided. The application of this theory to blood velocity estimation is then reviewed, and a number of signal processing strategies that have been applied to this problem are considered. Areas of new research including three-dimensional (3D) velocity estimation and the use of ultrasonic contrast agents are described in the final section.

14.3.1   Fundamental Concepts

In blood velocity estimation, the goal is not simply to estimate the mean target position and mean target velocity. The goal instead is to measure the velocity profile over the smallest region possible and to repeat this measurement quickly and accurately over the entire target. Therefore, the joint optimization of spatial, velocity, and temporal resolution is critical. In addition to the mean velocity, diagnostically useful information is contained in the volume of blood flowing through various vessels, spatial variations in the velocity profile, and the presence of turbulence. While current methods have proven extremely valuable in the assessment of the velocity profile over an entire vessel, improved *spatial resolution* is required in several diagnostic situations. Improved *velocity resolution* is also desirable for a number of clinical applications. Blood velocity estimation algorithms implemented in current systems also suffer from a velocity ambiguity due to aliasing.

14.3.1.1 Unique Features of the Operating Environment

A number of features make blood flow estimation distinct from typical radar and sonar target estimation situations. The combination of factors associated with the beam formation system, properties of the intervening medium, and properties of the target medium lead to a difficult and unique operating environment. Figure 14.14 summarizes the operating environment of an ultrasonic blood velocity estimation system, and Table 14.2 summarizes the key parameters.

14.3.1.1.1 Beam formation — data acquisition system

The transducer bandwidth is limited. Most current transducers are limited to a 50 to 75% fractional bandwidth due to their finite dimensions and a variety of electrical and mechanical properties. This

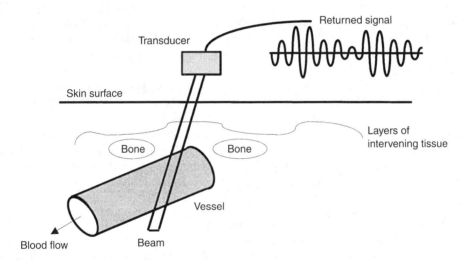

FIGURE 14.14   Operating environment for the estimation of blood velocity.

TABLE 14.2   Important Parameters

Typical transducer center frequency	2–10 MHz
Maximum transducer fractional bandwidth	50–75%
Speed of sound c	1500–1600 m/sec
Acoustic wavelength ($c = 1540$)	0.154–1.54 mm
Phased-array size	$>32 \cdot$ wavelength
Sample volume size	mm^3
Blood velocity	Normal; up to 1 m/sec
	Pathological: up to 8 m/sec
Vessel wall echo/blood echo	20–40 dB
Diameter of a red blood cell	8.5 μm
Thickness of a red blood cell	2.4 μm
Volume of a red blood cell	87 ± 6 mm^3
Volume concentration of cells (hematocrit)	45%
Maximum concentration without cell deformation	58%

limits the form of the transmitted signal. The transmitted pulse is typically a short pulse with a **carrier frequency**, which is the center frequency in the spectrum of the transmitted signal.

Federal agencies monitor four distinct intensity levels. The levels are TASA, TASP, TPSA, and TPSP, where T represents temporal, S represents spatial, A represents average, and P represents peak. Therefore, the use of long bursts requires a proportionate reduction in the transmitted peak power. This may limit the signal-to-noise ratio (SNR) obtained with a long transmitted burst due to the weak reflections from the complex set of targets within the body.

14.3.1.1.2 *Intervening medium*

Acoustic windows, which are locations for placement of a transducer to successfully interrogate particular organs, are limited in number and size. Due to the presence of bone and air, the number of usable acoustic windows is extremely limited. The reflection of acoustic energy from bone is only 3 dB below that of a perfect reflector [Wells, 1977]. Therefore, transducers cannot typically surround a desired imaging site. In many cases, it is difficult to find a single small access window. This limits the use of inverse techniques.

Intervening tissue produces acoustic refraction and reflection. Energy is reflected at unpredictable angles.

The **clutter**-to-signal ratio is very high. Clutter is the returned signal from stationary or slowly moving tissue, which can be 40 dB above the returned signal from blood. Movement of the vessel walls and valves during the cardiac cycle introduces a high-amplitude, low-frequency signal. This is typically considered to be unwanted noise, and a high-pass filter is used to eliminate the estimated wall frequencies.

The sampling rate is restricted. The speed of sound in tissue is low ($\sim$1540 m/sec), and each transmitted pulse must reach the target and return before the returned signal is recorded. Thus the sampling rate is restricted, and the aliasing limit is often exceeded.

The total observation time is limited (due to low acoustic velocity). In order to estimate the velocity of blood in all locations in a 2D field in real time, the estimate for each region must be based on the return from a limited number of pulses because of the low speed of sound.

Frequency-dependent attenuation affects the signal. Tissue acts as a low-pass transmission filter; the scattering functions as a high-pass filter. The received signal is therefore a distorted version of the transmitted signal. In order to estimate the effective filter function, the type and extent of each tissue type encountered by the wave must be known. Also, extension of the bandwidth of the transmitted signal to higher frequencies increases absorption, requiring higher power levels that can increase health concerns.

14.3.1.1.3 *Target scattering medium (red blood cells)*

Multiple groups of scatterers are present. The target medium consists of multiple volumes of diffuse moving scatterers with velocity vectors that vary in magnitude and direction. The target medium is spread in space and velocity. The goal is to estimate the velocity over the smallest region possible.

There is a limited period of statistical stationarity. The underlying cardiac process can only be considered to be stationary for a limited time. This time was estimated to be 10 msec for the arterial system by Hatle and Angelsen [1985]. If an observation interval greater than this period is used, the average scatterer velocity cannot be considered to be constant.

14.3.1.2 Overview of Ultrasonic Flow Estimation Systems

Current ultrasonic imaging systems operate in a pulse-echo (PE) or continuous-wave (CW) intensity mapping mode. In pulse-echo mode, a very short pulse is transmitted, and the reflected signal is analyzed. For a continuous-wave system, a lower-intensity signal is continuously transmitted into the body, and the reflected energy is analyzed. In both types of systems, an acoustic wave is launched along a specific path into the body, and the return from this wave is processed as a function of time. The return is due to reflected waves from structures along the line of sight, combined with unwanted noise. Spatial selectivity is provided by beam formation performed on burst transmission and reception. Steering of the beam to a particular angle and creating a narrow beam width at the depth of interest are accomplished by an effective lens applied to the ultrasonic transducer. This lens may be produced by a contoured material, or it may be simulated by phased pulses applied to a transducer array. The spatial weighting pattern will ultimately be the product of the effective lens on transmission and reception. The returned signal from the formed beam can be used to map the backscattered intensity into a two-dimensional gray-scale image, or to estimate target velocity. *We shall focus on the use of this information to estimate the velocity of red blood cells moving through the body.*

14.3.1.2.1 Single sample volume doppler instruments

One type of system uses the Doppler effect to estimate velocity in a single volume of blood, known as the sample volume, which is designated by the system operator. The Doppler shift frequency from a moving target can be shown to equal $2f_c v/c$, where f_c is the transducer center frequency in Hertz, c is the speed of sound within tissue, and v is the velocity component of the blood cells toward or away from the transducer. These "Doppler" systems transmit a train of long pulses with a well-defined carrier frequency and measure the Doppler shift in the returned signal. The spectrum of Doppler frequencies is proportional to the distribution of velocities present in the sample volume. The sample volume is on a cubic millimeter scale for typical pulse-echo systems operating in the frequency range of 2–10 MHz. Therefore, a thorough cardiac or peripheral vascular examination requires a long period. In these systems, 64–128 temporal samples are acquired for each estimate. The spectrum of these samples is typically computed using a fast Fourier transform (FFT) technique [Kay and Marple, 1981]. The range of velocities present within the sample volume can then be estimated. The spectrum is scaled to represent velocity and plotted on the vertical axis. Subsequent spectral estimates are then calculated and plotted vertically adjacent to the first estimate.

14.3.1.2.2 Color flow mapping

In color flow mapping, a pseudo-color velocity display is overlaid on a 2D gray-scale image. Simultaneous amplitude and velocity information is thus available for a 2D sector area of the body. The clinical advantage is a reduction in the examination time and the ability to visualize the velocity profile as a 2D map. Figure 14.15 shows a typical color flow map of ovarian blood flow combined with the Doppler spectrum of the region indicated by the small graphic sample volume. The color flow map shows color-encoded velocities superimposed on the gray-scale image with the velocity magnitude indicated by the color bar on the side of the image. Motion toward the transducer is shown in yellow and red, and motion away from the transducer is shown in blue and green, with the range of colors representing a range of velocities to a maximum of 6 cm/sec in each direction. Velocities above this limit would produce aliasing for the parameters used in optimizing the instrument for the display of ovarian flow. A velocity of 0 m/sec

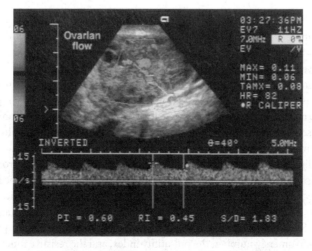

FIGURE 14.15   Flow map and Doppler spectrum for ovarian blood flow.

would be indicated by black, as shown at the center of the color bar. Early discussions of the implement-ation of color flow mapping systems can be found in Curry and White [1978] and Nowicki and Reid [1981].

The lower portion of the image presents an intensity-modulated display of instantaneous Doppler components along the vertical axis. As time progresses, the display is translated along the horizontal axis to generate a Doppler time history for the selected region of interest (provided by Acuson Corporation, Mountain View, California).

Limitations of color flow instruments result in part from the transmission of a narrowband (long) pulse that is needed for velocity estimation but degrades spatial resolution and prevents mapping of the spatial-velocity profile. Due to the velocity gradient in each blood vessel, the transmission of a long pulse also degrades the velocity resolution. This is caused by the simultaneous examination of blood cells moving at different velocities and the resulting mixing of regions of the scattering medium, which can be distinctly resolved on a conventional B-mode image. Since the limited speed of acoustic propagation velocity limits the sampling rate, a second problem is aliasing of the Doppler frequency. Third, information regarding the presence of velocity gradients and turbulence is desired and is not currently available. Finally, estimation of blood velocity based on the Doppler shift provides only an estimate of the axial velocity, which is the movement toward or away from the transducer, and cannot be used to estimate movement across the transducer beam. It is the 3D velocity magnitude that is of clinical interest.

For a color flow map, the velocity estimation technique is based on estimation of the mean Doppler shift using signal-processing techniques optimized for rapid (real-time) estimation of velocity in each region of the image. The transmitted pulse is typically a burst of 4 to 8 cycles of the carrier frequency. Data acquisition for use in velocity estimation is interleaved with the acquisition of information for the gray-scale image. Each frame of acquired data samples is used to generate one update of the image display. An azimuthal line is a line that describes the direction of the beam from the transducer to the target. A typical 2D ultrasound scanner uses 128 azimuthal lines per frame and 30 frames per second to generate a gray-scale image. Data acquisition for the velocity estimator used in color flow imaging requires an additional 4 to 18 transducer firings per azimuthal line and therefore reduces both the number of azimuthal lines and the number of frames per second. If the number of lines per frame is decreased, spatial undersampling or a reduced examination area results. If the number of frames per second is decreased, temporal undersampling results, and the display becomes difficult to interpret.

The number of data samples available for each color flow velocity estimate is reduced to 4–18 in comparison with the 64–128 data samples available to estimate velocity in a single sample volume Doppler mode. This reduction, required to estimate velocity over the 2D image, produces a large increase in the estimator variance.

14.3.1.3 Fluid Dynamics and the Cardiovascular System

In order to predict and adequately assess blood flow profiles within the body, the fluid dynamics of the cardiovascular system will be briefly reviewed. The idealized case known as Poiseuille flow will be considered first, allowed by a summary of the factors that disturb Poiseuille flow.

A Poiseuille flow model is appropriate in a long rigid circular pipe at a large distance from the entrance. The velocity in this case is described by the equation $v/v_0 = 1 - (r/a)^2$, where v represents the velocity parallel to the wall, v_0 represents the center-line velocity, r is the radial distance variable, and a is the radius of the tube. In this case, the mean velocity is half the center-line velocity, and the volume flow rate is given by the mean velocity multiplied by the cross-sectional area of the vessel.

For the actual conditions within the arterial system, Poiseuille flow is only an approximation. The actual arterial geometry is tortuous and individualistic, and the resulting flow is perturbed by entrance effects and reflections. Reflections are produced by vascular branches and the geometric taper of the arterial diameter. In addition, spatial variations in vessel elasticity influence the amplitude and wave velocity of the arterial pulse. Several parameters can be used to characterize the velocity profile, including the Reynolds number, the Womersly number, the pulsatility index, and the resistive index. The pulsatility and resistive indices are frequently estimated during a clinical examination.

The Reynolds number is denoted Re and measures the ratio of fluid inertia to the viscous forces acting on the fluid. The Reynolds number is defined by $Re = Dv'/\mu_k$, where v' is the average cross-sectional velocity μ_k is the kinematic viscosity, and D is the vessel diameter. *Kinematic viscosity* is defined as the fluid viscosity divided by the fluid density. When the Reynolds number is high, fluid inertia dominates. This is true in the aorta and larger arteries, and bursts of turbulence are possible. When the number is low, viscous effects dominate.

The Womersly number is used to describe the effect introduced by the unsteady, pulsatile nature of the flow. This parameter, defined by $a(\omega/\mu_k)^{1/2}$, where ω represents radian frequency of the wave, governs propagation along an elastic, fluid-filled tube. When the Womersly number is small, the instantaneous profile will be parabolic in shape, the flow is viscous dominated, and the profile is oscillatory and Poiseuille in nature. When the Womersly number is large, the flow will be blunt, inviscid, and have thin wall layers [Nicholas and O'Rourke, 1990].

The pulsatility index represents the ratio of the unsteady and steady velocity components of the flow. This shows the magnitude of the velocity changes that occur during acceleration and deceleration of blood constituents. Since the arterial pulse decreases in magnitude as it travels, this index is maximum in the aorta. The pulsatility index is given by the difference between the peak systolic and minimum diastolic values divided by the average value over one cardiac cycle. The Pourcelot, or resistance, index is the peak-to-peak swing in velocity from systole to diastole divided by the peak systolic value [Nichols and O'Rourke, 1990].

14.3.1.3.1 Blood velocity profiles

Specific factors that influence the blood velocity profile include the entrance effect, vessel curvature, skewing, stenosis, acceleration, secondary flows, and turbulence. These effects are briefly introduced in this section.

The entrance effect is a result of fluid flow passing from a large tube or chamber into a smaller tube. The velocity distribution at the entrance becomes blunt. At a distance known as the entry length, the fully developed parabolic profile is restored, where the entry length is given by $0.06Re \cdot (2a)$ [Nerem, 1985]. Distal to this point the profile is independent of distance.

If the vessel is curved, there will also be an entrance effect. The blunt profile in this case is skewed, with the peak velocity closer to the inner wall of curvature. When the fully developed profile occurs downstream, the distribution will again be skewed, with the maximal velocity toward the outer wall of curvature. Skewing also occurs at a bifurcation where proximal flow divides into daughter vessels. The higher-velocity components, which occurred at the center of the parent vessel, are then closer to the flow divider, and the velocity distribution in the daughter vessels is skewed toward the divider.

Stenosis, a localized narrowing of the vessel diameter, dampens the pulsatility of the flow and pressure waveforms. The downstream flow profile depends on the shape and degree of stenosis. Acceleration adds a flat component to the velocity profile. It is responsible for the flat profile during systole, as well as the negative flat component near the walls in the deceleration phase.

Secondary flows are swirling components which are superimposed on the main velocity profile. These occur at bends and branches, although regions of secondary flow can break away from the vessel wall and are then known as separated flow. These regions reattach to the wall at a point downstream.

One definition of turbulent flow is flow that demonstrates a random fluctuation in the magnitude and direction of velocity as a function of space and time. The intensity of turbulence is calculated using the magnitude of the fluctuating velocities. The relative intensity of turbulence is given by $I_t = u_{rms}/u_{mean}$, where urms represents the root-mean-square value of the fluctuating portion of the velocity, and u_{mean} represents the nonfluctuating mean velocity [Hinze, 1975]).

14.3.1.4 Clinical Applications and Their Requirements

Blood flow measurement with ultrasound is used in estimating the velocity and volume of flow within the heart and peripheral arteries and veins. Normal blood vessels vary in diameter up to a maximum of 2 cm, although most vessels examined with ultrasound have a diameter of 1 to 10 mm. Motion of the vessel wall results in a diameter change of 5 to 10% during a cardiac cycle.

14.3.1.4.1   Carotid arteries (common, internal, external)

The evaluation of flow in the carotid arteries is of great clinical interest due to their importance in supplying blood to the brain, their proximity to the skin, and the wealth of experience that has been developed in characterizing vascular pathology through an evaluation of flow. The size of the carotid arteries is moderate; they narrow quickly from a maximum diameter of 0.8 cm. The shape of carotid flow waveforms over the cardiac cycle can be related to the pathophysiology of the circulation. Numerous attempts have been made to characterize the parameters of carotid waveforms and to compare these parameters in normal and stenotic cases. A number of indices have been used to summarize the information contained in these waveforms. The normal range of the Pourcelot index is 0.55 to 0.75. Many researchers have shown that accurate detection of a minor stenosis requires accurate quantitation of the entire Doppler spectrum and remains very difficult with current technology. The presence of a stenosis causes spectral broadening with the introduction of lower frequency or velocity components.

14.3.1.4.2   Cardiology

Blood velocity measurement in cardiology requires analysis of information at depths up to 18 cm. A relatively low center frequency (e.g., 2.5 to 3.5 MHz) typically is used in order to reduce attenuation. Areas commonly studied and the maximum rate of flow include the following [Hatle, 1985]:

Normal Adult Maximal Velocity (m/sec)	
Mitral flow	0.9
Tricuspid flow	0.5
Pulmonary artery	0.75
Left ventricle	0.9

14.3.1.4.3   Aorta

Aortic flow exhibits a blunt profile with entrance region characteristics. The entrance length is approximately 30 cm. The vessel diameter is approximately 2 cm. The mean Reynolds number is 2500 [Nerem, 1985], although the peak Reynolds number in the ascending aorta can range from 4300 to 8900, and the peak Reynolds number in the abdominal aorta is in the range of 400 to 1100 [Nichols and O'Rourke, 1990]. The maximal velocity is on the order of 1.35 m/sec. The flow is skewed in the aortic arch with a higher velocity at the inner wall. The flow is unsteady and laminar with possible turbulent bursts at peak systole.

14.3.1.4.4   Peripheral arteries

The peak systolic velocity [Hatsukami et al., 1992] in centimeters per second and standard deviation of the velocity measurement technique are provided below for selected arteries.

Artery	Peak systolic velocity (cm/sec)	Standard deviation
Proximal external iliac	99	22
Distal external iliac	96	13
Proximal common femoral	89	16
Distal common femoral	71	15
Proximal popliteal	53	9
Distal popliteal	53	24
Proximal peroneal	46	14
Distal peroneal	44	12

Nearly all the vessels above normally show some flow reversal during early diastole. A value of the pulsatility index of 5 or more in a limb artery is considered to be normal.

14.3.2 Velocity Estimation Techniques

Prior to the basic overview of theoretical approaches to target velocity estimation, it is necessary to understand a few basic features of the received signal from blood scatterers. It is the statistical correlation of the received signal in space and time that provides the opportunity to use a variety of velocity estimation strategies. Velocity estimation based on analysis of the frequency shift or the temporal correlation can be justified by these statistical properties.

Blood velocity mapping has unique features due to the substantial viscosity of blood and the spatial limitations imposed by the vessel walls. Because of these properties, groups of red blood cells can be tracked over a significant distance. Blood consists of a viscous incompressible fluid containing an average volume concentration of red blood cells of 45%, although this concentration varies randomly through the blood medium. The red blood cells are primarily responsible for producing the scattered wave, due to the difference in their acoustic properties in comparison with plasma. Recent research into the characteristics of blood has led to stochastic models for its properties as a function of time and space [Atkinson and Berry, 1974; Shung et al., 1976, 1992; Angelson, 1980; Mo and Cobbold, 1986]. The scattered signal from an insonified spatial volume is a random process that varies with the fluctuations in the density of scatterers in the insonified area, the shear rate within the vessel, and the hematocrit [Atkinson and Berry, 1974; Mo and Cobbold, 1986; Ferrara and Algazi, 1994a,b].

Since the concentration of cells varies randomly through the vessel, the magnitude of the returned signal varies when the group of scatterers being insonified changes. The returned amplitude from one spatial region is independent of the amplitude of the signal from adjacent spatial areas. As blood flows through a vessel, it transports cells whose backscattered signals can be tracked to estimate flow velocities.

Between the transmission of one pulse and the next, the scatterers move a small distance within the vessel. As shown in Figure 14.16, a group of cells with a particular concentration which are originally located at depth D_1 at time T_1 move to depth D_2 at time T_2. The resulting change in axial depth produces a change in the delay of the signal returning to the transducer from each group of scatterers. This change in delay of the radiofrequency (RF) signal can be estimated in several ways. As shown in Figure 14.17, the returned signal from a set of sequential pulses then shows a random amplitude that can be used to estimate the velocity. Motion is detected using signal-processing techniques that estimate the shift of the signal between pulses.

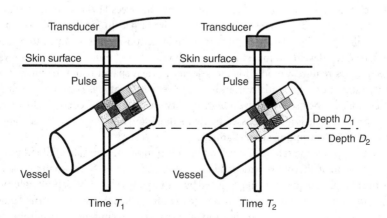

FIGURE 14.16 Random concentration of red blood cells within a vessel at times T_1 and T_2, where the change in depth from D_1 to D_2 would be used to estimate velocity.

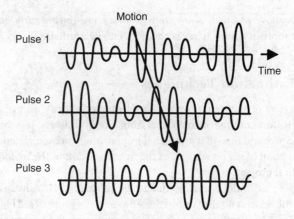

FIGURE 14.17 Received RF signal from three transmitted pulses, with a random amplitude which can be used to estimate the axial movement of blood between pulses. Motion is shown by the shift in the signal with a recognizable amplitude.

14.3.2.1 Clutter

In addition to the desired signal from the blood scatterers, the received signal contains clutter echoes returned from the surrounding tissue. An important component of this clutter signal arises from slowly moving vessel walls. The wall motion produces Doppler frequency shifts typically below 1 kHz, while the desired information from the blood cells exists in frequencies up to 15 kHz. Due to the smooth structure of the walls, energy is scattered coherently, and the clutter signal can be 40 dB above the scattered signal from blood. High-pass filters have been developed to remove the unwanted signal from the surrounding vessel walls.

14.3.2.2 Classic Theory of Velocity Estimation

Most current commercial ultrasound systems transmit a train of long pulses with a carrier frequency of 2 to 10 MHz and estimate velocity using the Doppler shift of the reflected signal. The transmission of a train of short pulses and new signal-processing strategies may improve the spatial resolution and quality of the resulting velocity estimate. In order to provide a basis for discussion and comparison of these techniques, the problem of blood velocity estimation is considered in this subsection from the view of classic velocity estimation theory typically applied to radar and sonar problems.

Important differences exist between classic detection and estimation for radar and sonar and the application of such techniques to medical ultrasound. The Van Trees [1971] approach is based on joint estimation of the Doppler shift and position over the entire target. In medical ultrasound, the velocity is estimated in small regions of a large target, where the target position is assumed to be known. While classic theories have been developed for estimation of all velocities within a large target by Van Trees and others, such techniques require a model for the velocity in each spatial region of interest. For the case of blood velocity estimation, the spatial variation in the velocity profile is complex, and it is difficult to postulate a model that can be used to derive a high-quality estimate. The theory of velocity estimation in the presence of spread targets is also discussed by Kennedy [1969] and Price [1968] as it applies to radar astronomy and dispersive communication channels.

It is the desire to improve the spatial and velocity resolution of the estimate of blood velocity that has motivated the evaluation of alternative wideband estimation techniques. Narrowband velocity estimation techniques use the Doppler frequency shift produced by the moving cells with a sample volume that is fixed in space. Wideband estimation techniques incorporate the change in delay of the returned pulse due to the motion of the moving cells. Within the classification of narrowband techniques are a number of estimation strategies to be detailed below. These include the fast Fourier transform (FFT), finite derivative estimation, the autocorrelator, and modern spectral estimation techniques, including autoregressive strategies. Within

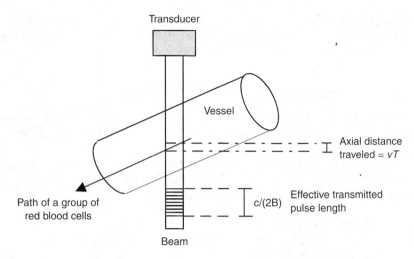

Transducer

Vessel

Axial distance
traveled = vT

c/(2B)

Effective transmitted
pulse length

Path of a group of
red blood cells

Beam

FIGURE 14.18 Comparison of the axial distance traveled and the effective length of the transmitted pulse.

the classification of wideband techniques are cross-correlation strategies and the wideband **maximum likelihood** estimator (WMLE).

For improving the spatial mapping of blood velocity within the body, the transmission of short pulses is desirable. Therefore, it is of interest to assess the quality of velocity estimates made using narrowband and wideband estimators with transmitted signals of varying lengths. If $(2v/c)BT \ll 1$, where v represents the axial velocity of the target, c represents the speed of the wave in tissue, B represents the transmitted signal bandwidth, and T represents the total time interval used in estimating velocity within an individual region, then the change in delay produced by the motion of the red blood cells can be ignored [(Van Trees, 1971].

This inequality is interpreted for the physical conditions of medical ultrasound in Figure 14.18. As shown in Figure 14.18, the value vT represents the axial distance traveled by the target while it is observed by the transducer beam, and $c/(2B)$ represents the effective length of the signal that is used to observe the moving cells. If $vT \ll c/(2B)$, the shift in the position of a group of red blood cells during their travel though the ultrasonic beam is not a detectable fraction of the signal length. This leads to two important restrictions on estimation techniques. First, under the "narrowband" condition of transmission of a long (narrowband) pulse, motion of a group of cells through the beam can only be estimated using the Doppler frequency shift. Second, if the inequality is not satisfied and therefore the transmitted signal is short (wideband), faster-moving red blood cells leave the region of interest, and the use of a narrowband estimation technique produces a biased velocity estimate. Thus two strategies can be used to estimate velocity. A long (narrowband) pulse can transmitted, and the signal from a fixed depth then can be used to estimate velocity. Alternatively, a short (wideband) signal can be transmitted in order to improve spatial resolution, and the estimator used to determine the velocity must move along with the red blood cells.

The inequality is now evaluated for typical parameters. When the angle between the axis of the beam and the axis of the vessel is 45 degrees, the axial distance traveled by the red blood cells while they cross the beam is equivalent to the lateral beam width. Using an axial distance vT of 0.75 mm, which is a reasonable lateral beam width, and an acoustic velocity of 1540 m/sec, the bandwidth of the transmitted pulse must be much less than 1.026 MHz for the narrowband approximation to be valid.

Due to practical advantages in the implementation of the smaller bandwidth required by **baseband signal**s, the center frequency of the signal is often removed before velocity estimation. The processing required for the extraction of the baseband signal is shown in Figure 14.19. The returned signal from the transducer is amplified and coherently demodulated, through multiplication by the carrier frequency, and then a low-pass filter is applied to remove the signal sideband frequencies and noise. The remaining signal is the **complex envelope**. A high-pass filter is then applied to the signal from each fixed depth to remove the unwanted echoes from stationary tissue. The output of this processing is denoted as $I_k(t)$ for the in-phase signal from the kth pulse as a function of time and $Q_k(t)$ for the quadrature signal from the kth pulse.

14.3.2.3 Narrowband Estimation

Narrowband estimation techniques that estimate velocity for blood at a fixed depth are described in this subsection. Both the classic Doppler technique, which frequently is used in single-sample volume systems, and the autocorrelator, which frequently is used in color flow mapping systems, are included, as well as a finite derivative estimator and an autoregressive estimator, which have been the subject of previous research. The autocorrelator is used in real-time color flow mapping systems due to the ease of implementation and the relatively small bias and variance.

14.3.2.3.1 Classic Doppler Estimation

If the carrier frequency is removed by coherently demodulating the signal, the change in delay of the RF signal becomes a change in the phase of the baseband signal. The Doppler shift frequency from a moving target equals $2f_c v/c$. With a center frequency of 5 MHz, sound velocity of 1540 m/sec, and blood velocity of 1 m/sec, the resulting frequency shift is 6493.5 Hz. For the estimation of blood velocity, the Doppler shift is not detectable using a single short pulse, and therefore, the signal from a fixed depth and a train of pulses is acquired.

A pulse-echo Doppler processing block diagram is shown in Figure 14.20. The baseband signal, from Figure 14.19, is shown as the input to this processing block. The received signal from each pulse is multiplied by a time window that is typically equal to the length of the transmitted pulse and integrated to produce a single data sample from each pulse. The set of data samples from a train of pulses is then Fourier-transformed, with the resulting frequency spectrum related to the axial velocity using the Doppler relationship.

Estimation of velocity using the Fourier transform of the signal from a fixed depth suffers from the limitations of all narrowband estimators, in that the variance of the estimate increases when a short pulse is transmitted. In addition, the velocity resolution produced using the Fourier transform is inversely

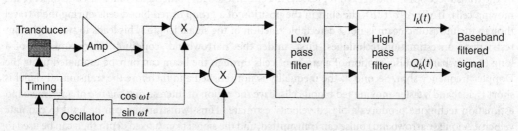

FIGURE 14.19 Block diagram of the system architecture required to generate the baseband signal used by several estimation techniques.

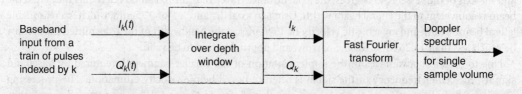

FIGURE 14.20 Block diagram of the system architecture required to estimate the Doppler spectrum from a set of baseband samples from a fixed depth.

proportional to the length of the data window. Therefore, if 64 pulses with a pulse repetition frequency of 5 kHz are used in the spectral estimate, the frequency resolution is on the order of 78.125 Hz (5000/64). The velocity resolution for a carrier frequency of 5 MHz and speed of sound of 1540 m/sec is then on the order of 1.2 cm/sec, determined from the Doppler relationship. Increasing the data window only improves the velocity resolution if the majority of the red blood cells have not left the sample volume and the flow conditions have not produced a decorrelation of the signal. It is this relationship between the data window and velocity resolution, a fundamental feature of Fourier transform techniques, that has motivated the use of autoregressive estimators. The frequency and velocity resolution are not fundamentally constrained by the data window using these modern spectral estimators introduced below.

14.3.2.3.2 Autoregressive estimation (AR)

In addition to the classic techniques discussed previously, higher-order modern spectral estimation techniques have been used in an attempt to improve the velocity resolution of the estimate. These techniques are again narrowband estimation techniques, since the data samples used in computing the estimate are obtained from a fixed depth. The challenges encountered in applying such techniques to blood velocity estimation include the selection of an appropriate order which adequately models the data sequence while providing the opportunity for real-time velocity estimation and determination of the length of the data sequence to be used in the estimation process.

The goal in autogressive velocity estimation is to model the frequency content of the received signal by a set of coefficients which cold be used to reconstruct the signal spectrum. The coefficients $a(m)$ represent the AR parameters of the AR(p) process, where p is the number of poles in the model for the signal. Estimation of the AR parameters has been accomplished using the Burg and Levinson-Durban recursion methods. The spectrum $P(f)$ is then estimated using the following equation:

$$P(f) = k \left| 1 + \sum_{m=1}^{p} a(m) \exp[-i2\pi mf] \right|^{-2}$$

The poles of the AR transfer function which lie within the unit circle can then be determined based on these parameters, and the velocity associated with each pole is determined by the Doppler equation.

Both autoregressive and autoregressive moving-average estimation techniques have been applied to single-sample-volume Doppler estimation. Order selection for single-sample-volume AR estimators is discussed in Kaluzinski [1989]. Second-order autoregressive estimation has been applied to color flow mapping by Loupas and McDicken [1990] and Ahn and Park [1991]. Although two poles are not sufficient to model the data sequence, the parameters of a higher-order process cannot be estimated in real time. In addition, the estimation of parameters of a higher-order process using the limited number of data points available in color flow mapping produces a large variance. Loupas and McDicken have used the two poles to model the signal returned from blood. Ahn and Park have used one pole to model the received signal from blood and the second pole to model the stationary signal from the surrounding tissue.

While AR techniques are useful in modeling the stationary tissue and blood and in providing a high-resolution estimate of multiple velocity components, several problems have been encountered in the practical application to blood velocity estimation. First, the order required to adequately model any region of the vessel can change when stationary tissue is present in the sample volume or when the range of velocity components in the sample volume increases. In addition, the performance of an AR estimate degrades rapidly in the presence of white noise, particularly with a small number of data samples.

14.3.2.3.3 Autocorrelator

Kasai et al. [1985] and Barber et al. [1985] discussed a narrowband mean velocity estimation structure for use in color flow mapping. The phase of the signal correlation at a lag of one transmitted period is estimated and used in an inverse tangent calculation of the estimated mean Doppler shift f_{mean} of the returned signal. A block diagram of the autocorrelator is shown in Figure 14.21. The baseband signal is first integrated over a short depth window. The phase of the correlation at a lag of one pulse period is then

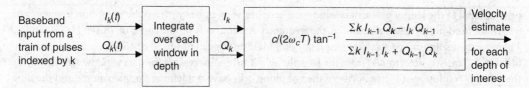

FIGURE 14.21   Block diagram of the system architecture required to estimate the mean Doppler shift for each depth location using the autocorrelator.

estimated as the inverse tangent of the imaginary part of the correlation divided by the real part of the correlation. The estimated mean velocity v_{mean} of the scattering medium is then determined by scaling the estimated Doppler shift by several factors, including the expected center frequency of the returned signal.

The autocorrelator structure can be derived from the definition of instantaneous frequency, from the phase of the correlation at a lag of one period, or as the first-order autoregressive estimate of the mean frequency of a baseband signal. The contributions of uncorrelated noise should average to zero in both the numerator and denominator of the autocorrelator. This is an advantage because the autocorrelation estimate is unbiased when the input signal includes the desired flow signal and noise. Alternatively, in the absence of a moving target, the input to the autocorrelator may consist only of white noise. Under these conditions, both the numerator and denominator can average to values near zero, and the resulting output of the autocorrelator has a very large variance. This estimation structure must therefore be used with a power threshold that can determine the presence or absence of a signal from blood flow and set the output of the estimator to zero when this motion is absent.

The variance of the autocorrelation estimate increases with the transmitted bandwidth, and therefore, the performance is degraded by transmitting a short pulse.

14.3.2.3.4 Finite derivative estimator (FDE)

A second approach to mean velocity or frequency estimation is based on a finite implementation of a derivative operator. The finite derivative estimator is derived based on the first and second moments of the spectrum. The basis for this estimator comes from the definition of the spectral centroid:

$$v_{\text{mean}} = \frac{\int \omega S(\omega)\mathrm{d}\omega}{\int S(\omega)\mathrm{d}\omega} \tag{14.27}$$

The mean velocity is given by v_{mean}, which is a scaled version of the mean frequency, where the scaling constant is given by k' and $S(\omega)$ represents the power spectral density. Letting $R_r(\cdot)$ represent the complex signal correlation and t represent the difference between the two times used in the correlation estimate, Equation 14.27 is equivalent to

$$v_{\text{mean}} = k' \frac{[(\partial/\partial\tau)R_r(\tau)|_{\tau=0}]}{R_r(0)} \tag{14.28}$$

Writing the baseband signal as the sum $I(t) + jQ(t)$ and letting E indicate the statistical expectation, Brody and Meindl ([974] have shown that the mean velocity estimate can be rewritten as

$$v_{\text{mean}} = \frac{k' E\{(\partial/\partial t)[I(t)]Q(t) - (\partial/\partial t)[Q(t)]I(t)\}}{E[I^2(t) + Q^2(t)]} \tag{14.29}$$

The estimate of this quantity requires estimation of the derivative of the in-phase portion I(t) and quadrature portion $Q(t)$ of the signal. For an analog, continuous-time implementation, the bias and variance were evaluated by Brody and Meindl [1974]. The discrete case has been studied by Kristoffersen [1986]. The differentiation has been implemented in the discrete case as a finite difference or as a finite impulse response differentiation filter. The estimator is biased by noise, since the denominator represents power in the returned signal. Therefore, for nonzero noise power, the averaged noise power in the denominator will not be zero mean and will constitute a bias. The variance of the finite derivative estimator depends on the shape and bandwidth of the Doppler spectrum, as well as on the observation interval.

14.3.2.4 Wideband Estimation Techniques

It is desirable to transmit a short ultrasonic pulse in order to examine blood flow in small regions individually. For these short pulses, the narrowband approximation is not valid, and the estimation techniques used should track the motion of the red blood cells as they move to a new position over time. Estimation techniques that track the motion of the red blood cells are known as wideband estimation techniques and include cross-correlation techniques, the wideband maximum likelihood estimator and high time bandwidth estimation techniques. A thorough review of time-domain estimation techniques to estimate tissue motion is presented in Hein and O'Brien [1993].

14.3.2.4.1 Cross-correlation estimator

The use of time shift to estimate signal parameters has been studied extensively in radar. If the transmitted signal is known, a maximum likelihood (ML) solution for the estimation of delay has been discussed by Van Trees [1971] and others. If the signal shape is not known, the use of cross-correlation for delay estimation has been discussed by Helstrom [1968] and Knapp and Carter [1976]). If information regarding the statistics of the signal and noise are available, an MLE based on cross-correlation has been proposed by Knapp and Carter [1976] known as the generalized correlation method for the estimation of time delay.

Several researchers have applied cross-correlation analysis to medical ultrasound. Bonnefous and Pesque [1986], Embree and O'Brien [1986], Foster et al. [1990], and Trahey et al. [1987] have studied the estimation of mean velocity based on the change in delay due to target movement. This analysis has assumed the shape of the transmitted signal to be unknown, and a cross-correlation technique has been used to estimate the difference in delay between successive pulses. This differential delay has then been used to estimate target velocity, where the velocity estimate is now based on the change in delay of the signal over an axial window, by maximizing the cross-correlation of the returned signal over all possible target velocities. Cross-correlation processing is typically performed on the radiofrequency (RF) signal, and a typical cross-correlation block diagram is shown in Figure 14.22. A high-pass filter is first applied to the signal from a fixed depth to remove the unwanted return from stationary tissue. One advantage of this strategy is that the variance is now inversely proportional to bandwidth of the transmitted signal rather than proportional.

14.3.2.4.2 Wideband Maximum Likelihood Estimator (WMLE)

Wideband maximum likelihood estimation is a baseband strategy with performance properties that are similar to cross-correlation. The estimate of the velocity of the blood cells is jointly based on the shift in the signal envelope and the shift in the carrier frequency of the returned signal. This estimator can be derived using a model for the signal that is expected to be reflected from the moving blood medium after the signal passes through intervening tissue. The processing of the signal can be interpreted as a filter matched to

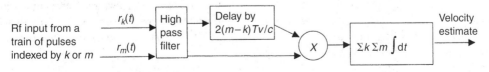

FIGURE 14.22 Block diagram of the system architecture required to estimate the velocity at each depth using a cross-correlation estimator.

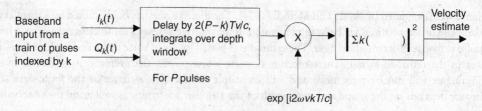

FIGURE 14.23 Block diagram of the system architecture required to estimate the velocity at each depth using the wideband MLE.

the expected signal. A diagram of the processing required for the wideband maximum likelihood estimator is shown in Figure 14.23 [Ferrara and Algazi, 1991]. Assume that P pulses were transmitted. Required processing involves the delay of the signal from the $(P - k)$th pulse by an amount equal to $2v/ckT$, which corresponds to the movement of the cells between pulses for a specific v, followed by multiplication by a frequency which corresponds to the expected Doppler shift frequency of the baseband returned signal. The result of this multiplication is summed for all pulses, and the maximum likelihood velocity is then the velocity which produces the largest output from this estimator structure.

14.3.2.4.3 Estimation using high-time-bandwidth signals

Several researchers have also investigated the use of long wideband signals including "chirp" modulated signals and pseduo-random noise for the estimation of blood velocity. These signals are transmitted continuously (or with a short "flyback" time). Since these signals require continual transmission, the instantaneous power level must be reduced in order to achieve safe average power levels.

Bertram [1979] concluded that transmission of a "chirp" appears to give inferior precision for range measurement and inferior resolution of closely spaced multiple targets than a conventional pulse-echo system applied to a similar transducer. Multiple targets confuse the analysis. Using a simple sawtooth waveform, it is not possible to differentiate a stationary target at one range from a moving target at a different range. This problem could possibly be overcome with increasing and decreasing frequency intervals. Axial resolution is independent of the modulation rate, dependent only on the spectral frequency range (which is limited).

The limitations of systems that have transmitted a long pulse of random noise and correlated the return with the transmitted signal include reverberations from outside the sample volume which degrade the signal-to-noise ratio (the federally required reduction in peak transmitted power also reduces SNR), limited signal bandwidth due to frequency-dependent attenuation in tissue, and the finite transducer bandwidth [Cooper and McGillem, 1972; Bendick and Newhouse, 1974].

14.3.3 New Directions

Areas of research interest, including estimation of the 3D velocity magnitude, volume flow estimation, the use of high-frequency catheter-based transducers, mapping blood flow within malignant tumors, a new display mode known as color Doppler energy, and the use of contrast agents, are summarized in this subsection.

Estimation of the 3D velocity magnitude and beam vessel angle: Continued research designed to provide an estimate of the 3D magnitude of the flow velocity includes the use of crossed-beam Doppler systems [Wang and Yao, 1982; Overbeck et al., 1992] and tracking of speckle in two and three dimensions [Trahey et al., 1987]. Mapping of the velocity estimate in two and three dimensions, resulting in a 3D color flow map has been described by Carson et al. [1992], Picot et al. [1993], and Cosgrove et al. [1990].

Volume flow estimation: Along with the peak velocity, instantaneous velocity profile, and velocity indices, a parameter of clinical interest is the volume of flow through vessels as a function of time. Estimation strategies for the determination of the volume of flow through a vessel have been described by Embree and O'Brien [1990], Gill [1979], Hottinger and Meindl [1979], and Uematsu [1981].

Intravascular ultrasound: It has been shown that intravascular ultrasonic imaging can provide information about the composition of healthy tissue and atheroma as well as anatomic data. A number of researchers have now shown that using frequencies of 30 MHz or above, individual layers and tissue types can be differentiated [de Kroon et al., 1991a,b; Lockwood et al., 1991]. Although obvious changes in the vessel wall, such as dense fibrosis and calcification, have been identified with lower-frequency transducers, more subtle changes have been difficult to detect. Recent research has indicated that the character of plaque may be a more reliable predictor of subsequent cerebrovascular symptoms than the degree of vessel narrowing or the presence of ulceration [Merritt et al., 1992]. Therefore, the recognition of subtle differences in tissue type may be extremely valuable. One signal-processing challenge in imaging the vascular wall at frequencies of 30 MHz or above is the removal of the unwanted echo from red blood cells, which is a strong interfering signal at high frequencies.

Vascular changes associated with tumors: Three-dimensional color flow mapping of the vascular structure is proposed to provide new information for the differentiation of benign and malignant masses. Judah Folkman and associates first recognized the importance of tumor vascularity in 1971 [Folkman et al., 1971]. They hypothesized that the increased cell population required for the growth of a malignant tumor must be preceded by the production of new vessels. Subsequent work has shown that the walls of these vessels are deficient in muscular elements, and this deficiency results in a low impedance to flow [Gammill et al., 1976]. This change can be detected by an increase in diastolic flow and a change in the resistive index.

More recently, Less et al. [1991] have shown that the vascular architecture of solid mammary tumors has several distinct differences from normal tissues, at least in the microvasculature. A type of network exists that exhibits fluctuations in both the diameter and length of the vessel with increasing branch order. Current color flow mapping systems with a center frequency of 5 MHz or above have been able to detect abnormal flow with varying degrees of clinical sensitivity from 40 to 82% [Belcaro et al., 1988; Balu-Maestro et al., 1991; Luska et al., 1992]. Researchers using traditional Doppler systems have also reported a range of clinical sensitivity, with a general reporting of high sensitivity but moderate to low specificity. Burns et al., [1982] studied the signal from benign and malignant masses with 10-MHz CW Doppler. They hypothesized, and confirmed through angiography, that the tumors under study were fed by multiple small arteries, with a mean flow velocity below 10 cm/sec. Carson et al. [1992] compared 10-MHz CW Doppler to 5- and 7.5-MHz color flow mapping and concluded that while 3D reconstruction of the vasculature could provide significant additional information, color flow mapping systems must increase their ability to detect slow flow in small vessels in order to effectively map the vasculature.

Ultrasound contrast agents: The introduction of substances that enhance the ultrasonic echo signal from blood primarily through the production of microbubbles is of growing interest in ultrasonic flow measurement. The increased echo power may have a significant impact in contrast echocardiography, where acquisition of the signal from the coronary arteries has been difficult. In addition, such agents have been used to increase the backscattered signal from small vessels in masses that are suspected to be malignant. Contrast agents have been developed using sonicated albumen, saccharide microbubbles, and gelatin-encapsulated microbubbles.

Research to improve the sensitivity of flow measurement systems to low-velocity flow and small volumes of flow, with the goal of mapping the vasculature architecture, includes the use of ultrasonic contrast agents with conventional Doppler signal processing [Hartley et al., 1993], as well as the detection of the second harmonic of the transducer center frequency [Shrope and Newhouse, 1993].

Color Doppler energy: During 1993, a new format for the presentation of the returned signal from the blood scattering medium was introduced and termed color Doppler energy (CDE) or color power imaging (CPI). In this format, the backscattered signal is filtered to remove the signal from stationary tissue, and the remaining energy in the backscattered signal is color encoded and displayed as an overlay on the gray-scale image. The advantage of this signal-processing technique is the sensitivity to very low flow velocities.

Defining Terms

Baseband signal: The received signal after the center frequency component (carrier frequency) has been removed by demodulation.

Carrier frequency: The center frequency in the spectrum of the transmitted signal.

Clutter: An unwanted fixed signal component generated by stationary targets typically outside the region of interest (such as vessel walls).

Complex envelope: A signal expressed by the product of the carrier, a high-frequency component, and other lower-frequency components that comprise the envelope. The envelope is usually expressed in complex form.

Maximum likelihood: A statistical estimation technique that maximizes the probability of the occurrence of an event to estimate a parameter. ML estimate is the minimum variance, unbiased estimate.

References

Ahn Y. and Park S. 1991. Estimation of mean frequency and variance of ultrasonic Doppler signal by using second-order autoregressive model. *IEEE Trans. Ultrason. Ferroelec. Freq. Cont.* 38: 172.

Angelson B. 1980. Theoretical study of the scattering of ultrasound from blood. *IEEE Trans. Biomed. Eng.* 27: 61.

Atkinson P. and Berry M.V. 1974. Random noise in ultrasonic echoes diffracted by blood. *J. Phys. A: Math. Nucl. Gen.* 7: 1293.

Balu-Maestro C., Bruneton J.N., Giudicelli T. et al. 1991. Color Doppler in breast tumor pathology. *J. Radiol.* 72: 579.

Barber W., Eberhard J.W., and Karr S. 1985. A new time domain technique for velocity measurements using Doppler ultrasound. *IEEE Trans. Biomed. Eng.* 32: 213.

Belcaro G., Laurora G., Ricci A. et al. 1988. Evaluation of flow in nodular tumors of the breast by Doppler and duplex scanning. *Acta Chir. Belg.* 88: 323.

Bertram C.D. 1979. Distance resolution with the FM-CW ultrasonic echo-ranging system. *Ultrasound Med. Biol.* 61.

Bonnefous O. and Pesque P. 1986. Time domain formulation of pulse-Doppler ultrasound and blood velocity estimators by cross correlation. *Ultrason. Imag.* 8: 73.

Brody W. and Meindl J. 1974. Theoretical analysis of the CW Doppler ultrasonic flowmeter. *IEEE Trans. Biomed. Eng.* 21: 183.

Burns P.N., Halliwell M., Wells P.N.T., and Webb A.J. 1982. Ultrasonic Doppler studies of the breast. *Ultrasound Med. Biol.* 8: 127.

Carson P.L., Adler D.D., Fowlkes J.B. et al. 1992. Enhanced color flow imaging of breast cancer vasculature: continuous wave Doppler and three-dimensional display. *J. Ultrasound Med.* 11: 77.

Cosgrove D.O., Bamber J.C., Davey J.B. et al. 1990. Color Doppler signals from breast tumors: work in progress. *Radiology* 176: 175.

Curry G.R. and White D.N. 1978. Color coded ultrasonic differential velocity arterial scanner. *Ultrasound Med. Biol.* 4: 27.

de Kroon M.G.M., Slager C.J., Gussenhoven W.J. et al. 1991. Cyclic changes of blood echogenicity in high-frequency ultrasound. *Ultrasound Med. Biol.* 17: 723.

de Kroon M.G.M., van der Wal L.F., Gussenhoven W.J. et al. 1991. Backscatter directivity and integrated backscatter power of arterial tissue. *Int. J. Cardiac. Imag.* 6: 265.

Embree P.M. and O'Brien W.D. Jr. 1990. Volumetric blood flow via time-domain correlation: experimental verification. *IEEE Trans. Ultrason. Ferroelec. Freq. Cont.* 37: 176.

Ferrara K.W. and Algazi V.R. 1994a. A statistical analysis of the received signal from blood during laminar flow. *IEEE Trans. Ultrason. Ferroelec. Freq. Cont.* 41: 185.

Ferrara K.W. and Algazi V.R. 1994b. A theoretical and experimental analysis of the received signal from disturbed blood flow. *IEEE Trans. Ultrason. Ferroelec. Freq. Cont.* 41: 172.

Ferrara K.W. and Algazi V.R. 1991. A new wideband spread target maximum likelihood estimator for blood velocity estimation: I. Theory. *IEEE Trans. Ultrason. Ferroelec. Freq. Cont.* 38: 1.

Folkman J., Nerler E., Abernathy C., and Williams G. 1971. Isolation of a tumor factor responsible for angiogenesis. *J. Exp. Med.* 33: 275.

Foster S.G., Embree P.M., and O'Brien W.D. Jr. 1990. Flow velocity profile via time-domain correlation: error analysis and computer simulation. *IEEE Trans. Ultrason. Ferroelec. Freq. Cont.* 37: 164.

Gammill S.L., Stapkey K.B., and Himmellarb E.H. 1976. Roenigenology — pathology correlative study of neovascularay. *AJR* 126: 376.

Gill R.W. 1979. Pulsed Doppler with B-mode imaging for quantitative blood flow measurement. *Ultrasound Med. Biol.* 5: 223.

Hartley C.J., Cheirif J., Collier K.R., and Bravenec J.S. 1993. Doppler quantification of echo-contrast injections *in vivo*. *Ultrasound Med. Biol.* 19: 269.

Hatle L. and Angelsen B. 1985. *Doppler Ultrasound in Cardiology*, 3rd ed. Philadelphia, Lea and Febiger.

Hatsukami T.S., Primozich J., Zierler R.E., and Strandness D.E. 1992. Color Doppler characteristics in normal lower extremity arteries. *Ultrasound Med. Biol.* 18(2): 167.

Hein I. and O'Brien W. 1993. Current time domain methods for assessing tissue motion. *IEEE Trans. Ultrason. Ferroelec. Freq. Cont.* 40(2): 84.

Helstrom C.W. 1968. *Statistical Theory of Signal Detection*. London, Pergamon Press.

Hinze J.O. 1975. *Turbulence*. New York, McGraw-Hill.

Hottinger C.F. and Meindl J.D. 1979. Blood flow measurement using the attenuation compensated volume flowmeter. *Ultrason. Imag.* 1: 1.

Kaluzinski K. 1989. Order selection in Doppler blood flow signal spectral analysis using autoregressive modelling. *Med. Biol. Eng. Com.* 27: 89.

Kasai C., Namekawa K., Koyano A., and Omoto R. 1985. Real-time two-dimensional blood flow imaging using an autocorrelation technique. *IEEE Trans. Sonics Ultrason.* 32.

Kay S. and Marple S.L. 1981. Spectrum analysis. A modern perspective. *Proc. IEEE* 69: 1380.

Kennedy R.S. 1969. *Fading Dispersive Channel Theory*. New York, Wiley Interscience.

Knapp C.H. and Carter G.C. 1976. The generalized correlation method for estimation of time delay. *IEEE Trans. Acoust. Speech Signal Proc.* 24: 320.

Kristoffersen K. and Angelsen B.J. 1985. A comparison between mean frequency estimators for multigated Doppler systems with serial signal processing. *IEEE Trans. Biomed. Eng.* 32: 645.

Less J.R., Skalak T.C., Sevick E.M., and Jain R.K. 1991. Microvascular architecture in a mammary carcinoma: branching patterns and vessel dimensions. *Cancer Res.* 51: 265.

Lockwood G.R., Ryan L.K., Hunt J.W., and Foster F.S. 1991. Measurement of the ultrasonic properties of vascular tissues and blood from 35–65 MHz. *Ultrasound Med. Biol.* 17: 653.

Loupas T. and McDicken W.N. 1990. Low-order AR models for mean and maximum frequency estimation in the context of Doppler color flow mapping. *IEEE Trans. Ultrason. Ferroelec. Freq. Cont.* 37: 590.

Luska G., Lott D., Risch U., and von Boetticher H. 1992. The findings of color Doppler sonography in breast tumors. *Rofo Forts auf dem Gebiete der Rontgens und der Neuen Bildg Verf* 156: 142.

Merritt C. and Bluth E. 1992. The future of carotid sonography. *AJR* 158: 37.

Mo L. and Cobbold R. 1986. A stochastic model of the backscattered Doppler ultrasound from blood. *IEEE Trans. Biomed. Eng.* 33: 20.

Nerem R.M. 1985. Fluid dynamic considerations in the application of ultrasound flowmetry. In S.A. Altobelli, W.F. Voyles, and E.R. Greene (Eds.), *Cardiovascular Ultrasonic Flowmetry*. New York, Elsevier.

Nichols W.W. and O'Rourke M.F. 1990. *McDonald's Blood Flow in Arteries: Theoretic, Experimental and Clinical principles*. Philadelphia, Lea and Febiger.

Nowicki A. and Reid J.M. 1981. An infinite gate pulse Doppler. *Ultrasound Med. Biol.* 7: 1.

Overbeck J.R., Beach K.W., and Strandness D.E. Jr. 1992. Vector Doppler: accurate measurement of blood velocity in two dimensions. *Ultrasound Med. Biol.* 18: 19.

Picot P.A., Rickey D.W. and Mitchell R. et al. 1993. Three dimensional color Doppler mapping. *Ultrasound Med. Biol.* 19: 95.

Price R. 1968. Detectors for radar astronomy. In J. Evans and T. Hagfors (Eds.), *Radar Astronomy*. New York, McGraw-Hill.

Schrope B.A. and Newhouse V.L. 1993. Second harmonic ultrasound blood perfusion measurement. *Ultrasound Med. Biol.* 19: 567.

Shung K.K., Sigelman R.A., and Reid J.M. 1976. Scattering of ultrasound by blood. *IEEE Trans. Biomed. Eng.* 23: 460.

Shung K.K., Cloutier G., and Lim C.C. 1992. The effects of hematocrit, shear rate, and turbulence on ultrasonic Doppler spectrum from blood. *IEEE Trans. Biomed. Eng.* 39: 462.

Trahey G.E., Allison J.W., and Von Ramm O.T. 1987. Angle independent ultrasonic detection of blood flow. *IEEE Trans. Biomed. Eng.* 34: 964.

Uematsu S. 1981. Determination of volume of arterial blood flow by an ultrasonic device. *J. Clin. Ultrason.* 9: 209.

Van Trees H.L. 1971. *Detection, Estimation and Modulation Theory*, Part III. New York, Wiley.

Wang W. and Yao L. 1982. A double beam Doppler ultrasound method for quantitative blood flow velocity measurement. *Ultrasound Med. Biol.* 421.

Wells P.N.T. 1977. *Biomedical Ultrasonics*. London, Academic Press.

Further Information

The bimonthly journal *IEEE Transactions on Ultrasonics Ferroelectrics and Frequency* Control reports engineering advances in the area of ultrasonic flow measurement. For subscription information, contact IEEE Service Center, 445 Hoes Lane, P.O. Box 1331, Piscataway, NJ 08855-1331. Phone (800) 678-IEEE. The journal and the yearly conference proceedings of the IEEE Ultrasonic Symposium are published by the IEEE Ultrasonic Ferroelectrics and Frequency Control Society. Membership information can be obtained from the IEEE address above or from K. Ferrara, Riverside Research Institute, 330 West 42nd Street, New York, NY 10036.

The journal *Ultrasound in Medicine and Biology*, published 10 times per year, includes new developments in ultrasound signal processing and the clinical application of these developments. For subscription information, contact Pergamon Press, Inc., 660 White Plains Road, Tarrytown, NY 10591-5153. The American Institute of Ultrasound Medicine sponsors a yearly meeting which reviews new developments in ultrasound instrumentation and the clinical applications. For information, please contact American Institute of Ultrasound in Medicine, 11200 Rockville Pike, Suite 205, Rockville, MD 20852-3139; phone: (800) 638-5352.

15

Magnetic Resonance Microscopy

15.1 Basic Principles **15**-2
  Spatial Encoding and Decoding • Image Contrast
15.2 Resolution Limits **15**-4
  Intrinsic Resolution Limit • Digital Resolution Limit •
  Practical Resolution Limit
15.3 Instrumentation **15**-6
  Radiofrequency Coils • Magnetic Field Gradient Coils
15.4 Applications **15**-9
References **15**-11
Further Information **15**-14

Xiaohong Zhou
G. Allan Johnson
Duke University Medical Center

Visualization of internal structures of opaque biologic objects is essential in many biomedical studies. Limited by the penetration depth of the probing sources (photons and electrons) and the lack of endogenous contrast, conventional forms of microscopy such as optical microscopy and electron microscopy require tissues to be sectioned into thin slices and stained with organic chemicals or heavy-metal compounds prior to examination. These invasive and destructive procedures, as well as the harmful radiation in the case of electron microscopy, make it difficult to obtain three-dimensional information and virtually impossible to study biologic tissues *in vivo*.

Magnetic resonance (MR) microscopy is a new form of microscopy that overcomes the aforementioned limitations. Operating in the radiofrequency (RF) range, MR microscopy allows biologic samples to be examined in the living state without bleaching or damage by ionizing radiation and in fresh and fixed specimens after minimal preparation. It also can use a number of endogenous contrast mechanisms that are directly related to tissue biochemistry, physiology, and pathology. Additionally, MR microscopy is digital and three-dimensional; internal structures of opaque tissues can be quantitatively mapped out in three dimensions to accurately reveal their histopathologic status. These unique properties provide new opportunities for biomedical scientists to attack problems that have been difficult to investigate using conventional techniques.

Conceptually, MR microscopy is an extension of magnetic resonance imaging (MRI) to the microscopic domain, generating images with spatial resolution better than 100 mm [Lauterbur, 1984]. As such, MR microscopy is challenged by a new set of theoretical and technical problems [Johnson et al., 1992]. For example, to improve isotropic resolution from 1 to 10 mm, signal-to-noise ratio (SNR) per voxel must be increased by a million times to maintain the same image quality. In order to do so, almost every component of hardware must be optimized to the fullest extent, pulse sequences have to be carefully designed to minimize any potential signal loss, and special software and dedicated computation facilities must be involved to handle large image arrays (e.g., 256^3). Over the past decade, development of MR microscopy has focused mainly on these issues. Persistent efforts by many researchers have recently lead to images with isotropic resolution of the order of $\sim$10 μm [Cho et al., 1992; Jacobs and Fraser, 1994; Johnson et al., 1992; Zhou and Lauterbur, 1992]. The significant resolution improvement opens up a broad range of applications, from histology to cancer biology and from toxicology to plant biology [Johnson et al., 1992]. In this chapter we will first discuss the basic principles of MR microscopy, with special attention to such issues as resolution limits and sensitivity improvements. Then we will give an overview of the instrumentation. Finally, we will provide some examples to demonstrate the applications.

15.1 Basic Principles

15.1.1 Spatial Encoding and Decoding

Any digital imaging systems involve two processes. First, spatially resolved information must be encoded into a measurable signal, and second, the spatially encoded signal must be decoded to produce an image. In MR microscopy, the spatial encoding process is accomplished by acquiring nuclear magnetic resonance (NMR) signals under the influence of three orthogonal magnetic field gradients. There are many ways that a gradient can interact with a spin system. If the gradient is applied during a frequency-selective RF pulse, then the NMR signal arises only from a thin slab along the gradient direction. Thus a slice is selected from a three-dimensional (3D) object. If the gradient is applied during the acquisition of an NMR signal, the signal will consist of a range of spatially dependent frequencies given by

$$\omega(\vec{r}) = \gamma B_0 + \gamma \vec{G} \cdot \vec{r} \tag{15.1}$$

where γ is gyromagnetic ratio, B_0 is the static magnetic field, $\vec{G}$ is the magnetic field gradient, and $\vec{r}$ is the spatial variable. In this way, the spatial information along $\vec{G}$ direction is encoded into the signal as frequency variations. This method of encoding is called frequency encoding, and the gradient is referred to as a frequency-encoding gradient (or read-out gradient). If the gradient is applied for a fixed amount of time t_{pe} before the signal acquisition, then the phase of the signal, instead of the frequency, becomes spatially dependent, as given by

$$\phi(\vec{r}) = \int_0^{t_{pe}} \omega(\vec{r}) \mathrm{d}t = \phi_0 + \int_0^{t_{pe}} \gamma \vec{G} \cdot \vec{r} \, \mathrm{d}t \tag{15.2}$$

where ϕ_0 is the phase originated from the static magnetic field. This encoding method is known as phase encoding, and the gradient is called a phase-encoding gradient.

Based on the three basic spatial encoding approaches, many imaging schemes can be synthesized. For two-dimensional (2D) imaging, a slice-selection gradient is first applied to confine the NMR signal in a slice. Spatial encoding within the slice is then accomplished by frequency encoding and by phase encoding. For 3D imaging, the slice-selection gradient is replaced by either a frequency-encoding or a phase-encoding gradient. If all spatial directions are frequency-encoded, the encoding scheme is called projection acquisition, and the corresponding decoding method is called projection reconstruction [Lai and Lauterbur, 1981; Lauterbur, 1973]. If one of the spatial dimensions is frequency encoded while the rest are phase encoded, the method is known as Fourier imaging, and the image can be reconstructed simply by a multidimensional Fourier transform [Edelstein et al., 1980; Kumar et al., 1975]. Although other methods do exist, projection reconstruction and Fourier imaging are the two most popular in MR microscopy.

Projection reconstruction is particularly useful for spin systems with short apparent T_2 values, such as protons in lung and liver. Since the T_2 of most tissues decreases as static magnetic field increases, the advantage of projection reconstruction is more obvious at high magnetic fields. Another advantage of projection reconstruction is its superior SNR to Fourier imaging. This advantage has been theoretically analyzed and experimentally demonstrated in a number of independent studies [Callaghan and Eccles, 1987; Gewalt et al., 1993; Zhou and Lauterbur, 1992]. Recently, it also has been shown that projection reconstruction is less sensitive to motion and motion artifacts can be effectively reduced using sinograms [Glover and Noll, 1993; Glover and Pauly, 1992; Gmitro and Alexander, 1993]. Unlike projection reconstruction, data acquisition in Fourier imaging generates Fourier coefficients of the image in a cartesian coordinate. Since multidimensional fast Fourier transform algorithms can be applied directly to the raw data, Fourier imaging is computationally more efficient than projection reconstruction. This advantage is most evident when reconstructing 3D images with large arrays (e.g., 2563). In addition, Fourier transform imaging is less prone to image artifacts arising from various off-resonance effects and is more robust in applications such as chemical shift imaging [Brown et al., 1982] and flow imaging [Moran, 1982].

15.1.2 Image Contrast

A variety of contrast mechanisms can be exploited in MR microscopy, including spin density (r), spin–spin relaxation time (T_1), spin-lattice relaxation time (T_2), apparent T_2 relaxation time (T_2), diffusion coefficient (D), flow and chemical shift (d). One of the contrasts can be highlighted by varying data-acquisition parameters or by choosing different pulse sequences. Table 15.1 summarizes the pulse sequences and data-acquisition parameters to obtain each of the preceding contrasts.

In high-field MR microscopy ($>1.5T$), T_2 and diffusion contrast are strongly coupled together. An increasing number of evidences indicate that the apparent T_2 contrast observed in high-field MR microscopy is largely due to microscopic magnetic susceptibility variations [Majumdar and Gore, 1988; Zhong and Gore, 1991]. The magnetic susceptibility difference produces strong local magnetic field gradients. Molecular diffusion through the induced gradients causes significant signal loss. In addition, the large external magnetic field gradients required for spatial encoding further increase the diffusion-induced signal loss. Since the signal loss has similar dependence on echo time (TE) to T_2-related loss, the diffusion contrast mechanism is involved in virtually all T_2-weighted images. This unique contrast mechanism provides a direct means to probe the microscopic tissue heterogeneities and forms the basis for many histopathologic studies [Benveniste et al., 1992; Zhou et al., 1994].

Chemical shift is another unique contrast mechanism. Changes in chemical shift can directly reveal tissue metabolic and histopathologic stages. This mechanism exists in many spin systems such as ^{1}H, ^{31}P, and ^{13}C. Recently, Lean et al. [1993] showed that based on proton chemical shifts, MR microscopy can detect tissue pathologic changes with superior sensitivity to optical microscopy in a number of tumor models. A major limitation for chemical-shift MR microscopy is the rather poor spatial resolution, since most spin species other than water protons are of considerably low concentration and sensitivity. In addition, the long data-acquisition time required to resolve both spatial and spectral information also appears as an obstacle.

TABLE 15.1 Choice of Acquisition Parameters for Different Image Contrasts

Contrast	TR[b]	TE[b]	Pulse sequences[a]
r	3–5 $T_{1,max}$	$\ll T_{2,min}$	SE, GE
T_1	$-T_{1,avg}$	$\ll T_{2,min}$	SE, GE
T_2	3–5 $T_{1,max}$	$\sim T_{2,avg}$	SE, FSE
T_2^*	3–5 $T_{1,max}$	$\sim T_{s,avg}^*$	GE
D[c]	3–5 $T_{1,max}$	$\ll T_{2,min}$	Diffusion-weighted SE, GE, or FSE

[a] SE: spin-echo; GE: gradient echo; FSE: fast spin echo.
[b] Subscripts min, max and avg stand for minimum, maximum and average values, respectively.
[c] A pair of diffusion weighting gradients must be used.

15.2 Resolution Limits

15.2.1 Intrinsic Resolution Limit

Intrinsic resolution is defined as the width of the point-spread function originated from physics laws. In MR microscopy, the intrinsic resolution arises from two sources: natural linewidth broadening and diffusion [Callaghan and Eccles, 1988; Cho et al., 1988; House, 1984].

In most conventional pulse sequences, natural linewidth broadening affects the resolution limit only in the frequency-encoding direction. In some special cases, such as fast spin echo [Hennig et al., 1986] and echo planar imaging [Mansfield and Maudsley, 1977], natural linewidth broadening also imposes resolution limits in the phase-encoding direction [Zhou et al., 1993]. The natural linewidth resolution limit, defined by

$$\Delta r_{\text{n.l.w.}} = \frac{2}{\gamma G T_2} \tag{15.3}$$

is determined by the T_2 relaxation time and can be improved using a stronger gradient $\acute{G}$. To obtain 1 mm resolution from a specimen with $T_2 = 50$ msec, the gradient should be at least 14.9 G/cm. This gradient requirement is well within the range of most MR microscopes.

Molecular diffusion affects the spatial resolution in a number of ways. The bounded diffusion is responsible for many interesting phenomena known as edge enhancements [Callaghan et al., 1993; Hills et al., 1990; Hyslop and Lauterbur, 1991; Putz et al., 1991]. They are observable only at the microscopic resolution and are potentially useful to detect microscopic boundaries. The unbounded diffusion, on the other hand, causes signal attenuation, line broadening, and phase misregistration. All these effects originate from an incoherent and irreversible phase-dispersion. The root-mean-square value of the phase dispersion is

$$\sigma = \gamma \left\{ 2D \int_0^t \left[\int_{t'}^t G(t'') \, \mathrm{d}t'' \right]^2 \, \mathrm{d}t' \right\}^{1/2} \tag{15.4}$$

where t' and t are pulse-sequence-dependent time variables defined by Ahn and Cho [1989]. Because of the phase uncertainty, an intrinsic resolution limit along the phase encoding direction arises:

$$\Delta r_{\text{pe}} = \frac{\sigma}{\gamma \int_0^t G_{\text{pe}}(t') \, \mathrm{d}t'} \tag{15.5}$$

For a rectangularly shaped phase-encoding gradient, the preceding equation can be reduced to a very simple form:

$$\Delta r_{\text{pe}} = \sqrt{\frac{2}{3} D t_{\text{pe}}} \tag{15.6}$$

This simple result indicates that the diffusion resolution limit in the phase-encoded direction is determined only by the phase-encoding time t_{pe} (D is a constant for a chosen sample). This is so because the phase uncertainty is introduced only during the phase-encoding period. Once the spins are phase-encoded, they always carry the same spatial information no matter where they diffuse to. In the frequency-encoding direction, diffusion imposes resolution limits by broadening the point-spread function. Unlike natural linewidth broadening, broadening caused by diffusion is pulse-sequence-dependent. For the simplest pulse sequence, a 3D projection acquisition using free induction decays, the full width at half maximum

[Callaghan and Eccles, 1988; McFarland, 1992; Zhou, 1992] is

$$\Delta r_{\text{fr}} = 8 \left[\frac{D(\ln 2)^2}{3\gamma\, G_{\text{fr}}} \right]^{1/3} \tag{15.7}$$

Compared with the case of the natural linewidth broadening (Equation 15.3), the resolution limit caused by diffusion varies slowly with the frequency-encoding gradient G_{fr}. Therefore, to improve resolution by a same factor, a much larger gradient is required. With the currently achievable gradient strength, the diffusion resolution limit is estimated to be 5 to 10 μm.

15.2.2 Digital Resolution Limit

When the requirements imposed by intrinsic resolution limits are satisfied, image resolution is largely determined by the voxel size, provided that SNR is sufficient and the amplitude of physiologic motion is limited to a voxel. The voxel size, also known as digital resolution, can be calculated from the following equations:

Frequency-encoding direction:

$$\Delta x \equiv \frac{L_x}{N_x} = \frac{\Delta\nu}{2\pi\,\gamma\, G_x N_x} \tag{15.8}$$

Phase-encoding direction:

$$\Delta y \equiv \frac{L_y}{N_y} = \frac{\Delta\phi}{\gamma\, G_y t_{\text{pe}}} \tag{15.9}$$

where L is the field of view, N is the number of data points or the linear matrix size, G is the gradient strength, $\Delta\nu$ is the receiver bandwidth, $\Delta\phi$ is the phase range of the phase-encoding data (e.g., if the data cover a phase range from $-\pi$ to $+\pi$, then $\Delta\phi = 2\pi$), and the subscripts x and y represent frequency- and phase-encoding directions, respectively. To obtain a high digital resolution, L should be kept minimal, while N maximal. In practice, the minimal field of view and the maximal data points are constrained by other experimental parameters. In the frequency-encoding direction, decreasing field of view results in an increase in gradient amplitude at a constant receiver bandwidth or a decrease in the bandwidth for a constant gradient (Equation 15.8). Since the receiver bandwidth must be large enough to keep the acquisition of NMR signals within a certain time window, the largest available gradient strength thus imposes the digital resolution limit. In the phase-encoding direction, $\Delta\phi$ is fixed at 2π in most experiments, and the maximum t_{pe} value is refrained by the echo time. Thus digital resolution is also determined by the maximum available gradient, as indicated by Equation 15.9. It has been estimated that in order to achieve 1 mm resolution with a phase-encoding time of 4 msec, the required gradient strength is as high as 587 G/cm. This gradient requirement is beyond the range of current MR microscopes. Fortunately, the requirement is fully relaxed in projection acquisition where no phase encoding is involved.

15.2.3 Practical Resolution Limit

The intrinsic resolution limits predict that MR microscopy can theoretically reach the micron regime. To realize the resolution, one must overcome several technical obstacles. These obstacles, or practical resolution limits, include insufficient SNR, long data-acquisition times, and physiologic motion. At the current stage of development, these practical limitations are considerably more important than other resolution limits discussed earlier and actually determine the true image resolution.

SNR is of paramount importance in MR microscopy. As resolution improves, the total number of spins per voxel decreases drastically, resulting in a cubic decrease in signal intensity. When the voxel signal intensity becomes comparable with noise level, structures become unresolvable even if the digital resolution and intrinsic resolution are adequate.

SNR in a voxel depends on many factors. The relationship between SNR and common experimental variables is given by

$$\text{SNR} \propto \frac{B_1 B_0^2 \sqrt{n}}{\sqrt{4kT \Delta \nu (R_{\text{coil}} + R_{\text{sample}})}} \tag{15.10}$$

where B_1 is the RF magnetic field, B_0 is the static magnetic field, n is the number of average, T is the temperature, $\Delta \nu$ is the bandwidth, k is the Boltzmann constant, and R_{coil} and R_{sample} are the coil and sample resistance, respectively. When small RF coils are used, R_{sample} is negligible. Since R_{coil} is proportional to due to skin effects, the overall SNR increases as $B_0^{7/4}$. This result strongly suggests that MR microscopy be performed at high magnetic field. Another way to improve SNR is to increase the B_1 field. This is accomplished by reducing the size of RF coils [McFarland and Mortara, 1992; Peck et al., 1990; Schoeniger et al., 1991; Zhou and Lauterbur, 1992]. Although increasing B_0 and B_1 is the most common approach to attacking the SNR problem, other methods such as signal averaging, pulse-sequence optimization, and post data processing are also useful in MR microscopy. For example, diffusion-induced signal loss can be effectively minimized using diffusion-reduced-gradient (DRG) echo pulse sequences [Cho et al., 1992]. Various forms of projection acquisition techniques [Gewalt et al., 1993; Hedges, 1984; McFarland and Mortara, 1992; Zhou and Lauterbur, 1992], as well as new k-space sampling schemes [Zhou et al., 1993], also have proved useful in SNR improvements. Recently, Black et al. [1993] used high-temperature superconducting materials for coil fabrication to simultaneously reduce coil resistance R_{coil} and coil temperature T. This novel approach can provide up to 70-fold SNR increase, equivalent to the SNR gain by increasing the magnetic field strength 11 times.

Long data-acquisition time is another practical limitation. Large image arrays, long repetition times (TR), and signal averaging all contribute to the overall acquisition time. For instance, a T_2-weighted image with a 256^3 image array requires a total acquisition time of more than 18 h (assuming TR = 500 msec and $n = 2$). Such a long acquisition time is unacceptable for most applications. To reduce the acquisition time while still maintaining the desired contrast, fast-imaging pulse sequences such as echo-planar imaging (EPI) [Mansfield and Maudsley, 1977], driven equilibrium Fourier transform (DEFT) [Maki et al., 1988], fast low angle shot (FLASH) [Haase et al., 1986], gradient refocused acquisition at steady state (GRASS) [Karis et al., 1987], and rapid acquisition with relaxation enhancement (RARE) [Hennig et al., 1986] have been developed and applied to MR microscopy. The RARE pulse sequence, or fast spin-echo (FSE) [Mulkern et al., 1990], is particularly useful in high-field MR microscopy because of its insensitivity to magnetic susceptibility effects as well as the reduced diffusion loss [Zhou et al., 1993]. Using fast spin-echo techniques, a 256^3 image has been acquired in less than 2 h [Zhou et al., 1993].

For *in vivo* studies, the true image resolution is also limited by physiologic motion [Hedges, 1984; Wood and Henkelman, 1985]. Techniques to minimize the motion effects have been largely focused on pulse sequences and post data processing algorithms, including navigator echoes [Ehman and Felmlee, 1989], motion compensation using even echo or moment nulling gradients, projection acquisition [Glover and Noll, 1993], and various kinds of ghost-image decomposition techniques [Xiang and Henkelman, 1991]. It should be noted, however, that by refining animal handling techniques and using synchronized data acquisition, physiologic motion effects can be effectively avoided and very high quality images can be obtained [Hedlund et al., 1986; Johnson et al., 1992].

15.3 Instrumentation

An MR microscope consists of a high-field magnet (>1.5 T), a set of gradient coils, an RF coil (or RF coils), and the associated RF systems, gradient power supplies, and computers. Among these components,

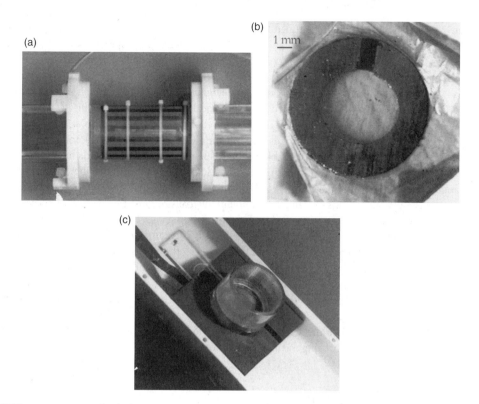

FIGURE 15.1   A range of radiofrequency coils are used in MR microscopy. (a) A quadrature birdcage coil scaled to the appropriate diameter for rats (6 cm) is used for whole-body imaging. (b) Resonant coils have been constructed on microwave substrate that can be surgically implanted to provide both localization and improved SNR. (c) MR microscopy of specimens is accomplished with a modified Helmholz coil providing good filling factors, high B homogeneity, and ease of access.

RF coils and gradient coils are often customized for specific applications in order to achieve optimal performance. Some general guidelines to design customized RF coils and gradient coils are presented below.

15.3.1   Radiofrequency Coils

Many types of RF coils can be used in MR microscopy (Figure 15.1). The choice of a particular coil configuration is determined by specific task and specimen size. If possible, the smallest coil size should always be chosen in order to obtain the highest SNR. For *ex-vivo* studies of tissue specimens, solenoid coils are a common choice because of their superior B_1 field homogeneity, high sensitivity, as well as simplicity in fabrication. Using a 2.9 mm solenoid coil (5 turn), Zhou and Lauterbur [1992] have achieved the highest ever reported spatial resolution at 6.4 μm^3. Solenoid coil configurations are also used by others to obtain images with similar resolution ($\sim$10 μm) [Cho et al., 1988; Hedges, 1984; McFarland and Mortara, 1992; Schoeniger et al., 1991]. Recently, several researchers began to develop microscopic solenoid coils with a size of a few hundred microns [McFarland and Mortara, 1992; Peck et al., 1990]. Fabrication of these microcoils often requires special techniques, such as light lithography and electron-beam lithography.

The direction of the B_1 field generated by a solenoid coil prevents the coil from being coaxially placed in the magnet. Thus accessing and positioning samples are difficult. To solve this problem, Banson et al. [1992] devised a unique Helmholtz coil that consists of two separate loops. Each loop is made from a microwave laminate with a dielectric material sandwiched between two copper foils. By making use of the distributed capacitance, the coil can be tuned to a desired frequency. Since the two loops of the coil are mechanically separated, samples can be easily slid into the gap between the loops without any obstruction. Under certain circumstances, the Helmholtz coil can outperform an optimally designed solenoid coil with similar dimensions.

For *in vivo* studies, although volume coils such as solenoid coils and birdcage coils can be employed, most high-resolution experiments are carried out using local RF coils, including surface coils [Banson et al., 1992; Rudin, 1987] and implanted coils [Farmer et al., 1989; Hollett et al., 1987; Zhou et al., 1994]. Surface coils can effectively reduce coil size and simultaneously limit the field of view to a small region of interest. They can be easily adaptable to the shape of samples and provide high sensitivity in the surface region. The problem of inhomogeneous B_1 fields can be minimized using composite pulses [Hetherington et al., 1986] or adiabatic pulses [Ugurbil et al., 1987]. To obtain high-resolution images from regions distant from the surface, surgically implantable coils become the method of choice. These coils not only give better SNR than optimized surface coils [Zhou et al., 1992] but also provide accurate and consistent localization. The latter advantage is particularly useful for time-course studies on dynamic processes such as the development of pathology and monitoring the effects of therapeutic drugs.

The recent advent of high-temperature superconducting (HTS) RF coils has brought new excitement to MR microscopy [Black et al., 1993]. The substantial improvement, as discussed earlier, makes signal averaging unnecessary. Using these coils, the total imaging time will be solely determined by the efficiency to traverse the k-space. Although much research is yet to be done in this new area, combination of the HTS coils with fast-imaging algorithms will most likely provide a unique way to fully realize the potential of MR microscopy and eventually bring the technique into routine use.

15.3.2 Magnetic Field Gradient Coils

As discussed previously, high spatial resolution requires magnetic field gradients. The gradient strength increases proportional to the coil current and inversely proportional to the coil size. Since increasing current generates many undesirable effects (overheating, mechanical vibrations, eddy current, etc.), strong magnetic field gradient is almost exclusively achieved by reducing the coil diameter.

Design of magnetic field gradient coils for MR microscopy is a classic problem. Based on Maxwell equations, ideal surface current density can be calculated for a chosen geometry of the conducting surface. Two conducting surfaces are mostly used: a cylindrical surface parallel to the axis of the magnet and a cylindrical surface perpendicular to the axis. The ideal surface current density distributions for these two geometries are illustrated in Figure 15.2 [Suits and Wilken, 1989]. After the ideal surface current density distribution is obtained, design of gradient coils is reduced to a problem of using discrete conductors with a finite length to approximate the continuous current distribution function. The error in the approximation determines the gradient linearity. Recent advancements in computer-based fabrication and etching techniques have made it feasible to produce complicated current density distributions. Using these techniques, nonlinear terms up to the eleventh order can be eliminated over a predefined cylindrical volume.

Another issue in gradient coil design involves minimizing the gradient rise time so that fast-imaging techniques can be implemented successfully and short echo times can be achieved to minimize signal loss for short T_2 specimens. The gradient rise time relies on three factors: the inductance over resistance ratio of the gradient coil, the time constant of the feedback circuit of the gradient power supply, and the decay rate of eddy current triggered by gradient switching. The time constant attributed to inductive resistance (L/R) is relatively short (<100 μsec) for most microscopy gradient coils, and the inductive resistance from the power supply can be easily adjusted to match the time constant of the coil. However, considering the high magnetic field gradient strength used in MR microscopy, eddy currents can be a serious problem. This problem is even worsened when the gradient coils are closely placed in a narrow magnet bore. To minimize the eddy currents, modern design of gradient coils uses an extra set of coils so that the eddy currents can be actively cancelled [Mansfield and Chapman, 1986]. Under close to optimal conditions,

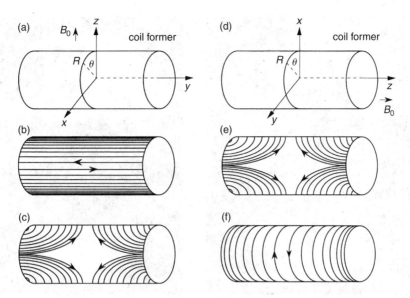

FIGURE 15.2 (a) Ideal surface current distributions to generate linear magnetic field gradients when the gradient coil former is parallel to the magnet bore: (b) for x gradient and (c) for z gradient. The analytical expressions for the current density distribution functions are $J_x = KG_x[R\cos\theta(\sin\theta i - \cos\theta j) - z\sin\theta k]$ and $J_z = KG_z Z[\sin\theta_i - \cos\theta_j]$. The y gradient can be obtained by rotating J_x 90°. (b) Ideal surface current distributions to generate linear magnetic field gradients when the gradient coil former is perpendicular to the magnet bore: (e) for x gradient and (f) for y gradient. The analytical expressions for the current density distribution functions are $J_x = KG_x R(\sin 2\theta_j)$ and $J_y = KG_y(-R\cos^2\theta_i + y\sin j + 0.5R\sin 2\theta_k)$. The z gradient can be obtained by rotating J_x 45°. (The graphs are adapted based on Suits, B.H. and Wilken, D.E. [1989]. *J. Phys. E: Sci. Instrum.* 22: 565.)

a rise time of <150 μsec can be achieved with a maximum gradient of 82 G/cm in a set of 8 cm coils [Johnson et al., 1992].

Although the majority of microscopic MR images are obtained using cylindrical gradient coils, surface gradient coils have been used recently in several studies [Cho et al., 1992]. Similar to surface RF coils, surface gradient coils can be easily adapted to the shape of samples and are capable of producing strong magnetic field gradient in limited areas. The surface gradient coils also provide more free space in the magnet, allowing easy access to samples. A major problem with surface gradient coils is the gradient nonlinearity. But when the region of interest is small, high-quality images can still be obtained with negligible distortions.

15.4 Applications

MR microscopy has a broad range of applications. We include here several examples. Figure 15.3 illustrates an application of MR microscopy in *ex vivo* histology. In this study, a fixed sheep heart with experimentally-induced infarct is imaged at $2T$ using 3D fast-spin-echo techniques with T_1 (Figure 15.3a) and T_2 (Figure 15.3b) contrasts. The infarct region is clearly detected in both images. The region of infarct can be segmented from the rest of the tissue and its volume can be accurately measured. Since the image is three-dimensional, the tissue pathology can be examined in any arbitrary orientation. The nondestructive nature of MR microscopy also allows the same specimen to be restudied using other techniques as well as using other contrast mechanisms of MR microscopy. Obtaining this dimension of information from conventional histologic studies would be virtually impossible.

The *in vivo* capability of MR microscopy for toxicologic studies is illustrated in Figure 15.4. In this study [Farmer et al., 1989], the effect of mercuric chloride in rat kidney is monitored in a single animal. Therefore, development of tissue pathology over a time period is directly observed without the unnecessary

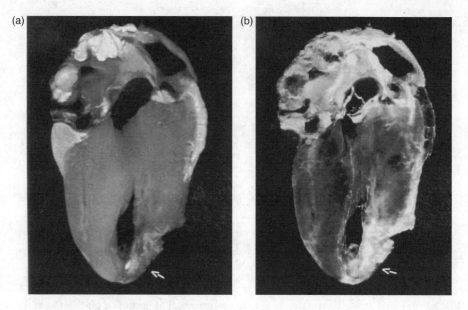

FIGURE 15.3 Selected sections of 3D isotropic images of a sheep heart with experimentally induced infarct show the utility of MRM in pathology studies. A 3D FSE sequence has been designed to allow rapid acquisition of either (a) T_1-weighted or (b) T_2-weighted images giving two separate "stains" for the pathology. Arrows indicate areas of necrosis.

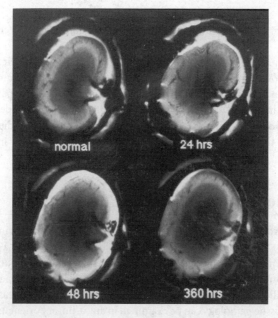

FIGURE 15.4 Implanted RF coils allow *in vivo* studies of deep structures with much higher spatial resolution by limiting the field of view during excitation and by increasing the SNR over volume coils. An added benefit is the ability to accurately localize the same region during a time course study. Shown here is the same region of a kidney at four different time points following exposure to mercuric chloride. Note the description of boundaries between the several zones of the kidney in the early part of the study followed by regeneration of the boundaries upon repair.

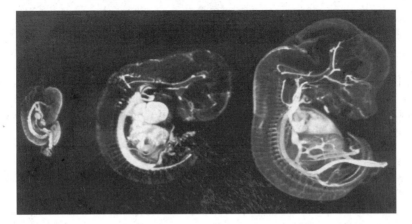

FIGURE 15.5 Isotropic 3D images of fixed mouse embryos at three stages of development have been volume rendered to allow visualization of the developing vascular anatomy.

interference arising from interanimal variabilities. Since the kidney was the only region of interest in this study, a surgically implanted coil was chosen to optimize SNR and to obtain consistent localization. Figure 15.4 shows four images obtained from the same animal at different time points to show the progression and regression of the $HgCl_2$-induced renal pathology. Tissue damage is first observed 24 h after the animal was treated by the chemical, as evident by the blurring between the cortex and the outer medulla. The degree of damage is greater in the image obtained at 48 h. Finally, at 360 h, the blurred boundary between the two tissue regions completely disappeared, indicating full recovery of the organ. The capability to monitor tissue pathologic changes *in vivo*, as illustrated in this example, bodes well for a broad range of applications in pharmacology, toxicology, and pathology.

Development biology is another area where MR microscopy has found an increasing number of applications, Jacobs and Fraser [1994] used MR microscopy to follow cell movements and lineages in developing frog embryos. In their study, 3D images of the developing embryo were obtained on a time scale faster than the cell division time and analyzed forward and backward in time to reconstruct full cell divisions and cell movements. By labeling a 16-cell embryo with an exogenous contrast agent (Gd-DTPA), they successfully followed the progression from early cleavage and blastula stage through gastrulation, neurulation, and finally to tail bud stage. More important, they found that external ectodermal and internal mesodermal tissues extend at different rates during amphibian gastrulation and neurulation. This and many other key events in vertebrate embryogenesis would be very difficult to observe with optical microscopy. Another example in developmental biology is given in Figure 15.5. Using 3D high-field (9.4-T) MR microscopy with large image arrays (256^3), Smith et al. [1993] studied the early development of the circulatory system of mouse embryos. With the aid of a T_1 contrast agent made from bovine serum albumin and Gd-DTPA, vasculature such as ventricles, atria, aorta, cardinal sinuses, basilar arteries, and thoracic arteries are clearly identified in mouse embryos at between 9.5 and 12.5 days of gestation. The ability to study embryonic development in a noninvasive fashion provided great opportunities to explore many problems in transgenic studies, gene targeting, and *in situ* hybridization.

In less than 10 yr, MR microscopy has grown from a scientific curiosity to a tool with a wide range of applications. Although many theoretical and experimental problems still exist at the present time, there is no doubt that MR microscopy will soon make a significant impact in many areas of basic research and clinical diagnosis.

References

Ahn, C.B. and Cho, Z.H. (1989). A generalized formulation of diffusion effects in mm resolution nuclear magnetic resonance imaging. *Med. Phys.* 16: 22.

Banson, M.B., Cofer, G.P., Black, R.D., and Johnson, G.A. (1992a). A probe for specimen magnetic resonance microscopy. *Invest. Radiol.* 27: 157.

Banson, M.L., Cofer, G.P., Hedlund, L.W., and Johnson, G.A. (1992b). Surface coil imaging of rat spine at 7.0 T. *Magn. Reson. Imag.* 10: 929.

Benveniste, H., Hedlund, L.W., and Johnson, G.A. (1992). Mechanism of detection of acute cerebral ischemia in rats by diffusion-weighted magnetic resonance microscopy. *Stroke* 23: 746.

Black, R.D., Early, T.A., Roemer, P.B. et al. (1993). A high-temperature superconducting receiver for NMR microscopy. *Science* 259: 793.

Brown, T.R., Kincaid, B.M., and Ugurbil, K. (1982). NMR chemical shift imaging in three dimensions. *Proc. Natl Acad. Sci. USA* 79: 3523.

Callaghan, P.T. and Eccles, C.D. (1987). Sensitivity and resolution in NMR imaging. *J. Magn. Reson.* 71: 426.

Callaghan, P.T. and Eccles, C.D. (1988). Diffusion-limited resolution in nuclear magnetic resonance microscopy. *J. Magn. Reson.* 78: 1.

Callaghan, P.T., Coy, A., Forde, L.C., and Rofe, C.J. (1993). Diffusive relaxation and edge enhancement in NMR microscopy. *J. Magn. Reson. Ser. A* 101: 347.

Cho, Z.H., Ahn, C.B., Juh, S.C. et al. (1988). Nuclear magnetic resonance microscopy with 4 mm resolution: theoretical study and experimental results. *Med. Phys.* 15: 815.

Cho, Z.H., Yi, J.H., and Friedenberg, R.M. (1992). NMR microscopy and ultra-high resolution NMR imaging. *Rev. Magn. Reson. Med.* 4: 221.

Edelstein, W.A., Hutchison, J.M.S., Johnson, G., and Redpath, T. (1980). Spin warp NMR imaging and applications to human whole-body imaging. *Phys. Med. Biol.* 25: 751.

Ehman, R.L. and Felmlee, J.P. (1989). Adaptive technique for high-definition MR imaging of moving structures. *Radiology* 173: 255.

Farmer, T.H.R., Johnson, G.A., Cofer, G.P. et al. (1989). Implanted coil MR microscopy of renal pathology. *Magn. Reson. Med.* 10: 310.

Gewalt, S.L., Glover, G.H., MacFall, J.R. et al. (1993). MR microscopy of the rat lung using projection reconstruction. *Magn. Reson. Med.* 29: 99.

Glover, G.H. and Noll, D.C. (1993). Consistent projection reconstruction techniques for MRI. *Magn. Reson. Med.* 29: 345.

Glover, G.H. and Pauly, J.M. (1992). Projection reconstruction techniques for suppression of motion artifacts. *Magn. Reson. Med.* 28: 275.

Gmitro, A. and Alexander, A.L. (1993). Use of a projection reconstruction method to decrease motion sensitivity in diffusion-weighted MRI. *Magn. Reson. Med.* 29: 835.

Haase, A., Frahm, J., Matthaei, D. et al. (1986). FLASH imaging: rapid NMR imaging using low flip angle pulses. *J. Magn. Reson.* 67: 258.

Hedges, H.K. (1984). Nuclear magnetic resonance microscopy. Ph.D. dissertation, State University of New York at Stony Brook.

Hedlund, L.W., Dietz, J., Nassar, R. et al. (1986). A ventilator for magnetic resonance imaging. *Invest. Radiol.* 21: 18.

Hennig, J., Nauerth, A., and Friedburg, H. (1986). RARE imaging: a fast imaging method for clinical MR. *Magn. Reson. Med.* 3: 823.

Hetherington, H.P., Wishart, D., Fitzpatrick, S.M. et al. (1986). The application of composite pulses to surface coil NMR. *J. Magn. Reson.* 66: 313.

Hills, B.P., Wright, K.M., and Belton, P.S. (1990). The effects of restricted diffusion in nuclear magnetic resonance microscopy. *Magn. Reson. Imag.* 8: 755.

Hollett, M.D., Cofer, G.P., and Johnson, G.A. (1987). *In situ* magnetic resonance microscopy. *Invest. Radiol.* 22: 965.

House, W.V. (1984). NMR microscopy. *IEEE Trans. Nucl. Sci.* NS-31: 570.

Hyslop, W.B. and Lauterbur, P.C. (1991). Effects of restricted diffusion on microscopic NMR imaging. *J. Magn. Reson.* 94: 501.

Jacobs, R.E. and Fraser, S.E. (1994). Magnetic resonance microscopy of embryonic cell lineages and movements. *Science* 263: 681.

Johnson, G.A., Hedlund, L.W., Cofer, G.P., and Suddarth, S.A. (1992). Magnetic resonance microscopy in the life sciences. *Rev. Magn. Reson. Med.* 4: 187.

Karis, J.P., Johnson, G.A., and Glover, G.H. (1987). Signal to noise improvements in three dimensional NMR microscopy using limited angle excitation. *J. Magn. Reson.* 71: 24.

Kumar, A., Welti, D., and Ernst, R.R. (1975). NMR Fourier zeugmatography. *J. Magn. Reson.* 18: 69.

Lai, C.M. and Lauterbur, P.C. (1981). True three-dimensional image reconstruction by nuclear magnetic resonance zeugmatography. *Phys. Med. Biol.* 26: 851.

Lauterbur, P.C. (1973). Image formation by induced local interactions: examples employing nuclear magnetic resonance. *Nature* 242: 190.

Lauterbur, P.C. (1984). New direction in NMR imaging. *IEEE Trans. Nucl. Sci.* NS-31: 1010.

Lean, C.L., Russell, P., Delbridge, L. et al. (1993). Metastatic follicular thyroid diagnosed by 1H MRS. *Proc. Soc. Magn. Reson. Med.* 1: 71.

Majumdar, S. and Gore, J.C. (1988). Studies of diffusion in random fields produced by variations in susceptibility. *J. Magn. Reson.* 78: 41.

Maki, J.H., Johnson, G.A., Cofer, G.P., and MacFall, J.R. (1988). SNR improvement in NMR microscopy using DEFT. *J. Magn. Reson.* 80: 482.

Mansfield, P. and Chapman, B. (1986). Active magnetic screening of gradient coils in NMR imaging. *J. Magn. Reson.* 66: 573.

Mansfield, P. and Maudsley, A.A. (1977). Planar spin imaging by NMR. *J. Magn. Reson.* 27: 129.

McFarland, E.W. (1992). Time independent point-spread function for MR microscopy. *Magn. Reson. Imag.* 10: 269.

McFarland, E.W. and Mortara, A. (1992). Three-dimensional NMR microscopy: improving SNR with temperature and microcoils. *Magn. Reson. Imag.* 10: 279.

Moran, P.R. (1982). A flow velocity zeugmatographic interlace for NMR imaging in humans. *Magn. Reson. Imag.* 1: 197.

Mulkern, R.V., Wong, S.T.S., Winalski, C., and Jolesz, F.A. (1990). Contrast manipulation and artifact assessment of 2D and 3D RARE sequences. *Magn. Reson. Imag.* 8: 557.

Peck, T.L., Magin, R.L., and Lauterbur, P.C. (1990). Microdomain magnetic resonance imaging. *Proc. Soc. Magn. Reson. Med.* 1: 207.

Putz, B., Barsky, D., and Schulten, K. (1991). Edge enhancement by diffusion: microscopic magnetic resonance imaging of an ultrathin glass capillary. *Chem. Phys.* 183: 391.

Rudin, M. (1987). MR microscopy on rats *in vivo* at 4.7 T using surface coils. *Magn. Reson. Med.* 5: 443.

Schoeniger, J.S., Aiken, N.R., and Blackband, S.J. (1991). NMR microscopy of single neurons. *Proc. Soc. Magn. Reson. Med.* 2: 880.

Smith, B.R., Johnson, G.A., Groman, E.V., and Linney, E. (1993). Contrast enhancement of normal and abnormal mouse embryo vasculature. *Proc. Soc. Magn. Reson. Med.* 1: 303.

Suits, B.H. and Wilken, D.E. (1989). Improving magnetic field gradient coils for NMR imaging. *J. Phys. E: Sci. Instrum.* 22: 565.

Ugurbil, K., Garwood, M., and Bendall, R. (1987). Amplitude- and frequency-modulated pulses to achieve 90° plane rotation with inhomogeneous B_1 fields. *J. Magn. Reson.* 72: 177.

Wood, M.L. and Henkelman, R.M. (1985). NMR image artifacts from periodic motion. *Med. Phys.* 12: 143.

Xiang, Q.-S. and Henkelman, R.M. (1991). Motion artifact reduction with three-point ghost phase cancellation. *J. Magn. Reson. Imag.* 1: 633.

Zhong, J. and Gore, J.C. (1991). Studies of restricted diffusion in heterogeneous media containing variations in susceptibility. *Magn. Reson. Med.* 19: 276.

Zhou, Z. (1992). Nuclear magnetic resonance microscopy: new theoretical and technical developments. Ph.D. dissertation, University of Illinois at Urbana-Champaign.

Zhou, X. and Lauterbur, P.C. (1992). NMR microscopy using projection reconstruction. In Blümich, B. and Kuhn, W. (eds.), *Magnetic Resonance Microscopy*, pp 1–27. Weinheim, Germany, VCH.

Zhou, X., Cofer, G.P., Mills, G.I., and Johnson, G.A. (1992). An inductively coupled probe for MR microscopy at 7 T. *Proc. Soc. Magn. Reson. Med.* 1: 971.

Zhou, X., Cofer, G.P., Suddarth, S.A., and Johnson, G.A. (1993). High-field MR microscopy using fast spin-echoes. *Magn. Reson. Med.* 31: 60.

Zhou, X., Liang, Z.-P., Cofer, G.P. et al. (1993). An FSE pulse sequence with circular sampling for MR microscopy. *Proc. Soc. Magn. Reson. Med.* 1: 297.

Zhou, X., Maronpot, R.R., Mills, G.I. et al. (1994). Studies on bromobenzene-induced hepatotoxicity using *in vivo* MR microscopy. *Magn. Reson. Med.* 31: 619.

Further Information

A detailed description of the physics of NMR and MRI can be found in Principles of Magnetic Resonance, by C.S., Slichter (3rd edition, Springer-Verlag, 1989), in NMR Imaging in Biology and Medicine, by P. Morris (Clarendon Press, 1986), and in Principles of Magnetic Resonance Microscopy, by P.T., Callaghan (Oxford Press, 1991). The latter two books also contain detailed discussions on instrumentation, data acquisition, and image reconstruction for conventional and microscopic magnetic resonance imaging.

Magnetic Resonance Microscopy, edited by Blümich and Kuhn (VCH, 1992), is particularly helpful to understand various aspects of MR microscopy, both methodology and applications. Each chapter of the book covers a specific topic and is written by experts in the field.

Proceedings of the Society of Magnetic Resonance (formerly Society of Magnetic Resonance in Medicine, Berkeley, California), published annually, documents the most recent developments in the field of MR microscopy. Magnetic Resonance in Medicine, Journal of Magnetic Resonance Imaging, and Magnetic Resonance Imaging, all monthly journals, contain original research articles and are good sources for up-to-date developments.

16

Positron-Emission Tomography (PET)

16.1 Radiopharmaceuticals **16**-1
Nuclear Reactor-Produced Radionuclides •
Accelerator-Produced Radionuclides • Generator-Produced
Radionuclides • Radiopharmaceuticals • PET
Radionuclides

Acknowledgments.. **16**-7

References **16**-7

16.2 Instrumentation **16**-8
Background • PET Theory • PET Detectors • Physical
Factors Affecting Resolution • Random Coincidences •
Tomographic Reconstruction • Sensitivity • Statistical
Properties of PET

Thomas F. Budinger
Henry F. VanBrocklin
University of California-Berkeley

Acknowledgments.. **16**-16
References **16**-16

16.1 Radiopharmaceuticals

Thomas F. Budinger and Henry F. VanBrocklin

Since the discovery of artificial radioactivity a half century ago, radiotracers, radionuclides, and radionuclide compounds have played a vital role in biology and medicine. Common to all is radionuclide (radioactive isotope) production. This section describes the basic ideas involved in radionuclide production and gives examples of the applications of radionuclides. The field of radiopharmaceutical chemistry has fallen into subspecialties of positron-emission tomography (PET) chemistry and general radiopharmaceutical chemistry, including specialists in technetium chemistry, taking advantage of the imaging attributes of technetium-99m.

The two general methods of radionuclide production are neutron addition (activation) from neutron reactors to make neutron-rich radionuclides which decay to give off electrons and gamma rays and charged-particle accelerators (linacs and cyclotrons) which usually produce neutron-deficient isotopes that decay by electron capture and emission of x-rays, gamma rays, and positrons. The production of artificial radionuclides is governed by the number of neutrons or charged particles hitting an appropriate target per time, the cross section for the particular reaction, the number of atoms in the target, and the half-life of the artificial radionuclide:

$$A(t) = \frac{N\sigma\phi}{3.7 \times 10^{10}} \left(1 - e^{0.693t/T_{1/2}}\right) \tag{16.1}$$

where $A(t)$ is the produced activity in number of atoms per second, N is the number of target nuclei, σ is the cross section (probability that the neutron or charged particles will interact with the nucleus to form the artificial radioisotope) for the reaction, ϕ is the flux of charged particles, and $T_{1/2}$ is the half-life of the product. Note that N is the target mass divided by the atomic weight and multiplied by Avogadro's number (6.024×10^{23}) and σ is measured in cm^2. The usual flux is about 10^{14} neutrons per sec or, for charged particles, 10 to 100 mA, which is equivalent to 6.25×10^{13} to 6.25×10^{14} charged particles per second.

16.1.1 Nuclear Reactor-Produced Radionuclides

Thermal neutrons of the order of 10^{14} neutrons/sec/cm^2 are produced in a nuclear reactor usually during a controlled nuclear fission of uranium, though thorium or plutonium are also used. High specific activity neutron-rich radionuclides are produced usually through the (n, g), (n, p), or (n, a) reactions (Figure 16.1a). The product nuclides usually decay by b — followed by g. Most of the reactor-produced radionuclides are produced by the (n, g) reaction. The final step in the production of a radionuclide consists of the separation of the product nuclide from the target container by chemical or physical means.

An alternative method for producing isotopes from a reactor is to separate the fission fragments from the spent fuel rods. This is the leading source of ^{99}Mo for medical applications. The following two methods of ^{99}Mo production are examples of carrier-added and no-carrier-added radionuclide synthesis, respectively. In Figure 16.1a, the ^{99}Mo is production from ^{98}Mo. Only a small fraction of the ^{98}Mo nuclei will be converted to ^{99}Mo. Therefore, at the end of neutron bombardment, there is a mixture of both isotopes. These are inseparable by conventional chemical separation techniques, and both isotopes would participate equally well in chemical reactions. The ^{99}Mo from fission of ^{238}U would not contain any other isotopes of Mo and is considered carrier-free. Thus radioisotopes produced by any means having the same atomic number as the target material would be considered carrier-added. Medical tracer techniques obviate the need for carrier-free isotopes.

16.1.2 Accelerator-Produced Radionuclides

Cyclotrons and linear accelerators (linacs) are sources of beams of protons, deuterons, or helium ions that bombarded targets to produce neutron-deficient (proton-rich) radionuclides (Figure 16.1b). The neutron-deficient radionuclides produced through these reactions are shown in Table 16.1. These product nuclides (usually carrier-free) decay either by electron capture or by positron emission tomography or both, followed by g emission. In Table 16.2, most of the useful charged-particle reactions are listed.

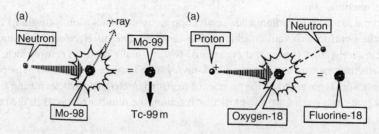

FIGURE 16.1   (a) High specific activity neutron-excess radionuclides are produced usually through the (n, g), (n, p) or (n, a) reactions. The product nuclides usually decay b — followed by g. Most of the reactor produced radionuclides are produced by the (n, g) reaction. (b) Cyclotrons and linear accelerators (linacs) are sources of beams of protons, deuterons, or helium ions which bombard targets to produce neutron-deficient radionuclides.

TABLE 16.1   Radionuclides Used in Biomedicine

Radionuclide	Half-life	Application(s)
Arsenic-74*	17.9 d	A positron emitting chemical analog of phosphorus
Barium-128*	2.4 d	Parent in the generator system for producing the positron emitting ^{128}Cs, a potassium analog
Beryllium-7*	53.37 d	Berylliosis studies
Bromine-77	57 h	Radioimmunotherapy
Bromin-82	35.3 h	Used in metabolic studies and studies of estrogen receptor content
Carbon-11*	20.3 min	Positron emitter for metabolism imaging
Cobalt-57*	270 d	Calibration of imaging instruments
Copper-62	9.8 min	Heart perfusion
Copper-64	12.8 h	Used as a clinical diagnostic agent for cancer and metabolic disorders
Copper-67	58.5 h	Radioimmunotherapy
Chromium-51	27.8 d	Used to assess red blood cell survival
Fluorine-18	109.7 min	Positron emitter used in glucose analogs uptake and neuroreceptor imaging
Gallium-68	68 min	Required in calibrating PET tomographs. Potential antibody level
Germanium-68*	287 d	Parent in the generator system for producing the positron emitting ^{68}Ga
Indium-111*	2.8 d	Radioimmunotherapy
Iodine-122	3.76 min	Positron emitter for blood flow studies
Iodine-123*	13.3 h	SPECT brain imaging agent
Iodine-124*	4.2 d	Radioimmunotherapy, positron emitter
Iodine-125	60.2 d	Used as a potential cancer therapeutic agent
Iodine-131	8.1 d	Used to diagnose and treat thyroid disorders including cancer
Iron-52*	8.2 h	Used as an iron tracer, positron emitter for bone-marrow imaging
Magnesium-28*	21.2 h	Magnesium tracer which decays to 2.3 in aluminum-28
Magnese-52m	5.6 d	Flow tracer for heart muscle
Mercury-195m*	40 h	Parent in the generator system for producing ^{195}mAu, which is used in cardiac blood pool studies
Molybdenum-99	67 h	Used to produce technetium-99m, the most commonly used radioisotope in clinical nuclear medicine
Nitrogen-13*	9.9 min	Positron emitter used as ^{13}NH for heart perfusion studies
Osmium-191	15 d	Decays to iridium-191 used for cardiac studies
Oxygen-15*	123 s	Positron emitter used for blood flow studies as H152O
Palladium-103	17 d	Used in the treatment of prostate cancer
Phosphorus-32	14.3 d	Used in cancer treatment, cell metabolism and kinetics, molecular biology, genetics research, biochemistry, microbiology, enzymology, and as a starter to make many basic chemicals and research products
Rhenium-188	17 h	Used for treatment of medullary thyroid carcinoma and alleviation of pain in bone metastases
Rubidium-82*	1.2 min	Positron emitter used for heart perfusion studies
Ruthemiun-97*	2.9 d	Hepatobiliary function, tumor and inflammation localization
Samarium-145	340 d	Treatment of ocular cancer
Samarium-153	46.8 h	Used to radiolabel various molecules as cancer therapeutic agents and to alleviate bone cancer pain
Scandium-47	3.4 d	Radioimmunotherapy
Scandium-47*	3.4 d	Used in the therapy of cancer
Strontium-82*	64.0 d	Parent in the generator system for producing the positron emitting ^{82}Rb, a potassium analogue
Strontium-85	64 d	Used to study bone formation metabolism
Strontium-89	52 d	Used to alleviate metastatic bone pain
Sulfur-35	87.9 d	Used in studies of cell metabolism and kinetics, molecular biology, genetics research, biochemistry, microbiology, enzymology, and as a start to make many basic chemicals and research products
Technetium-99m	6 h	The most widely used radiopharmaceutical in nuclear medicine and produced from molybdenum-99
Thalium-201*	74 h	Cardiac imaging agent
Tin-117m	14.0 d	Palliative treatment of bone cancer pain

(Continued)

TABLE 16.1 (Continued) Radionuclides Used in Biomedicine

Radionuclide	Half-life	Application(s)
Tritium (hydrogen-3)	12.3 yr	Used to make tritiated water which is used as a starter for thousands of different research products and basic chemicals; used for life science and drug metabolism studies to ensure the safety of potential new drugs
Tungsten-178*	21.5 d	Parent in generator system for producing ^{178}Ta, short-lived scanning agent
Tungsten-188	69 d	Decays to rhenium-188 for treatment of cancer and rheumatoid arthritis
Vanadium-48*	16.0 d	Nutrition and environmental studies
Xenon-122*	20 h	Parent in the generator system for producing the positron emitting ^{122}I
Xenon-127*	36.4 d	Used in lung ventilation studies
Xenon-133	5.3 d	Used in lung ventilation and perfusion studies
Yttrium-88*	106.6 d	Radioimmunotherapy
Yttrium-90	64 h	Used to radiolabel various molecules as cancer therapeutic agents
Zinc-62*	9.13 h	Parent in the generator system for producing the positron emitting ^{62}Cu
Zirconium-89*	78.4 h	Radioimmunotherapy, positron emitter

* Produced by accelerated charged particles. Others are produced by neutron reactors.

Sestamibi

$$^{99m}TcO_4^- + (CH_3)_2C(OMe)CH_2NC]_4CuBF_4$$

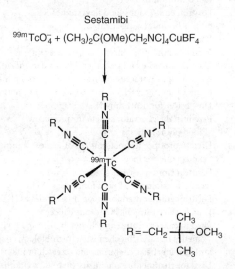

FIGURE 16.2 ^{99m}Tc-Sestamibi is a radiopharmaceutical used to evaluate myocardial perfusion or in the diagnosis of cancer using both computed tomography and scintigraphy techniques.

TABLE 16.2 Important Reactions for Cyclotron-Produced Radioisotopes

1.	p, n	7.	p, pn
2.	$p, 2n$	8.	$p, 2p$
3.	d, n	9.	d, p
4.	$d, 2n$	10.	$d, ^4$He
5.	$d, ^4$He	11.	p, d
6.	$d, ^4$Hen	12.	^{4}He, n
13.	^{3}He, p		

The heat produced by the beam current on the target material can interfere with isotope production and requires efficient heat-removal strategies using extremely stable heat-conducting target materials such as metal foils, electroplates metals, metal powders, metal oxides, and salts melted on duralmin plate. All the modern targets use circulating cold deionized water and chilled helium gas to aid in cooling the target body and window foils. Cyclotrons used in medical studies have ^{11}C, ^{13}N, ^{15}O, and ^{18}F production capabilities that deliver the product nuclides on demand through computer-executed commands. The radionuclide is remotely transferred into a lead-shielded hot cell for processing. The resulting radionuclides are manipulated using microscale radiochemical techniques: small-scale synthetic methodology, ion-exchange chromatography, solvent extraction, electrochemical synthesis, distillation, simple filtration, paper chromatography, and isotopic carrier precipitation. Various relevant radiochemical techniques have been published in standard texts.

16.1.3   Generator-Produced Radionuclides

If the reactor, cyclotron, or natural product radionuclide of long half-life decays to a daughter with nuclear characteristics appropriate for medical application, the system is called a medical radionuclide generator. There are several advantages afforded by generator-produced isotopes. These generators represent a convenient source of short-lived medical isotopes without the need for an on-site reactor or particle accelerator. Generators provide delivery of the radionuclide on demand at a site remote from the production facility. They are a source of both gamma- and positron-emitting isotopes.

The most common medical radionuclide generator is the ^{99}Mo Æ ^{99m}Tc system, the source of ^{99m}Tc, a gamma-emitting isotope currently used in 70% of the clinical nuclear medicine studies. The ^{99}Mo has a 67-h half-life, giving this generator a useful life of about a week. Another common generator is the ^{68}Ge Æ ^{68}Ga system. Germanium (half-life is 287 d) is accelerator-produced in high-energy accelerators (e.g., BLIP, LAMPF, TRIUMF) through the alpha-particle bombardment of ^{66}Zn. The 68Ge decays to ^{68}Ga, a positron emitter, which has a 68-min half-life. Gallium generators can last for several months.

The generator operation is fairly straightforward. In general, the parent isotope is bound to a solid chemical matrix (e.g., alumina column, anionic resin, Donux resin). As the parent decays, the daughter nuclide grows in. The column is then flushed ("milked") with a suitable solution (e.g., saline, hydrochloric acid) that elutes the daughter and leaves the remaining parent absorbed on the column. The eluent may be injected directly or processed into a radiopharmaceutical.

16.1.4   Radiopharmaceuticals

^{99m}Tc is removed from the generator in the form of TcO$_4^-$ (pertechnetate). This species can be injected directly for imaging or incorporated into a variety of useful radiopharmaceuticals. The labeling of ^{99m}Tc usually involves reduction complexation/chelation. ^{99m}Tc-Sestamibi (Figure 16.2) is a radiopharmaceutical used to evaluate myocardial perfusion or to diagnose cancer. There are several reduction methods employed, including Sn(II) reduction in NaHCO$_3$ at pH of 8 and other reduction and complexation reactions such as S$_2$O$_3$ + HCl, FeCl$_3$ + ascorbic acid, LiBH$_4$, Zn + HCl, HCl, Fe(II), Sn(II)F$_2$, Sn(II) citrate, and Sn(II) tartrate reduction and complexation, electrolytic reduction, and *in vivo* labeling of red cells following Sn(II) pyrophosphate or Sn(II) DTPA administration. ^{131}I, ^{125}I, and ^{123}I labeling requires special reagents or conditions such as chloramine-T, widely used for protein labeling at 7.5 pH; peroxidase + H$_2$O$_2$ widely used for radioassay tracers; isotopic exchange for imaging tracers; excitation labeling as in ^{123}Xe Æ ^{123}I diazotization plus iodination for primary amines; conjugation labeling with Bolton Hunter agent (N-succinimidyl 3-[4-hydroxy 5-(^{131,125,123}I)iodophenyl] propionate); hydroboration plus iodination; electrophilic destannylation; microdiffusion with fresh iodine vapor; and other methods. Radiopharmaceuticals in common use for brain perfusion studies are N-isopropyl-p [^{123}I] iodoamphetamine and ^{99m}Tc-labeled hexamethylpropyleneamine.

16.1.5   PET Radionuclides

For ^{11}C, ^{13}N, ^{15}O, and ^{18}F, the modes of production of short-lived positron emitters can dictate the chemical form of the product, as shown in Table 16.3. Online chemistry is used to make various PET agents and precursors. For example, ^{11}C cyanide, an important precursor for synthesis of other labeled compounds, is produced in the cyclotron target by first bombarding N$_2$ + 5% H$_2$ gas target with 20-MeV

TABLE 16.3   Major Positron-Emitting
Radionuclides Produced by Accelerated Protons

Radionuclide	Half-Life	Reaction
Carbon-11	20 min	$^{12}C\,(p, pn)\,^{11}C$
		$^{14}N\,(p, \alpha)\,^{11}C$
Nitrogen-12	10 min	$^{16}O\,(p, \alpha)\,^{13}N$
		$^{13}C\,(p, n)\,^{13}N$
Oxygen-15	2 min	$^{15}N\,(p, n)\,^{15}C$
		$^{14}N\,(d, n)\,^{15}O$
Fluorine-18	110 min	$^{18}O\,(p, n)\,^{18}F$
		$^{20}Ne\,(d, \alpha)\,^{18}F$

Note: $A(x,\ y)B$: A is target, x is the bombarding
particle, y is the radiation product, and B id the
isotope produced.

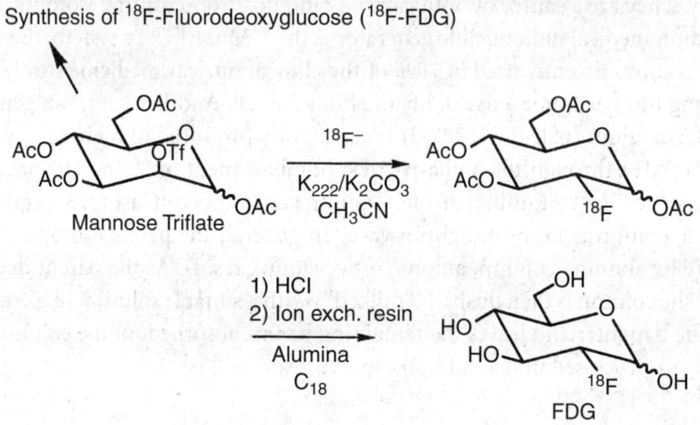

FIGURE 16.3   Schematic for the chemical production of deoxyglucose labeled with fluorine-18. Here K_{222} refers to Kryptofix and C_{18} denotes a reverse-phase high-pressure liquid chromatography column.

protons. The product is carbon-labeled methane, $11CH_4$, which when combined with ammonia and passed over a platinum wool catalyst at $1000°C$ becomes $11CN^-$, which is subsequently trapped in NaOH.

Molecular oxygen is produced by bombarding a gas target of $14N_2 + 2\%\ O_2$ with deuterons (6 to 8 MeV). A number of products (e.g., $15O_2$, $C15O_2$, $N15O_2$, $15O_3$, and $H_2 15O$) are trapped by soda lime followed by charcoal to give $15O_2$ as the product. However, if an activated charcoal trap at $900°C$ is used before the soda lime trap, the $15O_2$ will be converted to $C15O$. The specific strategies for other online PET agents is given in Rayudu [1990].

Fluorine-18 (^{18}F) is a very versatile positron emitting isotope. With a 2-h half-life and two forms (F^+ and F^-), one can develop several synthetic methods for incorporating ^{18}F into medically useful compounds [Kilbourn, 1990]. Additionally, fluorine forms strong bonds with carbon and is roughly the same size as a hydrogen atom, imparting metabolic and chemical stability of the molecules without drastically altering biologic activity. The most commonly produced ^{18}F radiopharmaceutical is 2-deoxy-2-[^{18}F]fluoroglucose (FDG). This radiotracer mimics part of the glucose metabolic pathway and has shown both hypo- and hypermetabolic abnormalities in cardiology, oncology, and neurology. The synthetic pathway for the production of FDG is shown in Figure 16.3.

The production of positron radiopharmaceuticals requires the rapid incorporation of the isotope into the desired molecule. Chemical techniques and synthetic strategies have been developed to facilitate these reactions. Many of these synthetic manipulations require hands-on operations by a highly trained chemist. Additionally, since positrons give off 2- to 511-keV gamma rays upon annihilation, proximity to the source can increase one's personal dose. The demand for the routine production of positron radiopharmaceuticals such as FDG has led to the development of remote synthetic devices. These devices can be human-controlled (i.e., flipping switches to open air-actuated valves), computer-controlled, or robotic. A sophisticated computer-controlled chemistry synthesis unit has been assembled for the fully automated production of ^{18}FDG [Padgett, 1989]. A computer-controlled robot has been programmed to produce 6a-[^{18}F]fluoroestradiol for breast cancer imaging [Brodack et al., 1986; Mathias et al., 1987]. Both these types of units increase the availability and reduce the cost of short-lived radiopharmaceutical production through greater reliability and reduced need for a highly trained staff. Additionally, these automated devices reduce personnel radiation exposure. These and other devices are being designed with greater versatility in mind to allow a variety of radiopharmaceuticals to be produced just by changing the programming and the required reagents.

These PET radionuclides have been incorporated into a wide variety of medically useful radiopharmaceuticals through a number of synthetic techniques. The development of PET scanner technology has added a new dimension to synthetic chemistry by challenging radiochemists to devise labeling and purification strategies that proceed on the order of minutes rather than hours or days as in conventional synthetic chemistry. To meet this challenge, radiochemists are developing new target systems to improve isotope production and sophisticated synthetic units to streamline routine production of commonly desired radiotracers as well as preparing short-lived radiopharmaceuticals for many applications.

Acknowledgments

This work was supported in part by the Director, Office of Energy Research, Office of Health and Environmental Research, Medical Applications and Biophysical Research Division of the U.S. Department of Energy, under contract No. DE-AC03-SF00098, and in part by NIH Grant HL25840.

References

Brodack, J.W., Dence, C.S., Kilbourn, M.R., and Welch, M.J. (1988). Robotic production of 2-deoxy-2-[^{18}F]fluoro-d-glucose: aroutine method of synthesis using tetrabutylammonium [^{18}F]fluoride. *Int. J. Radiat. Appl. Instrum. Part A: Appl. Radiat. Isotopes* 39: 699.

Brodack, J.W., Kilbourn, M.R., Welch, M.J., and Katzenellenbogen, J.A. (1986). Application of robotics to radiopharmaceutical preparation: controlled synthesis of fluorine-18 16 alpha-fluoroestradiol-17 beta. *J. Nucl. Med.* 27: 714.

Hupf, H.B. (1976). Production and purification of radionuclides. In *Radiopharmacy*. New York, Wiley.

Kilbourn, M.R. (1990). *Fluorine-18 Labeling of Radiopharmaceuticals*. Washington, National Academy Press.

Lamb, J. and Kramer, H.H. (1983). Commercial production of radioisotopes for nuclear medicine. In *Radiotracers for Medical Applications*, pp. 17–62. Boca Raton, FL, CRC Press.

Mathias, C.J., Welch, M.J., Katzenellenbogen, J.A. et al. (1987). Characterization of the uptake of 16 alpha-([^{18}F]fluoro)-17 beta-estradiol in DMBA-induced mammary tumors. *Int. J. Radiat. Appl. Instrum. Part B: Nucl. Med. Biol.* 14: 15.

Padgett, H.C., Schmidt, D.G., Luxen, A. et al. (1989). Computed-controlled radiochemical synthesis: a chemistry process control unit for the automated production of radiochemicals. *Int. J. Radiat. Appl. Instrum. Part A: Appl. Radiat. Isotopes* 40: 433.

Rayudu, G.V. (1990). Production of radionuclides for medicine. *Semin. Nucl. Med.* 20: 100.

Sorenson, J.A. and Phelps, M.E. (1987). *Physics in Nuclear Medicine*. New York, Grune & Stratton.

Steigman, J. and Eckerman, W.C. (1992). *The Chemistry of Technetium in Medicine*. Washington, National Academy Press.

Stocklin, G. (1992). Tracers for metabolic imaging of brain and heart: radiochemistry and radiopharmacology. *Eur. J. Nucl. Med.* 19: 527.

16.2 Instrumentation

Thomas F. Budinger

16.2.1 Background

The history of positron-emission tomography (PET) can be traced to the early 1950s, when workers in Boston first realized the medical imaging possibilities of a particular class of radioactive substances. It was recognized then that the high-energy photons produced by annihilation of the positron from positron-emitting isotopes could be used to describe, in three dimensions, the physiologic distribution of "tagged" chemical compounds. After two decades of moderate technological developments by a few research centers, widespread interest and broadly based research activity began in earnest following the development of sophisticated reconstruction algorithms and improvements in detector technology. By the mid-1980s, PET had become a tool for medical diagnosis and for dynamic studies of human metabolism.

Today, because of its million-fold sensitivity advantage over magnetic resonance imaging (MRI) in tracer studies and its chemical specificity, PET is used to study neuroreceptors in the brain and other body tissues. In contrast, MRI has exquisite resolution for anatomic (Figure 16.4) and flow studies as well as unique attributes of evaluating chemical composition of tissue but in the millimolar range rather than the nanomolar range of much of the receptor proteins in the body. Clinical studies include tumors of the brain, breast, lungs, lower gastrointestinal tract, and other sites. Additional clinical uses include Alzheimer's disease, Parkinson's disease, epilepsy, and coronary artery disease affecting heart muscle metabolism and flow. Its use has added immeasurably to our current understanding of flow, oxygen utilization, and the metabolic changes that accompany disease and that change during brain stimulation and cognitive activation.

16.2.2 PET Theory

PET imaging begins with the injection of a metabolically active tracer — a biologic molecule that carries with it a positron-emitting isotope (e.g., ^{11}C, ^{13}N, ^{15}O, or ^{18}F). Over a few minutes, the isotope accumulates in an area of the body for which the molecule has an affinity. As an example, glucose labeled with 11C, or a glucose analogue labeled with ^{18}F, accumulates in the brain or tumors, where glucose is used as the primary source of energy. The radioactive nuclei then decay by positron emission. In positron (positive electron) emission, a nuclear proton changes into a positive electron and a neutron. The atom maintains its atomic mass but decreases its atomic number by 1. The ejected positron combines with an electron almost instantaneously, and these two particles undergo the process of annihilation. The energy associated with

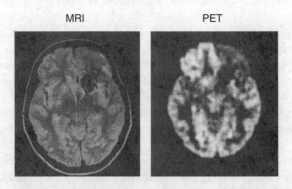

MRI   PET

FIGURE 16.4   The MRI image shows the arteriovenous malformation (AVM) as an area of signal loss due to blood flow. The PET image shows the AVM as a region devoid of glucose metabolism and also shows decreased metabolism in the adjacent frontal cortex. This is a metabolic effect of the AVM on the brain and may explain some of the patient's symptoms.

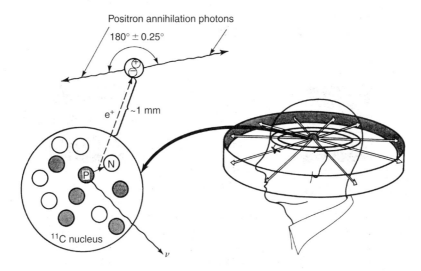

FIGURE 16.5 The physical basis of positron-emission tomography. Positrons emitted by "tagged" metabolically active molecules annihilate nearby electrons and give rise to a pair of high-energy photons. The photons fly off in nearly opposite directions and thus serve to pinpoint their source. The biologic activity of the tagged molecule can be used to investigate a number of physiologic functions, both normal and pathologic.

the masses of the positron and electron particles is 1.022 MeV in accordance with the energy E to mass m equivalence $E = mc^2$, where c is the velocity of light. This energy is divided equally between two photons that fly away from one another at a 180-degree angle. Each photon has an energy of 511 keV. These high-energy gamma rays emerge from the body in opposite directions, to be detected by an array of detectors that surround the patient (Figure 16.5). When two photons are recorded simultaneously by a pair of detectors, the annihilation event that gave rise to them must have occurred somewhere along the line connecting the detectors. Of course, if one of the photons is scattered, then the line of coincidence will be incorrect. After 100,000 or more annihilation events are detected, the distribution of the positron-emitting tracer is calculated by tomographic reconstruction procedures. PET reconstructs a two-dimensional (2D) image from the one-dimensional projections seen at different angles. Three-dimensional (3D) reconstructions also can be done using 2D projections from multiple angles.

16.2.3 PET Detectors

Efficient detection of the annihilation photons from positron emitters is usually provided by the combination of a crystal, which converts the high-energy photons to visible-light photons, and a photomultiplier tube that produces an amplified electric current pulse proportional to the amount of light photons interacting with the photocathode. The fact that imaging system sensitivity is proportional to the square of the detector efficiency leads to a very important requirement that the detector be nearly 100% efficient. Thus other detector systems such as plastic scintillators or gas-filled wire chambers, with typical individual efficiencies of 20% or less, would result in a coincident efficiency of only 4% or less.

Most modern PET cameras are multilayered with 15 to 47 levels or transaxial layers to be reconstructed (Figure 16.6). The lead shields prevent activity from the patient from causing spurious counts in the tomograph ring, while the tungsten septa reject some of the events in which one (or both) of the 511-keV photons suffer a Compton scatter in the patient. The sensitivity of this design is improved by collection of data from cross-planes (Figure 16.6). The arrangement of scintillators and phototubes is shown in Figure 16.7.

The "individually coupled" design is capable of very high resolution, and because the design is very parallel (all the photomultiplier tubes and scintillator crystals operate independently), it is capable of very high data throughput. The disadvantages of this type of design are the requirement for many expensive

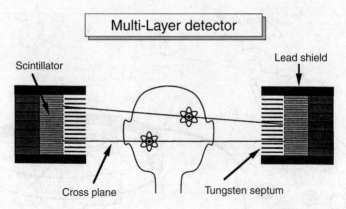

FIGURE 16.6 Most modern PET cameras are multilayered with 15 to 47 levels or transaxial layers to be reconstructed. The lead shields prevent activity from the patient from causing spurious counts in the tomograph ring, while the tungsten septa reject some of the events in which one (or both) of the 511-keV photons suffer a Compton scatter in the patient. The sensitivity of this design is improved by collection of data from cross-planes.

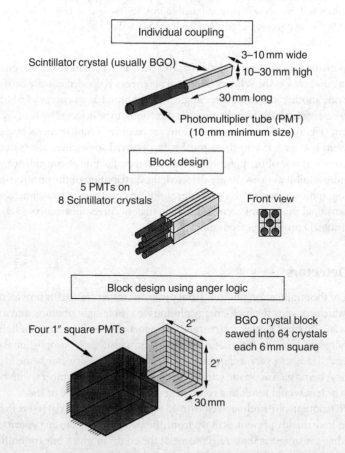

FIGURE 16.7 The arrangement of scintillators and phototubes is shown. The "individually coupled" design is capable of very high resolution, and because the design is very parallel (all the photomultiplier tubes and scintillator crystals operate independently), it is capable of very high data throughput. A block detector couples several photomultiplier tubes to a bank of scintillator crystals and uses a coding scheme to determine the crystal of interaction. In the two-layer block, five photomultiplier tubes are coupled to eight scintillator crystals.

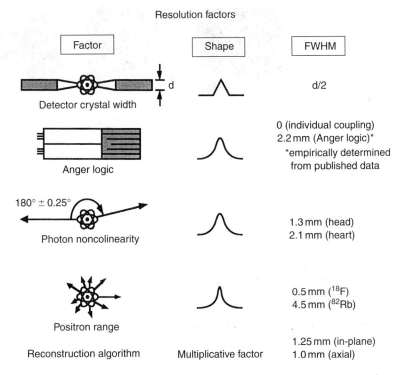

FIGURE 16.8 Factors contributing to the resolution of the PET tomograph. The contribution most accessible to further reduction is the size of the detector crystals.

photomultiplier tubes and, additionally, that connecting round photomultiplier tubes to rectangular scintillation crystals leads to problems of packing rectangular crystals and circular phototubes of sufficiently small diameter to form a solid ring.

The contemporary method of packing many scintillators for 511 keV around the patient is to use what is called a block detector design. A block detector couples several photomultiplier tubes to a bank of scintillator crystals and uses a coding scheme to determine the crystal of interaction. In the two-layer block (Figure 16.7), five photomultiplier tubes are coupled to eight scintillator crystals. Whenever one of the outside four photomultiplier tubes fires, a 511-keV photon has interacted in one of the two crystals attached to that photomultiplier tube, and the center photomultiplier tube is then used to determine whether it was the inner or outer crystal. This is known as a digital coding scheme, since each photomultiplier tube is either "hit" or "not hit" and the crystal of interaction is determined by a "digital" mapping of the hit pattern. Block detector designs are much less expensive and practical to form into a multilayer camera. However, errors in the decoding scheme reduce the spatial resolution, and since the entire block is "dead" whenever one of its member crystals is struck by a photon, the dead time is worse than with individual coupling. The electronics necessary to decode the output of the block are straightforward but more complex than that needed for the individually coupled design.

Most block detector coding schemes use an analog coding scheme, where the ratio of light output is used to determine the crystal of interaction. In the example above, four photomultiplier tubes are coupled to a block of BGO that has been partially sawed through to form 64 "individual" crystals. The depth of the cuts are critical; that is, deep cuts tend to focus the scintillation light onto the face of a single photomultiplier tube, while shallow cuts tend to spread the light over all four photomultiplier tubes. This type of coding scheme is more difficult to implement than digital coding, since analog light ratios place more stringent requirements on the photomultiplier tube linearity and uniformity as well as scintillator crystal uniformity. However, most commercial PET cameras use an analog coding scheme because it is much less expensive due to the lower number of photomultiplier tubes required.

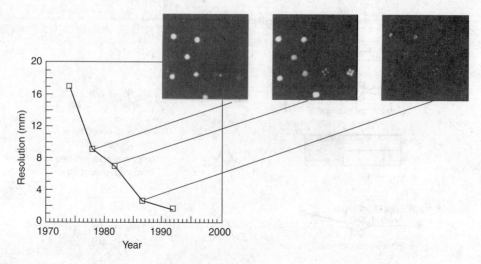

FIGURE 16.9 The evolution of resolution. Over the past decade, the resolving power of PET has improved from about 9 to 2.6 mm. This improvement is graphically illustrated by the increasing success with which one is able to resolve "hot spots" of an artificial sample that are detected and imaged by the tomographs.

16.2.4 Physical Factors Affecting Resolution

The factors that affect the spatial resolution of PET tomographs are shown in Figure 16.8. The size of the detector is critical in determining the system's geometric resolution. If the block design is used, there is a degradation in this geometric resolution by 2.2 mm for BGO. The degradation is probably due to the limited light output of BGO and the ratio of crystals (cuts) per phototube.

The angle between the paths of the annihilation photons can deviated from 180 degrees as a result of some residual kinetic motion (Fermi motion) at the time of annihilation. The effect on resolution of this deviation increases as the detector ring diameter increases so that eventually this factor can have a significant effect.

The distance the positron travels after being emitted from the nucleus and before annihilation causes a deterioration in spatial resolution. This distance depends on the particular nuclide. For example, the range of blurring for ^{18}F, the isotope used for many of the current PET studies, is quite small compared with that of the other isotopes. Combining values for these factors for the PET-600 tomograph, we can estimate a detector-pair spatial resolution of 2.0 mm and a reconstructed image resolution of 2.6 mm. The measured resolution of this system is 2.6 mm, but most commercially available tomographs use a block detector design (Figure 16.7), and the resolution of these systems is above 5 mm. The evolution of resolution improvement is shown in Figure 16.9.

The resolution evolutions discussed above pertain to results for the center or axis of the tomograph. The resolution at the edge of the object (e.g., patient) will be less by a significant amount due to two factors. First, the path of the photon from an "off-center" annihilation event typically traverses more than one detector crystal, as shown in Figure 16.10. This results in an elongation of the resolution spread function along the radius of the transaxial plane. The loss of resolution is dependent on the crystal density and the diameter of the tomograph detector ring. For a 60-cm diameter system, the resolution can deteriorate by a factor of 2 from the axis to 10 cm.

The coincidence circuitry must be able to determine coincident events with 10- to 20-nsec resolution for each crystal–crystal combination (i.e., chord). The timing requirement is set jointly by the time of flight across the detector ring (4 nsec) and the crystal-to-crystal resolving time (typically 3 nsec). The most stringent requirement, however, is the vast number of chords in which coincidences must be determined (over 1.5 million in a 24-layer camera with septa in place and 18 million with the septa removed).

It is obviously impractical to have an individual coincidence circuit for each chord, so tomograph builders use parallel organization to solve this problem. A typical method is to use a high-speed clock

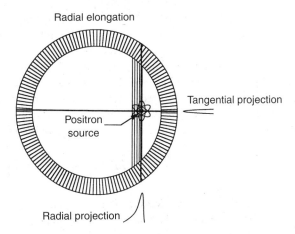

Radial elongation

Tangential projection

Positron source

Radial projection

FIGURE 16.10   Resolution astigmatism in detecting off-center events. Because annihilation photons can penetrate crystals to different depths, the resolution is not equal in all directions, particularly at the edge of the imaging field. This problem of astigmatism will be taken into account in future PET instrumentation.

(typically 200 MHz) to mark the arrival time of each 511-keV photon and a digital coincidence processor to search for coincident pairs of detected photons based on this time marker. This search can be done extremely quickly by having multiple sorters working in parallel.

The maximum event rate is also quite important, especially in septaless systems. The maximum rate in a single detector crystals is limited by the dead time due to the scintillator fluorescent lifetime (typically 1 msec per event), but as the remainder of the scintillator crystals are available, the instrument has much higher event rates (e.g., number of crystals ¥ 1 msec). Combining crystals together to form contiguous blocks reduces the maximum event rate because the fluorescent lifetime applies to the entire block and a fraction of the tomograph is dead after each event.

16.2.5   Random Coincidences

If two annihilation events occurs within the time resolution of the tomograph (e.g., 10 nsec), then random coincident "events" add erroneous background activity to the tomograph and are significant at high event rates. These can be corrected for on a chord-by-chord basis. The noncoincidence event rate of each crystal pair is measured by observing the rate of events beyond the coincident timing window. The random rate for the particular chord R_{ij} corresponding to a crystal pair is

$$R_{ij} = r_i \times r_j \times 2\tau \quad R_{ij} = R_{ij} \tag{16.2}$$

where r_i and r_j are the event rates of crystal i and crystal j, and τ is the coincidence window width. As the activity in the subject increases, the event rate in each detector increases. Thus the random event rate will increase as the square of the activity.

16.2.6   Tomographic Reconstruction

Before reconstruction, each projection ray or chord receives three corrections: crystal efficiency, attenuation, and random efficiency. The efficiency for each chord is computed by dividing the observed count rate for that chord by the average court rate for chords with a similar geometry (i.e., length). This is typically done daily using a transmission source without the patient or object in place. Once the patient is in position in the camera, a transmission scan is taken, and the attenuation factor for each chord is computed by dividing its transmission count rate by its efficiency count rate. The patient is then injected with the isotope, and an emission scan is taken, during which time the random count rate is also measured. For each chord, the random event rate is subtracted from the emission rate, and the difference is divided by the attenuation factor and the chord efficiency. (The detector efficiency is divided twice because two separate detection's measurements are made — transmission and emission.) The resulting value is reconstructed, usually with the filtered backprojection algorithm. This is the same algorithm used in x-ray computed tomography (CT) and in projection MRI. The corrected projection data are formatted onto parallel- or fan-beam data sets for each angle. These are modified by a high-pass filter and backprojected.

The process of PET reconstruction is linear and shown by operators successively operating on the projection P:

$$A = \sum_\theta BPF^{-1}RF(P) \tag{16.3}$$

where A is the image, F is the Fourier transform, R is the ramp-shaped high-pass filter, F^{-1} is the inverse Fourier transform, BP is the backprojection operation, and θ denotes the superposition operation.

The alternative class of reconstruction algorithms involves iterative solutions to the classic inverse problem:

$$P = FA \tag{16.4}$$

where P is the projection matrix, A is the matrix of true data being sought, and F is the projection operation. The inverse is

$$A = F^{-1}P \tag{16.4a}$$

which is computed by iteratively estimating the data A' and modifying the estimate by comparison of the calculated projection set P' with the true observed projections P. The expectation-maximization algorithm solves the inverse problem by updating each pixel value ai in accord with

$$a_1^{k+1} = \sum P_j \frac{a_j^k f_{ij}}{\sum_i a_l^k f_{ij}} \tag{16.5}$$

where P is the measured projection, f_{ij} is the probability a source at pixel i will be detected in projection detector j, and k is the iteration.

16.2.7 Sensitivity

The sensitivity is a measure of how efficiently the tomograph detects coincident events and has units of count rate per unit activity concentration. It is measured by placing a known concentration of radionuclide in a water-filled 20-cm-diameter cylinder in the field of view. This cylinder, known as a phantom, is placed in the tomograph, and the coincidence event rate is measured. High sensitivity is important because emission imaging involves counting each event, and the resulting data are as much as 1000 times less than experienced in x-ray CT. Most tomographs have high individual detection efficiency for 511-keV photons impinging on the detector (>90%), so the sensitivity is mostly determined by geometric factors, that is, the solid angle subtended by the tomograph:

$$S = \frac{A\varepsilon^2 \gamma \times 3.7 \times 10^4}{4\pi r^2} \text{(events/sec)/(mCi/cc)} \tag{16.6}$$

where:

   r = radius of tomograph
   A = area of detector material seen by each point in the object ($2\pi r$ ¥ axial aperture)
   ε = efficiency of scintillator
   γ = attenuation factor

For a single layer, the sensitivity of a tomograph of 90 cm diameter (2-cm axial crystals) will be 15,000 events/sec/mCi/ml for a disk of activity 20 cm in diameter and 1 cm thick. For a 20-cm-diameter cylinder, the sensitivity will be the same for a single layer with shields or septa that limit the off-slice activity from entering the collimators. However, modern multislice instruments use septa that allow activity from adjacent planes to be detected, thus increasing the solid angle and therefore the sensitivity. This increase comes at some cost due to increase in scatter. The improvement in sensitivity is by a factor of 7, but after correction for the noise, the improvement is 4. The noise equivalent sensitivity S_{NE} is given by

$$S_{NE} = \frac{(\text{true events})^2}{\text{true} \times \text{scatter} \times \text{random}} \tag{16.7}$$

16.2.8   Statistical Properties of PET

The ability to map quantitatively the spatial distribution of a positron-emitting isotope depends on adequate spatial resolution to avoid blurring. In addition, sufficient data must be acquired to allow a

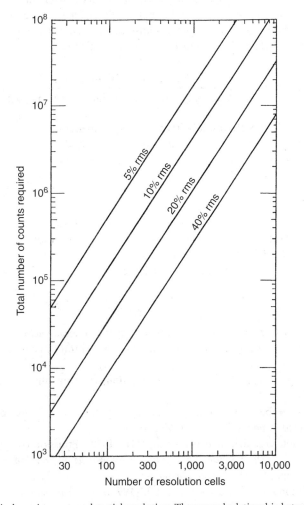

FIGURE 16.11   Statistical requirements and spatial resolution. The general relationship between the detected number of events and the number of resolution elements in an image is graphed for various levels of precision. These are relations for planes of constant thickness.

statistically reliable estimation of the tracer concentration. The amount of available data depends on the biomedical accumulation, the imaging system sensitivity, and the dose of injected radioactivity. The propagation of errors due to the reconstruction process results in an increase in the noise over that expected for an independent signal, for example, by a factor proportional to the square root of the number of resolution elements (true pixels) across the image. The formula that deals with the general case of emission reconstruction (PET or SPECT) is

$$\% \text{ uncertainty} = \frac{1.2 \times 100(\text{total no. of events})^{3/4}}{(\text{total no. of events})^{1/2}} \qquad (16.8)$$

The statistical requirements are closely related to the spatial resolution, as shown in Figure 16.11.

For a given accuracy or a signal-to-noise ratio for a uniform distribution, the ratio of the number of events needed in a high-resolution system to that needed in a low-resolution system is proportional to the 3/2 power of the ratio of the number of effective resolution elements in the two systems. Equation 16.8 and Figure 16.11 should be used not with the total pixels in the image but with the effective resolution cells. The number of effective resolution cells is the sum of the occupied resolution elements weighted by the activity within each element. Suppose, however, that the activity is mainly in a few resolution cells (e.g., 100 events per cell) and the remainder of the 10,000 cells have a background of 1 event per cell. The curves of Figure 16.11 would suggest unacceptable statistics; however, in this case, the effective number of resolution cells is below 100. The relevant equation for this situation is

$$\% \text{ uncertainty} = \frac{1.2 \times 100(\text{no. of resolutiion cells})^{3/4}}{(\text{avg. no. of events per resolution cell in target})^{3/4}} \qquad (16.9)$$

The better resolution gives improved results without the requirement for a drastic increase in the number of detected events is that the improved resolution increases contrast. (It is well known that the number of events needed to detect an object is inversely related to the square of the contrast.)

Acknowledgments

This work was supported in part by the Director, Office of Energy Research, Office of Health and Environmental Research, Medical Applications and Biophysical Research Division of the U.S. Department of Energy under contract No. DE-AC03-SF00098 and in part by NIH Grant HL25840. I wish to thank Drs. Stephen Derenzo and William Moses, who contributed material to this presentation.

References

[1] Anger, H.O. (1963). Gamma-ray and positron scintillator camera. *Nucleonics* 21: 56.

[2] Bailey, D.L. (1992). 3D acquisition and reconstruction in positron emission tomography. *Ann. Nucl. Med.* 6: 123.

[3] Brownell, G.L. and Sweet, W.H. (1953). Localization of brain tumors with positron emitters. *Nucleonics* 11: 40.

[4] Budinger, T.F., Greenberg, W.L., Derenzo, S.E. et al. (1978). Quantitative potentials of dynamic emission computed tomography. *J. Nucl. Med.* 19: 309.

[5] Budinger, T.F., Gullberg, G.T., and Huesman, R.H. (1979). Emission computed tomography. In G.T. Herman (ed.), *Topics in Applied Physics: Image Reconstruction from Projections: Implementation and Applications*, pp. 147–246. Berlin, Springer-Verlag.

[6] Cherry, S.R., Dahlbom M., and Hoffman, E.J. (1991). 3D PET using a conventional multislice tomograph without septa. *J. Comput. Assist. Tomogr.* 15: 655.

[7] Daube-Witherspoon, M.E. and Muehllehner G. (1987). Treatment of axial data in three-dimensional PET. *J. Nucl. Med.* 28: 1717.

[8] Derenzo, S.E., Huesman, R.H., Cahoon, J.L. et al. (1988). A positron tomograph with 600 BGO crystals and 2.6 mm resolution. *IEEE Trans. Nucl. Sci.* 35: 659.

[9] Kinahan, P.E. and Rogers, J.G. (1989). Analytic 3D image reconstruction using all detected events. *IEEE Trans. Nucl. Sci.* 36: 964–968.

[10] Shepp, L.A. and Vardi Y. (1982). Maximum likelihood reconstruction for emission tomography. *IEEE Trans. Med. Imaging* 1: 113.

[11] Ter-Pogossian, M.M., Phelps, M.E., Hoffman, E.J. et al. (1975). A positron-emission transaxial tomograph for nuclear imaging (PETT). *Radiology* 114: 89.

17

Electrical Impedance Tomography

17.1 The Electrical Impedance of Tissue **17**-1
17.2 Conduction in Human Tissues **17**-1
17.3 Determination of the Impedance Distribution **17**-3
   Data Collection • Image Reconstruction • Multifrequency
   Measurements
17.4 Areas of Clinical Application **17**-10
   Possible Biomedical Applications
17.5 Summary and Future Developments **17**-11
Defining Terms **17**-11
References **17**-12
Further Information **17**-13

D.C. Barber
University of Sheffield

17.1 The Electrical Impedance of Tissue

The specific conductance (**conductivity**) of human tissues varies from 15.4 mS/cm for cerebrospinal fluid to 0.06 mS/cm for bone. The difference in the value of conductivity is large between different tissues (Table 17.1). Cross-sectional images of the distribution of conductivity, or alternatively specific resistance (**resistivity**), should show good contrast. The aim of electrical impedance tomography (**EIT**) is to produce such images. It has been shown [Kohn and Vogelius, 1984a,b; Sylvester and Uhlmann, 1986] that for reasonable isotropic distributions of conductivity it is possible in principle to reconstruct conductivity images from electrical measurements made on the surface of an object. Electrical impedance tomography (EIT) is the technique of producing these images. In fact, human tissue is not simply conductive. There is evidence that many tissues also demonstrate a capacitive component of current flow and therefore, it is appropriate to speak of the specific admittance (**admittivity**) or specific impedance (**impedivity**) of tissue rather than the conductivity; hence the use of the world impedance in electrical impedance tomography.

17.2 Conduction in Human Tissues

Tissue consists of cells with conducting contents surrounded by insulating membranes embedded in a conducting medium. Inside and outside the cell wall is conducting fluid. At low frequencies of applied current, the current cannot pass through the membranes, and conduction is through the extracellular space. At high frequencies, current can flow through the membranes, which act as capacitors. A simple

TABLE 17.1 Values of Specific
Conductance for Human Tissues

Tissue	Conductivity, mS/cm
Cerebrospinal fluid	15.4
Blood	6.7
Liver	2.8
Skeletal muscle	8.0 (Longitudinal)
	0.6 (Transverse)
Cardiac muscle	6.3 (Longitudinal)
	2.3 (Transverse)
Neural tissue	1.7
Gray matter	3.5
White matter	1.5
Lung	1.0 (Expiration)
	0.4 (Inspiration)
Fat	0.36
Bone	0.06

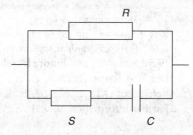

FIGURE 17.1 The Cole-Cole model of tissue impedance.

model of bulk tissue impedance based on this structure, which was proposed by Cole and Cole [1941], is shown in Figure 17.1.

Clearly, this model as it stands is too simple, since an actual tissue sample would be better represented as a large network of interconnected modules of this form. However, it has been shown that this model fits experimental data if the values of the components, especially the capacitance, are made a power function of the applied frequency ω. An equation which describes the behavior of tissue impedance as a function of frequency reasonably well is

$$Z = Z_\infty + \frac{Z_0 - Z_\infty}{1 + (j(f/f_c))^\alpha} \qquad (17.1)$$

where Z_0 and Z_∞ are the (complex) limiting values of tissue impedance low and high frequency and f_c is a characteristic frequency. The value of α allows for the frequency dependency of the components of the model and is tissue dependent. Numerical values for *in vivo* human tissues are not well established.

Making measurements of the real and imaginary components of tissue impedivity over a range of frequencies will allow the components in this model to be extracted. Since it is known that tissue structure alters in disease and that R, S, C are dependent on structure, it should be possible to use such measurements to distinguish different types of tissue and different disease conditions. It is worth noting that although maximum accuracy in the determination of the model components can be obtained if both real and imaginary components are available, in principle, knowledge of the resistive component alone should enable the values to be determined, provided an adequate range of frequencies is used. This can have practical consequences for data collection, since accurate measurement of the capacitive component can prove difficult.

Although on a microscopic scale tissue is almost certainly electrically isotropic, on a macroscopic scale this is not so for some tissues because of their anisotropic physical structure. Muscle tissue is a prime example (see Table 17.1), where the bulk conductivity along the direction of the fibers is significantly higher than across the fibers. Although unique solutions for conductivity are possible for isotropic conductors, it can be shown that for **anisotropic conductors** unique solutions for conductivity do not exist. There are sets of different anisotropic conductivity distributions that give the same surface voltage distributions and which therefore cannot be distinguished by these measurements. It is not yet clear how limiting anisotropy is to electrical impedance tomography. Clearly, if sufficient data could be obtained to resolve down to the microscopic level (this is not possible practically), then tissue becomes isotropic. Moreover, the tissue distribution of conductivity, including anisotropy, often can be modeled as a network of conductors, and it is known that a unique solution will always exist for such a network. In practice, use of some prior knowledge about the anisotropy of tissue may remove the ambiguities of conductivity distribution associated with anisotropy. The degree to which anisotropy might inhibit useful image reconstruction is still an open question.

17.3   Determination of the Impedance Distribution

The distribution of electrical potential within an isotropic conducting object through which a low-frequency current is flowing is given by

$$\nabla(\sigma \nabla \phi) = 0 \tag{17.2}$$

where ϕ is the potential distribution within the object and σ is the distribution of conductivity (generally admittivity) within the object. If the conductivity is uniform, this reduces to Laplace's equation. Strictly speaking, this equation is only correct for direct current, but for the frequencies of alternating current used in EIT (up to 1 MHz) and the sizes of objects being imaged, it can be assumed that this equation continues to describe the instantaneous distribution of potential within the conducting object. If this equation is solved for a given conductivity distribution and current distribution through the surface of the object, the potential distribution developed on the surface of the object may be determined. The distribution of potential will depend on several things. It will depend on the pattern of current applied and the shape of the object. It will also depend on the internal conductivity of the object, and it is this that needs to be determined. In theory, the current may be applied in a continuous and nonuniform pattern at every point across the surface. In practice, current is applied to an object through electrodes attached to the surface of the object. Theoretically, potential may be measured at every point on the surface of the object. Again, voltage on the surface of the object is measured in practice using electrodes (possibly different from those used to apply current) attached to the surface of the object. There will be a relationship, the forward solution, between an **applied current pattern** j_i, the conductivity distribution σ, and the surface potential distribution ϕ_i which can be formally represented as

$$\phi_i = R(j_i, \sigma) \tag{17.3}$$

If σ and j_i are known, ϕ_i can be computed. For one current pattern j_i, knowledge of ϕ_i is not in general sufficient to uniquely determine σ. However, by applying a complete set of independent current patterns, it becomes possible to obtain sufficient information to determine σ, at least in the isotropic case. This is the inverse solution. In practice, measurements of surface potential or voltage can only be made at a finite number of positions, corresponding to electrodes placed on the surface of the object. This also means that only a finite number of independent current patterns can be applied. For N electrodes, $N - 1$ independent current patterns can be defined and $N(N - 1)/2$ independent measurements made. This latter number determines the limit of image resolution achievable with N electrodes. In practice, it may not be possible to collect all possible independent measurements. Since only a finite number of current patterns and measurements is available, the set of equations represented by Equation 17.3 can be rewritten as

$$v = A_c c \qquad (17.4)$$

where v is now a concatenated vector of all voltage values for all current patterns, c is a vector of conductivity values, representing the conductivity distribution divided into uniform image **pixels**, and A_c a matrix representing the transformation of this conductivity vector into the voltage vector. Since A_c depends on the conductivity distribution, this equation is nonlinear. Although formally the preceding equation can be solved for c by inverting A_c, the nonlinear nature of this equation means that this cannot be done in a single step. An iterative procedure will therefore be needed to obtain c.

Examination of the physics of current flow shows that current tends to take the easiest path possible in its passage through the object. If the conductivity at some point is changed, the current path redistributes in such a way that the effects of this change are minimized. The practical effect of this is that it is possible to have fairly large changes in conductivity within the object which only produce relatively small changes in voltage at the surface of the object. The converse of this is that when reconstructing the conductivity distribution, small errors on the measured voltage data, both random and systematic, can translate into large errors in the estimate of the conductivity distribution. This effect forms, and will continue to form, a limit to the quality of reconstructed conductivity images in terms of resolution, accuracy, and sensitivity.

Any measurement of voltage must always be referred to a reference point. Usually this is one of the electrodes, which is given the nominal value of 0 V. The voltage on all other electrodes is determined by measuring the voltage difference between each electrode and the reference electrode. Alternatively, voltage differences may be measured between pairs of electrodes. A common approach is to measure the voltage between adjacent pairs of electrodes (Figure 17.2). Clearly, the measurement scheme affects the form of A_c. Choice of the pattern of applied currents and the voltage measurement scheme used can affect the accuracy with which images of conductivity can be reconstructed.

Electrical impedance tomography (EIT) is not a mature technology. However, it has been the subject of intensive research over the past few years, and this work is still continuing. Nearly all the research effort has been devoted to exploring the different possible ways of collecting data and producing images of tissue resistivity, with the aim of optimizing image reconstruction in terms of image accuracy, spatial resolution, and sensitivity.

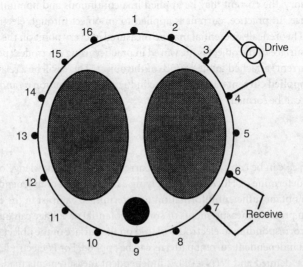

FIGURE 17.2 Idealized electrode positions around a conducting object with typical drive and measurement electrode pairs indicated.

Very few areas of medical application have been explored in any great depth, although in a number of cases preliminary work has been carried out. Although most current interest is in the use of EIT for medical imaging, there is also some interest in its use in geophysical measurements and some industrial uses. A recent detailed review of the state of Electrical Impedance Tomography is given in Boone et al. [1997].

17.3.1 Data Collection

17.3.1.1 Basic Requirements

Data are collected by applying a current to the object through electrodes connected to the surface of the object and then making measurements of the voltage on the object surface through the same or other electrodes. Although conceptually simple, technically this can be difficult. Great attention must be paid to the reduction of noise and the elimination of any voltage offsets on the measurements. The currents applied are alternating currents usually in the range 10 kHz to 1 MHz. Since tissue has a complex impedance, the voltage signals will contain in-phase and out-of-phase components. In principle, both of these can be measured. In practice, measurement of the out-of-phase (the capacitive) component is significantly more difficult because of the presence of unwanted (stray) capacitances between various parts of the voltage measurement system, including the leads from the data-collection apparatus to the electrodes. These stray capacitances can lead to appreciable leakage currents, especially at the higher frequencies, which translate into systematic errors on the voltage measurements. The signal measured on an electrode, or between a pair of electrodes, oscillates at the same frequency as the applied current. The magnitude of this signal (usually separated into real and imaginary components) is determined, typically by demodulation and integration. The frequency of the demodulated signal is much less than the frequency of the applied signal, and the effects of stray capacitances on this signal are generally negligible. This realization has led some workers to propose that the signal demodulation and detection system be mounted as close to the electrodes as possible, ideally at the electrode site itself, and some systems have been developed that use this approach, although none with sufficient miniaturization of the electronics to be practical in a clinical setting. This solution is not in itself free of problems, but this approach is likely to be of increasing importance if the frequency range of applied currents is to be extended beyond 1 MHz, necessary if the value of the complex impedance is to be adequately explored as a function of frequency.

Various data-collection schemes have been proposed. Most data are collected from a two-dimensional (2D) configuration of electrodes, either from 2D objects or around the border of a plane normal to the principal axis of a cylindrical (in the general sense) object where that plane intersects the object surface. The simplest data-collection protocol is to apply a current between a pair of electrodes (often an adjacent pair) and measure the voltage difference between other adjacent pairs (see Figure 17.2). Although in principle voltage could be measured on electrodes though which current is simultaneously flowing, the presence of an electrode impedance, generally unknown, between the electrode and the body surface means that the voltage measured is not actually that on the body surface. Various means have been suggested for either measuring the electrode impedance in some way or including it as an unknown in the image-reconstruction process. However, in many systems, measurements from electrodes through which current is flowing are simply ignored. Electrode impedance is generally not considered to be a problem when making voltage measurements on electrodes through which current is not flowing, provided a voltmeter with sufficiently high input impedance is used, although, since the input impedance is always finite, every attempt should be made to keep the electrode impedance as low as possible. Using the same electrode for driving current and making voltage measurements, even at different times in the data collection cycle, means that at some point in the data-collection apparatus wires carrying current and wires carrying voltage signals will be brought close together in a switching system, leading to the possibility of leakage currents. There is a good argument for using separate sets of electrodes for driving and measuring to reduce this problem. Paulson et al. [1992] have also proposed this approach and also have noted that it can aid in the modeling of the forward solution (see Image Reconstruction). Brown et al. [1994] have used this approach in making multi-frequency measurements.

Clearly, the magnitude of the voltage measured will depend on the magnitude of the current applied. If a constant-current drive is used, this must be able to deliver a known current to a variety of input impedances with a stability of better than 0.1%. This is technically demanding. The best approach to this problem is to measure the current being applied, which can easily be done to this accuracy. These measurements are then used to normalize the voltage data.

The current application and data-collection regime will depend on the reconstruction algorithm used. Several EIT systems apply current in a distributed manner, with currents of various magnitudes being applied to several or all of the electrodes. These **optimal currents** (see Image Reconstruction) must be specified accurately, and again, it is technically difficult to ensure that the correct current is applied at each electrode. Although there are significant theoretical advantages to using **distributed current** patterns, the increased technical problems associated with this approach, and the higher noise levels associated with the increase in electronic complexity, may outweigh these advantages.

Although most EIT at present is 2D in the sense given above, it is intrinsically a three-dimensional (3D) imaging procedure, since current cannot be constrained to flow in a plane through a 3D object. 3D data collection does not pose any further problems apart from increased complexity due to the need for more electrodes. Whereas most data-collection systems to date have been based on 16 or 32 electrodes, 3D systems will require four times or more electrodes distributed over the surface of the object if adequate resolution is to be maintained. Technically, this will require "belts" or "vests" of electrodes that can be rapidly applied [McAdams et al., 1994]. Some of these are already available, and the application of an adequate number of electrodes should not prove insuperable provided electrode-mounted electronics are not required. Metherell et al. [1996] describe a three-dimensional data collection system and reconstruction algorithm and note the improved accuracy of three-dimensional images compared to two-dimensional images constructed using data collected from three-dimensional objects.

17.3.1.2 Performance of Existing Systems

Several research groups have produced EIT systems for laboratory use [Brown and Seagar, 1987; Rigaud et al., 1990; Smith 1990; Gisser et al., 1991; Jossinet and Trillaud, 1992; Lidgey et al., 1992; Riu et al., 1992; Brown et al., 1994; Cook et al., 1994; Cusick et al., 1994; Zhu et al., 1994] and some clinical trials. The complexity of the systems largely depends on whether current is applied via a pair of electrodes (usually adjacent) or whether through many electrodes simultaneously. The former systems are much simpler in design and construction and can deliver higher signal-to-noise ratios. The Sheffield Mark II system [Smith, 1990] used 16 electrodes and was capable of providing signal-to-noise ratios of up to 17 dB at 25 datasets per second. The average image resolution achievable across the image was 15% of the image diameter. In general, multi-frequency systems have not yet delivered similar performance, but are being continuously improved.

Spatial resolution and noise levels are the most important constraints on possible clinical applications of EIT. As images are formed through a reconstruction process the values of these parameters will depend critically on the quality of the data collected and the reconstruction process used. However practical limitations to the number of electrodes which can be used and the ill-posed nature of the reconstruction problem make it unlikely that high quality images, comparable to other medical imaging modalities, can be produced. The impact of this on diagnostic performance still needs to be evaluated.

17.3.2 Image Reconstruction

17.3.2.1 Basics of Reconstruction

Although several different approaches to image reconstruction have been tried [Wexler et al., 1985; Yorkey, 1986; Barber and Seagar, 1987, Kim et al., 1987; Hua et al., 1988; Breckon, 1990; Cheny et al., 1990; Zadecoochak et al., 1991; Kotre et al., 1992; Bayford et al., 1994; Morucci et al., 1994], the most accurate approaches are based broadly on the following algorithm. For a given set of current patterns, a forward transform is set up for determining the voltages v produced form the conductivity distribution c (Equation 17.4). A_c is dependent on c, so it is necessary to assume an initial starting conductivity distribution c_0. This is usually taken to be uniform. Using A_c, the expected voltages v_0 are calculated and compared with the actual measured voltages v_m. Unless c_0 is correct (which it will not be initially), v_0 and v_m will differ. It can be shown that an improved estimate of c is given by

$$\Delta c = (S_c^t S_c)^{-1} S_c^t (v_0 - v_m) \tag{17.5}$$

$$c_1 = c_0 + \Delta c \tag{17.6}$$

where S_c is the differential of A_c with respect to c, the sensitivity matrix and S_c^t is the transpose of S_c. The improved value of c is then used in the next iteration to compute an improved estimate of v_m, that is, v_1. This iterative process is continued until some appropriate endpoint is reached. Although convergence is not guaranteed, in practice, convergence to the correct c in the absence of noise can be expected, provided a good starting value is chosen. Uniform conductivity seems to be a reasonable choice. In the presence of noise on the measurements, iteration is stopped when the difference between v and v_m is within the margin of error set by the known noise on the data.

There are some practical difficulties associated with this approach. One is that large changes in c may only produce small changes in v, and this will be reflected in the structure of S_c, making $S_c^t S_c$ very difficult to invert reliably. Various methods of regularization have been used, with varying degrees of success, to achieve stable inversion of this matrix although the greater the regularization applied the poorer the resolution that can be achieved. A more difficult practical problem is that for convergence to be possible the computed voltages v must be equal to the measured voltages v_m when the correct conductivity values are used in the forward calculation. Although in a few idealized cases analytical solutions of the forward problem are possible, in general, numerical solutions must be used. Techniques such as the finite-element method (FEM) have been developed to solve problems of this type numerically. However, the accuracy of these methods has to be carefully examined [Paulson et al., 1992] and, while they are adequate for many applications, may not be adequate for the EIT reconstruction problem, especially in the case of 3D objects. Accuracies of rather better than 1% appear to be required if image artifacts are to be minimized. Consider a situation in which the actual distortion of conductivity is uniform. Then the initial v should be equal to the v_m to an accuracy less than the magnitude of the noise. If this is not the case, then the algorithm will alter the conductivity distribution from uniform, which will clearly result in error. While the required accuracies have been approached under ideal conditions, there is only a limited amount of evidence at present to suggest that they can be achieved with data taken from human subjects.

17.3.2.2 Optimal Current Patterns

So far little has been said about the form of the current patterns applied to the object except that a set of independent patterns is needed. The simplest current patterns to use are those given by passing current into the object through one electrode and extracting current through a second electrode (a bipolar pattern). This pattern has the virtue of simplicity and ease of application. However, other current patterns are possible. Current can be passed simultaneously through many electrodes, with different amounts passing through each electrode. Indeed, an infinite number of patterns are possible, the only limiting condition being that the magnitude of the current flowing into the conducting object equals the magnitude of the current flowing out of the object. Isaacson [1986] has shown that for any conducting object there is a set of optimal current patterns and has provided an algorithm to compute them even if the conductivity distribution is initially unknown. Isaacson showed that by using optimal patterns, significant improvements in sensitivity could be obtained compared with simpler two-electrode current patterns. However, the additional computation and hardware required to use optimal current patterns compared with fixed, nonoptimal patterns is considerable.

Use of suboptimal patterns close to optimum also will produce significant gains. In general, the optimal patterns are very different from the patterns produced in the simple two-electrode case. The optimal patterns are often cosine-like patterns of current amplitude distributed around the object boundary rather than being localized at a pair of points, as in the two-electrode case. Since the currents are passed simultaneously through many electrodes, it is tempting to try and use the same electrodes for voltage measurements. This produces two problems. As noted above, measurement of voltage on an electrode through which an electric current is passing is compromised by the presence of electrode resistance, which causes a generally unknown voltage drop across the electrode, whereas voltage can be accurately measured on an electrode through which current is not flowing using a voltmeter of high input impedance. In addition, it has proved difficult to model current flow around an electrode through which current is flowing with sufficient accuracy to allow the reliable calculation of voltage on that electrode, which is needed for accurate reconstruction. It seems that separate electrodes should be used for voltage measurements with distributed current systems.

Theoretically, distributed (near-) optimal current systems have some advantages. As each of the optimal current patterns is applied, it is possible to determine if the voltage patterns produced contain any useful information or if they are simply noise. Since the patterns can be generated and applied in order of decreasing significance, it is possible to terminate application of further current patterns when no further information can be obtained. A consequence of this is that SNRs can be maximized for a given total data-collection time. With **bipolar current patterns** this option is not available. All patterns must be applied. Provided the SNR in the data is sufficiently good and only a limited number of electrodes are used, this may not be too important, and the extra effort involved in generating the optimal or near-optimal patterns may not be justified. However, as the number of electrodes is increased, the use of optimal patterns becomes more significant. It also has been suggested that the distributed nature of the optimal patterns makes the forward problem less sensitive to modeling errors. Although there is currently no firm evidence for this, this seems a reasonable assertion.

17.3.2.3 Three-Dimensional Imaging

Most published work so far on image reconstruction has concentrated on solving the 2D problem. However, real medical objects, that is, patients, are three-dimensional. Theoretically, as the dimensionality of the object increases, reconstruction should become better conditioned. However, unlike 3D x-ray images, which can be constructed from a set of independent 2D images, EIT data from 3D objects cannot be so decomposed and data from over the whole surface of the object is required for 3D reconstruction. The principles of reconstruction in 3D are identical to the 2D situation although practically the problem is quite formidable, principally because of the need to solve the forward problem in three dimensions. Some early work on 3D imaging was presented by Goble and Isaacson [1990]. More recently Metherall et al. [1996] have shown images using data collected from human subjects.

17.3.2.4 Single-Step Reconstruction

The complete reconstruction problem is nonlinear and requires iteration. However, each step in the iterative process is linear. Images reconstructed using only the first step of iteration effectively treat image formation as a liner process, an assumption approximately justified for small changes in conductivity from uniform. In the case the functions A_c and S_c often can be precomputed with reasonable accuracy because they usually are computed for the case of uniform conductivity. Although the solution cannot be correct, since the nonlinearity is not taken into account, it may be useful, and first-step linear approximations have gained some popularity. Cheney et al. [1990] have published some results from a first-step process using optimal currents. Most, if not all, of the clinical images produced to date have used a single-step reconstruction algorithm [Barber and Seagar, 1987; Barber and Brown, 1990]. Although this algorithm uses very nonoptimal current patterns, this has not so far been a limitation because of the high quality of data collected and the limited number of electrodes used (16). With larger numbers of electrodes, this conclusion may need to be revised.

17.3.2.5 Differential Imaging

Ideally, the aim of EIT is to reconstruct images of the absolute distribution of conductivity (or admittivity). These images are known as absolute (or static) images. However, this requires that the forward problem can be solved to an high degree of accuracy, and this can be difficult. The magnitude of the voltage signal measured on an electrode or between electrodes will depend on the body shape, the electrode shape and position, and the internal conductivity distribution. The signal magnitude is in fact dominated by the first two effects rather than by conductivity. However, if a change in conductivity occurs within the object, then it can often be assumed that the change in surface voltage is dominated by this conductivity change. In differential (or dynamic) imaging, the aim is to image changes in conductivity rather than absolute values. If the voltage difference between a pair of (usually adjacent) electrodes before a conductivity change occurs is g_1 and the value after change occurs is g_2, then a normalized data value is defined as

$$\Delta g_n = 2\frac{g_1 - g_2}{g_1 + g_2} = \frac{\Delta g}{g_{\text{mean}}} \tag{17.7}$$

Many of the effects of body shape (including interpreting the data as coming from a 2D object when in fact it is from a 3D object) and electrode placing at least partially cancel out in this definition. The values of the normalized data are determined largely by the conductivity changes. It can be argued that the relationship between the (normalized) changes in conductivity Δc_n and the normalized changes in boundary data Δg_n is given by

$$\Delta g_n = F\Delta c_n \tag{17.8}$$

where F is a sensitivity matrix which it can be shown is much less sensitive to object shape end electrode positions than the sensitivity matrix of Equation 17.5. Although images produced using this algorithm are not completely free of artifact that is the only algorithm which has reliably produced images using data taken from human subjects. Metherall et al. [1996] used a version of this algorithm for 3D imaging and Brown et al. [1994] for multi-frequency imaging, in this case imaging changes in conductivity with frequency. The principle disadvantage of this algorithm is that it can only image changes in conductivity, which must be either natural or induced. Figure 17.3 shows a typical differential image. This represents the changes in the conductivity of the lungs between expiration and inspiration.

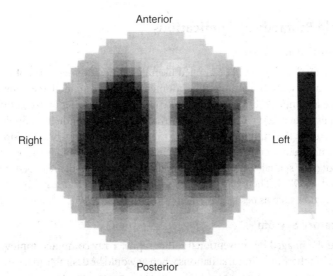

FIGURE 17.3 A differential conductivity image representing the changes in conductivity in going from maximum inspiration (breathing in) to maximum expiration (breathing out). Increasing blackness represents increasing conductivity.

17.3.3 Multifrequency Measurements

Differential algorithms can only image changes in conductivity. Absolute distributions of conductivity cannot be produced using these methods. In addition, any gross movement of the electrodes, either because they have to be removed and replaced or even because of significant patient movement, make the use of this technique difficult for long-term measurements of changes. As an alternative to changes in time, differential algorithms can image changes in conductivity with frequency. Brown et al. [1994] have shown that if measurements are made over a range of frequencies and differential images produced using data from the lowest frequency and the other frequencies in turn, these images can be used to compute parametric images representing the distribution of combinations of the circuit values in Figure 17.1. For example, images representing the ratio of S to R, a measure of the ratio of intracellular to extracellular volume, can be produced, as well as images of $f_o = 1/2p(RC + SC)$, the tissue characteristic frequency. Although not images of the absolute distribution of conductivity, they are images of absolute tissue properties. Since these properties are related to tissue structure, they should produce images with useful contrast. Data sufficient to reconstruct an image can be collected in a time short enough to preclude significant patient movement, which means these images are robust against movement artifacts. Changes of these parameters with time can still be observed.

17.4   Areas of Clinical Application

There is no doubt that the clinical strengths of EIT relate to its ability to be considered as a functional imaging modality that carries no hazard and can therefore be used for monitoring purposes. The best spatial resolution that might become available will still be much worse than anatomic imaging methods such as magnetic resonance imaging and x-ray computed tomography. However, EIT is able to image small changes in tissue conductivity such as those associated with blood perfusion, lung ventilation, and fluid shifts. Clinical applications seek to take advantage of the ability of EIT to follow rapid changes in physiologic function.

There are several areas in clinical medicine where electrical impedance tomography might provide advantages over existing techniques. These have been received elsewhere [Brown et al., 1985; Dawids, 1987; Holder and Brown, 1990; Boone et al., 1997].

17.4.1   Possible Biomedical Applications

17.4.1.1   Gastrointestinal System

A priori, it seems likely that EIT could be applied usefully to measurement of motor activity in the gut. Electrodes can be applied with ease around the abdomen, and there are no large bony structures likely to seriously violate the assumption of constant initial conductivity. During motor activity, such as gastric emptying or peristalsis, there are relatively large movements of the conducting fluids within the bowel. The quantity of interest is the timing of activity, for example, the rate at which the stomach empties, and the absolute impedance change and its exact location in space area of secondary importance. The principal limitations of EIT of poor spatial resolution and amplitude measurement are largely circumvented in this application [Avill et al., 1987]. There has also been some interest in the measurement of other aspects of gastro-intestinal function such as oesophageal activity [Erol et al., 1995].

17.4.1.2   Respiratory System

Lung pathology can be imaged by conventional radiography, x-ray computed tomography, or magnetic resonance imaging, but there are clinical situations where it would be desirable to have a portable means of imaging regional lung ventilation which could, if necessary, generate repeated images over time. Validation studies have shown that overall ventilation can be measured with good accuracy [Harris et al., 1988]. More recent work [Hampshire et al., 1995] suggests that multifrequency measurements may be useful in the diagnosis of some lung disorders.

17.4.1.3 EIT Imaging of Changes in Blood Volume

The conductivity of blood is about 6.7 mS/cm, which is approximately three times that of most intrathoracic tissues. It therefore seems possible that EIT images related to blood flow could be accomplished. The imaged quantity will be the change in conductivity due to replacement of tissue by blood (or vice versa) as a result of the pulsatile flow through the thorax. This may be relatively large in the cardiac ventricles but will be smaller in the peripheral lung fields.

The most interesting possibility is that of detecting pulmonary embolus (PE). If a blood clot is present in the lung, the lung beyond the clot will not be perfused, and under favorable circumstances, this may be visualized using a gated blood volume image of the lung. In combination with a ventilation image, which should show normal ventilation in this region, pulmonary embolism could be diagnosed. Some data [Leathard et al., 1994] indicate that PE can be visualized in human subjects. Although more sensitive methods already exist for detecting PE, the noninvasiveness and bedside availability of EIT mean that treatment of the patient could be monitored over the period following the occurrence of the embolism, an important aim, since the use of anticoagulants, the principal treatment for PE, needs to be minimized in postoperative patients, a common class of patients presenting with this complication.

17.5 Summary and Future Developments

Electrical Impedance Tomography is still an emerging technology. In its development, several novel and difficult measurement and image-reconstruction problems have had to be addressed. Most of these have been satisfactorily solved. The current generation of EIT imaging systems are multifrequency, with some capable of 3D imaging. These should be capable of greater quantitative accuracy and be less prone to image artifact and are likely to find a practical role in clinical diagnosis. Although there are still many technical problems to be answered and many clinical applications to be addressed, the technology may be close to coming of age.

Defining Terms

Absolute imaging: Imaging the actual distribution of conductivity.

Admittivity: The specific admittance of an electrically conducting material. For simple biomedical materials such as saline with no reactive component of resistance, this is, the same as conductivity.

Anisotropic conductor: A material in which the conductivity is dependent on the direction in which it is measured through the material.

Applied current pattern: In EIT, the electric current is applied to the surface of the conducting object via electrodes placed on the surface of the object. The spatial distribution of current flow through the surface of the object is the applied current pattern.

Bipolar current pattern: A current pattern applied between a single pair of electrodes.

Conductivity: The specific conductance of an electrically conducting material. The inverse of resistivity.

Differential imaging: An EIT imaging technique that specifically images changes in conductivity.

Distributed current: A current pattern applied through more than two electrodes.

Dynamic imaging: The same as differential imaging.

EIT: Electrical impedance tomography.

Forward transform or problem or solution: The operation, real or computational, that maps or transforms the conductivity distribution to surface voltages.

Impedivity: The specific impedance of an electrically conducting material. The inverse of admittivity. For simple biomedical materials such as saline with no reactive component of resistance, this is the same as resistivity.

Inverse transform or problem or solution: The computational operation that maps voltage measurements on the surface of the object to the conductivity distribution.

Optimal current: One of a set of a current patterns computed for a particular conductivity distribution that produce data with maximum possible SNR.

Pixel: The conductivity distribution is usually represented as a set of connected piecewise uniform patches. Each of these patches is a pixel. The pixel may take any shape, but square or triangular shapes are most common.

Resistivity: The specific electrical resistance of an electrical conducting material. The inverse of conductivity.

Static imaging: The same as absolute imaging.

References

Avill, R.F., Mangnall, R.F., Bird, N.C. et al. (1987). Applied potential tomography: a new non-invasive technique for measuring gastric emptying. *Gastroenterology* 92: 1019.

Barber, D.C. and Brown, B.H. (1990). Progress in electrical impedance tomography. In Colton, D., Ewing, R., and Rundell, W. (Eds), *Inverse Problems in Partial Differential Equations*, pp. 149–162. New York, SIAM.

Barber, D.C. and Seagar, A.D. (1987). Fast reconstruction of resistive images. *Clin. Phys. Physiol. Meas.* 8: 47.

Bayford, R. (1994). Ph.D. thesis. Middlesex University, U.K.

Boone, K., Barber, D., and Brown, B. (1997). Imaging with electricity: report of the European concerted action on impedance tomography. *J. Med. Eng. Tech.* 21: 201–232.

Breckon, W.R. (1990). Image Reconstruction in Electrical Impedance Tomography. Ph.D. thesis, School of Computing and Mathematical Sciences, Oxford Polytechnic, Oxford, U.K.

Brown, B.H., Barber, D.C., and Seagar, A.D. (1985). Applied potential tomography: possible clinical applications. *Clin. Phys. Physiol. Meas.* 6: 109.

Brown, B.H., Barber, D.C., Wang, W. et al. (1994). Multifrequency imaging and modelling of respiratory related electrical impedance changes. *Physiol. Meas.* 15: A1.

Brown, D.C. and Seagar, A.D. (1987). The Sheffield data collection system. *Clin. Phys. Physiol. Meas.* 8(suppl A): 91–98.

Cheney, M.D., Isaacson, D., Newell, J. et al. (1990). Noser: An algorithm for solving the inverse conductivity problem. *Int. J. Imag. Syst. Tech.* 2: 60.

Cole, K.S. and Cole, R.H. (1941). Dispersion and absorption in dielectrics: I. Alternating current characteristics. *J. Chem. Phys.* 9: 431.

Cook, R.D., Saulnier, G.J., Gisser, D.G., Goble, J., Newell, J.C., and Isaacson, D. (1994). ACT3: a high-speed high-precision electrical impedance tomograph. *IEEE Trans. Biomed. Eng.*, 41: 713–722.

Cusick, G., Holder, D.S., Birkett, A., and Boone, K.G. (1994). A system for impedance imaging of epilepsy in ambulatory human subjects. *Innovation Technol. Biol. Med.* 15(suppl 1): 34–39.

Dawids, S.G. (1987). Evaluation of applied potential tomography: a clinician's view. *Clin. Phys. Physiol. Meas.* 8: 175.

Erol, R.A., Smallwood, R.H., Brown, B.H., Cherian, P., and Bardham, K.D. (1995). Detecting oesophageal-related changes using electrical impedance tomography. *Physiol. Meas.* 16(suppl 3A): 143–152.

Gisser, D.G., Newell, J.C., Salunier, G., Hochgraf, C., Cook, R.D., and Goble, J.C. (1991). Analog electronics for a high-speed high-precision electrical impedance tomograph. *Proc. IEEE EMBS* 13: 23–24.

Goble, J. and Isaacson, D. (1990). Fast reconstruction algorithms for three-dimensional electrical tomo-graphy. *In IEEE EMBS Proceedings of the 12th Annual International Conference*, Philadelphia, pp. 285–286.

Hampshire, A.R., Smallwood, R.H., Brown, B.H., and Primhak, R.A. (1995). Multifrequency and parametric EIT images of neonatal lungs. *Physiol. Meas.* 16(suppl 3A): 175–189.

Harris, N.D., Sugget, A.J., Barber, D.C., and Brown, B.H. (1988). Applied potential tomography: a new technique for monitoring pulmonary function. *Clin. Phys. Physiol. Meas.* 9: 79.

Holder, D.S. and Brown, B.H. (1990). Biomedical applications of EIT: A critical review. In D. Holder (Ed.), *Clinical and Physiological Applications of Electrical Impedance* Tomography, pp. 6–41. London, UCL Press.

Hua, P., Webster, J.G., and Tompkins, W.J. (1988). A regularized electrical impedance tomography reconstruction algorithm. *Clin. Phys. Physiol. Meas.* 9(suppl A): 137–141.

Isaacson, D. (1986). Distinguishability of conductivities by electric current computed tomography. *IEEE Trans. Med. Imag.* 5: 91.

Jossinet, J. and Trillaud, C. (1992). Imaging the complex impedance in electrical impedance tomography. *Clin. Phys. Physiol. Meas.* 13: 47.

Kim, H. and Woo, H.W. (1987). A prototype system and reconstruction algorithms for electrical impedance technique in medical imaging. *Clin. Phys. Physiol. Meas.* 8: 63.

Kohn, R.V. and Vogelius, M. (1984a). Determining the conductivity by boundary measurement. *Commun. Pure Appl. Math.* 37: 289.

Kohn, R.V. and Vogelius, M. (1984b). Identification of an unknown conductivity by means of the boundary. *SIAM-AMS Proc.* 14: 113.

Koire, C.J. (1992). EIT image reconstruction using sensitivity coefficient weighted backprojection. *Physiol. Meas.* 15(suppl 2A): 125–136.

Leathard, A.D., Brown, B.H., Campbell, J. et al. (1994). A comparison of ventilatory and cardiac related changes in EIT images of normal human lungs and of lungs with pulmonary embolism. *Physiol. Meas.* 15: A137.

Lidgey, F.J., Zhu, Q.S., McLeod, C.N., and Breckon, W. (1992). Electrode current determination from programmable current sources. *Clin. Phys. Physiol. Meas.* 13(suppl A): 43–46.

McAdams, E.T., McLaughlin, J.A., and Anderson, J.Mc.C. (1994). Multielectrode systems for electrical impedance tomography. *Physiol. Meas.* 15: A101.

Metherall, P., Barber, D.C., Smallwood, R.H., and Brown, B.H. (1996). Three-dimensional electrical impedance tomography. *Physiol. Meas.* 15: A101.

Morucci, J.P., Marsili, P.M., Granie, M., Dai, W.W., and Shi, Y. (1994). Direct sensitivity matrix approach for fast reconstruction in electrical impedance tomography. *Physiol. Meas.* 15(suppl 2A): 107–114.

Riu, P.J., Rosell, J., Lozano, A., and Pallas-Areny, R.A. (1992). Broadband system for multi-frequency static imaging in electrical impedance tomography. *Clin. Phys. Physiol. Meas.* 13: 61.

Smith, R.W.M. (1990). Design of a Real-Time Impedance Imaging System for Medical Applications. Ph.D. thesis, University of Sheffield, U.K.

Sylvester, J. and Uhlmann, G. (1986). A uniqueness theorem for an inverse boundary value problem in electrical prospection. *Commun. Pure Appl. Math.* 39: 91.

Wexler, A., Fry, B., and Neuman, M.R. (1985). Impedance-computed tomography: algorithm and system. *Appl. Opt.* 24: 3985.

Yorkey, T.J. (1986). Comparing Reconstruction Algorithms for Electrical Impedance Imaging. Ph.D. thesis, University of Wisconsin, Madison, WI.

Zadehkoochak, M., Blott, B.H., Hames, T.K., and George, R.E. (1991). Special expansion in electrical impedance tomography. *J. Phys. D: Appl. Phys.* 24: 1911–1916.

Zhu, Q.S., McLeod, C.N., Denyer, C.W., Lidgey, F.L., and Lionheart, W.R.B. (1994). Development of a real-time adaptive current tomograph. *Clin. Phys. Physiol. Meas.* 15(suppl 2A): 37–43.

Further Information

All the following conferences were funded by the European commission under the biomedical engineering program. The first two were directly funded as exploratory workshops, the remainder as part of a Concerted Action on Electrical Impedance Tomography. Electrical Impedance Tomography — Applied Potential Tomography. 1987. Proceedings of a conference held in Sheffield, U.K., 1986. Published in *Clin. Phys.*

Physiol. Meas. 8: Suppl.A. Electrical Impedance Tomography — Applied Potential Tomography. 1988. Proceedings of a conference held in Lyon, France, November 1987. Published in *Clin. Phys. Physiol. Meas.* 9: Suppl.A. Electrical Impedance Tomography. 1991. Proceedings of a conference held in Copenhagen, Denmark, July 1990. Published by *Medical Physics*, University of Sheffield, U.K. Electrical Impedance Tomography. 1992. Proceedings of a conference held in York, U.K., July 1991. Published in *Clin. Phys. Physiol. Meas.* 13: Suppl.A. Clinical and Physiologic Applications of Electrical Impedance Tomography. 1993. Proceedings of a conference held at the Royal Society, London, U.K. April 1992. Ed. D.S. Holder, UCL Press, London. Electrical Impedance Tomography. 1994. Proceedings of a conference held in Barcelona, Spain, 1993. Published in *Clin. Phys. Physiol. Meas.* 15: Suppl.A.

18

Medical Applications of Virtual Reality Technology

18.1 Overview of Virtual Reality Technology............... **18**-2
Instrumented Clothing • Head-Mounted Display (HMD) •
3D Spatialized Sound • Other VR Interface Technology
18.2 VR Application Examples **18**-5
VR Applications
18.3 Current Status of Virtual Reality Technology.......... **18**-6
18.4 Overview of Medical Applications of Virtual Reality
Technology **18**-7
Surgical Training and Surgical Planning • Medical
Education, Modeling, and Nonsurgical Training •
Anatomical Imaging and Medical Image Fusion •
Ergonomics, Rehabilitation, and Disabilities • Telesurgery
and Telemedicine • Behavioral Evaluation and Intervention
18.5 Summary **18**-17
Defining Terms **18**-17
References **18**-18
Further Information **18**-23

Walter Greenleaf
Tom Piantanida
Greenleaf Medical

Virtual reality (VR) is the term commonly used to describe a novel human–computer interface that enables users to interact with computers in a radically different way. VR consists of a computer-generated, multi-dimensional environment and interface tools that allow users to:

1. Immerse themselves in the environment
2. Navigate within the environment
3. Interact with objects and other inhabitants in the environment

The experience of entering this environment — this computer-generated virtual world — is compelling. To enter, the user usually dons a helmet containing a head-mounted display (HMD) that incorporates a sensor to track the wearer's movement and location. The user may also wear sensor-clad clothing that likewise tracks movement and location. The sensors communicate position and location data to a computer, which updates the image of the virtual world accordingly. By employing this garb, the user "breaks through" the computer screen and becomes completely immersed in this multi-dimensional world. Thus immersed, one can walk through a virtual house, drive a virtual car, or run a marathon in a park still under design. Recent advances in computer processor speed and graphics make it possible for even desk-top computers to create highly realistic environments. The practical applications are far reaching. Today, using VR, architects design office buildings, NASA controls robots at remote locations, and physicians plan and practice difficult operations.

Virtual reality is quickly finding wide acceptance in the medical community as researchers and clinicians alike become aware of its potential benefits. Several pioneer research groups have already demonstrated improved clinical performance using VR imaging, planning, and control techniques.

18.1   Overview of Virtual Reality Technology

The term "Virtual Reality" describes the experience of interacting with data from within the computer-generated data set. The computer-generated data set may be completely synthetic or remotely sensed, such as x-ray, magnetic resonance imaging (MRI), positron emission tomography (PET), etc., images. Interaction with the data is natural and intuitive and occurs from a first-person perspective. From a system perspective, VR technology can be segmented as shown in Figure 18.1. The computer-generated environment, or virtual world content consists of a 3D graphic model, typically implemented as a spatially organized, object-oriented database; each object in the database represents an object in the virtual world.

A separate modeling program is used to create the individual objects for the virtual world. For greater realism, texture maps are used to create visual surface detail.

The data set is manipulated using a real-time dynamics generator that allows objects to be moved within the world according to natural laws such as gravity and inertia, or according to other variables such as spring-rate and flexibility that are specified for each particular experience by application-specific programming. The dynamics generator also tracks the position and orientation of the user's head and hand using input peripherals such as a head tracker and DataGlove. Powerful renderers are applied to present 3D images and 3D spatialized sound in real time to the observer.

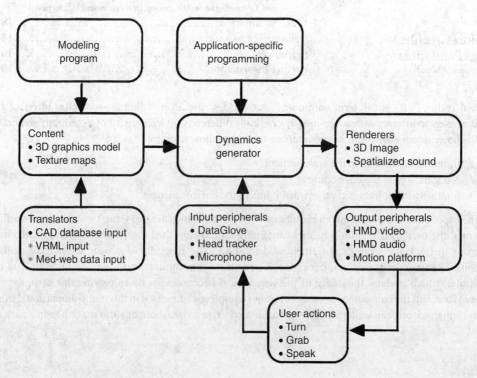

FIGURE 18.1   A complete VR system.

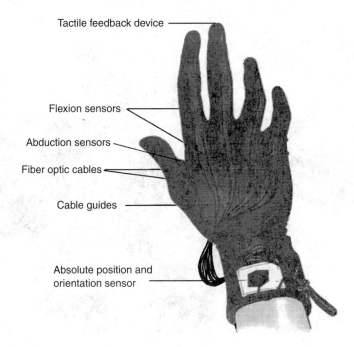

FIGURE 18.2   The DataGlove™, a VR control device.

The common method of working with a computer (the mouse/keyboard/monitor paradigm), based as it is, on a two-dimensional desk-top metaphor, is inappropriate for the multi-dimensional virtual world. Therefore, one long-term challenge for VR developers has been to replace the conventional computer interface with one that is more natural, intuitive, and allows the computer — not the user — to carry a greater proportion of the interface burden. Not surprisingly, this search for a more practical multi-dimensional metaphor for interacting with computers and computer-generated artificial environments has spawned the development of a new generation of computer interface hardware. Ideally, the interface hardware should consist of two components (1) sensors for controlling the virtual world and (2) effectors for providing feedback to the user. To date, three new computer-interface mechanisms, not all of which manifest the ideal sensor/effector duality, have evolved: Instrumented Clothing, the Head Mounted Display (HMD), and 3D Sound Systems.

18.1.1 Instrumented Clothing

The DataGlove™ and DataSuit™ use dramatic new methods to measure human motion dynamically in real time. The clothing is instrumented with sensors that track the full range of motion of specific activities of the person wearing the Glove or Suit, for example as the wearer bends, moves, grasps, or waves.

The DataGlove is a thin lycra glove with bend-sensors running along its dorsal surface. When the joints of the hand bend, the sensors bend and the angular movement is recorded by the sensors. These recordings are digitized and forwarded to the computer, which calculates the angle at which each joint is bent. On screen, an image of the hand moves in real time, reflecting the movements of the hand in the DataGlove and immediately replicating even the most subtle actions.

The DataGlove is often used in conjunction with an absolute position and orientation sensor that allows the computer to determine the three-space coordinates, as well as the orientation of the hand and fingers. A similar sensor can be used with the DataSuit and is nearly always used with an HMD.

The DataSuit is a customized body suit fitted with the same sophisticated bend-sensors found in the DataGlove. While the DataGlove is currently in production as both a VR interface and as a data-collection instrument, the DataSuit is available only as a custom device. As noted, DataGlove and DataSuit are

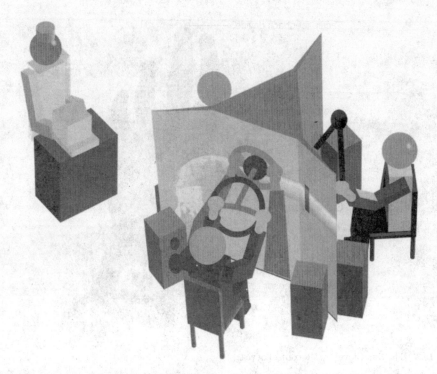

FIGURE 18.3   VR-based rehabilitation workstation.

utilized as general purpose computer interface devices for VR. There are several potential applications of this new technology for clinical and therapeutic medicine.

18.1.2   Head-Mounted Display (HMD)

The best-known sensor/effector system in VR is a head-mounted display (HMD). It supports first-person immersion by generating an image for each eye, which, in some HMDs, may provide stereoscopic vision. Most lower cost HMDs ($6000 range) use LCD displays; others use small cathode ray tubes (CRTs). The more expensive HMDs ($60,000 and up) use optical fibers to pipe the images from remotely mounted CRTs. An HMD requires a position/orientation sensor in addition to the visual display. Some displays, for example the binocular omni orientational monitors (BOOM) System [Bolas, 1994], may be head-mounted or may be used as a remote window into a virtual world.

18.1.3   3D Spatialized Sound

The impression of immersion within a virtual environment is greatly enhanced by inclusion of 3D spatialized sound [Durlach, 1994; Hendrix and Barfield, 1996]. Stereo-pan effects alone are inadequate since they tend to sound as if they are originating inside the head. Research into 3D audio has shown the importance of modeling the head and pinea and using this model as part of the 3D sound generation. A head related transfer function (HRTF) can be used to generate the proper acoustics [Begault and Wenzel, 1992; Wenzel, 1994]. A number of problems remain, such as the "cone of confusion" wherein sounds behind the head are perceived to be in front of the head [Wenzel, 1992].

18.1.4   Other VR Interface Technology

A sense of motion can be generated in a VR system by a motion platform. These have been used in flight simulators to provide cues that the mind integrates with visual and spatialized sound cues to generate perception of velocity and acceleration.

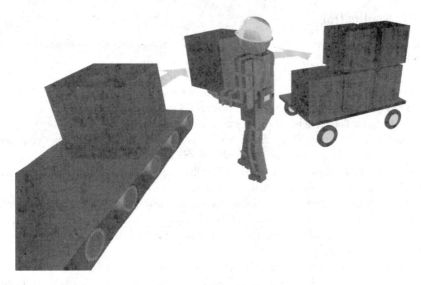

FIGURE 18.4 DataSuit™ for ergonomic and sports medicine applications.

Haptics is the science of touch. Haptic interfaces generate perception of touch and resistance in VR. Most systems to date have focused on providing force feedback to enable users to sense the inertial qualities of virtual objects, and/or kinesthetic feedback to specify the location of a virtual object in the world [Salisbury and Srinivasan, 1996, 1997]. A few prototype systems exist that generate tactile stimulation, which allow users to feel the surface qualities of virtual objects [Minsky and Lederman, 1996]. Many of the haptic systems developed thus far consist of exo-skeletons that provide position sensing as well as active force application [Burdea et al., 1992].

Some preliminary work has been conducted on generating the sense of temperature in VR. Small electrical heat pumps have been developed that produce sensations of heat and cold as part of the simulated environment [Caldwell and Gosney, 1993; Ino et al., 1993].

Olfaction is another sense that provides important cues in the real world. Consider, for example, a surgeon or dentist examining a patient for a potential bacterial infection. Inflammation and swelling may be present, but a major deciding factor is the odor of the lesion. Very early in the history of virtual reality, Mort Heilig patented his Sensorama Simulator, which incorporated olfactory, as well as visual, auditory, and motion cues (U.S. Patent 3850870, 1961). Recently, another pioneer of virtual reality, Myron Kreuger [1994, 1995a,b], has been developing virtual olfaction systems for use in medical training applications. The addition of virtual olfactory cues to medical training systems should greatly enhance both the realism and effectiveness of training.

18.2 VR Application Examples

Virtual reality had been researched for years in government laboratories and universities, but because of the enormous computing power demands and associated high costs, applications have been slow to migrate from the research world to other areas. Continual improvements in the price/performance ratio of graphic computer systems, however, have made VR technology more affordable and, thus, used more commonly in a wider range of application areas. In fact, there is even a strong "Garage VR" movement — groups of interested parties sharing information on how to build extremely low-cost VR systems using inexpensive off-the-shelf components [Jacobs, 1994]. These home-made systems are often inefficient, uncomfortable to use (sometimes painful), and slow, but they exist as a strong testament to a fervent interest in VR technology.

18.2.1   VR Applications

Applications today are diverse and represent dramatic improvements over conventional visualization and planning techniques:

Public entertainment: VR made its first major inroads in the area of public entertainment, with ventures ranging from shopping mall game simulators to low-cost VR games for the home. Major growth continues in home VR systems, partially as a result of 3D games on the Internet.

Computer-aided design: Using VR to create "virtual prototypes" in software allows engineers to test potential products in the design phase, even collaboratively over computer networks, without investing time or money for conventional hard models. All of the major automobile manufacturers and many aircraft manufacturers rely heavily on virtual prototyping.

Military: With VR, the military's solitary cab-based systems have evolved to extensive networked simulations involving a variety of equipment and situations. There is an apocryphal story that General Norman Schwartzkopf was selected to lead the Desert Storm operation on the basis of his extensive experience with simulations of the Middle East battle arena.

Architecture/construction: VR allows architects and engineers and their clients to "walk through" structural blueprints. Designs may be understood more clearly by clients who often have difficulty comprehending them even with conventional cardboard models. Atlanta, Georgia credits its VR model for winning it the site of the 1996 Olympics, while San Diego is using a VR model of a planned convention center addition to compete for the next convention of the Republican Party.

Data visualization: By allowing navigation through an abstract "world" of data, VR helps users rapidly visualize relationships within complex, multi-dimensional data structures. This is particularly important in financial-market data, where VR supports faster decision-making. VR is commonly associated with exotic "fully immersive applications" because of the overdramatized media coverage on helmets, body suits, entertainment simulators, and the like. Equally important are the "Window into World" applications where the user or operator is allowed to interact effectively with "virtual" data, either locally or remotely.

18.3   Current Status of Virtual Reality Technology

The commercial market for VR, while taking advantage of advances in VR technology at large, is nonetheless contending with the lack of integrated systems and the frequent turnover of equipment suppliers. Over the last few years, VR users in academia and industry have developed different strategies for circumventing these problems. In academic settings, researchers buy peripherals and software from separate companies and configure their own systems to maintain the greatest application versatility. In industry, however, expensive, state-of-the-art VR systems are vertically integrated to address problems peculiar to the industry.

Each solution is either too costly or too risky for most medical organizations. What is required is a VR system tailored to the needs of the medical community. Unfortunately, few companies offer integrated systems that are applicable to the VR medical market. This situation is likely to change in the next few years as VR-integration companies develop to fill this void.

At the same time, the nature of the commercial VR medical market is changing as the price of high-performance graphics systems continues to decline. High-resolution graphics monitors are becoming more cost-effective even for markets that rely solely on desktop computers. Technical advances are also occurring in networking, visual photo-realism, tracker latency through predictive algorithms, and variable-resolution image generators. Improved database access methods are underway. Hardware advances, such as eye gear that provide an increased field of view with high-resolution, untethered VR systems and inexpensive intuitive input devices, for example, DataGloves, have lagged behind advances in computational, communications, and display capabilities.

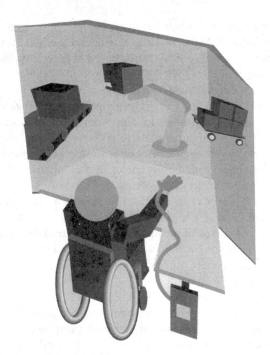

FIGURE 18.5   VR system used as a disability solution.

18.4   Overview of Medical Applications of Virtual Reality Technology

Within the medical community, the first wave of VR development efforts have evolved into six key categories:

1. Surgical training and surgical planning
2. Medical education, modeling, and nonsurgical training
3. Anatomical imaging and medical image fusion
4. Ergonomics, rehabilitation, and disabilities
5. Telesurgery and telemedicine
6. Behavioral evaluation and intervention

The potential of VR through education and information dissemination indicates there will be few areas of medicine not taking advantage of this improved computer interface. However, the latent potential of VR lies in its capacity to be used to manipulate and combine heterogeneous multi-dimensional data sets from many sources, for example, MRI, PET, and x-ray images. This feature is most significant and continues to transform the traditional applications environment.

18.4.1   Surgical Training and Surgical Planning

Various projects are underway to utilize VR and imaging technology to plan, simulate, and customize invasive (as well as minimally invasive) surgical procedures. One example of a VR surgical-planning and training system is the computer-based workstation developed by Ciné-Med of Woodbury, Connecticut [McGovern, 1994]. The goal was to develop a realistic, interactive training workstation that helps surgeons make a more seamless transition from surgical simulation to the actual surgical event.

Ciné-Med focused on television-controlled endosurgical procedures because of the intensive training required for endosurgery and the adaptability of endosurgery to high quality imaging. Surgeons can gain clinical expertise by training on this highly realistic and functional surgical simulator. Ciné-Med's computer environment includes life-like virtual organs that react much like their real counterparts, and sophisticated details such as the actual surgical instruments that provide system input/output (I/O). To further enhance training, the simulator allows the instructor to adapt clinical instruction to advance the technical expertise of learners. Surgical anomalies and emergency situations can be replicated to allow practicing surgeons to experiment and gain technical expertise on a wide range of surgical problems using the computer model before using an animal model. Since the steps of the procedure can be repeated and replayed at a later time, the learning environment surpasses other skills-training modalities.

The current prototype simulates the environment of laparoscopic cholecystectomy for use as a surgical training device. Development began with the creation of an accurate anatomic landscape, including the liver, the gallbladder, and related structures. Appropriate surgical instruments are used for the system I/O and inserted into a fiberglass replica of a human torso. Four surgical incisional ports are assigned for three scissors grip instruments and camera zoom control. The instruments, retrofitted with switching devices, read and relay the opening and closing of the tips, with position trackers located within the simulator. The virtual surgical instruments are graphically generated on a display monitor where they interact with fully textural, anatomically correct, three-dimensional virtual organs. The organs are created as independent objects and conform to object-oriented programming.

To replicate physical properties, each virtual organ must be assigned appropriate values to dictate its reaction when contacted by a virtual surgical instrument. Collision algorithms are established to define when the virtual organ is touched by a virtual surgical instrument. Additionally, with the creation of spontaneous objects resulting from the dissection of a virtual organ, each new object is calculated to have independent physical properties using artificial intelligence (AI) subroutines. Collision algorithms drive the programmed creation of spontaneous objects.

To reproduce the patient's physiological reactions during the surgical procedure, the simulation employs an expert system. This software sub-system generates patient reactions and probable outcomes derived from surgical stimuli, for example, bleeding control, heart rate failure, and, in the extreme, a death outcome. The acceptable value ranges of these factors are programmed to be constantly updated by the expert system while important data is displayed on the monitor.

Three-dimensional graphical representation of a patient's anatomy is a challenge for accurate surgical planning. Technological progress has been seen in the visualization of bone, brain, and soft tissue. Heretofore, three-dimensional modeling of soft tissue has been difficult and often inaccurate owing to the intricacies of the internal organ, its vasculature, ducts, volume, and connective tissues.

As an extension of this surgical simulator, a functional surgical planning device using VR technology is under development that will enable surgeons to operate on an actual patient, in virtual reality, prior to the actual operation. With the advent of technological advances in anatomic imaging, the parallel development of a surgical planning device incorporating real-time interaction with computer graphics that mimic a patient's anatomy is possible. Identification of anatomical structures to be modeled constitutes the initial phase for development of the surgical planning device. A spiral CAT scanning device records multiple slices of the anatomy during a single breath inhalation by the patient. Pin-registered layers of the anatomy are thus provided for the computer to read.

Individual anatomical structures are defined at the scan level according to gray scale. Once the anatomical structures are identified and labeled, the scans are stacked and connected. The result is a volumetric polygonal model of the patient's actual anatomy. A polygon-reduction program is initiated to create a wire frame that can be successfully texture-mapped and interacted with in real time. As each slice of the CAT scan is stacked and linked together, the result is a fully volumetric, graphic representation of the human anatomy. Since the model, at this point, is unmanageable by the graphics workstation because of the volume polygons, a polygon-reduction program is initiated to eliminate excessive polygons.

Key to the planning device is development of a user-friendly software program that will allow the radiologist to define anatomical structures, incorporate them into graphical representations, and assign physiological parameters to the anatomy. Surgeons will then be able to diagnose, plan, and prescribe appropriate therapy to their patients using a trial run of a computerized simulation.

Several VR-based systems currently under development allow real-time tracking of surgical instrumentation and simultaneous display and manipulation of three-dimensional anatomy corresponding to the simulated procedure [Hon, 1994; McGovern, 1994; Edmond et al., 1997]. With this design surgeons can practice procedures and experience the possible complications and variations in anatomy encountered during surgery. Ranging from advanced imaging technologies for endoscopic surgery to routine hip replacements, these new developments will have a tremendous impact on improving surgical morbidity and mortality. According to Merril [1993, 1994], studies show that doctors are more likely to make errors performing their first few to several dozen diagnostic and therapeutic surgical procedures. Merril claims that operative risk could be substantially reduced by the development of a simulator that allows transference of skills from the simulation to the actual point of patient contact.

A preliminary test of Meril's claim was achieved by Taffinder and colleagues [1998]. Following the observations by McDougall et al. [1996] that 2D representations of anatomic imagery are insufficient to develop the eye–hand coordination of surgeons, Taffinder et al. conducted randomized, controlled studies of psychomotor skills developed either through the use of the Minimally Invasive Surgical Trainer-Virtual Reality (MIST-VR) Laparoscopic Simulator or through a standard laparoscopic-surgery training course. They used the MIST-VR Laparoscopic Simulator to compare the psychomotor skills of experienced surgeons, surgeon trainees, and nonsurgeons. When task speed and the number of correctional movements were compared across subjects, experienced surgeons surpassed trainees and nonsurgeons. Taffinder and colleagues also noted that among trainees, training on the VR system improved efficiency and reduced errors, but did not increase the speed of the laparoscopic procedures.

To increase the realism of medical simulators, software tools have been developed to create "virtual tissues" that reflect the physical characteristics of physiological tissues. This technology operates in real-time using three-dimensional graphics, on a high speed computer platform. Recent advances in creating virtual tissues have occurred as force feedback is incorporated into more VR systems and the computational overhead of finite-element analysis is reduced [see, e.g., Grabowski, 1998; McInerney and Terzopoulos, 1996]. Bro-Nielsen and Cotin [1996] have been developing tissue models that incorporate appropriate real-time volumetric deformation in response to applied forces. Their goal was to provide surgeons with the same "hands-on" feel in VR that they experience in actual surgery. They used mass-spring systems [Bro-Nielsen, 1997] to simplify finite-element analysis, significantly reduced computational overhead, and thereby achieving near-real-time performance. While advancing the state of the art considerably toward the real-time, hands-on objective, much more work remains to be done.

In another study of the effectiveness of force-feedback in surgical simulations, Baur et al. [1998] reported on the use of VIRGY, a VR endoscopic surgery simulator. VIRGY provides both visual and force feedback to the user, through the use of the Pantoscope [Baumann, 1996]. Because the Pantoscope is a remote-center-of-motion force-reflecting system, Baur et al. were able to hide the system beneath the skin of the endoscope mannequin. Force reflection of tissue interactions, including probing and cutting, was controlled by nearest neighbor propagation of look-up table values to circumvent the computational overhead inherent in finite element analysis. Surgeons were asked to assess the tissue feel achieved through this simulation.

Evaluation of another surgical simulator system was carried out by Weghorst et al. [1998]. This evaluation involved the use of the Madigan Endoscopic Sinus Surgery (ESS) Simulator (see Edmond et al. [1997] for a full description), developed jointly by the U.S. Army, Lockheed-Martin, and the Human Interface Technology Laboratory at the University of Washington. The ESS Simulator, which was designed to train otolaryngologists to perform paranasal endoscopic procedures, incorporates 3D models of the naso-pharyngeal anatomy derived from the National Library of Medicine's Virtual Human Data Base. It employs two 6-DOF force-reflecting instruments developed by the Immersion Corporation to simulate the endoscope and 11 surgical instruments used in paranasal surgery.

Weghorst and colleagues pitted three groups of subjects against each other in a test of the effectiveness of the ESS Simulator: non-MDs, non-ENT MDs, and ENTs with various levels of experience. Training aids, in the form of circular hoops projected onto the simulated nasal anatomy, identified the desired endoscope trajectory; targets identified anatomical injection sites; and text labels identified anatomical landmarks. Successive approximations to the actual task involved training first on an abstract, geometric model of the nasal anatomy with superimposed training aids (Level 1); next on real nasal anatomy with superimposed training aids (Level 2); and finally, on real nasal anatomy without training aids (Level 3).

Results of the evaluation indicated that, in general, ENTs performed better than non-ENTs on Level 1 and 2 tasks, and that among the ENTs, those with more ESS experience scored higher than those who had performed fewer ESS procedures. The researchers also found that deviations from the optimum endoscope path differentiated ENT and non-ENT subjects. In post-training questionnaires, ENTs rated the realism of the simulation as high and confirmed the validity and usefulness of training on the ESS Simulator.

While the ESS Simulator described above requires a 200 MHz Pentium PC and a 4-CPU SGI Oxyx with Reality Engine 2 graphics to synthesize the virtual nasal cavity, a current trend in surgical simulation is toward lower-end simulation platforms. As computational power of PCs continues to escalate, simulations are increasingly being ported to or developed on relatively inexpensive computers. Tseng et al. [1998] used an Intel-based PC as the basis of their laparoscopic surgery simulator. This device incorporates a 5-DOF force-reflecting effector, a monitor for viewing the end-effector, and a speech-recognition system for changing viewpoint. The system detects collisions between the end effector and virtual tissues, and is capable of producing tissue deformation through one of several models including a finite element model, a displacement model, or a transmission line model. Computational power is provided by dual Pentium Pro 200 MHz CPUs and a Realizm Graphics Accelerator Board.

18.4.2 Medical Education, Modeling, and Nonsurgical Training

Researchers at the University of California — San Diego are exploring the value of hybridizing elements of VR, multimedia (MM), and communications technologies into a unified educational paradigm [Hoffman, 1994; Hoffman et al., 1995; Hoffman et al., 1997]. The goal is to develop powerful tools that extend the flexibility and effectiveness of medical teaching and promote lifelong learning. To this end, they have undertaken a multi-year initiative, named the "VR-MM Synthesis Project." Based on instructional design and user-need (rather than technology per se), they have planned a linked 3-computer array representing the Data Communications Gateway, the Electronic Medical Record System, and the Simulation Environment. This system supports medical students, surgical residents, and clinical faculty running applications ranging from full surgical simulation to basic anatomical exploration and review, all via a common interface. The plan also supports integration of learning and telecommunications resources (such as interactive MM libraries, online textbooks, databases of medical literature, decision support systems, electronic mail, and access to electronic medical records).

The first application brought to fruition in the VR-MM Synthesis Project is an anatomical instructional-aid system called Anatomic VisualizeR [Hoffman et al., 1997] that uses anatomical models derived from the Visible Human Project of the National Library of Medicine. Using the "Guided Lessons" paradigm of Anatomical VisualizeR, the student enters a 3D workspace that contains a "Study Guide." The student uses the study guide to navigate through the 3D workspace, downloading anatomical models of interest, as well as supporting resources like diagrammatic representations, photographic material, and text. Manipulation of the anatomical models is encouraged to provide the student with an intuitive understanding of anatomical relationships. The study guide also incorporates other instructional material necessary for the completion of a given lesson.

Another advanced medical training system based on VR technology is VMET — the virtual medical trainer — jointly developed by the Research Triangle Institute and Advanced Simulation Corp. [Kizakevich et al., 1998]. VMET was developed to provide training in trauma care. The VMET trauma patient simulator (VMET-TPS), which was designed to comply with civilian guidelines for both Basic Trauma Life Support and Advanced Trauma Life Support, incorporates models of (1) physiological systems and functions, (2) dynamic consequences of trauma to these physiological systems, and (3) medical intervention effects on these physiological systems.

VMET provides a multisensory simulation of a trauma patient, including visible, audible, and behavioral aspects of the trauma patient. To maintain cost-effectiveness, VMET is constrained to providing "virtual spaces" at the site of several injuries, including a penetrating chest wound, a penetrating arm wound, laceration to the arm, and a thigh contusion. Within the virtual spaces, the trainee can experience the physiological effects of the injury and of his intervention in real time, as the physiological engine updates the condition of the wound.

VMET-TPS was designed to train military personnel in trauma care, so it places emphasis on the medical technology currently and foreseeably available to the military. However, VMET-TPS will find applications in civilian teaching hospitals, as well. Partially because of the cost-constraint requirements of the project, the price of VMET should be within reach of many trauma centers.

In another task-specific program at the Fraunhofer Institute, researchers have been developing an ultrasonic probe training system based on VR components called the UltraTrainer [Stallkamp and Walper, 1998]. UltraTrainer uses a Silicon Graphics workstation and monitor to present images drawn from a database of real ultrasonograms, a Polhemus tracker to determine the position of the user's hand, a joystick representation of the ultrasound probe, and an ultrasound phantom to provide probe position/orientation feedback to the trainee. In using the UltraTrainer, the trainee moves the ultrasound probe against the phantom, which is used in this system as a representation of the virtual patient's body. On the monitor, the trainee sees an image of the probe in relation to the phantom, showing the trainee the position and orientation of the probe with respect to the virtual patient.

The Polhemus tracker determines and records the real-space position of the virtual ultrasound probe, and this tracker information is then used to extract stored ultrasonograms from a database of images. An ultrasonic image of the appropriate virtual scanfield is presented on the monitor in accordance with the position of the virtual probe on the phantom. As the probe is moved on the phantom, new virtual scanfields are extracted from the database and presented on the monitor. The UltraTrainer is able to present sequential virtual scanfields rapidly enough for the trainee to perceive the virtual ultrasonography as occurring in real time.

Planned improvements to the UltraTrainer include a larger database of stored sonograms that can be customized for different medical specialties, and a reduction in cost by porting the system to a PC and by using a less expensive tracking system. These improvements should allow the UltraTrainer to be accessed by a broader range of users and to move from the laboratory to the classroom, or even to the home.

Three groups of researchers have taken different approaches to developing VR-based training systems for needle insertion, each based on feedback to a different sensory system. At Georgetown University, Lathan and associates [1998] have produced a spine biopsy simulator based on visual feedback; a team from Ohio State University and the Ohio Supercomputer Center have demonstrated an epidural needle insertion simulator based on force feedback [Heimenz et al., 1998]; and Computer Aided Surgery in New York has developed a blind needle biopsy placement simulator that uses 3D auditory feedback [Wenger and Karron, 1998]. Each of these innovative systems draws on technological advances in VR. In the aggregate, they disclose that, given appropriate cognitive constructs, humans are capable of using diverse sensory input to learn very demanding tasks. Imagine how effective VR could be in training complex tasks if all of the sensory information could be integrated in a single system. That is currently one of the goals of the VR community.

18.4.3 Anatomical Imaging and Medical Image Fusion

An anatomically keyed display with real-time data fusion is currently in use at NYU Medical Center's Department of Neurosurgery. The system allows both preoperative planning and real-time tumor visualization [Kall, 1994; Kelly, 1994]. The technology offers a technique for surgeons to plan and simulate the surgical procedure beforehand in order to reach deep-seated or centrally located brain tumors. The imaging method (volumetric stereotaxis) gathers, stores, and reformats imaging-derived, three-dimensional volumetric information that defines an intracranial lesion (tumor) with respect to the surgical field.

Computer-generated information is displayed intraoperatively on computer monitors in the operating room and on a "heads up" display mounted on the operating microscope. These images provide surgeons with a CT (computed tomography) and MRI defined map of the surgical field area scaled to actual size and location. This guides the surgeon in finding and defining the boundaries of brain tumors. The computer-generated images are indexed to the surgical field by means of a robotics-controlled stereotactic frame which positions the patient's tumor within a defined targeting area. Simulated systems using VR models are being advocated for high risk techniques, such as the alignment of radiation sources to treat cancerous tumors. Where registration of virtual and real anatomical features is not an issue, other display technologies can be employed. Two recent examples, based on totally different display modalities, are described later.

Parsons and Rolland [1998] developed a nonintrusive display technique that projects images of virtual inclusions such as tumors, cysts, or abscesses, or other medical image data into the surgeon's field of view on demand. The system relies on retroreflective material, perhaps used as a backing for the surgeon's glove or on a surgical instrument, to provide an imaging surface upon which can be presented images extracted from 2D data sources, for example MRI scans. The surgeon can access the data by placing the retroreflective screen, for example, his gloved hand, in the path of an imaging beam. The image of the virtual MRI scan, for example, will appear superimposed along the surgeon's line of sight. Although image registration is not currently possible with this real-time display system, the system does provide a means for the clinician to access critical information without turning to view a monitor or other screen.

For displaying volumetric data, Senger [1998] devised a system based on the FakeSpace Immersive Workbench™ and position-tracked StereoGraphics CrystalEyes™ that presents stereoscopic images derived from CT, MRI, and the Visible Human data sets. The viewer can interact with the immersive data structure through the use of a position/orientation sensed probe. The probe can be used first to identify a region of interest within the anatomical data set and then to segment the data so that particular anatomical features are highlighted. The probe can also be used to "inject" digital stain into the data set and to direct the propagation of the stain into structures that meet predetermined parameters, such as voxel density, opacity, etc. Through the use of the probe, the vasculature, fascia, bone, etc. may be selectively stained. This imaging system takes advantage of the recent advances in VR hardware and software, the advent of programs such as the National Library of Medicine's Visible Human Project, and significant cost reductions in computational power to make it feasible for medical researchers to create accurate, interactive 3D human anatomical atlases.

Suzuki and colleagues [1998] have pushed virtual anatomical imaging a step further by including the temporal domain. In 1987, Suzuki, Itou, and Okamura developed a 3D human atlas based on serial MRI scans. Originally designed to be resident on a PC, the 3D Human Atlas has been upgraded during the last decade to take advantage of major advances in computer graphics. The latest atlas is based on composite super-conducting MRI scans at 4 mm intervals at 4 mm pitch of young male and female humans. In addition to volume and surface rendering, this atlas is also capable of dynamic cardiac imaging.

Rendered on a Silicon Graphics Onyx Reality Engine, this atlas presents volumetric images at approximately 10 frames per second. The user interface allows sectioning of the anatomical data along any plane, as well as extracting organ surface information. Organs can be manipulated individually and rendered transparent to enable the user to view hidden structures. By rendering the surface of the heart transparent, it is possible to view the chambers of the heart in 4D at approximately 8 frames per second. Suzuki and colleagues plan to distribute the atlas over the internet so that users throughout the world will be able to access it.

Distribution of volumetric medical imagery over the Internet through the world wide web (WWW) has already been examined by Hendin and colleagues [1998]. These authors relied on the virtual reality modeling language (VRML) and VRMLscript to display and interact with the medial data sets, and they used a Java graphical user interface (GUI) to preserve platform independence. They conclude that it is currently feasible to share and interact with medical image data over the WWW.

Similarly, Silverstein et al. [1998] have demonstrated a system for interacting with 3D radiologic image data over the Internet. While they conclude that the Web-based system is effective for transmitting useful imagery to remote colleagues for diagnosis and pretreatment planning, it does not supplant the requirement that a knowledgeable radiologist examine the 2D tomographic images. This raises the question of the effectiveness of the display and interaction with virtual medical images. The perceived effectiveness of VR-based anatomical imaging systems similar to those described earlier, has been assessed by Oyama and colleagues [1998]. They created virtual environments consisting of 3D images of cancerous lesions and surrounding tissue, derived from CT or MRI scans, and presented these environments to clinicians in one of three modes. The cancers were from the brain, breast, lung, stomach, liver, and colon, and the presentation modes were either as surface-rendered images, real-time volume-rendered images, or editable real-time volume-rendered images. Clinicians had to rate the effectiveness of the three modes in providing them with information about (1) the location of the cancer, (2) the shape of the cancer, (3) the shape of fine vessels, (4) the degree of infiltration of surrounding organs, and (5) the relationship between the cancer and normal organs. In each of the five categories, the clinicians rated the editable real-time volume-rendered images as superior to the other modes of presentation. From the study, the authors conclude that real-time surface rendering, while applicable to many areas of medicine, is not suitable for use in cancer diagnosis.

18.4.4 Ergonomics, Rehabilitation, and Disabilities

Virtual reality offers the possibility to better shape a rehabilitative program to an individual patient. Greenleaf [1994] has theorized that the rehabilitation process can be enhanced through the use of VR technology. The group is currently developing a VR-based rehabilitation workstation that will be used to (1) decompose rehabilitation into small, incremental functional steps to facilitate the rehabilitation process; and (2) make the rehabilitation process more realistic and less boring, thus enhancing motivation and recovery of function.

DataGlove and DataSuit technologies were originally developed as control devices for VR, but through improvements they are now being applied to the field of functional evaluation of movement and to rehabilitation in a variety of ways. One system, for example, uses a glove device coupled with a force feedback system — The Rutgers Master (RM-I) — to rehabilitate a damaged hand or to diagnose a range of hand problems [Burdea et al., 1995, 1997]. The rehabilitation system developed by Burdea and colleagues uses programmable force feedback to control the level of effort required to accomplish rehabilitative tasks. This system measures finger-specific forces while the patient performs one of several rehabilitative tasks, including ball squeezing, DigiKey exercises, and peg insertion.

Another system under development — The RM II — incorporates tactile feedback to a glove system to produce feeling in the fingers when virtual objects are "touched" [Burdea, 1994]. In order to facilitate accurate goniometric assessment, improvements to the resolution of the standard DataGlove have been developed [Greenleaf, 1992]. The improved DataGlove allows highly accurate measurement of dynamic range of motion of the fingers and wrist and is in use at research centers such as Johns Hopkins and Loma Linda University to measure and analyze functional movements.

Adjacent to rehabilitation evaluation systems are systems utilizing the same measurement technology to provide ergonomic evaluation and injury prevention. Workplace ergonomics has already received a boost from new VR technologies that enable customized workstations tailored to individual requirements [Greenleaf, 1994]. In another area, surgical room ergonomics for medical personnel and patients is projected to reduce the hostile and complicated interface among patients, health care providers, and surgical spaces [Kaplan, 1994].

Motion analysis software (MAS) can assess and analyze upper extremity function from dynamic measurement data acquired by the improved DataGlove. This technology not only provides highly objective measurement, but also ensures more accurate methods for collecting data and performing quantitative analyses for physicians, therapists, and ergonomics specialists involved in job site evaluation and design. The DataGlove/MAS technology is contributing to a greater understanding of upper extremity biomechanics and kinesiology. Basic DataGlove technology coupled with VR media will offer numerous opportunities for the rehabilitation sector of the medical market, not the least of which is the positive implication for enhancing patient recovery by making the process more realistic and participatory.

One exciting aspect of VR technology is the inherent ability to enable individuals with physical disabilities to accomplish tasks and have experiences otherwise denied to them. The strategies currently employed for disability-related VR research include head-mounted displays; position/orientation sensing; tactile feedback; eye tracking; 3D sound systems; data input devices; image generation; and optics. For physically disabled persons, VR will provide a new link to capabilities and experiences heretofore unattainable, such as:

- An individual with cerebral palsy who is confined to a wheelchair can operate a telephone switchboard, play hand ball, and dance [Greenleaf, 1994] within a virtual environment.
- Patients with spinal cord injury or CNS dysfunction can relearn limb movements through adaptive visual feedback in virtual environments [Steffin, 1997].
- Disabled individuals can be in one location while their "virtual being" is in a totally different location. This opens all manner of possibilities for participating in work, study, or leisure activities anywhere in the world without leaving home.
- Physically disabled individuals could interact with real world activities through robotic devices they control from within the virtual world.
- Blind persons could practice and plan in advance navigating through or among buildings if the accesses represented in a virtual world were made up of three-dimensional sound images and tactile stimuli [Max and Gonzalez, 1997].

One novel application of VR technology to disabilities has been demonstrated by Inman [1994a,b; 1996] who trained handicapped children to operate wheelchairs without the inherent dangers of such training. Inman trained children with cerebral palsy or orthopedic impairments to navigate virtual worlds that contained simulated physical conditions that they would encounter in the real world. By training in a virtual environment, the children acquired an appreciation of the dynamics of their wheelchairs and of the dangers that they might encounter in the real world, but in a safe setting. The safety aspect of VR training is impossible to achieve with other training technologies.

VR will also enable persons with disabilities to experience situations and sensations not accessible in a physical world. Learning and working environments can be tailored to specific needs with VR. For example, since the virtual world can be superimposed over the real world, a learner could move progressively from a highly supported mode of performing a task in the virtual world, through to performing it unassisted in the real world. One project, "Wheelchair VR" [Trimble, 1992], is a highly specialized architectural software being developed to aid in the design of barrier-free building for persons with disabilities.

VR also presents unique opportunities for retraining persons who have incurred neuropsychological deficits. The cognitive deficits associated with neurophysiological insults are often difficult to assess and for this and other reasons, not readily amenable to treatment. Several groups have begun to investigate the use of VR in the assessment and retraining of persons with neuropsychological cognitive impairments. Pugnetti and colleagues [1995a,b, 1996] have begun to develop VR-based scenarios based on standardized tests of cognitive function, for example, card-sorting tasks. Because the tester has essentially absolute control over the cognitive environment in which the test is administered, the effects of environmental distractors can be both assessed and controlled. Initial tests by the Italian group suggests that VR-based cognitive tests offer great promise for both evaluation and retraining of brain-injury-associated cognitive deficits.

Other groups have been developing cognitive tests based on mental rotation of virtual objects [Buchwalter and Rizzo, 1997; Rizzo and Buchwalter, 1997] or spatial memory of virtual buildings [Attree et al., 1996]. Although VR technology shows promise in both the assessment and treatment of persons with acquired cognitive deficits, Buchwalter and Rizzo find that the technology is currently too cumbersome, too unfamiliar, and has too many side effects to allow many patients to benefit from its use.

Attree and associates, however, have begun to develop a taxonomy of VR applications in cognitive rehabilitation. Their study examined the differences between active and passive navigation of virtual environments. They report that active navigation improves spatial memory of the route through the virtual environment, while passive navigation improves object recognition for landmarks within the virtual environment. This report sends a clear message that VR is capable of improving cognitive function, but that much more work is required to understand how the technology interacts with the human psyche.

One researcher who is actively pursuing this understanding is Dorothy Strickland [1995, 1996], who has developed a virtual environment for working with autistic children. Strickland's premise is that VR technology allows precise control of visual and auditory stimuli within virtual environments. Frequently, autistic children find the magnitude of environmental stimuli overwhelming, so it is difficult for them to focus. Strickland has developed a sparse virtual environment into which stimuli can be introduced as the autistic child becomes capable of handling more environmental stimulation. Essentially, she produces successive approximations to a real environment at a rate that the autistic child can tolerate. Her work has shown that autistic children can benefit greatly by exposure to successively richer environments and that the advances that they make in virtual environments transfer to the real world.

Max and Burke [1997], also using VR with autistic children, report that contrary to expectations, their patients were able to focus on the virtual environment, rather than "fidgeting" as they are prone to do in other environments. These researchers also found that in the absence of competing acoustic stimuli, autistic children were drawn to loud music and shunned soft choral music. These findings may provide important insights into the etiology of autism that could not be observed in the "real world" setting.

18.4.5 Telesurgery and Telemedicine

Telepresence is the "sister field" of VR. Classically defined as the ability to act and interact in an off-site environment by making use of VR technology, telepresence is emerging as an area of development in its own right. Telemedicine (the telepresence of medical experts) is being explored as a way to reduce the cost of medical practice and to bring expertise into remote areas [Burrow, 1994; Rosen, 1994; Rovetta et al., 1997; Rissam et al., 1998].

Telesurgery is a fertile area for development. On the verge of realization, telesurgery (remote surgery) will help resolve issues that can complicate or compromise surgery, among them:

- The patient is too ill or injured to be moved for surgery
- A specialist surgeon is located at some distance from the patient requiring specialized attention
- Accident victims may have a better chance of survival if immediate, on-the-scene surgery can be performed remotely by an emergency room surgeon at a local hospital
- Soldiers wounded in battle could undergo surgery on the battlefield by a surgeon located elsewhere

The surgeon really does operate — on flesh, not a computer animation. And while the distance aspect of remote surgery is a provocative one, telepresence is proving an aid in nonremote surgery as well. It can help surgeons gain dexterity over conventional methods of manipulation. This is expected to be particularly important in laparoscopic surgery. For example, suturing and knot-tying will be as easy to see in laparoscopic surgery as it is in open surgery because telepresence enables the surgery to look and feel like open surgery.

As developed at SRI International [Satava 1992; Hill et al., 1995, 1998], telepresence not only offers a compelling sense of reality for the surgeon, but also allows the surgeon to perform the surgery according to the usual methods and procedures. There is nothing new to learn. Hand motions are quick and precise. The visual field, instrument motion, and force feedback can all be scaled to make microsurgery easier than it would be if the surgeon were at the patient's side. While the current technology has been implemented in prototype, SRI and Telesurgical Corporation, based in Redwood City, California, are collaborating to develop a full system based on this novel concept.

The system uses color video cameras to image the surgical field in stereo, which the remote surgeon views with stereo shutter glasses. The remote surgeon grasps a pair of force-reflecting 6-DOF remote manipulators linked to a slaved pair of end effectors in the surgical field. Coordinated visual, auditory, and haptic feedback from the end effectors provides the remote surgeon with a compelling sense of presence at the surgical site.

Because the remote manipulators and end effectors are only linked electronically, the gain between them can be adjusted to provide the remote surgeon with microsurgically precise movement of the slaved instruments with relatively gross movement of the master manipulators. Researchers at SRI have demonstrated the microsurgery capabilities of this system by performing microvascular surgery on rats.

Again, because only an electronic link exists between manipulator and end effector, separation of the remote surgeon and the surgical field can be on a global scale. To demonstrate this global remote surgery capability, Rovetta and colleagues [1998] established Internet and ISDN networks between Monterey, California, and Milan, Italy, and used these networks to remotely control a surgical robot. By manipulating controls in Monterey, Professor Rovetta was able to perform simulated biopsies on liver, prostate, and breasts in his laboratory in Milan, Italy. Using both an Internet and ISDN network facilitated the transmission of large amounts of image data and robotic control signals in a timely manner.

Prior to the telesurgery demonstration between Monterey and Milan, Rovetta and colleagues [1997] established a link between European hospitals and hospitals in Africa as part of the Telehealth in Africa Program of the European Collaboration Group for Telemedicine. Among the objectives of this program was a demonstration of the feasibility of transmitting large amounts of medical data including x-ray and other diagnostic images, case histories, and diagnostic analyses. Once established, the data link could be used for teleconsulting and teletraining.

Teleconsulting is becoming commonplace. Within the last year, the U.S. Department of Veteran Affairs has established a network to link rural and urban Vet Centers. This network, which will initially link 20 Vet Centers, will provide teleconsultation for chronic disease screening, trauma outreach, and psychosocial care. In Europe, where telemedicine is making great strides, the Telemedical Information Society has been established [see Marsh, 1998, for additional information]. At the International Telemedical Information Society '98 Conference held in Amsterdam in April 1998, a number of important issues pertaining to teleconsultation were addressed. Among these were discussions about the appropriate network for telemedicine, for example, the WWW, ATM, and privacy and liability issues.

Privacy, that is security of transmitted medical information, will be a continuing problem as hackers hone their ability to circumvent Internet security [Radesovich, 1997]. Aslan and colleagues [1998] have examined the practicality of using 128-bit encryption for securing the transmission of medical images. Using software called Photomailer™, Aslan at Duke Medical Center and his colleagues at Boston University Medical Center and Johns Hopkins encrypted 60 medical images and transmitted them over the Internet. They then attempted to access the encrypted images without Photomailer™ installed on the receiving computer. They reported complete success and insignificant increases in processing time with the encrypting software installed.

18.4.6 Behavioral Evaluation and Intervention

VR technology has been successfully applied to a number of behavioral conditions over the last few years. Among the greatest breakthroughs attained through the use of this technology is the relief of akinesia, a symptom of Parkinsonism wherein a patient has progressively greater difficulty initiating and sustaining walking. The condition can be mitigated by treatment with drugs such as L-dopa, a precursor of the natural neural transmitters dopamine, but usually not without unwanted side effects. Now, collaborators at the Human Interface Technology Laboratory at the University of Washington, along with the University's Department of Rehabilitation Medicine and the San Francisco Parkinson's Institute, are using virtual imagery to simulate an effect called kinesia paradoxa, or the triggering of normal walking behavior in akinetic Parkinson's patients [Weghorst, 1994].

Using a commercial, field-multiplexed, "heads-up" video display, the research team has developed an approach that elicits near-normal walking by presenting collimated virtual images of objects and abstract visual cues moving through the patient's visual field at speeds that emulate normal walking. The combination of image collimation and animation speed reinforces the illusion of space-stabilized visual cues at the patient's feet. This novel, VR-assisted technology may also prove to be therapeutically useful for other movement disorders.

In the area of phobia intervention, Lamson [1994, 1997] and Lamson and Meisner [1994] has investigated the diagnostic and treatment possibilities of VR immersion on anxiety, panic, and phobia of heights. By immersing both patients and controls in computer-generated situations, the researchers were able to expose the subjects to anxiety provoking situations (such as jumping from a height) in a controlled manner. Experimental results indicated a significant subject habituation and desensitization through this approach, and the approach appears clinically useful.

The effectiveness of VR as a treatment for acrophobia has been critically examined by Rothbaum and associates [1995a,b]. They used a procedure in which phobic patients were immersed in virtual environments that could be altered to present graded fear-inducing situations. Patient responses were monitored and used to modify the virtual threats accordingly. Rothbaum et al. report that the ability to present graded exposure to aversive environments through the use of VR technology provides a very effective means of overcoming acrophobia. Transfer to the real world was quite good.

The use of VR technology in the treatment of phobias has expanded in recent years to include fear of flying [Rothbaum et al., 1996; North et al., 1997], arachnophobia [Carlin et al., 1997], and sexual dysfunction [Optale et al., 1998]. In each of these areas, patients attained a significant reduction in their phobias through graded exposure to fear-provoking virtual environments. In the treatment of arachnophobia, Carlin and associates devised a clever synthesis of real and virtual environments to desensitize patients to spiders. Patients viewed virtual spiders while at the same time touching the simulated fuzziness of a spider. The tactile aspect of the exposure was produced by having the patient touch a toupé.

Before leaving the subject of VR treatment of phobias, a word of caution is necessary. Bloom [1997] has examined the application of VR technology to the treatment of psychiatric disorders and sounds a note of warning. Bloom notes the advances made in the treatment of anxiety disorders, but also points out that there are examples of physiological and psychological side effects from immersion in VR. While the major side effects tend to be physiological, mainly simulator sickness and Sopite Syndrome (malaise, lethargy), psychological maladaptations, such as ". . . unpredictable modifications in perceptions of social context . . ." and ". . . fragmentation of self" [Bloom, 1997] reportedly occur.

18.5   Summary

VR tools and techniques are being developed rapidly in the scientific, engineering, and medical areas. This technology will directly affect medical practice. Computer simulation will allow physicians to practice surgical procedures in a virtual environment in which there is no risk to patients, and where mistakes can be recognized and rectified immediately by the computer. Procedures can be reviewed from new, insightful perspectives that are not possible in the real world.

The innovators in medical VR will be called upon to refine technical efficiency and increase physical and psychological comfort and capability, while keeping an eye on reducing costs for health care. The mandate is complex, but like VR technology itself, the possibilities are very exciting. While the possibilities — and the need — for medical VR are immense, approaches and solutions using new VR-based applications require diligent, cooperative efforts among technology developers, medical practitioners, and medical consumers to establish where future requirements and demand will lie.

Defining Terms

For an excellent treatment of the state-of-the-art of VR and its taxonomy, see the ACM SIGGRAPH publication "Computer Graphics," Vol. 26, #3, August 1992. It covers the U.S. Government's National Science Foundation invitational workshop on Interactive Systems Program, March 23 to 24, 1992, which served to identify and recommend future research directions in the area of virtual environments. A more in-depth exposition of VR taxonomy can be found in the MIT Journal "Presence," Vol. 1 #2.

References

Aslan, P., Lee, B., Kuo, R., Babayan, R.K., Kavoussi, L.R., Pavlin, K.A., and Preminger, G.M. (1998). Secured Medical Imaging Over the Internet. *Medicine Meets Virtual Reality: Art, Science, Technology: Healthcare (R)Evolution* (pp. 74–78). IOS Press, San Diego, CA.

Attree, E.A., Brooks, B.M., Rose, F.D., Andrews, T.K., Leadbetter, A.G., and Clifford, B.R. (1996). Memory Processes and Virtual Environments: I Can't Remember What Was There, But I Can Remember How I Got There. Implications for Persons with Disabilities. *Proceedings of the European Conference on Disability, Virtual Reality, and Associated Technology* (pp. 117–121).

Begault, D.R. and Wenzel, E.M. (1992). Techniques and Applications for Binaural Sound Manipulation in Human–Machine Interfaces. *International Journal of Aviation Psychology* 2, 1–22.

Bloom, R.W. (1997). Psychiatric Therapeutic Applications of Virtual Reality Technology (VRT): Research Prospectus and Phenomenological Critique. *Medicine Meets Virtual Reality: Global Healthcare Grid* (pp. 11–16). IOS Press, San Diego, CA.

Bolas, M.T. (1994). Human Factors in the Design of an Immersive Display. *IEEE Computer Graphics and Applications* 14, 55–59.

Buchwalter, J.G. and Rizzo, A.A. (1997). Virtual Reality and the Neuropsychological Assessment of Persons with Neurologically Based Cognitive Impairments. *Medicine Meets Virtual Reality: Global Healthcare Grid* (pp. 17–21). IOS Press, San Diego, CA.

Burdea, G., Zhuang, J., Roskos, E., Silver, D., and Langrana, N. (1992). A Portable Dextrous Master with Force Feedback. *Presence* 1, 18–28.

Burdea, G., Goratowski, R., and Langrana, N. (1995). Tactile Sensing Glove for Computerized Hand Diagnosis. *Journal of Medicine and Virtual Reality* 1, 40–44.

Burdea, G., Deshpande, S., Popescu, V., Langrana, N., Gomez, D., DiPaolo, D., and Kanter, M. (1997). Computerized Hand Diagnostic/Rehabilitation System Using a Force Feedback Glove. *Medicine Meets Virtual Reality: Global Healthcare Grid* (pp. 141–150). IOS Press, San Diego, CA.

Burrow, M. (1994). A Telemedicine Testbed for Developing and Evaluating Telerobotic Tools for Rural Health Care. *Medicine Meets Virtual Reality II: Interactive Technology & Healthcare: Visionary Applications for Simulation Visualization Robotics* (pp. 15–18). Aligned Management Associates, San Diego, CA.

Caldwell, G. and Gosney, C. (1993). Enhanced Tactile Feedback (Tele-Taction) Using a Multi-Functional Sensory System. *Proceedings of the IEEE International Conference on Robotics and Automation*, 955–960.

Carlin, A.S., Hoffman, H.G., and Weghorst, S. (1997). Virtual Reality and Tactile Augmentation in the Treatment of Spider Phobia: A Case Study. *Behavior Research and Therapy* 35, 153–158.

Durlach, N.I., Shinn-Cunningham, B.G., and Held, R.M. (1993). Supernormal Auditory Localization. I. General Background. *Presence: Teleoperators and Virtual Environments* 2, 89–103.

Edmond, C.V., Heskamp, D., Sluis, D., Stredney, D., Sessanna, D., Weit, G., Yagel, R., Weghorst, S., Openheimer, P., Miller, J., Levin, M., and Rosenberg, L. (1997). ENT Endoscopic Surgical Training Simulator. *Medicine Meets Virtual Reality: Global Healthcare Grid* (pp. 518–528). IOS Press, San Diego, CA.

Grabowski, H.A. (1998). Generating Finite Element Models from Volumetric Medical Images. *Medicine Meets Virtual Reality: Art, Science, Technology: Healthcare (R)Evolution* (pp. 355–356). IOS Press, San Diego, CA.

Greenleaf, W. (1992). DataGlove, DataSuit and Virtual Reality. *Virtual Reality and Persons with Disabilities: Proceedings of the 7th Annual Conference* (pp. 21–24). March 18–21, 1992. Los Angeles, CA. Northridge, CA. California State University. 1992. Available from: Office of Disabled Student Services, California State University, Northridge. 18111 Nordhoff Street — DVSS. Northridge, CA 91330.

Greenleaf, W.J. (1994). DataGlove and DataSuit: Virtual Reality Technology Applied to the Measurement of Human Movement. *Medicine Meets Virtual Reality II: Interactive Technology & Healthcare: Visionary*

Applications for Simulation Visualization Robotics (pp. 63–69). Aligned Management Associates, San Diego, CA.

Hendin, O., John, N.W., and Shochet, O. (1998). Medical Volume Rendering over the WWW Using VRML and JAVA. *Medicine Meets Virtual Reality: Art, Science, Technology: Healthcare (R)Evolution* (pp. 34–40). IOS Press, San Diego, CA.

Hendrix, C. and Barfield, W. (1996). The Sense of Presence Within Audio Virtual Environments. *Presence* 5, 295–301.

Hiemenz, L., Stredney, D., and Schmalbrock, P. (1998). Development of a Force-Feedback Model for an Epidural Needle Insertion Simulator: Surgical Simulation. *Medicine Meets Virtual Reality: Art, Science, Technology: Healthcare (R)Evolution* (pp. 272–277). IOS Press, San Diego, CA.

Hill, J.W., Jensen, J.F., Green, P.S., and Shah, A.S. (1995). Two-Handed Tele-Presence Surgery Demonstration System. *Proceedings of the ANS Sixth Annual Topical Meeting on Robotics and Remote Systems*, Vol. 2, (pp. 713–720), Monterey, CA.

Hill, J.W., Holst, P.A., Jensen, J.F., Goldman, J., Gorfu, Y., and Ploeger, D.W. (1998). Telepresence Interface with Applications to Microsurgery and Surgical Simulation. *Medicine Meets Virtual Reality: Art, Science, Technology: Healthcare (R)Evolution* (pp. 96–102). IOS Press, San Diego, CA.

Hoffman, H.M. (1994). Virtual Reality and the Medical Curriculum: Integrating Extant and Emerging Technologies. *Medicine Meets Virtual Reality II: Interactive Technology & Healthcare: Visionary Applications for Simulation Visualization Robotics* (pp. 73–76). Aligned Management Associates, San Diego, CA.

Hoffman, H.M., Irwin, A.E., Ligon, R., Murray, M., and Tohsaku, C. (1995). Virtual Reality–Multimedia Synthesis: Next Generation Learning Environments for Medical Education. *Journal of Biocommunications* 22, 2–7.

Hoffman, H.M., Murray, M., Danks, M., Prayaga, R., Irwin, A., and Vu, D. (1997). A Flexible and Extensible Object-Oriented 3D Architecture: Application in the Development of Virtual Anatomy Lessons. *Medicine Meets Virtual Reality: Global Healthcare Grid* (pp. 461–466). IOS Press, San Diego, CA.

Holler, E. and Breitwieser, H. (1994). Telepresence Systems for Application in Minimally Invasive Surgery. *Medicine Meets Virtual Reality II: Interactive Technology & Healthcare: Visionary Applications for Simulation Visualization Robotics* (pp. 77–80). Aligned Management Associates, San Diego, CA.

Hon, D. (1994). Ixion's Laparoscopic Surgical Skills Simulator. *Medicine Meets Virtual Reality II: Interactive Technology & Healthcare: Visionary Applications for Simulation Visualization Robotics* (pp. 81–83). Aligned Management Associates, San Diego, CA.

Inman, D.P. (1994a). Use of Virtual Reality to Teach Students with Orthopedic Impairments to Drive Motorized Wheelchairs. Paper presented at the Fourth Annual Fall Conference of the Oregon Department of Education, Office of Special Education, Portland, Oregon.

Inman, D.P. (1994b). Virtual Reality Wheelchair Drivers' Training for Children with Cerebral Palsy. Paper presented to the New York Virtual Reality Expo '94, New York, NY.

Inman, D.P. (1996). Use of Virtual Reality and Computerization in Wheelchair Training. Paper presented to Shriner's Hospital for Crippled Children, Portland, OR.

Ino, S., Shimizu, S., Odagawa, T., Sato, M., Takahashi, M., Izumi, T., and Ifukube, T. (1993). A Tactile Display for Presenting Quality of Materials by Changing the Temperature of Skin Surface. *Proceedings of the Second IEEE International Workshop on Robot and Human Communication* (pp. 220–224).

Jacobs, L. (1994). *Garage Virtual Reality*. Sams Publications, Indianapolis, IN.

Johnson, A.D. (1994). Tactile Feedback Enhancement to Laparoscopic Tools. [abstract]. In *Medicine Meets Virtual Reality II: Interactive Technology & Healthcare: Visionary Applications for Simulation Visualization Robotics* (p. 92). Aligned Management Associates, San Diego, CA.

Kall, B.A., Kelly, P.J., Stiving, S.O., and Goerss, S.J. (1994). Integrated Multimodality Visualization in Stereotactic Neurologic Surgery. *Medicine Meets Virtual Reality II: Interactive Technology & Healthcare: Visionary Applications for Simulation Visualization Robotics* (pp. 93–94). Aligned Management Associates, San Diego, CA.

Kaplan, K.L. (1994). Project Description: Surgical Room of the Future. *Medicine Meets Virtual Reality II: Interactive Technology & Healthcare: Visionary Applications for Simulation Visualization Robotics* (pp. 95–98). Aligned Management Associates, San Diego, CA.

Kelly, P.J. (1994). Quantitative Virtual Reality Surgical Simulation, Minimally Invasive Stereotactic Neurosurgery and Frameless Stereotactic Technologies. *Medicine Meets Virtual Reality II: Interactive Technology & Healthcare: Visionary Applications for Simulation Visualization Robotics* (pp. 103–108). Aligned Management Associates, San Diego, CA.

Kizakevich, P.N., McCartney, M.L., Nissman, D.B., Starko, K., and Smith, N.T. (1998). Virtual Medical Trainer. *Medicine Meets Virtual Reality: Art, Science, Technology: Healthcare (R)Evolution* (pp. 309–315). IOS Press, San Diego, CA.

Kreuger, M. (1994). Olfactory Stimuli in Medical Virtual Reality Applications. *Proceedings: Virtual Reality in Medicine — The Cutting Edge* (pp. 32–33). Sig-Advanced Applications, Inc., New York.

Kreuger, M. (1995a). Olfactory Stimuli in Virtual Reality for Medical Applications. *Interactive Technology and the New Paradigm for Healthcare* (pp. 180–181). IOS Press, Washington, D.C.

Kreuger, M. (1995b). Olfactory Stimuli in Virtual Reality Medical Training. *Proceedings: Virtual Reality in Medicine and Developers' Expo.*

Kuhnapfel, U.G. (1994). Realtime Graphical Computer Simulation for Endoscopic Surgery. *Medicine Meets Virtual Reality II: Interactive Technology & Healthcare: Visionary Applications for Simulation Visualization Robotics* (pp. 114–116). Aligned Management Associates, San Diego, CA.

Lamson, R. (1994) Virtual Therapy of Anxiety Disorders. *CyberEdge Journal* 4, 1–28.

Lamson, R. (1995). Clinical Application of Virtual Therapy to Psychiatric Disorders. *Medicine Meets Virtual Reality III.* IOS Press, San Diego, CA.

Lamson, R. (1997). *Virtual Therapy.* Polytechnic International Press, Montreal.

Lamson, R. and Meisner, M. (1994). The Effects of Virtual Reality Immersion in the Treatment of Anxiety, Panic, & Phobia of Heights. *Virtual Reality and Persons with Disabilities: Proceedings of the 2nd Annual International Conference;* 1994 June 8–10. San Francisco, CA. Sponsored by the Center on Disabilities, California State University, Northridge. 18111 Nordhoff Street — DVSS. Northridge, CA.

Lathan, C., Cleary, K., and Greco, R. (1998). Development and Evaluation of a Spine Biopsy Simulator. Surgical Simulation. *Medicine Meets Virtual Reality: Art, Science, Technology: Healthcare (R)Evolution* (pp. 375–376). IOS Press, San Diego, CA.

Loftin, R.B., Ota, D., Saito, T., and Voss, M. (1994). A Virtual Environment for Laparoscopic Surgical Training. *Medicine Meets Virtual Reality II: Interactive Technology & Healthcare: Visionary Applications for Simulation Visualization Robotics* (pp. 121–123). Aligned Management Associates, San Diego, CA.

Marsh, A. (1998). Special Double Issue: The Telemedical Information Society. *Future Generation Computer Systems,* Vol. 14. Elsevier, Amsterdam.

Max, M.L. and Burke, J.C. (1997). Virtual Reality for Autism Communication and Education, with Lessons for Medical Training Simulators. *Medicine Meets Virtual Reality: Global Healthcare Grid* (pp. 46–53). IOS Press, San Diego, CA.

Max, M.L. and Gonzalez, J.R. (1997). Blind Persons Navigating in Virtual Reality (VR): Hearing and Feeling Communicates "Reality." *Medicine Meets Virtual Reality: Global Healthcare Grid* (pp. 54–59). IOS Press, San Diego, CA.

McGovern, K.T. and McGovern, L.T. (1994). Virtual Clinic: A Virtual Reality Surgical Simulator. *Virtual Reality World* 2, 41–44.

McInerney, T. and Terzopoulos, D. (1996). Deformable Models in Medical Image Analysis. *Medical Image Analysis* 1, 91–108.

Merril, J.R. (1993). Surgery on the Cutting Edge. *Virtual Reality World* 1, 34–38.

Merril, J.R. (1994). Presentation Material: Medicine Meets Virtual Reality II. [abstract] *Medicine Meets Virtual Reality II: Interactive Technology & Healthcare: Visionary Applications for Simulation Visualization Robotics* (pp. 158–159). Aligned Management Associates, San Diego, CA.

Minsky, M. and Lederman, S.J. (1996). Simulated Haptic Textures: Roughness. Symposium on Haptic Interfaces for Virtual Environment and Teleoperator Systems. ASME International Mechanical Engineering Congress and Exposition. *Proceedings of the ASME Dynamic Systems and Control Division*, DSC-Vol. 58 (pp. 451–458).

North, M.M., North, S.M., and Coble, J.R. (1997). Virtual Reality Therapy for Fear of Flying. *American Journal of Psychiatry* 154, 130.

Optale, G., Munari, A., Nasta, A., Pianon, C., Verde, J.B., and Viggiano, G. (1998).Virtual Reality Techniques in the Treatment of Impotence and Premature Ejaculation. *Medicine Meets Virtual Reality: Art, Science, Technology: Healthcare (R)Evolution* (pp. 186–192). IOS Press, San Diego, CA.

Oyama, H., Wakao, F., and Takahira, Y. (1998). The Clinical Advantages of Editable Real-Time Volume Rendering in a Medical Virtual Environment: VolMed. *Medicine Meets Virtual Reality: Art, Science, Technology: Healthcare (R)Evolution* (pp. 341–345). IOS Press, San Diego, CA.

Parsons, J. and Rolland, J.P. (1998). A Non-Intrusive Display Technique for Providing Real-Time Data within a Surgeon's Critical Area of Interest. *Medicine Meets Virtual Reality: Art, Science, Technology: Healthcare (R)Evolution* (pp. 246–251). IOS Press, San Diego, CA.

Peifer, J. (1994). Virtual Environment for Eye Surgery Simulation. *Medicine Meets Virtual Reality II: Interactive Technology & Healthcare: Visionary Applications for Simulation Visualization Robotics* (pp. 166–173). Aligned Management Associates, San Diego, CA.

Preminger, G.M. (1994). Advanced Imaging Technologies for Endoscopic Surgery. *Medicine Meets Virtual Reality II: Interactive Technology & Healthcare: Visionary Applications for Simulation Visualization Robotics* (pp. 177–178). Aligned Management Associates, San Diego, CA.

Pugnetti, L. (1994). Recovery Diagnostics and Monitoring in Virtual Environments. Virtual Reality in Rehabilitation, Research, Experience and Perspectives. *Proceedings of the 1st International Congress on Virtual Reality in Rehabilitation.* 1994 June 13–18. Gubbio, Italy.

Pugnetti, L., Mendozzi, L., Motta, A., Cattaneo, A., Barbieri, E., and Brancotti, S. (1995a). Evaluation and Retraining of Adults' Cognitive Impairments: Which Role for Virtual Reality Technology? *Computers in Biology and Medicine* 25, 213–227.

Pugnetti, L., Mendozzi, L., Motta, A., Cattaneo, A., Barbieri, E., Brancotti, S., and Cazzullo, C.L. (1995b). Immersive Virtual Reality to Assist Retraining of Acquired Cognitive Deficits: First Results with a Dedicated System. *Interactive Technology and the New Paradigm for Healthcare.* (pp. 455–456). IOS Press, Washington, D.C.

Pugnetti, L., Mendozzi, L., Barbieri, E., Rose, F.D., and Attree, E.A. (1996). Nervous System Correlates of Virtual Reality Experience. *Proceedings of the European Conference on Disability, Virtual Reality and Associated Technology* (pp. 239–246).

Rabinowitz, W.M., Maxwell, J., Shao, Y., and Wei, M. (1993). Sound Localization Cues for a Magnified Head: Implications from Sound Diffraction about a Rigid Sphere. *Presence: Teleoperators and Virtual Environments* 2, 125–129.

Radesovich, L. (1997). Hackers Prove 56-bit DES is Not Enough. *InfoWorld* 18, 27.

Rissam, H.S., Kishore, S., Bhatia, M.L., and Trehan, N. (1998). Trans-Telephonic Electro-Cardiographic Monitoring (TTEM) — First Indian Experience. *Medicine Meets Virtual Reality: Art, Science, Technology: Healthcare (R)Evolution* (pp. 361–363). IOS Press, San Diego, CA.

Rizzo, A.A. and Buckwalter, J.G. (1997). The Status of Virtual Reality for the Cognitive Rehabilitation of Persons with Neurological Disorders and Acquired Brain Injury. *Medicine Meets Virtual Reality: Global Healthcare Grid* (pp. 22–33). IOS Press, San Diego, CA.

Rosen, J. (1994). The Role of Telemedicine and Telepresence in Reducing Health Care Costs. *Medicine Meets Virtual Reality II: Interactive Technology & Healthcare: Visionary Applications for Simulation Visualization Robotics* (pp. 187–194). Aligned Management Associates, San Diego, CA.

Rothbaum, B.O., Hodges, L.F., Kooper, I.R., Opdyke, D., Williford, J.S., and North, M. (1995a). Virtual Reality Graded Exposure in the Treatment of Acrophobia: A Case Report. *Behavior Therapy* 26, 547–554.

Rothbaum, B.O., Hodges, L.F., Kooper, I.R., Opdyke, D., Williford, J.S., and North, M. (1995b). Effectiveness of Computer Generated Graded Exposure in the Treatment of Achrophobia. *American Journal of Psychiatry* 152, 626–628.

Rothbaum, B.O., Hodges, B.F., Watson, B.A., Kessler, G.D., and Opdyke, D. (1996). Virtual Reality Exposure Therapy in the Treatment of Fear of Flying: A Case Report. *Behavior Research and Therapy* 34, 477–481.

Rovetta, A., Falcone, F., Sala, R., and Garavaldi, M.E. (1997). Telehealth in Africa. *Medicine Meets Virtual Reality: Global Healthcare Grid* (pp. 277–285). IOS Press, San Diego, CA.

Rovetta, A., Sala, R., Bressanelli, M., Garavaldi, M.E., Lorini, F., Pegoraro, R., and Canina, M. (1998). Demonstration of Surgical Telerobotics and Virtual Telepresence by Internet + ISDN From Monterey (USA) to Milan (Italy). *Medicine Meets Virtual Reality: Art, Science, Technology: Healthcare (R)Evolution* (pp. 79–83). IOS Press, San Diego, CA.

Salisbury, J.K. and Srinivasan, M. (1996). *Proceedings of the First PHANToM User's Group Workshop*. MIT Press, Cambridge, MA.

Salisbury, J.K. and Srinivasan, M. (1997). *Proceedings of the Second PHANToM User's Group Workshop*. MIT Press, Cambridge, MA.

Satava, R.M. (1992). Robotics, Telepresence and Virtual Reality: A Critical Analysis of the Future of Surgery. *Minimally Invasive Therapy* 1, 357–363.

Schraft, R.D., Neugebauer, J.G., and Wapler, M. (1994). Virtual Reality for Improved Control in Endoscopic Surgery. *Medicine Meets Virtual Reality II: Interactive Technology & Healthcare: Visionary Applications for Simulation Visualization Robotics* (pp. 233–236). Aligned Management Associates, San Diego, CA.

Senger, S. (1998). An Immersive Environment for the Direct Visualization and Segmentation of Volumetric Data Sets. *Medicine Meets Virtual Reality: Art, Science, Technology: Healthcare (R)Evolution* (pp. 7–12). IOS Press, San Diego, CA.

Shimoga, K.B., Khosla, P.K., and Sclabassi, R.J. (1994). Teleneurosurgery: An Approach to Enhance the Dexterity of Neurosurgeons. *Medicine Meets Virtual Reality II: Interactive Technology & Healthcare: Visionary Applications for Simulation Visualization Robotics* (p. 203). Aligned Management Associates, San Diego, CA.

Stallkamp, J. and Walper, M. (1998). UltraTrainer — A Training System for Medical Ultrasound Examination. *Medicine Meets Virtual Reality: Art, Science, Technology: Healthcare (R)Evolution* (pp. 298–301). IOS Press, San Diego, CA.

Steffin, M. (1997). Computer Assisted Therapy for Multiple Sclerosis and Spinal Cord Injury Patients: Application of Virtual Reality. *Medicine Meets Virtual Reality: Global Healthcare Grid* (pp. 64–72). IOS Press, San Diego, CA.

Strickland, D.C. (1995). *Virtual Reality Training for Autism*. North Carolina State University, College of Engineering Updates, May 1995.

Strickland, D.C. (1996). Virtual Reality Helps Children with Autism. *Presence* 5, 319–329.

Suzuki, N., Ito, M., and Okamura, T. (1987). Morphological Reference System of Human Structure Using Computer Graphics. *World Congress on Medical Physics and Biomedical Engineering*, San Antonio, TX.

Suzuki, N., Takatsu, A., Hattori, A., Ezumi, T., Oda, S., Yanai, T., and Tominaga, H. (1998). 3D and 4D Atlas System of Living Human Body Structure. *Medicine Meets Virtual Reality: Art, Science, Technology: Healthcare (R)Evolution* (pp. 131–136). IOS Press, San Diego, CA.

Szabo, Z., Hunter, J.G., Berci, G. et al. (1994). Choreographed Instrument Movements During Laparoscopic Surgery: Needle Driving, Knot Tying and Anastomosis Techniques. *Medicine Meets Virtual Reality II: Interactive Technology & Healthcare: Visionary Applications for Simulation Visualization Robotics* (pp. 216–217). Aligned Management Associates, San Diego, CA.

Tendick, F., Jennings, R.W., Tharp, G., and Stark, L. (1993). Sensing and Manipulation Problems in Endoscopic Surgery: Experiment, Analysis, and Observation. *Presence: Teleoperators and Virtual Environments* 2, 66–81.

Trimble, J., Morris, T., and Crandall, R. (1992). Virtual Reality. *TeamRehab Report* 3, 33–37.

Wang, Y. and Sackier, J. (1994). Robotically Enhanced Surgery. *Medicine Meets Virtual Reality II: Interactive Technology & Healthcare: Visionary Applications for Simulation Visualization Robotics* (pp. 218–220). Aligned Management Associates, San Diego, CA.

Weghorst, S., Airola, C., Openheimer, P., Edmond, C.V., Patience, T., Heskamp, D., and Miller, J. (1998). Validation of the Madigan ESS Simulator. *Medicine Meets Virtual Reality: Art, Science, Technology: Healthcare (R)Evolution* (pp. 399–405). IOS Press, San Diego, CA.

Weghorst, S., Prothero, J., and Furness, T. (1994). Virtual Images in the Treatment of Parkinson's Disease Akinesia. *Medicine Meets Virtual Reality II: Interactive Technology & Healthcare: Visionary Applications for Simulation Visualization Robotics* (pp. 242–243). Aligned Management Associates, San Diego, CA.

Wenger, K. and Karron, D.B. (1998). Audio-Guided Blind Biopsy Needle Placement. *Medicine Meets Virtual Reality: Art, Science, Technology: Healthcare (R)Evolution* (pp. 90–95). IOS Press, San Diego, CA.

Wenzel, E.M. (1992) Localization in Virtual Acoustic Displays. *Presence* 1, 80–107.

Wenzel. E.M. (1994). Spatial Sound and Sonification. In G. Kramer (Ed.) *Auditory Display: Sonification, Audification, and Auditory Interfaces* (pp. 127–150). Addison-Wesley, Reading, MA.

Further Information

Burdea, G. and Coiffet, P. *Virtual Reality Technology*. John Wiley & Sons, New York.

HITL (Human Interface Technology Laboratory), University of Washington, FJ-15, Seattle, WA 98195.

UNC Laboratory, University of North Carolina, Chapel Hill, Computer Science Department, Chapel Hill, NC 27599-3175.

Presence: Teleoperators & Virtual Environments. Professional Tech Papers and Journal, MIT Press Journals, 55 Hayward St, Cambridge MA 02142.

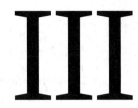

Infrared Imaging

Nicholas A. Diakides
Advanced Concepts Analysis, Inc.

19 Advances in Medical Infrared Imaging
Nicholas Diakides, Mary Diakides, Jasper Lupo, Jeffrey L. Paul, Raymond Balcerak . . **19**-1

20 The Historical Development of Thermometry and Thermal Imaging in Medicine
E. Francis Ring, Bryan F. Jones **20**-1

21 Physiology of Thermal Signals
David D. Pascoe, James B. Mercer, Lois de Weerd **21**-1

22 Quantitative Active Dynamic Thermal IR-Imaging and Thermal Tomography in Medical Diagnostics
Antoni Nowakowski **22**-1

23 Thermal Texture Maps (TTM): Concept, Theory, and Applications
Zhongqi Liu, Chen Wang, Hairong Qi, Yune Yuan, Yi Zeng, Z.R. Li,
Yulin Zhou, Wen Yu, Wang Wei **23**-1

24 IR Imagers as Fever Monitoring Devices: Physics, Physiology, and Clinical Accuracy
E.Y.K. Ng, G.J.L. Kaw **24**-1

25 Infrared Imaging of the Breast — An Overview
William C. Amalu, William B. Hobbins, Jonathan F. Head, Robert L. Elliot **25**-1

26 Functional Infrared Imaging of the Breast: Historical Perspectives, Current Application, and Future Considerations
J.R. Keyserlingk, P.D. Ahlgren, E. Yu, N. Belliveau, M. Yassa **26-1**

27 Detecting Breast Cancer from Thermal Infrared Images by Asymmetry Analysis
Hairong Qi, Phani Teja Kuruganti, Wesley E. Snyder **27-1**

28 Advanced Thermal Image Processing
B. Wiecek, M. Strzelecki, T. Jakubowska, M. Wysocki, C. Drews-Peszynski **28-1**

29 Biometrics: Face Recognition in Thermal Infrared
I. Pavlidis, P. Tsiamyrtzis, P. Buddharaju, C. Manohar **29-1**

30 Infrared Imaging for Tissue Characterization and Function
Moinuddin Hassan, Victor Chernomordik, Abby Vogel, David Hattery, Israel Gannot, Richard F. Little, Robert Yarchoan, Amir H. Gandjbakhche **30-1**

31 Thermal Imaging in Diseases of the Skeletal and Neuromuscular Systems
E. Francis Ring, Kurt Ammer **31-1**

32 Functional Infrared Imaging in Clinical Applications
Arcangelo Merla, Gian Luca Romani **32-1**

33 Thermal Imaging in Surgery
Paul Campbell, Roderick Thomas **33-1**

34 Infrared Imaging Applied to Dentistry
Barton M. Gratt **34-1**

35 Use of Infrared Imaging in Veterinary Medicine
Ram C. Purohit, Tracy A. Turner, David D. Pascoe **35-1**

36 Standard Procedures for Infrared Imaging in Medicine
Kurt Ammer, E. Francis Ring **36-1**

37 Infrared Detectors and Detector Arrays
Paul Norton, Stuart Horn, Joseph G. Pellegrino, Philip Perconti **37-1**

38 Infrared Camera Characterization
Joseph G. Pellegrino, Jason Zeibel, Ronald G. Driggers, Philip Perconti **38-1**

39 Infrared Camera and Optics for Medical Applications
Michael W. Grenn, Jay Vizgaitis, Joseph G. Pellegrino, Philip Perconti **39-1**

THE EVOLUTION OF TECHNOLOGICAL ADVANCES in infrared sensor technology, image processing, "smart" algorithms, knowledge-based databases and their overall system integration has resulted in new methods of research and use in medical infrared imaging. The development of infrared cameras with focal plane arrays not requiring cooling added a new dimension to this modality. New detector materials with improved thermal sensitivity are now available and production of high-density focal plane arrays (640×480) have been achieved. Advance read-out circuitry using on-chip signal processing is in common use. These breakthroughs permit low-cost and easy-to-use camera systems with thermal sensitivity less than 50 milli-kelvin degrees, as well as spatial resolution of 25 to 50 μm, given the appropriate optics. Another important factor is the emerging interest in the development of smart image processing algorithms to enhance the interpretation of thermal signatures. In the clinical area, new research addresses the key issues of diagnostic sensitivity and specificity of infrared imaging. Efforts are underway to achieve quantitative clinical data interpretation in standardized diagnostic procedures. For this purpose, clinical protocols are emphasized.

New concepts such as dynamic thermal imaging and thermal texture mapping (thermal tomography) and thermal multi-spectral imaging are being implemented in clinical environments. Other areas like three-dimensional infrared are being investigated.

Some of these new ideas, concepts, and technologies are covered in this section. We have assembled a set of chapters which range in content from historical background, concepts, clinical applications, standards, and infrared technology.

Chapter 19 deals with worldwide advances in and a guide to thermal imaging systems for medical applications. Chapter 20 presents an historical perspective and the evolution of thermal imaging. Chapter 21 deals with the physiological basis of the thermal signature and its interpretation in a medical setting. Chapters 22 and 23 cover innovative concepts such as dynamic thermal imaging and thermal tomography which enhance the clinical utility leading to improved diagnostic capability. Chapters 24 discusses the physics of thermal radiation theory and the pathophysiology as related to infrared imaging. Chapters 25 and 26 expose the fundamentals of infrared breast imaging, equipment considerations, early detection and the use of infrared imaging in a multi-modality setting. Chapters 27 and 28 are on innovative image processing techniques for the early detection of breast cancer. Chapter 29 presents biometrics, a novel method for facial recognition. Today, this technology is of utmost importance in the area of homeland security and other applications. Chapter 30 deals with infrared monitoring of therapies multi-spectral optical imaging in Kaposi's Sarcoma investigations at NIH. Chapters 31 to 34 deal with the use of infrared in various clinical applications: surgery, dental, skeletal and neuromuscular diseases, as well as the quantification of the TAU image technique in the relevance and stage of a disease. Chapter 35 is on infrared imaging in veterinary medicine. Chapter 36 discusses the complexities and importance of standardization, calibration and protocols for effective and reproducible results. Chapters 37 to 39 are comprehensive chapters on technology and hardware including detectors, detector materials, uncooled focal plane arrays, high performance systems, camera characterization, electronics for on-chip image processing, optics and cost reduction designs.

This section will be of interest to both the medical and biomedical engineering communities. It could provide many opportunities for developing and conducting multi-disciplinary research in many areas of medical infrared imaging. These range from clinical quantification, to intelligent image processing for enhancement of the interpretation of images, and for further development of user-friendly high resolution thermal cameras. These would enable the wide use of infrared imaging as a viable, non-invasive, low cost first-line detection modality.

Acknowledgments

I would like to acknowledge each and every author in this section for their excellent contributions. I am aware of their busy schedules and I appreciate the time they dedicated to the first Infrared Imaging Section to be contained in a *CRC Biomedical Engineering Handbook*.

19

Advances in Medical Infrared Imaging

19.1 Introduction.. **19**-1
19.2 Worldwide Use of Infrared Imaging in Medicine...... **19**-3
   United States of America and Canada • China • Japan •
   Korea • United Kingdom • Germany • Austria • Poland
   • Italy
19.3 Infrared Imaging in Breast Cancer...................... **19**-5
   The Image Processing and Medical Applications • Website
   and Database • Sensor Technology for Medical Applications
19.4 Guide to Thermal Imaging Systems for Medical
   Applications **19**-8
   Introduction • Background • Applications and Image
   Formats • Dynamic Range • Resolution and Sensitivity •
   Calibration • Single Band Imagers • Emerging and Future
   Camera Technology • Summary Specifications
19.5 Summary, Conclusions, and Recommendations **19**-12
References **19**-13

Nicholas Diakides
Mary Diakides
Advanced Concepts Analysis, Inc.

Jasper Lupo
Applied Research Associates, Inc.

Jeffrey L. Paul
Raymond Balcerak
*Defense Advanced Research
Projects Agency*

19.1 Introduction

Infrared (IR) imaging in medicine has been used in the past but without the advantage of 21st century technology. In 1994, under the Department of Defense (DOD) grants jointly funded by the Office of the Secretary of Defense (OSD-S&T), the Defense Advanced Research Projeects Agency (DARPA) and the Army Research Office (ARO), a concerted effort was initiated to re-visit this subject. Specifically, it was to explore the potential of integrating advanced IR technology with "smart" image processing for use in medicine. The major challenges for acceptance of this modality by the medical community were investigated. It was found that the following issues were of prime importance (1) standardization and quantification of clinical data; (2) better understanding of the pathophysiological nature of thermal signatures; (3) wider publication and exposure of medical IR imaging in conferences and leading journals; (4) characterization of thermal signatures through an interactive web-based database; and (5) training in both image acquisition and interpretation.

In the last ten years, significant progress has been made internationally by advancing a thrust for new initiatives worldwide for clinical quantification, international collaboration, and providing a forum for coordination, discussion, and publication through the following activities (1) medical infrared imaging symposia, workshops, and tracks at IEEE/Engineering in Medicine and Biology Society (EMBS) conferences from 1994 to 2004; (2) three Engineering in Medicine and Biology Magazines (EMBS), Special Issues dedicated to this topic [1–3]; (3) The DOD "From Tanks to Tumors" Workshop [4]. The products of these efforts are documented in final government technical reports [5–8] and IEEE/EMBS Conference Proceedings (1994 to 2004).

Early infrared cameras used a small number of detector elements (1 to 180 individual detectors) which required cryogenic cooling in order to operate effectively without noise. The camera design incorporated a scanning mechanism with mirrors to form the image. Electrical contact was made to each individual detector — a very laborious and time intensive task. The signal leads were brought out of the cryogenic envelope and each individual signal was combined. The processing was performed outside of the focal plane array. This type of camera was heavy in weight, high in power consumption, and very expensive to manufacture. Hence, the technology focused on producing a more efficient, lower-cost system which ultimately led to the un-cooled focal plane array (FPA) type cameras. In the focal plane array camera, the detectors are fabricated in large arrays which eliminates the need for scanning. Electrical contact is made simultaneously to the detector array thus reducing significantly the number of leads through vacuum. Furthermore, the uncooled focal plane array has the potential to accommodate on-chip processing, thus leading to faster operation and fewer leads.

Presently, infrared imaging is used in many different medical applications. The most prominent of these are oncology (breast, skin, etc.), vascular disorders (diabetes DVT, etc.), pain, surgery, tissue viability, monitoring the efficacy of drugs and therapies; respiratory (recently introduced for testing of SARS).

There are various methods used to acquire infrared images: Static, Dynamic, Passive, and Active — Dynamic Area Telethermometry (DAT), subtraction, etc. [9], Thermal Texture Mapping (TTM),

TABLE 19.1 Medical applications and methods

Applications	IR Imaging Methods
Oncology (breast, skin, etc)	Static (classical)
Pain (management/control)	Dynamic (DAT, subtraction, etc.)
Vascular Disorders (diabetes, DVT)	Dynamic (Active)
Arthritis / Rheumatism	Thermal Texture Mapping (TTM)
Neurology	Multispectral/Hyperspectral
Surgery (open heart, transplant, etc.)	Multi-modality
Ophthalmic (cataract removal)	Sensor Fusion
Tissue Viability (burns, etc.)	
Dermatological Disorders	
Monitoring Efficacy of drugs and therapies	
Thyroid	
Dentistry	
Respiratory (allergies, SARS)	
Sports and Rehabilitation Medicine	

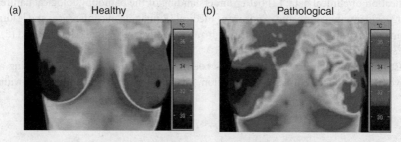

FIGURE 19.1 An application of infrared technique for breast screening. (a) Healthy; (b) Pathological breast.

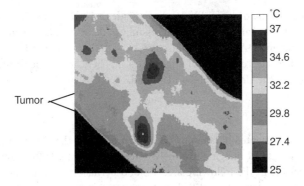

FIGURE 19.2 An application of infrared technique for cancer research.

Multispectral/Hyperspectral, Multi-modality, and Sensor Fusion. A list of current applications and infrared imaging methods are listed in Table 19.1. Figure 19.1 and Figure 19.2 illustrate thermal signatures of breast screening and Kaposi Sarcoma.

19.2 Worldwide Use of Infrared Imaging in Medicine

19.2.1 United States of America and Canada

Infrared imaging is beginning to be reconsidered in the Unites States, largely due to new infrared technology, advanced image processing, powerful, high speed computers, and exposure of existing research. This is evidenced by the increased number of publications available in open literature and national databases such as "Index Medicus" and "Medline" (National Library of Medicine) on this modality. Currently, there are several academic institutions with research initiatives in infrared imaging. Some of the most prominent are the following: NIH, Johns Hopkins University, University of Houston, University of Texas. NIH has several ongoing programs: vascular disorders (diabetes, Deep Venous Thrombosis), monitoring angiogenesis activity — Kaposi Sarcoma, pain-reflex sympathetic dystrophy, monitoring the efficacy of radiation therapy, organ transplant — perfusion, multi-spectral imaging.

Johns Hopkins University does research in microcirculation, monitoring angiogenic activity in Kaposi Sarcoma and breast screening, laparoscopic IR images — renal disease.

The University of Houston just created an infrared imaging laboratory to investigate with IR the facial thermal characteristics for such applications as lie detection and other behavioral issues (fatigue, anxiety, and fear, etc.).

There are two medical centers specializing in breast cancer research and treatment which use infrared routinely as part of their first line detection system, which also includes mammography and clinical exam. These are: Elliott-Elliott-Head Breast Cancer and Treatment Center, Baton Rouge, LA. And Ville Marie Oncology Research Center, Montreal, Canada. Their centers are fully equipped with all state-of-the-art imaging equipment. These centers are members of the coalition team for the development of a "knowledge-based" database of thermal signatures of the breast with "ground-truth" validation.

19.2.2 China

China has a long-standing interest in infrared imaging. More recently, the novel method Thermal Texture Mapping (TTM) has added increased specificity to static imaging. It is known that this method is widely used in this country, but unfortunately there is no formal literature about this important work. This is urgently needed in order for TTM to be exposed and accepted as a viable, effective method by the international community. The clinical results obtained through this method should be published in open literature of medical journals and international conference proceedings. Despite the lack of the availability of this documentation, introduction of TTM has been made to The National Institutes of Health (NIH). They are now using this method and its camera successfully in detection and treatment in Kaposi Sarcoma (associated with AIDS patients). After further discussions with them, interest has also been shown for its use in the area of breast cancer (detection of angiogenesis). There are further possibilities for high level research for this method in the United States and abroad.

19.2.3 Japan

Infrared imaging is widely accepted in Japan by the government and the medical community. More than 1500 hospitals and clinics use IR imaging routinely. The government sets the standards and reimburses clinical tests. Their focus is in the following areas: blood perfusion, breast cancer, dermatology, pain, neurology, surgery (open-heart, orthopedic, dental, cosmetic), sport medicine, and oriental medicine. The main research is performed at the following universities: University of Tokyo — organ transplant; Tokyo Medical and Dental University (skin temperature characterization and thermal properties); Toho University (neurological operation); Cancer Institute hospital (breast cancer). In addition, around forty other medical institutions are using infrared for breast cancer screening.

19.2.4 Korea

Began involvement in IR imaging during the early 1990s. More than 450 systems being used in hospitals and medical centers. Primary clinical applications are neurology, back pain/treatment, surgery, and oriental medicine. Yonsei College of Medicine is one of the leading institutions in medical IR imaging research along with three others.

19.2.5 United Kingdom

The University of Glamorgan is the center of IR imaging; the School of Computing has a thermal physiology laboratory which focuses in the following areas: medical infrared research, standardization, training (university diploma), "SPORTI" Project funded by the European Union Organization. The objective of this effort is to develop a reference database of normal, thermal signatures from healthy subjects.

The Royal National Hospital of Rheumatic Diseases specializes in rheumatic disorders, occupational health (Raynaud's Disease, Carpal Tunnel Syndrome, and Sports Medicine).

The Royal Free University College Medical School Hospital specializes in vascular disorders (diabetes, DVT, etc.), optimization of IR imaging techniques, and Raynaud's Phenomenon).

19.2.6 Germany

University of Leipzig uses infrared for open-heart surgery, perfusion and micro-circulation. There are several private clinics and other hospitals that use infrared imaging in various applications.

EvoBus-Daimler Chrysler uses infrared imaging for screening all their employees for wellness/health assessment (occupational health).

InfraMedic, AG, conducts breast cancer screening of women from 20 to 85 years old for the government under a two year grant. Infrared is the sole modality used. Their screening method is called Infrared Regulation Imaging (IRI) (see Figure 19.1).

19.2.7 Austria

Ludwig Bolzman Research Institute for Physical Diagnostics has done research in infrared for many years and it publishes the "Thermology International" (a quarterly journal of IR clinical research and instrumentation). This journal contains papers from many Thermology Societies. A recent issue contains the results of a survey of 2003 international papers dedicated to Thermology [10].

The General Hospital, University of Vienna, does research mainly in angiology (study of blood and lymph vessels) diabetic foot (pedobarography).

19.2.8 Poland

There has been a more recent rapid increase in the use of infrared imaging for medicine in Poland since the Polish market for IR cameras was opened up. There are more than fifty cameras being used in the following medical centers: Warsaw University, Technical University of Gdansk, Poznan University. Lodz University, Katowice University and the Military Clinical Hospital. The research activities are focused on the following areas.

Active Infrared Imaging, open-heart surgery, quantitative assessment of skin burns, ophthalmology, dentistry, allergic diseases, neurological disorders, plastic surgery, thermal image database for healthy and pathological cases, and multi-spectral imaging (IR, visual, x-ray, ultrasound).

In 1986 the Eurotherm Committee was created by members of the European Community to promote co-operation in the thermal sciences by gathering scientist and engineers working in the area of Thermology. This organization focuses on quantitative infrared thermography and periodically holds conferences and seminars in this field [11].

19.2.9 Italy

Much of the clinical use of IR imaging is done under the public health system, besides private clinics. The ongoing clinical work is in the following areas: dermatology (melanoma), neurology, rheumatology, anaesthesiology, reproductive medicine, and sports medicine. The University of G. d'Annunzio, Chieti, has an imaging laboratory purely for research on infrared applications. It collaborates on these projects with other universities throughout Italy.

There are other places, such as Australia, Norway, South America, Russia, etc. that have ongoing research as well.

19.3 Infrared Imaging in Breast Cancer

In the United States, breast cancer is a national concern. There are 192,000 cases a year; it is estimated that there are 1 million women with undetected breast cancer; presently, the figure of women affected is 1.8 million; 45,000 women die per year. The cost burden of the U.S. healthcare is estimated at $18 billion per year. The cost for early stage detection is $12,000 per patient and for late detection it is $345,000 per patient. Hence, early detection would potentially save $12B dollars annually — as well as many lives. As a result, the U.S. Congress created "The Congressionally Directed Medical Research Program for Breast Cancer." Clinical infrared has not as yet been supported through this funding. Effort is being directed toward including infrared. Since 1982, the FDA has approved infrared imaging (Thermography) as an adjunct modality to mammography for breast cancer as shown in Table 19.2.

Ideal characteristics for an early breast cancer detection method as defined by the Congressionally Directed Medical Research Programs on Breast Cancer are listed in Table 19.3. Infrared imaging meets these requirements with the exception of the detection of early lesions at 1,000 to 10,000 cells which has not yet been fully determined.

A program is underway in the United States to develop a prototype web-based database with a collection of approximately 2000 patient thermal signatures to be categorized into three categories: normal, equivocal, and suspicious for developing algorithms for screening and early detection of tumor development.

The origin of this program can be traced back to a 1994 multi-agency DOD grant sponsored by the Director for Research in the Office of the Director, Defense Research and Engineering, the Defense Advanced Research Projects Agency, and the Army Research Office. This grant funded a study to determine the applicability of advanced military technology to the detection of breast cancer — particularly thermal

TABLE 19.2   Imaging for breast cancer detection∗

Film-screen mammography
Full-field digital mammography
Computer-aided detection
Ultrasound
Magnetic resonance imaging (MRI)
Positron emission tomography (PET)
Thermography
Electrical impedance imaging

∙Food and Drug Administration
Reference: *Mammography and Beyond,* Institute of Medicine,
National Academy Press, 2001.

TABLE 19.3   Ideal characteristics for an early breast cancer detection method

Detects early lesion (1,000–10,000 cells)
Available to population (48 million U.S. women age 40–70 yrs)
High sensitivity ⎫
High Specificity ⎭ in all age groups
Inexpensive
Noninvasive
Easily trainable and with high quality assurance
Decreases mortality

imaging and automatic target recognition. The study produced two reports, one in 1995 and another in 1998; these studies identified technology, concepts, and ongoing activity that would have direct relevance to a rigorous application of infrared. Rigor was the essential ingredient to further progress. The U.S. effort had been dormant since the 1970s because of the limitations imposed by poor sensors, simplistic imaging processing, lack of automatic target recognition, and inadequate computing power. This was complicated by the fact that the virtues of infrared had been overstated by a few developers.

In 1999, the Director for Research in the Office of the Director, Defense Research and Engineering and the Deputy Assistant Secretary of the Army for Installations and Environment; Environmental Safety and Occupational Health formulated a technology transfer program that would facilitate the use of advanced military technology and processes to breast cancer screening. Funds were provided by the Army and the project was funded through the Office of Naval Research (ONR).

A major milestone in the U.S. program was the Tanks to Tumors workshop held in Arlington, VA, December 4 to 5, 2001. The workshop was co-sponsored by Office of the Director, Defense Research and Engineering, Space and Sensor Technology Directorate; the Deputy Assistant Secretary of the Army for Environment, Safety and Occupational Health; the Defense Advanced Research Projects Agency; and the Army Research Office. The purpose was to explore means for exploiting the technological opportunities in the integration of image processing, web-based database management and development, and infrared sensor technology for the early detection of breast cancer. A second objective was to provide guidance to a program. The government speakers noted that significant military advances in thermal imaging, and automatic target recognition coupled with medical understanding of abnormal vascularity (angiogenesis) offer the prospect of automated detection from one to two years earlier than other, more costly and invasive screening methods.

There were compelling reasons for both military and civilian researchers to attend (1) recognition of breast cancer as a major occupational health issue by key personnel such as Raymond Fatz, Deputy Assistant Secretary of the Army for Installations and Environment; Environmental Safety and Occupational Health; (2) growing use of thermal imaging in military and civilian medicine (especially abroad); (3) maturation of military technology in automatic target recognition (ATR), ATR evaluation, and low cost thermal imaging; (4) emerging transfer opportunities to and from the military. In particular, ATR assessment technology has developed image data management, dissemination, collaboration, and assessment tools for use by government and industrial developers of ATR software used to find military targets in thermal imagery. Such tools seem naturally suited for adaptation to the creation and use of a national database for infrared breast cancer imagery and the evaluation of screening algorithms that would assist physicians in detecting the disease early. Finally, recent infrared theories developed by civilian physicians indicate that the abnormal vascularity (angiogenisis) associated with the formation of breast tumors may be detected easily by infrared cameras from 1 to 5 years before any other technique. Early detection has been shown to be the key to high survival probability.

The workshop involved specialists and leaders from the military R&D, academic, and medical communities. Together they covered a multidisciplinary range of topics: military infrared sensor technology, automatic target recognition (ATR), smart image processing, database management, interactive web-based data management, infrared imaging for screening of breast cancer, and related medical topics. Three panels of experts considered (1) Image Processing and Medical Applications; (2) Website and Database; (3) Sensor Technology for Medical Applications. A subject area expert led each. The deliberations of each group were presented in a briefing to the plenary session of the final day. Their outputs were quite general; they still apply to the current program and are discussed below for the benefit of all future U.S. efforts.

19.3.1   The Image Processing and Medical Applications

This group focused on the algorithms (ATR approaches) and how to evaluate and use them. It advised that the clinical methods of collection must be able to support the most common ATR approaches, for example, single frame, change detection, multi-look, and anomaly detection. They also provided detailed draft guidelines for controlled problem sets for ATR evaluation. Although they thought a multi-sensor approach would pay dividends, they stressed the need to quantify algorithm performance in a methodical way, starting with approaches that work with single infrared images.

19.3.2   Website and Database

This panel concerned itself with the collection and management of an infrared image database for breast cancer. It looked particularly at issues of data standards and security. It concluded that the OSD supported Virtual Distributed Laboratory (VDL), created within the OSD ATR Evaluation Program, is a very good model for the medical data repository to include collaborative software, image management software, evaluation concepts, data standards, security, bandwidth, and storage capacity. It also advised that camera calibration concepts and phantom targets be provided to help baseline performance and eliminate unknowns. It noted that privacy regulations would have to be dealt with in order to post the human data but suggested that this would complicate but not impede the formation of the database.

19.3.3   Sensor Technology for Medical Applications

The sensor panel started by pointing out that, if angiogenesis is a reliable early indicator of risk, then thermal imaging is ideally suited to detection at that stage. Current sensor performance is fully adequate. The group discussed calibration issues associated with hardware design and concluded that internal reference is desirable to insure that temperature differences are being measured accurately. However, they questioned the need for absolute temperature measurement; the plenary group offered no counter to this. This group also looked at the economics of thermal imaging, and concluded that recent military developments in uncooled thermal imaging systems at DARPA and the Army Night Vision and Electronic Sensing Division would allow the proliferation of infrared cameras costing at most a few thousand dollars each. They cited China's installation of over 60 such cameras. The panel challenged ATR and algorithm developers to look at software methods to help simplify the sensor hardware, for example, frame to frame change detection to replace mechanical stabilization.

Infrared imaging for medical uses is a multidisciplinary technology and must include experts from very different fields if its full potential is to be realized. The Tanks to Tumors workshop is a model for future U.S. efforts. It succeeded in bringing several different communities together — medical, military, academic, industrial, and engineering. These experts worked together to determine how the United States might adopt thermal imaging diagnostic technology in an orderly and demonstrable way for the early detection of breast cancer and other conditions. The panel recommendations will serve to guide the transition of military technology developments in ATR, the VDL, and IR sensors, to the civilian medical community. The result will be a new tool in the war against breast cancer — a major benefit to the military and civilian population. Detailed proceedings of this workshop are available from ACA, Falls Church, VA.

19.4   Guide to Thermal Imaging Systems for Medical Applications

19.4.1   Introduction

The purpose of this section is to provide the physician with an overview of the key features of thermal imaging systems and a brief discussion of the marketplace. It assumes that the reader is somewhat familiar with thermal imaging theory and terminology as well as the fundamentals of digital imaging. It contains a brief, modestly technical guide to buying sensor hardware, and a short list of active websites that can introduce the buyer to the current marketplace. It is intended primarily to aid the newcomer, however, advanced workers may also find some of these websites useful in seeking custom or cutting edge capabilities in their quest to better understand the thermal phenomenology of breast cancer.

19.4.2   Background

As discussed elsewhere, the last decade has seen a resurgence of interest in thermal imaging for the early detection of breast cancer and other medical applications, both civilian and military. There was a brief period in the 1970s when thermal imaging became the subject of medical interest. That interest waned due to the combination of high prices and modest to marginal performance. Dramatic progress has been made in the intervening years; prices have dropped thanks to burgeoning military, domestic, and industrial use; performance has improved significantly; and new technology has emerged from Defense investments. Imaging electronics, digitization, image manipulation software, and automatic detection algorithms have emerged. Cameras can be had for prices that range from about $3,000 on up. Cameras under $10,000 can provide a significant capability for screening and data collection. The camera field is highly competitive; it is possible to rent, lease, or buy cameras from numerous vendors and manufacturers.

19.4.3   Applications and Image Formats

Currently, thermal imaging is being used for research and development into the phenomenology of breast cancer detection, and for screening and cuing in the multimodal diagnosis and tracking of breast cancer in patients. The least stressful and most affordable is the latter. Here, two types of formats can be of general utility: uncalibrated still pictures and simple uncalibrated video. Such formats can be stored and archived for future viewing. Use of such imagery for rigorous research and development is not recommended. Furthermore, there may be legal issues associated with the recording and collection of such imagery unless it is applied merely as a screening aid to the doctor rather than as a primary diagnostic tool. In other words, such imagery would provide the doctor with anecdotal support in future review of a patient's record. In this mode, the thermal imagery has the same diagnostic relevance as a stethoscope or endoscope, neither of which is routinely recorded in the doctor's office. Imagery so obtained would not carry the same diagnostic weight as a mammogram. Still cameras and video imagers of this kind are quite affordable and compact. The can be kept in a drawer or cabinet and be used for thermal viewing of many types of conditions including tumors, fractures, skin anomalies, circulation, and drug affects, to name a few. The marketplace is saturated with imagers under $10,000 that can provide adequate resolution and sensitivity for informal "eyeballing" the thermal features of interest. Virtually any image or video format is adequate for this kind of use.

For medical R&D, in which still imagery is to be archived, shared, and used for the testing of software and medical theories, or to explore phenomenology, it is important to collect calibrated still imagery in lossless archival formats (e.g., the so-called "raw" format that many digital cameras offer). It is thus desirable to purchase or rent a radiometric still camera with uncompressed standard formats or "raw" output that preserves the thermal calibration. This kind imagery allows the medical center to put its collected thermal imagery into a standard format for distribution to the Virtual Distributed Laboratory and other interested medical centers. There are image manipulation software packages that can transform the imagery if need be. On the other hand, the data can be transmitted in any number of uncompressed formats and transformed by the data collection center. The use of standard formats is critical if medical research centers are to share common databases. There is no obvious need yet for video in R&D for breast cancer, although thermal video is being studied for many medical applications where dynamic phenomena are of interest.

19.4.4 Dynamic Range

The ability of a camera to preserve fine temperature detail in the presence of large scene temperature range is determined by its dynamic range. Dynamic range is determined by the camera's image digitization and formation electronics. Take care to use a camera that allocates an adequate number of bits to the digitization of the images. Most commercially available cameras use 12 bits or more per pixel. This is quite adequate to preserve fine detail in images of the human body. However, when collecting images, make sure there is nothing in the field of view of the camera that is dramatically cooler or hotter than the subject; that is, avoid scene temperature differences of more than roughly 30°C (e.g., lamps, refrigerators, or radiators in the background could cause trouble). This is analogous to trying to use a visible digital camera to capture a picture of a person standing next to headlights — electronic circuits may bloom or sacrifice detail of the scene near the bright lights. Although 12-bit digitization should preserve fine temperature differences at a 30°C delta, large temperature differences generally stress the image formation circuitry, and undesired artifacts may appear. Nevertheless, it is relatively easy to design a collection environment with a modest temperature range. A simple way to do this is to simply fill the camera field of view with the human subject. Experiment with the imaging arrangement before collecting a large body of imagery for archiving.

19.4.5 Resolution and Sensitivity

The two most important parameters for a thermal sensor are its sensitivity and resolution. The sensitivity is measured in degrees Celsius. Modest sensitivity is on the order of a tenth of a degree Celsius. Good sensitivity sensors can detect temperature differences up to 4 times lower or 0.025°C. This sensitivity is deemed valuable for medical diagnosis, since local temperature variations caused by tumors and angiogenesis are usually higher than this. The temperature resolution is analogous to the number of colors in a computer display or color photograph. The better the resolution, the smoother the temperature transitions will be. If the subject has sudden temperature gradients, those will be attributable to the subject and not to the camera.

The spatial resolution of the sensor is determined primarily by the size of the imaging chip or pixel count. This parameter is exactly analogous to the world of proliferating digital photography. Just as a 4 megapixel digital camera can make sharper photos than a 2 megapixel camera, pixel count is a key element in the design of a medical camera. There are quite economical thermal cameras on the market with 320 × 240 pixels, and the images from such cameras can be quite adequate for informal screening; imagery may appear to be grainy if magnified unless the viewing area or field of view is reduced. By way of example, if the image is of the full chest area, about 18 inches, then a 320 pixel camera will provide the ability to resolve spatial features of about a sixteenth of an inch. If only the left breast is imaged, spatial features as low as 1/32 inch can be resolved. On the other hand, a 640×480 camera can cut these feature sizes in half. Good sensitivity and pixel count ensures that the medical images will contain useful thermal and spatial detail. In summary, although 320×240 imagery is quite adequate, larger pixel counts can provide more freedom for casual use, and are essential for R&D in medical centers. Although the military is developing megapixel arrays, they are not commercially available. Larger pixel counts have advantages for consumer digital photography and military applications, but there is no identified, clear need at this time for megapixel arrays in breast cancer detection. Avoid the quest for larger pixel counts unless there is a clear need. Temperature resolution should be a tenth of a degree or better.

19.4.6 Calibration

Another key feature is temperature calibration. Many thermal imaging systems are designed to detect temperature differences, not to map calibrated temperature. A camera that maps the actual surface temperature is a radiographic sensor. A reasonably good job of screening for tumors can be accomplished by only mapping local temperature differences. This application would amount to a third eye for the physician, aiding him in finding asymmetries and temperature anomalies — hot or cold spots. For example, checking circulation with thermal imaging amounts to looking for cold spots relative to the normally warm torso. However, if the physician intends to share his imagery with other doctors, or use the imagery for research, it is advisable to use a calibrated camera so that the meaning of the thermal differences can be quantified and separated from display settings and digital compression artifacts. For example, viewing the same image on two different computer displays may result in different assessments. But, if the imagery is calibrated so that each color or brightness is associated with a specific temperature, then doctors can be sure that they viewing relevant imagery and accurate temperatures, not image artifacts.

It is critical that the calibration be stable and accurate enough to match the temperature sensitivity of the camera. Here caution is advised. Many radiometric cameras on the market are designed for industrial applications where large temperature differences are expected and the temperature of the object is well over $100°C$; for example, the temperature difference may be $5°C$ at $600°C$. In breast cancer, the temperature differences of interest are about a tenth of a degree at about $37°C$. Therefore, the calibration method must be relevant for those parameters. Since the dynamic range of the breast cancer application is very small, the calibration method is simplified. More important are the temporal stability, temperature resolution, and accuracy of the calibration. Useful calibration parameters are: of $0.1°C$ resolution at $37°C$, stability of $0.1°C/h$ (drift), and accuracy of $\pm0.3°C$. This means that the camera can measure a temperature difference of $0.1°C$ with an accuracy of $\pm0.3°C$ at body temperature. For example, suppose the breast is at $36.5°C$; the camera might read $36.7°C$.

Two methods of calibration are available — internal and external. External calibration devices are available from numerous sources. They are traceable to NIST and meet the above requirements. Prices are under $3000 for compact, portable devices. The drawback with external calibration is that it involves a second piece of equipment and more complex procedure for use. The thermal camera must be calibrated just prior to use and calibration imagery recorded, or the calibration source must be placed in the image while data is collected. The latter method is more reliable but it complicates the collection geometry.

Internal calibration is preferable because it simplifies the entire data collection process. However, radiometric still cameras with the above specifications are more expensive than uncalibrated cameras by $3000 to $5000.

19.4.7 Single Band Imagers

Today there are thermal imaging sensors with suitable performance parameters. There are two distinct spectral bands that provide adequate thermal sensitivity for medical use: the medium wave infrared band (MWIR) covers the electromagnetic spectrum from 3 to 5 μm in wavelength, approximately; the long wave infrared band (LWIR) covers the wavelength spectrum from about 8 to 12 μm. There are advocates for both bands, and neither band offers a clear advantage over the other for medical applications, although the LWIR is rapidly becoming the most economical sensor technology. Some experimenters believe that there is merit to using both bands.

MWIR cameras are widely available and generally have more pixels, hence higher resolution for the same price. Phenomenology in this band has been quite effective in detecting small tumors and temperature asymmetries. MWIR sensors must be cooled to cryogenic temperatures as low as 77 K. Thermoelectric coolers are used for some MWIR sensors; they operate at 175 to 220 K depending on the design of the imaging chip. MWIR sensors not only respond to emitted radiation from thermal sources but they also sense radiation from broadband visible sources such as the sun. Images in this band can contain structure caused by reflected light rather than emitted radiation. Some care must be taken to minimize reflected light from broadband sources including incandescent light bulbs and sunlight. Unwanted light can cause shadows, reflections, and bright spots in the imagery. Care should be taken to avoid direct illumination of the subject by wideband artificial sources and sunlight. It is advisable to experiment with lighting geometries and sources before collecting data for the record. Moisturizing creams, sweat, and other skin surface coatings should also be avoided.

The cost of LWIR cameras has dropped dramatically since the advent of uncooled thermal imaging arrays. This is a dramatic difference between the current state of the art and what was available in the 1970s. Now, LWIR cameras are being proliferated and can be competitive in price and performance to the thermoelectrically cooled MWIR. Uncooled thermal cameras are compact and have good resolution and sensitivity. Cameras with 320×240 pixels can be purchased for well under \$10,000. This year, sensors with 640×480 pixels have hit the market. Sensors in this band are far less likely to be affected by shadows, lighting, and reflections. Nevertheless, it is advisable to experiment with viewing geometry, ambient lighting, and skin condition before collecting data for the record and for dissemination.

19.4.8 Emerging and Future Camera Technology

There are emerging developments that may soon provide for a richer set of observable phenomena in the thermography for breast cancer. Some researchers are already simultaneously collecting imagery in both the MWIR and LWIR bands. This is normally accomplished using two cameras at the same time. Dual band imagery arguably provides software and physicians with a richer set of observables. Developers of automatic screening algorithms are exploring schemes that compare the images in the two bands and emphasize the common elements of both to get greater confidence in detecting tumors. More sophisticated software (based on neural networks) learns what is important in both bands. New dual band technology has emerged from recent investments by the Defense Advanced Research Projects Agency (DARPA). Uncooled detector arrays have been demonstrated that operate in both bands simultaneously. It is likely that larger or well-endowed medical centers can order custom imagers with this capability this year. Contact the Materials Technology Office at DARPA for further information.

Spectroscopic (hyperspectral) imaging in the thermal bands is also an important research topic. Investigators are looking for phenomenology that manifests itself in fine spectral detail. Since flesh is a thermally absorptive and scattering medium, it may be possible to detect unique signatures that help detect tumors. Interested parties should ask vendors if such cameras are available for lease or purchase.

Some researchers are using multiple views and color to attempt to enhance tomographic imaging processes and to image to greater depths using physical models of the flesh and its thermal profiles at different wavelengths. Contact the principal investigators directly.

19.4.9 Summary Specifications

Table 19.4 summarizes the key parameters and their nominal values to use in shopping for a camera.

How to begin. Those who are new to thermal phenomenology should carefully study the material in this handbook. Medical centers, researchers, and physicians seeking to purchase cameras and enter the field may wish to contact the authors or leading investigators mentioned in this handbook for advice before looking for sensor hardware. The participants in the Tanks to Tumors workshop and the MedATR program may already have the answers. If possible, compare advice from two or more of these experts before moving on; the experts do not agree on everything. They are currently using sensors and software suitable for building the VDL database. They may also be aware of public domain image screening software. Once advice has been collected, the potential buyer should begin shopping at the one or more of the websites listed in this section. Do not rely on the website alone. Most vendors provide contact information so that the purchaser may discuss imaging needs with a consultant. Take advantage of these advisory services to shop around and survey the field. Researchers may also wish to contact government and university experts before deciding on a camera. Finally, many of the vendors below offer custom sensor design services. Some vendors may be willing to lease or loan equipment for evaluation. High-end, leading edge researchers may need to contact component developers at companies such as Raytheon, DRS, BAE, or SOFRADIR to see if the state of the art supports their specific needs.

Supplier Websites: The reader is advised that all references to brand names or specific manufacturers do not connote an endorsement of the vendor, producer, or its products. Likewise, the list is not a complete survey; we apologize for any omissions.

http://www.infrared-camera-rentals.com/
http://www.electrophysics.com/Browse/Brw_AllProductLineCategory.asp
http://www.cantronic.com/ir860.html
http://www.nationalinfrared.com/Medical_Imaging.php
http://www.flirthermography.com/cameras/all_cameras.asp
http://www.mikroninst.com/
http://www.baesystems.com/newsroom/2005/jan/310105news4.htm
http://www.indigosystems.com/product/rental.html
http://www.indigosystems.com/
http://www.raytheoninfrared.com/productcatalog/
http://x26.com/Night_Vision_Thermal_Links.html
http://www.infraredsolutions.com/
http://www.isgfire.com/
http://www.infrared.com/
http://www.sofradir.com/
http://www.infrared-detectors.com/
http://www.drs.com/products/index.cfm?gID=21&cID=39
http://www.flir.com/ (radiometric cameras)

19.5 Summary, Conclusions, and Recommendations

Today, medical infrared is being backed by more clinical research worldwide where state-of-the-art equipment is being used. Focus must be placed on the quantification of clinical data, standardization, effective

TABLE 19.4 Summary of Key Camera Parameters

	Application: recording	Application: informal
Format	Digital stills	Video or stills
Compression	None	As provided by mfr
Digitization (dynamic range)	12 bits or more	12 bits nominal
Pixels (array size)	320×240 up to 640×480	320×240
Sensitivity	$0.04°C$, $0.1°C$ max.	$0.1°C$
Calibration accuracy	$\pm 0.3°C$	Not required
Calibration range	Room and body temperature	Not required
Calibration resolution	$0.1°C$	Not required
Spectral band	MWIR or LWIR	MWIR or LWIR

training with high quality assurance, collaborations, and more publications in leading peer reviewed medical journals.

For an effective integration of 21st century technologies for IR imaging we need to focus on the following areas:

- IR cameras and systems
- Advanced image processing
- Image analysis techniques
- High speed computers
- Computer-aided detection (CAD)
- Knowledge-based databases
- Telemedicine

Other areas of importance are:

- Effective clinical use
- Protocol-based image acquisition
- Image interpretation
- System operation and calibration
- Training
- Better understanding of the pathophysiological nature of thermal signatures
- Quantification of clinical data

In conclusion, this noninvasive, non-ionizing imaging modality can provide added value to the present multiimaging clinical setting. This functional image measures metabolic activity in the tissue and thus can noninvasively detect abnormalities very early. It is well known that early detection leads to enhanced survivability and great reduction in health care costs. With these becoming exorbitant, this would be of great value. Besides its usefulness at this stage, a second critical benefit is that it has the capability to non-invasively monitor the efficacy of therapies [12].

References

[1] Diakides, N.A. (Guest Editor): Special Issue on Medical Infrared Imaging, *IEEE/Engineering in Medicine and Biology*, 17, 17–18, 1998.

[2] Diakides, N.A. (Guest Editor): Special Issue on Medical Infrared Imaging, *IEEE/Engineering in Medicine and Biology*, 19, 28–29, 2000.

[3] Diakides, N.A. (Guest Editor): Special Issue on Medical Infrared Imaging, *IEEE/Engineering in Medicine and Biology*, 21, 32–33, 2002.

[4] Paul, J.L. and Lupo, J.C., "From Tanks to Tumors: Applications of Infrared Imaging and Automatic Target Recognition Image Processing for Early Detection of Breast Cancer," Special Issue on Medical Infrared Imaging, *IEEE/Engineering in Medicine and Biology*, 21, 34–35, 2002.

[5] Diakides, N.A., "Medical Applications of IR Focal Plane Arrays," Final Progress Report, U.S. Army Research Office, Contract DAAH04-94-C-0020, Mar. 1998.

[6] Diakides, N.A., "Application of Army IR Technology to Medical IR Imaging." Technical Report, U.S. Army Research Office Contract DAAH04-96-C-0086 (TCN 97-143), Aug. 1999.

[7] Diakides, N.A., "Exploitation of Infrared Imaging for Medicine," Final Progress Report, U.S. Army Research Office, Contract DAAG55-98-0035, Jan. 2001.

[8] Diakides, N.A., "Medical IR Imaging and Image Processing," Final Report, U.S. Army Research Office, Contract DAAH04-96-C-0086 (TNC 01041), Oct. 2003.

[9] Anbar, M., *Quantitative Dynamic Telethermometry in Medical Diagnosis and Management*, CRC Press, 1994.

[10] Ammer, K. (Ed. in Chief), *Journal of Thermology*, International, 14, 2004.

[11] Balageas, D., Busse, G., Carlomagno, C., and Wiecek, B. (Eds.), *Proceedings of Quantitative Infrared Thermography 4*, Technical University of Lodz, 1998.

[12] Hassan, M. et al., "Quantitative Assessment of Tumor Vasculature and Response to Therapy in Kaposi's Sarcoma Using Functional Noninvasive Imaging," *Technology in Cancer Research and Treatment*, 3, 451–457, Adenine Press (2004).

20

The Historical Development of Thermometry and Thermal Imaging in Medicine

E. Francis Ring
Bryan F. Jones
University of Glamorgan

Fever was the most frequently occurring condition in early medical observation. From the early days of Hippocrates, when it is said that wet mud was used on the skin to observe fast drying over a tumorous swelling, physicians have recognised the importance of a raised temperature. For centuries, this remained a subjective skill, and the concept of measuring temperature was not developed until the 16th Century. Galileo made his famous thermoscope from a glass tube, which functioned as an unsealed thermometer. It was affected by atmospheric pressure as a result.

In modern terms we now describe heat transfer by three main modes. The first is conduction, requiring contact between the object and the sensor to enable the flow of thermal energy. The second mode of heat transfer is convection where the flow of a hot mass transfers thermal energy. The third is radiation. The latter two led to remote detection methods.

Thermometry developed slowly from Galileo's experiments. There were Florentine and Venetian glassblowers in Italy who made sealed glass containers of various shapes, which were tied onto the body surface. The temperature of an object was assessed by the rising or falling of small beads or seeds within the fluid inside the container. Huygens, Roemer, and Fahrenheit all proposed the need for a calibrated scale in the late 17th and early 18th century. Celsius did propose a centigrade scale based on ice and boiling water. He strangely suggested that boiling water should be zero, and melting ice 100 on his scale. It was the Danish biologist Linnaeus in 1750 who proposed the reversal of this scale, as it is known today. Although International Standards have given the term Celsius to the 0 to 100 scale today, strictly speaking it would be historically accurate to refer to degrees Linnaeus or centigrade [1].

The Clinical thermometer, which has been universally used in medicine for over 130 years, was developed by Dr. Carl Wunderlich in 1868. This is essentially a maximum thermometer with a limited scale around the normal internal body temperature of 37°C or 98.4°F. Wunderlich's treatise on body temperature in health and disease is a masterpiece of painstaking work over many years. He charted the progress of all his patients daily, and sometimes two or three times during the day. His thesis was written in German for Leipzig University and was also translated into English in the late 19th century [2]. The significance of body temperature lies in the fact that humans are homeotherms who are capable of maintaining a constant temperature that is different from that of the surroundings. This is essential to the preservation of a relatively constant environment within the body known as homeostasis. Changes in temperature of more than a few degrees either way is a clear indicator of a bodily dysfunction; temperature variations outside this range may disrupt the essential chemical processes in the body.

Today, there has been a move away from glass thermometers in many countries, giving rise to more disposable thermocouple systems for routine clinical use.

Liquid crystal sensors for temperature became available in usable form in the 1960s. Originally the crystalline substances were painted on the skin that had previously been coated with black paint. Three of four colours became visible if the paint was at the critical temperature range for the subject. Micro-encapsulation of these substances, that are primarily cholesteric esters, resulted in plastic sheet detectors. Later these sheets were mounted on a soft latex base to mould to the skin under air pressure using a cushion with a rigid clear window. Polaroid photography was then used to record the colour pattern while the sensor remained in contact. The system was re-usable and inexpensive. However, sensitivity declined over 1–2 years from the date of manufacture, and many different pictures were required to obtain a subjective pattern of skin temperature [3].

Convection currents of heat emitted by the human body have been imaged by a technique called Schlieren Photography. The change in refractive index with density in the warm air around the body is made visible by special illumination. This method has been used to monitor heat loss in experimental subjects, especially in the design of protective clothing for people working in extreme physical environments.

Heat transfer by radiation is of great value in medicine. The human body surface requires variable degrees of heat exchange with the environment as part of the normal thermo-regulatory process. Most of this heat transfer occurs in the infrared, which can be imaged by electronic thermal imaging [4]. Infrared radiation was discovered in 1800 when Sir William Herschel performed his famous experiment to measure heat beyond the visible spectrum. Nearly 200 years before, Italian observers had noted the presence of reflected heat. John Della Porta in 1698 observed that when a candle was lit and placed before a large silver bowl in church, that he could sense the heat on his face. When he altered the positions of the candle, bowl, and his face, the sensation of heat was lost.

William Herschel, in a series of careful experiments, showed that not only was there a "dark heat" present, but that heat itself behaved like light, it could be reflected and refracted under the right conditions. William's only son, John Herschel, repeated some experiments after his father's death, and successfully made an image using solar radiation. This he called a "thermogram," a term still in use today to describe an image made by thermal radiation. John Herschel's thermogram was made by focussing solar radiation with a lens onto to a suspension of carbon particles in alcohol. This process is known as evaporography [5].

A major development came in the early 1940s with the first electronic sensor for infrared radiation. Rudimentary night vision systems were produced towards the end of the Second World War for use by snipers. The electrons from near-infrared cathodes were directed onto visible phosphors which converted the infrared radiation to visible light. Sniperscope devices, based on this principle, were provided for soldiers in the Pacific in 1945, but found little use.

At about the same time, another device was made from indium antimonide; this was mounted at the base of a small Dewar vessel to allow cooling with liquid nitrogen. A cumbersome device such as this, which required a constant supply of liquid nitrogen, was clearly impractical for battlefield use but could be used with only minor inconvenience in a hospital. The first medical images taken with a British prototype system, the "Pyroscan," were made at The Middlesex Hospital in London and The Royal National Hospital for Rheumatic Diseases in Bath between 1959 and 1961. By modern standards, these thermograms were very crude.

In the meantime, the cascade image tube, that had been pioneered during World War II in Germany, had been developed by RCA into a multi-alkali photocathode tube whose performance exceeded expectations. These strides in technology were motivated by military needs in Vietnam; they were classified and, therefore, unavailable to clinicians. However, a mark 2 Pyroscan was made for medical use in 1962, with improved images. The mechanical scanning was slow and each image needed from 2 to 5 min to record. The final picture was written line by line on electro-sensitive paper. In the seventies, the U.S. Military sponsored the development of a multi-element detector array that was to form the basis of a real-time framing imager. This led to the targeting and navigation system known as Forward Looking InfraRed (FLIR) systems which had the added advantage of being able to detect warm objects through smoke and fog.

During this time the potential for thermal imaging in medicine was being explored in an increasing number of centres. Earlier work by the American physiologist J. Hardy had shown that the human skin, regardless of colour, is a highly efficient radiator with an emissivity of 0.98 which is close to that of a perfect black body. Even so, the normal temperature of skin in the region of 20 to 30°C generated low intensities of infrared radiation at about 10 μm wavelength [6]. The detection of such low intensities at these wavelengths presented a considerable challenge to the technology of the day. Cancer detection was a high priority subject and hopes that this new technique would be a tool for screening breast cancer provided the motivation to develop detectors. Many centres across Europe, the United States, and Japan became involved. In the United Kingdom, a British surgeon, K. Lloyd Williams showed that many tumours are hot and the hotter the tumour, the worse the prognosis. By this time, the images were displayed on a cathode ray screen in black and white. Image processing by computer had not arrived, so much discussion was given to schemes to score the images subjectively, and to look for hot spots and asymmetry of temperature in the breast. This was confounded by changes in the breast through the menstrual cycle in younger women. The use of false colour thermograms was only possible by photography at this time. A series of bright isotherms were manually ranged across the temperature span of the image, each being exposed through a different colour filter, and superimposed on a single frame of film.

Improvements in infrared technology were forging ahead at the behest of the U.S. Military during the seventies. At Fort Belvoir, some of the first monolithic laser diode arrays were designed and produced with a capability of generating 500 W pulses at 15 kHz at room temperature. These lasers were able to image objects at distances of 3 km. Attention then turned to solid state, gas, and tunable lasers which were used in a wide range of applications.

By the mid-seventies, computer technology made a widespread impact with the introduction of smaller mini and microcomputers at affordable prices. The first "personal" computer systems had arrived. In Bath, a special system for nuclear medicine made in Sweden was adapted for thermal imaging. A colour screen was provided to display the digitised image. The processor was a PDP8, and the program was loaded every day from paper-tape. With computerisation many problems began to be resolved. The images were archived in digital form, standard regions of interest could be selected, and temperature measurements obtained from the images. Manufacturers of thermal imaging equipment slowly adapted to the call for quantification and some sold thermal radiation calibration sources to their customers to aid the standardisation of technique. Workshops that had started in the late 1960s became a regular feature, and the European Thermographic Association was formed with a major conference in Amsterdam in 1974. Apart from a range of physiological and medical applications groups were formed to formulate guidelines for good practice. This included the requirements for patient preparation, conditions for thermal imaging and criteria for the use of thermal imaging in medicine and pharmacology [7,8]. At the IEEE EMBS conference in Amsterdam some twenty years later in 1996, Dr. N. Diakides facilitated the production of a CD ROM of the early, seminal papers on infrared imaging in medicine that had been published in *ACTA Thermographica* and the *Journal of Thermology*. This CD was sponsored by the U.S. Office of Technology Applications, Ballistic Missile Defence Organisation and the U.S. National Technology Transfer Center Washington Operations and is available from the authors at the Medical Imaging Research Group at the University of Glamorgan, U.K. [9]. The archive of papers may also be search online at the Medical Imaging Group's web site [9].

A thermal index was devised in Bath to provide clinicians with a simplified measure of inflammation [10]. A normal range of values was established for ankles, elbows, hands, and knees, with raised values obtained in osteoarthritic joints and higher values still in Rheumatoid Arthritis. A series of clinical trials with non-steroid, anti-inflammatory, oral drugs, and steroid analogues for joint injection was published using the index to document the course of treatment [11].

Improvements in thermal imaging cameras have had a major impact, both on image quality and speed of image capture. Early single element detectors were dependent on optical mechanical scanning. Both spatial and thermal image resolutions were inversely dependent on scanning speed. The Bofors and some American imagers scanned at 1 to 4 frames per sec. AGA cameras were faster at 16 frames per sec, and used interlacing to smooth the image. Multi-element arrays were developed in the United Kingdom and were employed in cameras made by EMI and Rank. Alignment of the elements was critical, and a poorly aligned array produced characteristic banding in the image. Prof. Tom Elliott F.R.S. solved this problem when he designed and produced the first significant detector for faster high-resolution images that subsequently became known as the Signal PRocessing In The Element (Sprite) detector. Rank Taylor Hobson used the Sprite in the high-resolution system called Talytherm. This camera also had a high specification Infrared zoom lens, with a macro attachment. Superb images of sweat pore function, eyes with contact lenses, and skin pathology were recorded with this system.

With the end of the cold war, the greatly improved military technology was declassified and its use for medical applications was encouraged. As a result, the first focal plane array detectors came from the multi-element arrays, with increasing numbers of pixel/elements, yielding high resolution at video frame rates. Uncooled bolometer arrays have also been shown to be adequate for many medical applications. Without the need for electronic cooling systems these cameras are almost maintenance free. Good software with enhancement and analysis is now expected in thermal imaging. Many commercial systems use general imaging software, which is primarily designed for industrial users of the technique. A few dedicated medical software packages have been produced, which can even enhance the images from the older cameras. CTHERM is one such package that is a robust and almost universally usable programme for medical thermography [9]. As standardisation of image capture and analysis becomes more widely accepted, the ability to manage the images and, if necessary, to transmit them over an intranet or internet for communication becomes paramount. Future developments will enable the operator of thermal imaging to use reference images and reference data as a diagnostic aid. This, however, depends on the level of standardisation that can be provided by the manufacturers, and by the operators themselves in the performance of their technique [12].

Modern thermal imaging is already digital and quantifiable, and ready for the integration into anticipated hospital and clinical computer networks.

References

[1] Ring, E.F.J., *The History of Thermal Imaging in the Thermal Image in Medicine and Biology*, eds. Ammer, K. and Ring, E.F.J., pp. 13–20. Uhlen Verlag, Vienna, 1995.

[2] Wunderlich, C.A., *On the Temperature in Diseases, A Manual of Medical Thermometry.* Translated from the second German edition by Bathurst Woodman, W., The New Sydenham Society, London, 1871.

[3] Flesch, U., Thermographic techniques with liquid crystals in medicine, In *Recent Advances in Medical Thermology*, eds. Ring, E.F.J. and Phillips, B., pp. 283–299. Plenum Press, New York, London, 1984.

[4] Houdas, Y. and Ring, E.F.J., *Human Body Temperature, its Measurement and Regulation*, Plenum Press, New York, London, 1982.

[5] Ring, E.F.J., The discovery of infrared radiation in 1800. *Imaging Science Journal*, 48, 1–8, 2000.

[6] Jones, B.F., A Reappraisal of Infrared Thermal Image Analysis in Medicine. *IEEE Transactions on Medical Imaging*, 17, 1019–1027, 1998.

[7] Engel, J.M., Cosh, J.A., Ring, E.F.J. et al., Thermography in locomotor diseases: recommended procedure. *European Journal of Rheumatology and Inflammation*, 2, 299–306, 1979.

[8] Ring, E.F.J., Engel, J.M., and Page-Thomas, D.P., Thermological methods in clinical pharmacology, *International Journal of Clinical Pharmacology*, 22, 20–24, 1984.

[9] CTHERM website www.medimaging.org

[10] Collins, A.J., Ring, E.J.F., Cash, J.A., and Brown, P.A., Quantification of thermography in arthritis using multi-isothermal analysis: I. The thermographic index. *Annals of the Rheumatic Diseases*, 33, 113–115, 1974.

[11] Bacon, P.A., Ring, E.F.J., and Collins, A.J., Thermography in the assessment of antirheumatic agents. In *Rheumatoid Arthritis*, eds. Gordon and Hazleman. pp. 105–110. Elsevier/North Holland Biochemical Press, Amsterdam, 1977.

[12] Ring, E.F.J. and Ammer, K., The technique of infrared imaging in medicine, *Thermology International*, 10, 7–14, 2000.

21

Physiology of Thermal Signals

21.1 Overview **21**-1
21.2 Skin Thermal Properties in Response to Stress **21**-2
21.3 Regulation of Skin Blood Flow for Heat Transfers **21**-3
21.4 Heat Transfer Modeling Equations for
      Microcirculation **21**-4
21.5 Cutaneous Circulation Measurement Techniques..... **21**-5
      Procedures and Techniques • Dyes and Stains •
      Plethysmography • Doppler Measurement • Clearance
      Measurement • Thermal Skin Measurement •
      Measurement Techniques and Procedures Summary
21.6 Objective Thermography................................ **21**-7
      Efficiency of Heat Transport in the Skin of the Hand
      (Example 21.1) • Effect of a Reduced Blood Flow
      (Example 21.2) • Median Nerve Block in the Hand
      (Example 21.3) • Infrared-Thermography and Laser
      Doppler Mapping of Skin Blood Flow (Example 21.4) • Use
      of Dynamic IR-Thermography to Highlight Perforating
      Vessels (Example 21.5) • Reperfusion of Transplanted Tissue
      (Example 21.6) • Sports Medicine Injury (Example 21.7) •
      Conclusions
Acknowledgments... **21**-17
References **21**-18

David D. Pascoe
Auburn University

James B. Mercer
University of Tromsø

Lois de Weerd
*University Hospital of
North Norway*

21.1 Overview

William Herschel first recognized heat emitted in the infrared (IR) wave spectrum in the 1800s. Medical infrared, popularly known as IR-thermography has utilized this heat signature since the 1960s to measure and map skin temperatures. Our understanding of the regulation of skin blood flow, heat transfers through the tissue layers, and skin temperatures has radically changed during these past 40 years, allowing us to better interpret and evaluate these thermographic measurements. During this same period of time, improved camera sensitivity coupled with advances in focal plan array technology and new developments in computerized systems with assisted image analysis have improved the quality of the noncontact, non-invasive thermal map or thermogram [1–3]. In a recent electronic literature search in Medline using the keywords "thermography" and "thermogram" more than 5000 hits were found [4]. In 2003 alone, there were 494 medical references, 188 basic science, 148 applied science (14 combined with Laser Doppler and

28 combined with ultrasound research), and 47 in biology including veterinary medicine [5]. Further databases and references for medical thermography since 1987 are available [6].

This review will highlight some of the literature and applications of thermography in medical and physiological settings. More specifically, infrared thermography and the structure and functions of skin thermal microcirculation can provide a better understanding of (1) thermoregulation and skin thermal patterns (e.g., comfort zone, influences of heat, cold, and exercise stressors, etc.), (2) assess skin blood perfusion (e.g., skin grafts), (3) observe and diagnose vascular pathologies that manifest thermal disturbances in the cutaneous circulation, (4) evaluate thermal therapies, and (5) monitor patient/subject/athlete's recovery as evidenced by the resumption of normal thermal patterns during the rehabilitation process for some musculoskeletal injuries.

At the outset, it needs to be stressed that an IR image is a visual map of the skin surface temperature that can provide accurate thermal measurement but cannot quantify measurements of blood flow to the skin tissue. It is also important to stress that recorded skin temperatures may represent heat transferred from within the core through various tissue layers to the skin that may be the result of conductive or radiant heat provided from an external thermal stressor. In order to interpret thermographic images and thermal measurement, a basic understanding of physiological mechanisms of skin blood flow and factors that influence heat transfers to the skin must be considered to evaluate this dynamic process. With this understanding, objective data from IR thermography can add valuable information and complement other methodologies in the scientific inquiry and medical practices.

21.2   Skin Thermal Properties in Response to Stress

The thermal properties of the skin surface can change dramatically to maintain our core temperature within a narrowly defined survival range (cardiac arrest at 25°C to cell denaturation at 45°C) [7]. This remarkable task is accomplished despite a large variability in temperatures both from the hostile environment and internal production of heat from metabolism. Further perturbations to core and skin temperature may result from thermal stressors associated with injury, fever, hormonal milieu, and disease. The skin responds to these thermal challenges by regulating skin perfusion.

During heat exposure or intense exercise, skin blood flow can be increased to provide greater heat dissipating capacity. The thermal properties of the skin combined with increased cutaneous circulation operate as a very efficient radiator of heat (emitted radiant heat of 0.98 compared to a blackbody source of 1.0) [8]. Evaporative cooling of sweat on the skin surface further enhances this heat dissipating process. Under hyperthermic conditions, the skin masterfully combines anatomical structure and physiological function to protect and defend the organism from potentially lethal thermal stressors by regulating heat transfers between core, skin, and environment. When exposed to a cold environment, the skin surface nearly eliminates blood flow and becomes an excellent insulator. Under these hypothermic conditions, our skin functions to conserve our body's core temperature. It accomplishes this by reducing convective heat transfers, minimizing heat losses from the core and lessening the possibility of excessive cooling from the environment.

The ability of the skin to substantially increase blood flow, far in excess of the tissue's metabolic needs, alludes to the tissue's role and potential in heat transfer mechanisms. The nutritive needs of skin tissue has been estimated at 0.2 ml/min per cubic centimeter of skin [9], which is considerably lower than the maximal rate of 24 ml/min per cubic centimeter of skin (estimated from total forearm circulatory measurement during heat stress) [10]. If one were to approximate skin tissue as 8% of the forearm, then skin blood would equate to 250 to 300 ml/100 ml of skin per minute [11]. Applying this flow rate to an estimated skin surface of 1.8 m^2 (average individual), suggests that approximately 8 liters of blood flow could be diverted to the skin to dissipate heat at rate of 1750 W to the environment [12,13]. This increased blood flow required for heat transfers from active muscle tissue and skin blood flow for thermoregulation is made available through the redistribution of blood flow (splanchnic circulatory beds, renal tissues) and increases in cardiac output [14]. The increased cardiac output has been suggested to account for two-thirds of the increased blood flow needs, while redistribution provides the remaining one-third [15]. Several good reviews are available regarding cutaneous blood flow, cardiovascular function, and thermal stress [14–19].

21.3 Regulation of Skin Blood Flow for Heat Transfers

In the 1870s, Goltz, Ostromov, and others injected atropine and pilocaprine into the skin to help elucidate the sympathetic neural innervation of the skin tissue for temperature, pressure, pain, and the activation of the sweat glands [20]. The reflex neural regulation of skin blood flow relies on both sympathetic vasoconstrictor and vasodilator controls to modulate internal heat temperature transfers to the skin. The vasoconstrictor system is responsible for eliminating nearly all of the blood flow to the skin during exposure to cold. When exposed to thermal neutral conditions, the vasoconstrictor system maintains the vasomotor tone of the skin vasculature from which small changes in skin blood flow can elicit large changes in heat dissipation. Under these conditions, the core temperature is maintained; mean skin temperature is stable, but dependent upon the extraneous influences of radiant heat, humidity, forced convective airflow, and clothing. A naked individual in a closed room with ambient air temperature between 27 and 28°C can retain thermal equilibrium without shivering or sweating [21]. Slightly dressed individuals are comfortable in a neutral environment with temperatures between 20 and 25°C. This thermoneutral zone provides the basis for the clinical testing standards for room temperatures being set at 18–25°C during infrared thermographic studies. Controlling room test conditions is important when measuring skin temperature responses as changes in ambient temperatures can alter the fraction of flow shared between the musculature and skin [19]. Under the influence of whole body hyperthermic conditions, removal of the vasomotor vasoconstrictor tone can account for 10–20% of cutaneous vasodilation, while the vasodilator system provides the remaining skin blood flow regulation [10]. Alterations in the threshold (onset of vascular response and sweating) and sensitivity (level of response) in vasodilation blood flow control can be related to an individual's level of heat acclimation [22], exercise training [22], circadian rhythm [23,24], and women's reproductive hormonal status [10]. Recent literature suggests that some observed shifts in the reflex control are the result of female reproductive hormones. Both estrogen and progesterone have been linked to menopausal hot flashes [10].

Skin blood flow research has identified differences in reflex sympathetic nerve activation for various skin surface regions. In 1956, Gaskell demonstrated that sympathetic neural activation in the acral regions (digits, lips, ears, cheeks, and palmer surfaces of hands and feet) is controlled by adrenergic vasoconstrictor nerve activity [20]. In contrast, I.C. Roddie in 1957 demonstrated that in nonacral regions, the adrenergic vasoconstrictor activity accounts for less than 25% of the control mechanism [25]. In the nonacral region, the sympathetic nervous system has both adrenergic (vasoconstriction) and nonadrenergic (vasodilator) components. While the vasodilator activity in the nonacral region is well accepted, the vasoconstrictor regulation is not fully understood and awaits the identification of neural cotransmitters that mediate the reductions in blood flow. For a more in-depth discussion of regional sympathetic reflex regulation, see Charkoudian [10] and Johnson and Proppe [13].

A further distinction in blood flow regulation can be found in the existence of arteriovenous anastamoses (AVA) that are principally found in acral tissues but not commonly found in nonacral tissues of the legs, arms, and chest regions [10,26,27]. The AVAs are thick walled, low resistance vessels that provide a direct blood flow route from arterioles to the venules. The arterioles and AVA, under sympathetic adrenergic vasoconstrictor control, modulate and substantially control flow rates to the skin vascular plexuses in these areas. When constricted, blood flow into subcutaneous venous plexus is reduced to a very low level (minimal heat loss); while, when dilated, extremely rapid flow of warm blood into the venous plexus is allowed (maximal heat loss). The skin sites where these vessels are found are among those where skin blood flow changes are discernible to the IR-thermographer. While the AVA are most active during heat stress, their thick walls and high velocity flow rates do not support their significant role in heat transfers to adjoining skin tissue [12].

Localized cooling of the skin surface can cause skin blood flow vasoconstriction induced by the stimulation of the nonadrenergic sympathetic nerves. This localized cooling or challenge can be used as a diagnostic tool by infrared thermographers to identify clinically significant alterations in skin blood flow response. Using a cold challenge test, Francis Ring developed a vasopasticity test for Raynaud's syndrome based on the temperature gradient in the hand following a cold water immersion (20°C for 60 sec) [28]. Challenge testing and IR imaging has also been used to evaluate blood flow thermal patterns in patients with carpal tunnel syndrome pre- and post-surgery [29]. Skin blood flow vasodilation in response to local heating is stimulated by the release of sensory nerve neuropeptides or the nonneural stimulation of the cutaneous arteriole by nitric oxide. Thermographic imagers have exploited this localized warming response to provide a skin blood flow challenge [10].

As stated earlier, conditions of thermal stress from heat exposure and increased metabolic heat from exercise necessitate increases in skin blood flow to transfer the heat to the environment. This could have serious blood pressure consequences if it were not for baroreflex modulation of skin blood flow in regulating both sympathetic vasoconstriction and vasodilation [30,31]. With mild heat stress for 1 h (38 and 46°C, 42% relative humidity), cardiac output was not significantly impacted [32–34]. When exposing the individual to longer duration bouts and higher temperatures, significant changes in cardiac output have been observed. During these hyperthermic bouts, skin blood flow will withdraw vasodilation in nonacral regions in response to situations that displace blood volumes to the legs (lower body negative pressure or upright tilting) [35]. In contrast, under normothermic conditions, skin blood flow will demonstrate a sympathetic vasoconstriction to these same blood volume situations. Thus, it appears that the baroreceptor response can activate either sympathetic pathway. Withdrawing vasodilation under normothermic conditions was not an option in this inactive system [36].

In summary, skin blood flow during whole body thermal stress is regulated by neural reflex control via sympathetic vasoconstriction and vasodilation. There are structural (AVA) and neural mechanisms (vasoconstriction vs. vasodilation) differences between the acral and nonacral regions. During local thermal stress, stimulation of the sensory afferent nerve, nitric oxide stimulation of cutaneous arteriole, and inhibition of sympathetic vasoconstrictor system regulate changes in local blood flow. During thermal stress and increased heat from exercise metabolism, the skin blood flow can be dramatically increased. This increase in skin blood flow is matched to increased cardiac output and peripheral resistance to maintain blood pressure.

21.4   Heat Transfer Modeling Equations for Microcirculation

The capacity and ability of blood to transfer heat through various tissue layers to the skin can be predicted from models. These models are based on calculations from tissue conductivity, tissue density, tissue specific heat, local tissue temperature, metabolic or externally derived heat sources, and blood velocity. Many current models were derived from the 1948 Pennes model of blood perfusion, often referred to as the "bioheat equation" [9]. The bioheat equation calculates volumetric heat that is equated to the proportional volumetric rate of blood perfusion. The Pennes model assumed that thermal equilibrium occurs in the capillaries and venous temperatures were equal to local tissue temperatures. Both of these assumptions have been challenged in more recent modeling research. The assumption of thermal equilibrium within capillaries was challenged by the work of Chato [37] and Chen and Holmes in 1980 [38]. Based on this vascular modeling for heat transfer, thermal equilibrium occurred in "thermally significant blood vessels" that are approximately 50 to 75 μm in diameter and located prior to the capillary plexus. These thermally significant blood vessels derive from a tree-like structure of branching vessels that are closely spaced in countercurrent pairs. For a historical perspective of heat transfer bioengineering, see Chato in Reference 37 and for a review of heat transfers and microvascular modeling, see Baish in Reference 39.

This modeling literature provides a conceptual understanding of the thermal response of skin when altered by disease, injury, or external thermal stressors to skin temperatures (environment or application of cold or hot thermal sources, convective airflow, or exercise). From tissue modeling, we know that tissue is only slightly influenced by the deep tissue blood supply but is strongly influenced by the cutaneous circulation. With the use of infrared thermography, the skin temperatures can be accurately quantified and the thermal pattern mapped. However, these temperatures cannot be assumed to represent thermal conditions at the source of the thermal stress. Furthermore, the thermal pattern only provides a visual map of the skin surface in which heat is dissipated throughout the skin's multiple microvascular plexuses.

21.5 Cutaneous Circulation Measurement Techniques

A brief review of some of the techniques and procedures that have been employed to reveal skin tissue structure, rates and variability of perfusion, and factors that provide regulatory control of blood flow are provided. This serves to inform the reader as to how these measurement techniques have molded our understanding of skin structure and function. It is also important to recognize the advantages and disadvantages each technique brings to our experimental investigations. It is the opinion of the authors that IR thermography can provide complimentary data to information obtained from these other methodologies.

21.5.1 Procedures and Techniques

Visual and microscopic views of skin have provided scientists with a structural layout of skin layers and blood flow. Despite our understanding of the structural organization, we still struggle to understand the regulation and functioning of the skin as influenced by the multitude of external and internal stressors. Since ancient times, documents have recorded visible observations made regarding changes to skin color and temperature that underscore some of the skin's functions. These observations include increased skin color and temperature when someone is hyperthermic, skin flushing when embarrassed, and the appearance of skin reddening when the skin is scratched. In contrast, decreases of skin color and temperature are observed during hypothermia, when blood flow is occluded, or during times of circulatory shock. In addition to observations, testing procedures and techniques have been employed in search of an understanding of skin function. Skin blood flow has provided one of the greatest challenges and has been notoriously difficult to record quantitatively in terms of ml/min per gram of skin tissue.

21.5.2 Dyes and Stains

Stains and dyes have been a useful tool to investigate the structure of various histological tissue preparations. In 1889 Overton used Florescin, a yellow dye that glows in visible light, to visualize the lipid bilayer membrane structure [40]. Florescin is still used today to illuminate the blood vessel in various tissues. In the early 1900s, August Krogh was able to identify perfused capillaries by staining them with writer's ink before the tissue was excised and observed under the microscope. Using a different approach to observe the structure of skin blood flow, Michael Salmon in the 1930s developed a radio-opaque preservative mixture that was injected into fresh cadavers and produced detailed pictures of the arterial blood flow to skin tissue regions which were mapped for the entire skin surface [41]. Scientists have also used Evans Blue Dye to investigate changes in blood volume by calculating the dilution factor of pre- and post-samples. Evans Blue and Pontamine Sky Blue dyes have also been used to investigate skin microvascular permeability and leakage as induced by various stimuli [42]. A more recent staining technique involves the use of an IR absorbing dye, indocyanine green (ICG). The dye ICG fluoresces with invisible IR light when captured by special cameras sensitive to these light wavelengths. Recent publications have suggested that ICG video angiographies provide qualitative and quantitative data from which clinicians may assess tissue blood flow in burn wounds [43,44].

21.5.3 Plethysmography

The rationale for venous occlusion plethysmography (VOP) is that a partially inflated cuff around a limb exceeds the pressure of venous blood flow but does not interfere with arterial blood flow to the limb.

This can be effectively accomplished when the cuff is inflated to a pressure just below diastolic arterial pressure. Consequently, portions of the limb distal to the cuff will swell as blood accumulates. The original VOP technology relied on measuring the rate of swelling as indicated by the displacement volume of the water-filled chamber around the limb. Later, gauges were used to record changes in limb circumference as the limb expanded. Either way, the geometric forces allows one to express the changes in terms of a starting volume, thus scales are labeled as ml/min per 100 ml in the illustrations of VOP data. Unfortunately, the 100 ml reference quantity refers to the whole limb (not the quantity of the skin) and the VOP technique provides discontinuous measurement, usually four measurements per minute. Currently, VOP represents the most reliable quantitative measure of skin blood flow. More recently, a modified plethysmography technique has been developed that equates changes in blood flow to the changes in electrical impedance, when a mild current is introduced into the blood flow and recorded by serially placed electrodes along the limb.

21.5.4 Doppler Measurement

The Doppler Effect describes the shift in wave length frequency or pitch that result when sound or light from any portion of the electromagnetic spectrum are influenced by the distance and directional movement of the object. Both ultrasound and laser Doppler techniques rely on this physical principle to make the skin blood flow measurement. A continuous wave Doppler ultrasound emits a high frequency sound wave from which reflected or echo sounds can be used to calculate the direction of flow and velocity of moving objects (circulating blood cells). When ultrasound equipment is pulsated, the depth of the circulatory flow vessel can be identified. The blood flow is assessed in Doppler units or volts and can be continuously monitored over a small surface area. Similar measurements can be made with the laser Doppler technique, but neither technique is able to yield quantitative blood flow values except through reference data obtained by VOP.

21.5.5 Clearance Measurement

In the 1930s, scientists relied on the thermal conductance method for determining blood flow in tissues. This methodology was based on measurement of heat dissipation in blood flow downstream from a known heat source (thermocouple). The accuracy of the methodology was assumed through strong correlations made with direct drop counting from isolated sheep spleens. However, these blood flow measurements had problems related to trauma associated with the obstruction and insertion of the thermocouple. During the 1950s and 1960s, injection of small amounts of radioactive isotopes was used in an attempt to better quantify skin blood flow [45]. In order to accurately measure skin blood flow, the isotopes had to be freely diffusible and able to cross the capillary endothelium to enter the blood stream. The blood flow measurement (ml blood flow per 100 g of tissue) obtained through this methodology was not reproducible and subjects were exposed to injected radioactive isotope substances.

21.5.6 Thermal Skin Measurement

Physicians and parents have often relied upon touching a child's forehead to identify a fever or elevated temperature. While this is a crude measure of skin temperature, it has demonstrated practical importance. The development of the thermistor has provided quantifiable measurements of the skin surface. This has been extensively used in research related to thermoregulation and in research in which the skin temperature for a particular physiological perturbation must be quantified. Mean skin temperature formulas have been developed in which various regional temperatures (3 to 15 sites) are combined or a weighted mean based on the DuBois formula for surface area is calculated from the regions measured. When measuring skin temperatures under the influence of colder environments, skin temperature distribution is heterogeneous, especially in the acral regions [46]. Under these conditions, the various placements of the thermistor will provide different temperature measurement that may not be indicative of the mean skin temperature for that region. In contrast, the skin surface temperature is more homogeneous under warm environmental conditions. To provide an accurate measurement, physiologists investigating mean skin temperatures have modified the number of thermistors required during testing as dictated by environmental temperatures [46]. Thermistor attachment to the skin surface is problematic as it creates a microenvironment between the probe, skin, and adhering tape and exerts a pressure on the site. Furthermore, one site placement of the thermistor cannot represent variable responses under conditions and within regions that demonstrate heterogeneous temperature distributions.

Infrared thermography provides a thermal map of the skin surface area by measuring the radiant heat that is emitted. Current IR thermography machines provide accurate skin surface temperatures ($<0.05°C$) that are noninvasive, noncontact measurements through the use of stable detectors. These systems produce high speed–high resolution images from which thermal data can be pictorially and quantitatively stored and analyzed. While IR radiation begins at wavelengths of 0.7 μm, current IR thermographic imagers are operating at either the mid-range (3–5 μm) or long range (8–14 μm) wavelengths [1–3]. At these wavelengths the skin's ability to emit the radiant heat is 0.98 on a scale of 1.0 for a perfect radiator, blackbody surface [8]. IR-thermographers sometimes rely on "challenge tests" in which the skin thermal response is evaluated after cold or hot water immersion, convective airflow, or an exercise bout that alters skin blood flow. Under these thermally challenging conditions, the clinical importance of abnormalities of skin blood flow may be more apparent. However, one must also recognize that as the heat is being transferred through the various layers of skin, some of the heat is dissipated into the adjoining tissues. The heat decay as the blood traverses the layers of tissue and its dispersion pattern within the circulatory plexus of the skin may disguise the origin of the tissue producing the abnormal thermal response.

21.5.7 Measurement Techniques and Procedures Summary

Since ancient times, significant progress has been made in the quest to understand the anatomy and physiology of skin blood flow and the thermal heat transfers that are dissipated to the skin surface. Current measurement technologies are unable to quantify skin blood flow per skin tissue area (ml/min per 100 ml skin). At this time, our best estimations of skin blood flow come from venous occlusion plethysmography. VOP provides discontinuous blood flow measurements based on tissue perfusion of a whole limb extremity. In recent years, laser Doppler blood flow measures have been popular when investigating more localized tissue areas, but this technique must be calibrated through the data obtained by plethysmography. In the quest to understand skin surface heat transfers, noncontact IR thermography provides researchers with accurate measures of skin temperature for specific locations and thermal maps of regions of interest. Thermographic images provide spatial and temporal changes in skin temperature that are representative of spatial and temporal changes in perfusion. However, the scientist and clinician should be aware of blood–skin heat transfer properties prior to interpreting and evaluating the thermal responses of skin perfusion or investigating pathologies that are thermally transferred to the skin.

21.6 Objective Thermography

The main focus of this section is to present some specific examples to show that IR thermal imaging is a useful, objective tool for medical and physiological-based investigations. Although IR thermal imaging cannot determine quantitative measurements of blood flow, this imaging can quantify skin thermal measurement that can be correlated to qualitative evaluations of skin blood flow. As with any technique, it is imperative for the IR thermographer to understand the anatomical and dynamic physiological features (e.g., vasomotor activity) of the blood vessels involved in skin circulation in order to interpret skin temperature responses. This is particularly important in situations where skin blood flow and temperature are responding to some external or internal thermal stress (e.g., clinician's cold challenge testing, exercise, environment, etc.) or nonthermal stimuli (e.g., disease, injury, medications, etc.). When properly assessed, skin temperature can provide researchers, scientists, and physicians with valuable information about the blood flow and thermal regulation of organs and tissues (see Example 21.6.1 to Example 21.6.7).

21.6.1   Efficiency of Heat Transport in the Skin of the Hand (Example 21.1)

The AVA are specialized vascular structures within acral regions. At normal body temperature, sympathetic vasoconstrictor nerves keep these anastomoses closed. However, when the body becomes overheated, sympathetic discharge is greatly reduced so that the anastomoses dilate allowing large quantities of warm blood to flow into the subcutaneous venous plexus, thereby promoting heat loss from the body (Figure 21.1a). In thermal physiology, hands and feet are well recognized as effective thermal windows. By controlling the amount of blood perfusing through these extremities, the temperature of the skin surface can change over a wide range of temperatures. It is at such peripheral sites that the effect of changes in blood flow, and therefore skin temperature are most clearly discernable.

The following example demonstrates how efficient skin blood flow in the hand is dissipating a large incoming radiant heat load. The radiant heat load was provided by a Hydrosun® type 501 water-filtered infrared-A (wIRA) irradiator. The Hydrosun® allows a local regional heating of skin tissue with a higher penetration depth than that of conventional IR therapy. The unique principle of operation involves the use of a hermetically sealed water filter in the radiation path to absorb those IR wavelengths emitted by conventional IR lamps which would otherwise harm the skin (OH-group at 0.94, 1.18, 1.38, and 1.87 μm). The total effective radiation from the Hydrosun® lamp was 400 mW/cm^2, which is about three times the intensity of the IR-A radiation from the sun. Throughout the time course of the experiment (Figure 21.1a), sequential digital IR-thermal images were taken every 2 sec. With the image analysis software, five points within the radiation field of each image were selected for temperature measurement and used to construct temperature curves shown in Figure 21.1b.

In the experiment (Figure 21.1b) a rubber mat with an emissivity close to 1.0 was irradiated with the Hydrosun® wIRA lamp for a period of 25 min at a standard distance of 25 cm. At this distance the circular irradiation field had a diameter of about 16 cm. Since the rubber material has a high emissivity it rapidly absorbs heat from the lamp. As can be seen from the time course of the five temperature curves in Figure 21.2 (five fixed measuring points within the radiation field), the center of the irradiated rubber mat rapidly reached temperatures over 90°C during the first 10 min of irradiation. After the first 10 min of irradiation, the hand of a healthy 54-year-old male subject was abruptly placed on the irradiated rubber mat and kept there for a further 10 min, before being removed. When the hand was placed onto the irradiation field, three of the five fixed temperature-measuring sites now measured skin temperature on the dorsal skin surface. Based on the temperature curves in Figure 21.1b, skin temperature on the surface of the hand directed toward the irradiator never rose higher than 40°C, while the two remaining temperature-measuring points on the rubber mat remained at their original high values. The patient suffered no thermal discomfort from placing his hand on the 'hot' rubber mat, even though the temperature of the center of the rubber mat was more than 90°C before the hand was placed on it. This was presumably due to a combination of the low heat capacity of the rubber material combined with a high rate of skin blood flow that is capable of rapidly dissipating heat. The visual data created from the IR-thermal images coupled with the temperature curves which were calculated from sequential IR-thermal images clearly demonstrates the large heat transporting capacity of the skin.

21.6.2   Effect of a Reduced Blood Flow (Example 21.2)

During exposure to cold, heat loss from the extremities is minimized by reducing blood flow (vasoconstriction). In cool environments, this vasomotor tone results in a heterogeneous distribution of skin surface temperatures; while in a warm environment the skin surface becomes more homogeneous (see Figure 21.2a). The importance of the integrity of blood flow in a limb as a whole can also be demonstrated at room temperature by totally cutting off the blood supply to the limb with the aid of a pressure cuff. This is demonstrated in the experiment shown in Figure 21.2b. In this experiment, skin surface on the back of the left hand of a 60-year-old healthy male subject was irradiated for a 10-min period with a wIRA lamp (see description in Section 21.6.1). The fingers were not heated. The heating was repeated twice. In the upper panel (Figure 21.2b) intact blood supply is demonstrated. In the lower panel (Figure 21.2b),

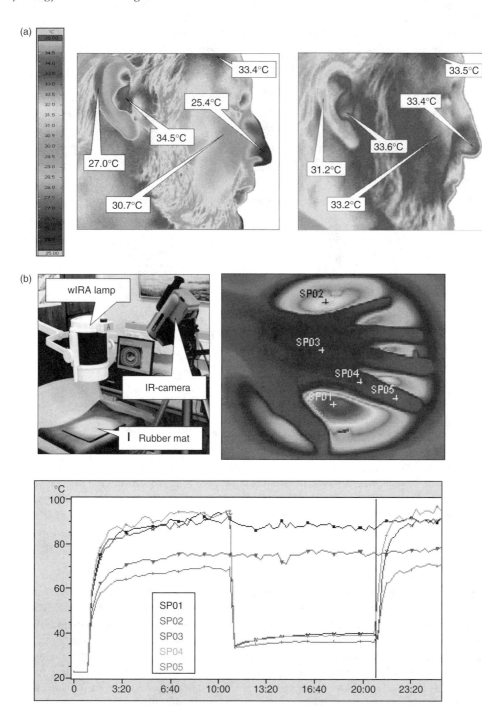

FIGURE 21.1 (See color insert following, page **29**-16.) (a) A Thermogram of a healthy 52-year-old male subject in a cold environment (ca. 15°C; left panel) and in a warm environment (ca. 25°C; right panel). In the cold environment arteriovenous anastomoses in the nose and the auricle region of the ears are closed, resulting in low skin temperatures at these sites. Also note reduced blood flow in the cheeks but not on the forehead, where the blood vessels in the skin are unable to vasoconstrict. (b) Efficiency of skin blood flow as a heat transporter. The photograph in the upper left panel shows a rubber mat being heated with a water-filtered infrared-A irradiator at high intensity (400 mW/cm²) for a period of 20 min. In the lower panel the time course of surface temperature of the mat at five selected spots as measured by an IR-camera is given. During the last 10 min of the 20-min heating period, the left hand of a healthy 54-year-old male subject was placed on the mat.Note that skin surface temperature of the hand remains below 39°C.

(a)   30 min equilibration in cool environment (20°C, 30% rh)

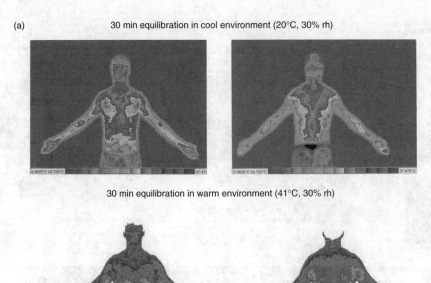

30 min equilibration in warm environment (41°C, 30% rh)

Range of temperature (°C) within regions at two climatic conditions.

	Anterior torso	Posterior torso	Anterior arms	Posterior arms	Palmer hands	Dorsal hands
Cool 20°C	5.0	5.1	6.3	4.5	5.2	4.0
Warm 41°C	3.0	3.2	3.2	3.6	4.0	3.5

FIGURE 21.2 (See color insert.) (a) A The thermoregulatory response of the torso when exposed to a cool or warm environment. Note the heterogeneous temperature distribution in the cool environment as opposed to the more homogeneous temperature distribution in the warm environment. Different colors represent different temperatures. One might recognize the difficulty related to choosing one point (thermocouple data) as the reference value in a region.

thermal response to heating of the limb while blood flow was totally restricted using a blood pressure cuff is presented. The time course of the temperature curves shown in the upper panel of Figure 21.2b demonstrates a gradual increase in skin temperature, eventually stabilizing just below 39°C. The finger skin temperature on the heated hand only showed a minor increase during the heating period. When the lamp was switched off the accumulated heat was rapidly dissipated and skin temperature of the heated area returned to the preheating level. In the lower panel the experiment was repeated, but as the heater was turned on, a pressure cuff placed around the upper arm was inflated to above systolic pressure to totally cut off blood supply to the arm. As can be seen, the rate of rise of skin temperature over the heated skin area was quite rapid, soon reaching a level deemed to be uncomfortably hot, after which the heater was turned off (at this stage the pressure cuff was still inflated). During the heating period finger skin temperature on the same hand steadily decreased (i.e., the fingers were passively cooling due to lack of circulation). After the heater was turned off the temperature of the back of the left hand also began to decrease indicating a passive cooling. When the pressure cuff was reopened and blood flow to the arm reestablished, the rate of cooling on the back of the hand increased (active cooling) and the skin temperature of the cooled fingers also rapidly returned to normal.

While the same result could have been gained by using other methods to measure skin temperature, such as thermocouples, the visual effect gained by using IR thermography provides much more information

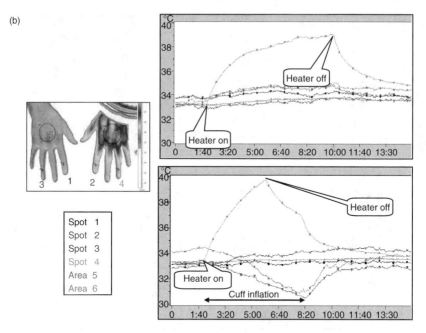

FIGURE 21.2 (Continued.) (b) Skin heating with and without intact circulation in a 65-year-old healthy male subject. The two panels on the right show the time course of 6 selected measuring sites (4 spot measurements and 2 area measurements) of skin temperatures as determined by IR-thermography before, during, and after a period in which the skin surface on the back of the left hand was heated with a water-filtered infrared-A irradiator at high intensity (400 mW/cm^2) in two separate experiments. The results shown in the upper right panel were performed under a situation with a normal intact blood circulation, while the results shown in the lower left panel were made during total occlusion of circulation in the right arm by means of an inflated pressure cuff placed around the upper arm. The time of occlusion is indicated. The IR-thermogram on the left was taken just prior to the end of the heating period in the experiment described in the upper panel. The location of the temperature measurement sites on the hand (4 spot measurements [Spot 1–Spot 4] and the average temperature within a circle [Area 5 and Area 6]) are indicated on the thermogram.

than a single point measurement. Various points or areas of interest can be investigated during and after the experimental procedures. Modern digital image processing software provides endless possibilities, especially with systems allowing the recording of sequential IR-images. Today modern fire-wire technology permits one to record IR-images at very high frequencies (100 Hz and greater).

21.6.3 Median Nerve Block in the Hand (Example 21.3)

The nervous supply to the hand is via three main nerves: radial, ulnar, and median nerve. The approximate distribution of the sensory innervation by these nerves is shown in Figure 21.3a. With a sudden removal (or disruption) of the sympathetic discharge to one of the main nerves, a maximal vasodilatation of blood vessels in the area supplied by the nerve is observed. Such a vasodilatation will result in a significant increase in skin blood flow to that area and therefore in a rise in skin temperature. The IR-thermogram in Figure 21.3b shows such a response. The subject is a 40-year-old female suffering from excessive sweating in the palms of her hands, a condition known as hyperhidrosis palmaris. Excessive sweating causes cooling of the skin surface. The blue color in Figure 21.3b represents areas of excessive sweating as well as areas of lowest skin temperature. Hyperhidrosis palmaris is treated by subcutaneous injections of Botulinum Toxin. The skin in the palm of the hand is very sensitive and anesthesia is therefore required. A very effective way to provide adequate anesthesia is the median nerve block. At the level of the wrist, a local anesthetic is injected around the median nerve and blocks the nervous activity in the median nerve.

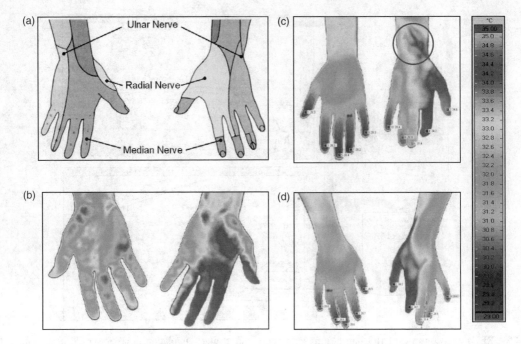

FIGURE 21.3 (See color insert.) (a) The distribution of cutaneous nerves to the hand. (b) IR-thermogram of a 40-year-old female patient following a successful nerve block of the left median nerve. (c) and (d) IR-thermograms of the hands of a 36-year-old female patient whose left wrist (middle of the red circle) was punctured with a sharp object resulting in partial nerve damage (motor and sensory loss). The strong vasodilatory response resulting from partially severed nerves can be easily seen.

The resulting increase in skin temperature on the palmar side of the left hand after such an injection is clearly seen in Figure 21.3b. One sees that part of the thumb and half of the fourth finger show no increase in temperature, closely matching the predicted area of distribution for this nerve in Figure 21.3a. Although a median nerve block was applied to the right hand, neither vasodilatation nor a change in skin temperature was seen. The Botulinum Toxin injections on this side were painful. The placement of the anesthetic was therefore incorrect, and as a result, normal nervous activity in the right hand was observed. In Figure 21.3c,d, the thermograms show the hands of a 36-year-old female patient. Her left wrist (middle of the red circle) was punctured with a sharp object, resulting in partial nerve damage. The strong vasodilatory response, due to the nerve damage, results in an increased skin temperature as shown in Figure 21.3d.

The diagnosis of acute nerve damage can be a challenge for a surgeon. In the acute situation, pain makes a proper physical examination often impossible. To evaluate the extent of the nerve injury, cooperation of the patient is necessary and the use of local anesthesia can mask the extent of the injury. IR-thermography proves to be a helpful, noninvasive diagnostic tool by visualizing changes in skin temperature and, indirectly blood flow to the skin, due to the nerve injury.

21.6.4 Infrared-Thermography and Laser Doppler Mapping of Skin Blood Flow (Example 21.4)

As mentioned in the introduction above, one of the drawbacks of using IR-thermography to indirectly indicate changes in skin blood flow is being able to decide, for example, if an increase in skin temperature is due to a parallel increase in skin blood flow. One way to verify whether observed skin temperature changes are related to changes in skin blood flow is to combine IR-thermography with a more direct measurement technique of skin blood flow. Laser Doppler can ascertain the direction of skin blood flow

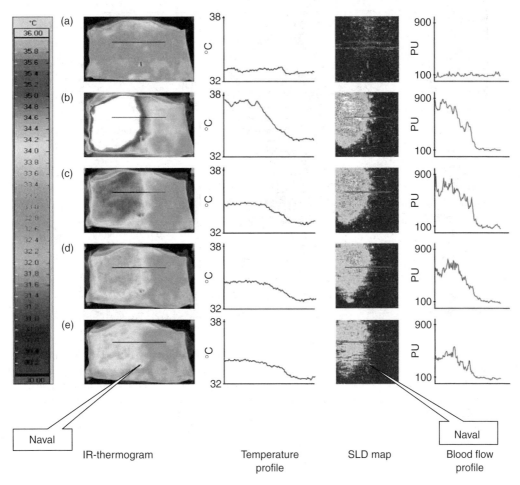

IR-thermogram   Temperature profile   SLD map   Blood flow profile

FIGURE 21.4 (See color insert.) IR-thermograms, temperature profiles, scanning laser Doppler scans (SLD), and blood flow profiles (perfusion units PU) of the abdominal area of a 44-year-old healthy female subject before (a), immediately after (b), and 5 min (c), 10 min (d) and 20 min (e) after a 20 min heating of the right side of the abdomen with a water-filtered infrared-A irradiation lamp. The blue horizontal lines in the IR-thermograms indicate the position of the temperature profiles.The red horizontal lines in the SLD scans indicate the position of the blood flow profiles. In IR-thermogram (b) the white color indicates skin temperatures greater than 36°C.

but these measurements are restricted to small surfaces and blood flow is not quantified but reported as changes in Doppler units or volts [45]. With IR-thermography rapid changes in skin temperature over a large area can be easily measured. Laser-Doppler mapping involves a scanning technique using a lower power laser beam in a raster pattern and requires time to complete a scan (up to minutes depending on the size of the scanned area). During the time it takes to complete a scan it is possible that the skin blood flow has changed in the skin area examined at the start compared to the skin area being examined at the end of each scan. This is most likely to happen in dynamic situations where skin blood flow is rapidly changing. Despite this draw back, the use of IR-thermography and laser Doppler mapping can provide a complimentary investigative view of this dynamic process.

In Figure 21.4, both IR-thermography and scanning laser Doppler mapping have been simultaneously used to examine a healthy 44-year-old female subject. In this experiment the subject was submitted to a 20 min heating of the right side of the abdomen using a water filtered IR-A irradiation lamp (see Section 21.6.1). During the period of heating, the left side of the abdomen was covered with a drape to prevent this side of the body from being heated. At predetermined intervals prior to, during, and

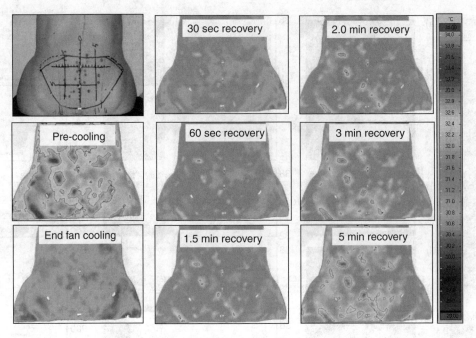

FIGURE 21.5 (See color insert.) Abdominal cooling in a 32-year-old female patient prior to breast reconstruction surgery. In this procedure skin and fat tissue from the abdominal area was used to reconstruct a new breast. The localization of suitable perforating vessels for reconnection to the mammary artery is an important part of the surgical procedure. In this sequence of thermograms the patient was first subjected to a mild cooling of the abdominal skin (2 min fan cooling). IR-thermograms of the skin over the entire abdominal area were taken prior to, immediately after, and at various time intervals during the recovery period following the cooling period. To help highlight the perforating vessels, an outline function has been employed in which all skin areas having a temperature greater than 32.5°C are enclosed in solid lines.

after the heating period both IR-thermal images and laser Doppler mapping images were recorded, the latter with a MoorLDI™ laser Doppler imager (LDI-1), Moor Instruments, England. As can be seen in Figure 21.5, the wIRA heating lamp causes a large increase in skin temperature on the irradiated side of the abdomen. After the end of the heating period, the temperature of the heated area gradually decreases. These changes nicely correspond with the laser Doppler mapping images. A semi quantitative value of blood flow (perfusion units) for each LDI image was also calculated (right panels in Figure 21.5). Each blood flow profile corresponds well with their respective temperature profiles.

21.6.5 Use of Dynamic IR-Thermography to Highlight Perforating Vessels (Example 21.5)

The procedure of dynamic thermography involves promoting changes in skin blood flow by local heating or cooling. In the example shown in Figure 21.5, a mild cooling (2 min period of fan cooling) of the skin overlying the abdominal area of a 36-year-old female patient prior to undergoing breast reconstruction surgery was performed in order to highlight perforating blood vessels [41]. These blood vessels originate in deeper lying tissue and course their way toward the skin surface, although they may not necessarily reach the skin surface. By invoking a local cooling, a temporary vasoconstrictor response is initiated in skin blood vessels. Blood flow in the perforating blood vessels is little affected and following the end of the cooling period they rapidly contribute to the skin rewarming. During the rewarming process the localization of the "hot-spots" caused by these perforating vessels becomes more diffuse as heat from them spreads into neighboring tissue. This technique allows one to more easily identify so-called perforator vessels of the medial and lateral branches of the deep inferior epigastric artery, one or more of which will be selected for reconnection to the internal mammary artery (the usual recipient vessel) during reconstruction of a new breast from this abdominal tissue.

21.6.6 Reperfusion of Transplanted Tissue (Example 21.6)

With the development of microvascular surgery it has become possible to connect (anastomose) blood r. Transplantation of tissue from one place to another on) or from one individual to another (allologous e. The technique requires high surgical skills. During letely severed and the blood vessels to the transplant ent blood vessels will supply blood to the transplant own example of allologous transplantation. Here, a kidney to provide normal renal function. Nowadays, in trauma surgery and cancer surgery. The successful for its survival. A nonsuccessful operation causes inefficient use of resources stress. IR-thermography r monitoring the reperfusion status of transplanted

t of the overall care plan for patients faced with a removal of the breast. The deep inferior epigastric ologous breast reconstruction today. The technique or reconstruction of a new breast (Figure 21.6). The pplied by many blood vessels. By using this tissue , the blood supply to this tissue is reduced to one to 1.5 mm. A critical period during the operative flap to the recipient vessels. The blood vessels of nmary vessels to provide blood supply to the flap. is dependent on the viability of the microvascular Figure 21.6 were taken at various time intervals after undergoing autologous breast reconstruction with a

) with no blood supply to the dissected flap, and as rming of the flap after anastomoses to the recipient ion on the blood circulation in the transplanted flap. nosis, the rewarming response was found to be rapid g response often made an extra venous anastomosis common problem). In such cases, IR-thermography provides an excellent method to quickly verify improvement in the blood flow status in the flap. In addition, in the days following surgery, examination of the skin temperatures using IR-thermography of the newly reconstructed breast was found to be a quick and easy way to monitor its blood flow status. The peripheral areas of the new breast can suffer from diminished blood circulation. Improvement in blood circulation could be seen during post surgery.

21.6.7 Sports Medicine Injury (Example 21.7)

Thermal images of an injury sustained by an 18-year-old American football player after a helmet impacted the superior portion of his right shoulder. X-ray and MRI immediately post game showed no structural damage. IR images were taken 12 h post injury in a controlled environment (22°C, 30% rh, after 20 min equilibration). Upon examination, the athlete was unable to lift his right arm above shoulder level. Note the disruption in the thermal pattern in the right side torso view (T4 spinal region on left side of image)

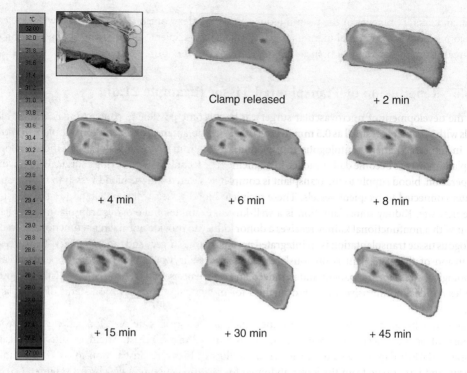

FIGURE 21.6 (See color insert.) Infrared thermal images of an abdominal skin flap during breast reconstruction surgery. The sequence of IR-thermal images demonstrates the return of heat to the excised skin flap following reestablishing its blood supply (anastomizing of a mammary artery and vein to a single branch of the deep inferior epigastric artery and a concomitant vein). Prior to this procedure the excised skin flap had been without a blood supply for about 50 min and consequently cooled down. The photograph in the upper left panel shows the skin flap in position on the chest wall prior to being shaped into a new breast.

and the very cold temperatures and pattern extending down the left arm. After 3 weeks of rehabilitation, the weakness experienced in the shoulder and arm was resolved. IR imaging confirmed a return to normal symmetrical thermal pattern in the back torso and warmer arm temperatures.

21.6.8 Conclusions

As pointed out in the introduction to this section the main objective of this article is to try and persuade those who are not familiar with IR-thermography that this technology can provide objective data, which makes clinical sense. The reader has to be aware that the examples presented above only represent a tiny fraction of the possibilities that this technology provides. It is important to realize that an IR-thermal image of a skin area under examination will more often not provide the examiner with a satisfactory result. It is important to keep in mind that blood flow is a very dynamic event and in many situations useful clinical information can only be obtained by manipulating skin blood flow, for example by local cooling. Thus, the need to have a basic understanding of the physiological mechanisms behind the control of skin blood flow cannot be overemphasized. One also has to realize that this technology should be thought of as an aid to making a clinical diagnosis and in many cases should, if possible, be combined with other complementary techniques. For example, IR-thermography does not have the ability to pinpoint the location of a tumor in the breast. Consequently, IR-thermography's role is in addition to mammography, ultrasound and physical examination, not in lieu of. IR-thermography does not replace mammography and mammography does not replace IR-thermography, the tests complement each other.

12 h post injury   Post 3 weeks rehabilitation

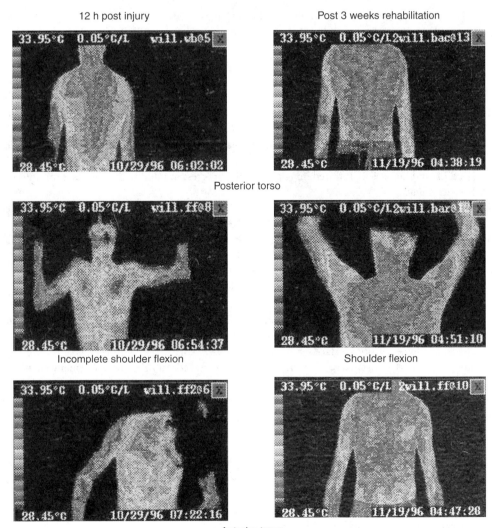

Posterior torso

Incomplete shoulder flexion   Shoulder flexion

Anterior torso

FIGURE 21.7   (See color insert.) An American football player who suffered a helmet impact to the right shoulder (left side of image). The athlete was unable to flex his arm above shoulder level. Note the asymmetrical torso pattern in the posterior torso.

Acknowledgments

Examples of IR images from patients and volunteers (Figure 21.1, Figure 21.2b, Figure 21.3 to Figure 21.7) from the Department of Medical Physiology, Faculty of Medicine, University of Tromsø, Norway and the Department of Clinical Physiology, Hillerød Hospital, Hillerød, Denmark. The IR images in these examples were taken using two different IR-cameras: A Nikon Laird S270 cooled camera and a FLIR ThermaCAM® PM695 uncooled bolometer. The respective image analysis software used was ThermaCAM researcher ver. 2.1 and PicWin-IRIS, (EBS Systemtechnik GmbH, Munich, Germany). The studies described in Example 21.1 and Example 21.2 were carried out at the Department of Clinical Physiology, Hillerød Hospital, Hillerød, Denmark in collaboration with consultant Dr Stig Pors Nielsen. The assistance of Master student Lise Bøe Setså in the studies described in Example 21.5 and Example 21.6 is also acknowledged. Examples of IR images (Figure 21.2a and Figure 21.8) come from the Thermal Lab,

Auburn University, Alabama, United States, utilizing a Computerized Thermal Imager 2000. We would like to acknowledge the assistance of JohnEric Smith and Estevam Strecker in these projects.

References

[1] Jones B.F. and Plassmann P. Digital infrared thermal imaging of human skin. *IEEE Eng. Med. Biol.* 21, 41–48, 2002.

[2] Otsuka K., Okada S., Hassan M., and Togawa T. Imaging of skin thermal properties with estimation of ambient radiation temperature. *IEEE Eng. Med. Biol.* 21, 65–71, 2002.

[3] Head J.F. and Elliott R.L. Infrared imaging: making progress in fulfilling its medical promise. *IEEE Eng. Med. Biol.* 21, 80–85, 2002.

[4] Park J.Y., Kim S.D., Kim S.H., Lim D.J., and Cho T.H. The role of thermography in clinical practice: review of the literature. *Thermol. Int.* 13, 77–78, 2003.

[5] Ammer K. Thermology 2003 — a computer-assisted literature survey with a focus on nonmedical applications of thermal imaging. *Thermol. Int.* 14, 5–36, 2004.

[6] Abernathy M. and Abernathy T.B. *International Bibliography of Medical Thermology.* Vol. 2, Washington DC, American College of Thermology, Georgetown University Medical Center, 1987.

[7] Pascoe D.D., Bellinger T.A., and McCluskey B.S. Clothing and exercise II: influence of clothing during exercise/work in environmental extremes. *Sports Med.* 18, 94–108, 1994.

[8] Flesch, U. Physics of skin-surface temperature. In *Thermology Methods.* Engel J.M., Flesch U., and Stüttgen G. (eds), translated by Biederman–Thorson M.A. Federal Republic of Germany Weinheim, pp. 21–37, 1985.

[9] Pennes H.H. Analysis of tissue and arterial blood temperatures in resting human forearm. *J. Appl. Physiol.* 1, 93–102, 1948.

[10] Charkoudian N. Skin blood flow in adult thermoregulation: how it works, when it does not, and why. *Mayo Clin. Proc.* 78, 603–612, 2003.

[11] Greenfield A.D.M. The circulation through the skin. In *Handbook of Physiology — Circulation.* Hamilton W.P. (ed.), Washington DC, American Physiological Society, Sec. 3, Vol. 2 (Chapter 39), pp. 1325–1351, 1963.

[12] Johnson J.M., Brenglemann G.L., Hales J.R.S., Vanhoutte M., and Wenger C.B. Regulation of the cutaneous circulation. *Fed. Proc.* 45, 2841–2850, 1986.

[13] Johnson J.M. and Proppe D.W. Cardiovascular adjustments to heat stress. In *Handbook of Physiology — Environmental Physiology.* Fregly M.J. and Blatteis C.M. (eds), Oxford, Oxford University Press/American Physiological Society, pp. 215–243, 1996.

[14] Rowell L.B. Human cardiovascular adjustments to exercise and thermal stress. *Physiol. Rev.* 54, 75–159, 1974.

[15] Rowell L.B. Cardiovascular adjustments in thermal stress. In *Handbook of Physiology. Section 2 Cardiovascular System, Vol. 3 Peripheral Circulation and ORgan Flow,* J.T. Shepard and F.M. Abboud (Eds), Bethesda MD, American Physiological Society, pp. 967–1024, 1983.

[16] Rowell L.B. *Human Circulation: Regulation During Physiological Stress.* New York, Oxford University Press, 1986.

[17] Sawka M.N. and Wenger C.B. Physiological responses to acute exercise–heat stress. In *Human Performance Physiology and Environmental Medicine at Terrestrial Extremes.* Pandolf K.B., Sawka M.N., and Gonzales R.R. (eds), Indianapolis, IN, Benchmark Press, pp. 97–151, 1988.

[18] Johnson J.M. Circulation to the skin. In *Textbook of Physiology.* Patton H.D., Fuchs A.F., Hille B., Scher A.M., and Steiner R. (eds), Philadelphia, W.B. Saunders Co. Vol. 2, (Chapter 45), 1989.

[19] Johnson J.M. Exercise and the cutaneous circulation. *Exercise Sports Sci. Rev.,* 20, 59–97, 1992.

[20] Garrison F.H. *Contributions to the History of Medicine.* New York, Hafner Publishing Co., Inc., p. 311, 1966.

[21] Kirsh K.A. Physiology of skin-surface temperature. In *Thermology Methods*. Engel J.M., Flesch U., and Stüttgen G. (eds), translated by Biederman–Thorson M.A., Federal Republic of Germany/Weinheim, pp. 1–9, 1985.

[22] Roberts M.P., Wenger C.B., Stölwik, and Nadel E.R. Skin blood flow and sweating changes following exercise training and heat acclimation. *J. Appl. Physiol.* 43, 133–137, 1977.

[23] Stephenson L.A. and Kolka M.A. Menstrual cycle phase and time of day alter reference signal controlling arm blood flow and sweating. *Am. J. Physiol.* 249, R186–R192, 1985.

[24] Aoki K., Stephens D.P., and Johnson J.M. Diurnal variations in cutaneous vasodilator and vasoconstrictor systems during heat stress. *Am. J. Physiol. Regul. Integr. Comp. Physiol.* 281, R591–R595, 2001.

[25] Rodie I.C., Shepard J.T., and Whelan R.F. Evidence from venous oxygen saturation that the increase in arm blood flow during body heating is confined to the skin *J. Physiol.* 134, 444–450, 1956.

[26] Gaskell P. Are there sympathetic vasodilator nerves in the vessels of the hands? *J. Physiol.* 131, 647–656, 1956.

[27] Fox R.H. and Edholm O.G. Nervous control of the cutaneous circulation. *J. Appl. Physiol.* 57, 1688–1695, 1984.

[28] Ring E.E.J. Cold stress testing in the hand. In *The Thermal Image in Medicine and Biology*. Ammer K. and Ring E.E.J. (eds), Wein, Uhlen-Verlag, pp. 237–240, 1995.

[29] Pascoe D., Purohit R., Shanley L.A., and Herrick R.T. Pre and post operative thermographic evaluations of CTS. In *The Thermal Image in Medicine and Biology*. Ammer K. and Ring E.E.J. (eds), Wein, Uhlen-Verlag, pp. 188–190, 1995.

[30] Faithfull N.S., Reinhold P.R., van den Berg A.P., van Roon G.C., Van der Zee J., and Wike-Hooley J.L. Cardiovascular challenges during whole body hyperthermia treatment of advanced malignancy. *Eur. J. Appl. Physiol.* 53, 274–281, 1984.

[31] Finberg J.P.M., Katz M., Gazit H., and Berlyne G.M. Plasma rennin activity after acute heat exposure in non-acclimatized and naturally acclimatized man. *J. Appl. Physiol.* 36, 519–523, 1974.

[32] Carlsen A., Gustafson A., and Werko L. Hemodynamic influence of warm and dry environment in man with and without rheumatic heart disease. *Acta Med. Scand.* 169, 411–417, 1961.

[33] Damato A.N., Lau S.H., Stein E., Haft J.I., Kosowsky B., and Cohen S.J. Cardiovascular response to acute thermal stress (hot dry environment) in unacclimatized normal subjects. *Am. Heart J.* 76, 769–774, 1968.

[34] Sancetta S.M., Kramer J., and Husni E. The effects of "dry" heat on the circulation of man. I. General hemodynamics. *Am. Heart J.* 56, 212–221, 1958.

[35] Crandall C.G., Johnson J.M., Kosiba W.A., and Kellogg D.L. Jr. Baroreceptor control of the cutaneous active vasodilator system. *J. Appl. Physiol.* 81, 2192–2198, 1996.

[36] Kellogg D.L. Jr, Johnson J.M., and Kosiba, W.A. Baroreflex control of the cutaneous active vasodilator system in humans. *Cir. Res.* 66, 1420–1426, 1990.

[37] Chato J.C. A view of the history of heat transfer in bioengineering. In *Advances in Heat Transfer*. Cho Y.J. (Ed.), Academic Press, Inc/Harcourt Brace Jovanovich Publishers, Boston, Vol. 22, pp. 1–19, May 1981.

[38] Chen M.M. and Holmes K.R. Microvascular contributions in tissue heat transfer. In *Thermal Characteristics of Tumors: Applications in Detection and Treatment*. Jain R.K. and Guillino P.M. (eds), *Ann. N.Y. Acad Sci.* 335, 137, 1980.

[39] Baish J.W. Microvascular heat transfer. In *The Biomedical Engineering Handbook*. Bronzino J.D. (ed.), Boca Raton, FL, CRC Press/IEEE Press, Vol. 2, 98, pp. 1–14, 2000.

[40] Hille B. Membranes and ions: introduction to physiology of excitable cells. In *Textbook of Physiology*. Patton H.D., Fuchs A.F., Hille B., Scher A.M. and Steiner R. (eds), Philadelphia, W.B. Saunders Co., pp. 2–4, 1989.

[41] Taylor G.I. and Tempest M.N. (eds), *Michael Salmon: Arteries of the Skin*. London, Churchill Livingstone, 1988.

[42] He S. and Walls A.F. Human mast cell trypase: a stimulus of micorvascular leakage and mast cell activation. *Eur. J. Pharmacol.* 328, 89–97, 1997.

[43] Kalmolz L.P., Haslik A.H., Donner A., Winter W., Meissl G., and Frey M. Indocyanine green video angiographics help identify burns requiring operating. *Burns* 29, 785–791, 2003.

[44] Flock S.T. and Jacques S.L. Thermal damage of blood vessels in a rat skin-flap window chamber using indocyanine green and pulsated alexandrite laser: a feasibility study. *Lasers Med. Sci.* 8, 185–196, 1993.

[45] Ryan T.J., Jolles B., and Holti G. *Methods in Microcirculation Studies.* London, HK Lewis and Co., Ltd, 1972.

[46] Olsen B.W. How many sites are necessary to estimate a mean skin temperature? In *Thermal Physiology.* Hales J.R.S. (ed.), New York, Raven Press, pp. 33–38, 1984.

22

Quantitative Active Dynamic Thermal IR-Imaging and Thermal Tomography in Medical Diagnostics

22.1 Introduction... **22**-1
    Thermal Tomography
22.2 Thermal Properties of Biological Tissues **22**-3
22.3 Thermal Models and Equivalent/Synthetic Parameters **22**-7
22.4 Measurement Procedures **22**-8
22.5 Measurement Equipment **22**-11
22.6 Procedures of Data and Image Processing **22**-12
    Pulsed Thermography • Active Dynamic Thermal
    IR-Imaging • Pulse Phase Thermography • Thermal
    Tomography
22.7 Experiments and Applications **22**-17
    Organization of Experiments • Results and Discussion •
    Skin Burns • Clinics • Cardiac Surgery • Clinics
22.8 Conclusions **22**-25
Acknowledgments... **22**-27
References **22**-27

Antoni Nowakowski
Gdansk University of Technology

22.1 Introduction

Static infrared (IR) thermal imaging has a number of attractive properties for its practical applications in industry and medicine. The technique is noninvasive and harmless as there is no direct contact of the diagnostic tool to an object under test, the data acquisition is simple and the equipment is transportable and well adapted to mass screening applications. There are also some fundamental limitations concerning this technique. Only processes characterized by changes in temperature distribution on external surfaces directly accessible by an IR camera can be observed. The absolute value of temperature measurement is usually not very accurate due to generally limited knowledge of the emission coefficient. Many harmful processes are not inducting any changes in surface temperature, for example, in industrial applications material corrosion or cracks are usually not visible in IR thermographs, in medicine in mammography inspection a cyst may mask cancer, etc. For such cases active dynamic thermal imaging methods with sources of external excitations are helpful. Therefore the nondestructive evaluation (NDE) of materials using active dynamic thermal IR-imaging is extensively studied; see, for example, proceedings of QIRT [1]. The method is already well developed in some of industrial applications but in medicine this technique is almost unknown.

Active dynamic thermal (ADT) IR-imaging, known in industry either as *infrared-nondestructive testing* (IR-NDT), or as thermographic nondestructive testing (TNDT or just NDT), is under intensive development during at least the last 20 years [1,2]. The concept of material testing by active thermography is based on delivery of external energy to a specimen and observation of the thermal response. In ADT imaging only thermal transients are studied. Such approach allows visualization of material subsurface abnormalities or failures and has already gained high recognition in technical applications [1,2]. In medicine it was applied probably for the first time also around 20 years ago [3,4]. Microwave excitation was applied to evidence breast cancer. Unfortunately, after early experiments the research was suspended, probably due to poor control of microwave energy dissipation. Again some proposals to use ADT in medicine have been published at the end of the last years of the 20th century [5–7].

The visualization of affected regions needs some extra efforts therefore the role and practical importance of the use of synthetic pictures in ADT for medical applications should be underlined [8–10]. In this case equivalent thermal model parameters are defined and calculated for objective quantitative data visualization and evaluation.

Potential role of medical applications of ADT is clearly visible from experiments on phantoms, and *in vivo* on animals as well as in clinical applications [11,12].

22.1.1 Thermal Tomography

Another concept based on ADT is *thermal tomography* (TT). Vavilow et al. [13–15] dealing with IR-NDT, proposed this term almost 20 years ago. Even today, the concept is not new this modality may be regarded as being still at the early development stage in technical applications, especially taking into account the limited number of practical applications published up to now. The first proposals to apply the concept of thermal tomography in medicine are just under intensive development in the Department of Biomedical Engineering TUG [16–18]. The main differences comparing TT to simple ADT arise due to necessity of advanced reconstruction procedures applied for determination of internal structure of tested objects.

Tomography is known in medical diagnostics as the most advanced technology for visualization of tested object internal structures. X-rays — CT (computed tomography), NMR — MRI (nuclear magnetic resonance imaging), US — ultrasound imaging, SPECT (single-photon emission computed tomography), PET (positron-emission tomography) are the modalities of already established position in medical diagnostics. There are three additional tomography modalities, still in the phase of intensive research and development — optical tomography (OT), electroimpedance tomography (EIT), and TT. Here we concentrate our notice on ADT and TT. The aim of this chapter is discussion of potential applications of the both modalities in medical diagnostics and analysis of existing limitations.

General concept of tomography requires collection of data received in so-called projections — measurements performed for a specific direction of applied excitation; data from all projections form a scan. Having a model of a tested object the inverse problem is solved showing internal structure of the object. In the oldest tomographic modality — CT — the measurement procedure requires irradiation of a tested object from different directions (projections), all possible projections giving one scan. Then, basing on realistic model of a tested object, a reconstruction procedure based on solving the inverse problem allows visualization of external structure of the object. In early systems, a 2D picture of internal organs was shown; nowadays more complex acquisition systems allow visualization of 3D cases. More or less similar procedures are applied in all other tomography modalities, including TT, OT, and EIT. The main advantages of TT, OT, and EIT technologies are fully safe interaction with tested objects (organisms) and relatively low cost of instrumentation.

The concept and problems of validity in medical diagnostics of ADT imaging as well as of TT are here discussed. In both cases practically the same instrumentation is applied and only the data treatment and object reconstruction differs. Also, the sources of errors influencing quality of measurements and limiting accuracy of reconstruction data are the same. Main limitations are due to the necessity of using proper thermal models of living tissues, which are influenced by physiological processes from one side and are not very accurate due to hardly controlled experiment conditions from the other side.

The main element allowing quantitative evaluation of tested objects is the use of realistic thermal equivalent models. The measurement procedure requires use of heat sources, which should be applied to the object under test (OUT). Thermal response at the surface of OUT to external excitation is recorded using IR camera. Usually the natural recovery to initial conditions gives reliable data for further analysis. The dynamic response recorded as a series of IR pictures allows reconstruction of properties of the OUT equivalent thermal model. Either thermal properties of the model elements (for defined structure of OUT) or the internal structure (for known material thermal properties) may be determined and recognized. The main problem is correlation of thermal and physiological properties of living tissues, which may strongly differ for *ex vivo* and *in vivo* data. Practical measurement results from phantoms and *in vivo* animal experiments as well as from clinical applications of ADT performed in the Department of Biomedical Engineering Gdansk University of Technology (TUG), Poland and in co-operating clinics of the Medical University of Gdansk are taken into account for illustration of this chapter. The studies in this field are concentrated on applications of burns, skin transplants, cancer visualization, and open-heart surgery, evaluation and diagnostics [19–26].

In following subchapters all elements of the ADT and TT procedures are described. First, thermal tissue properties are defined. Then basic elements of thermal model construction are described. Following is description of the experiment of active dynamic thermography based on OUT excitation (pulse) and infrared recording. Finally the procedures of model identification are described basing on phantom and *in vivo* experiments. Some clinical applications illustrate practical value of the described modalities.

22.2   Thermal Properties of Biological Tissues

What is the basic difference between IR-thermography (IRT) and ADT and TT?

In IRT, main information is the absolute value of temperature, T, and distribution of thermal fields, $T(x, y)$. Therefore regions of high temperature (hot spots) or low temperature (cold spots) are determined giving usually data of important diagnostic value. Unfortunately the accuracy of temperature measurements is limited. It is mainly due to limited accuracy of IR cameras; due to limited knowledge of the emission coefficient, as individual features of living tissues may be strongly diversified; finally due to hardly controlled conditions of the environment, what may strongly influence temperature distribution at the surface and its absolute values. Additionally surface temperature does not always properly reflects complicated processes, which may exist underneath or in the tissue bulk or which may be masked by fat or other biological structures.

In ADT and TT basic thermal properties of tissues are quantitatively determined; the absolute value of temperature practically is not interesting. Only thermal flows are important. We ask the question — how fast are thermal processes? In ADT, specific equivalent parameters are defined and visualized. In TT directly either spatial distribution of thermal conductivity is of major importance or for known tissue properties the geometry of the structure is determined.

Basic thermal properties (Figures of Merit) of materials and tissues important in ADT and in TT are following:

- k — Thermal conductivity — (W m^{-1} K^{-1}), it describes ability of a material (tissue) to conduct heat in the steady state conditions
- c_p — Specific heat — (J kg^{-1} K^{-1}), describes ability of a material to store the heat energy. It is defined by the amount of heat energy necessary to raise the temperature of a unit mass by 1 K
- ρ — Density of material — (kg m^{-3})
- ρc_p — Volumetric specific heat — (J m^{-3} K^{-1})
- α — Thermal diffusivity — (m^2 sec^{-1}); is defined as

$$\alpha = \frac{k}{\rho \cdot c_p} \tag{22.1}$$

Volumetric specific heat and thermal conductivity are responsible for thermal transients described by the equation

$$\frac{\partial T}{\partial t} = \alpha \nabla^2 T \tag{22.2}$$

For one directional heat flow (what describes the case of infinite plate structures composed of uniform layers and uniformly excited at the surface) this may be rewritten in the form:

$$\frac{\partial T}{\partial t} = \frac{k}{\rho \cdot c_p} \cdot \frac{\partial^2 T}{\partial x^2} \tag{22.3}$$

Thermal diffusivity describes heat flow and is equivalent to the reciprocal of the time constant τ describing the electrical RC circuit:

$$\alpha = \frac{k}{\rho \cdot c_p} \leftrightarrow \frac{1}{\tau} = \frac{1}{RC} \tag{22.4}$$

Basing on this analogy, materials are frequently described by equivalent thermal model composed of thermal resistivity R_{th} and thermal capacity C_{th}, which are responsible for the value of the thermal time constant, τ_{th},

$$\tau_{th} = R_{th} C_{th} \tag{22.5}$$

Those are the most frequently used equivalent parameters. Determination of such parameters is easy basing on measurements of thermal transients and using fitting procedures for determination of the applied model parameters.

Additionally one may define thermal inertia as $k \cdot \rho \cdot c_p$.

Useful may be also introducing the definition of thermal effusivity β, defined as the root-square of the thermal inertia — (J m^{-2} K^{-1} sec$^{-1/2}$) or (W sec$^{1/2}$ m^{-2} K^{-1}).

$$\beta^2 = k \cdot \rho \cdot c_p \tag{22.6}$$

Importance of IRT and ADT/TT in medical diagnostics is complementary. Regions of abnormal vascularization are detected in IRT as *hot spots* in the cases of intensive metabolic processes or as *cold spots* for regions of affected vascularization or necrosis. The same places may represent higher or lower thermal conductivity, but this is not a rule. Thermal properties of tissues may differ significantly depending on the vascularization, physical structure, water content, and so on. Knowledge of thermal properties and geometry of tested objects may be used in medical diagnostics if correlation of thermal properties and specific physiological features are known. Important is character of the data allowing objective quantitative description of tissues or organs.

The main advantage of thermal tissue parameter characterization comparing to absolute temperature measurements is relatively low dependence on external conditions, for example, ambient temperature, what usually is of a great importance in IRT. The main disadvantage is still limited knowledge of thermal tissue properties and very complicated structure of biological organs. Although the first results of thermal tissue properties have been published at the end of 19th century, the main data, still broadly cited, were collected around 30 years ago [27–30]. Unfortunately, literature data of thermal tissue properties should be treated as not very reliable, because measurement conditions are not always known [31], *in vivo* and *ex vivo* data are mixed, etc. Table 22.1 illustrates this problem. Detailed description of measurement methods of biological tissue thermal parameters is given in References 18, 31, and 32.

In Table 22.2 basic thermal tissue properties — mean values of data given by different studies and for different tissues taken *in vitro* at 37°C — are collected [18].

It has to be underlined that thermal tissue properties are temperature dependent (typically around 0.2–1 %/°C). In most of ADT and TT measurements this effect may be neglected as being not significant for data interpretation, as possible temperature differences are usually limited. The differences of temperature in *in vivo* experiments may be usually neglected as not important at all. Also there is a strong influence of water content and blood perfusion, see, for example, results of Valvano et al., 1985 in Reference 33. Usually effective thermal conductivity and diffusivity are applied to overcome this problem in modeling of thermal processes. Additionally, in subtle analysis one should remember that some tissues might be anisotropic [18,31].

For mixture of N substances, each characterized by thermal conductivity $k_1, \ldots, k_N$, the effective thermal conductivity is the mean value of the volumetric content of components:

$$k_{tk} = \frac{\sum_{i=1}^{N} k_i \cdot V_i}{\sum_{i=1}^{N} V_i} = \rho_{tk} \sum_{i=1}^{N} k_i \frac{m_i}{m_{tk}} \cdot \frac{1}{\rho_i} \tag{22.7}$$

where the index tk concerns all tissue, and the index i — ith component. Analogically, one may calculate effective specific heat either as the mean value of mass components

$$c_{wtk} = \frac{\sum_{i=1}^{N} c_{wi} \cdot m_i}{\sum_{i=1}^{N} m_i} \tag{22.8}$$

TABLE 22.1 Thermal Properties of Muscle Tissue

Muscle	Conditions	Author	Thermal conductivity (W m^{-1} K^{-1})	Diffusivity (m^2 sec^{-1})
Heart	37°C	Bowman (1981)	0.492–0.562	No data
Heart	37°C	Valvano et al. (1985)	0.537	1.47×10^{-7}
Heart	5–20°C	Cooper, Trezek (1972)	No data	$1.41–1.57 \times 10^{-7}$
Heart (dog)	*In vivo*	Chen et al. (1981)	0.49	No data
Heart (dog)	37°C	Valvano et al. (1985)	0.536	1.51×10^{-7}
Heart (dog)	21°C	Bowman et al. (1974)	No data	$1.47–1.55 \times 10^{-7}$
Heart (swine)	38°C	Valvano et al. (1986)	0.533	No data
Skeletal	37°C	Bowman (1981)	0.449-0,546	No data
Skeletal (dog)	No data	Bowman et al. (1974)	No data	1.83×10^{-7}
Skeletal (cow)	30°C	Cherneeva (1956)	No data	1.25×10^{-7}
Skeletal (cow)	24–38°C	Poppendiek (1966)	0.528	No data
Skeletal (swine)	30°C	Cherneeva (1956)	No data	1.25×10^{-7}
Skeletal (ship)	21°C	Balasubramaniam, Bowman (1977)	No data	$1.51–1.67 \times 10^{-7}$

TABLE 22.2   Mean Values of Thermal Tissue Properties Taken *In Vitro*

Parameter unit of measure symbol	Density (kg m^{-3}) ρ	Thermal conductivity [W/(m K)] k	Specific heat [J/(kg K)] c	Volumetric specific heat [J/(m^3 K)] $\rho \cdot c\,(\times 10^6)$	Diffusivity (m^2 sec^{-1}) $\alpha(\times 10^{-7})$	Effusivity [J/(m^2 K sec$^{1/2}$)] β
Soft tissues						
Heart muscle	1060	0.49–0.56	3720	3.94	1.24–1.42	1390–1490
Skeletal muscle	1045	0.45–0.55	3750	3.92	1.15–1.4	1330–1470
Brain	1035	0.50–0.58	3650	3.78	1.32–1.54	1375–1480
Kidney	1050	0.51	3700	3.89	1.31	1410
Liver	1060	0.53	3500	3.71	1.27–1.43	1320–1400
Lung	1050	0.30–0.55	3100	3.26	0.92–1.69	990–1340
Eye	1020	0.59	4200	4.28	1.38	1590
Skin superficial layer	1150	0.27	3600	4.14	0.65	1060
Fat under skin	920	0.22	2600	2.39	0.92	725
Hard tissues						
Tooth-enamel	3000	0.9	720	2.16	4.17	1400
Tooth-dentine	2200	0.45	1300	2.86	1.57	1130
Cancellous bone	1990	0.4	1330	2.65	1.4–1.89	990–1150
Trabecular bone	1920	0.3	2100	4.03	0.92–1.26	1220–1430
Marrow	1000	0.22	2700	2.70	0.82	770
Fluids						
Blood; 44% HCT	1060	0.49	3600	3.82	1.28	1370
Plasma	1027	0.58	3900	4.01	1.45	1520

Source: From Hryciuk M., Ph.D. Dissertation — Investigation of layered biological object structure using thermal excitation (in Polish), *Politechnika Gdanska*, 2003. Shitzer A. and Eberhart R.C., *Heat Transfer in Medicine and Biology*, Plenum Press, 1985.

TABLE 22.3   Thermal Properties for the Equivalent Three-Component Model

Quantity unit Symbol	Density [kg/m^3] ρ	Thermal conductivity [W/(m K)] K see Reference 28		Specific heat [J/(kg K)] c_w	Specific heat (volumetric) [J/(m^{3}K)] $\rho \cdot c_w\,(\times 10^6)$
Water	1000	0.628	0.6	4200	4.2
Fat	815	0.231	0.22	2300	1.87
Proteins	1540	0.117	0.195	1090	1.68

Source: From Marks R.M. and Bartan S.P., *The Physical Nature of the Skin*, MTP Press, Boston, 1998.

or as the mean value of volumetric components

$$\rho_{tk} c_{wtk} = \frac{\sum_{i=1}^{N} \rho_i c_{wi} \cdot V_i}{\sum_{i=1}^{N} V_i} \tag{22.9}$$

Marks and Burton [34] propose a thermal model, composed of three components — water, fat, and proteins — using the values collected in the Table 22.3. Though, it was suggested that more realistic values of thermal conductivity are given by Bowman [18,28].

22.3   Thermal Models and Equivalent/Synthetic Parameters

Basic analysis of existing thermal processes in correlation with physiological processes is necessary to understand significance of thermal flows in medical diagnostics. Thermal models are very useful to study such problems. It should be underlined that ADT and TT are based on analysis of thermal models of tested objects. Solution of the so-called direct problem while external excitation (determination of temperature distribution in time and space for assumed boundary conditions and known model parameters) involves simulation of temperature distribution in defined object under test. It allows study on thermal tomography concept, simulation of heat exchange and flows using optimal excitation methods, analysis of theoretical, and practical limitations of proposed methods, etc.

Direct problems may be properly solved only for realistic thermal models. Having such a model, one can compare the results of experiments and can try to solve the reverse problem. This responds to the question — what is the distribution of thermal properties in the internal structure of a human body? Such knowledge may be directly used in clinical diagnostics if the correlation of thermal and physiological properties is high.

In biologic applications solution of the direct problem is basic to see relationship between excitation and temperature distribution at the surface of a tested object, what is a measurable quantity. This requires solution of the heat flow in 3D space. Equation 22.10, representing the general parabolic heat flow [35] describes this problem mathematically:

$$\text{div}\left(k \cdot \text{grad}\, T\right) - c_{\text{p}}\rho \frac{\partial T}{\partial t} = -q\left(P,\, t\right) \tag{22.10}$$

where T is the temperature in K; k the thermal conductivity in W m^{-1} K^{-1}, c_{p} the specific heat in J g^{-1} K^{-1}; ρ the material (tissue) density in g m^{-3}, t the time in sec, and $q(P,\, t)$ is the volumetric density of generating or dissipated power in W m^{-3}. For biologic tissues Pennes [36] defined "the biologic heat flow equation":

$$c_{\text{p}}\rho \frac{\partial T(x, y, z, t)}{\partial t} = k\nabla^2 T(x, y, z, t) + q_{\text{b}} + q_{\text{m}} + q_{\text{ex}} \tag{22.11}$$

where $T(x, y, z, t)$ is the temperature distribution at the moment t, q_{b} (W/m^3) the heat power density delivered or dissipated by blood, q_{m} the heat power density delivered by metabolism, and q_{ex} is the heat power density delivered by external sources. Solving of this equation, including all processes influencing tissue temperature, is very complicated and analytically even impossible. Generally there are three approaches in analysis and solving of heat transfers and distribution of temperature.

The first one is analytic, usually very simplified description of an object, typically using the Fourier series method. Analytical solutions of heat flows are known only for very simple structures of well-defined shapes, what usually is not the case acceptable for analysis of biological objects. The simplest solution assumes one directional flow of energy, as it is for multilayer, infinite structures, thermally uniformly excited. Distribution of temperature, if several sources exist, may be solved assuming the superposition method.

The second option is the use numerical methods, usually based on finite element method (FEM); to model more complicated structures. There are several commercial software packages broadly known and used for solving problems of heat flows, usually combining a mechanical part, including generator of a model mesh as well as modules solving specific thermal problems, for example References 37 and 38. Also general mathematical programs, as Matlab [39] or Mathematica [40], contain proper tools allowing thermal analysis. FEM methods allow solution of 3D heat flow problems in time. Functional variability of thermal properties and nonlinear parametric description of tested objects may be easy taken into consideration. Again, there are basic limitations concerning the dimension of a problem to be solved (complexity and number of model elements), which should be taken into account from the point of view of the computational costs.

The solution of the Equation 22.10 and Equation 22.11 may be given in the explicit form:

$$T_n^{i+1} = \frac{\Delta t}{\rho c_p V_n} \left[\sum_m k_{nm} T_m^i + \left(\frac{\rho c_w V_n}{\Delta t} - \sum_m k_{nm} T_m^i \right) + q_n V_n \right] \tag{22.12}$$

or in the implicit form:

$$T_n^{i+1} - T_n^i = \frac{\Delta t}{\rho c_p V_n} \left[\sum_m k_{nm} \left(T_m^{i+1} - T_n^i \right) + q_n V_n \right] \tag{22.13}$$

where i indicates moment of time, Δt is the time step, n the position in space (node number), V_n the volume of the n node, m indicates neighboring nodes, k_{nm} is thermal conductivity between the nodes n and m, T_n^i the temperature of a node at the beginning of a time step, T_n^{i+1} the temperature of a node at the end of the time step, and q_n is the power density representing generation of heat per unit volume at the nth node. Each node represents a specific part of the modeled structure defined by mass, dimensions, and physical properties. The node is assumed to be thermally uniform and isotropic. Boundary conditions may be assumed discretional, depending on real conditions of experiments to be performed (under analysis). Usually adiabatic or isothermic conditions and a value of excitation power are assumed. The boundary conditions, the value of excitation power as well as individual properties of any node may be modified with time!

In the explicit method the temperature of each node is determined at the end of the time step, taking into account the heat balance based on temperature, heat generation, and thermal properties at the beginning of the time step. Assuming neither proper time step nor model geometry may effect in lack of stable solution or poor accuracy of analysis.

In the implicit method, the increase of temperature in each node is calculated from the heat balance resulting from temperatures, heat generation, and thermal properties during the time step. The solution is stable. The duration of a time step may be modified in the adaptation procedure assuming several conditions, for example, maximum rise of temperature in any of nodes. Increase of iteration steps followed by the need of many possible modifications of parameters during iterations may lead to unacceptable rise of the computation time. Still, the mesh geometry may influence accuracy of analysis.

The numerical modeling is preferable in cases where solution of the direct problem may be sufficient, for example, in analysis of methods of investigation, because it allows easy and accurate modifications of important factors influencing measurements. The forward problem may be solved for any configuration of mesh and tissue as well as excitation parameters. Unfortunately, limited knowledge of living tissue properties is reducing possibility of using simulation methods for reliable *in vivo* case analysis.

The third approach is to build simple equivalent models of tested tissues or organs based on such synthetic parameters as thermal resistivity (conductivity) and thermal capacity. This solution, as the simplest one, seems to be the most useful practically. A medical doctor may accept relatively simple, still reliable description, based on synthetic parameters easily determined for such simple models. As an example, thermal structure of the skin may be represented by three equivalent layers described by the $R_{th}(1–3)C_{th}(1–3)$ model. Values of such simple model parameters may be relatively easily determined from experimental data using fitting procedures and well correlated to physical phenomena, for example, depth of burns. This is also probably the easiest method to be applied for solving the inverse problem and therefore the best offer for modern computer technology based diagnostic tools. Also, correlation of model parameters coefficients is not as complicated as in the case of the FEM approach.

22.4 Measurement Procedures

Study of heat transfer enables quantification of thermo-physical material properties such as thermal diffusivity or conductivity and finally detection of subsurface defects. The main drawback of thermal measurement methods is limitation in number of contact sensors distributed within a tested object or

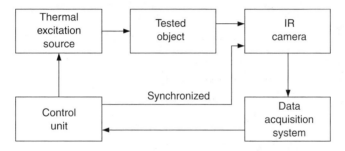

FIGURE 22.1   Schematic diagram of ADT and TT instrumentation.

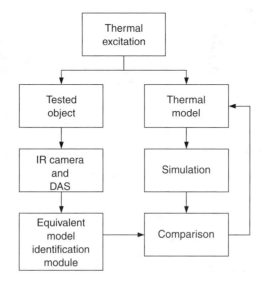

FIGURE 22.2   Model-based identification of a tested structure (object).

application of IR-methods of temperature measurements, allowing observation of the surface temperature distribution only, what in both cases results in limited accuracy of analysis.

The ADT and TT are based on IR technology. The general concept of measurements performed in such applications is shown in Figure 22.1. External thermal excitation source (heating or cooling) is applied to a tested object (TO). First, steady state temperature distribution on TO surface is registered using the IR camera. The next step requires thermal excitation application, and registration of temperature transients on the TO surface. The control unit synchronizes the processes of excitation and registration. All data are stored in the data acquisition system (DAS) for further computer analysis.

To allow quantitative evaluation of TO properties, the procedures of both, ADT and TT, are based on determination of thermal models of TO. Typical procedure of model parameter estimation is shown in Figure 22.2. For the measurement structure shown in Figure 22.1 an equivalent model of TO must be assumed (developed and applied in the procedure). In this case usually a simple model, for example, the three layers $R_{th}(1-3)C_{th}(1-3)$, is applied. Thermal excitation (from a physical source as well as simulated for the assumed model), applied simultaneously to TO and to its model, results in thermal transients, registered at the surface of TO by the IR camera (applied and simulated for the model). For each pixel, the registered temperature course is identified (typically the least square approximation — LSA and exponential model for thermal transients are applied). The result (measured thermal course) is compared with the simulated transient and if necessary the thermal model is modified to fit to experimental results.

The registration process is illustrated in Figure 22.3. An example for a pulse excitation and registration of temperature only during the recovery phase (in this case — cooling, after heating excitation) is shown.

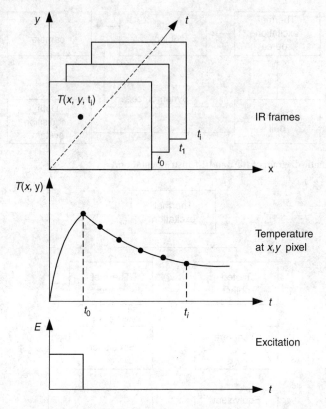

FIGURE 22.3 Registration procedure — after thermal excitation (here heating), a series of IR frames are recorded in controlled moments, starting just at the moment of switching the excitation off; temperature of each pixel is recorded to calculate time constants specific in each pixel.

This is a typical case of practical measurements using optical excitation. Each pixel showing the temperature distribution at the TO surface is represented by an equivalent model, therefore single excitation and registration of transient temperatures at the position x, y allows identification of the structure *in depth*, resulting in 3D picture of TO.

There are several procedures of nondestructive evaluation of defects by observation of temperature changes of an inspected sample surface using IR-imaging [2]:

1. Continuous heating of a tested object and observation of surface temperature changes during thermal stimulation (step heating, long pulse); the main drawback of the method is limited possibility of quantitative measurements. The information may be similar to classical static thermography with enhancement of specific defects.
2. Sinusoidal heating and synchronized observation of temperature distribution during stimulation (lock-in technique); this is the most accurate NDT-ADT method but not practical in medical applications as the experiment is rather difficult and time consuming.
3. Pulse excitation (e.g., heating using optical excitation, air fan for cooling, etc.) and observation during the heating and/or the cooling phases. Several procedures are possible, as pulsed ADT, multi-frequency binary sequences (MFBS) technique, pulse phase thermography (PPT), and other. The description in the following text is concentrating on a single pulse excitation, because this experiment is relatively simple, fast and of accuracy acceptable in medical applications. The time of excitation may be set short enough to eliminate biofeedback interactions, which are otherwise difficult in interpretation.

22.5   Measurement Equipment

Typical measurement set is shown in Figure 22.4. The main elements of the set are shown: an IR camera; a fast data acquisition system; a set of excitation sources with a synchronized driving unit.

The better are the camera properties the higher accuracy measurements are possible, what is a condition for proper reconstruction of thermal properties of TO. Minimal technical requirements for an IR camera are: repetition rate 30 frames/sec; MRTD better than 0.1°C; LW — long wavelengths range preferable; FOV dependent on application — typically in clinical conditions measurements taken from around 1 m distance to a patient are advisable. Still application of a cooled FPA camera with higher registration speed and better MRTD would be advisable. SW cameras may be used for other than optical excitations or for analysis of the recovery phase only (time when the excitation is switched off).

Very important is the use of proper excitation sources. Application of optical halogen lamps, laser sources, microwave applicators, even ultrasound generators for heating and air fans or cold sprays for cooling, and some other has been noted [41–44]. As a heating source, an optical or IR lamp, a laser beam, a microwave generator, or an ultrasonic generator can be used. Electromagnetic or mechanical irradiation generated by a source (usually distant) is illuminating a tested object and generating a heating wave proportional to the irradiation energy and to the absorption rate, specific for a tested object material and varying with wavelength of excitation. Microwave irradiation, ultrasonic excitation or electric current flow might generate heat inside a specimen proportional to its dielectric or mechanical properties. For the microwave excitation the main role in the heating process plays the electrical conductivity of a tested object. For the ultrasonic excitation the thermo-elastic effect and mechanical hysteresis are responsible for temperature changes proportional to the applied stress tensor. For the optical irradiation the absorption coefficient is describing the rate of energy converted into heat.

In ADT, the basic information is connected with time dependent reaction of tested structures therefore it is very important to know the switching properties of the heating or cooling sources, especially the raising and the falling time of generated pulses. Dynamic properties of heating or cooling sources must be taken into account during modeling the different shapes of excitation. Some extra measures should be practically adopted, for example, to avoid the interaction between a lamp, which is self-heated during experiments, and a tested object; sometimes a special shutter is needed to assure proper shape of a heating signal. For microwave excitation the applicator must be directly connected to a tested object therefore a time for mechanical removing of an applicator from the heated object to allow thermographic observation is additionally needed what practically eliminates application of such sources in medical applications.

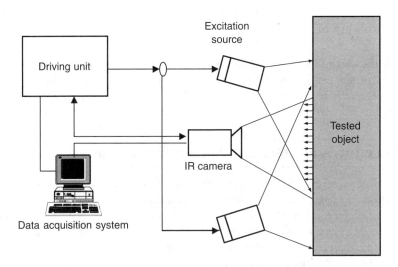

FIGURE 22.4   Measurement set — tested object is exposed to external thermal excitation; the IR camera, synchronically with excitation records, surface temperature distribution in time.

TABLE 22.4 Wavelengths and Penetration Depths of the Microwave Source 2.45 GHz for Typical Tissue with Low and High Water Content

Water content	λ — In air (cm)	λ — In tissue (cm)	σ — Tissue conductivity (S/m)	Penetration depth (cm)
High (muscle, skin)	12.2	1.76	2.21	1.70
Low (fat, bones)	12.2	5.21	0.96–2.13	11.2

Source: Duek A.F., *Physical Properties of Tissue*, Academic Press, London, 1990.

There are several conclusions regarding application of different sources of thermal excitation:

1. We are dealing with biological objects; therefore heating should be limited to a safe level, not exceeding 42°C; while cooling temperature of a living tissue should not be lower than 4°C.
2. Thermal excitation should be as uniform as possible; nonuniform excitation results in decrease of accuracy and misinterpretation of measurement data. It is relatively easy to fulfil this condition for optical excitation but very difficult for ultrasonic or microwave methods, even using specially developed applicators.
3. The other important factor is the depth of heat penetration. For different sources of excitation the energy penetration can vary from superficial only absorption to millimeters for some laser beams or even up to a few centimeters for microwave excitation. Ultrasounds are not applicable for biological tissues but of rigid structures only. As an example the data concerning microwave penetration are shown in the Table 22.4. High heat penetration may be very interesting for discrimination of deep regions; unfortunately control of microwave energy absorption practically is impossible being dependent on tissue electrical properties. This feature makes the use of microwave sources in medical applications very problematic.
4. Temperature interactions should be limited to periods not affected by biological feedback; additionally to assure proper data treatment special care should be devoted to fast switching the excitation power on and off. For optical sources mechanical shutters are advisable, as electrical switching is effective in the visible range but also other elements as, for example, housing may be heated to a level influencing sensitive IR camera.
5. Noncontact methods, as optical, seem to be especially appreciated, as septic conditions are easy to be secured.
6. Concluding — optical excitation for heating and air fan for cooling seem to be the best options for daily practice in medical diagnostics.

Even ADT is not so sensitive to external conditions as the classical IRT still there are several conditions to be assured. Generally, patients should be prepared for experiments and all "golden standards" valid for classical thermography here should be also applied [46].

22.6 Procedures of Data and Image Processing

Depending on the method of excitation several procedures may be adopted to process the measurement data and then to extract diagnostic information. Here we concentrate only on pulse excitation as is at it is shown in Figure 22.3. Measurements of transients during the heating and the cooling phases allow further use of procedures developed for pulsed thermography (PT), ADT IR-imaging, pulse phase thermography (PPT), and TT. In all four cases, excitation and registration of thermal transients is performed in the same way using IR camera. Visualization data differ as it is expressed respectively by thermal contrast images in PT; thermal time constants in ADT and phase shift images in PPT, finally thermal conductivity distribution in TT.

22.6.1 Pulsed Thermography

Pulsed thermography applies calculation of *the maximal thermal contrast index* — $C(t)$ [2].

$$C(t) = \frac{T_d(t) - T_d(0)}{T_s(t) - T_s(0)} \tag{22.14}$$

where T is the temperature, t the time; for $t = 0$ the sample temperature is maximal, d, s are the subscripts indicating the defect and the sample. With given number of temperature images acquired during PT, the thermal contrast image may be expressed also as

$$C(x, y, t) = \frac{T(x, y, t) - T(x_0, y_0, t)}{T(x_0, y_0, t)} \tag{22.15}$$

where x, y is the pixel coordinates and x_0, y_0 the pixel coordinates of the reference point in the chosen defect area.

To calculate contrast images, a defect template or a reference point should be defined. In medical applications, it is almost impossible to indicate such templates therefore to overcome this limitation estimation of the behavior of living tissues in PT conditions is possible. As an example, heat transfer caused by blood flow is different in normal and affected (e.g., cancerous) tissues. During the heating process the affected tissues usually are heated more than the normal tissues, what is caused by reduced thermoregulation. Further image processing (segmentation) allows discrimination of so-called *hot spots* and *cold spots* images. Another possibility is to define *the normalized differential PT index* (NDPTI) [47]:

$$\text{NDPTI}(x, y, t) = \frac{T(x, y, 0) - T(x, y, t)}{T(x, y, 0) + T(x, y, t)} \tag{22.16}$$

Automatic processing requires definition of thresholds, which can extract only "hot spots" or "cold spots" in the image (i.e., pixels with a value lower than the threshold will compose an image background, while pixels with a value equal or greater than the threshold will compose — "hot spots"). Because popular indexes are constructed to indicate higher probability of detected elements by a higher index value (low values — "cold spots"; high values — "hot spots") it is possible to calculate a negative NDPTI image, too.

$$\text{NPTI}(x, y, t) = 1 - \text{NDPTI}(x, y, t) = \frac{2 * T(x, y, t)}{T(x, y, 0) + T(x, y, t)} \tag{22.17}$$

The signal to noise ratio (SNR) of this technique is rather small. It can be improved by averaging images, repeating the pulse excitation with time interval long enough for proper cooling.

As an example Figure 22.5a is a photograph of the burns caused by fire. Figure 22.5b,c show fields of IIa/b degree burn evidenced at the first and the second day after the accident. The effect of treatment is also very well visible comparing the results of measurements done day by day. In the related example the burn area was small enough to avoid grafting.

(a) 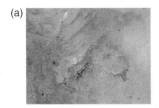 (b) 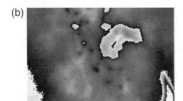 (c)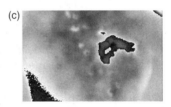

FIGURE 22.5 Patient with burn wound, first day after the accident — photograph of the burn (a), NDPTI image of the same field (b), and the NDPTI image at the second day (c)

22.6.2 Active Dynamic Thermal IR-Imaging

The ADT is based on comparison of measurements with a simple multilayer thermal model described by Equation 22.4 and Equation 22.5 giving a simplified description of parametric images of thermal time constants, which values are correlated with internal structure of tested objects [11,48]. Recorded in time thermal transients at a given pixel are described by exponential models. Here, the two exponential models are describing the process of natural cooling after switching the heating pulse off.

$$T(t) = T_{min} + \Delta T_1 e^{-t/\tau_{1c}} + \Delta T_2 e^{-t/\tau_{2c}} \tag{22.18}$$

Model based identification of a tested structure (object) is performed as it is shown in Figure 22.2. The recorded thermal response is fitted to a model. In many cases the two exponential description is fully sufficient for practical applications. As an example, typical transient in time for a single pixel (e.g., from Figure 22.5) is shown in Figure 22.6, with fitting procedure applied to one and two exponential models.

The two exponential models, as Equation 22.18, are fully sufficient for the data of accuracy available in the performed experiment. Some more pictures and examples of the ADT procedure are shown in following paragraphs, especially in skin burn evaluation [49,50]. It should be underlined that time constants for the heating phase τ_h and for the cooling phase τ_c usually are different due to different heat flow paths.

22.6.3 Pulse Phase Thermography

The procedure of PPT [2,51] is based on Fourier transform. The sequence of infrared images is obtained as in conventional PT experiments, Figure 22.7. Next, for each pixel (x, y) in every of N images the temporal evolution $g_i(t)$ is extracted and then the discrete Fourier transform is performed using the formula:

$$F_i(f) = \frac{1}{N} \sum_{n=0}^{N-1} g_i(t) \exp\left(\frac{-j2\pi f t}{N}\right) = \text{Re}_i(f) + j\text{Im}_i(f)$$

$$\varphi_i(f) = \text{atan}\left(\frac{\text{Im}_i(f)}{\text{Re}_i(f)}\right); \qquad A_i(f) = \sqrt{\text{Re}_i(f)^2 + \text{Im}_i(f)^2} \tag{22.19}$$

More valuable diagnostic information is given in the phase shift; therefore this parameter is of major interest.

Interesting characteristics of PPT are evident since it combines the speed of PT with the features of lock-in approach (the phase and the magnitude image). The condition to get reliable results is application of fast and very high quality IR cameras.

As this method was not applied in medicine, yet, we do not show any examples, but extensive discussion of the validity of the procedure may be found in Reference 51.

22.6.4 Thermal Tomography

Thermal tomography should allow tomographic visualization of 3D structures, solving the real inverse problem — find distribution of thermal conductivity inside a tested object. This attempt is fully successful in the case of skin burn evaluation [16–18], giving a powerful tool in hands of medical doctors allowing reliable quantitative evaluation of the burn depth [52–54]. Other applications are under intensive research [55–57].

In TT the first step is determination of thermal properties of a tested object, necessary for development of its thermal equivalent model, to be applied for further data treatment. A typical procedure allowing the model parameters determination is shown in Figure 22.8. The forward problem is solved and assumed model parameters are modified to satisfy a chosen criterion for model and measurement data comparison.

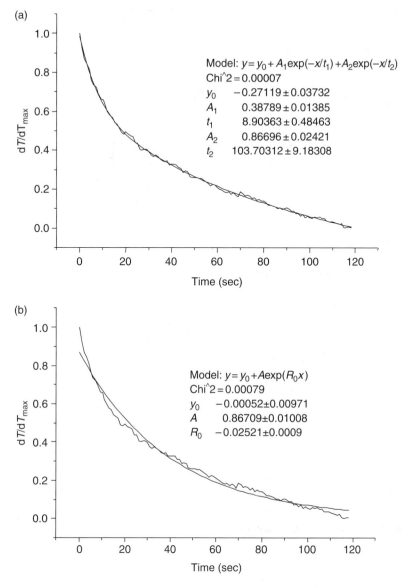

FIGURE 22.6 Fitting of the models to the measurement data — 5-parameter model (a) and 3-parameter model (b).

The second step is organization of an active dynamic thermography experiment and registration of thermal transients forced by external excitation.

The next step requires advanced calculations to solve the inverse problem. The information of the correlation of the calculated figure of merit with a specific diagnostic feature is necessary to take a proper diagnostic decision based on the performed measurements. The decision function is directed to determine the internal thermal structure of the tested object basing on thermal transients at its surface. In this case, a real inverse problem has to be solved. We perform this procedure using Matlab scripts [17,18]. As the result a multilayer structure of different thermal properties may be reconstructed. To solve this problem additional assumptions, as number of layers, values of thermal properties or dimensions, are necessary because in general the problem is mathematically ill posed and nonlinear.

The method allows, under some conditions, not only to calculate the thermal effusivity, but also to reconstruct thermal diffusivity distribution in a layered structure. It is done using the nonlinear least

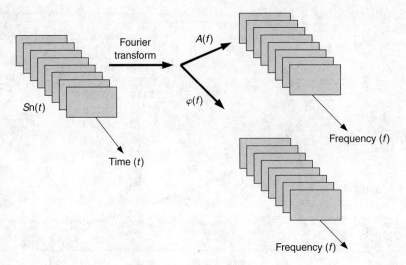

FIGURE 22.7 Procedure of calculation of synthetic pictures in PPT.

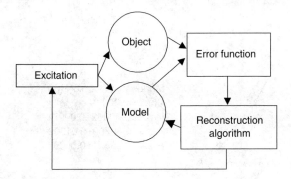

FIGURE 22.8 Determination of model parameters, based on comparison of measurement and simulation data, valid for all kind of tomography.

square optimization algorithm in inversion of direct problem:

$$\left.\begin{array}{l} T_0(x) \\ T_{exc} \\ \Phi(0, t) \\ k(0) \end{array}\right\} \implies \alpha(x) \tag{22.20}$$

where $T_0(x)$ is the initial temperature distribution in the object, T_{exc} the temperature of the heater, $\Phi(0, t)$ the heat flux at the surface, and $k(0)$ is the thermal conductivity of the outermost layer. In medical diagnostics of burn depth determination the problem is defined in a discrete form allowing determination of the parameter D, describing the depth of specific thermal properties, for example, depth of the burned tissue (the unknown parameter is local thickness of the tested object $d = D \cdot \Delta x$):

$$\left.\begin{array}{l} T_m^1, \quad m = 1 \cdots M \\ \Phi_{exc} \\ T_1^p, \quad p = 1 \cdots P \\ [k_m, \rho c_m]|_{m \leq D} = [k_{rub}, \rho c_{rub}] \\ [k_m, \rho c_m]|_{D < m < M} = [k_{air}, \rho c_{air}] \end{array}\right\} \implies D \tag{22.21}$$

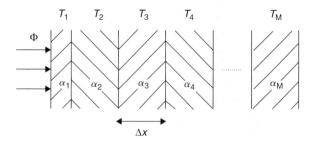

FIGURE 22.9   Spatial discretization of the properties of a multilayer object under test.

where the upper indexes describe the time domain and lower — the space domain. The inverse problem allows solution for which the direct simulation of temperature distribution is closest to the experiment results. This is by solving the problem, which is set by the goal function $F(D)$:

$$F(D) = \sum_{p=1}^{P}(T_{\text{dir}}^{p}(D) - T_{\text{meas}}^{p})^{2} \xrightarrow{D} \min \tag{22.22}$$

where T_{dir}^{p} is the surface temperature for simulation performed for assumed value of the parameter D and T_{meas}^{p} the values measured. In the following examples the Matlab *lsqnonlin* function was adopted to solve this problem basing on modified interior-reflective Newton method [18]. Description of multilayer structures is also possible and may be defined in the form illustrated in Figure 22.9 [18,54]. One directional flow of heat energy is assumed.

What should be underlined is that the TT procedure requires advanced calculations and very reliable data, both from measurements as well as for modeling. Comparing to ADT this is much more demanding method, therefore it seems that typical for ADT description using thermal time constants at present stage of development seems to be easier accepted by medical staff.

22.7   Experiments and Applications

There are three groups of study performed:

1. On phantoms, for evaluation of technical aspects of instrumentation to be applied for *in vivo* experiments
2. On animals, *in vivo* experiments, for reference data
3. Clinical, for evaluation of the practical meaning of applied procedures

As the ADT as well as TT methods are new in medical diagnostics here we show some results of animal *in vivo* experiments and a few clinical cases. Described applications concern burns diagnostics and evaluation of cardiosurgery interventions. Results of phantom experiments and some other clinical applications were described in other cited publications, for example, References 22, 26, and 43.

22.7.1   Organization of Experiments

The clinical trials are done in *the Department of Plastic Surgery and Burns Treatment*, and in *the Department of Cardiac Surgery and Cardiology* of the Medical University of Gdansk. The leading medical personnel had all necessary legal rights for carrying the experiments, approved by the local ethical commission. All clinical experiments were done during normal diagnostic or treatment procedures, as the applied PT, ADT, and TT are noninvasive, aseptic, and safe. The excess of evoked surface temperature rise is around 2 to 4°C and the observation by the IR-camera is taken from a distance of 1 m. For skin temperature

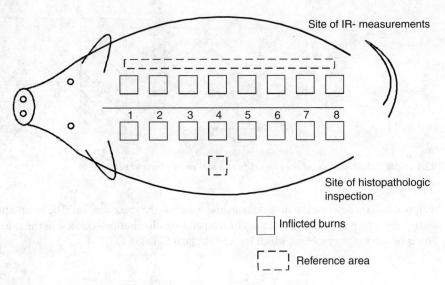

FIGURE 22.10   Location of experimental burns.

measurements illuminated area usually is kept wet using a thin layer of ointment to satisfy condition of constant evaporation from a tested surface and a constant value of emissivity coefficient. In cardiac surgery experiments with open chest, the surface of the heart is observed where the conditions of emissivity are regarded as constant. The IR-camera is located in a way not disturbing any activity of a surgeon.

The *in vivo* experiments on domestic pigs were performed in *the Department of Animal Physiology, Gdansk University*. The research program received a positive opinion of the institutional board of medical ethics. Housing and care of animals were in accordance with the national regulations concerning experiments on living animals. The choice of animals was intentional. No other animals have skin, blood, or heart properties so close to the human organs than pigs do [45]. Therefore, the experimental data carrying important medical information are of direct relationship to human organ properties.

Our burn experiments were based on the research of Singer et al. [58] and his methodology on standardized burn model. Following his experiment more than 120 paired sets of burns were inflicted on the back skin of 14 young domestic anesthetized pigs using aluminum and copper bars preheated in water in the range from 60 to 100°C. Typical distribution of burns is shown in Figure 22.10. Each pair was representing different conditions of injury giving a set of controlled burn depths. Additionally, each of measuring points was controlled by full-thickness skin biopsies and followed by histopathologic analysis of burn depth. The results of skin burn degree are in good accordance to the data given by Singer. The pigs were maintained under a surgical plane of anesthesia in conditioned environment of 24°C. The back skin was clipped before creation of burns. The total body surface area of the burns in each pig was approximately 4%. The animals were observed and treated against pain or discomfort.

After the "burns" experiment completed the same pigs were anesthetized, intubated and used for experimental myocardial infarction by closing the left descending artery. This experiment was lasting 5 h to evidence the nonreciprocal changes of the heart muscle. Full histopathology investigation was performed for objective evaluation of necrosis process.

Basic measurement set-up used in our experiments is composed of instruments shown in Figure 22.4. It is consisting the Agema 900 thermographic camera system; IR incandescent lamps of different power or a set of halogen lamps (up to 1000 W) with mechanical shutter or an air-cooling fan as thermal excitation sources; a control unit for driving the system. Additionally a specially designed meter of tissue thermal properties is used to determine the contact reference data necessary for reliable model of the skin or other tissue.

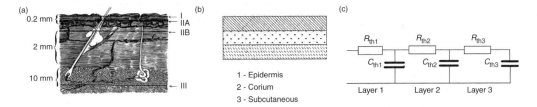

FIGURE 22.11   (a) Anatomy of the skin [59], (b) three-layer structural model, and (c) equivalent thermo-electric model.

The initial assumptions applied for reconstruction of a tested structure using ADT and TT procedures:

- Tested tissue is a 2- or 3D medium with two- or three-layer composite structure (e.g., for skin — epidermis, dermis, subcutaneous tissue); (but for simplicity and having limited performance instrumentation even one layer model may be useful for diagnostic use in tissue evaluation).
- Tissue properties are independent on its initial temperature.

For skin and under-skin tissues an equivalent three-layer thermal model was developed [11]. For the assumed model its effective parameters have been reconstructed basing on the results of transient thermal processes. For known thermal diffusivity and conductivity of specific tissues the local thickness of a two- or three-layer structure may be calculated. In the structural model, each layer should correspond to the anatomy structure of the skin (see Figure 22.11). But in the case of a well developed burn a two-layer model is sufficient as the skin is totally changed and the new structure is determined by the died burned layer and modified by injury internal structure of thermal properties drastically different comparing the pre-injury state.

22.7.2   Results and Discussion

The related results are divided into groups covering clinical measurements of skin burns and heart surgery and equivalent measurements on pigs. The animal experiments are especially valuable to show importance of the discussed methods. Such experiments assure conditions which may be regarded as reference because fully controlled interventions and objective histopathologic investigations have been performed in this case.

22.7.3   Skin Burns

22.7.3.1   *In Vivo* Experiments on Pigs

The measurements were performed approximately 0.5 h after the burn creation and were repeated after 2 and 5 h and every 24 h during 5 consecutive days after the injury. As the ADT and TT experiments are new in medicine there are several notices concerning methodology of experiments. Especially some biological factors are of high importance. The pigs are growing in extremely fast; therefore the conditions of measurements are constantly changed. Also the hairs grow anew changing the measurement conditions and cannot be clipped again as the area is affected by injury. This was especially important for direct contact measurements but was not influencing IR measurements. The position of animals in consecutive days was not always the same causing some problems with data interpretation. The results of biopsy and histopathologic observations are used as the reference data of the skin burn thickness. We indicated the same set of parameters as given by Singer, what is shown in Figure 22.12 for exemplary burns of one of the pigs. The affected thickness of skin is dependent on the temperature and time of the aluminum and copper bars application. The plots are showing relative thickness of a burn with respect to the thickness of the skin. Such normalization may be important as the skin is of different thickness along the body. All affected points have full histopathologic description. Here only one example

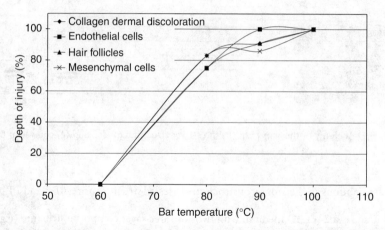

FIGURE 22.12 Relative thickness of the burned skin for several aluminum bar temperatures for time of application equal 30 sec — different indicators describing burns are listed (biopsy results).

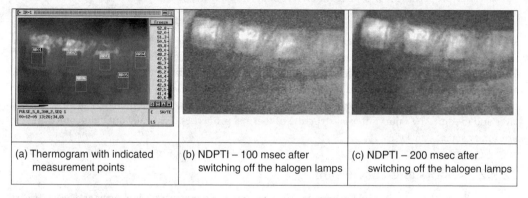

| (a) Thermogram with indicated measurement points | (b) NDPTI – 100 msec after switching off the halogen lamps | (c) NDPTI – 200 msec after switching off the halogen lamps |

FIGURE 22.13 (See color insert following page **29**-16.) Classical thermogram (a) and PT normalized differential thermography index pictures of burns (b) and (c).

is shown for points of the aluminum bar applications of different temperature but constant 30 sec time of application.

Some thermographic data of one of pigs taken 5 h after the burn injury are shown in Figure 22.13a [11]. A thermogram while heating is switched off with indicated six measurement areas is shown. Two bottom fields are uninjured reference points, four other are burns made using the aluminum bar — from the left: 100°C/30 sec; 100°C/10 sec and 90°C/30 sec; 80°C/30 sec. The set of halogen lamps was applied for PT and ADT experiment. The result of NDPTI pictures show temperature distribution 100 and 200 msec after the excitation Figure 22.13b,c. The burns are clearly visible and the relative temperature rise is very strongly correlated to the condition of the injury. For the indicated areas the mean value of temperature changes are calculated. This is shown for the first phase of cooling in Figure 22.14. The data might be fitted to thermal models giving ADT specific synthetic pictures of thermal time constants. The quality of the fitting procedure of measurement data to the equivalent model parameters is shown as an example in Figure 22.6a,b for one and two layer models.

There is a possibility to transform each of pixels into the equivalent model descriptor. In Figure 22.15a to Figure 22.15 f thermograms taken in consecutive days are transformed according to the formula $A \exp(-R_0 t)$. Distribution of the parameter — the thermal time constant — is shown.

Diagnostic importance of thermal transients is especially clearly visible in Figure 22.16 [18], where different injuries are responding differently to thermal excitation. The line mode of the IR-camera is here applied for fast data registration (>3000 scans/sec), allowing reduction of noise.

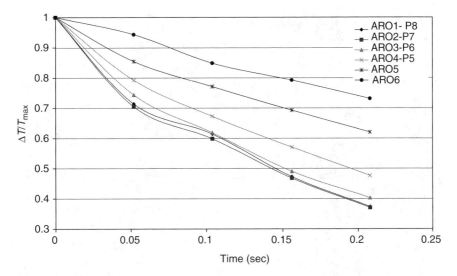

FIGURE 22.14 The normalized averaged temperature changes at the first phase after the excitation is switched off for indicated in Figure 22.13a points.

Basing on the same material TT procedure and reconstruction of thermal conductivity is also possible [18,54]. Assuming that we know the initial state of the object, the value of excitation flux, thermal response on the surface and spatial distribution of volumetric specific heat within the object it is possible to find the distribution of thermal conductivity:

$$\left.\begin{array}{l} T_m^1, m = 1, \ldots, M \\ \Phi_{exc} \\ T_1^p, p = 1, \ldots, P \\ \rho c_m, m = 1, \ldots, M \end{array}\right\} \Longrightarrow k_m, \quad m = 1, \ldots, M \tag{22.23}$$

The inverse problem defined by Equation 22.23 is highly justified due to practical reasons: the volumetric specific heat of biological tissues is much less dependent on water and fat content and other physiological factors than thermal conductivity is (especially effective thermal conductivity, which includes blood perfusion) [45]. Hence, the distribution of $\rho c(x)$ may be regarded with good approximation as known, and irregularities in thermal conductivity distribution should be searched for.

Figure 22.17 presents the results of minimization based on measurements taken during experiments with controlled degree burn fields as it was shown in Figure 22.16. The distribution of specific heat has been assumed identical with the healthy tissue, because of its low dependency on burn [18]. On the reconstructed thermal tomogram, a distinct layered structure of the skin can be seen, as well as the changes in its thermal structure caused by burns. The outermost two slices (0–0.2 mm) represent the epidermis and have thermal conductivity close to 0.3 W m^{-1} K^{-1}, which is almost not affected by burns. Fundamental changes in thermal properties induced by burns may be noticed in the next four slices (0.2–0.5 mm). From the anatomical point of view, this region represents the superficial plexus and adjacent layer of the dermis. As one can expect, for superficial burns we observe increase of k in this region, and decrease of k for severe burns. Based on this observation, quantitative classification criteria can be proposed [18].

For examination of skin burns is seems optimal to implement the expression 22.23. It allows obtaining thermal tomography images, which reflect pathologic changes in thermal conductivity distribution up to 2 to 3 mm.

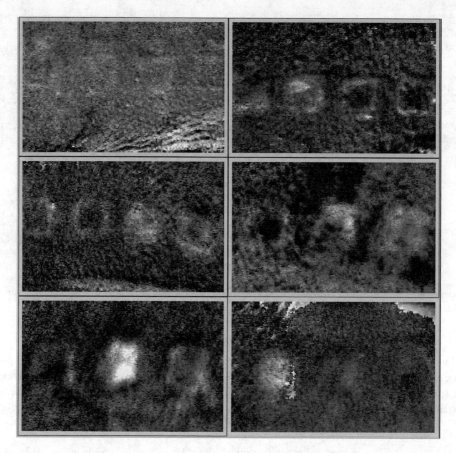

FIGURE 22.15 Thermal time constant representation for the same case as showed in Figure 22.13 and Figure 22.14 in consecutive days, starting from the moment of injury (upper left) and ending on the 5th day (bottom right). The placement of injures seems to be shifted due to different positions of the animal from day to day. Specific burn areas are easy recognizable. Additional studies are necessary for making full diagnostic medical recognition of injury, as there are two factors influencing each other — healing process and fast growth of the animal.

22.7.4 Clinics

We have examined around 100 patients with different skin injuries. Burn injuries were formed in different accidents as a result of flame action directly on skin, hands and faces, and on burning clothes, thorax. The investigations were performed during the first 5 days following an accident. To illustrate the clinical importance of the discussed methods an example of burns caused by an accident is shown in Figure 22.5. The well-determined area of the second-degree burn is evident. The next step — after rising more clinical data — will be quantitative classification based on data of the burn thickness. Long lasting effects of treatment and scars formation are still studied and not related here, yet. Already we claim that the value of the thermal time constant taken at the second day after the accident allows quantitative, objective discrimination between IIa and IIb burn [Renkielska, to be published].

22.7.5 Cardiac Surgery

22.7.5.1 *In Vivo* Experiments on Pigs

Understanding of thermal processes existing during the open chest heart operations is essential for proper surgical interventions, performed for saving the life. Experiments on pigs may be giving answers to several

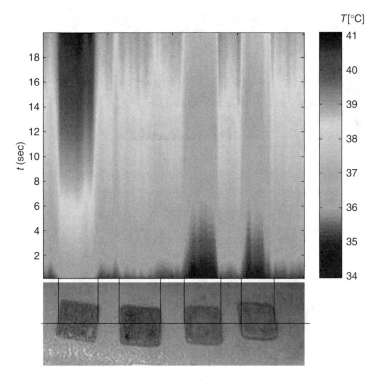

FIGURE 22.16   (See color insert.) Thermal transients of burn fields of degree: I, IIa, IIb, IIb.

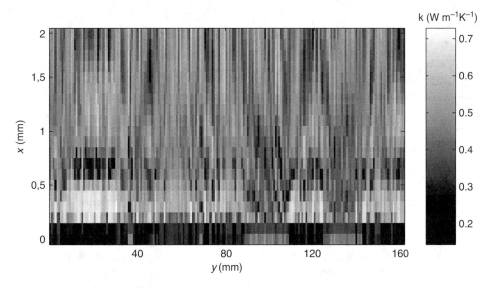

FIGURE 22.17   Results of the reconstruction of thermal conductivity distribution in burn fields.

important questions impossible to be responded in clinical situations. This especially may concern sudden heart temperature changes and proper interpretation of the causes.

Clamping the left descending artery and evoking a heart infarct performs the study. Temperature changes have been correlated with the histopathologic observations. The macroscopic thickness of the necrosis was evaluated. This was confirmed by the microscopic data. In Figure 22.18a anatomy of the

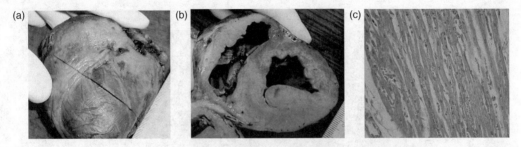

FIGURE 22.18 (See color insert.) Pig's heart after heart infarct evoked by the indicated clamp (a), the cross section of the heart with visible area of the stroke (the necrosis of the left ventricle wall — under the finger — is evidenced by darker shadow) (b) and the micro-histopathologic picture showing the cell necrosis (c).

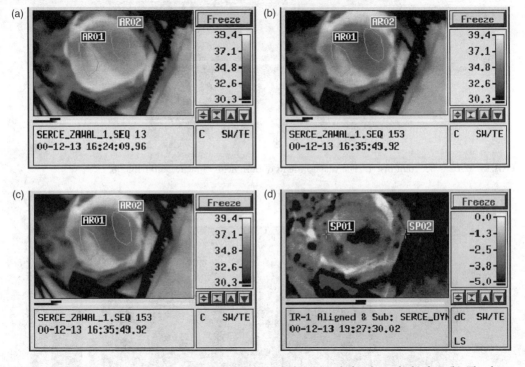

FIGURE 22.19 (See color insert.) Thermograms of the heart: before (a) and after the evoked infarct (b). The change of the PT/ADT pictures in time (indicated in the subscript of the thermogram) 0.5 h after the LAD clamping (the tissue is still alive) (c) and 3 h later (the necrosis is evidenced by the change of thermal properties of the tissue) (d).

heart with the clamp is shown. The cross-section line is visible. In the Figure 22.18b the macroscopic cross-section is shown and the evidence of tissue necrosis is by the microscopic histopathology is shown in Figure 22.18c. The widths of the left and right ventricle as well as septum were also measured. The mass of the necrosis tissue was calculated. The evident correlation between the thickness of the left and right ventricle walls and the thermographic data are found. Thermographic views of this heart are shown in Figure 22.19a,b respectively before and after application of the clamp. The left ventricle wall is cooling faster than the right one as the left ventricle wall thickness is bigger and the heating effect caused by the flowing blood (of the same temperature in both ventricles) is here weaker. The cooling process of the heart caused by stopping the blood flow in LAD is shown in Figure 22.20 — the mean temperature changes of the indicated in Figure 22.18a regions AR01 and AR02 are plotted.

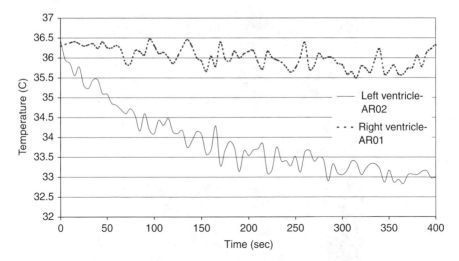

FIGURE 22.20   Temperature changes of the left and right ventricle after the LAD clamping related to Figure 22.19a,b.

The PT/ADT picture 0.5 h after the clamp was applied (Figure 22.19c) is still showing that thermal properties of the walls are unchanged even the temperature of the left ventricle wall is evidently decreased (Figure 22.19b). Progressing in time the necrosis process is changing thermal tissue properties what is clearly visible after 3 h in Figure 22.19d.

22.7.6   Clinics

Operation under extracorporeal circulation is normally a typical clinical situation. Two cases before and after CABG — coronary artery by-pass grafting — are shown for ADT in Figure 22.21a,b respectively. Areas of necrosis and of ischemia as well as volume of the healthy heart muscle were evaluated in respect to coronaroangiographic and radioisotope data showing high correlation. The observations performed before and after CABG show evident recovery of heart functioning. It is evidenced by smaller temperature rise after optical excitation of the heart in the same conditions. ADT shows the level and efficiency of revascularisation. The region of heart muscle dysfunction due to heart stroke was possible to be differentiated using both — normal thermography as well as ADT method — what leads to the conclusion that both modalities should be taken into account for diagnostics. The application of thermography for instant evaluation of the quality of the CABG intervention is prompt — the patency of the LIMA — LAD graft is unbeatable by any other method [60], but thermal tissue properties reflecting real state of the tissue is given only by ADT.

Application of all discussed modalities PT, ADT, PPT, and TT during the cardiosurgical interventions gives important indications how to improve surgical procedures.

22.8   Conclusions

The study shows that ADT as well as TT have been successfully used in medical applications giving not only qualitative improvement of diagnostics but in several applications allowing also quantitative evaluation of affected structures.

The importance of active dynamic thermal imaging and thermal tomography applied to burn evaluation and in the inspection of the open chest cardiology interventions was verified. Most probably there are also other attractive fields of medical applications of ADT and TT as, for example, cancer diagnostics [60]. ADT can by applied in medical procedures for monitoring the state of the skin and subdermal tissue structure during burns treatment giving objective, measurable ratings of the treatment procedure. The moment

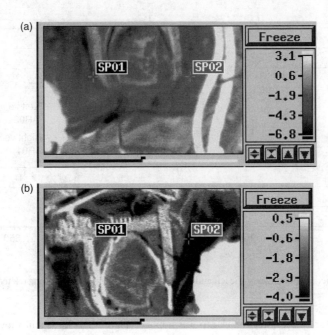

FIGURE 22.21 (See color insert.) ADT picture of clinical intervention — before the CABG (a) and after the operation (b). Important is more uniform temperature distribution after the operation proving that intervention was fully successful.

of thermal investigation after an accident is of the highest significance. The most valuable results are obtained during the first and the second days following an accident. The clinical valuable features of the method in skin burns evaluation are the early objective determination of the burn depth — up to two days after an accident and possibility of quantitative evaluation of burn surface and depth as well as objective classification of burn degree. Also, the monitoring role of the method in interoperation of cardiac protection seems to be unbeatable. Changes of tissue vascularisation are important for prediction of treatment progress. In all applications, the method is noncontact, noninvasive, clean and nonstressed, allows wide area of investigation and clear and objective documentation of diagnoses and treatment process.

The use of different excitation sources should be limited to those of the best measurement properties. Basing on the described experiments most handy are optical sources of irradiation but probably cooling may give even better results in terms of higher signal to noise ratio. The operation of such sources is safe, harmful, and easy. The distribution of light may be relatively uniform; the control of irradiated power is also easy.

The work in the field of ADT and TT is still under fast development. Important is extensive IR instrumentation progress giving radical imaging improvement. The problem to be solved is development of a method of noncontact automatic determination of basic properties of thermal parameters of affected tissue what is one of main tasks for the future. Special software is under development for objective and automatic generation of affected tissue depth maps. Important will be to find not only qualitative information but also application of quantitative measures; to describe ratings of the burn wounds or calculate the thickness of affected heart tissues. Still more experiments giving statistically significant knowledge are necessary.

One of important goals is combination of different modalities and application of automatic classification procedures for improved diagnostics. This requires some progress in standardization of IR imaging, which still is not offered in the DICOM standard. For sure, distant consultation of images and automatic data retrieval will be pushing proper work in this field.

Acknowledgments

The author thanks his co-workers and Ph.D. students, who participated in development of ADT & TT in medicine and who produced the presented data. Most of the reported *in vivo* experiments have been performed with the help of Dr M. Kaczmarek, Dr M. Hryciuk, A. Galikowski and others from the Department of Biomedical Engineering, Gdansk University of Technology. Participation of medical staff: Dr A. Renkielska and Dr J. Grudziński (from the Department of Plastic Surgery and Burns Treatment), Prof. J. Siebert (from the Department of Cardiac Surgery and Cardiology, Medical University of Gdansk) and others are highly appreciated. *In vivo* animal experiments have been performed at the Department of Animal Physiology, Gdansk University with the main assistance of Dr W. Stojek. Others are listed in the attached bibliography as coauthors of common publications. The work was supported by several grants from KBN (Polish Ministry of Science and Information).

References

[1] *Proc. Quantitative InfraRed Thermography:* Chatenay-Malabary-1992, Naples-94, Stuttgart-1996, Lodz-1998, Venice-2000, Reims-2002, and Brussels-2004. See also QIRT Journal, 2004.

[2] Maldague X.P.V. *Theory and Practice of Infrared Technology for Nondestructive Testing,* J. Wiley & Sons, Inc., New York, 2001.

[3] Van Denhaute E., Ranson W., Cornelis J., Barel A., and Steenhaut O., Contrast enhancement of IR thermographic images by microwave heating in biomedical applications, *Application mikro- und-optolelktronischer Systemelemente*, pp. 71–75, 1985.

[4] Steenhaut O., Van Denhaute E., and Cornelis J., Contrast enhancement in IR-thermography by application of microwave irradiation applied to tumor detection, *MECOMBE '86*, pp. 485–488, 1986.

[5] Nowakowski A. and Kaczmarek M., Dynamic thermography as a quantitative medical diagnostic tool, *Med. Biol. Eng. Comput. Incorporate Cell. Eng.* 37, Suppl. 1, Part 1, pp. 244–245, 1999.

[6] Kaczmarek M., Rumiński J., and Nowakowski A., Measurement of thermal properties of biological tissues — comparison of different thermal NDT techniques, *Proceedings of the Advanced Infrared Technology and Application*, Venice, 1999, pp. 322–329, 2001.

[7] Rumiński J., Kaczmarek M., and Nowakowski A., Data Visualization in dynamic thermography, *J. Med. Inform. Technol.*, v. 5, pp. IT29–IT36, 2000.

[8] Rumiński J., Nowakowski A., Kaczmarek M., and Hryciuk M., Model-based parametric images in dynamic thermography, *Polish J. Med. Phys. Eng.*, 6, pp. 159–164, 2000.

[9] Rumiński J., Kaczmarek M., and Nowakowski A., Medical active thermography — a new image reconstruction method, *Lecture Notes in Computer Science*, LNCS 2124, Springer, Berlin-Heidelberg, pp. 274–281, 2001.

[10] Nowakowski A., Kaczmarek M., and Rumiński J., Synthetic pictures in thermographic diagnostics, *Proceedings of the EMBS-BMES Conference*, CD, Houston, pp. 1131–1132, 2002.

[11] Nowakowski A., Kaczmarek M., Rumiński J., Hryciuk M., Renkielska A., Grudziński J., Siebert J., Jagielak D., Rogowski J., Roszak K., and Stojek W., Medical applications of model based dynamic thermography, Thermosense XIII, Orlando, *Proc. SPIE*, 4360, pp. 492–503, 2001.

[12] Sakagami T., Kubo S., Naganuma T., Inoue T., Matsuyama K., and Kaneko K., Development of a new diagnosis method for caries in human teeth based on thermal images under pulse heating, Thermosense XIII, Orlando, *Proc. SPIE*, 4360, pp. 511–515, 2001.

[13] Vavilov V., and Shirayev V., Thermal Tomograph — USSR Patent no. 1.266.308, 1985.

[14] Vavilov V.P, Kourtenkov D., Grinzato E., Bison P., Marinetti S., and Bressan C., Inversion of experimental data and thermal tomography using "Thermo Heat" and "Termidge" Software, *Proc. QIRT'94*, pp. 273–278, 1994.

[15] Vavilov V.P., 1D–2D–3D transition conditions in transient IR thermographic NDE, Seminar 64 — Quantitative Infra-Red Thermography — QIRT'2000, Reims, 74, 2000.

[16] Hryciuk M., Nowakowski A., and Renkielska A., Multi-layer thermal model of healthy and burned skin, *Proc. 2nd European Medical and Biological Engineering Conference*, EMBEC'02, Vol. 3, Pt. 2., pp. 1614–1617, Vienna, 2002.

[17] Nowakowski A., Kaczmarek M., and Hryciuk M., Tomografia Termiczna, pp. 615–696, in Chmielewski L., Kulikowski J.L., and Nowakowski A., *Obrazowanie Biomedyczne*, (Biomedical Imaging — *in Polish*) Biocybernetyka i Inżynieria Biomedyczna 2000, 8, Akademicka Oficyna Wydawnicza EXIT, Warszawa, 2003.

[18] Hryciuk M., Badanie struktury biologicznych obiektów warstwowych z wykorzystaniem pobudzenia cieplnego (Ph.D. Dissertation — Investigation of layered biological object structure using thermal excitation, *in Polish*), *Politechnika Gdanska*, 2003.

[19] Kaczmarek M., Nowakowski A., and Renkielska A., Rating burn wounds by dynamic thermography, in D. Balageas, J. Beaudoin, G. Busse, and G. Carlomagno, eds., *Quantitative InfraRed Thermography* 5, pp. 376–381, Reims, 2000.

[20] Kaczmarek M., Nowakowski A., Renkielska A., Grudziński J., and Stojek W., Investigation of skin burns based on active thermography, *Proc. 23rd Annual International Conference IEEE EMBS*, CD-ROM, Istanbul, 2001.

[21] Nowakowski A, Kaczmarek M., Wtorek J., Siebert J., Jagielak D., Roszak K., and Topolewicz J., Thermographic and electrical measurements for cardiac surgery inspection, *Proc. of 23rd Annual International Conference IEEE EMBS*, CD-ROM, Istanbul, 2001.

[22] Nowakowski A., Kaczmarek M., Hryciuk M., and Rumiński J., *Postępy termografii–aplikacje medyczne*, Wyd. Gdańskie (Advances of thermography–medical applications, *in Polish*), Gdańsk, 2001.

[23] Hryciuk M. and Nowakowski A., Multi-layer thermal model of healthy and burned skin, *Proc. 2nd European Medical and Biological Engineering Conference*, EMBEC'02, Vol. 3, Pt. 2., pp. 1614–1617, Vienna, 2002.

[24] Hryciuk M. and Nowakowski A., Evaluation of thermal diffusivity variations in multi-layered structures, *Proc. 6 QIRT*, Zagreb, pp. 267–274, 2003.

[25] Kaczmarek M. and Nowakowski A., Analysis of transient thermal processes for improved visualization of breast cancer using IR imaging, *Proc. IEEE EMBC*, Cancun, pp. 1113–1116, 2003.

[26] Kaczmarek M., Modelowanie właściwości tkanek żywych dla potrzeb termografii dynamicznej, (Ph.D. dissertation — Modeling of living tissue properties for dynamic thermography, *in Polish*) Politechnika Gdańska, 2003.

[27] Chato J.C., A method for the measurement of the thermal properties of biological materials, thermal problems in biotechnology, *ASME Symp.*, pp. 16–25, 1968.

[28] Bowman H.F., Cravalho E.G., and Woods M., Theory, measurement and application of thermal properties of biomaterials, *Ann. Rev. Biophys. Bioeng.*, No. 4, pp. 43–80, 1975.

[29] Chen M.M., Holmes K.R., and Rupinskas V., Pulse-decay method for measuring the thermal conductivity of living tissues, *J. Biomech. Eng.*, 103, pp. 253–260, 1981.

[30] Balasubramaniam T.A. and Bowman H.F., Thermal conductivity and thermal diffusivity of biomaterials: a simultaneous measurement technique, *J. Biomech. Eng.*, 99, pp. 148–154, 1977.

[31] Shitzer A. and Eberhart R.C., *Heat Transfer in Medicine and Biology*, Vol. 1, 2, Plenum Press, 1985.

[32] Balageas D.L., Characterization of living tissues from the measurement of thermal effusivity, *Innov. Tech. Biol. Med.*, Vol. 12, 1991.

[33] Valvano J.W., Cochran J.R., and Diller K.R., Thermal conductivity and diffusivity of biomaterials measured with self-heating thermistors, *Int. J. Thermophys.*, No. 6, pp. 301–311, 1985.

[34] Marks R.M. and Barton S.P., *The Physical Nature of the Skin*, Boston, MTP Press, 1998.

[35] Janna W.S., *Engineering Heat Transfer*, CRC Press, Washington DC, 2000.

[36] Pennes H.H., Analysis of tissue and arterial blood temperatures in the resting human forearm, *J. Appl. Physiol.*, No. 1, pp. 93–122, 1948.

[37] IDEAS operating manual.

[38] NASTRAN operating manual.

[39] Matlab operating manual.

[40] Mathematica operating manual.

[41] Salerno A., Dillenz A., Wu D., Rantala J., and Busse G., Progress in ultrasound lock-in thermography, *Proc. QIRT'98*, pp. 154–160, Lodz, 1998.

[42] Maldague X. and Marinetti S., Pulse phase thermography, *J. Appl. Phys.*, 79, No. 5, pp. 2694–2698, 1996.

[43] Nowakowski A., Kaczmarek M., and Dębicki P., Active thermography with microwave excitation, D. Balageas, J., Beaudoin, G., Busse, G., and Carlomagno, eds., *Quantitative InfraRed Thermography*, Vol. 5, pp. 387–392, 2000.

[44] Nowakowski A., Kaczmarek M., Renkielska A., Grudziński J., and Stojek J., Heating or cooling to increase contrast in thermographic diagnostics, *Proc. EMBS-BMES Conference*, CD, Houston, pp. 1137–1138, 2002.

[45] Duck A.F., *Physical Properties of Tissue*, Academic Press, London, 1990.

[46] Ring E.F.J., Standardization of Thermal Imaging Technique, *Thermology Oesterrich*, 3, pp. 11–13, 1993.

[47] Rumiński J., Kaczmarek M., Nowakowski A., Hryciuk M., and Werra W., Differential analysis of medical images in dynamic thermography, *Proc. V National Conference on Application of Mathematics in Biology and Medicine*, Zawoja, pp. 126–131, 1999.

[48] Nowakowski A., Kaczmarek M., and Rumiński J., Synthetic pictures in thermographic diagnostics, *Proc. EMBS-BMES Conf.* 2002, CD, pp. 1131–1132, Houston, 2002.

[49] Kaczmarek M., Nowakowski A., and Renkielska A., Rating burn wounds by dynamic thermography, D. Balageas, J. Beaudoin, G. Busse, and G. Carlomagno, eds., *Quantitative InfraRed Thermography*, Vol. 5, pp. 376–381, 2000.

[50] Kaczmarek M., Rumiński J., Nowakowski A., Renkielska A., Grudziński J., and Stojek W., In-vivo experiments for evaluation of new diagnostic procedures in medical thermography, *Proceedings of 6th International Conference on Quantitative Infrared thermography*, Proc. Quantitative Infrared Thermography 6-QIRT'02, pp. 260–266, Zagreb, 2003.

[51] Ibarra-Castanedo C. and Maldague X., Pulsed phase thermography reviewed, *QIRT J.*, 1, No. 1, p. 47–70, 2004.

[52] Hryciuk M. and Nowakowski A., Multilayer thermal model of healthy and burned skin, *Proc. 2nd European Medical and Biological Engineering Conference*, EMBEC'02, Vol. 3, Pt. 2., pp. 1614–1617, Vienna, 2002.

[53] Hryciuk M. and Nowakowski A., Evaluation of thermal diffusivity variations in multi-layered structures, *Proceedings of 6th International Conference on Quantitative Infrared thermography*, Proc. Quantitative Infrared Thermography 6-QIRT'02, pp. 267–274, Zagreb, 2003.

[54] Hryciuk M. and Nowakowski A., Formulation of inverse problem in thermal tomography for burns diagnostics, *Proc. SPIE*, 5505, pp. 11–18, 2004.

[55] Kaczmarek M., Rumiński J., and Nowakowski A., Data processing methods for dynamic medical thermography, *Proceedings of International Federation for Medical and Biological Engineering*, EMBEC'02, pp. 1098–1099, Vienna, 2002.

[56] Nowakowski A., Kaczmarek M., Siebert J., Rogowski J., Jagielak D., Roszak K., Topolewicz J., and Stojek W., Role of thermographic inspection in cardiosurgery, *Proc. Int. Federation for Medical and Biological Engineering*, EMBEC'02, pp. 1626–1627, Vienna, 2002.

[57] Kaczmarek M. and Nowakowski A., Analysis of transient thermal processes for improved visualization of breast cancer using IR imaging, *25th Annual International Conference of the IEEE Engineering in Medicine and Biology Society* "A New Beginning for Human Health," Cancun, Mexico, CD, 2003.

[58] Singer A.J., Berruti L., Thode HC J.R., and McClain S.A., Standardized burn model using a multiparametric histologic analysis of burn depth. *Academic Emergency Medicine*, 7:1, pp. 1–6, 2000.

[59] Eberhart C. *Heat Transfer in Medicine and Biology, Analysis and Applications*, Vol. 1. Plenum Press, London, 1985

[60] Kaczmarek M., Nowakowski A., Siebert J., and Rogowski J., Infrared thermography — applications in heart surgery, *Proc. SPIE*, 3730, pp. 184–188, 1999.

23

Thermal Texture Maps (TTM): Concept, Theory, and Applications

23.1 Introduction.. 23-2
23.2 Medical Evaluation of TTM — Present and Future ... 23-2
   The Development Status of TTM • Existing Problems and Expectations
23.3 TTM Theory and Application in Early Breast Cancer Diagnosis............................... 23-3
   Introduction • The Thermal–Electric Analog • Estimation of the Depth of the Heat Source • Experimental Results and Analysis
23.4 Relationship between Surface Temperature Distribution and Internal Heat Source Size of the *In Vitro* Tissue.. 23-7
   Introduction • Method • Experimental Design and Results • Discussion
23.5 A Comparative Study of Breast Disease Examination with Thermal Texture Mapping, Mammography, and Ultrasound 23-12
   Introduction • Material and Methods • Results • Discussion • The Value of TTM for Breast Diseases Differentiation
23.6 Clinical Study on Using Thermal Texture Mapping in SARS Diagnosis 23-16
   Introduction • The Pathology of SARS • SARS Diagnosis Principles Using CT and TTM • Study Design • Result Analysis and Performance Comparison
23.7 Study of Trilogy-Imaging Characteristics on TTM and Its Relationship with Malignancies 23-22
   Introduction • The Neuro-Endocrine–Immune Theory • Clinical Study of Correlation Between Trilogy-Imaging of TTM and Malignancies
23.8 Discussion 23-24
23.9 Summary, Conclusions, and Recommendations 23-25
Acknowledgments... 23-26
References 23-26

Zhongqi Liu
TTM Management Group

Chen Wang
TTM International

Hairong Qi
The University of Tennessee

Yune Yuan
China Army General Hospital

Yi Zeng
Central Disease Control of China

Z.R. Li
South China Normal University

Yulin Zhou
Wen Yu
Shanghai RuiJin Hospital

Wang Wei
Beijing You An Hospital

23.1   Introduction

Due to the progress of society and increasing health concerns, the health issue is becoming more and more important. However, thousands of years of practice in the medical field presented us with the fact that humans intend to play a passive role in the process of fighting diseases. We may keep track of some diseases by resorting to modern medicine. However, we are not content and still lag far behind in understanding the root of the disease, performing initial and early detection, as well as finding the linkage between the disease and the organization of the human body. Working on solutions to these issues have pushed forward the birth of an innovative health monitoring and treatment evaluation technology, thermal texture maps (TTM).

The TTM evaluation technology mainly concerns the study of functions of living cells. Unlike other imaging techniques such as computer tomography (CT) and magnetic resonance imaging (MRT) that primarily provide information on the anatomical structures, TTM is more sensitive and provides functional information not easily measured by other methods. In addition, this technology is based on the detection of heat radiation generated by metabolic activities of living cells, thus is noninvasive and environmental friendly.

In this chapter, we introduce the concept and theory of the TTM technology. We also present its applications in early detection of breast cancer, estimate of tumor size, comparative study of breast cancer detection with mammography and ultrasound, diagnosis of severe acute respiratory syndrome (SARS) patients, and the trilogy-imaging characteristics of TTM.

23.2   Medical Evaluation of TTM — Present and Future

23.2.1   The Development Status of TTM

Functional medical imaging technology has been the mainstream in the technological world during the past few decades. The end of 1990s witnessed a breakthrough brought by a group of scientists and engineers in China. Based on their extensive experience working with CT, MRI, and Ultrasound, they have initiated the development of a new generation functional imaging technology, TTMs, with which the metabolic activities within a human body can be detected and analyzed from the radiation heat generated by the human body cells. With a decade of efforts, they finally discovered the relationship between the surface temperature distribution and the internal heat source of the human body. Their research findings are supported by several years of clinical studies. In 1997, a patent application for the TTM technology was made to the Food and Drug Administration (FDA) of the United States as well as 93 other countries' patent offices for patent protection. The patent was granted by the United States on February 2, 2000.

A company named Bioyear Group was formed in 1995 in Beijing, China, dedicated to the research and development work on TTM. In 1997, the U.S.-based Bioyear company (now TTM International) was incorporated and the first thermal infrared (TIR) imaging scanner with slicing capability hit the market. Since then, a series of thermo-scanner imaging (TSI) products has been manufactured and shipped to Chinese hospitals. In 1998, a brand new TSI system that adopted uncooled infrared detector was shipped to China, the United States, and Canadian hospitals for clinical studies.

The first public announcement of the TTM technology in the United States took place at the special event "From Tanks to Tumors: A Workshop on the Application of IR Imaging and Automatic Target Recognition (ATR) Image Processing for Early Detection of Breast Cancer," held in Arlington, Virginia, United States, December 4–6, 2001 (see Chapter 1 for details). On July 4–6, 2002, at the IEEE International Symposium on Biomedical Imaging, TTM technology was first presented at a major international conference and has generated considerable interest in the audience. Since then, TTM technology has been discussed among researchers worldwide at the IEEE Engineering on Medicine and Biology Society Annual Conferences, in the format of training workshop, mini-symposium, as well as technical talks. In China, to speed up the pragmatic deployment of the TTM technology, a specially tailored conference, sponsored by the Chinese Ministry of Health, was held at the Xiangshan Science Conference Center in Beijing, 2003. To assess the usefulness of the TTM technology, the technical committee of the conference were members from the Academy of Science, Engineering, and Medicine, including professors and physicians from selective universities and medical centers.

To date, more than 100 medical units in China are equipped with TTM facilities. Since 2001, NIH has been using TTM technology for studies in skin cancers. In addition, TTM was used successfully during the SARS outbreak at the beginning of 2003. Significant results have been achieved then. At present, mass production of TTM scanners is under consideration in order to bring the technology to the benefit of human health as soon as possible.

23.2.2 Existing Problems and Expectations

The next improvement of TTM technology needs to be based on basic research in engineering and clinical studies. The important area of basic engineering research work should concentrate on the relationship between surface heat distribution and the estimation of single heat source's depth and size information under complicated situations. More importantly, this estimation needs to also consider multi heat sources condition. Some very encouraging preliminary results have been achieved in the definition of relationship between surface heat distribution and heat source size estimation.

Standard database generation is another factor to be considered for the improvement and evaluation of TTM technology. The healthy growth and benefits of TTM technology will certainly build on the standardization of training and operation. The engineering world should produce practical and simple mobile machines to satisfy multi-purpose requirements, also they should produce cost-effective machines for medium size hospitals.

Research and development in detector will certainly influence the advance of TTM technology in the future. As uncooled detectors and scanners are being manufactured with low cost, high sensitivity, high accuracy, and high stability, direct influence is expected on the popularization and improvement of the TTM technology.

23.3 TTM Theory and Application in Early Breast Cancer Diagnosis

23.3.1 Introduction

All objects at a temperature above absolute zero emit electromagnetic radiation spontaneously, called the natural thermal radiation [1]. The heat emanating on to the surface from the cancerous tissue and the surrounding blood flow can be quantified using the Pennes [2] bio-heat equation [3]. This equation includes the heat transfer due to conduction through the tissue, the volumetric metabolic heat generation of the tissue, and the volumetric blood perfusion rate whose strength is considered to be the arterio-venous temperature difference. In theory, given the heat emanating from the surface of the body measured by IR imaging, by solving the inverse heat transfer problem, we can obtain the heat pattern of various internal elements of the body. Different methods of solving the bio-heat transfer equation have been presented in literature [4,5].

Although it is possible to calculate the thermal radiation from a thermal body by thermodynamics, the complexity of the boundary conditions associated with the biological body makes this approach impractical.

23.3.2 The Thermal–Electric Analog

This section presents a new method for analyzing a thermal system based on an analogy to electrical circuit theory; referred to as thermal–electric analog [6]. We demonstrate how the analog can be used to estimate the depth of the heat source, and furthermore, help understand the metabolic activities undergoing within the human body. The method has been used in early breast cancer detection and has achieved high

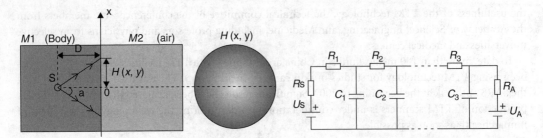

FIGURE 23.1   The thermal–electric analog (© 2005 IEEE).

sensitivity. Several breast cancer study cases are given to show the effectiveness of the method. Ongoing clinical study results are provided as well.

As the living cells within a biological body are constantly undergoing metabolic activities, the biochemical and the physical metabolic processes generate heat. Thus the amount of radiation on the surface of the human body can reflect its metabolic rate. The theory underlying conventional thermographic techniques as applied to cancer is that the change of the pulse distribution around a cancerous area and the rate of metabolism are greater than the general tissue, resulting in a higher temperature at the skin surface [6].

Even though the temperature of the skin surface can be measured, if the relationship between the surface temperature and the emissions from inside of the body cannot be established, the application of TIR imaging technique is still limited. Pennes' bio-heat equation models the process of heat transfer but has its limits in practice. Thus, a new method that does not require a direct solution to the inverse heat transfer problem, the thermal–electric analog, comes into light.

Figure 23.1 illustrates the analogy between thermodynamics systems and the electrical circuit, where the heat source S inside the human body can be simulated as a battery with voltage U_S, the heat loss inside the heat source can be simulated as the heat loss on a resistor R_S. The temperature of the heat source can then correspond to the voltage of the battery, and the heat current to the circuit current. Similarly, we can map the heat source in the air (outside the human body) as U_A, and the heat loss as R_A. The set of R_is and C_is corresponds to the unit heat resistance and heat capacity along each radiation line. The circuit in Figure 23.1 only shows the analogy for one radiation line. In the study of breast cancer, it is reasonable to assume that the medium between the heat source (S) and the surface is homogeneous. Therefore, the radiation pattern sensed by the IR camera at the surface should have a distribution like Gaussian as shown in Figure 23.1. The surface temperature $H(x)$ which corresponds to the output voltage can then be calculated by

$$H(x) = U_S - \frac{\sum_{i=1}^{n} R_i}{R_S + R_A + \sum_{i=1}^{n} R_i} \times (U_S - U_A)$$

and

$$n = \left\lfloor \frac{D}{R_o \cos a} \right\rfloor$$

where $\lfloor a \rfloor$ represents the largest integer less than a, n is the number of resistors used in the circuit, D is the depth of the heat source, and R_0 is the unit heat loss in a certain medium (or the heat resistance rate). Different parts of human body have different heat resistance rate, as shown in Table 23.1.

The thermal–electric analog provides a convenient way to estimate the depth of the heat source.

23.3.3 Estimation of the Depth of the Heat Source

The depth estimation is based on the assumption that we can use Gaussian to model the distribution of the surface temperature. A half power point is a useful property of Gaussian distribution. The property

TABLE 23.1 Heat Resistance Rate of
Different Body Parts

Body parts	Heat resistance rate (°C/cm)
Fatty tissue	0.1–0.15
Muscle	0.2
Bone	0.3–0.6

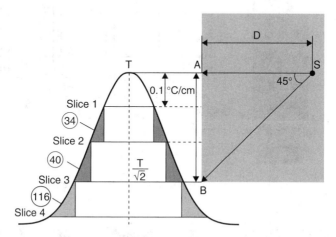

FIGURE 23.2 Illustration of half power point of Gaussian and the depth of the heat source (©2005 IEEE).

says that the half power point divides the area enclosed by the Gaussian into equally half. If we slice the Gaussian from top to bottom at a fixed interval as shown in Figure 23.2, the increment of the radius in the horizontal direction would not have dramatic change until the half power point is crossed. From Figure 23.2, we can see that the relative increment of the radius between the first slice and the second slice is 34 pixels, and 40 pixels between the second slice and the third slice, but 116 pixels between the third slice and the fourth slice. Therefore, the half power point is at the position of the third slice.

Suppose the temperature of the heat source is H_0. In the right triangle formed by SAB, the hypotenuse (SB) is equal to H_0 and the sides (SA = AB) should be equal to $0.707H_0$. The horizontal side (SA) is the depth of the heat source, and the vertical side (AB) is the temperature drop between the maximum value of the Gaussian and the half power point. In other words, if we can find the half power point, we can find the depth of the heat source.

Each slice of the Gaussian curve corresponds to a temperature deduction of 0.1 degree. For the application of breast cancer detection, based on the heat resistance rate of fat tissues, the 0.1 degree temperature drop corresponds to a distance of 1 cm. Therefore, by slicing (decreasing) the surface temperature at a certain degree per step, we can find the half power point with the accuracy at the level of centimeter.

23.3.4 Experimental Results and Analysis

Figure 23.3 shows a synthetic example of how slicing works. The image is taken from a piece of pork fat. An electric bulb is lit and inserted at the center of the pork fat as a heat source such that we can control the location of the heat source. The pseudo colormap is also shown in the figure. "White" represents the highest temperature and "black" represents the lowest temperature. First of all, an appropriate temperature needs to be found so that white pixels at the center of the pork fat will show up in the next slice. In this example, this appropriate temperature is 20.50°. Each following slicing process decreases the highest temperature in the color-map by 0.1 degree (e.g., the threshold is lowered by 0.1 degree), such that more white pixels can appear. If we come to a point where the increment of the white pixel is dramatic, the half power point

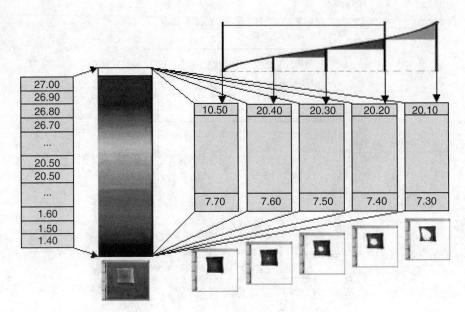

FIGURE 23.3   (See color insert following page **29**-16.) Simulation of slicing operation on pork fat (©2005 IEEE).

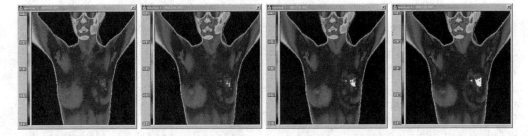

FIGURE 23.4   (See color insert.) Slicing of patient with lobular carcinoma in the left breast (©2005 IEEE).

is the slice before it. In the example, the fourth slice generates much more white pixels than the previous three slices. The depth of the bulb is 3 cm, which is the same as the ground truth. Note that the increment of the white pixel is measured by the increment of the radius of the white cluster.

Besides measuring the depth of the heat source, slicing can also reveal the growth pattern of the white pixels. Dissimilar tissues have different growth patterns. By observing this pattern, different tissues can be distinguished as well. For example, the pixels of lymph nodes and tumors should grow in a circular pattern, while the growth pattern of blood vessel is along the direction of the blood vessel.

A diagnosis protocol has been designed for early detection of breast cancer. Six steps are involved in this protocol:

- Step 1: Growth pattern of lymph nodes in the armpits
- Step 2: Size of the abnormal area
- Step 3: Appearance of the abnormal area
- Step 4: Vascular pattern
- Step 5: Nipples and areola pattern
- Step 6: Dynamic diagnosis with outside agents (antibiotic, etc.)

Take the first step as an example, if the lymph nodes in the armpits reveal one heat source with a depth less than 2 cm, one abnormal sign (+) will be recorded; if two heat sources appear with a depth less than

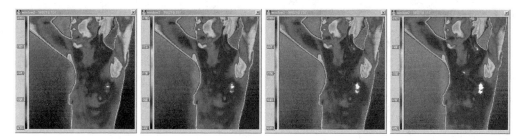

FIGURE 23.5   (See color insert.) Slicing of patient with ductal carcinoma in the left breast (©2005 IEEE).

2 cm and a bilateral temperature difference greater than 0.2 degree, then two abnormal signs (++) will be recorded, etc.

Figure 23.4 shows a patient with lobular carcinoma in the left breast. From slicing, we observe the following abnormal signs:

1. 2 cm tumor surrounded by four blood vessels (+ + +)
2. White pixels surround the nipple in three slices (+ + +)
3. Nipple bilateral temperature difference is 0.8 degree (+)

Figure 23.5 shows a patient diagnosed to have ductal carcinoma in her left breast. From slicing, we observe the following abnormal signs:

1. Lymph node bilateral temperature difference is 0.8 (++++)
2. The tumor is 2 cm from the surface (++)
3. The tumor is surrounded by five blood vessels (+++)
4. It takes less than three slices to have the white pixels surround the nipple (++)

23.4   Relationship between Surface Temperature Distribution and Internal Heat Source Size of the *In Vitro* Tissue

23.4.1   Introduction

In contrast to traditional anatomical imaging technologies, such as X-CT and ultrasound, thermography is a functional imaging modality. Thermography obtains skin temperature distribution through detecting thermal radiation emanating from the human body surface. Thermograph is the image of surface temperature distribution. The skin temperature can reflect the metabolic rate of the human body. The patterns of thermograph are affected by the activities of the tissues, organs, and vessels inside the body [6].

As a noncontact and noninvasive imaging modality, thermography is widely used in clinical practice. The FDA, Bureau of Medical Devices has approved the thermography procedures, including the screening for breast cancer, extra-cranial vessel disease (head and neck vessels), neuro-musculo-skeletal disorders, and vascular disease of the lower extremities [7].

As pointed out in [8], a shift should occur in the study of thermography from phenomenological to pathophysiological. Currently, the application of thermography is limited if only the skin temperature is obtained. It would be desirable to provide a method for revealing the relationship between the skin temperature and internal heat sources. In order to clinically effectively detect and diagnose cancers (especially in their early stages) and other diseases, the depth and size information of internal heat sources hidden in the abnormal patterns of thermographs need to be discovered.

23.4.2 Method

23.4.2.1 Heat Transfer Formulation

In the field of bio-heat transfer [9], the basic formulation is the bio-heat equation, originally proposed by Pennes [2],

$$\rho c \frac{\partial T}{\partial t} = \nabla \cdot (k\nabla T) + Q_{b} + Q_{m} \tag{23.1}$$

where T is the local temperature, ∇ is the Laplace operator, ρ, c, and k are the tissue density, specific heat, and the heat conductivity, respectively, Q_{b} is the Pennes perfusion term, and Q_{m} is the metabolic heat production.

Consider a simpler condition, in which the *in vitro* tissue in a stable state is heated by an internal heat source, then the bio-heat Equation 23.1 can be simplified to

$$\nabla \cdot (k\nabla T) = 0 \tag{23.2}$$

On the boundary, heat can be exchanged through radiation and convection with the environment. The convection on the boundary was considered as natural convection. And the radiation heat exchange can be induced from Stephan–Boltzman Law,

$$q_{r} = \sigma \varepsilon T_{s}^{4} - \sigma \varepsilon T_{0}^{4} \tag{23.3}$$

where q_{r} is the radiation heat exchange density, σ is the Stephan–Boltzman constant, ε is the surface emissivity, T_{s} is the surface temperature, and T_{0} is the environment temperature. In order to simplify the calculation, Equation 23.3 can be expressed as

$$q_{r} = h_{r}(T_{s} - T_{0}) \tag{23.4}$$

where h_{r} is the radiation heat exchange coefficient. Natural convection heat exchange is determined as

$$q_{c} = h_{c}(T_{s} - T_{0}) \tag{23.5}$$

where q_{c} is the convection heat exchange density, h_{c} is the convection heat exchange coefficient, and h_{c} can be calculated by an empirical formulation,

$$h_{c} = 1.57(T_{s} - T_{0})^{1/4} \tag{23.6}$$

The total heat exchange density q_{e} with environment on the boundary is the sum of the two heat exchange densities: the radiation heat exchange q_{r} and the convection heat exchange q_{c}.

$$q_{e} = q_{r} + q_{c} \tag{23.7}$$

Equation 23.2 can be solved only if the boundary conditions are complete and the solution is unique. However, the boundary conditions are very hard to be complete. Under the conditions described in Figure 23.6, that is, (1) the heat source is a sphere, (2) the *in vitro* tissue is isotropy, and (3) the *in vitro* tissue is a slab whose length and width is much larger than the sphere's radius, then some approximation can be made.

The first approximation is to assume that the solution to Equation 23.2 is a family of concentric spheres with the same center, that is, the center of the heat source. Using the spherical coordinate system,

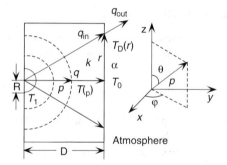

FIGURE 23.6 Conditions and approximation (©2005 IEEE).

Equation 23.2 can be expressed as

$$\frac{d}{d\rho}\left(\rho^2 \frac{dT}{d\rho}\right) = 0 \tag{23.8}$$

If the total heat emanating from the heat source is Q, the heat density of the spot at a distance ρ from the center of the heat source is

$$q = \frac{Q}{4\pi\rho^2} \tag{23.9}$$

The heat density also can be obtained through the Fourier's Law

$$\rho = -\frac{dT}{d\rho} \tag{23.10}$$

From Equation 23.8 and Equation 23.9, the temperature field function $T(\rho)$ can be induced after integration

$$T(\rho) = T_1 - \frac{Q}{4\pi}\frac{1}{k}\left(\frac{1}{R} - \frac{1}{\rho}\right) \tag{23.11}$$

where T_1 is the temperature of the heat source and R is the radius of the sphere.

The second approximation is to assume that at any spot of the boundary, heat density transferring from the internal heat source is fully exchanged with the environment, that is,

$$q_{in} = q_{out}$$

where

$$q_{in} = \frac{Q}{4\pi\rho^2} = k\frac{T_1 - T_D(r)}{\frac{\rho}{R}(\rho - R)}, \qquad q_{out} = h_r(T_D(r) - T_0) + h_c(T_D(r) - T_0) = \alpha(T_D(r) - T_0)$$

and α is the total heat exchange coefficient.

Finally the approximation solution of the boundary surface temperature distribution can be obtained

$$T_D(r) = T_0 + \frac{(T_1 - T_2)}{(\alpha/k)\cdot(\sqrt{D^2 + r^2}/R)\cdot(\sqrt{D^2 + r^2} - R) + 1} \tag{23.12}$$

where D is the distance from the surface to the center of the sphere.

In the following, the formulation of the approximation will be validated through experiments.

23.4.3 Experimental Design and Results

We design one experiment to validate the correctness of the approximation solution. The experimental setup is illustrated in Figure 23.7, in which three components are involved,

1. One piece of adipose hanged in the air, whose dimension is about 15 × 15 × 2 cm, served as the *in vitro* tissue
2. Four brass balls buried in the adipose, whose diameters are 5.07, 10.00, 15.44, and 19.77 mm, respectively, served as the internal heat source
3. One infrared camera (TSI-2 Bioyear Group, Inc. ± 0.1°) that captures the surface temperature distribution onto a 256 × 256 image

We first let the heater heat the brass ball through the heat conduction of brass bar. After about 2 h or so, the surface temperature distribution does not vary and reaches the stable state. Figure 23.8 shows the surface temperature distribution at the stable state.

Next, we generate the surface temperature distribution templates of the approximation solution corresponding to the four heat sources according to the experiment conditions as given in Table 23.2 and Figure 23.9 shows the generated templates.

Templates of the approximation solution are matched with the practical surface temperature distribution. We use the error energy Equation 23.13 and the normalized error energy Equation 23.14 to measure the closeness of the matching,

$$E = \sum\sum (mT - T)^2 \tag{23.13}$$

$$\tilde{E} = \frac{E}{\sum\sum T^2} \tag{23.14}$$

where mT is the surface temperature distribution template and T is the practical temperature distribution.

The matching results are given in Table 23.2 Both the error energy and the normalized error energy demonstrate quite low value, indicating the close match between the templates and the practical surface temperature distribution. It also validates the reasonability of the approximation solution.

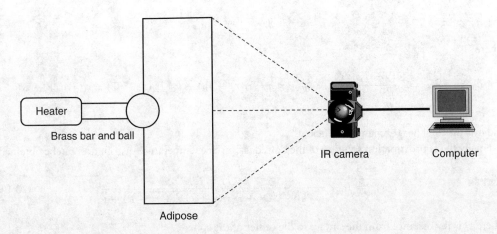

Heater

Brass bar and ball

IR camera   Computer

Adipose

FIGURE 23.7 Experimental setup (©2005 IEEE).

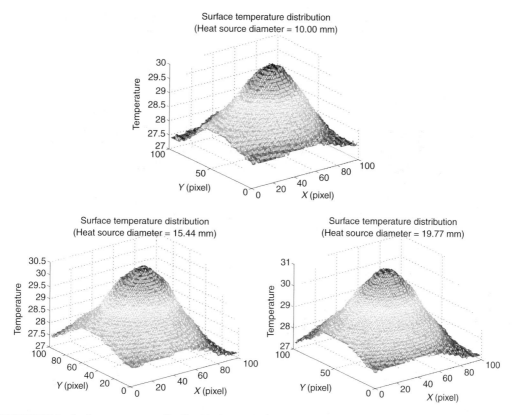

FIGURE 23.8 Surface temperature distribution (©2005 IEEE).

TABLE 23.2 Experimental Conditions

Adipose heat conductivity $k = 0.2W\ m^{-1}\ {}^{\circ}C^{-1}$			
$D = 20.00$ mm			
Heat source 1	Ball 2	Ball 3	Ball 4
Heat source diameter $2R$	5.07 mm	10.00 mm	15.44 mm	19.77 mm
Environment temperature T_0	26.9°C	27.4°C	27.0°C	27.1°C
Heat source temperature T_1	49.2°C	37.3°C	36.2°C	34.7°C

Source: From Z.Q. Liu and C. Wang. *Method and Apparatus for Thermal Radiation Imaging*, U.S. Patent 6,023,637. February 8, 2000.

23.4.4 Discussion

If a heat source is buried in the *in vitro* tissue, the tissue surface temperature distribution at the stable state will present a special pattern. The pattern of the temperature distribution reveals certain information about the internal heat source, such as the size. Through approximation, a simple relationship between surface temperature distribution and the size of the internal heat source is provided. The reasonability of the approximation is validated through the high degree of matching between the practical surface temperature distribution and the template generated by the approximation solution. It also validates the existence of the relationship between the surface temperature distribution and the internal heat source. Through this relationship, the internal heat source information can be obtained from the surface temperature distribution.

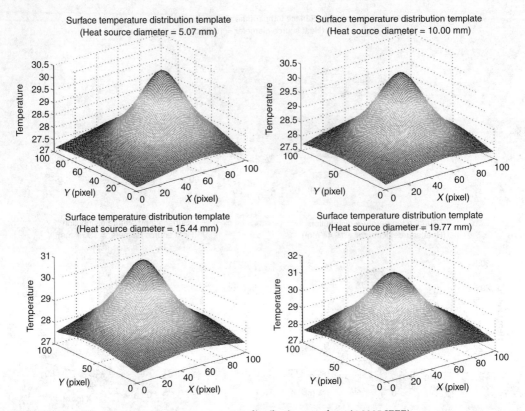

FIGURE 23.9   (See color insert.) Surface temperature distribution templates (©2005 IEEE).

TABLE 23.3   Error Energy and Normalized Error Energy

Heat source diameter (mm)	Error energy	Normalized error energy ($\times 10^{-5}$)
5.07	491.91	6.35
10.00	533.87	6.73
15.44	657.72	8.23
19.77	570.10	7.06

23.5 A Comparative Study of Breast Disease Examination with Thermal Texture Mapping, Mammography, and Ultrasound

23.5.1 Introduction

In recent years, the occurrence of breast cancer has been steadily increasing. Doctors around the world are likely to be searching for a new type of methodology and technique, that can be used for screening breast cancer more easily and more specifically. TTM system, as one of the functional diagnostic procedures, may detect the abnormal metabolism of body tissues at an early stage. A group of 38 females with breast abnormalities, who were prepared for surgery, underwent double blind study using TTM, ultrasound, and mammography with molybdenum target tube (MMT). The diagnosis results from these three imaging modalities are compared with the pathological results after surgery. TTM was used to explore the position in differentiation between the benign and malignant breast abnormalities.

23.5.2 Material and Methods

Females ranging from 20 to 78 years old, 38 in number were hospitalized in the surgery sections of the 301 and 307 Hospital between December 20, 2003 and March 20, 2004. The main symptom was palpable masses in their breasts. After receiving TTM, ultrasonography, and MMT, all patients underwent surgery. Histology of the tumor sample demonstrated malignancy in 25 patients and benignity in the others.

The apparatus used for the study is a TSI-21 TTM system manufactured by Bioyear Group, Inc. Its main parameters include a thermal resolution of 0.1°C, a scanning period of 5 sec or less, and a scanning distance between 1 and 3 m.

The room temperature was controlled between 20 and 24°C, and the patients were asked to remove their clothes or just cover the lower part of the body after having 10 min rest. Their hands should not touch the body. After focusing, the images of the head, the breast and the abdomen were taken anteroposteriorly, adding breast oblique pictures from both sides. The abnormal thermo-sources in the images were digitized from tomography and the temperatures were measured for evaluation purposes.

The examination items used by TTM for breast masses included endocrino-logical triple images (pituitary, thyroid, and pancreas), abnormal auxiliary thermo-source, abnormal breast thermo-source, abnormal vascular thermo-source, abnormal nipple thermo-source, and abnormal areola of nipple thermo-source. The thermo-sources were analyzed according to their morphology, structure, depth, and temperature measured. The diagnostic standards for malignant breast tumor include asymmetry thermo-point, abnormal symmetry angiography, temperature deviation in the thermography, the positive thermography in the thermo-tomography, and thermo-point in the attenuation images [6,10,11].

23.5.3 Results

The correlation rates between TTM, MMT, ultrasonography, and pathological results in the 38 cases are shown in Table 23.4. There were 25 cases of malignancy and 13 cases of benignity from pathological tests. The correlation rate of the malignant and benign cases between TTM with pathological findings is (100%, 96%), respectively, which is superior to the correlation rate between MMT and ultrasound with pathological findings, (88.88, 63.63%) and (90.47, 63.63%).

Since endocrine-logical triple images are the most important in differential diagnosis of malignant and benign breast diseases, we study them in more detail. Figure 23.10 shows three signatures of the endocrino-logical triple images with the positive rate being higher in malignant cases than in benign cases.

Figure 23.11 and Figure 23.12 illustrate a side-by-side comparison between TTM and MMT in the diagnosis of benign and malignant tumors confirmed by pathological results obtained from surgery. The first case (Figure 23.11) shows benign bumps with abnormal breast thermo-source that was regular morphology with less vascular around the nipple and the areola of the nipple thermo-source. The second case (Figure 23.12) shows malignant bumps with abnormal breast thermo-source that was irregular morphology and more vascular, accompanied with swollen auxiliary lymph node. TTM evaluation results for the benign and malignant breast diseases are detailed in Table 23.5.

TABLE 23.4 The Correlation Rate Between TTM, MMT, Ultrasound, and Pathological Results

Result	Pathology	TTM + (%)	TTM − (%)	MMT + (%)	MMT − (%)	Ultrasound + (%)	Ultrasound − (%)
Malignant	25	24 (96)	1 (4)	16 (89)	2 (11)	19 (91)	2 (9)
Benign	13	0	13 (100)	4 (36)	7 (64)	4 (36)	7 (64)
Total	38	38		29		32	

Note: +indicates malignancy and −indicates benignity.

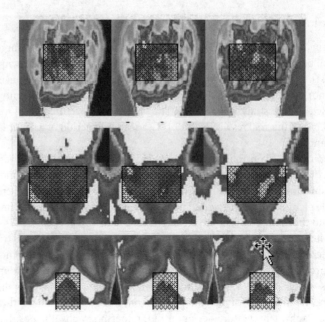

FIGURE 23.10 (See color insert.) Endocrine logical triple images of breast. From top to bottom, three signatures of the endocrine logical triple (©2005 IEEE).

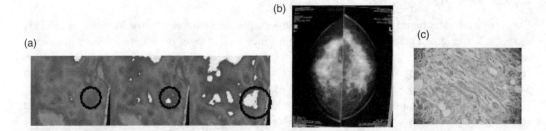

FIGURE 23.11 (See color insert.) Benign bumps compared between TTM and MMT, confirmed by pathology. (a) TTM image of January 16, 2004 indicates the slices of abnormal thermo-source in the out-upper quadrant on left breast. These slices of thermo-source show the regular morphology and less vascular. (b) MMT image of January 16, 2004 shows a 0.6 × 0.5 cm, clear-edged lump in the outboard on the left breast. (c) Pathology diagnosis of fatty tumor (©2005 IEEE).

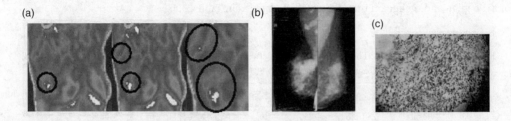

FIGURE 23.12 (See color insert.) Malignant bumps compared between TTM and MMT, confirmed by pathology. (a) TTM image of February 4, 2004 indicates the slices of abnormal breast thermo-source that were of irregular morphology, more vascular and higher heat values accompanied with swollen auxiliary lymph node. (b) MMT image taken of February 4, 2004 shows a blurred boundary mass with sand-grained calcification in the outboard on the right breast. (c) Pathology is infiltrated duct carcinoma (©2005 IEEE).

TABLE 23.5 TTM Evaluation Results for the Benign and Malignant Breast Diseases

TTM evaluation standard	Result	Malignant patient/(%)	Benign patient/(%)
Endocrinological Triple graphs	Positive	24/(96)	5/(38)
	Negative	1/(4)	8/(62)
Abnormal breast heat source	Positive	25/(100)	12/(92.4)
	Negative	0	1/(7.6)
Abnormal axillaries heat source	Positive	15/(60)	8/(61.5)
	Negative	10/(40)	5/(38.5)
Abnormal vascular heat source	Positive	23/(92)	4/(30.7)
	Negative	2/(8)	9/(69.3)
Abnormal nipple heat source	Positive	20/(80)	2/(18.4)
	Negative	5/(20)	11/(84.6)
Abnormal areola heat source	Positive	12/(48)	3/(23.1)
	Negative	13/(52)	10/(76.9)

23.5.4 Discussion

Mammographic imaging using x-ray tubes with molybdenum, known for its low radiation, clear film and diagnostic accuracy, has been widely accepted by the doctors in the clinic. Unfortunately, it is rather difficult to obtain clear pictures with MMT detecting abnormalities of dense breasts in adolescent females due to its weak penetration. In addition, it is not easy to obtain correct diagnosis of breast cancer in its early stages. There is speculation limit in special areas such as laterosuperior quadrant of the breasts and axilla. There are also other disadvantages such as high cost and radiation damage, which result in limited usage. Ultrasonography is useful for tumor localization and identification of cystic tumors, but not good at differentiation between malignant and benign abnormalities.

Traditional infrared scanners are simple, harmless, and sensitive at the early stages of the tumor; however the poor penetration and localization, and temperatures assessment being limited on the body's surfaces result in a higher false-positive rate. Compared with the traditional infrared scanner, TTM is not only capable of measuring depths and temperature values of thermo-source which improves the specificity of assaying, it is also capable of evaluating the patients' general conditions including detecting metastasis of the lymph node in the auxiliary and superclavicular areas as well as other organs.

23.5.4.1 The Mechanism of TTM Diagnostic Functions

Thermo-radiation that transferred heat energy from the inside to the surface of the body, reflects the subtle metabolism changes of living cells in the body. Using infrared scanners to receive signals from the heat radiation, TTM reconstructs a cell's metabolic extent map, which reflects the target organs or tissues by computerized processing of the data with specific regulations and measurements, and which measures the depths and temperature values of the thermo-source according to the thermo-deviations between normal and abnormal tissues, providing quantitative evidence for diagnosis [11].

Normal breasts are symmetrical, in which blood vessels are evenly distributed and metabolism of the acinic tissues is accordant with the adjacent structures. When cell differentiation is nearly mature, benign growth in the breasts is rather slow, resulting in little or no temperature difference between them. The metabolism of cancer cells is, on the other hand, very active, therefore its blood circulation is very rich. The cancer cells may develop several vasoactive agents such as bradykinin. The thermo energy transferred from the source of the dermis results in a high temperature area, that is, the thermo energy carried by the blood stream is transferred to the venous vessels in the superficial area and forms abnormal angio-images on the thermogram. There is no fat in the areola of nipple for heat isolation and the venous vessel plexus in the superficial area communicates with the ones in the deep area of the Haller's circle just behind the areola of nipple. Hence high temperature in the area shows significance in diagnosis of breast cancer.

23.5.5   The Value of TTM for Breast Diseases Differentiation

Jone reported that among more than 20,000 breast cancer cases from 1967 to 1972, the positive rates were 70% and nearly 90% in breast cancers in the I, II stages and III, IV stages, respectively [12]. The positive rate was 23% in 4,393 cases without symptoms with infrared scanner. Of the 1,028 positive cases, there were 2.4% cancer patients found using x-ray mammography, which was higher than the rate (0.7%) for the same test in the general survey of breast cancer [13]. In the meanwhile, at the 7th International Cancer Conference held by the American Cancer Association and the U.S. National Cancer Institute, Gerald D. Dodd reported that in a general survey of breast cancer for the female aged more than 40 years, 5% of those who were found have abnormal infrared results accounted for 15 to 20% of the total numbers, and to whom biopsy was suggested [14]. The study in this paper shows that TTM was found to be superior to MMT and ultrasonography for the detection of malignant cases from the benign cases.

Comparing TTM with other modern diagnostic techniques, TTM focuses on cell metabolism and provides both morphological evidence in anatomy and functional evidence in physiology, and reached concordance between the systematical examination and dynamic real-time examination. TTM was able to find more than 80% of micro-pathological changes in the tissues at its early stage [15,16]. Feig et al. [17] reported that infrared images are fourfold more sensitive than physical examination among 16,000 females who underwent general survey of breasts. Wallace [9] found that the detection rates were 0.27 and 1.9% in the x-ray mammography and infrared pictures, respectively. In 1980, Gautheriehe and Gros demonstrated that 1,245 females with all normal results including physical examination, mammogram, ultrasonography, and biopsy, but infrared confirmed more than one third of them as having breast cancer during the 5-year follow-up. It is concluded that breast thermography is not only an indicator of breast cancer, it may also detect breast abnormalities that develop quickly [18]. In 1983, Isard concluded that a combination of breast thermography and mammography raised the accuracy of diagnosis and reduced the amount of unnecessary surgery after exploring the characteristics of breast thermography and ultrasound [19]. As one of the functional diagnostic techniques, TTM is not only able to detect abnormal metabolism of the cells in the early stage with noninvasive techniques, it can also evaluate and analyze the depth, morphology and the thermo-values in real time. All but one in 38 cases coincided with the pathological results, and the diagnostic accuracy was 97.35%. It is concluded that TTM can be used to evaluate the sub-healthy conditions in humans as well as locate tumors at very early stages for the majority of breast diseases; especially those that develop very slowly, and is harmless to the human body, uses no environment pollutants.

23.6   Clinical Study on Using Thermal Texture Mapping in SARS Diagnosis

23.6.1   Introduction

Severe acute respiratory syndrome is a viral respiratory illness caused by a coronavirus, called SARS-associated coronavirus (SARS-CoV). Its first outbreak was recorded in Guang Dong Province of southern China in November 2002. In just a few months, the disease spread to 28 countries around the world. According to the World Health Organization (WHO) [20], during the SARS outbreak of 2003, a total of 8098 people worldwide became sick with SARS; of these, 774 died. This high infection rate and high fatality rate (1 out of 10.5 infected) are largely due to the limited understanding to the disease.

Scientists around the world have been trying to decode the genetic sequence of SARS in the hope of developing SARS antibody. However, till now, the most effective treatment still relies on good, intensive, and supportive care. Under this circumstance, early detection, early diagnosis, and immediate isolation are the keys to preventing another outbreak of SARS. Active image monitoring and analysis of the full clinical stages of illness are important for accurate diagnosis and treatment. Today, the standard diagnostic procedures are based on chest x-ray radiology exams and CT.

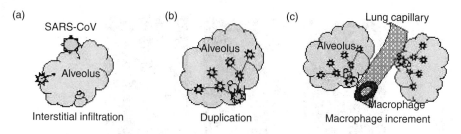

FIGURE 23.13   (See color insert.) SARS-CoV infection stages (©2005 IEEE).

In order to improve the process of diagnosing and monitoring SARS, a study has taken place in China that evaluates the clinical value of *infrared imaging* (IR) in the diagnosis of SARS. We use the term TTM [21] to represent the images captured from IR imaging.

Infrared imaging is a physiological test that measures the physiology of the blood flow and behavior of the nervous system by means of precise temperature measurement. Unlike imaging techniques such as x-ray radiology and CT that primarily provide information on the anatomical structures, IR imaging provides functional information not easily measured by other methods [20]. Compared to other imaging modalities, IR imaging is noninvasive, nonionizing, risk-free, patient-friendly, and inexpensive. It has the potential to provide more dynamic information of the patho-physiological abnormalities occurring in the human body at an early stage of disease development since the disease can affect a small area but can be fast growing making it appear as a high temperature spot in the TTM. The major shortcoming, however, is that it can only image the surface temperature and is principally a qualitative technique that can reveal little quantitative information about the size, shape, and depth information of the potential tumor. In this chapter, we present a new methodology which can estimate the depth information of lesion through surface temperature slicing. We evaluate the clinical value of IR imaging as a complementary tool to CT in SARS diagnosis.

Our study is conducted on a group of 111 patients that have been preconfirmed to be SARS patients by both clinical and laboratory diagnosis. Two imaging modalities, CT and IR, are used on each patient. The diagnostic results are cross-compared in order to study the clinical value of IR in the detection and monitoring of SARS.

23.6.2 The Pathology of SARS

Several studies have been conducted since SARS outbreak to help understand the pathology of SARS [22], which includes both parenchymal and interstitial abnormalities. Here, we divide the SARS infection process into three stages, interstitial infiltration, duplication, and macrophage increment.

In the early stage of SARS, the virus were mainly interstitial infiltrative as shown in Figure 23.13a. After penetrating into the alveoli, the SARS-CoV starts to duplicate itself in massive amount (Figure 23.13b) which eventually triggers the human immune system to react, causing proliferation of macrophages that could damage or block lung capillary, shown in Figure 23.13c.

In the following sections, we show how IR imaging can detect and monitor this abnormal metabolic activity of human body triggered by the invasion of SARS-CoV from different perspectives.

23.6.3 SARS Diagnosis Principles Using CT and TTM

It is considered, in general, that CT indications of SARS are in the density, appearance, and distribution of lesions. Density can show ground-glass opacity and consolidation. The shape of lesion could be focal, multi-focal, nodular, patchy, segmental, lobar, and in extensive conglomerated lesions. In addition, the lesions appear mostly in the lower lung areas and sub-pleural regions.

On the other hand, the TTM indications of SARS are in the discovery of abnormal heat patterns. This, combined with the depth estimation methodology discussed in Section 23.3.3, can be used to assist SARS

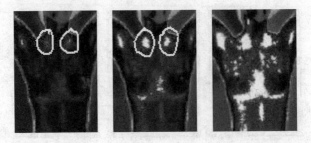

FIGURE 23.14   (See color insert.) TTM slicing of normal case (©2005 IEEE).

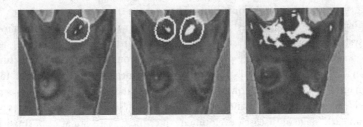

FIGURE 23.15   (See color insert.) TTM slicing of lung TB condition (©2005 IEEE).

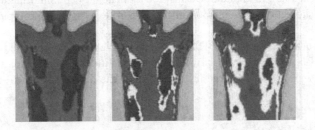

FIGURE 23.16   (See color insert.) TTM slicing of SARS patient 1 (©2005 IEEE).

diagnosis. A study of the human cardiovascular system shows a couple of blood vessel concentration areas, among which the place where the jugular veins, carotid arteries, subclavian artery/vein meet is one of the most concentrated, and correspondingly, the hottest. We refer to this area as subclavian area. Therefore, when slicing the TTM of a normal patient, the subclavian area should first appear as white since it has a higher temperature than other parts of the human body. Otherwise, some abnormal metabolic activities must exist. Figure 23.14 shows the slicing results of the TTM of a normal patient. We observe that both the left and right subclavian areas appear as white earlier than the lung area. This rule of thumb applies to regular lung diseases as well. Figure 23.15 shows the slicing results of the TTM of a patient with lung TB condition. We can see that in the slicing process, the subclavian area is still the first one that goes white (the hottest).

Figure 23.16 and Figure 23.17 show the slicing results of TTMs from two SARS patients. In both cases, we observe that the subclavian areas do not show as white until the slicing causes portions of the lung area to be white. This indicates some serious abnormities in the metabolic activity of the lung, which through clinical study, has been identified as one of the symptoms in the diagnosis of SARS.

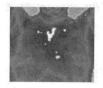 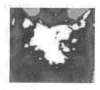

FIGURE 23.17   (See color insert.) TTM slicing of SARS patient 2 (©2005 IEEE).

At the initial and progress stages of SARS development, there is an increase in the thermal radiation of the lesions, and solid density heat structures normally appear over 3 cm deep from the surface of the skin that corresponds to the lesions found in CT.

In the later stages, the SARS patient may develop adult respiratory distress syndrome (ARDS), in which the main pathological abnormity is pulmonary edema. TTM would show the appearance of low thermal radiation zones and solid heat structures in lung areas, along with possible metabolic changes in the other organs.

At the recovery stage, there is normally decreased thermal radiation, with "cool zone" structures or "oval cold" solitary density structures that match lesions that display interstitial hyperplasia and compensatory emphysema, or cavities with purulence in the CT. TTM also shows decreased thermal radiation of the spleen, and increased thermal radiation of the spine.

23.6.4 Study Design

The study was conducted between March 10, 2003 and June 18, 2003 on 111 SARS patients (preconfirmed by both clinical and laboratory diagnosis) at Department of Communicable Diseases of Beijing You An Hospital, Beijing, China. All cases met the standard SARS diagnosis criteria set by the China Ministry of Health and the United States Center for Disease Control and Prevention (CDC). Among the 111 examined patients, 54 were male (24 cases between 12 and 30 years of age, 30 cases between 31 and 62 years of age, the average age being 34) and 57 were female (22 cases between 14 and 30 years of age, 35 cases between 31 and 68 years of age, the average age being 36). Out of the 111 cases, 98 claimed to have had close contact with another SARS patient or patients; their symptoms included fever (94.4%), nonproductive cough (92.7%), chest pain (83.3%), headache (55.6%), and Diarrhea (3%). Among the 111 patients, only 3 experienced no major symptoms. Laboratory tests of all the patients showed the following common symptoms (a) White blood cell count and lymphocyte count decreased during the earlier phases of the disease and (b) CD3, CD4, and CD8 T-cell counts were decreased — CD4 decreased most severely. T-cell counts were at their lowest 10 to 14 days after the symptoms started. The lower the T-cell count, the greater the severity of the SARS disease.

CT was performed for every patient upon admission into the hospital. Regular follow-up examinations were performed afterwards once every 4 to 6 days for a total of 80 to 90 days. TTM examinations were performed between May 19 and June 18, 2003 for all 111 cases. The CT was performed with a High-speed DX/I helical CT (HRCT) unit manufactured by GE Company with slice thickness and slice interval of 10 mm from lung apices to phrenic angles. The HRCT was performed with a 140 kV, 180 mA, with a slice thickness of 2 mm, and slice interval of 2 to 4 mm and bone algorithm reconstruction. The TTM examinations were performed in three positions; anterior, dorsal, and right lateral of body with a TSI-21M system manufactured by Bioyear Group, Inc. More than three senior radiologists and scientists assessed and reviewed all images.

23.6.5 Result Analysis and Performance Comparison

From the clinical study, we summarize our findings in the following three subsections.

23.6.5.1 Image Characterization of the Initial Stage of SARS

Small focal or multiple and extensive patches of infiltration density showed in 28 out of 111 cases, and among those 28, small focal opacity were more common (24/28, 85.7%). HRCT could show the lesion more clearly. It indicated that the focal ground glass opacity was common. TTM depicted abnormally increased thermal radiation and solitary density structures that correspond to lesions displayed in the HRCT, as well as an abnormal thermal radiation increase in the spleen and a decrease in the spine.

23.6.5.2 Imaging Characterization of the Progressive Stage of SARS

In this stage of SARS development, we found that (1) the uniform ground-glass-like density with ill-defined border and blood vessels (throughout the whole course of the continued follow-up observation) showed in 18 cases of 111 (16.2%), (2) the mainly ground-glass-like density with consolidation showed in 85 cases of 111 (76.6%), and (3) the mainly consolidation density with air-bronchogram image showed in 8 cases of 111 (7.2%).

Again, TTM dynamic manifestation depicted abnormally increased thermal radiation as well as solitary density structures that correspond to lesions displayed in the CT. The abnormal thermal radiation reached its highest level in the spleen. TTM also shows abnormity in the functions of other organs caused by SARS, or possibly by other, related or unrelated diseases.

23.6.5.3 Image Characterization of the Recovery Stage of SARS

In the *recovery stage* of SARS development, most of the patients exhibited normal images. Four (4) of the 111 cases showed pulmonary interstitial hyperplasia with multiple linear, reticular or honey-combed patterns. Some also displayed an increase in density of the subpleural arc line and thickened interlobular septa, or compensatory emphysema and reduced thoracic cage. Five (5) of the 111 cases showed focal or multi-cavity with purulence. TTM manifestations depicted abnormally low thermal radiation with "cool zone" structures that corresponded to lesions that displayed interstitial hyperplasia or compensatory emphysema, or "oval cold" solitary density structures that corresponded to cavities with purulent in the CT and radiograph. TTM continued to show a decrease in thermal radiation of the spleen and an increase in the thermal radiation of the spine.

23.6.5.4 Dynamic Evolution Imaging in SARS

Dynamic follow-up observations of changes in the images of SARS patients are indispensable, which is normally not necessary in other pneumonias. Imaging changes in SARS patients are not only dependent on the inherent development of the disease itself, but also on treatment management, treatment effects, age, previous health, etc. Among the 111 cases, some of the small patchy densities in the early stages progressed into extensive lesions in a very short time — roughly 24 to 48 h. Such dynamic change was largely consistent with worsening of the clinical condition. Diffusely scattered lesions in both lungs are suggestive of early ARDS. Progression from focal ground-glass-like density to extensive density with consolidation (CT) and appearance of low thermal radiation zone with abnormal solid density structure of heat (TTM) and signs of rapid development of the lesion are compatible with the clinical features of ARDS.

The decreased opacity showed resolution of the lesion, and eventual disappearance of low thermal radiation zone, along with decreased density of lesion structures and increased appearance of spine line and liver heat.

During the recovery stage, some patients displayed complicated pulmonary interstitial fibrosis or multiple abscess-like cavities. HRCT showed linear, reticular, and honeycomb-like densities. Radiographs cannot demonstrate detailed interstitial changes. Radiographic changes of lung markings are nonspecific for interstitial fibrosis. The low thermal radiation zone of TTM suggests the possibility of interstitial fibrosis.

23.6.5.5   Comparison of the Usage of CT and TTM in SARS Diagnosis

HRCT may demonstrate subtle focal lesions in the early stage of SARS, especially ground-glass-like density; corresponding TTM images may show solid density structures of lesions as well as other functional image information related with illness.

Figure 23.18 shows a side-by-side comparison of using TTM and CT in SARS diagnosis. The TTM slicing shows the abnormal heat pattern with the depth of heat source 6 cm from skin surface. In addition, the subclavian area has a lower temperature than that of the right lung since the lower part of the right lung becomes white first. The CT image of April 26, 2003 showed the right lung lesion of SARS in its progress stage. The CT image of May 23, 2003 showed right lung lesion of SARS in its recovery stage. TTM image of May 23, 2003 indicates the abnormal heat pattern of lower right lung lesion which is confirmed by the CT image of the same date.

During the treatment of SARS, it is necessary to monitor the chest condition, such as the distribution and extent of the lesion and the effect of treatment. Following the initial stage of the disease, TTM could become the main imaging modality of examination of SARS since it can show the general manifestation of the disease. In addition, it is convenient, less expensive, and requires less exposure to potentially harmful radiation. During the recovery stage, if there is any change towards possible pulmonary interstitial hyperplasia, HRCT and TTM should be used to reveal the details of the interstitial and functional low-thermal radiation zone. The different features of these two imaging modalities are summarized in Table 23.6.

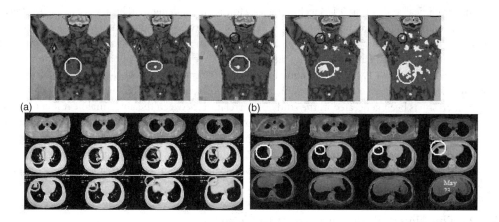

FIGURE 23.18   (See color insert.) Comparison between CT and TTM in SARS diagnosis — TTM image of May 23, 2003 indicates the abnormal heat pattern of lower right lung lesion which is confirmed by the CT image of the same date. *First row:* TTM slicing shows the abnormal heat pattern with the depth of heat source 6 cm from skin surface; in addition, the subclavian area has a lower temperature than that of the right lung. *Second row:* (a) CT image of April 26, 2003 showed right lung lesion of SARS progress stage; (b) CT image of May 23, 2003 showed right lung lesion of SARS recovery stage (©2005 IEEE).

TABLE 23.6   Performance
Comparison between CT and TTM

	CT	TTM
Radiation	Yes	No
Protection	Difficult	Easy
Exam time	25 min	5 min
Cost	High	Low
Environment risk	Yes	No
Mobility	Worst	Best
Consumption	30 KW	0.3 KW

The TTM, as a functional imaging modality, is able to quickly examine and assess the position, morphology, and progress of SARS lesions, in the meantime effectively monitoring treatment and patient recovery by providing information regarding the functional condition of the liver, spleen, kidney, and other organs.

The TTM can be used as first line imaging system for SARS screening, followed by CT, and TTM to carry out further differential diagnosis, including full course treatment monitoring. This combination of the two imaging systems should be the most beneficial for future prevention and treatment of SARS.

23.7 Study of Trilogy-Imaging Characteristics on TTM and Its Relationship with Malignancies

23.7.1 Introduction

The human body is a heat-radiant source under normal condition with balanced metabolism, and the heat is transmitted from the within the body to the surface. Once disease occurs at a site, such as a tumor, an inflammation, or hyper-functionalism and hypo-functionalism, the normal metabolism of regional cells in this site will change, reflected as the change of the heat radiance value. TTM can receive ultra-red radiance signal transmitted from cells during metabolism, and examine the exact intensity of different sites. The depth of abnormal heat foci can also be localized. See Section 23.3 for detail.

During the clinical study of the TTM technology, we found that independent heat foci can be discovered in the head (equivalent to occipital tuberosity), the neck (equivalent to thyroid gland), and the upper abdomen (equivalent to pancreas) in most of the patients with malignancies (these abnormal heat foci are not obvious in senile and advanced malignancy patients). We refer to this phenomenon as the *trilogy-imaging characteristics on* TTM. This phenomenon also exists in a small set of normal populations, and surprisingly, in this small set, 60% of the people have a family history of malignancy in direct relatives.

Great interest has been generated in the study of correlation between the abnormal heat foci (trilogy-imaging with TTM) and tumor. In our research, we examined 90 cancer patients and 32 normal controls with TTM. Their imaging characteristics were compared to elucidate the relationship between cancer patients and trilogy-imaging characteristics on TTM. Based on these study results, we can explore the mechanism of trilogy-imaging characteristics on TTM in cancer patients, and provide theoretic basis for further diagnosis.

23.7.2 The Neuro-Endocrine–Immune Theory

Due to its origin from neuro-endocrine system [23–27], we try to discuss the characteristics of trilogy-imaging on the basis of Neuro-Endocrine–Immune theory.

In 1977, Besedovsky first advised the Neuro-Endocrine–Immune network hypothesis. In the last two decades, many studies were performed at the *in vivo*, cellular and molecular levels; and results have shown the effectiveness of neurotransmitters and hormone molecules on the modulation of the immune system. On the other hand, the immune cell can produce neuro-endocrine hormone through some cytokines, which indicates that the neuro-endocrine and immune system constitutes a complex network, and the latter plays an important role in the regulation of normal activities of the whole body. However, can this theory explain the phenomenon of abnormal heat foci on TTM in the patients with malignancies?

Studies show that, in the status of malignancies, there are two kinds of antitumor immune responses, including specific ones and nonspecific ones, and many cytokines are involved in this process. At the same time, circulating cytokines can enter the brain through the third cerebral ventricle, binding the correspondent receptors, and exerting its effect on the central nervous system (CNS), to stimulate the production and release of neuropeptide, such as dopamine (DA) and epinephrine, as well as other local cytokines. In addition, the second messenger, such as cAMP, IP3, and DAG can be activated by cytokines and antigens. All the above show that cytokines can work on CNS, and indirectly affect the release of specific neuro-hormone (TRH, CRH, etc.) on pituitary gland, and finally regulate the endocrine system, manifested by the abnormal heat foci in the occipital tuberosity (hypothalamus), thyroidal gland and pancreas on TTM imaging. The compromised immune function in the senile and patients with advanced cancer can explain the unobvious heat foci in this population.

The exchange of the message in the above mentioned neuro-endocrine–immune network constitutes a regulative circuit: antigens (including tumor antigens) stimulate the release of the immune cytokines, and the latter work on the distant neuro-endocrine structure, then feed back to the CNS. The CNS can regulate the peripheral immune system through the release of hormones, peripheral neurotransmitters, and neuropeptides. In the animal models, the electronic activities and hormone shifting rate in neuro-endocrine system changes greatly after the activation of the immune system by antigen. This result provides strong support for the theory, that the imaging of TTM can confirm the modulation of neuro-endocrine–immune network and stress status indirectly.

23.7.3 Clinical Study of Correlation Between Trilogy-Imaging of TTM and Malignancies

23.7.3.1 Experiment 1

This study selected 90 cancer patients, aged between 35 and 75. Among them, 28 were diagnosed as having digestive tract cancers, 43 with breast cancer, 17 with lung cancer, and 2 with prostate cancer. All patients are from either Rui-Jin Hospital or Rui-Mei Health Center in Shanghai, China. To form the control data, 32 healthy volunteers from Rui-Mei Health Center, aged between 25 and 51, were chosen.

All the patients were asked to take off their clothes and rest in the room of examination of temperature 22 to 25° for heat balance. The TTM technique (TSI-2 type system, made in China) was then used to capture the thermal image from the standard position. Appropriate variables such as temperature scale, lens, and temperature window were set and topographic analysis was performed. The CES2000 software was used for statistical analysis.

Among the 90 cancer patients, 86 were diagnosed to have trilogy-imaging characteristics on TTM. Two patients with advanced cancer and 2 senile cancer patients did not have that characteristic. Table 23.7 shows the detailed statistics. TTM (+) is used to denote patients with trilogy imaging on TTM, and TTM (−) those without trilogy imaging on TTM.

We performed the chi-square test on the data. Statistical significance was reached ($P = 0.0000$), and H0 was refused if $\alpha = 0.0500$ is assumed. The percentage of the characteristics of trilogy imaging on TTM is higher in the cancer patients than in normal population.

In the 32 normal control patients, 9 volunteers had trilogy characteristic on TTM, among them, 6 (more than 66%) had cancer family history in direct relatives. Detailed statistics are listed in the following table.

	TTM (+)	TTM (−)
With cancer family history	6	3
Without cancer family history	3	20

We also performed chi-square test on the data. Statistical significance was reached ($P = 0.0003$), and H0 was refused if $\alpha = 0.0500$ is assumed. The percentage of the characteristics of trilogy imaging on TTM is higher in the people with a family history of cancer than those without.

TABLE 23.7   Chi-Square Value (Pearson Unadjusted) $= 62.2843, P = 0.0000$

	TTM(+)	TTM(−)
Cancer patients	86	4
Normal population	9	23

TABLE 23.8   TTM and Chi-Square Test Results

Results	TTM (+)	TTM (−)
Abnormal thyroid function (↑ or ↓)	1	0
Normal thyroid function	8	2

TABLE 23.9   The TTM Trilogy
Imaging Results of Six SLE Patients

Results	TTM (+)	TTM (−)
6 SLE Patients	0	6

23.7.3.2   Experiment 2 — Study of Correlation between Thyroid Function and Abnormal Heat Foci in Neck

TTM examination were received by histology-diagnosed cancer patients (4 males and 7 females, aged 38 to 71) received TTM examination. Among them, 3 were diagnosed with gastric and colon-rectal cancer, 6 with breast cancer, and 2 with lung cancer. Trilogy imaging occurs in 9 out of 11 (81.82%) cancer patients.

Thyroid examination was performed on the patients by isotope scan. Thyroid function including T3, T4, FT3, FT4 was assayed at the same time. Detailed statistics are listed in Table 23.8. The chi-square test is performed on the data. Correlation analysis of cross table data shows that $P = 1.0000$, and H0 is not refused according to $\alpha = 0.0500$, which indicates that abnormal heat foci might not be related to thyroid function.

23.7.3.3   Experiment 3 — Correlation Study of Autoimmune Diseases and Trilogy Imaging Characteristics

Totally 6 clear diagnosed SLE patients (all female, aged 22 to 43 [mean 29]) received TTM examination on March 2004. There is no relationship between the trilogy characteristics on TTM and the autoimmune disease. But these patients all received high dose corticoids, which may affect the results of TTM. The clinical data of previously untreated autoimmune disease patients will be collected for further research. Detailed statistical results are shown in Table 23.9.

23.8   Discussion

Through various clinical studies, we found that most of the patients with malignant cancers were related to trilogy-imaging characteristics on TTM (corresponding to occipital tuberosity in the head, thyroid gland in the neck, and pancreas in the upper abdomen). Interesting questions are raised, for example, are these characteristics representing function abnormality of these specific tissue or organ? Is there any theoretical basis behind the abnormal behavior? Based on their correspondent anatomic sites, we think it is associated with hypothalamus, thyroid gland, and pancreas.

We have conducted three clinical studies. Statistical results show that there is a high correlation between the trilogy-imaging characteristics of TTM and the malignancies. In the meanwhile, we also found, from the first clinical study, that a lot of the normal volunteers also manifest trilogy characteristics on TTM, and above 60% of these volunteers have direct family history in close relatives. How can we explain this phenomenon given that no clinical malignant parameters are found in these patients? Study shows that malignancy is a kind of genetic disease, determined by both genetic and environmental factors. The volunteers with family history may carry potential abnormal genes, which determines the evolution of malignant cells, and the abnormal protein expressed by these genes can induce immune response that further affects the neuro-endocrine system. Due to the long process of the formation and development of the tumor, the neuro-endocrine–immune network was already in stress status, hence forming the characteristic change of TTM imaging. Theoretically, specific antitumor immune response works in the early or even primitive period of the tumor development stage. We can discover the occipital tuberosity, cervical, and mid- or para-abdominal abnormal heat foci in the very early stage of the tumor, which will help us in the early diagnosis of the tumor if the results are proved by prospective studies.

Many studies have shown the effect of cytokines on neurohypothalamus-endocrine system. From the second clinical study, we found that the abnormal heat foci in the neck may not originate from the thyroid, and that the foci in abdomen may not originate from pancreas.

In addition, we have studied the manifestation of TTM trilogy imaging in cancer patients, and discovered that, in part of the patients, the abnormal heat foci present in a node form and concatenate with each other. This phenomenon also occurs in the unfixed site in chest.

According to the correspondent anatomic site of abnormal heat foci on TTM, we reviewed many references and propose a new possible hypothesis: *A tetralogy imaging originates from hypothalamus and cervical, thoracic and abdominal sympathetic ganglia.* This hypothesis is based on the following four arguments:

1. According to the neuro-endocrine–immune theory, hypothalamus can regulate sympathetic and parasympathetic nerve (the highest center of vegetable nerve), besides the modulation of the secretion of hormones of pituitary gland.
2. Cytokines can activate hypothalamus platform, especially hypothalamus–pituitary body–adrenal gland (HPA) axis (through IL-1).
3. Sympathetic trunk was distributed both on the neck and along the spine: cervical sympathetic trunk was localized posterior to cervical vessel sheath, anterior to transverse process; thoracic and lumbar sympathetic ganglia was localized along the spine. They are all activated by norepinephrine and other transmitters such as neuropeptide. Norepinephrine is mainly released from the sympathetic nerve end; it plays an important role on integrating the neuro-endocrine function and visceral automatic nerve reaction.
4. There is clear correspondence among the sites of four abnormal heat foci and the sites of hypothalamus, cervical sympathetic trunk and thoracic, lumbar sympathetic ganglia.

These imply that TTM signal abnormality was caused by hypothalamus, cervical sympathetic trunk and thoracic and lumbar sympathetic ganglia dysfunction, rather than hypothalamus–thyroid gland–pancreas platform we know before. This hypothesis is in consistence with the neuro-endocrine–immune theory. In immune mechanism, cytokines can affect hypothalamus, and play another important role, regulation of vegetable nerve function besides affecting endocrine. Hence, sympathetic trunk function is changed, manifesting of signal abnormality of malignancy platform on TTM. In animal models, immune response was first triggered by no toxic, no infectant and no newborn antigen. Results also showed that their endocrine system, automatic nerve system and catecholamine shifting rate were changed after the activation of the immune system.

23.9 Summary, Conclusions, and Recommendations

After ten years of R&D work, the TTM medical evaluation technology has gone through different phases; from merely a lab experiment, accepted by society and finally enters the initial stage of mass production. At the dawn of the new century, TTM technology will change the conventional model of medicine and lead human health to a completely new phase, the medical prediction phase. During this phase, efforts are dedicated to a new model of medicine, that is, active prediction and protection compared to conventional passive treatment, such that unhealthy elements can be restrained before the onset of diseases.

The TTM technique and the resulting apparatus have been patented [27]. Clinical study has shown increased sensitivity and specificity with the use of this method. The concept has been validated in China for several applications, including breast cancer detection, and ovarian cancer detection. About 400,000 patients were scanned using the TTM system in 5 years. Among them, 50,000 patients underwent breast scan. There are 103 breast cancer cases detected by TTM which were proved by biopsy. Among these 103 cases, 92 cases also went through mammography. Mammography missed 6 out of these 92 cases. Two of the missed tumor size is 2 mm. The concept is also in the process of validation in the United States/Canada, including the Ville Marie Breast Cancer Center in Canada (TTM's diagnosis agrees with Center's diagnosis on 198 cases out of 200 testing images), Elliott Mastology Center at Baton Rouge, LA, and NIH (Karposi Sarcoma/Angiogenesis).

Different from routine biochemical assays and imaging examinations, TTM is convenient, nontraumatic, and economical. At the same time, it can provide additional information of the status of immune function, in addition to the exact tumor image. The tumor platform of TTM is especially helpful to the patients with occulting history or susceptible to malignancy, probing for a health examination, and disease screening.

In addition, initial clinical studies also make us believe that tetralogy imaging may be more reasonable according to the nature of the cancer, which is caused by the activation of hypothalamus, cervical, thoracic, and abdominal sympathetic ganglia. Further research is needed for more accurate validation and quantification.

Acknowledgments

The authors are grateful to colleagues and many contributors for the very instructive suggestions and support of the clinical study which led to the much improved quality of the chapter.

- Section 23.4: Drs. X. W. Tang, H. S. Ding, and G. Z. Wang (Biomedical Engineering Department of Tsinghua University, Beijing, China).
- Section 23.5: Drs. Q. Wang, Y. Tan, L. Rong, S. S. Tai, L. J. Ye, W. T. Xiu, Y. J. Zhang, and M. Liu (Institute of Basic Medical Science, China Army General Hospital, Beijing, China), Prof. W. C. Qin (The 304 Hospital, Beijing China), Drs. X. W. Tang (Tsing Hua University), Dr. J. B. Liu (Beijing Long Fu Hospital), and Dr. J. Wu (TTM International Inc. USA).
- Section 23.6: Drs. W. Wang, D.Q. Ma, and C.W. Yuan (Beijing You An Hospital, China), Dr. Z.Y. Jin (Beijing Xie He Hospital, China), Dr. J. Wu (TTM International, Inc. USA), Drs. N. Patronas, A.H. Gandjdakhche, and M. Hassan (National Institute of Health), Dr. R. Xue (Johns Hopkins Medical Center), and Dr. J. Head (Mastology Institute, Baton Rouge, LA), Dr. N.A. Diakides and M. Diakides (Advanced Concepts Analysis, Inc., USA).

References

[1] B.F. Jones, "A reappraisal of the use of infrared thermal image analysis in medicine." *IEEE Trans. Med. Imag.*, 17: 1019–1027, 1998.

[2] H.H. Pennes, "Analysis of tissue and arterial blood temperature in resting human forearm." *J. Appl. Physiol.* 2: 93–122, 1948.

[3] E.Y.K. Ng and N.M. Sudarshan, *J. Med. Eng. Technol.* 25: 53–60, March/April 2001.

[4] C.L. Chan, "Boundary element method analysis for the bioheat transfer equation." *ASME J. Heat Transfer* 114: 358–365, 1992.

[5] T.R. Hsu, N.S. Sun, and G.G. Chen, "Finite element formulation for two dimensional inverse heat conduction analysis. "*ASME J. Heat Transfer* 114: 553–557, 1992.

[6] Z.Q. Liu and C. Wang. *Method and Apparatus for Thermal Radiation Imaging.* U.S. Patent 6,023,637, February 8, 2000.

[7] W. Cockburn, *Medical Thermal Imaging Facts and Myths.* Cockburn Health and Weilness, IRIE, 1999.

[8] M. Anbar, "Clinical thermal imaging today." *IEEE Eng. Med. Biol.* July/August: 25–33, 1998.

[9] J.D. Wallace, "Thermography examination of the breast." In *Early Breast Cancer: Detection and Treatment*. H.S. Gallagher (ed). New York: Wiley, 1975.

[10] Y. Ohashi and I. Uchida, "Application of dynamic thermography on breast cancer diagnosis." *IEEE Eng. Med. Biol.* July/August: 34–42, 1998.

[11] H. Qi, P.T. Kuruganti, and Z.Q. Liu, "Early detection of breast cancer using thermal texture maps." *IEEE International Symposium on Biomedical Imaging*, Washington, 2002.

[12] C.H. Jone, "Thermography of female breast." In *Diagnosis of Breast Disease*. C.A. Parsons (ed.) Baltimore: University Park Press, pp. 214–234, 1983.

[13] H.J. Isard, W. Becker, R. Shilo et al., "Breast thermography after four years 100 studies." *Am. J. Roentgenol.* 115: 811–821, 1972.

[14] L.J. Degroot et al., *Endocrinology.* 2nd ed. Vol. 1, Philadelphia, NB. Saunders Company, pp. 264–283, 1989.

[15] I. Fujimasa. "Pathophysiological expression and analysis of far infrared thermal images." *IEEE Eng. Med. Bio.* July/August: 34–42, 1998.

[16] J.F. Head, F. Wang, C.A. Lipari, and R. Elliott, "The important role of infrared imaging in breast cancer." *IEEE Eng. Med. Biol.* May/June: 52–57, 2000.

[17] S.A. Feig, G.S. Shaber, G.F. Schwartz et al., "Thermography, mammography, and clinical examination in breast cancer screening." *Radiology* 122: 123–127, 1977.

[18] M. Gautheriehe and Gros, "Breast thermography and cancer risk prediction." *Cancer* 45: 51–56, 1980

[19] H.J. Isard, "Other imaging techniques." *Cancer* 53: 658–664, 1984.

[20] NIAID Research on Severe Acute Respiratory Syndrome (SARS).http://www.niaid.nih.gov/factsheets/sars.htm

[21] X.R. Liu, J. Lu, Y.W. Wang, and X.W. Ni, "Physical analysis of intravascular low-reaction-lever laser irradiation therapy on improving the hemorheologic characteristics." *Proceedings of SPIE — The International Society for Optical Engineering*, Vol. 3863, pp. 465–467, 1999.

[22] J.M. Nicholls, L.L. Poon, K.C. Lee, W.F. Ng, S.T. Lai et al., "Lung pathology of fatal severe acute respiratory syndrome." *Lancet* 361: 1773–1778, May 24, 2003.

[23] H.D. Basedovsky and A. D. Rey, "Immun-neuro-endocrine interactions: facts and hypotheses." *Endocr. Rev.* 17: 64, 1996.

[24] L.J. Crofford, "Neuroendocrine influences." In *Primer on the Rheumatic Diseases*. J.H. Klippel (ed.) 11th ed. Georgia USA; Arthritis Foundation, pp. 80–83, 1997.

[25] K.S. Madden and D.L. Felten, "Experimental basis for neutral-immune interactions." *Phys. Rev.* 75: 77, 1995.

[26] P.T. Mandrup, J. Neurop, et al., "Cytokines and the endocrine system. 1. The immunoendocrine network." *Eur. J. Endoc.*, 133: 660, 1995.

[27] S. Reichlin, "Endocrine-immune interaction." In *Endocrinology*. L.J. Degroot. ed. Vol. 3, 3rd ed., Philadelphia: WB Saunders and Co Ltd, pp. 2964–2989, 1995.

24

IR Imagers as Fever Monitoring Devices: Physics, Physiology, and Clinical Accuracy

24.1 Introduction... 24-1
24.2 Physics of Thermal Radiation Theory................. 24-2
24.3 Pathophysiology 24-3
    Body vs. Skin Temperature • Human Body Heat Exchange •
    Fever • Infrared Thermography
24.4 Study Design 24-7
24.5 Linear Regression Analysis 24-9
24.6 Receiver Operating Curve (ROC) Analysis............ 24-10
24.7 Artificial Neural Networks (ANNs) Analysis 24-11
24.8 Results and Discussions 24-12
    General Linear Regression Analysis • General ROC Curve
    Analysis • Statistical Analysis on Data Sets E and F •
    General ANNs Analysis
24.9 Conclusions 24-17
Acknowledgments... 24-19
References 24-19

E.Y.K. Ng
Nanyang Technological University

G.J.L. Kaw
Tan Tock Seng Hospital

24.1 Introduction

The SARS is a new potentially fatal infectious viral respiratory illness caused by a novel coronavirus, named the SARS-associated coronavirus (SARS-CoV) (Ksiazek, 2003; Peris, 2003; Rota, 2003; de Jong, 1997). The main symptoms of SARS (Ksiazek, 2003) are high fever, dry cough, shortness of breath, and breathing difficulties. The first SARS outbreak occurred in Guangdong Province, China in November 2002. Aided by international air travel, it had spread worldwide by late February 2003. The first outbreak of SARS officially ended when World Health Organization (WHO) announced that the last human-to-human transmission of the coronavirus had been broken on June 5, 2003. From the data compiled by WHO in August 2003, there were 8437 cases of SARS in 29 countries of which 813 were fatal (CDC, 2004). Singapore is one of the more severely affected countries, which includes China (including Hong Kong and Taiwan), Canada, and Vietnam. The economic cost of the SARS outbreak has been high with disruption of commerce and health care. With the diminished number of overseas travelers, the tourism and airline industries were particularly affected.

Although SARS has been contained, there is a constant fear of reemergence of the virus. It has been proposed that the imposed ban on the exotic-animals trade is one of the main reasons that SARS has failed to stage a significant resurgence still April 2004 (Pottinger, 2004). Other reasons why the disease did not return in the winter of 2004 are open to debate. This winter, just four people were diagnosed with SARS, all in Guangdong province. By May 5, 2004 only nine more people (with one dead) were diagnosed with SARS in Beijing and Anhui. There has been a vast improvement in China's response to the recent SARS outbreak and at the time of writing, there has not been community spread of the disease. Despite intense research, the behavior of the SARS coronavirus is still unpredictable and the threat of SARS resurfacing and causing an epidemic still remains.

Officials at the WHO therefore worry that the disease still has the potential to resurface and create a health crisis as it did in 2003, when it caused serious atypical pneumonia killing 813 and disrupting commerce and health care in cities from Hong Kong to Hanoi and Singapore, Toronto to Taipei. For example, the diminished number of overseas travelers, the reduced number of airline flights, and other factors significantly damaged the relevant sectors, such as the tourism and airline industries in many countries.

In short, speculation that the virus had lain dormant in human during the warm months of summer and autumn, waiting to wreak havoc when temperatures dropped, appears to have been incorrect. Exactly how the virus burred itself out during the summer of 2003 remains a mystery. Bold policy measures, including travel alerts, quarantines, and public-hygiene campaigns, were critical in containing the disease and saving lives. There is still no cure or vaccines for SARS and the best that can be done to prevent another SARS outbreak is early detection to prevent the local and international spread of the SARS virus. Constant vigilance must be maintained. It is therefore important to have a reliable mass screening method for potential SARS patients at airports, seaports, immigration checkpoints, and hospitals.

It is thus important for the use of screening process at airports, seaports, immigration checkpoints, and hospitals for reliable mass blind screening of potential fever subjects, as these are crowded, mission critical facilities, and unfortunately terrific amplifiers for SARS transmission.

The cardinal symptom of SARS is fever. Because of the ability of infrared (IR) imaging systems to generate thermograms and measure temperature, it has been proposed that the use of these systems for the detection of elevated body temperature would be an efficient and accurate method for mass blind screening for potential SARS infected persons. The quality of the IR system depends on how well it fulfills its intended purpose, understanding of its limitation and degree of error involved. Some sources of uncertainty include drift, ambient temperature, humidity range, sunlight, nearby electrical sources, lighting, target distance, response time, etc. These variables may potentially cause both false negative and false positive readings without any outward indication that the data are flawed (Airport, 2003; Blackwell, 2003; Canadian, 2003).

The IR imager measures only the skin temperature. The skin temperature is lower than the normal core body temperature (98.6°F/36.9°C), due to well-studied heat evaporation, conduction, and convection principles (Ng and Sudharsan, 2001). It is thus important to establish an appropriate temperature baseline at the most practical site (such as forehead, eyes, or whole face, etc.) as the upper limit of normal for a healthy person. A temperature reading above the cut-off "baseline" reading signals a potential fever. When an elevated temperature is detected, the subject's body temperature is confirmed with an oral or aural thermometer. A truly febrile subject will be sent for medical assessment. Used in this manner, IR imagers can be the first line of defense in SARS screening.

24.2 Physics of Thermal Radiation Theory

Any object whose temperature is above absolute zero Kelvin emits radiation at a particular rate and with a distribution of wavelengths. This wavelength distribution is dependent on the temperature of the object and its spectral emissivity, $\varepsilon(\lambda)$. The spectral emissivity, which may also be considered as the radiation efficiency at a given wavelength, is in turn characterized by the radiation emission efficiency based on whether the body is a blackbody, greybody, or selective radiators. The blackbody is an ideal body. It is a perfect absorber that absorbs all incident radiation and is conversely a perfect radiator. This means that a blackbody absorbs and emits energy to the maximum that is theoretically possible at a given temperature. Within a given wavelength:

- $\varepsilon = 1$ for blackbody
- $\varepsilon = $ constant < 1 for greybody
- $0 \leq \varepsilon \leq 1$ for selective radiator

The radiative power (or energy) and its wavelength distribution are given by Planck radiation law (Burnay et al., 1988):

$$W(\lambda, T) = \frac{2\pi hc^2}{\lambda^4} \left[\exp\left(\frac{hc}{\lambda kT}\right) - 1 \right]^{-1} \text{Wcm}^{-2}\mu\text{m}^{-1} \tag{24.1}$$

or in number of photons emitted:

$$P(\lambda, T) = \frac{2\pi c}{\lambda^4} \left[\exp\left(\frac{hc}{\lambda kT}\right) - 1 \right]^{-1} \text{photons sec}^{-1}\,\text{cm}^{-2}\mu\text{m}^{-1} \tag{24.2}$$

where

h (Planck's constant) $= 6.6256 \times 10^{-34}$ Jsec
c (velocity of light in vacuum) $= 2.9979 \times 10^8$ msec^{-1}
k (Boltzmann's constant) $= 1.38054 \times 10^{-23}$ WsecK^{-1}
$\lambda = $ wavelength in μm
$T = $ temperature in K.

While infrared radiation is invisible to human eye, it can be detected and displayed by special IR cameras. These cameras detect the invisible infrared radiation emitted by an object and convert it to a monochrome or multicolored image on a monitor screen wherein the various shades or colors represent the thermal patterns across the surface of the object. The thermal imager is coupled with computer software, for the interpretation of the infrared images (thermal maps). Figure 24.1 illustrates an example of normal and febrile temperature profiles from a thermal imager (Flir, 2004). Temperature readings are also registered.

In general, thermal imagers offer an excellent means of making a qualitative determination of surface temperature, but there are many difficulties in obtaining an absolute measurement. The skin is the largest organ in the human body and helps to maintain the thermal equilibrium of the body and the environment through heat transfer processes. The study of the heat exchange processes of the body from the deep tissues to the skin and subsequently to the environment can provide information on pathology (Ng and Sudharsan, 2001; Ng and Chua, 2002; Ng and Kaw, 2004a,b).

24.3 Pathophysiology

24.3.1 Body vs. Skin Temperature

Heat is generated from energy released secondary to metabolic processes that are constantly taking place in the body. For example, the enthalpy change of reaction for average mixed foodstuffs (with balanced stoichiometric reaction) is -320 kcal/mole.

$$C_2H_6O \text{ (foodstuff)} + 3O_2 \quad \rightarrow \quad 3H_2O + 2CO_2 - 320 \text{ kcal/mole} \tag{24.3}$$

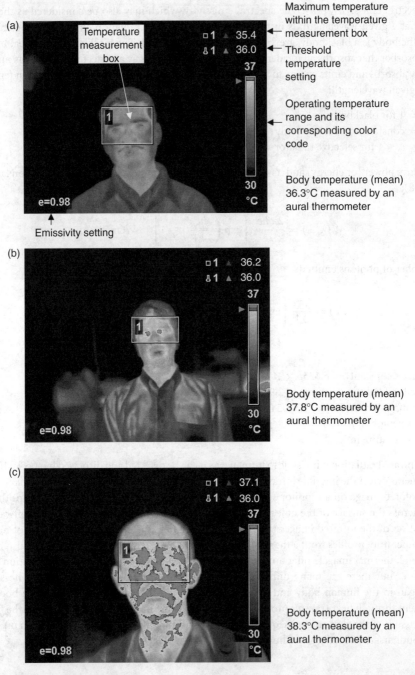

FIGURE 24.1   (See color insert following page **29**-16.) Examples of temperature profiles using thermal imager with temperature readings. (Taken from FLIR Systems http.//www.flir.com, accessed November, 2004. With permission.)

Part of this energy is conserved as transformation and the rest is released as heat that accumulates within the body, causing its temperature to rise. Following Newton's law of cooling, this heat can be readily dissipated into the environment as long as it is cooler than the body temperature. The body temperature is thus the difference between the amount of heat produced by metabolism within the body and the amount of heat lost to external environment (Ng and Sudharsan, 2004).

Heat generated by the body is first transported to the skin before dissipation into the environment (Figure 24.2). The skin has its own temperature, which will be termed skin temperature in this chapter. Temperature from different sites on the skin surface varies. This in turn varies from the core body temperature. The normal body temperature ranges from 36 to 38°C whilst the mean skin temperature is 33°C. The core temperature refers to the temperature within deep tissue (Houdas and Ring, 1982). It is relatively constant, despite changes in environmental conditions and the degree of physical activity. On the contrary, skin temperature fluctuates and is a function of the amount of heat flow into it. Therefore it is generally agreed that the core temperature is a better indicator of body temperature. However, the measurement of core temperature is generally more difficult and time consuming. Hence, it is not practical for mass-screening purposes. Some of the sites for body temperature measurement are:

1. Oral
2. Aural or Tympanic membrane (Core)
3. Rectal (Core)
4. Axillary (Core)
5. Esophageal (Core)
6. Pulmonary artery (Core)
7. Urinary bladder (Core)

24.3.2 Human Body Heat Exchange

Heat produced by the human body through metabolism is transported from the body to the skin and is subsequently dissipated to the environment via conduction, convection, radiation, and evaporation (Houdas and Ring, 1982). These methods of heat loss can be classified as "Dry" heat exchange with the environment. Within the body, heat is transferred by conduction through the tissue and convection through blood. Convection via the blood is a very efficient component of heat transfer within the body, thus making skin temperature predominantly determined by the blood flow to the skin. Apart from "Dry" heat exchange, heat is also lost by evaporation of sweat and respiration. Evaporation of sweat removes heat from the body. This is a surface process in which only the portion of sweat evaporated results in heat loss from the body. Evaporation also takes place in the respiratory tract. However, the heat loss from this site is minimal and insignificant. Figure 24.2 illustrates the heat exchange processes of the body, which will affect the skin temperature. The body and environment eventually reaches equilibrium. Nonetheless, there are pathological processes such as inflammation, tumors, etc. that can cause changes in the heat flux. Invasion of pyrogens (of which the SARS coronavirus is an example) can also cause the body temperature to change. This is discussed in the next section. In fact, temperature change is one of the earliest symptoms of a pathological process. This may be detected via the patterns produced on thermography.

24.3.3 Fever

Blatties (1998) defines fever specifically as the elevation of the core body temperature exhibited by most species in response to invasion by infectious agents. Fever is a non-systemic reaction designed to combat the effects of invading pathogens. A fever is the primary host defense response to restore health to the afflicted host. High fevers destroy temperature-sensitive enzymes and proteins and cause increase in ventilation, perspiration, and blood flow to the skin. A fever should be distinguished from hyperthermia. During hyperthermia, the rise in body temperature is the consequence of the passive gain of heat in excess of the capability of active thermolytic processes. The rise in body temperature during a fever is the result of the activation of thermogenic effectors. Many different substances (pyrogens) can cause fever. The consequence of infection and fever is a hot flushed skin and increased fluid loss.

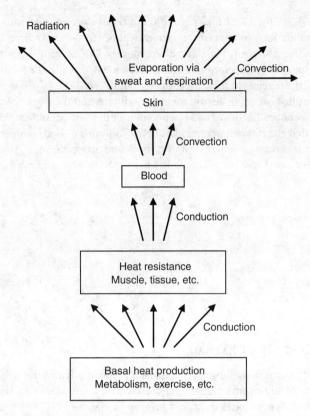

FIGURE 24.2   Human body heat exchange.

24.3.4   Infrared Thermography

As a diagnostic tool, thermography has several advantages in clinical use (Ng and Sudharsan, 2000). First, the physiological test equipment is completely passive, emits no harmful radiation, can be sited at a distance from the subject, and is noninvasive. Second, the test is ideal for detecting hot and cold spots, or areas of different emissivities on the skin surface since humans radiate infrared energy very efficiently. The emissivity of human skin is nearly 1.0. Third, the data collected can be recorded on photographic media, videotape, or sent to a computer for post processing. Finally, the equipment is highly portable, fully self-contained, and can be set up within minutes. It does not need any sources of illumination, thus making day and night imaging possible.

Although IR systems have many advantages for temperature screening, other than its cost, there are many variables that can affect its accuracy (Ng and Sudharsan, 2000). Ideally, the thermal imager should be operated in a stable indoor environment with stability of the operating ambient conditions within ±1°C. The thermal imager is ideally intended to operate in a stable indoor environment with operating ambient conditions and stability of ±1°C. The relative humidity range for the operating temperature range should also be from 40 to 75%. Environmental infrared sources such as sunlight, nearby electrical sources, and lighting can affect the accuracy of IR systems and should be minimized. The target should be located in an area free from draft and direct airflow.

The accuracy of the thermal imager is highly dependent on the skill and knowledge of the operator (Spring, 2003). Mishandling of the equipment will result in erroneous data. It is also important to understand that each make and model of IR equipment has different specifications and accuracies that can affect observed temperatures. Various scanners have different drift between self-corrections (Figure 24.3), uniformity within the field of view, minimum detectable temperature difference, error and stability of

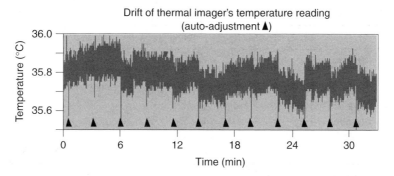

FIGURE 24.3 An example of the drift of a typical thermal imager's temperature reading between auto-adjustments. (Taken from Standards Technical Reference for *Thermal Imagers for Human Temperature Screening Part I: Requirements and Test Methods*, 2003. TR 15-1, Spring Singapore. ISBN 9971-67-963-9. With permission.)

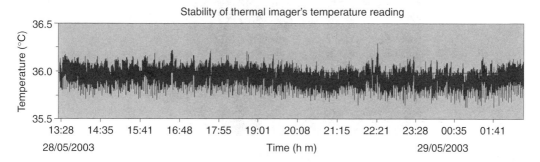

FIGURE 24.4 An example of the stability of a typical thermal imager's temperature reading. (Taken from Standard Technical Reference for *Thermal Imagers for Human Temperature Screening Part I: Requirements and Test Methods*, 2003. TR 15-1, Spring Singapore. ISBN 9971-67-963-9. With permission.)

threshold temperature (Figure 24.4), distance effect and minimum number of detector pixels in addition to different environmental requirements and subject conditions. For rapid and effective screening of a large number of people, it is essential that the thermal imager be capable of operating in a real time processing mode.

Disease processes can produce significant and unpredictable changes in body temperatures. Circulatory problems, previous injuries, and alcohol consumption can reduce body surface temperature. On the other hand, skin temperature can be increased by stress, physical exertion, the use of stimulants such as caffeine and nicotine, and inflammation secondary to trauma, or even sunburn. Heavy makeup, hormone replacement therapy, pregnancy and menstruation, can affect also skin temperature.

24.4 Study Design

The study was conducted in the Emergency Department of Tan Tock Seng Hospital (TTSH), the designated SARS hospital in Singapore and the Singapore Civil Defense Force Academy (SCDF). The total blind sample size collected was 502 with 85 febrile and 417 normal cases. Temperature readings were taken from the eye region (Ng and Kaw, 2004a,b). The breakdown of the sample is shown in Table 24.1.

The imager used by for the study in TTSH and SCDF was a handheld ThermaCAM S60 Flir system (Flir, 2004). The focal length from the subject to scanner was fixed at 2 m. The average temperature of the skin surface was measured from the field of view of the thermal imager with an appropriate adjustment for skin emissivity. Human skin emissivity may vary from site to site ranging from 0.94 to 0.99. Averaged

TABLE 24.1   The Sample Sizes for Eye Region

	Normal patients			Febrile patients			Total		
Descriptions	Male	Female	Total	Male	Female	Total	Male	Female	Total
TTSH									
2 weeks	190	72	262	36	12	48	227	83	310
2 days	14	6	20	12	4	16	26	10	36
3 days	20	13	33	13	8	21	33	21	54
SCDF	94	8	102	0	0	0	94	8	102
Total	318	99	417	61	24	85	380	122	502

Fever if average ear temperature $\geq 38°$C.

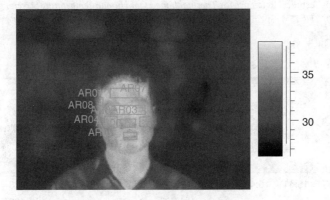

FIGURE 24.5   (See color insert.) Processed thermal image of the frontal profile.

aural temperature readings of both left and right ears were also taken using Braun Thermoscan IRT 3520+ (Ear, 2004). Thermal images from the TTSH (obtained over 2 weeks) sample were later processed using the ThermaCam Researcher 2002, computer software (Flir system, 2004). The following spots were logged and analyzed from the frontal profiles:

- Forehead
- Eye region
- Average cheeks
- Nose
- Mouth (closed)
- Average temple

Figure 24.5 shows an example of a processed thermal image of the frontal profile. A total of 187 (subjects) temperature readings were extracted from these spots. Among which, 21 were febrile cases and 166 were normal cases. This set of readings will be referred as data set E in this paper. The images were further processed to obtain readings from both frontal and side profiles from some of the subjects. Sixty-five sets of temperature readings with 10 febrile and 55 normal cases were extracted. This set of readings is referred to as data set F in the chapter. Figure 24.5 and Figure 24.6 presents an example of the processed thermal images of both frontal and side (left) profiles from the same subject. The following spots were logged from the subjects with frontal and side profiles:

- Forehead
- Eye region
- Average cheeks
- Nose

- Mouth (closed)
- Average temple
- Side face
- Ears
- Side temple

24.5   Linear Regression Analysis

Linear regression analysis (Dupont, 2002; Golberg, 2004) is a statistical method for obtaining the unique line that best fits a set of data points. The line of best fit is also known as the linear regression line. It uses the concept of "least squares," which minimizes the sum of square of the residuals or errors. S-Plus (version 6.1) software (2004) was used to perform the regression analysis. Different combinations of blind data from TTSH — 2 weeks, 2 days, and 3 days and SCDF were used for the regression analysis in order to increase the total sample size for comprehensive analysis. The mass screened data were given an alphabetical representation for easy reference and is summarized in Table 24.2. These alphabetical representations will be used synonymously with the actual data name in this chapter. For example, ABCD represents the combination of TTSH (2 weeks), TTSH (2 days), SCDF, and TTSH (3 days).

A linear regression analysis has two types of variable: dependent and independent variables. The independent variable used in the analysis is skin temperature (detected by the thermal imager) and the dependent variable is the core temperature (taken from the ear temperature readings). Figure 24.7 shows the regression line obtained using data set ABCD. The skin temperatures used here were extracted from the inner eye region.

Using the S-Plus software, a linear regression equation $y = \alpha + \beta x$ is generated where α is the intercept and β is the slope of the line. The linear regression equation in this case is $y = 24.0922 + 0.3695x$. The result of main interest here is the slope of the line β, which is 0.3695. This parameter indicates the strength of relationship between the skin temperature and body temperature and can be used to predict one variable

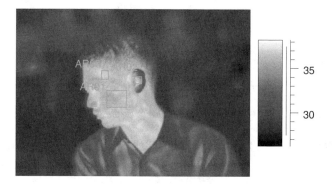

FIGURE 24.6   (See color insert.) Processed thermal images of the side profile.

TABLE 24.2   Alphabetical
Representations of Data

Data	Alphabetical representation
TTSH (2 weeks)	A
TTSH (2 days)	B
SCDF	C
TTSH (3 days)	D

from another. While the regression line explains a proportion of the variability in the dependent variable (y), the residuals indicate the amount of unexplained variability. The residual is thus a good indicator of the goodness of fit. A more general way of assessing the goodness of fit is to consider the proportion of the total variation explained by the model. This is usually done by considering the sum of squares explained by the regression as a percentage of the total sum of squares. This value is called R^2 and it assesses how well the model fits the overall data. R^2 has a value from 1 to 0 and a low value of R^2 indicates that even if a significant slope exists, the majority of the variability in body temperature is not explained by variation in the skin temperature and vice versa. Therefore, a high R^2 value is desirable. S-Plus software was used to predict the value of R^2.

24.6 Receiver Operating Curve (ROC) Analysis

The diagnostic performance of a test, or the ability of a test to discriminate diseased cases from normal cases is evaluated using ROC curve analysis (Shapiro, 1999; Ng, 2004; ROC, 2004). Perfect separation is rarely observed when we consider the result of a particular test in two populations, one population with a disease and the other without the disease. This is shown in Figure 24.8.

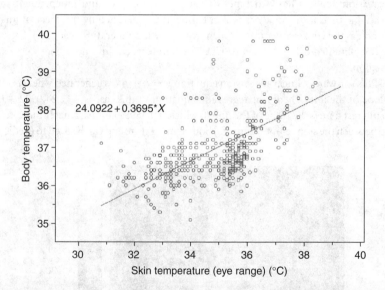

FIGURE 24.7   Linear regression line of body temperature vs. skin temperature (eye region). Data from ABCD set.

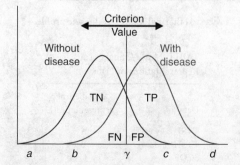

FIGURE 24.8   Test result.

It is common to define a threshold or decision limit γ and classify the patient as diseased if $A > \gamma$ and normal if $A < \gamma$ as illustrated in Figure 24.8. However, when defining a particular decision limit γ to discriminate between the two populations, some cases with the disease will be correctly classified as positive, True Positive (TP), but some cases with the disease will be classified as negative, False Negative (FN). On the other hand, some cases without the disease will be classified as positive, False Positive (FP), but some cases without the disease will be classified as negative, True Negative (TN). The following statistics can then be defined:

- *Sensitivity:* Probability that a test result will be positive when the disease is present (true positive rate, expressed as a percentage)
- *Specificity:* Probability that a test result will be negative when the disease is not present (true negative rate, expressed as a percentage)
- *Positive likelihood ratio:* Ratio between the probability of a positive test result given the presence of the disease and the probability of a positive test result given the absence of the disease
- *Negative likelihood ratio:* Ratio between the probability of a negative test result given the presence of the diseased and the probability of a negative test given the absence of the disease
- *Positive predictive value:* Probability that the disease is present when the test is positive (expressed as a percentage)
- *Negative predictive value:* Probability that the disease is not present when the test is negative (expressed as a percentage)
- *Accuracy:* The overall percentage of correct test results

Each decision limit γ gives a different set of results. Sensitivity and specificity can be used to estimate the decision limit. However, as γ decreases, sensitivity increases but specificity decreases and vice versa. It can be seen that there is a trade off between sensitivity and specificity as the decision limit varies. This implies that there must be an optimum decision limit γ with the highest accuracy, that is, the point with the best discrimination of the positive and negative cases. A useful graphical summary of discriminating accuracy is a plot of sensitivity vs. $(1 - \text{specificity})$ as γ varies. This is known as the ROC curve. MedCalc (version 7.4) software (ROC, 2004) was used for ROC curve analysis and a dichotomous variable with quantitative result must be input. The dichotomous variable selected was that of body temperature and the quantitative result used was skin temperature. Figure 24.9 shows the ROC curve of the ABD data set and Table 24.3 is the associated ROC report.

The cross-point marked on the ROC curve is the point with highest accuracy. From the ROC report, the optimum cutoff was also identified as the criterion with a $*$ marked at its side. This value is >34.6 in Table 24.3. Therefore 34.6°C is the recommended skin temperature cutoff from the ROC analysis. The ROC area was used to determine the ability of the test to discriminate febrile from normal cases and the value can be read off from the ROC report. From Table 24.3, the ROC area is 0.907. This means that a randomly selected individual from the febrile group has a test value larger than that for a randomly chosen individual from a normal group in 90.7% of the time. When the variables under study cannot distinguish between the two groups, the area will be equal to 0.5 (the ROC curve will coincide with the diagonal). When there is a perfect separation of the values of the two groups, the ROC area will be equals 1 (the ROC curve will reach the upper left corner of the plot). A larger ROC area is desirable as it implies that there is a better separation of the two groups of patients.

24.7 Artificial Neural Networks (ANNs) Analysis

Next, neural networks (NN) based mapping and classification have been used to analyze the temperature data collected from various sites on the face on both the frontal and side profiles (Ng and Kaw, 2004). Two networks namely single layer perception (SLP) back propagation (BP) and Kohonen self-organizing map (SOM) are experimented with different learning rules, transfer parameter settings, and the number of hidden neurons in order to decide networks that appear to perform reasonably well on both the

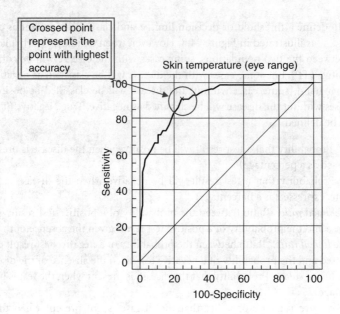

FIGURE 24.9   ROC curve of skin temperature (eye range) at body cutoff of 37.7°C. Data from ABD set.

training and testing data. Each network performance is measured informally on the basis of the RMS level. The best-trained network setting is subsequently saved in binary mode with a suitable filename. The performance of those two networks is evaluated more formally using a scoring system with the threshold of 0.5. Based on the score results, the threshold value is determined and used consistently. Once the evaluation of the two networks is completed, a good performance network is then selected.

24.8   Results and Discussions

24.8.1   General Linear Regression Analysis

The linear regression analysis was performed using S-Plus (version 6.1) software for different combinations of data collected from TTSH and SCDF. The best-fitted curve of body and skin temperatures (eye range) was plotted and their results were tabulated in Table 24.4.

The intercept α has no physical meaning and is of no actual interest in this chapter but is added in the result for completeness. The interest of regression analysis would be the regression ratio β and R^2. Comparing the original data sets A, B, C, and D, the regression ratio β is best for data set B: TTSH (2 days). The next best is data set D: TTSH (3 days) followed by those for data set A: TTSH (2 weeks). Data set C has the worse regression ratio. Similar trend had been observed for the value of R^2 with the exception of data set D being the highest followed by data set B. It was found that data set C has an exceptionally low β and R^2 values of 0.5133 and 0.1367. In other words, the body and skin temperatures (eye range) of data set C have very weak relationship. This is due to the fact that SCDF data has all nonfever (majority are young males with mean age of 23) data thereby making the sample bias. This observation was further proven by comparison made between data set AB, AC, and AD. Data set AC showed relatively low values for β and R^2. This was expected since data C already has low β and R^2 values. Comparison between data set ABC and ABD also indicated similar results. When data set C was added to data set ABD, forming data set ABCD, the results showed lower β and R^2 values as compared to those of data set ABD. This can be explained by the same reasoning.

On the contrary, data set BD has relatively high β and R^2 coefficients. This was attributed by high β and R^2 coefficients of the two individual sets of data. It thus suggested that data sets B and D possess a

TABLE 24.3 ROC Report of Skin Temperature (Eye Range — ABD Data Set) Using Body Temperature Cutoff of 37.7°C

Criterion	Sens. (95% C.I.)	Spec. (95% C.I.)	+LR	−LR
>30.8	100.0 (95.8–100.0)	0.0 (0.0–1.2)	1.00	
>30.8	100.0 (95.8–100.0)	0.6 (0.1–2.3)	1.01	0.00
>31.1	100.0 (95.8–100.0)	1.0 (0.2–2.8)	1.01	0.00
>31.4	100.0 (95.8–100.0)	1.3 (0.4–3.2)	1.01	0.00
>31.5	100.0 (95.8–100.0)	1.6 (0.5–3.7)	1.02	0.00
>31.6	100.0 (95.8–100.0)	2.2 (0.9–4.5)	1.02	0.00
>31.7	100.0 (95.8–100.0)	3.5 (1.8–6.2)	1.04	0.00
>31.8	100.0 (95.8–100.0)	4.5 (2.5–7.4)	1.05	0.00
>31.9	100.0 (95.8–100.0)	4.8 (2.7–7.8)	1.05	0.00
>32	100.0 (95.8–100.0)	6.1 (3.7–9.3)	1.06	0.00
>32.1	100.0 (95.8–100.0)	6.4 (3.9–9.7)	1.07	0.00
>32.3	100.0 (95.8–100.0)	6.7 (4.2–10.0)	1.07	0.00
>32.4	100.0 (95.8–100.0)	10.5 (7.3–14.4)	1.12	0.00
>32.5	100.0 (95.8–100.0)	12.4 (9.0–16.6)	1.14	0.00
>32.6	100.0 (95.8–100.0)	14.6 (10.9–19.1)	1.17	0.00
>32.7	100.0 (95.8–100.0)	16.9 (12.9–21.5)	1.20	0.00
>32.8	100.0 (95.8–100.0)	17.8 (13.8–22.5)	1.22	0.00
>32.9	100.0 (95.8–100.0)	21.7 (17.2–26.6)	1.28	0.00
>33	98.8 (93.7–99.8)	24.2 (19.6–29.3)	1.30	0.05
>33.1	98.8 (93.7–99.8)	28.3 (23.4–33.7)	1.38	0.04
>33.2	98.8 (93.7–99.8)	31.2 (26.1–36.7)	1.44	0.04
>33.3	98.8 (93.7–99.8)	36.6 (31.3–42.2)	1.56	0.03
>33.4	98.8 (93.7–99.8)	39.5 (34.0–45.1)	1.63	0.03
>33.5	98.8 (93.7–99.8)	43.0 (37.4–48.7)	1.73	0.03
>33.6	98.8 (93.7–99.8)	48.1 (42.4–53.8)	1.90	0.02
>33.7	98.8 (93.7–99.8)	53.5 (47.8–59.1)	2.13	0.02
>33.8	96.5 (90.1–99.2)	57.3 (51.6–62.9)	2.26	0.06
>33.9	96.5 (90.1–99.2)	58.6 (52.9–64.1)	2.33	0.06
>34	95.3 (88.5–98.7)	63.1 (57.5–68.4)	2.58	0.07
>34.1	94.2 (86.9–98.1)	65.3 (59.7–70.5)	2.71	0.09
>34.2	93.0 (85.4–97.4)	66.9 (61.4–72.1)	2.81	0.10
>34.3	93.0 (85.4–97.4)	68.8 (63.3–73.9)	2.98	0.10
>34.4	90.7 (82.5–95.9)	71.7 (66.3–76.6)	3.20	0.13
>34.5	90.7 (82.5–95.9)	72.9 (67.7–77.8)	3.35	0.13
>34.6[a]	90.7 (82.5–95.9)	75.8 (70.7–80.4)	3.75	0.12
>34.7	86.0 (76.9–92.6)	77.7 (72.7–82.2)	3.86	0.18
>34.8	82.6 (72.9–89.9)	80.6 (75.8–84.8)	4.25	0.22
>34.9	76.7 (66.4–85.2)	82.8 (78.2–86.8)	4.46	0.28
>35	74.4 (63.9–83.2)	84.1 (79.6–87.9)	4.67	0.30
>35.1	73.3 (62.6–82.2)	84.7 (80.2–88.5)	4.79	0.32
>35.2	73.3 (62.6–82.2)	86.6 (82.4–90.2)	5.48	0.31
>35.3	70.9 (60.1–80.2)	87.9 (83.8–91.3)	5.86	0.33
>35.4	70.9 (60.1–80.2)	88.9 (84.8–92.1)	6.36	0.33
>35.5	70.9 (60.1–80.2)	89.2 (85.2–92.4)	6.55	0.33
>35.6	66.3 (55.3–76.1)	89.2 (85.2–92.4)	6.12	0.38
>35.7	66.3 (55.3–76.1)	89.8 (85.9–92.9)	6.50	0.38
>35.8	66.3 (55.3–76.1)	90.1 (86.3–93.2)	6.71	0.37
>35.9	66.3 (55.3–76.1)	91.4 (87.7–94.3)	7.71	0.37
>36	62.8 (51.7–73.0)	93.0 (89.6–95.6)	8.96	0.40
>36.1	61.6 (50.5–71.9)	93.9 (90.7–96.3)	10.18	0.41
>36.2	59.3 (48.2–69.8)	95.2 (92.2–97.3)	12.41	0.43
>36.3	57.0 (45.8–67.6)	96.8 (94.2–98.5)	17.89	0.44
>36.4	53.5 (42.4–64.3)	97.5 (95.0–98.9)	20.99	0.48
>36.5	50.0 (39.0–61.0)	98.4 (96.3–99.5)	31.40	0.51
>36.6	39.5 (29.2–50.7)	98.4 (96.3–99.5)	24.83	0.61
>36.7	38.4 (28.1–49.5)	98.4 (96.3–99.5)	24.10	0.63

(Continued)

TABLE 24.3   (Continued) ROC Report of Skin Temperature

Criterion	Sens. (95% C.I.)	Spec. (95% C.I.)	+LR	−LR
>36.8	36.0 (26.0–47.1)	98.4 (96.3–99.5)	22.64	0.65
>36.9	31.4 (21.8–42.3)	98.4 (96.3–99.5)	19.72	0.70
>37	30.2 (20.8–41.1)	98.7 (96.8–99.6)	23.73	0.71
>37.1	26.7 (17.8–37.4)	99.0 (97.2–99.8)	27.99	0.74
>37.2	25.6 (16.8–36.1)	99.0 (97.2–99.8)	26.78	0.75
>37.3	22.1 (13.9–32.3)	99.7 (98.2–99.9)	69.37	0.78
>37.4	16.3 (9.2–25.8)	100.0 (98.8–100.0)	0.84	
⋮				
>38.3	3.5 (0.8–9.9)	100.0 (98.8–100.0)		0.97
>38.4	2.3 (0.3–8.2)	100.0 (98.8–100.0)		0.98
>39.1	1.2 (0.2–6.3)	100.0 (98.8–100.0)		0.99
>39.3	0.0 (0.0–4.2)	100.0 (98.8–100.0)		1.00

VARIABLE = Skin Temperature (Eye Range)
CLASSIFICATION VARIABLE
    Diagnosis
POSITIVE GROUP
    Diagnosis = 1
    Sample size = 86
NEGATIVE GROUP
    Diagnosis = 0
    Sample size = 314
Disease prevalence unknown.
Area under the ROC curve = 0.907
Standard error = 0.022
95% Confidence interval = 0.875 to 0.934
Sens. = Sensitivity
Spec. = Specificity
+LR = Positive likelihood ratio
−LR = Negative likelihood ratio
[a] = The optimum skin temperature cutoff

TABLE 24.4   Results of Linear Regression of Body and Skin Temperatures (Eye Range) for Various Data Sets

Description	A	B	C	D	AB	AC
Regression ratio β	0.5296	0.8127	0.5133	0.7240	0.4558	0.3158
Intercept α	18.8695	7.7702	18.4127	11.2713	21.3173	25.9282
R^2	0.4490	0.5969	0.1367	0.6797	0.4804	0.2462

Description	AD	BD	ABC	ABD	ABCD	—
Regression ratio β	0.4586	0.7194	0.3494	0.4369	0.3695	—
Intercept α	21.2088	11.3484	24.7844	21.9210	24.0922	—
R^2	0.4777	0.6292	0.3341	0.5016	0.3849	—

good relationship of body temperature with skin temperature (eye region). However, these two data sets have too few data points for their analysis to be meaningful. Even the combination of the two sets of data was still inadequate as there were only 90 cases. Results from the data sets of different sample sizes would also be expected to differ and it would be unfair to compare them. Having a larger sample size, would make the analysis more accurate and representative. Due to bias present in data set C, it was only right to exclude it from further analysis. Data set ABD was thus potentially the more representative set with a sample size of 400. It should also be noted that the individual data of set ABD were all collected using the same scanner settings and this consistency is important for the combination of data. From Table 24.4, the

TABLE 24.5   Results of ROC Analysis of Skin
Temperature (Eye Range) for Data Set ABD and ABCD

Cutoff at 37.5°C	ABD	ABCD
ROC area	0.908	0.854
Sensitivity (%)	67.4	56.8
Specificity (%)	90.6	97.1
False positive (%)	7.3	2.4
False negative (%)	7.5	8.2
Prevalence (%)	23.0	18.9
Accuracy (%)	85.3	89.4
Recommended Cutoff (°C)	34.6	35.9
Cutoff at 37.7°C		
ROC area	0.907	0.854
Sensitivity (%)	63.5	39.8
Specificity (%)	93.0	98.8
False positive (%)	5.5	1.0
False negative (%)	7.8	10.0
Prevalence (%)	21.3	16.5
Accuracy (%)	86.8	89.0
Recommended cutoff (°C)	34.6	35.9
Cutoff at 37.9°C		
ROC area	0.903	0.862
Sensitivity (%)	56.3	25.7
Specificity (%)	96.4	99.5
False positive (%)	3.0	0.4
False negative (%)	7.8	10.4
Prevalence (%)	17.8	13.9
Accuracy (%)	89.3	89.2
Recommended cutoff (°C)	34.6	36.2
Cutoff at 38.0°C		
ROC area	0.907	0.878
Sensitivity (%)	46.0	17.5
Specificity (%)	97.3	99.8
False positive (%)	2.3	0.2
False negative (%)	8.5	10.4
Prevalence (%)	15.8	12.5
Accuracy (%)	89.3	89.4
Recommended cutoff (°C)	35.5	36.1

β and R^2 value for data set ABD was 0.4369 and 0.5016 respectively. These were average values implying a reasonable relationship between body and skin temperatures (eye region), despite the presence of external variability such as environmental conditions, the patient's condition, and differing experience of operators obtaining the data.

24.8.2   General ROC Curve Analysis

ROC analysis has also been conducted for data set ABD and ABCD using MedCalc software. Skin temperatures measured from the eye region were used. The results using cutoff body temperature of 37.5, 37.7, 37.9, and 38.0°C are summarized in Table 24.5.

It can be seen from the results in Table 24.5 that sensitivity decreases and specificity increases as the cutoff decision limit, γ, increases. Similarly, increasing γ results in the false negative rate increasing and the false positive rate decreasing. Both the ROC areas of data set ABD and ABCD presented in Table 24.5 were high. This means that infrared thermography possesses great potential in differentiating subjects with elevated body temperature from normal cases during the blind mass screening of subjects. The accuracy of the ROC analysis for both sets of data was also high. This reinforces the potential of using an infrared system for the identification of a person with an elevated body temperature. The values of false positive and false negative of both sets of data at different cutoff have also shown promise of infrared thermography for screening febrile cases accurately from normal cases. The false positive and false negative values of both data sets at different cutoff temperatures shows that febrile subjects can be differentiated accurately from normal ones. As indicated in Table 24.5, these values generally fall below 10%. A low false positive rate implies that the infrared system has erroneously classified few normal cases as febrile cases. Similarly a low false negative rate would mean that the scanner has erroneously classified few febrile cases as normal cases. The latter could be avoided with a lower cutoff temperature.

24.8.3 Statistical Analysis on Data Sets E and F

Regression analysis was also performed on the data set F. This was to determine the site on the face with the best correlation with the core body temperature. The results are tabulated in Table 24.6.

Table 24.6 shows that the averaged (ave) temple readings have the highest values for both the β and R^2 coefficients. β and R^2 values for the side temple and eye region were also close to those of the ave temples. This suggested that the skin temperature measured from temple region offered a relatively better relationship with the body temperature. The eye region also shows a good correlation as its coefficients differed only slightly from the ave temple and side temple readings. However, there were only 65 samples in this data set. This may not be proven statistically significant. Table 24.7 tabulated the linear regression of body and skin temperatures of various sites on the face taken from the frontal profile (data set E) only. The sample size in this set of data was 187, which was more representative and thus the ROC analysis was performed for this sample.

Referring to Table 24.7, eye region has the highest β and R^2 values. Ave temples also have high β and R^2 values. Based on the results from the regression analysis, the skin temperature measured from eye

TABLE 24.6   Results of Regression Analysis Performed on Body and Skin Temperatures (Data Set F) Measured from Various Sites

Description	Regression ratio β	Intercept α	R^2
Frontal			
Forehead	0.4206	22.5443	0.3495
Eye range	0.5175	19.2068	0.4005
Ave cheeks	0.3896	23.8133	0.3582
Nose	0.1846	30.6197	0.1295
Mouth (closed)	0.2997	26.7337	0.1374
Ave temples	0.5490	18.1076	0.4532
Side			
Side face	0.4065	23.1397	0.4731
Ear	0.4880	20.0523	0.4205
Side temples	0.5407	18.2503	0.4509

TABLE 24.7   Results of Regression Analysis Performed on Body and Skin Temperatures (Data Set E) Measured from Different Sites on the Frontal Facial Profile

Description	Forehead	Eye range	Ave. cheeks	Nose	Mouth	Ave. temples
Regression ratio β	0.3962	0.4653	0.3446	0.2322	0.3044	0.4564
Intercept α	23.3745	20.9945	25.2887	29.0176	26.5577	21.2721
R^2	0.3292	0.3763	0.3543	0.2440	0.2131	0.3690

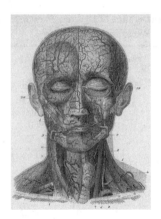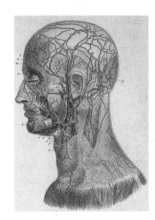

FIGURE 24.10   Diagrams showing superficial arterial and venous branches on the frontal and side profiles (Virtual, 2004).

region, has a good relationship with body temperature. A ROC analysis was performed for this data and the results are shown in Table 24.8.

From the ROC analysis, it was observed that sensitivity decreases and specificity increases as the cutoff decision limit, γ, increases. In other words, increasing γ leads to increasing of false negative rate and decreasing of false positive rate. The ROC areas for all the different sites at different cutoff temperatures were relatively high. This concludes that the current IR system can distinguish persons with elevated body temperature from normal subjects rather well from the skin temperatures measured at various sites as presented in Table 24.8. The ROC analysis showed that the skin temperatures of the ave temples resulted in a higher ROC area than those from eye region although the two sets of results were close. The only exception was observed at the cutoff of 37.7°C where the ROC area for eye region was higher than that of the ave temples. However, the results also suggested that the sensitivity and accuracy of the eye region for the entire cutoff temperature range were slightly higher. False negative rates were also lower for the eye region. False positive rates were low for both sets of data. It can be deduced from the regression and ROC analysis that the eye region has a slightly better overall performance for. Figure 24.10 shows that there are quite a few arteries around the eye. Thus, a small area of the skin near the eyes and nose offers the body temperature to be measured since the thin skin in this area has the highest amount of light energy thus making it a preferred point for brain temperature tunnel.

24.8.4   General ANNs Analysis

In the SLP-BP-NN experiment, different parameters are tested at each time to choose the best parameter for multilayer perception (MLP) evaluation in order to achieve a good score with different numbers of hidden neurons. In Kohonen SOM network, the 10×10 Kohonen layer has a better performance ($>97.3\%$) to classify the classes. Increasing the number of hidden neurons will improve the performance but the score will descend if the number of hidden neurons is exceeded. Thus, from the NN results, it shows that such type of NN (Ng and Chong, 2004) can be used as clinical decision support system for mass screening of febrile subjects.

24.9   Conclusions

From the results of the biostatistical analysis, the use of thermal imagers for the detection of persons with elevated body temperature during mass blind screening is very promising. The biostatistical analysis performed on readings from the eye region shows generally high ROC area values. ROC analysis performed on readings taken from other sites also showed high ROC area values. Since ROC area was used to

TABLE 24.8   Results of ROC Analysis for Skin Temperature of Different Sites on the Face of Frontal Profile. Data Set A Obtained from TTSH (2 Weeks).

	Forehead	Eye range	Ave. cheeks	Nose	Mouths	Ave. temples
Cutoff at 37.5°C						
ROC area	0.871	0.898	0.882	0.855	0.806	0.904
Sensitivity (%)	45.5	45.5	36.4	31.8	36.4	40.9
Specificity (%)	100	99.4	100	100	100	99.4
False positive (%)	0	0.5	0	0	0	0.5
False negative (%)	6.4	6.4	7.5	8.0	7.5	7.0
Prevalence (%)	11.8	11.8	11.8	11.8	11.8	11.8
Accuracy (%)	93.6	93.0	92.5	92.0	92.5	92.5
Recommended cutoff (°C)	34.7	34.6	34.1	34.4	33.4	34.9
Cutoff at 37.7°C						
ROC area	0.888	0.913	0.907	0.875	0.827	0.909
Sensitivity (%)	28.6	42.9	33.3	28.6	28.6	33.3
Specificity (%)	100	99.4	100	100	100	100
False positive (%)	0	0.5	0	0	0	0
False negative (%)	8.0	6.4	7.5	8.0	8.0	7.5
Prevalence (%)	11.2	11.2	11.2	11.2	11.2	11.2
Accuracy (%)	92.0	93.0	92.5	92.0	92.0	92.5
Recommended cutoff (°C)	34.7	34.6	34.1	34.4	33.4	34.9
Cutoff at 37.9°C						
ROC area	0.891	0.896	0.927	0.859	0.813	0.916
Sensitivity (%)	11.8	23.5	17.6	11.8	5.9	17.6
Specificity (%)	100	100	100	100	100	100
False positive (%)	0	0	0	0	0	0
False negative (%)	8.0	7.0	7.5	8.0	8.6	7.5
Prevalence (%)	9.1	9.1	9.1	9.1	9.1	9.1
Accuracy (%)	92.0	93.0	92.5	92.0	91.4	92.5
Recommended cutoff (°C)	35.0	34.6	34.8	34.4	34.1	35.2
Cutoff at 38.0°C						
ROC area	0.871	0.895	0.923	0.853	0.805	0.910
Sensitivity (%)	6.3	12.5	0	0	0	6.3
Specificity (%)	100	100	100	100	100	100
False positive (%)	0	0	0	0	0	0
False negative (%)	8.0	7.5	8.6	8.6	8.6	8.0
Prevalence (%)	8.6	8.6	8.6	8.6	8.6	8.6
Accuracy (%)	92.0	92.5	91.4	91.4	91.4	92.0
Recommended cutoff (°C)	35.3	34.8	34.9	34.4	34.1	35.2

determine how well infrared thermography could be applied to differentiate febrile from normal cases, it seemed that there was great potential in using this technology for deterring entry of SARS (with elevated body temperature) across the checkpoints.

Accurate detection of fever by thermal imager requires a body surface site that can correlate well for representation of body temperature physiologically. From the regression analysis, the best reading was taken from the eye range followed by the ave temples. The quick observation of the ROC results seemed that the readings taken from ave temples have higher ROC area. Further analysis showed that the accuracy and sensitivity of skin temperatures from eye range, however, has higher values than the ave temples for the entire cutoff. False negative rates of eye range are also lower than those of ave temples. Moreover, the human anatomy has suggested that the eye region has several arteries and potentially a good point for entry of the brain temperature tunnel too.

The aim of blind mass screening for SARS, is to have a speedy noninvasive and fairly accurate method of detecting people with elevated body temperature and at the same time minimize inconvenience and disruption to human traffic. Therefore, obtaining temperature readings from a site on the face would be most practical. The temples site for measuring skin surface of a person with fever is frequently met with the problem of the area being covered by hair or even accessories such as caps, hats, turban, and even tudung. Eye range provides a comparatively more practical site for this application.

The ROC analysis revealed that the thermal imager cutoff should be set to 34.6°C to detect aural temperatures of 37.5°C and above with respect to the associated environment. Similar cutoff of temperature for the thermal imagers has been found for detecting aural temperature above 37.7°C and 37.9°C. For detecting aural temperature of 38.0°C and above, the cutoff for thermal imager would have to be set at 35.5°C. Any temperature readings that exceed the thermal imager's cutoff would trigger the alarm and a thermometer would be used to verify the actual fever status of the subject.

The results of the ANN analysis further confirm that the use of thermal imagers for the detection of persons with elevated body temperature during mass blind screening is a very promising tool. Both BP and SOM can form an opinion about the type of network that is better to complement thermogram technology in fever diagnosis to drive better parameters for reducing the size of the neural network classifier while maintaining good classification accuracy. We observe that BP performs better than SOM neural network.

In order to ensure accurate collection of data, specific test procedures, and the physical requirements of the test sites will need to be standardized (Spring, 2003, 2004). Improper use of IR equipment, improper preparation of subjects, and improper collection of data can cause erroneous readings resulting in both false negative and false positive diagnosis. In summary, though IR thermography is promising for mass screening of potential SARS carriers, the technology must be applied with caution. Misapplication of the technology will not only waste resources, but can endanger the public safety by allowing infected persons to slip past and further spread the disease. The IR thermography applied for mass screening should therefore be used to complement and not replace the conventional thermometers (i.e., 2nd defense).

Acknowledgments

The first author would like to express utmost appreciation to research associates, Mr. Chang W.M. and Miss Ong C.F. for their efforts and hard works in collecting the data from the hospital and SCDF. He also want to express his thanks to members of the Ad-hoc Technical Reference Committee on Thermal Imagers under Medical Technology Standards Division by SPRING, and Ministry of Health, TTSH of National Health Group, Singapore for sharing of their views and interests on "Thermal Imagers for Fever Screening — Selection, Usage, and Testing." Gratitude is also extended to the people who have helped the authors to accomplish the project in one-way or another.

References

Airport SARS screener defective. (2003) *The Manila Times.* May 17.

Blatteis C.M. (1998) Physiology and pathophysiology of temperature regulation. *Temperature Regulation.* Chapter 10. 2nd ed. World Scientific Publishing, New Jersey.

Blackwell T. (2003) SARS scanners praised as placebo, Canada National Post, Wednesday, September 24, by tblackwell@nationalpost.com

Burnay S.G., Williams T.L., and Jones C.H. (1988) *Applications of Thermal Imaging.* IOP Publishing Ltd.

Canadian Coordinating Office for Health Technology Assessment. Pre-Assessment; The use of thermal imaging device in screening for fever 2003. URL: http://www.ccohta.ca (accessed 4th November 2004).

Centers for Disease Control and Prevention. Fact Sheet: Basic Information about SARS: http://www.cdc.gov/ncidod/sars/factsheet.htm (accessed 4th November 2004).

de Jong J.C., Claas E.C., Osterhaus A.D. et al. (1997) A pandemic warning? *Nature* 359: 544.

Dupont D.W. (2002). *Statistical Modelling for Biomedical Researchers: A Simple Introduction to the Analysis of Complex Data.* Cambridge University Press, Chapters 2 and 3.

Ear thermometer: URL: http://www.braun.com/global/products/healthwellness/earthermometers/thermoscan/models.html (accessed 4th November 2004).

FLIR Systems: http://www.flir.com (accessed 4th November 2004).

Golberg M.A. and Cho H.A. (2004) *Introduction to Regression Analysis.* WIT Press, Southampton, England.

Houdas Y. and Ring E.F.J. (1982) *Human Body Temperature — Its Measurement and Regulation.* Plenum Press, New York.

Ksiazek T.G., Erdman D., Goldsmith C.S., Zaki S.R., Peret T., Emery S., Tong S.Z. et al. (2003) A novel coronavirus associated with severe acute respiratory syndrome, *The New England Journal of Medicine* 348: 1953–1966.

Ng E.Y.K. and Sudharsan N.M. (2000) Can numerical simulation adjunct to thermography be an early detection tool? *Journal of Thermology International* 10: 119–127.

Ng E.Y.K. and Sudharsan N.M. (2001) Effect of blood flow, tumour and cold stress in a female breast: a novel time-accurate computer simulation. *International Journal of Engineering in Medicine* 215: 393–404.

Ng E.Y.K. and Chua L.T. (2002) Comparison of one- and two-dimensional programmes for predicting the state of skin burns. *International Journal of BURNS* 28: 27–34.

Ng E.Y.K., Kaw G., and Ng K. (2004a) Infrared thermography in identification of human elevated temperature with biostatistical and ROC analysis, *The International Society for Optical Engineering — ThermoSense XXVI — Symposium on Defense and Security*, 12–16 April at Orlando, FL, pp. 88–97.

Ng E.Y.K., Kaw G., and Chang W.M. (2004b) *Analysis of IR Thermal Imager for Mass Blind Fever Screening, Microvascular Research.* Reed Elsevier Science, Academic Press, New York, Vol. 68, pp. 104–109.

Ng E.Y.K. and Sudharsan N.M. (2004) Numerical modelling in conjunction with thermography as an adjunct tool for breast tumour detection, *BMC Cancer Medline Journal* 4: 1–26.

Ng E.Y.K. (2005) Is thermal scanner losing its bite in mass screening of fever due to SARS? Medical Physics, American Association of Physicists in Medicine, 32(1): 93–97.

Ng E.Y.K. and Chong C. (2005) ANN based mapping of febrile subjects in mass thermogram screening: facts and myths, *International Journal of Medical Engineering & Technology* (in-press).

Ng E.Y.K. and Kaw G. (2005) Classification of human facial and aural temperature using neural networks and IR fever scanner: a responsible second look, *Journal of Mechanics in Medicine and Biology* 5(1): 165–190.

Peris J., Lai S., Poon L. et al. (2003) Coronavirus as a possible cause of severe acute respiratory syndrome, *Lancet* 361: 1319–1325.

Pottinger, M. (2004) Medical science: why SARS didn't return? *Far Eastern Economic Review* 35–36, April 8. URL: www.feer.com (accessed 4th November 2004).

ROC MedCalc Software, Belgium (ver. 7.4): http://www.medcalc.be (accessed 4th October 2005).

Rota P.A., Oberste M.S., Monroe S.S. et al. (2003) Characterization of a novel coronavirus associated with severe acute respiratory syndrome, Sciencexpress: http://www.sciencemag.org/cgi/rapidpdf/ 1085952v1.pdf (accessed 4th November 2004).

Standards Technical Reference for *Thermal Imagers for Human Temperature Screening Part 1: Requirements and Test Methods*, 2003. TR 15-1, Spring Singapore. ISBN 9971-67-963-9.

Standards Technical Reference for *Thermal Imagers for Human Temperature Screening Part 2: Users' Implementation Guidelines*, 2004. TR 15-2, Spring Singapore. ISBN 9971-67-977-9.

Shapiro D.E. (1999). The interpretation of diagnostic tests. *Statistical Methods in Medical Research*, 8: 113–134.

S-Plus Software: http://www.insightful.com (accessed 4th November 2004).

Virtual hospital, Atlas of Human Anatomy, Translated by: Ronald A. Bergman and Adel K. Afifi: (accessed 4th November 2004). http://www.vh.org/adult/provider/anatomy/atlasofanatomy/plate17/ index.html

25

Infrared Imaging of the Breast — An Overview

Prologue **25-1**
25.1 Introduction.. **25-2**
25.2 Fundamentals of Infrared Breast Imaging **25-2**
  Physics • Equipment Considerations • Laboratory and
  Patient Preparation Protocols • Imaging • Special Tests •
  Image Interpretation
25.3 Correlation between Pathology and Infrared Imaging **25-7**
25.4 The Role of Infrared Imaging in the Detection of
  Cancer **25-8**
25.5 Infrared Imaging as a Risk Indicator **25-10**
25.6 Infrared Imaging as a Prognostic Indicator **25-11**
25.7 Breast Cancer Detection and Demonstration Project . **25-12**
  Poor Study Design • Untrained Personnel and Protocol
  Violations
25.8 Mammography and Infrared Imaging **25-14**
25.9 Current Status of Breast Cancer Detection **25-15**
25.10 Future Advancements in Infrared Imaging **25-16**
25.11 Conclusion **25-17**
References **25-17**

William C. Amalu
*Pacific Chiropractic and Research
Center*

William B. Hobbins
Women's Breast Health Center

Jonathan F. Head
*Elliott-Elliott-Head Breast Cancer
Research and Treatment Center*

Robert L. Elliott
*Elliott-Elliott-Head Breast Cancer
Research and Treatment Center*

Prologue

The use of infrared imaging in health care is not a recent phenomenon. Its utilization in breast cancer screening, however, is seeing renewed interest. This attention is fueled by research that clearly demonstrates the value of this procedure and the tremendous impact it has on the mortality of breast cancer.

Infrared imaging of the breast has undergone extensive research since the late 1950s. Over 800 papers can be found in the indexed medical literature. In this database, well over 300,000 women have been included as study participants. The number of participants in many studies are very large and range from 10,000 to 85,000 women. Some of these studies have followed patients up to 12 years in order to establish the technology's ability as a risk marker.

With strict standardized interpretation protocols having been established for over 15 years, infrared imaging of the breast has obtained an average sensitivity and specificity of 90%. As a future risk indicator for breast cancer, a persistent abnormal thermogram caries a 22 times higher risk and is 10 times more significant than a first order family history of the disease. Studies clearly show that an abnormal infrared image is the single most important risk marker for the existence of or future development of breast cancer.

25.1 Introduction

The first recorded use of thermobiological diagnostics can be found in the writings of Hippocrates around 480 BC [1]. A mud slurry spread over the patient was observed for areas that would dry first and was thought to indicate underlying organ pathology. Since this time, continued research and clinical observations proved that certain temperatures related to the human body were indeed indicative of normal and abnormal physiologic processes.

In the 1950s, military research into infrared monitoring systems for nighttime troop movements ushered in a new era in thermal diagnostics. Once declassified in the mid-1950s, infrared imaging technology was made available for medical purposes. The first diagnostic use of infrared imaging came in 1956 when Lawson discovered that the skin temperature over a cancer in the breast was higher than that of normal tissue [2–4]. He also showed that the venous blood draining the cancer is often warmer than its arterial supply.

The Department of Health Education and Welfare released a position paper in 1972 in which the director, Thomas Tiernery, wrote, "The medical consultants indicate that thermography, in its present state of development, is beyond the experimental state as a diagnostic procedure in the following 4 areas: (1) Pathology of the female breast..." On January 29, 1982, the Food and Drug Administration published its approval and classification of thermography as an adjunctive diagnostic screening procedure for the detection of breast cancer. Since the late 1970s, numerous medical centers and independent clinics have used thermography for a variety of diagnostic purposes.

Since Lawson's groundbreaking research, infrared imaging has been used for over 40 years as an adjunctive screening procedure in the evaluation of the breast. In this time significant advances have been made in infrared detection systems and the application of sophisticated computerized image processing.

25.2 Fundamentals of Infrared Breast Imaging

Clinical infrared imaging is a procedure that detects, records, and produces an image of a patient's skin surface temperatures and thermal patterns. The image produced resembles the likeness of the anatomic area under study. The procedure uses equipment that can provide both qualitative and quantitative representations of these temperature patterns.

Infrared imaging does not entail the use of ionizing radiation, venous access, or other invasive procedures; therefore, the examination poses no harm to the patient. Classified as a functional imaging technology, infrared imaging of the breast provides information on the normal and abnormal physiologic functioning of the sensory and sympathetic nervous systems, vascular system, and local inflammatory processes.

25.2.1 Physics

All objects with a temperature above absolute zero (-273 K) emit infrared radiation from their surface. The Stefan-Boltzmann Law defines the relation between radiated energy and temperature by stating that the total radiation emitted by an object is directly proportional to the object's area and emissivity and the fourth power of its absolute temperature. Since the emissivity of human skin is extremely high (within 1% of that of a black body), measurements of infrared radiation emitted by the skin can be converted directly into accurate temperature values. This makes infrared imaging an ideal procedure to evaluate surface temperatures of the body.

25.2.2 Equipment Considerations

Infrared rays are found in the electromagnetic spectrum within the wavelengths of 0.75 μm to 1 mm. Human skin emits infrared radiation mainly in the 2–20 μm wavelength range, with an average peak at 9–10 μm [5]. With the application of Plank's equation and Wein's Law, it is found that approximately 90% of emitted infrared radiation in humans is in the longer wavelengths (6–14 μm).

There are many important technical aspects to consider when choosing an appropriate clinical infrared imaging system (the majority of which is outside the scope of this chapter). However, minimum equipment standards have been established from research studies, applied infrared physics, and human anatomic and physiologic parameters [6,7]. Absolute, spatial, and temperature resolution along with thermal stability and adequate computerized image processing are just a few of the critical specifications to take into account. However, the most fundamental consideration in the selection of clinical infrared imaging equipment is the wavelength sensitivity of the infrared detector. The decision on which area in the infrared spectrum to select a detector from depends on the object one wants to investigate and the environmental conditions in which the detection is taking place. Considering that the object in question is the human body, Plank's equation leads us to select a detector in the 6–14 μm region. Assessment of skin temperature by infrared measurement in the 3–5 μm region is less reliable due to the emissivity of human skin being farther from that of a blackbody in that region [8,9]. The environment under which the examination takes place is well controlled, but not free from possible sources of detection errors. Imaging room environmental artifacts such as reflectance can cause errors when shorter wavelength detectors (under 7 μm) are used [10]. Consequently, the optimum infrared detector to use in imaging the breast, and the body as a whole, would have a sensitivity in the longer wavelengths spanning the 9–10 μm range [7–14].

The problems encountered with first generation infrared camera systems, such as incorrect detector sensitivity (shorter wavelengths), thermal drift, calibration, analog interface, and so on, have been solved for almost two decades. Modern computerized infrared imaging systems have the ability to discern minute variations in thermal emissions while producing extremely high-resolution images that can undergo digital manipulation by sophisticated computerized analytical processing.

25.2.3 Laboratory and Patient Preparation Protocols

In order to produce diagnostic quality infrared images, certain laboratory and patient preparation protocols must be strictly adhered to. Infrared imaging must be performed in a controlled environment. The primary reason for this is the nature of human physiology. Changes from a different external (noncontrolled room) environment, clothing, and the like, produce thermal artifacts. In order to properly prepare the patient for imaging, the patient should be instructed to refrain from sun exposure, stimulation or treatment of the breasts, cosmetics, lotions, antiperspirants, deodorants, exercise, and bathing before the exam.

The imaging room must be temperature and humidity-controlled and maintained between 18 and 23°C, and kept to within 1°C of change during the examination. This temperature range insures that the patient is not placed in an environment in which their physiology is stressed into a state of shivering or perspiring. The room should also be free from drafts and infrared sources of heat (i.e., sunlight and incandescent lighting). In keeping with a physiologically neutral temperature environment, the floor should be carpeted or the patient must wear shoes in order to prevent increased physiologic stress.

Lastly, the patient must undergo 15 min of waist-up nude acclimation in order to reach a condition in which the body is at thermal equilibrium with the environment. At this point, further changes in the surface temperatures of the body occur very slowly and uniformly; thus, not affecting changes in homologous anatomic regions. Thermal artifacts from clothing or the outside environment are also removed at this time. The last 5 min of this acclimation period is usually spent with the patient placing their hands on top of their head in order to facilitate an improved anatomic presentation of the breasts for imaging. Depending

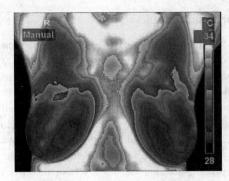

FIGURE 25.1   (See color insert following page **29**-16.) Bilateral frontal.

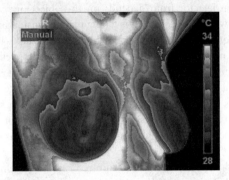

FIGURE 25.2   (See color insert.) Right oblique.

on the patient's individual anatomy, certain positioning maneuvers may need to be implemented such that all of the pertinent surfaces of the breasts may be imaged. In summary, adherence to proper patient and laboratory protocols is absolutely necessary to produce a physiologically neutral image, free from artifact and ready for interpretation.

25.2.4 Imaging

The actual process of imaging is undertaken with the intent to adequately detect the infrared emissions from the pertinent surface areas of the breasts. As with mammography, a minimum series of images is needed in order to facilitate adequate coverage. The series includes the bilateral frontal breast along with the right and left oblique views (a right and left single breast close-up view may also be included). The bilateral frontal view acts as a scout image to give a baseline impression of both breasts. The oblique views (approximately 45° to the detector) expose the lateral and medial quadrants of the breasts for analysis. The optional close-up views maximize the use of the detector allowing for the highest thermal and spatial resolution image of each breast. This series of images takes into consideration the infrared analyses of curved surfaces and adequately provides for an accurate analysis of all the pertinent surface areas of the breasts (see Figure 25.1 to Figure 25.5).

Positioning of the patient prior to imaging facilitates acclimation of the surface areas and ease of imaging. Placing the patient in a seated or standing posture during the acclimation period is ideal to facilitate these needs. In the seated position, the patient places their arms on the arm rests away from the body to allow for proper acclimation. When positioning the patient in front of the camera, the use of a rotating chair or having the patient stand makes for uncomplicated positioning for the necessary views.

Because of differing anatomy from patient to patient, special views may be necessary to adequately detect the infrared emissions from the pertinent surface areas of the breasts. The most common problem

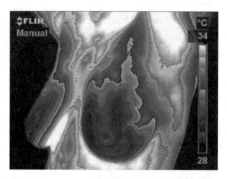

FIGURE 25.3   (See color insert.) Left oblique.

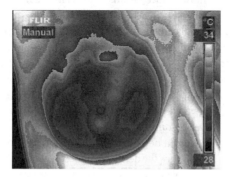

FIGURE 25.4   (See color insert.) Right close-up.

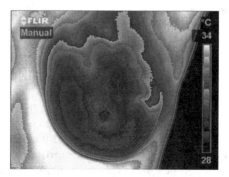

FIGURE 25.5   (See color insert.) Left close-up.

encountered is inadequate viewing of the inferior quadrants due to nipple ptosis. This is easily remedied by adding "lift views." Once the baseline images are taken, the patient is asked to "lift" each breast from the Tail of Spence exposing the inferior quadrants for detection. Additional images are then taken in this position in order to maintain the surface areas covered in the standard views.

25.2.5 Special Tests

In the past, an optional set of views may have been added to the baseline images. Additional views would be taken after the patient placed their hands in ice cold water as a thermoregulatory cold challenge. It was hoped that this dynamic methodology would increase the sensitivity and specificity of the thermographic procedure.

In order to understand the hopes placed on this test, one needs to understand the underlying physiologic mechanisms of the procedure. The most common and accepted method of applied thermoregulatory challenge involves ice water immersion of the hands or feet (previous studies investigating the use of fans or alcohol spray noted concerns over the creation of thermal artifacts along with the methods causing a limited superficial effect). The mechanism is purely neurovascular and involves a primitive survival reflex initiated from peripheral neural receptors and conveyed to the central nervous system. To protect the body from hypothermia, the reflex invokes a sympathetically mediated blood vessel constriction in the periphery in an attempt to maintain the normal core temperature set point. This stress test is intended to increase the sensitivity of the thermogram by attempting to identify nonresponding blood vessels such as those involved in angiogenesis associated with neoplasm. Blood vessels produced by cancerous tumors are simple endothelial tubes devoid of a muscular layer and the neural regulation afforded to embryologic vessels. As such, these new vessels would fail to constrict in response to a sympathetic stimulus. In the normal breast, test results would produce an image of relative cooling with attenuation of vascular diameter. A breast harboring a malignancy would theoretically remain unchanged in temperature or demonstrate hyperthermia with vascular dilation. However, to date it has not been found that the stress test offers any advantage over the baseline images [15].

For well over a decade, leading experts and researchers in the field of infrared breast imaging have discontinued the use of the cold challenge. Yet, in a 2004 detailed review of the literature combined with an investigational study, Amalu [15] explored the validity of the cold challenge test. Results from 23 patients with histologically confirmed breast cancers along with 500 noncancer cases were presented demonstrating positive and negative responses to the challenge. From the combined literature review and study analysis it was found that the test did not alter the clinical decision-making process for following up suspicious thermograms, nor did it enhance the detection of occult cancers found in normal thermograms. In summary, it was found that there was no evidence to support the use of the cold challenge. The study noted insufficient evidence to warrant its use as a mandated test with all women undergoing infrared breast imaging. It also warned that it would be incorrect to consider a breast thermogram "substandard" if a cold challenge was not included. In conclusion, Amalu stated that "Until further studies are performed and ample evidence can be presented to the contrary, a review of the available data indicates that infrared imaging of the breast can be performed excluding the cold challenge without any known loss of sensitivity or specificity in the detection of breast cancers."

25.2.6 Image Interpretation

Early methods of interpretation of infrared breast images was based solely on qualitative (subjective) criteria. The images were read for variations in vascular patterning with no regard to temperature variations between the breasts (Tricore method) [16]. This lead to wide variations in the outcomes of studies preformed with inexperienced interpreters. Research throughout the 1970s proved that when both qualitative and quantitative data were incorporated in the interpretations, an increase in sensitivity and specificity was realized. In the early 1980s, a standardized method of thermovascular analysis was proposed. The interpretation was composed of 20 discrete vascular and temperature attributes in the breast [17,18]. This method of analysis was based on previous research and large scale studies comprising tens of thousands of patients. Using this methodology, thermograms would be graded into 1 of 5 TH (thermobiological) classifications. Based on the combined vascular patterning and temperatures across the two breasts, the images would be graded as TH1 (normal nonvascular), TH2 (normal vascular), TH3 (equivocal), TH4 (abnormal), or TH5 (severely abnormal) (see Figure 25.6 and Figure 25.7). The use of this standardized interpretation method significantly increased infrared imaging's sensitivity, specificity, positive and negative predictive value, and inter/intra-examiner interpretation reliability. Continued patient observations and research over the past two decades have caused changes in some of the thermovascular values; thus, keeping the interpretation system up-to-date. Variations in this methodology have also been adopted with great success. However, it is recognized that, as with any other imaging procedure, specialized training and experience produces the highest level of screening success.

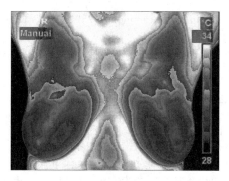

FIGURE 25.6   (See color insert.) TH1 (normal non-vascular).

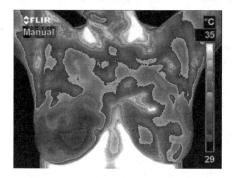

FIGURE 25.7   (See color insert.) Left TH5 (severely abnormal).

25.3   Correlation between Pathology and Infrared Imaging

The empirical evidence that an underlying breast cancer alters regional skin surface temperatures was investigated early on. In 1963, Lawson and Chughtai, two McGill University surgeons, published an elegant intra-operative study demonstrating that the increase in regional skin surface temperature associated with breast cancer was related to venous convection [19]. This early quantitative experiment added credence to previous research suggesting that infrared findings were linked to increased vascularity.

Infrared imaging of the breast may also have critical prognostic significance since it may correlate with a variety of pathologic prognostic features such as tumor size, tumor grade, lymph node status, and markers of tumor growth [20]. Continued research is underway investigating the pathologic basis for these infrared findings. One possibility is increased blood flow due to vascular proliferation (assessed by quantifying the microvascular density [MVD]) as a result of tumor associated angiogenesis. Although in one study [21], the MVD did not correlate with abnormal infrared findings. However, the imaging method used in that study consisted of contact plate technology (liquid crystal thermography [LCT]), which is not capable of modern computerized analysis. Consequently, LCT does not possess the discrimination and digital processing necessary to begin to correlate histological and discrete vascular changes [22].

In 1993, Head and Elliott reported that improved images from second generation infrared systems allowed more objective and quantitative analysis [20], and indicated that growth-rate related prognostic indicators were strongly associated with the infrared image interpretation.

In a 1994 detailed review of the potential of infrared imaging [23], Anbar suggested that the previous empirical observation that small tumors were capable of producing notable infrared changes could be due to enhanced perfusion over a substantial area of the breast surface via regional tumor induced nitric oxide (NO) vasodilatation. NO is synthesized by nitric oxide synthase (NOS), found both as a constitutive form of NOS, especially in endothelial cells, and as an inducible form of NOS, especially in macrophages

[24]. NOS has been demonstrated in breast carcinoma [25] using tissue immunohistochemistry, and is associated with a high tumor grade.

Nitric oxide is a molecule with potent vasodilating properties. It is a simple highly reactive free radical that readily oxidizes to form nitrite or nitrate ions. It diffuses easily through both hydrophilic and hydrophobic media. Thus, once produced, NO diffuses throughout the surrounding tissues, inside and outside the vascular system, and induces a variety of biochemical changes depending on the specific receptors involved. NO exerts its influence by binding to receptor sites in the endothelium of arteries or arterioles. This causes inhibition of sympathetic vasoconstriction. The end result is NO induced vasodilatation, which in turn may produce an asymmetrical thermovascular infrared image.

The largest body of evidence surrounding the physiologic mechanism by which infrared imaging detects precancerous and malignant states of the breast lies in the recruitment of existing blood vessels and the formation of new ones (angiogenesis). The process of angiogenesis begins with the release of angiogenesis factors (AF) from precancerous or cancerous cells. In the early stages of tumor growth, the majority of neoplasms exhibit a lower cellular metabolic demand. As such, the release of AF causes the existing vessels to resist constriction in order to maintain a steady supply of nutrients to the growing mass. As the tumor increases in size the need for nutrients becomes greater. AF begins to exert its influence by opening the dormant vessels in the breast. Once this blood supply becomes too little to maintain the growth of the neoplasm, AF causes the formation of new blood vessels. These new vessels are simple endothelial tubes connecting the tumor to existing nearby arteries and arterioles. This augmented blood supply produces the increase in heat and vascular asymmetry seen in infrared images.

The concept of angiogenesis, as an integral part of early breast cancer, was emphasized in 1996 by Guido and Schnitt. Their observations suggested that it is an early event in the development of breast cancer and may occur before tumor cells acquire the ability to invade the surrounding stroma and even before there is morphologic evidence of an *in situ* carcinoma [26]. In 1996, in his highly reviewed textbook entitled *Atlas of Mammography — New Early Signs in Breast Cancer*, Gamagami studied angiogenesis by infrared imaging and reported that hypervascularity and hyperthermia could be shown in 86% of nonpalpable breast cancers. He also noted that in 15% of these cases infrared imaging helped to detect cancers that were not visible on mammography [27].

The greatest evidence supporting the underlying principle by which infrared imaging detects precancerous growths and cancerous tumors surrounds the well documented recruitment of existing vascularity and angiogenesis, which is necessary to maintain the increased metabolism of malignant cellular growth and multiplication. The biomedical engineering evidence of infrared imaging's value, both in model *in vitro* and clinically *in vivo* studies of various tissue growths, normal and neoplastic, has been established [28–34].

25.4   The Role of Infrared Imaging in the Detection of Cancer

In order to determine the value of infrared imaging, two viewpoints must be considered: first, the sensitivity of thermograms taken preoperatively in patients with known breast carcinoma; and second, the incidence of normal and abnormal thermograms in asymptomatic populations (specificity) and the presence or absence of malignancy in each of these groups.

In 1965, Gershon-Cohen et al. [35], a radiologist and researcher from the Albert Einstein Medical Center, introduced infrared imaging to the United States [35]. Using a Barnes thermograph, he reported on 4000 cases with a sensitivity of 94% and a false-positive rate of 6%. This data was included in a review of the then current status of infrared imaging published in 1968 in *CA — A Cancer Journal for Physicians* [36].

In prospective studies, Hoffman first reported on thermography in a gynecologic practice. He detected 23 carcinomas in 1924 patients (a detection rate of 12.5 per 1000), with an 8.4% false-negative (91.6% sensitivity) and a 7.4% false-positive (92.6% specificity) rate [37].

Stark and Way [38] screened 4621 asymptomatic women, 35% of whom were under 35 years of age, and detected 24 cancers (detection rate of 7.6 per 1000), with a sensitivity and specificity of 98.3 and 93.5%, respectively.

In a study comprising 25,000 patients screened and 1,878 histologically proven breast cancers, Amalric and Spitalier reported on their results with infrared imaging. From this group a false-negative and false-positive rate of 9% (91% sensitivity and specificity) was found [39].

In a mobile unit examination of rural Wisconsin, Hobbins screened 37,506 women using thermography. He reported the detection of 5.7 cancers per 1,000 women screened with a 12% false-negative and 14% false-positive rate. His findings also corroborated with others that thermography is the sole early initial signal in 10% of breast cancers [17,40].

Reporting his Radiology division's experience with 10,000 thermographic studies done concomitantly with mammography over a 3-year period, Isard reiterated a number of important concepts including the remarkable thermal and vascular stability of the infrared image from year to year in the otherwise healthy patient and the importance of recognizing any significant change [41]. In his experience, combining these modalities increased the sensitivity rate of detection by approximately 10%; thus, underlining the complementarity of these procedures since each one did not always suspect the same lesion. It was Isard's conclusion that, had there been a preliminary selection of his group of 4393 asymptomatic patients by infrared imaging, mammographic examination would have been restricted to the 1028 patients with abnormal infrared imaging, or 23% of this cohort. This would have resulted in a cancer detection rate of 24.1 per 1000 combined infrared and mammographic examinations as contrasted to the expected 7 per 1000 by mammographic screening alone. He concluded that since infrared imaging is an innocuous examination, it could be utilized to focus attention upon asymptomatic women who should be examined more intensely. Isard emphasized that, like mammography and other breast imaging techniques, infrared imaging does not diagnose cancer, but merely indicates the presence of an abnormality.

Spitalier and associates screened 61,000 women using thermography over a 10-year period. The false-negative and positive rate was found to be 11% (89% sensitivity and specificity). Thermography also detected 91% of the nonpalpable cancers (Grade T0: tumors less than 1 cm in size). The authors noted that of all the patients with cancer, thermography alone was the first alarm in 60% of the cases [42].

Two small-scale studies by Moskowitz (150 patients) [43] and Treatt (515 patients) [44] reported on the sensitivity and reliability of infrared imaging. Both used unknown experts to review the images of breast cancer patients. While Moskowitz excluded unreadable images, data from Threatt's study indicated that less than 30% of the images produced were considered good, the rest being substandard. Both of these studies produced poor results; however, this could be expected considering the lack of adherence to accepted imaging methods and protocols. The greatest error in these studies is found in the methods used to analyze the images. The type of image analysis consisted of the sole use of abnormal vascular pattern recognition. At the time these studies were performed, the accepted method of infrared image interpretation consisted of a combined vascular pattern and quantitative analysis of temperature variations across the breasts. Consequently, the data obtained from these studies is highly questionable. Their findings were also inconsistent with numerous previous large-scale multicenter trials. The authors suggested that for infrared imaging to be truly effective as a screening tool, there needed to be a more objective means of interpretation and proposed that this would be facilitated by computerized evaluation. This statement is interesting considering that recognized quantitative and qualitative reading protocols (including computer analysis) were being used at the time.

In a unique study comprising 39,802 women screened over a 3-year period, Haberman and associates used thermography and physical examination to determine if mammography was recommended. They reported an 85% sensitivity and 70% specificity for thermography. Haberman cautioned that the findings of thermographic specificity could not be extrapolated from this study as it was well documented that long-term observation (8 to 10 years or more) is necessary to determine a true false-positive rate. The authors noted that 30% of the cancers found would not have been detected if it were not for thermography [45].

Gros and Gautherie reported on a large scale study comprising 85,000 patients screened. Culmination of the data resulted in a 90% sensitivity and 88% specificity for thermography [46–49].

In a large-scale multicenter review of nearly 70,000 women screened, Jones reported a false-negative and false-positive rate of 13% (87% sensitivity) and 15% (85% sensitivity) respectively for thermography [50].

In a study performed in 1986, Usuki reported on the relation of thermographic findings in breast cancer diagnosis. He noted an 88% sensitivity for thermography in the detection of breast cancers [51].

Parisky and associates published a study from a multicenter 4-year clinical trial using infrared imaging to evaluate mammographically suspicious lesions. Data from a blinded subject set was obtained in 769 women with 875 biopsied lesions resulting in 187 malignant and 688 benign findings. The index of suspicion resulted in a 97% sensitivity in the detection of breast cancers [52].

In a study comparing clinical examination, mammography, and thermography in the diagnosis of breast cancer, three groups of patients were used: 4,716 patients with confirmed carcinoma, 3,305 patients with histologically diagnosed benign breast disease, and 8,757 general patients (16,778 total participants). This paper also compared clinical examination and mammography to other well-known studies in the literature including the National Cancer Institute (NCI)-sponsored Breast Cancer Detection and Demonstration Projects. In this study, clinical examination had an average sensitivity of 75% in detecting all tumors and 50% in cancers less than 2 cm in size. This rate is exceptionally good when compared to many other studies at between 35 and 66% sensitivity. Mammography was found to have an average 80% sensitivity and 73% specificity. Thermography had an average sensitivity of 88% (85% in tumors less than 1 cm in size) and a specificity of 85%. An abnormal thermogram was found to have a 94% predictive value. From the findings in this study, the authors suggested that "none of the techniques available for screening for breast carcinoma and evaluating patients with breast related symptoms is sufficiently accurate to be used alone. For the best results, a multimodal approach should be used" [53].

In a series of 4,000 confirmed breast cancers, Thomassin and associates observed 130 subclinical carcinomas ranging in diameter of 3 to 5 mm. Both mammography and thermography were used alone and in combination. Of the 130 cancers, 10% were detected by mammography only, 50% by thermography alone, and 40% by both techniques. Thus, there was a thermal alarm in 90% of the patients and the only sign in 50% of the cases [54].

In a simple review of over 15 large-scale studies from 1967 to 1998, infrared imaging of the breast has showed an average sensitivity and specificity of 90%. With continued technological advances in infrared imaging in the past decade, some studies are showing even higher sensitivity and specificity values. However, until further large-scale studies are performed, these findings remain in question.

25.5 Infrared Imaging as a Risk Indicator

As early as 1976, at the Third International Symposium on Detection and Prevention of Cancer held in New York, thermal imaging was established by consensus as the highest risk marker for the possibility of the presence of an undetected breast cancer. It had also been shown to predict such a subsequent occurrence [55–57]. The Wisconsin Breast Cancer Detection Foundation presented a summary of its findings in this area, which has remained undisputed [58]. This, combined with other reports, has confirmed that an abnormal infrared image is the highest risk indicator for the future development of breast cancer and is 10 times as significant as a first order family history of the disease [48].

In a study of 10,000 women screened, Gautherie found that, when applied to asymptomatic women, thermography was very useful in assessing the risk of cancer by dividing patients into low and high risk categories. This was based on an objective evaluation of each patient's thermograms using an improved reading protocol that incorporated 20 thermopathological factors [59].

A screening of 61,000 women using thermography was performed by Spitalier over a 10-year period. The authors concluded that "in patients having no clinical or radiographic suspicion of malignancy, a persistently abnormal breast thermogram represents the highest known risk factor for the future development of breast cancer" [42].

From a patient base of 58,000 women screened with thermography, Gros and associates followed 1527 patients with initially healthy breasts and abnormal thermograms for 12 years. Of this group, 44%

developed malignancies within 5 years. The study concluded that "an abnormal thermogram is the single most important marker of high risk for the future development of breast cancer" [49].

Spitalier and associates followed 1416 patients with isolated abnormal breast thermograms. It was found that a persistently abnormal thermogram, as an isolated phenomenon, is associated with an actuarial breast cancer risk of 26% at 5 years. Within this study, 165 patients with nonpalpable cancers were observed. In 53% of these patients, thermography was the only test which was positive at the time of initial evaluation. It was concluded that (1) A persistently abnormal thermogram, even in the absence of any other sign of malignancy, is associated with a high risk of developing cancer, (2) This isolated abnormal also carries with it a high risk of developing interval cancer, and as such the patient should be examined more frequently than the customary 12 months, (3) Most patients diagnosed as having minimal breast cancer have abnormal thermograms as the first warning sign [60,61].

In a study by Gautherie and associates, the effectiveness of thermography in terms of survival benefit was discussed. The authors analyzed the survival rates of 106 patients in whom the diagnosis of breast cancer was established as a result of the follow-up of thermographic abnormalities found on the initial examination when the breasts were apparently healthy (negative physical and mammographic findings). The control group consisted of 372 breast cancer patients. The patients in both groups were subjected to identical treatment and followed for 5 years. A 61% increase in survival was noted in the patients who were followed-up due to initial thermographic abnormalities. The authors summarized the study by stating that "the findings clearly establish that the early identification of women at high risk of breast cancer based on the objective thermal assessment of breast health results in a dramatic survival benefit" [62,63].

Infrared imaging provides a reflection of functional tumor induced angiogenesis and metabolic activity rather than structurally based parameters (i.e., tumor size, architectural distortion, microcalcifications). Recent advances in cancer research have determined that the biological activity of a neoplasm is far more significant an indicator of aggressiveness than the size of the tumor. As a direct reflection of the biological activity in the breast, infrared imaging has been found to provide a significant biological risk marker for cancer.

25.6   Infrared Imaging as a Prognostic Indicator

Studies exploring the biology of cancers have shown that the amount of thermovascular activity in the breast is directly proportional to the aggressiveness of the tumor. As such, infrared imaging provides the clinician with an invaluable tool in prognosis and treatment monitoring.

In a study of 209 breast cancers, Dilhuydy and associates found a positive correlation between the degree of infrared abnormalities and the existence of positive axillary lymph nodes. It was reported that the amount of thermovascular activity seen in the breast was directly related to the prognosis. The study concluded that infrared imaging provides a highly significant factor in prognosis and that it should be included in the pretherapeutic assessment of a breast cancer [64].

Amalric and Spitalier reported on 25,000 patients screened and 1,878 histologically proven breast cancers investigated with infrared imaging. The study noted that the amount of infrared activity in the breast was directly proportional to the survival of the patient. The "hot" cancers showed a significantly poorer prognosis with a 24% survival rate at 3 years. A much better prognosis with an 80% survival rate at 3 years was seen in the more biologically inactive or "cooler" cancers. The study also noted a positive association between the amount of thermal activity in the breast and the presence of positive axillary nodes [65].

Reporting on a study of breast cancer doubling times and infrared imaging, Fournier noted significant changes in the thermovascular appearance of the images. The shorter the tumor doubling time, the more thermographic pathological signs were evident. It was concluded that infrared imaging served as a warning signal for the faster-growing breast cancers [66].

A retrospective analysis of 100 normal patients, 100 living cancer patients, and 126 deceased cancer patients was published by Head. Infrared imaging was found to be abnormal in 28% of the normal patients, compared to 65% of the living cancer patients and 88% of the deceased cancer patients. Known prognostic indicators related to tumor growth rate were compared to the results of the infrared images. The concentration of tumor ferritin, the proportion of cells in DNA synthesis and proliferating, and the expression of the proliferation-associated tumor antigen Ki-67 were all found to be associated with an abnormal infrared image. It was concluded that "The strong relationships of thermographic results with these three growth rate-related prognostic indicators suggest that breast cancer patients with abnormal thermograms have faster-growing tumors that are more likely to have metastasized and to recur with a shorter disease-free interval" [20].

In a paper by Gros and Gautherie, the use of infrared imaging in the prognosis of treated breast cancers was investigated. The authors considered infrared imaging to be absolutely necessary for assessing pretherapeutic prognosis or carrying out the follow-up of breast cancers treated by exclusive radiotherapy. They noted that before treatment, infrared imaging yields evidence of the cancer growth rate (aggressiveness) and contributes to the therapeutic choice. It also indicates the success of radiosterilization or the suspicion of a possible recurrence or radio-resistance. The authors also noted a weaker 5-year survival with infrared images that showed an increase in thermal signals [67].

In a recent study by Keyserlingk, 20 women with core biopsy-proven locally advanced breast cancer underwent infrared imaging before and after chemohormonotherapy. All 20 patients were found to have abnormal thermovascular signs prior to treatment. Upon completion of the final round of chemotherapy, each patient underwent curative-intent surgery. Prior to surgery, all 20 patients showed improvement in their initial infrared scores. The amount of improvement in the infrared images was found to be directly related to the decrease in tumor size. A complete normalization of prechemotherapy infrared scores was seen in five patients. In these same patients there was no histological evidence of cancer remaining in the breast. In summary, the authors stated that "Further research will determine whether lingering infrared detected angiogenesis following treatment reflects tumor aggressiveness and ultimately prognosis, as well as early tumor resistance, thus providing an additional early signal for the need of a therapeutic adjustment" [68].

25.7   Breast Cancer Detection and Demonstration Project

The breast cancer detection and demonstration project (BCDDP) is the most frequently quoted reason for the decreased interest in infrared imaging. The BCDDP was a large-scale study performed from 1973 through 1979, which collected data from many centers around the United States. Three methods of breast cancer detection were studied: physical examination, mammography, and infrared imaging.

Just before the onset of the BCDDP, two important papers appeared in the literature. In 1972, Gerald D. Dodd of the University of Texas Department of Diagnostic Radiology presented an update on infrared imaging in breast cancer diagnosis at the 7th National Cancer Conference sponsored by the National Cancer Society and the National Cancer Institute [69]. In his presentation, he suggested that infrared imaging would be best employed as a screening agent for mammography. He proposed that in any general survey of the female population aged 40 and over, 15 to 20% of these subjects would have positive infrared imaging and would require mammograms. Of these, approximately 5% would be recommended for biopsy. He concluded that infrared imaging would serve to eliminate 80 to 85% of the potential mammograms. Dodd also reiterated that the procedure was not competitive with mammography and, reporting the Texas Medical School's experience with infrared imaging, noted that it was capable of detecting approximately 85% of all breast cancers. Dodd's ideas would later help to fuel the premise and attitudes incorporated into the BCDDP.

Three years later, J.D. Wallace presented to another Cancer Conference, sponsored by the American College of Radiology, the American Cancer Society, and the Cancer Control Program of the National Cancer Institute, an update on infrared imaging of the breast [70]. The author's analysis suggested that the incidence of breast cancer detection per 1000 patients screened could increase from 2.72 when using mammography to 19 when using infrared imaging. He then underlined that infrared imaging poses no radiation burden on the patient, requires no physical contact and, being an innocuous technique, could concentrate the sought population by a significant factor selecting those patients who required further investigation. He concluded that, "the resulting infrared image contains only a small amount of information as compared to the mammogram, so that the reading of the infrared image is a substantially simpler task."

Unfortunately, this rather simplistic and cavalier attitude toward the generation and interpretation of infrared images was prevalent when it was hastily added and then prematurely dismissed from the BCDDP, which was just getting underway. Exaggerated expectations led to the ill-founded premise that infrared imaging might replace mammography rather than complement it. A detailed review of the Report of the Working Group of the BCDDP, published in 1979, is essential to understand the subsequent evolution of infrared imaging [71].

The work scope of this project was issued by the NCI on the 26th of March 1973 with six objectives, the second being to determine if a negative infrared image was sufficient to preclude the use of clinical examination and mammography in the detection of breast cancer. The Working Group, reporting on results of the first 4 years of this project, gave a short history regarding infrared imaging in breast cancer detection. They wrote that, as of the sixties, there was intense interest in determining the suitability of infrared imaging for large-scale applications, and mass screening was one possibility. The need for technological improvement was recognized and the authors stated that efforts had been made to refine the technique. One of the important objectives behind these efforts had been to achieve a sufficiently high sensitivity and specificity for infrared imaging in order to make it useful as a prescreening device in selecting patients for referral for mammographic examination. It was thought that, if successful, the incorporation of this technology would result in a relatively small proportion of women having mammography (a technique that had caused concern at that time because of the carcinogenic effects of radiation). The Working Group indicated that the sensitivity and specificity of infrared imaging readings, with clinical data emanating from interinstitutional studies, were close to the corresponding results for physical examination and mammography. They noted that these three modalities selected different subgroups of breast cancers, and for this reason further evaluation of infrared imaging as a screening device in a controlled clinical trial was recommended.

25.7.1 Poor Study Design

While the Working Group describes in detail the importance of quality control of mammography, the entire protocol for infrared imaging was summarized in one paragraph and simply indicated that infrared imaging was conducted by a BCDDP trained technician. The detailed extensive results from this report, consisting of over 50 tables, included only one that referred to infrared imaging showing that it had detected only 41% of the breast cancers during the first screening while the residual were either normal or unknown. There is no breakdown as far as these two latter groups were concerned. Since 28% of the first screening and 32% of the second screening were picked up by mammography alone, infrared imaging was dropped from any further evaluation and consideration. The report stated that it was impossible to determine whether abnormal infrared images could be predictive of interval cancers (cancers developing between screenings) since they did not collect this data.

By the same token, the Working Group was unable to conclude, with their limited experience, whether the findings were related to the then available technology of infrared imaging or with its application. They did, however, conclude that the decision to dismiss infrared imaging should not be taken as a determination of the future of this technique, rather that the procedure continued to be of interest because it does not entail the risk of radiation exposure. In the Working Group's final recommendation, they state that "infrared imaging does not appear to be suitable as a substitute for mammography for routine screening in the BCDDP." The report admitted that several individual programs of the BCDDP had results that were more favorable than what was reported for the BCDDP as a whole. They encouraged investment in the development and testing of infrared imaging under carefully controlled study conditions and suggested that high priority be given to these studies. They noted that a few suitable sites appeared to be available within the BCDDP participants and proposed that developmental studies should be solicited from sites with sufficient experience.

25.7.2   Untrained Personnel and Protocol Violations

JoAnn Haberman, who was a participant in this project [72], provided further insight into the relatively simplistic regard assigned to infrared imaging during this program. The author reiterated that expertize in mammography was an absolute requirement for the awarding of a contract to establish a screening center. However, the situation was just the opposite with regard to infrared imaging — no experience was required at all. When the 27 demonstration project centers opened their doors, only 5 had any preexisting expertize in infrared imaging. Of the remaining screening centers, there was no experience at all in this technology. Finally, more than 18 months after the project had begun, the NCI established centers where radiologists and their technicians could obtain sufficient training in infrared imaging. Unfortunately, only 11 of the demonstration project directors considered this training of sufficient importance to send their technologists to learn proper infrared technique. The imaging sites also disregarded environmental controls. Many of the project sites were mobile imaging vans, which had poor heating and cooling capabilities and often kept their doors open in the front and rear to permit an easy flow of patients. This, combined with a lack of adherence to protocols and preimaging patient acclimation, lead to unreadable images.

In summary, with regard to infrared imaging, the BCDDP was plagued with problems and seriously flawed in five critical areas (1) The study was initiated with an incorrect premise that infrared imaging might replace mammography. A functional imaging procedure that detects metabolic thermovascular aberrations cannot replace a test that looks for specific areas of structural changes in the breast, (2) Completely untrained technicians were used to perform the scans, (3) The study used radiologists who had no experience or knowledge in reading infrared images, (4) Proper laboratory environmental controls were completely ignored. In fact, many of the research sites were mobile trailers with extreme variations in internal temperatures, (5) No standardized reading protocol had yet been established for infrared imaging. It was not until the early 1980s that established and standardized reading protocols were adopted. Considering these facts, the BCDDP could not have properly evaluated infrared imaging. Since the termination of the BCDDP, a considerable amount of published research has demonstrated the true value of this technology.

25.8   Mammography and Infrared Imaging

From a scientific standpoint, mammography and infrared imaging are completely different screening tests. As a structural imaging procedure, mammography cannot be compared to a functional imaging technology such as infrared imaging. While mammography attempts to detect architectural tissue shadows, infrared imaging observes for changes in the subtle metabolic milieu of the breast. Even though mammography and infrared imaging examine completely different aspects of the breast, research has been performed that allows for a statistical comparison of the two technologies. Since a review of the research on infrared imaging has been covered, data on the current state of mammography is presented.

In a study by Rosenberg, 183,134 screening mammograms were reviewed for changes in sensitivity due to age, breast density, ethnicity, and estrogen replacement therapy. Out of these screening mammograms 807 cancers were discovered at screening. The results showed that the sensitivity for mammography was 54% in women younger than 40, 77% in women aged 40–49, 78% in women aged 50–64, and 81% in women older than 64 years. Sensitivity was 68% in women with dense breasts and 74% in estrogen replacement therapy users [73].

Investigating the cumulative risk of a false-positive result in mammographic screening, Elmore and associates performed a 10-year retrospective study of 2400 women, 40 to 69 years of age. A total of 9762 mammograms were investigated. It was found that a woman had an estimated 49.1% cumulative risk of having a false-positive result after 10 mammograms. Even though no breast cancer was present, over one-third of the women screened were required to have additional evaluations [74].

In a review of the literature, Head investigated the sensitivity, specificity, positive predictive value, and negative predictive values for mammography and infrared imaging. The averaged reported performance for mammography was: 86% sensitivity, 79% specificity, 28% positive predictive value, and 92% negative predictive value. For infrared imaging the averaged performance was: 86% sensitivity, 89% specificity, 23% positive predictive value, and 99.4% negative predictive value [75].

Pisano, along with a large investigational group, provided a detailed report on the Digital Mammographic Imaging Screening Trial (DMIST). The study investigated the diagnostic performance of digital versus film mammography in breast cancer screening. Both digital and film mammograms were taken on 42,760 asymptomatic women presenting for screening mammography. Data was gathered from 33 sites in the United States and Canada. Digital mammography was found to be more accurate in women under age 50 and in women whose breasts were radiographically dense. The sensitivity for both film and digital mammography was found to be 69% [76].

Keyserlingk and associates published a retrospective study reviewing the relative ability of clinical examinations, mammography, and infrared imaging to detect 100 new cases of ductal carcinoma *in situ*, stage I and 2 breast cancers. Results from the study found that the sensitivity for clinical examination alone was 61%, mammography alone was 66%, and infrared imaging alone was 83%. When suspicious and equivocal mammograms were combined the sensitivity was increased to 85%. A sensitivity of 95% was found when suspicious and equivocal mammograms were combined with abnormal infrared images. However, when clinical examination, mammography, and infrared images were combined a sensitivity of 98% was reached 77].

From a review of the cumulative literature database, it can be found that the average sensitivity and specificity for mammography is 80 and 79% respectively for women over the age of 50 [78–80]. A significant decrease in sensitivity and specificity is seen in women below this age. This same research also shows that mammography routinely misses interval cancers (cancers that form between screening exams) [81], which may be detected by infrared imaging. Taking into consideration all the available data, mammography leaves much to be desired as the current gold standard for breast cancer screening. As a stand alone screening procedure, it is suggested that mammography may not be the best choice. In the same light, infrared imaging should also not be used alone as a screening test. The two technologies are of a complimentary nature. Neither used alone are sufficient, but when combined each builds on the deficiencies of the other. In reviewing the literature it seems evident that a multimodal approach to breast cancer screening would serve women best. A combination of clinical examination, mammography, and infrared imaging would provide the greatest potential for breast conservation and survival.

25.9   Current Status of Breast Cancer Detection

Current first-line breast cancer detection strategy still depends essentially on clinical examination and mammography. The limitations of the former, with its reported sensitivity rate often below 65% [77,82] is well-recognized, and even the proposed value of self-breast examination is being contested [83]. While mammography is accepted as the most cost-effective imaging modality, its contribution continues to be challenged with persistent false-negative rates ranging up to 30% [73,76,84,85]; with decreasing sensitivity in younger patients and those on estrogen replacement therapy [73,86]. In addition, there is recent data suggesting that denser and less informative mammography images are precisely those associated with an increased cancer risk [86]. Echoing some of the shortcomings of the BCDDP7 concerning their study design and infrared imaging, Moskowitz indicated that mammography is also not a procedure to be performed by the inexperienced technician or radiologist [88].

With the current emphasis on earlier detection, there is now renewed interest in the parallel development of complimentary imaging techniques that can also exploit the precocious metabolic, immunological, and vascular changes associated with early tumor growth. While promising, techniques such as scintimammography [89], doppler ultrasound [90], and MRI [91] are associated with a number of disadvantages that include exam duration, limited accessibility, need of intravenous access, patient discomfort, restricted imaging area, difficult interpretation, and limited availability of the technology. Like ultrasound, they are more suited to use as second-line options to pursue the already abnormal screening evaluations. While practical, this stepwise approach currently results in the nonrecognition, and thus delayed utilization of second-line technology in approximately 10% of established breast cancers [88]. This is consistent with a study published by Keyserlingk [77].

As an addition to the breast health screening process, infrared imaging has a significant role to play. Owing to infrared imaging's unique ability to image the metabolic aspects of the breast, extremely early warning signals (up to 10 years before any other detection method) have been observed in long-term studies. It is for this reason that an abnormal infrared image is the single most important marker of high risk for the existence of or future development of breast cancer. This, combined with the proven sensitivity, specificity, and prognostic value of the technology, places infrared imaging as one of the major frontline methods of breast cancer screening.

25.10 Future Advancements in Infrared Imaging

Modern high-resolution uncooled focal plane array cameras coupled with high speed computers running sophisticated image analysis software are commonplace in today's top infrared imaging centers. However, research in this field continues to produce technological advancements in image acquisition and digital processing.

Research is currently underway investigating the possible subtle alterations in the blood supply of the breast during the earliest stages of malignancy. Evidence suggests that there may be a normal vasomotor oscillation frequency in the arterial structures of the human body. It is theorized that there may be disturbances in this normal oscillatory rate when a malignancy is forming. Research using infrared detection systems capturing 200 frames per second with a sensitivity of 0.009 of a degree centigrade may be able to monitor alterations in this vasomotor frequency band.

Another unique methodology is investigating the possibility of using infrared emission data to extrapolate depth and location of a metabolic heat source within the body. In the case of cancer, the increased tissue metabolism resulting from rapid cellular multiplication and growth generates heat. With this new approach in infrared detection, it is theorized that an analysis based on an analogy to electrical circuit theory — termed the thermal-electric analog — may possibly be used to determine the depth and location of the heat source.

The most promising of all the advances in medical infrared imaging are the adaptations being used from military developments in the technology. Hardware advances in narrow band filtering hold promise in providing multispectral and hyperspectral images. One of the most intriguing applications of mutispectral/hyperspectral imaging may include real-time intraoperative cytology. Investigations are also underway utilizing smart processing, also known as artificial intelligence. This comes in the form of post-image processing of the raw data from the infrared sensor array. Some of the leading-edge processing currently under study include automated target recognition (ATR), artificial neural networks (ANN), and threshold algorithms to mention only a few. The use of ATR and threshold algorithms are dependent on a reliable normative database. The images are processed based on what the system has learned as normal and compares the new image to that database. Unlike ATR and threshold algorithms, ANN uses data summation to produce pattern recognition. This is extremely important when it comes to the complex thermovascular patterns seen in infrared breast imaging. Ultimately, these advancements will lead to a decrease in operator dependence and a substantial increase in both objectivity and accuracy.

New breast cancer treatments are also exploring methods of targeting the angiogenic process. Due to a tumor's dependence on a constant blood supply to maintain growth, antiangiogenesis therapy is becoming one of the most promising therapeutic strategies and has been found to be pivotal in the new paradigm for consideration of breast cancer development and treatment [92]. The future may see infrared imaging and antiangiogenesis therapy combined as the state of the art in the biological assessment and treatment of breast cancer.

These and other new methodologies in medical infrared imaging are being investigated and may prove to be significant advancements. However, a great deal of research will need to be performed before new technologies can be adopted for medical use.

25.11 Conclusion

The large patient populations and long survey periods in many of the above clinical studies yield a high significance to the various statistical data obtained. This is especially true for the contribution of infrared imaging to early cancer diagnosis, as an invaluable marker of high-risk populations, and in therapeutic decision making.

Currently available high-resolution digital infrared imaging technology benefits greatly from enhanced image production, computerized image processing and analysis, and standardized image interpretation protocols. Over 40 years of research and 800 indexed papers encompassing well over 300,000 women participants has demonstrated infrared imaging's abilities in the early detection of breast cancer. Infrared imaging has distinguished itself as the earliest detection technology for breast cancer. It has the ability to signal an alarm that a cancer may be forming up to 10 years before any other procedure can detect it. In 7 out of 10 cases, infrared imaging will detect signs of a cancer before it is seen on a mammogram. Clinical trials have also shown that infrared imaging significantly augments the long-term survival rates of its recipients by as much as 61%. And when used as part of a multimodal approach (clinical examination, mammography, and infrared imaging) 95% of all early stage cancers will be detected. Ongoing research into the thermal characteristics of breast pathologies will continue to investigate the relationships between neoangiogenesis, chemical mediators, and the neoplastic process.

It is unfortunate, but many clinicians still hesitate to consider infrared imaging as a useful tool in spite of the considerable research database, steady improvements in both infrared technology and image analysis, and continued efforts on the part of the infrared imaging societies. This attitude may be due in part to the average clinician's unfamiliarity with the physical and biological basis of infrared imaging. The other methods of cancer investigations refer directly to topics of medical teaching. For instance, radiography and ultrasonography refer to structural anatomy. Infrared imaging, however, is based on thermodynamics and thermokinetics, which are unfamiliar to most clinicians; though man is experiencing heat production and exchange in every situation he undergoes or creates.

Considering the contribution that infrared imaging has demonstrated thus far in the field of early breast cancer detection, all possibilities should be considered for promoting further technical, biological, and clinical research along with the incorporation of the technology into common clinical use.

References

[1] Adams, F., *The Genuine Works of Hippocrates*, Williams and Wilkins, Baltimore, 1939.

[2] Lawson, R.N., Implications of surface temperatures in the diagnosis of breast cancer. *Can. Med. Assoc. J.*, 75, 309, 1956.

[3] Lawson, R.N., Thermography — a new tool in the investigation of breast lesions. *Can. Serv. Med.*, 13, 517, 1957.

[4] Lawson, R.N., A new infrared imaging device. *Can. Med. Assoc. J.*, 79, 402, 1958.

[5] Archer, F. and Gros, C., Classification thermographique des cancers mammaires. *Bulletin du Cancer*, 58, 351, 1971.

[6] Amalu, W. et al., Standards and protocols in clinical thermographic imaging. *International Academy of Clinical Thermology*, September 2002.

[7] Kurbitz, G., Design criteria for radiometric thermal-imaging devices, in *Thermological Methods*, VCH mbH, pp. 94–100, 1985.

[8] Houdas, Y. and Ring E.F.J., Models of thermoregulation, in *Human Temperature: Its Measurement and Regulation*, Plenum Press, New York, pp. 136–141.

[9] Flesch, U., Physics of skin-surface temperature, in *Thermological Methods*, VCH mbH, pp. 21–33, 1985.

[10] Anbar M., *Quantitative Dynamic Telethermometry in Medical Diagnosis and Management*, CRC Press, Boca Raton, FL, p. 106, 1994.

[11] Anbar, M., Potential artifacts in infrared thermographic measurements. *Thermology*, 3, 273, 1991.

[12] Friedrich, K. (Optic research laboratory, Carl Zeiss — West Germany), Assessment criteria for infrared thermography systems. *Acta Thermogr.*, 5, 68–72.

[13] Engel, J.M., Thermography in locomotor diseases. *Acta Thermogr.*, 5, 11–13.

[14] Cuthbertson, G.M., The development of IR imaging in the United Kingdom, in *The Thermal Image in Medicine and Biology*, Uhlen-Verlag, Wien, pp. 21–32, 1995.

[15] Amalu, W., The validity of the thermoregulatory stress test in infrared imaging of the breast, *Presented at the 31st annual symposium of the American Academy of Thermology*, Auburn University, Alabama, 2004.

[16] Gautherie, M., Kotewicz, A., and Gueblez, P., Accurate and objective evaluation of breastthermograms: basic principles and new advances with special reference to an improved computer-assisted scoring system, in *Thermal assessment of Breast Health*, MTP Press Limited, pp. 72–97, 1983.

[17] Hobbins, W.B., Abnormal thermogram — significance in breast cancer. *Interamer. J. Rad.*, 12, 337, 1987.

[18] Gautherie, M., New protocol for the evaluation of breast thermograms, in *Thermological Methods*, VCH mbH, pp. 227–235, 1985.

[19] Lawson, R.N. and Chughtai, M.S., Breast cancer and body temperatures. *Can. Med. Assoc. J.*, 88, 68, 1963.

[20] Head, J.F., Wang, F., and Elliott, R.L., Breast thermography is a noninvasive prognostic procedure that predicts tumor growth rate in breast cancer patients. *Ann. NY Acad. Sci.*, 698, 153, 1993.

[21] Sterns, E.E., Zee, B., Sen Gupta, J. and Saunders, F.W., Thermography: its relation to pathologic characteristics, vascularity, proliferative rate and survival of patients with invasive ductal carcinoma of the breast. *Cancer*, 77, 1324, 1996.

[22] Head, J.F. and Elliott, R.L., Breast thermography. *Cancer*, 79, 186, 1995.

[23] Anbar M., *Quantitative Dynamic Telethermometry in Medical Diagnosis and Management*, CRC Press, pp. 84–94, 1994.

[24] Rodenberg, D.A., Chaet, M.S., Bass, R.C. et al., Nitric oxide: an overview. *Am. J. Surg.* 170, 292, 1995.

[25] Thomsen, L.L., Miles, D.W., Happerfield, L. et al., Nitric oxide synthase activity in human breast cancer. *Br. J. Cancer*, 72, 41, 1995.

[26] Guidi, A.J. and Schnitt, S.J., Angiogenesis in pre-invasive lesions of the breast. *The Breast J.*, 2, 364, 1996.

[27] Gamagami, P., Indirect signs of breast cancer: Angiogenesis study, in *Atlas of Mammography*, Blackwell Science, Cambridge, MA, pp. 231–26, 1996.

[28] Love, T., Thermography as an indicator of blood perfusion. *Proc. NY Acad. Sci. J.*, 335, 429, 1980.

[29] Chato, J., Measurement of thermal properties of growing tumors. *Proc. N.Y. Acad. Sci.*, 335, 67, 1980.

[30] Draper, J., Skin temperature distribution over veins and tumors. *Phys. Med. Biol.*, 16, 645, 1971.

[31] Jain, R. and Gullino, P., Thermal characteristics of tumors: applications in detection and treatment. *Ann. NY Acad. Sci.*, 335, 1, 1980.

[32] Gautherie, M., Thermopathology of breast cancer; measurement and analysis of *in vivo* temperature and blood flow. *Ann. NY Acad. Sci.*, 365, 383, 1980.

[33] Gautherie, M., Thermobiological assessment of benign and malignant breast diseases. *Am. J. Obstet. Gynecol.*, 147, 861, 1983.

[34] Gamigami, P., *Atlas of Mammography: New Early Signs in Breast Cancer*, Blackwell Science, 1996.

[35] Gershen-Cohen, J., Haberman, J., and Brueschke, E., Medical thermography: a summary of current status. *Radiol. Clin. North Am.*, 3, 403, 1965.

[36] Haberman, J., The present status of mammary thermography. *CA: A Cancer Journal for Clinicians*, 18, 314,1968.

[37] Hoffman, R., Thermography in the detection of breast malignancy. *Am. J. Obstet. Gynecol.*, 98, 681, 1967.

[38] Stark, A. and Way, S., The screening of well women for the early detection of breast cancer using clinical examination with thermography and mammography. *Cancer*, 33, 1671, 1974.

[39] Amalric, D. et al., Value and interest of dynamic telethermography in detection of breast cancer. *Acta Thermographica*, 1, 89–96.

[40] Hobbins, W., Mass breast cancer screening. *Proceedings, Third International Symposium on Detection and Prevention of Breast Cancer*, New York, NY, p. 637, 1976.

[41] Isard, H.J., Becker, W., Shilo, R. et al., Breast thermography after four years and 10,000 studies. *Am. J. Roentgenol.*, 115, 811, 1972.

[42] Spitalier, H., Giraud, D. et al., Does infrared thermography truly have a role in present-day breast cancer management? *Biomedical Thermology*, Alan R. Liss, New York, NY, 269–278, 1982.

[43] Moskowitz, M., Milbrath, J., Gartside, P. et al., Lack of efficacy of thermography as a screening tool for minimal and stage I breast cancer. *N. Engl. J. Med.*, 295, 249, 1976.

[44] Threatt, B., Norbeck, J.M., Ullman, N.S. et al., Thermography and breast cancer: an analysis of a blind reading. *Ann. NY Acad. Sci.*, 335, 501,1980.

[45] Haberman, J., Francis, J. and Love, T., Screening a rural population for breast cancer using thermography and physical examination techniques. *Ann. NY Acad. Sci.*, 335, 492, 1980.

[46] Sciarra, J., Breast cancer: strategies for early detection, in *Thermal Assessment of Breast Health (Proceedings of the International Conference on Thermal Assessment of Breast Health)*, MTP Press Ltd, pp. 117–129, 1983.

[47] Gautherie, M., Thermobiological assessment of benign and malignant breast diseases. *Am. J. Obstet. Gynecol.*, 147, 861, 1983.

[48] Louis, K., Walter, J., and Gautherie, M., Long-term assessment of breast cancer risk by thermal imaging, in *Biomedical Thermology*, Alan R. Liss Inc., pp. 279–301, 1982.

[49] Gros, C. and Gautherie, M., Breast thermography and cancer risk prediction. *Cancer*, 45, 51, 1980.

[50] Jones, C.H., Thermography of the female breast, in *Diagnosis of Breast Disease*, C.A. Parsons (Ed.), University Park Press, Baltimore, pp. 214–234, 1983.

[51] Useki, H., Evaluation of the thermographic diagnosis of breast disease: relation of thermographic findings and pathologic findings of cancer growth. *Nippon Gan Chiryo Gakkai Shi*, 23, 2687, 1988.

[52] Parisky, Y.R., Sardi, A. et al., Efficacy of computerized infrared imaging analysis to evaluate mammographically suspicious lesions. *AJR*, 180, 263, 2003.

[53] Nyirjesy, I., Ayme, Y. et al., Clinical evaluation, mammography, and thermography in the diagnosis of breast carcinoma. *Thermology*, 1, 170, 1986.

[54] Thomassin, L., Giraud, D. et al., Detection of subclinical breast cancers by infrared thermo-graphy, in *Recent Advances in Medical Thermology (Proceedings of the Third International Congress of Thermology)*, Plenum Press, New York, NY, pp. 575–579, 1984.

[55] Amalric, R., Gautherie, M., Hobbins, W., and Stark, A., The future of women with an isolated abnormal infrared thermogram. *La Nouvelle Presse Medicale*, 10, 3153, 1981.

[56] Gautherie, M. and Gros, C., Contribution of infrared thermography to early diagnosis, pre-therapeutic prognosis, and post-irradiation follow-up of breast carcinomas. Laboratory of Electroradiology, Faculty of Medicine, Louis Pasteur University, Strasbourg, France, 1976.

[57] Hobbins, W., Significance of an "isolated" abnormal thermogram. *La Nouvelle Presse Medicale*, 10, 3155, 1981.

[58] Hobbins, W., Thermography, highest risk marker in breast cancer. *Proceedings of the Gynecological Society for the Study of Breast Disease*, pp. 267–282, 1977.

[59] Gauthrie, M., Improved system for the objective evaluation of breast thermograms, in *Biomedical Thermology*. Alan R. Liss, Inc., New York, NY, pp. 897–905, 1982.

[60] Amalric, R., Giraud, D. et al., Combined diagnosis of small breast cancer. *Acta Thermogr.*, 1984.

[61] Spitalier, J., Amalric, D. et al., The Importance of infrared thermography in the early suspicion and detection of minimal breast cancer, *in Thermal Assessment of Breast Health*, MTP Press Ltd., pp. 173–179, 1983.

[62] Gautherie, M. et al., Thermobiological assessment of benign and malignant breast diseases. *Am. J. Obstet. Gynecol.*, 147, 861, 1983.

[63] Jay, E. and Karpman, H., Computerized breast thermography, in *Thermal Assessment of Breast Health*, MTP Press Ltd., pp. 98–109, 1983.

[64] Dilhuydy, M.H. et al., The importance of thermography in the prognostic evaluation of breast cancers. *Acta Thermogr.*, 130–136.

[65] Amalric, D. et al., Value and interest of dynamic telethermography in detection of breast cancer. *Acta Thermogr.*, 89–96.

[66] Fournier, V.D., Kubli, F. et al., Infrared thermography and breast cancer doubling time. *Acta Thermogr.*, 107–111.

[67] Gros, D., Gautherie, M., and Warter, F., Thermographic prognosis of treated breast cancers. *Acta Thermogr.*, 11–14.

[68] Keyserlingk, J.R., Ahlgren P.D. et al., Preliminary evaluation of high resolution functional infrared imaging to monitor pre-operative chemohormonotherapy-induced changes in neo-angiogenesis in patients with locally advanced breast cancer. Ville Marie Oncology Center/St. Mary's Hospital, Montreal, Canada. In submission for publication, 2003.

[69] Dodd, G.D., Thermography in breast cancer diagnosis, in *Abstracts for the Seventh National Cancer Conference Proceedings*. Lippincott Philadelphia, Los Angeles, CA, 267, 1972.

[70] Wallace, J.D., Thermographic examination of the breast: An assessment of its present capabilities, in *Early Breast Cancer: Detection and Treatment*, Gallagher, H.S. (Ed.). American College of Radiology, Wiley, New York, pp. 13–19, 1975.

[71] Report of the Working Group to Review the National Cancer Institute Breast Cancer Detection Demonstration Projects. *J. Natl Cancer Inst.*, 62, 641, 1979.

[72] Haberman, J., An overview of breast thermography in the United States, in *Medical Thermography*, Margaret Abernathy and Sumio Uematsu (Eds.), American Academy of Thermology, Washington, pp. 218–223, 1986.

[73] Rosenberg, R.D., Hunt, W.C. et al., Effects of age, breast density, ethnicity, and estrogen replacement therapy on screening mammographic sensitivity and cancer stage at diagnosis: Review of 183,134 screening mammograms in Albuquerque, New Mexico. *Radiology*, 209, 511, 1998.

[74] Elmore, J. et al., Ten-year risk of false positive screening mammograms and clinical breast examinations. *N. Engl. J. Med.*, 338, 1089, 1998.

[75] Head, J.F., Lipari, C.A., and Elliott, R.L., Comparison of mammography, and breast infrared imaging: sensitivity, specificity, false negatives, false positives, positive predictive value and negative predictive value. *IEEE*, 1999.

[76] Pisano, E.D., Gatsonis, C. et al, Diagnostic performance of digital versus film mammography for breast-cancer screening. *N. Engl. J. Med.*, 353, October, 2005.

[77] Keyserlignk, J.R., Ahlgren, P.D. et al., Infrared imaging of the breast; initial reappraisal using high-resolution digital technology in 100 successive cases of stage 1 and 2 breast cancer. *Breast J.*, 4, 1998.

[78] Schell, M.J., Bird, R.D., and Desrochers, D.A., Reassessment of breast cancers missed during routine screening mammography. *Am. J. Roentgenol.*, 177, 535, 2001.

[79] Poplack, S.P., Tosteson, A.N., Grove, M. et al., The practice of mammography in 53,803 women from the New Hampshire mammography network. *Radiology*, 217, 832, 2000.

[80] Pullon, S. and McLeod, D., The early detection and diagnosis of breast cancer: a literature review. General Practice Department, Wellington School of Medicine, December 1996.

[81] Gilliland, F.D., Joste, N., Stauber, P.M. et al., Biologic characteristics of interval and screen-detected breast cancers. *J. Natl Cancer Inst.*, 92, 743, 2000.

[82] Sickles, E.A., Mammographic features of "early" breast cancer. *Am. J. Roentgenol.*, 143, 461, 1984.

[83] Thomas, D.B., Gao, D.L., Self, S.G. et al., Randomized trial of breast self-examination in Shanghai: methodology and preliminary results. *J. Natl Cancer Inst.*, 5, 355, 1997.

[84] Moskowitz, M., Screening for breast cancer. How effective are our tests? *CA Cancer J. Clin.*, 33, 26, 1983.

[85] Elmore, J.G., Wells, C.F., Carol, M.P. et al., Variability in radiologists interpretation of mammograms. *N. Engl. J. Med.*, 331, 1493, 1994

[86] Laya, M.B., Effect on estrogen replacement therapy on the specificity and sensitivity of screening mammography. *J. Natl Cancer Inst.*, 88, 643, 1996.

[87] Boyd, N.F., Byng, J.W., Jong, R.A. et al., Quantitative classification of mammographic densities and breast cancer risk. *J. Natl Cancer Inst.*, 87, 670, 1995.

[88] Moskowitz, M., Breast imaging, in *Cancer of the Breast*, Donegan, W.L. and Spratt, J.S. (Eds.), Saunders, New York, pp. 206–239, 1995.

[89] Khalkhali, I., Cutrone, J.A. et al., Scintimammography: the complementary role of Tc-99m sestamibi prone breast imaging for the diagnosis of breast carcinoma. *Radiology*, 196, 421, 1995.

[90] Kedar, R.P., Cosgrove, D.O. et al., Breast carcinoma: measurement of tumor response in primary medical therapy with color doppler flow imaging. *Radiology*, 190, 825, 1994.

[91] Weinreb, J.C. and Newstead, G., MR imaging of the breast. *Radiology*, 196, 593, 1995.

[92] Love, S.M. and Barsky, S.H., Breast cancer: an interactive paradigm. *Breast J.*, 3, 171, 1996.

26

Functional Infrared Imaging of the Breast: Historical Perspectives, Current Application, and Future Considerations

26.1 Historical Perspectives...................................... **26**-2
    Pre-Breast Cancer Detection Demonstration Projects Era •
    The Breast Cancer Detection Demonstration Projects Era •
    Post-Breast Cancer Detection Demonstration Projects Era
26.2 The Ville Marie Multi-Disciplinary Breast Center
    Experience with High-Resolution Digital Infrared
    Imaging to Detect and Monitor Breast Cancer **26**-7
    Infrared Imaging as Part of a First-Line Multi-Imaging
    Strategy to Promote Early Detection of Breast Cancer •
    Preliminary Evaluation of Digital High-Resolution Functional
    Infrared Imaging to Monitor Pre-Operative
    Chemohormonotherapy-Induced Changes in
    Neo-Angiogenesis in Patients with Advanced Breast Cancer •
    Results
26.3 Future Considerations Concerning
    Infrared Imaging....................................... **26**-25
References **26**-29

J.R. Keyserlingk
P.D. Ahlgren
E. Yu
N. Belliveau
M. Yassa
Ville Marie Oncology Center

There is general consensus that earlier detection of breast cancer should result in improved survival. For the last two decades, first-line breast imaging has relied primarily on mammography. Despite better equipment and regulation, particularly with the recent introduction of digital mammography, variability in interpretation and tissue density can affect mammography accuracy. To promote earlier diagnosis, a number of adjuvant functional imaging techniques have recently been introduced, including Doppler ultrasound and gadolinium-enhanced magnetic resonance imaging (MRI) that can detect cancer-induced regional neovascularity. While valuable modalities, problems relating to complexity, accessibility, cost, and in most cases the need for intravenous access make them unsuitable as components of a first-line imaging strategy.

In order to re-assess the potential contribution of infrared (IR) imaging as a first-line component of a multi-imaging strategy, using currently available technology, we will first review the history of its introduction and early clinical application, including the results of the Breast Cancer Demonstration Projects (BCDDP). We will then review the Ville Marie Multi-Disciplinary Breast Center's more recent experience with currently available high-resolution computerized IR technology to assess IR imaging both as a complement to clinical exam and mammography in the early detection of breast cancer and also as a tool to monitor the effects of pre-operative chemohormonotherapy in advanced breast cancer. Our goal is to show that high-resolution IR imaging provides additional safe, practical, cost effective, and objective information in both of these instances when produced by strict protocol and interpreted by sufficiently trained breast physicians. Finally, we will comment on its further evolution.

26.1 Historical Perspectives

26.1.1 Pre-Breast Cancer Detection Demonstration Projects Era

In 1961 in the *Lancet*, Williams and Handley [1] using a rudimentary hand-held thermopile, reported that 54 of 57 of their breast cancer patients were detectable by IR imaging, and "among these were cases in which the clinical diagnosis was in much doubt." The authors reported that the majority of these cancers had a temperature increase of 1 to 2°C, and that the IR imaging permitted excellent discrimination between benign and malignant processes. Their protocol at the Middlesex Hospital consisted of having the patient strip to the waist and be exposed to the ambient temperature for 15 min.

The authors demonstrated a precocious understanding of the significance of IR imaging by introducing the concept that increased cooling to 18°C further enhanced the temperature discrepancy between cancer and the normal breast. In a follow-up article the subsequent year, Handley [2] demonstrated a close correlation between the increased thermal pattern and increased recurrence rate. While only four of 35 cancer patients with a 1 to 2°C discrepancy recurred, five of the six patients with over 3°C rise developed recurrent cancer, suggesting already that the prognosis could be gauged by the amount of rise of temperature in the overlying skin.

In 1963, Lawson and Chughtai [3], two McGill University surgeons, published an elegant intra-operative study demonstrating that the increase in regional temperature associated with breast cancer was related to venous convection. This quantitative experiment added credence to Handley's suggestion that IR findings were related to both increased venous flow and increased metabolism.

In 1965, Gershon-Cohen [4], a radiologist and researcher from the Albert Einstein Medical Center, introduced IR imaging to the United States. Using a Barnes thermograph that required 15 min to produce a single IR image, he reported 4000 cases with a remarkable true positive rate of 94% and a false positive rate of 6%. This data was included in a review of the then current status of infrared imaging published in 1968 in *CA — A Cancer Journal for Physicians* [5]. The author, JoAnn Haberman, a radiologist from Temple University School of Medicine, reported the local experience with IR imaging, which produced a true positive rate of 84% compared with a concomitant true positive rate of 80% for mammography. In addition, she compiled 16,409 IR imaging cases from the literature between 1964 and 1968 revealing an overall true positive rate of 87% and a false positive rate of 13%.

A similar contemporary review compiled by Jones, consisting of nearly 70,000 cases, revealed an identical true positive rate of 85% and an identical false positive rate of 13%. Furthermore, Jones [6] reported on over 20,000 IR imagings from the Royal Marsden Hospital between 1967 and 1972, and noted that approximately 70% of Stage I and Stage II cancers and up to 90% of Stage III and Stage IV cancers had abnormal IR features. These reports resulted in an unbridled enthusiasm for IR imaging as a front-line detection modality for breast cancer.

Sensing a potential misuse of this promising but unregulated imaging modality, Isard made some sobering comments in 1972 [7] in a publication of the *American Journal of Roentengology*, where he emphasized that, like other imaging techniques, IR imaging does not diagnose cancer but merely indicates the presence of an abnormality. Reporting his Radiology division's experience with 10,000 IR studies done concomitantly with mammography between 1967 and 1970, he reiterated a number of important concepts, including the remarkable stability of the IR image from year to year in the otherwise healthy patient, and the importance of recognizing any significant change. Infrared imaging detected 60% of occult cancers in his experience, vs. 80% with mammography. The combination of both these modalities increased the sensitivity by approximately 10%, thus underlining the complimentarity of both of these processes, since each one did not always suspect the same lesion.

It was Isard's conclusion that, had there been a preliminary selection of his group of 4393 asymptomatic patients by IR imaging, mammography examination would have been restricted to the 1028 patients with abnormal IR imaging (23% of this cohort). This would have resulted in a cancer detection rate of 24.1 per 1000 mammographic examinations, as contrasted to the expected 7 per 1000 by mammographic screening. He concluded that since IR imaging is an innocuous examination, it could be utilized to focus attention upon asymptomatic women who should be examined more intensely.

In 1972, Gerald D. Dodd [8] of the Department of Diagnostic Radiology of the University of Texas presented an update on IR imaging in breast cancer diagnosis at the Seventh National Cancer Conference sponsored by the National Cancer Society, and the National Cancer Institute. He also suggested that IR imaging would be best employed as a screening agent for mammography and proposed that in any general survey of the female population age 40 and over, 15–20% would have positive IR imaging and would require mammograms. Of these, approximately 5% would be recommended for biopsy. He concluded that IR imaging would serve to eliminate 80–85% of the potential mammograms. Reporting the Texas Medical School's experience with IR imaging, he reiterated that IR was capable of detecting approximately 85% of all breast cancers. The false positive rate of 15–20% did not concern the author, who stated that these were false positives only in the sense that there was no corroborative evidence of breast cancer at the time of the examination and that they could serve to identify a high-risk population.

Feig et al. [9], reported the respective abilities of clinical exam, mammography, and IR imaging to detect breast cancer in 16,000 self-selected women. While only 39% of the initial series of overall established cancer patients had an abnormal IR imaging, this increased to 75% in his later cohort, reflecting an improved methodology. Of particular interest was the ability of IR imaging to detect 54% of the smallest tumors, four times that of clinical examination. This potential important finding was not elaborated, but it could reflect IR's ability to detect vascular changes that are sometimes more apparent at the initiation of tumor genesis. The authors suggested that the potential of IR imaging to select high-risk groups for follow-up screening merited further investigation.

Wallace [10] presented an update on IR imaging of the breast to another contemporary Cancer Conference sponsored by the American College of Radiology, the American Cancer Society, and the Cancer Control Programme of the National Cancer Institute. The analysis suggested that the incidence of breast cancer detection per 1000 screenees could increase from 2.72 when using mammography to 19 when using IR imaging. He then underlined that IR imaging poses no radiation burden on the patient, requires no physical contact, and, being an innocuous technique, could concentrate the sought population by a significant factor, selecting those patients that required further investigation. He concluded that "the resulting IR image contains only a small amount of information as compared to the mammogram, so that the reading of the IR image is a substantially simpler task."

Unfortunately, this rather simplistic and cavalier attitude toward the acquisition and interpretation of IR imaging was widely prevalent when it was hastily added to the BCDDP, which was just getting underway. Rather than assess, in a controlled manner, its potential as a complementary first-line detection modality, it was hastily introduced into the BCDDP as apotential replacement for mammography and clinical exam.

26.1.2 The Breast Cancer Detection Demonstration Projects Era

A detailed review of the Report of the Working Group of the BCDDP is essential to understand the subsequent evolution of IR imaging [11]. The scope of this project was issued by the National Cancer

Institute (NCI) on March 26, 1973, with six objectives, the second being to determine if a negative IR imaging was sufficient to preclude the use of clinical examination and mammography in the detection of breast cancer. The Working Group, reporting on results of the first 4 years of this project, gave a short history regarding IR imaging in breast cancer detection. They reported that as of the 1960s, there was intense interest in determining the suitability of IR imaging for large-scale applications, and mass screening was one possibility. The need for technological improvement was recognized and the authors stated that efforts had been made to refine the technique. One of the important objectives behind these efforts had been to achieve a sufficiently high sensitivity and specificity for IR imaging under screening conditions to make it useful as a prescreening device in selecting patients who would then be referred for mammographic examination. It was thought that if successful, this technology would result in a relatively small proportion of women having mammography, a technique that caused concern because of the carcinogenic effects of radiation. The Working Group indicated that the sensitivity and specificity of IR imaging readings from clinical data emanating from interinstitutional studies were close to the corresponding results for physical examination and for mammography. While they noted that these three modalities selected different subgroups of breast cancers, further evaluation of IR imaging as a potential stand-alone screening device in a controlled clinical trial was recommended.

The authors of the BCDDP Working Group generated a detailed review of mammography and efforts to improve its quality control in image quality and reduction in radiation. They recalled that in the 1960s, the Cancer Control Board of the U.S. Public Health Service had financed a national mammography training programme for radiologists and their technologists. Weekly courses in mammography were taught at approximately ten institutions throughout the country with material supplied by the American College of Radiology. In 1975, shortly after the beginning of this project, the NCI had already funded seven institutions in the United States in a 3-year effort aimed at reorienting radiologists and their technologists in more advanced mammographic techniques and interpretation for the detection of early breast cancer.

In the interim, the American College of Radiology and many interested mammographers and technologists had presented local postgraduate refresher courses and workshops on mammography. Every year for the previous 16 years, the American College of Radiology had supported, planned and coordinated week-long conferences and workshops aimed at optimizing mammography to promote the earlier detection and treatment of breast cancer. It was recognized that the well-known primary and secondary mammographic signs of a malignant condition, such as ill-defined mass, skin thickening, skin retraction, marked fibrosis and architectural distortion, obliteration of the retromammary space, and enlarged visible axillary lymph nodes, could detect an established breast cancer. However, the authors emphasized that more subtle radiographic signs that occur in minimal, clinically occult, and early cancers, such as localized punctate calcifications, focal areas of duct prominence, and minor architectural distortion, could lead to an earlier diagnosis even when the carcinoma was not infiltrating, which was a rare finding when previous mammographic techniques were used.

The authors reiterated that the reproduction of early mammography signs required a constant high-quality technique for fine image detail, careful comparison of the two breasts during interpretation, and the search for areas of bilateral, parenchymal asymmetry that could reflect underlying cancer. The BCDDP Working Group report stated that mammographies were conducted by trained technicians and that, while some projects utilized radiological technicians for the initial interpretation, most used either a radiologist or a combination of technician and radiologist. Quality control for mammography consisted of reviews by the project radiologists and site visits by consultants to identify problems in procedures and the quality of the films.

On the other hand, the entire protocol for IR imaging within this study was summarized in one paragraph, and it indicated that IR imaging was conducted by a BCDDP trained technician. Initial interpretation was made mostly by technicians; some projects used technicians plus radiologists and a few used radiologists and/or physicians with other specialties for all readings. Quality control relied on review of procedures and interpretations by the project physicians. Positive physical exams and mammographies were reported in various degrees of certainty about malignancy or as suspicious-benign; IR imaging was reported simply as normal or abnormal. While the protocol for the BCDDP required that the three clinical components of this study (physical examination, IR imaging, and mammography) be conducted separately, and initial findings and recommendations be reported independently, it was not possible for the Working Group to assess the extent to which this protocol was adhered to or to evaluate the quality of the examinations.

The detailed extensive results from this Working Group report consisted of over 50 tables. There was, however, only one table that referred to IR imaging, showing that it had detected 41% of the breast cancers during the first screening, while the residuals were either normal or unknown. There is no breakdown as far as these two latter groups were concerned. Since 28% of the first screening and 32% of the second screening were picked up by mammography alone, IR imaging was dropped from any further evaluation and consideration. The report stated that it was impossible to determine whether abnormal IR imaging could be predictive of interval (developing between screenings) cancers, since these data were not collected.

By the same token, the Working Group was unable to conclude, with their limited experience, whether the findings were related to the then existing technology of IR imaging or with its application. They did, however, indicate that the decision to dismiss IR imaging should not be taken as a determination of the future of this technique, rather that the procedure continued to be of interest because it does not entail the risk of radiation exposure. In the Working Group's final recommendation, they state that "infrared imaging does not appear to be suitable as a substitute for mammography for routine screening in the BCDDP" but could not comment on its role as a complementary modality. The report admitted that several individual programs of the BCDDP had results that were more favorable than for the BCDDP as a whole. They also insisted that high priority be given to development and testing of IR imaging under carefully controlled study conditions. They noted that a few suitable sites appeared to be available among the BCDDP and proposed that developmental studies should be solicited from the sites with sufficient experience.

Further insight into the inadequate quality control assigned to IR imaging during this program was provided by Haberman, a participant in that project [12]. The author reiterated that, while proven expertise in mammography was an absolute requirement for the awarding of a contract to establish a Screening Center, the situation was just the opposite as regards to IR imaging. As no experience was required, when the 27 demonstration projects opened their doors, only five of the centers had pre-existing expertise in IR imaging. Of the remaining screening centers, there was no experience at all in this technology. Finally, more than 18 months after the BCDDP project had begun operating, the NCI, recognizing this problem, established centers where radiologists and their technicians could obtain further training in IR imaging. Unfortunately, only 11 of the demonstration project directors considered this training of sufficient importance to send their technologists. In some centers, it was reported that there was no effort to cool the patient prior to examination. In other centers, there was complete lack of standardization, and a casual attitude prevailed with reference to interpretation of results. While quality control of this imaging technology could be considered lacking, it was nevertheless subjected to the same stringent statistical analysis as was mammography and clinical breast examination.

26.1.3 Post-Breast Cancer Detection Demonstration Projects Era

Two small-scale studies carried out in the 1970s by Moskowitz [13] and Threatt [14] reported on the sensitivity and reliability of IR imaging. Both used "experts" to review the images of breast cancer patients. While Moskowitz excluded unreadable images, data from Threatt's study indicated that less than 30% of the images produced were considered good, with the rest being substandard. Both these studies produced poor results, inconsistent with numerous previous multicenter trials, particularly that of Stark [15] who, 16 years earlier, reported an 81% detection rate for preclinical cancers.

Threatt noted that IR imaging demonstrated an increasing accuracy as cancers increased in size or aggressiveness, as did the other testing modalities (i.e., physical examination and mammography). The author also suggested that computerized pattern recognition would help solve the reproducibility problems sometimes associated with this technology and that further investigation was warranted. Moskowitz also suggested that for IR imaging to be truly effective as a screening tool, there needed to be more objective means of interpretation. He proposed that this would be much facilitated by computerized evaluation.

In a frequently cited article, Sterns and Cardis [16] reviewed their group's limited experience with IR in 1982. While there were only 11 cancer cases in this trial, they were concerned about a sensitivity of 60% and a false positive rate of IR of 12%. While there was no mention of training, they concluded, based on a surprisingly low false positive rate of clinical exam of only 1.4%, that IR could not be recommended for breast diagnosis or as an indication for mammography.

Thirteen years later, reviewing the then status of breast imaging, Moskowitz [17] challenged the findings of the recent Canadian National Breast Screening Study (NBSS) that questioned the value of mammography, much in the same way that the Working Group of the BCDDP questioned IR imaging 20 years previously. Using arguments that could have qualified the disappointing results of the IR imaging used in the BCDDP study, the author explained the poor results of mammography in the NBSS on the basis of inadequate technical quality. He concluded that only 68% of the women received satisfactory breast imaging.

In addition to the usual causes of poor technical quality, failure to use the medial lateral oblique view resulted in exclusion of the tail of Spence and of much of the upper outer quadrant in many of the subjects screened. There was also a low interobserver agreement in the reading of mammographies, which resulted in a potential diagnostic delay. His review stated that of all noncontrast, nondigital radiological procedures, mammography required the greatest attention to meticulous detail for the training of technologists, selection of the film, contrast monitoring of processing, choosing of equipment, and positioning of the patient. For mammography to be of value, it required dedicated equipment, a dedicated room, dedicated film, and the need to be performed and interpreted by dedicated people. Echoing some of the criticisms that could be pertinent to the BCDDP's use of IR imaging, he indicated that mammography is not a procedure to be performed by the untutored. In rejecting any lack of quality control of IR imaging during the BCDDP studies by stating that "most of the investigators in the BCDDP did undergo a period of training." The author once again suggested that the potential of IR imaging would only increase if there was better standardization of technology and better-designed clinical trials.

Despite its initial promise, this challenge was not taken up by the medical community, who systematically lost interest in this technique, primarily due to the nebulous BCDDP experience. Nevertheless, during the 1980s, a number of isolated reports continued to appear, most emphasizing the risk factors associated with abnormal IR imaging. In *Cancer* in 1980, Gautherie and Gros [18] reported their experience with a group of 1245 women who had a mildly abnormal infrared image along with either normal or benign disease by conventional means, including physical exam, mammography, ultrasonography, and fine needle aspiration or biopsy. They noted that within 5 years, more than one-third of this group had histologically confirmed cancers. They concluded that IR imaging is useful not only as a predictor of breast cancer risk but also to identify the more rapidly growing neoplasms.

The following year, Amalric et al. [19], expanded on this concept by reporting that 10 to 15% of patients undergoing IR imaging will be found to be mildly abnormal when the remainder of the examination is essentially unremarkable. They noted that among these "false positive" cases, up to 38% will eventually develop breast cancer when followed closely. In 1981, Mariel [20] carried out a study in France on 655 patients and noted an 82% sensitivity. Two years later, Isard [21] discussed the unique characteristics and respective roles of IR imaging and ultrasonography and concluded that, when used in conjunction with mammography in a multi-imaging strategy, their potential advantages included enhanced diagnostic accuracy, reduction of unnecessary surgery, and improved prognostic ability. The author emphasized that neither of these techniques should be used as a sole screening modalitiy for breast cancer in asymptomatic women, but rather as a complementary modality to mammography.

In 1984, Nyirjesy [22] reported in *Obstetrics and Gynecology* a 76% sensitivity for IR imaging of 8767 patients. The same year, Bothmann [23] reported a sensitivity of 68% from a study carried out in Germany on 2702 patients. In 1986, Useki [24] published the results of a Japanese study indicating an 88% sensitivity.

Despite newly available IR technology, due in large part to military research and development, as well as compelling statistics of over 70,000 documented cases showing the contribution of functional IR imaging in a hitherto structurally based strategy to detect breast cancer, few North American centers have shown an interest, and fewer still have published their experience. This is surprising in view of the current consensus regarding the importance of vascular-related events associated with tumor initiation and growth that finally provide a plausible explanation for the IR findings associated with the early development of smaller tumors. The questionable results of the BCDDP and a few small-scale studies are still being referred to by a dwindling authorship that even mention the existence of this imaging modality. This has resulted in a generation of imagers that have neither knowledge of nor training in IR imaging. However, there are a few isolated centers that have continued to develop an expertise in this modality and have published their results.

In 1993, Head et al. [25] reported that improved images of the second generation of IR systems allowed more objective and quantitative visual analysis. They also reported that growth-rate-related prognostic indicators were strongly associated with the IR results [26]. In 1996, Gamagami [27] studied angiogenesis by IR imaging and reported that hypervascularity and hyperthermia could be shown in 86% of nonpalpable breast cancers. He also noted that in 15% of these cases, this technique helped to detect cancers that were not visible on mammography.

The concept of angiogenesis, suggested by Gamagami as an integral part of early breast cancer, was reiterated in 1996 by Guidi and Schnitt [28], whose observations suggested that angiogenesis is an early event in the development of breast cancer. They noted that it may occur before tumor cells acquire the ability to invade the surrounding stroma and even before there is morphologic evidence of an *in situ* carcinoma.

In contemporary publications, Anbar [29,30], using an elegant biochemical and immunological cascade, suggested that the empirical observation that small tumors capable of producing notable IR changes could be due to enhanced perfusion over a substantial area of breast surface via tumor-induced nitric oxide vasodilatation. He introduced the importance of dynamic area telethermometry to validate IR's full potential.

Parisky and his colleagues working out of six radiology centers [31] published an interesting report in Radiology in 2003 relating to the efficacy of computerized infrared imaging analysis of mammographically suspicious lesions. They reported a 97% sensitivity, a 14% specificity, and a 95% negative predictive value when IR was used to help determine the risk factors relating to mammographically noted abnormal lesions in 875 patients undergoing biopsy. They concluded that infrared imaging offers a safe, noninvasive procedure that would be valuable as an adjunct to mammography determining whether a lesion is benign or malignant.

26.2 The Ville Marie Multi-Disciplinary Breast Center Experience with High-Resolution Digital Infrared Imaging to Detect and Monitor Breast Cancer

26.2.1 Infrared Imaging as Part of a First-Line Multi-Imaging Strategy to Promote Early Detection of Breast Cancer

There is still a general consensus that the crucial strategy for the first-line detection of breast cancer depends essentially on clinical examination and mammography. Limitation of the former, with its reported sensitivity rate below 65% is well recognized [32], and even the proposed value of breast self-examination is now being contested [33]. With the current emphasis on earlier detection, there is an increasing reliance on better imaging. Mammography is still considered as our most reliable and cost-effective imaging modality [17]. However, variable inter-reader interpretation [34] and tissue density, now proposed as a risk factor itself [35] and seen in both younger patients and those on hormonal replacement [36], prompted us to reassess currently available IR technology spearheaded by military research and development, as a first-line component of a multi-imaging breast cancer detection strategy (Figure 26.1).

This modality is capable of quantifying minute temperature variations and qualifying abnormal vascular patterns, probably associated with regional angiogenesis, neovascularization (Figure 26.2), and nitric oxide-induced regional vasodilatation [29], frequently associated with tumor initiation and progression, and potentially an early predictor of tumor growth rate [26,28]. We evaluated a new fully integrated high-resolution computerized IR imaging station to complement mammography units. To validate its

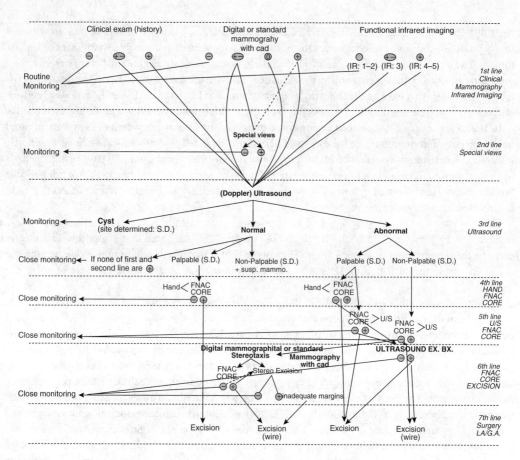

FIGURE 26.1 Ville Marie breast center: clinical and multi-imaging breast cancer detection strategy.

reported ability to help detect early tumor-related regional metabolic and vascular changes [27], we limited our initial review to a series of 100 successive cases of breast cancer who filled the following three criteria (a) minimal evaluation included a clinical exam, mammography, and IR imaging; (b) definitive surgical management constituted the preliminary therapeutic modality carried out at one of our affiliated institutions; and (c) the final staging consisted of either noninvasive cancer ($n = 4$), Stage I ($n = 42$), or Stage II ($n = 54$) invasive breast cancer.

While 94% of these patients were referred to our Multidisciplinary Breast Center for the first time, 65% from family physicians and 29% from specialists, the remaining 6% had their diagnosis of breast cancer at a follow-up visit. Age at diagnosis ranged from 31 to 84 years, with a mean age of 53. The mean histologic tumor size was 2.5 cm. Lymphatic, vascular, or neural invasion was noted in 18% of patients; and concomitant noninvasive cancer was present, along with the invasive component, in 64%. One-third of the 89 patients had axillary lymph node dissection, one-third had involved nodes, and 38% of the tumors were histologic Grade III.

While most of these patients underwent standard four-view mammography, with additional views when indicated, using a GE DMR apparatus at our center, in 17 cases we relied on recent and adequate quality outside films. Mammograms were interpreted by our examining physician and radiologist, both having access to the clinical findings. Lesions were considered suspicious if either of them noted findings indicative of carcinoma. The remainder were considered either contributory but equivocal or nonspecific. A nonspecific mammography required concordance with our examining physician, radiologist, and the authors.

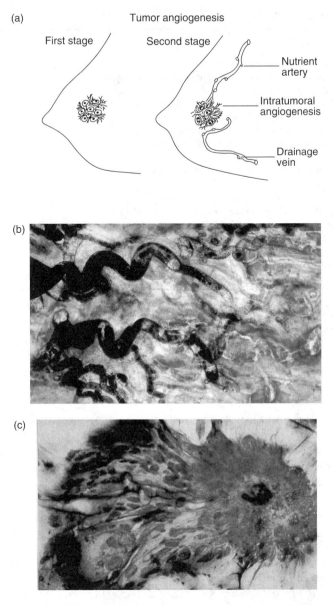

FIGURE 26.2 (See color insert following page **29**-16.) (a) Tumor angiogenesis. (b) High nuclear grade ductal carcinoma *in situ* with numerous blood vessels (angiogenesis) (Tabar). (c) Invasive ductal carcinoma with central necrosis and angiogenesis (Tabar).

Our integrated IR station at that time consisted of a scanning-mirror optical system containing a mercury–cadmium–telleride detector (Bales Scientific, CA) with a spatial resolution of 600 optical lines, a central processing unit providing multitasking capabilities, and a high-resolution color monitor capable of displaying 1024 × 768 resolution points and up to 110 colors or shades of gray per image. IR imaging took place in a draft-free thermally controlled room, maintained at between 18 and 20°C, after a 5 min equilibration period during which the patient sat disrobed with her hands locked over her head. We requested that the patients refrain from alcohol, coffee, smoking, exercise, deodorant, and lotions 3 h prior to testing.

Four images (an anterior, an under-surface, and two lateral views), were generated simultaneously on the video screen. The examining physician would digitally adjust them to minimize noise and enhance

TABLE 26.1   Ville Marie Infrared (IR) Grading Scale

Abnormal signs

1. Significant vascular asymmetry.[a]
2. Vascular anarchy consisting of unusual tortuous or serpiginous vessels that form clusters, loops, abnormal arborization, or aberrant patterns.
3. A 1°C focal increase in temperature (ΔT) when compared to the contralateral site and when associated with the area of clinical abnormality.[a]
4. A 2°C focal ΔT versus the contralateral site.[a]
5. A 3°C focal ΔT versus the rest of the ipsilateral breast when not present on the contralateral site.[a]
6. Global breast ΔT of 1.5°C versus the contralateral breast.[a]

Infrared scale

IR1 = Absence of any vascular pattern to mild vascular symmetry.
IR2 = Significant but symmetrical vascular pattern to moderate vascular asymmetry, particularly if stable.
IR3 = One abnormal sign.
IR4 = Two abnormal signs.
IR5 = Three abnormal signs.

[a] Unless stable on serial imaging or due to known non-cancer causes (e.g., abcess or receent benign surgery).
Infrared Imaging takes place in a draft free, thermally controlled room maintained between 18 and 20°C, after a 5 min equilibration period during which the patient is disrobed with her hands locked over her head. Patients are asked to refrain from alcohol, coffee, smoking, exercise, deodorant, and lotions 3 h prior to testing.

detection of more subtle abnormalities prior to exact on-screen computerized temperature reading and IR grading. Images were then electronically stored on retrievable laser discs. Our original Ville Marie grading scale relies on pertinent clinical information, comparing IR images of both breasts with previous images. An abnormal IR image required the presence of at least one abnormal sign (Table 26.1). To assess the false-positive rate, we reviewed, using similar criteria, our last 100 consecutive patients who underwent an open breast biopsy that produced a benign histology. We used the Carefile Data Analysis Program to evaluate the detection rate of variable combinations of clinical exam, mammography, and IR imaging.

Of this series, 61% presented with a suspicious palpable abnormality, while the remainder had either an equivocal (34%) or a nonspecific clinical exam (5%). Similarly, mammography was considered suspicious for cancer in 66%, while 19% were contributory but equivocal, and 15% were considered nonspecific. Infrared imaging revealed minor variations (IR-1 or IR-2) in 17% of our patients while the remaining 83% had at least one (34%), two (37%), or three (12%) abnormal IR signs. Of the 39 patients with either a nonspecific or equivocal clinical exam, 31 had at least one abnormal IR sign, with this modality providing pertinent indication of a potential abnormality in 14 of these patients who, in addition, had an equivocal or nonspecific mammography.

Among the 15 patients with a nonspecific mammography, there were 10 patients (mean age of 48; 5 years younger than the full sample) who had an abnormal IR image. This abnormal finding constituted a particularly important indicator in six of these patients who also had only equivocal clinical findings. While 61% of our series presented with a suspicious clinical exam, the additional information provided by the 66 suspicious mammographies resulted in an 83% detection rate. The combination of only suspicious mammograms and abnormal IR imaging increased the sensitivity to 93%, with a further increase to 98% when suspicious clinical exams were also considered (Figure 26.3).

The mean histologically measured tumor size for those cases undetected by mammography was 1.66 cm. while those undetected by IR imaging averaged 1.28 cm. In a concurrent series of 100 consecutive eligible patients who had an open biopsy that produced benign histology, 19% had an abnormal IR image while 30% had an abnormal pre-operative mammography that was the only indication for surgery in 16 cases.

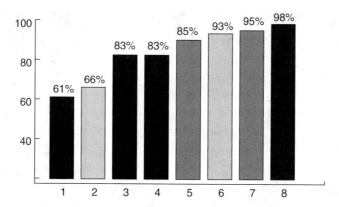

FIGURE 26.3 Relative contribution of clinical exam, mammography, and IR imaging to detect breast cancer in the Ville Marie Breast Center series. In this series, adding infrared imaging to both suspicious and equivocal mammographies increased the detection rate. (1) Suspicious clinical exam; (2) Suspicious mammography; (3) Suspicious clinical exam or suspicious mammography; (4) Abnormal infrared imaging; (5) Suspicious or equivocal mammography; (6) Abnormal infrared imaging or suspicious mammography; (7) Abnormal infrared imaging or equivocal or suspicious mammography; and (8) Abnormal infrared imaging or suspicious mammography or suspicious clinical exam.

The 83% sensitivity of IR imaging in this series is higher than the 70% rate for similar Stage I and II patients tested from the Royal Marsden Hospital two decades earlier [6]. Although our results might reflect an increased index of suspicion associated with a referred population, this factor should apply equally to both clinical exam and mammography, maintaining the validity of our evaluation. Additional factors could include our standard protocol, our physicians' prior experience with IR imaging, their involvement in both image production and interpretation, as well as their access to much improved image acquisition and precision (Figure 26.4).

While most previous IR cameras had 8-bit (one part in 256) resolution, current cameras are capable of one part in 4096 resolution, providing enough dynamic range to capture all images with 0.05°C discrimination without the need for range switching. With the advancement of video display and enhanced gray and colors, multiple high-resolution views can be compared simultaneously on the same monitor. Faster computers now allow processing functions such as image subtraction and digital filtering techniques for image enhancement. New algorithms provide soft tissue imaging by characterizing dynamic heat-flow patterns. These and other innovations have made vast improvements in the medical IR technology available today.

The detection rate in a series where half the tumors were under 2 cm, would suggest that tumor-induced thermal patterns detected by currently available IR technology are more dependent on early vascular and metabolic changes. These changes possibly are induced by regional nitric oxide diffusion and ferritin interaction, rather than strictly on tumor size [29]. This hypothesis agrees with the concept that angiogenesis may precede any morphological changes [28]. Although both initial clinical exam and mammography are crucial in signaling the need for further investigation, equivocal and nonspecific findings can still result in a combined delayed detection rate of 10% [17].

When eliminating the dubious contribution of our 34 equivocal clinical exams and 19 equivocal mammograms, which is disconcerting to both physician and patient, the alternative information provided by IR imaging increased the index of concern of the remaining suspicious mammograms by 27% and the combination of suspicious clinical exams or suspicious mammograms by 15% (Figure 26.3). An imaging-only strategy, consisting of both suspicious and equivocal mammography and abnormal IR imaging, also detected 95% of these tumors, even without the input of the clinical exam. Infrared imaging's most tangible contribution in this series was to signal an abnormality in a younger cohort of breast cancer patients who had noncontributory mammograms and also nonspecific clinical exams who conceivably would not have been passed on for second-line evaluation.

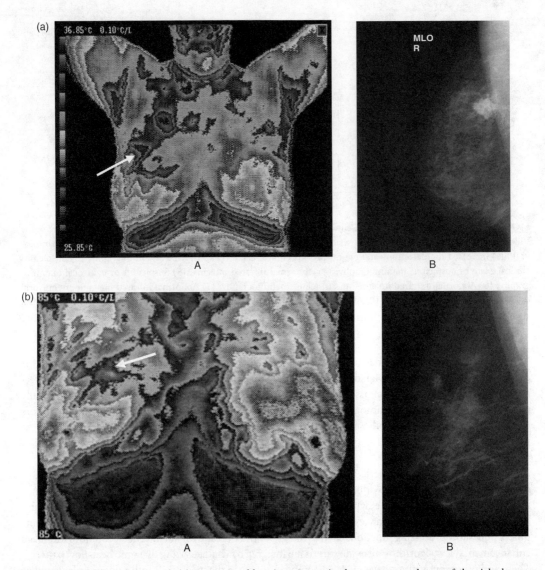

FIGURE 26.4 (See color insert.) (a) A 46-year old patient: Lump in the upper central area of the right breast. *Infrared imaging* (A): Significant vascular asymmetry (SVA) in the upper central area of the right breast (IR-3). *Mammography* (B): Corresponding speculated opacity. *Surgical histology:* 2 cm infiltrating ductal carcinoma with negative sentinel nodes. (b) A 44-year old patient. *Infrared imaging* (A): Revealed a significant vascular asymmetry in the upper central and inner quadrants of the right breast with a ΔT of 1.8°C (IR-4.8). *Corresponding mammography* (B): Reveals a spiculated lesion in the upper central portion of the right breast. *Surgical histology:* 0.7 cm infiltrating ductal carcinoma. Patient underwent adjuvant brachytherapy.

While 17% of these tumors were undetected by IR imaging, either due to insufficient production or detection of metabolic or vascular changes, the 19% false positive rate in histologically proven benign conditions, in part a reflection of our current grading system, suggests sufficient specificity for this modality to be used in an adjuvant setting.

Our validation of prior data would also suggest that IR imaging, based more on process than structural changes and requiring neither contact, compression, radiation, nor venous access, can provide pertinent and practical complementary information to both clinical exam and mammography, our current first-line detection modalities. Quality-controlled abnormal IR imaging heightened our index of suspicion

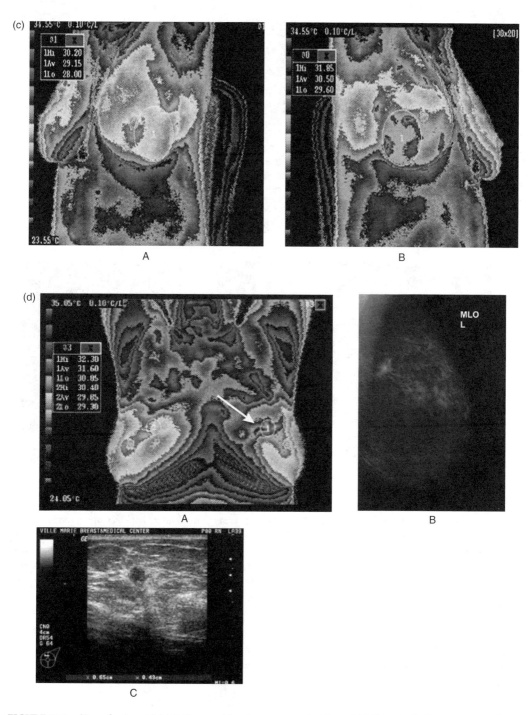

FIGURE 26.4 (See color insert.) (c) A 52-year old patient presented with a mild fullness in the lower outer quadrant of the right breast. *Infrared imaging* (A): Left breast (B): right breast reveals extensive significant vascular asymmetry with a ΔT of 1.35°C (IR-5.3). A 2 cm cancer was found in the lower outer area of the right breast. (d) A 37-year old patient. *Infrared image* (A): Significant vascular asymmetry in the upper inner quadrant of the left breast with a ΔT of 1.75°C (IR-4) (mod IR-4.75). *Mammography* (B): Corresponding spiculated lesion. *Ultrasound* (C): 6 mm lesion. *Surgical histology*: 0.7 cm infiltrating ductal carcinoma.

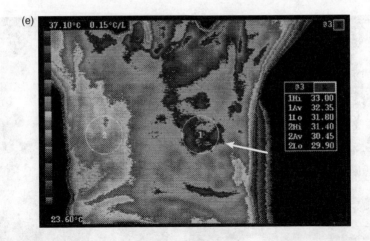

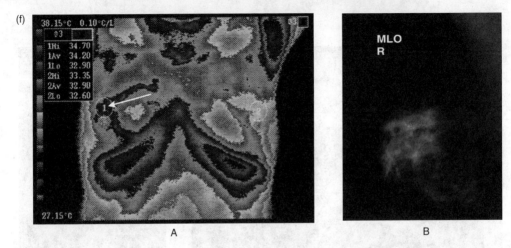

A   B

FIGURE 26.4 (See color insert.) (e) An 82-year old patient. *Infrared imaging anterior view:* Significant vascular asymmetry and a ΔT of 1.90°C (IR-4) in the left subareolar area. *Corresponding mammography:* (not included) asymmetrical density in the left areolar area. *Surgical histology:* Left subareolar 1 cm infiltrating ductal carcinoma.(f) A 34-year old patient with a palpable fullness in the supra-areolar area of the right breast. *Infrared imaging*(A): Extensive significant vascular asymmetry and a ΔT of 1.3°C in the right supra areolar area (IR-4) (mod IR-5.3). *Mammography* (B): Scattered and clustered central microcalcifications. *Surgical histology:* After total right mastectomy and TRAM flap: multifocal DCIS and infiltrating ductal CA centered over a 3 cm area of the supra areolar area.

in cases where clinical or mammographic findings were equivocal or nonspecific, thus signaling further investigation rather than observation or close monitoring (Figure 26.5) and to minimize possibility of further delay (Figure 26.6).

26.2.2 Preliminary Evaluation of Digital High-Resolution Functional Infrared Imaging to Monitor Pre-Operative Chemohormonotherapy-Induced Changes in Neo-Angiogenesis in Patients with Advanced Breast Cancer

Approximately 10% of our current breast cancer patients present with sufficient tumor load to be classified as having locally advanced breast cancer (LABC). This heterogeneous subset of patients, usually diagnosed

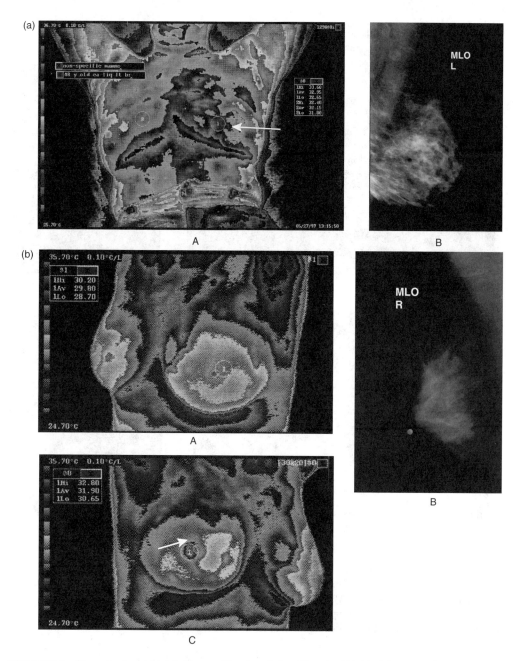

FIGURE 26.5 (See color insert.) (a) A 48-year old patient *Infrared imaging* (A): Significant vascular asymmetry and a ΔT of 0.8°C (IR-3) in the lower inner quadrant of the left breast. *Corresponding mammography* (B): A nonspecific density. *Surgical histology*: 1.6 cm left lower inner quadrant infiltrating ductal carcinoma. (b) A 40-year old patient. *Infrared imaging* (A): left breast (B) right breast: focal hot spot in the right subareolar area on a background of increased vascular activity with a ΔT of 1.1°C (IR-4). *Corresponding mammography* (C): Reveals dense tissue bilaterally. *Surgical histology*: reveals a 1 cm right infiltrating ductal carcinoma and positive lymph nodes.

with either stage T3 or T4 lesions without evidence of metastasis, and thus judged as potential surgical candidates, constitutes a formidable therapeutic challenge. Pre-operative or neo-adjuvant chemotherapy (PCT), hormonotherapy or both, preferably delivered within a clinical trial, is the current favored treatment strategy.

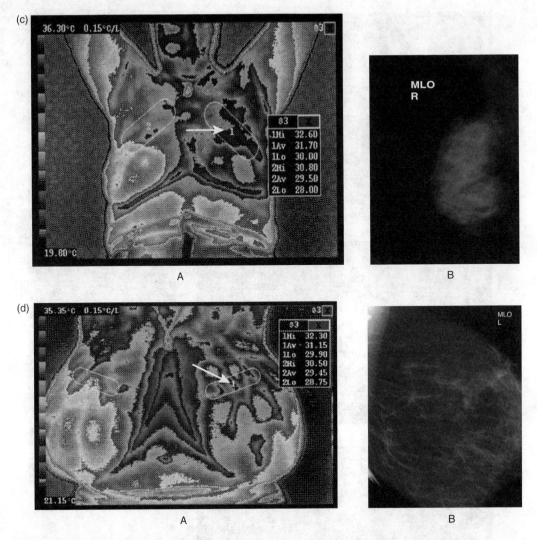

FIGURE 26.5   (See color insert.) (c) A 51-year old patient. *Infrared imaging* (A): Significant vascular asymmetry and a ΔT of 2.2°C (IR-5) in the upper central area of the left breast. *Corresponding mammography* (B): Mild scattered densities. *Surgical histology:* 2.5 cm infiltrating ductal carcinoma in the upper central area of the left breast. (d) A 44-year old patient. *Infrared imaging* (A): Significant vascular asymmetry and a ΔT of 1.58°C (IR-4) in the upper inner quadrant of the left breast. *Corresponding mammography* (B): A nonspecific corresponding density. *Surgical histology:* A 0.9 cm left upper inner quadrant infiltrating ductal carcinoma.

Pre-operative chemotherapy offers a number of advantages, including ensuring improved drug access to the primary tumor site by avoiding surgical scarring, the possibility of complete or partial tumor reduction that could down-size the extent of surgery and also the ability to better plan breast reconstruction when the initial tumor load suggests the need for a possible total mastectomy. In addition, there is sufficient data to suggest that the absence of any residual tumor cells in the surgical pathology specimen following PTC confers the best prognosis, while those patients achieving at least a partial clinical response as measured by at least a 50% reduction in the tumor's largest diameter often can aspire to a better survival than nonresponders [37]. While current clinical parameters do not always reflect actual PCT-induced tumor changes, there is sufficient correlation to make measuring the early clinical response to PTC an important element in assessing the efficacy of any chosen regimen. Unfortunately, the currently available conventional

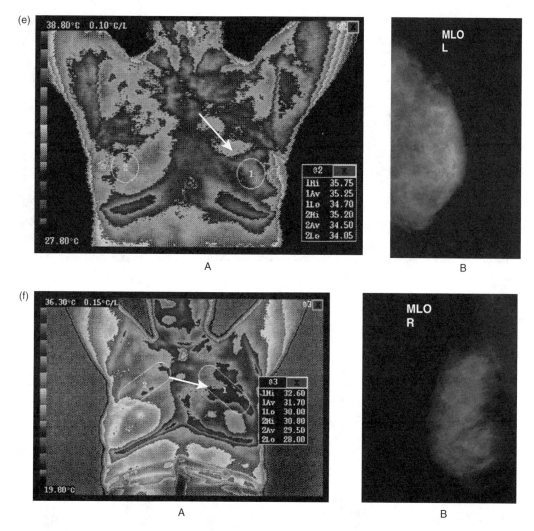

FIGURE 26.5 (See color insert.) (e) A 45-year old patient with a nodule in central area of left breast. *Infrared imaging* (A): Extensive significant vascular asymmetry (SVA) in the central inner area of the left breast with a ΔT of 0.75°C (IR-3) (mod IR-4.75). *Mammography* (B): Non-contributory. *Surgical histology:* 1.5 cm infiltrating ductal carcinoma with necrosis in the central inner area and 3 + axillary nodes. (f) A 51-year old patient. *Infrared imaging* (A): Extensive significant vascular asymmetry and a ΔT of 2.2° (IR-5) (mod IR-6.2) in the upper central area of the left breast. *Corresponding mammography* (B) scattered densities. *Surgical histology:* 2.5 cm infiltrating ductal carcinoma in the upper central area of the left breast.

monitoring tools, such as palpation combined with structural/anatomic imaging such as mammography and ultrasound have a limited ability to precisely measure the initial tumor load, and even less to reflect the effect of PCT [34].

These relatively rudimentary tools are dependent on often-imprecise anatomical and structural parameters. A more effective selection of often quite aggressive therapeutic agents and ideal duration of their use could be enhanced by the introduction of a convenient, safe, and accessible modality that could provide an alternative and serial measurement of their therapeutic efficacy.

There is thus currently a flurry of interest to assess the potential of different functional imaging modalities that could possibly monitor tumor changes looking at metabolic and vascular features to fill the void. Detecting early metabolic changes associated early tumor initiation and growth using positron emission

(g)

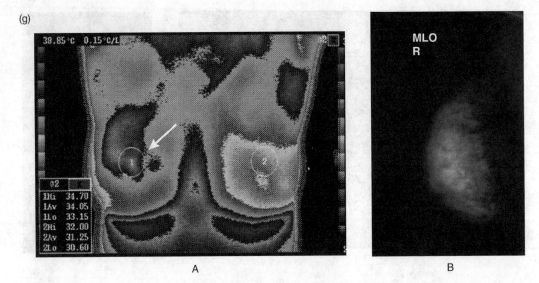

FIGURE 26.5 (See color insert.) (g) A 74-year old patient. *Infrared imaging* (A): significant vascular asymmetry in the upper central portion of the right breast with a ΔT of 2.8°C (IR-5) (Mod VM IR: 6.8). *Corresponding mammography* (B): Bilateral extensive density. *Surgical histology*: 1 cm right central quadrant infiltrating ductal carcinoma.

(a)

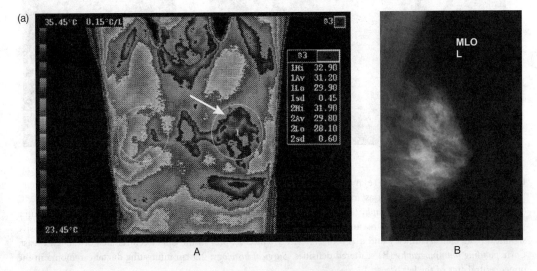

FIGURE 26.6 (See color insert.) (a) A 66-year old patient. Initially seen 2 years prior to diagnosis of left breast cancer for probable fibrocystic disorder (FCD) and scattered cysts, mostly on the left side. *Initial infrared imaging* (A): Extensive significant vascular asymmetry left breast and a near global ΔT of 1.4°C (IR-4) (Mod IR: 5.4). *Initial mammography* (B): Scattered opacities and ultrasound and cytologies were consistent with FCD. Two years later a 1.7 cm cancer was found in the central portion of the left breast.

tomography [38,39], MRI, and Sestamibi scanning are all potential candidates to help monitor PCT-related effects. Unfortunately, they are all hampered by limited access for serial use, duration of the exam, costs, and the need of intravenous access. High-resolution digital infrared imaging, on the other hand, a convenient functional imaging modality free of these inconveniences and requiring neither radiation, nuclear material, contact, nor compression, can be used repeatedly without safety issues. There is ample data indicating its ability to effectively and reliably detect, in a multi-imaging strategy, neoangiogenesis

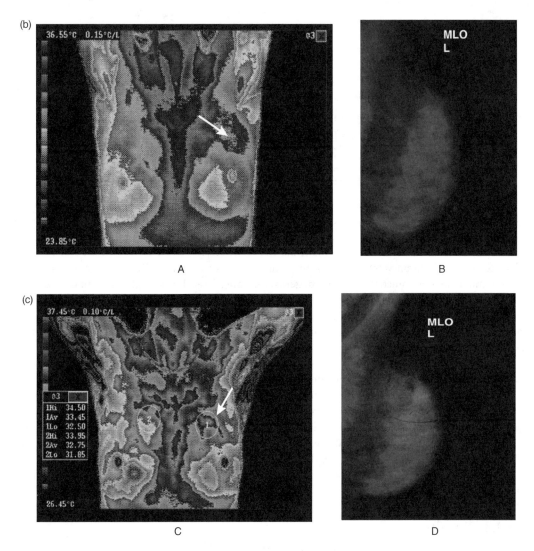

FIGURE 26.6 (See color insert.) (b) A 49-year old patient. *Infrared imaging* 1997 (A): Significant vascular asymmetry in the upper central aspect of the left breast (IR-3) *Corresponding mammography* 1997 (B): Dense tissue (contd. 6B2) (c) Patient presents 2 years later with a lump in the upper central portion of the left breast. *Corresponding infrared imaging* (C): Still reveals significant vascular asymmetry and a ΔT of 0.7°C (IR-3) (Mod VM IR″: 3.7). *Corresponding mammography* (D): Now reveals an opacity in the upper aspect of the left breast. *Surgical histology*: 1 cm infiltrating ductal carcinoma.

related to early tumor growth [40]. The premise of our review is that this same phenomenon should even be more obvious when using IR as a monitoring tool in patients with tumors associated with extensive vascular activity as seen in LABC.

To evaluate the ability of our high-resolution digital IR imaging station and a modified Ville Marie scoring system to monitor the functional impact of PCT, 20 successive patients with LABC underwent prospective IR imaging, both prior to and after completion of PCT, usually lasting between 3 and 6 months, which was then followed by curative-intent surgery [41]. Ages ranged between 32 and 82 with a mean of 55. Half of the patients were under 50. Patients presented with T2, T3, or inflammatory carcinoma were all free of any distant disease, thus remaining post-PCT surgical candidates. IR was done at the initial clinical evaluation and prior to core biopsy, often ultrasound guided to ensure optimal specimen harvesting,

TABLE 26.2   Modified Ville Marie Infrared Scoring Scale

IR-1	Absence of any vascular pattern to mild vascular symmetry
IR-2	Symmetrical vascular pattern to moderate vascular asymmetry, particularly if stable or due to known non-cancer causes (eg.: infection, abscess, recent or prior surgery or anatomical asymmetry). Local clinically related vascular assymetry
IR-3	Regional significant vascular asymmetry (SVA)
IR-4	Extensive SVA, involving at least 1/3 of the breast area

Add the temperature difference (ΔT) in degrees centigrade between the involved area and the corresponding area of the non-involved contralateral breast to calculate final IR score

which was used to document invasive carcinoma. Both sets of IR images were acquired according to our published protocol [38] using the same integrated infrared station described in our previous section.

We used a modification of the original Ville Marie IR scale (Table 26.2) where IR-1 reflects the absence of any significant vascular pattern to minimal vascular symmetry; IR-2 encompasses symmetrical to moderately asymmetrical vascular patterns, including focal clinically related significant vascular asymmetry; IR-3 implies a regional significant vascular asymmetry (SVA) while an extensive SVA, occupying more than a third of the involved breast, constitutes an IR-4. Mean temperature difference (ΔT) in degrees centigrade between the area of focal, regional or extensive SVA and the corresponding area of the noninvolved breast is then added, resulting in the final IR score.

Conventional clinical response to PCT was done by measuring the maximum tumor diameter in centimeters, both before beginning and after completion of PCT.

Induction PCT in 10 patients, 8 on a clinical trial (NSABP B-27 or B-57) consisted of 4 cycles of adriamycin (A) 60 mg/m^2 and cyclophosphamide (C) 600 mg/m^2, with or without additional taxotere (T) 100 mg/m^2, or 6 cycles of AT every 21 days. Eight other patients received AC with additional 5 FU (1000 mg/m^2) and methotrexate (300 mg/m^2). Tamoxifen, given to select patients along with the chemotherapy, was used as sole induction therapy in two elderly patients.

Values in both clinical size and IR scoring both before and after chemotherapy were compared using a paired t-test.

26.2.3   Results

All 20 patients in this series with LABC presented with an abnormal IR image (IR $\geq$ 3). The pre-induction PCT mean IR score was 5.5 (range: 4.4 to 6.9). Infrared imaging revealed a decrease in the IR score in all 20 patients following PCT, ranging from 1 to 5 with a mean of 3.1 ($p < .05$). This decrease following PCT reflected the change in the clinical maximum tumor dimension, which decreased from a mean of 5.2 cm prior to PCT to 2.2 cm ($p < .05$) following PCT in the two-thirds of our series who presented with a measurable tumor. Four of the complete pathological responders in this series saw their IR score revert to normal (<3) following PCT (Figure 26.7) while a fifth had a post-PCT IR score of 3.6. An additional seven patients had a final post-PCT IR score that reflected the final tumor size as measured at surgery (Figure 26.8).

Locally advanced breast cancer is considered an aggressive process that is typically associated with extensive neo-angiogenesis required to sustain rapid and continued tumor growth [27]. Functional IR imaging provided a vivid real-time visual reflection of this invasive process in all our patients. The dramatic IR findings associated with LABC, often occupying more than a third of the breast, are further emphasized by the comparative absence of any significant vascular findings in the uninvolved breast. These images thus provided a new parameter and baseline to complement the traditional structurally based imaging, particularly for the seven patients with clinically nonmeasurable LABC.

The significant reduction in the mean IR score following PCT is primarily an indication of its effect on neo-angiogenesis. While this reduction can sometimes correspond to tumor size, as it did in half of

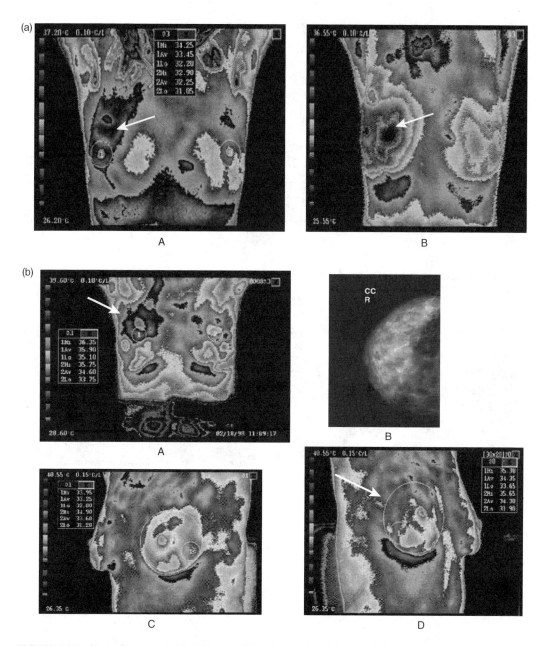

FIGURE 26.7 (See color insert.) (a) A 52-year old patient. *Infrared imaging* (A): Extensive vascular asymmetry (SVA) in the right breast with a ΔT of 1.2°C (IR-5.2). The patient was started on pre-operative chemotherapy (PCT). *Post-PCT infrared imaging* (B): Resolution of previously noted SVA (IR-2). *Surgical histology*: no residual carcinoma in the resected right breast specimen. (b) A 32-year old patient. *Infrared imaging* (A): Extensive significant vascular asymmetry and tortuous vascular pattern and a ΔT of 1.3°C (IR-5.3) in the right breast. *Corresponding mammography* (B): Scattered densities. Patient was started on pre-operative chemotherapy (PCT). *Post-PCT infrared image* (C — left breast; D — right breast): Notable resolution of SVA, with a whole breast ΔT of 0.7°C (IR-2). *Surgical histology*: No residual right carcinoma and chemotherapy induced changes.

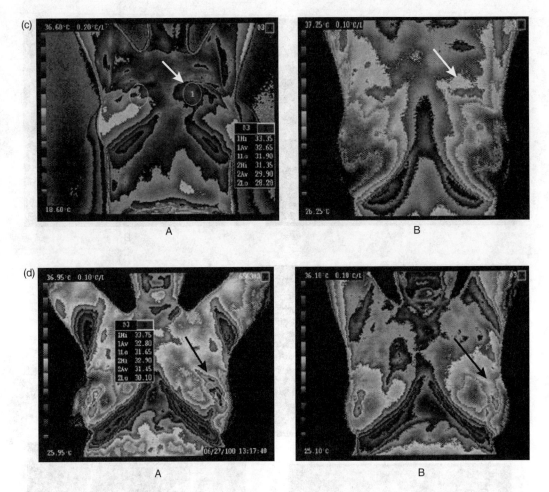

FIGURE 26.7 (See color insert.) (c) A 47-year old patient. *Infrared imaging* (A): Extensive significant vascular asymmetry in the inner half of the left breast with a ΔT of 2°C (IR-6.0). The patient was started on pre-operative chemotherapy (PCT). *Post-PCT infrared imaging* (B): no residual asymmetry (IR-1). *Surgical histology*: No viable residual carcinoma, with chemotherapy induced dense fibrosis surrounding nonviable tumor cells. (d) A 56-year old patient. *Pre-chemotherapy infrared imaging* (A): Significant vascular asymmetry overlying the central portion of the left breast with a ΔT of 1.35°C (IR-4.35). The patient was given pre-operative chemotherapy (PCT). *Post-PCT infrared* (C): mild bilateral vascular symmetry (IR-). *Surgical histology*: no residual tumor.

this series, IR's main contribution concerns functional parameters that can both precede and linger after structural tumor-induced changes occur. Because IR-detected regional angiogenesis responded slightly slower to PCT than did the anatomical parameters in nine patients underscores the fundamental difference between functional imaging such as IR and structural dependent parameters such as clinical tumor dimensions currently used to assess PCT response. IR has the advantage of not being dependent on a minimal tumor size but rather on the tumor's very early necessity to develop an extensive network to survive and proliferate. This would be the basis of IR's ability to sometimes detect tumor growth earlier than can structurally based modalities. The slight discrepancy between the resolving IR score and the anatomical findings in nine of our patients could suggest that this extensive vascular network, most evident in LABC, requires more time to dismantle in some patients. It could reflect the variable volume of angiogenesis, the inability of PCT to affect it, and thus possibly constitute a prognostic factor. This feature could also result from a deficiency in our proposed scoring scale.

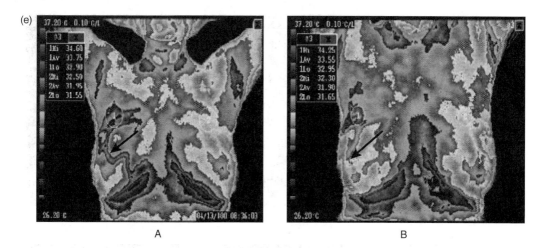

A   B

FIGURE 26.7 (See color insert.) (e) A 54-year old patient. *Infrared image* (A): extensive significant vascular asymmetry right breast with a rT of 2.8°C (IR-6.8). Received pre-operative chemotherapy (PCT). *Post-PCT infrared* (B): Mild local residual vascular asymmetry with a rT of 1.65°C (IR-3.65). *Surgical pathology*: No residual viable carcinoma.

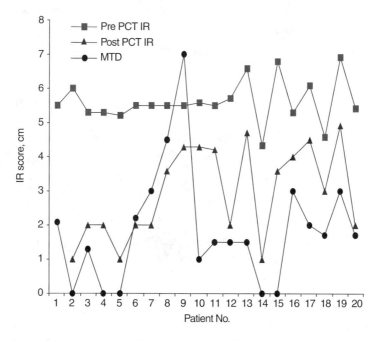

FIGURE 26.8 (See color insert.) Pre-PCT and Post-PCT IR Score and histological maximum tumor dimension (MTD).

Further study and follow-up are needed to better evaluate whether the sequential utilization of this practical imaging modality can provide additional pertinent information regarding the efficacy of our current and new therapeutic strategies, particularly in view of the increasing number with anti-angiogenesis properties, and whether lingering IR-reflected neo-angiogenesis following PCT ultimately reflects on prognosis.

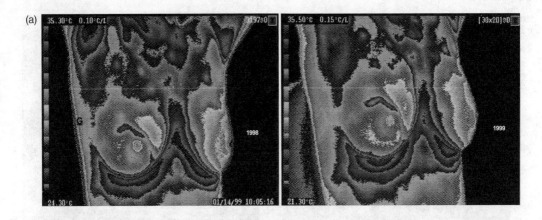

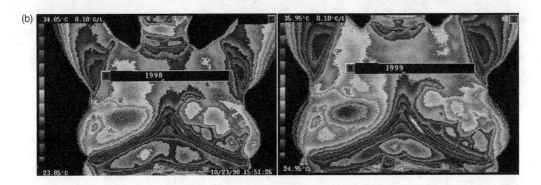

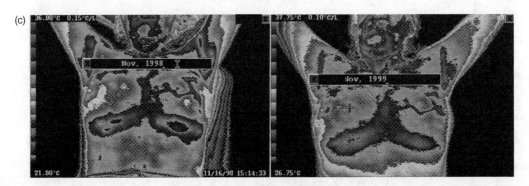

FIGURE 26.9 (See color insert.) (a) A stable vascular distribution in the lower inner quadrant of the left breast over a 12-month period. *Infrared imaging* of the breast usually remains remarkably stable in the absence of any on going developing significant pathology. It is important in grading these images to determine if the findings are to be considered evolving and important or stable and possibly relating to the patient's vascular anatomy. (b) An identical vascular distribution of the left breast over a 12-month period. (c) A stable vascular distribution in both breasts over a 12-month period.

26.3 Future Considerations Concerning Infrared Imaging

Mammography, our current standard first-line imaging modality only reflects an abnormality that could then prompt the alert clinician to intervene rather than to observe. This decision is crucial since it is at this first level that sensitivity and specificity are most vulnerable. There is a clear consensus that we have not yet developed the ideal breast cancer imaging technique and this is reflected in the flurry of

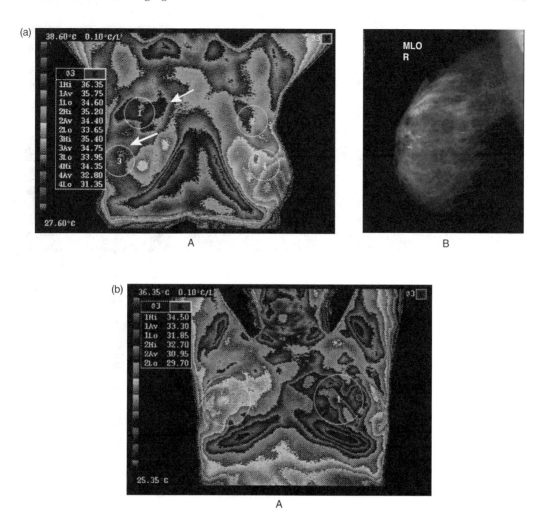

FIGURE 26.10 (See color insert.) (a) A 50-year old patient. *Infrared imaging* (A): Significant vascular asymmetry and a ΔT of 3.4°C (IR-5) in the right breast. *Corresponding mammography* (B): Increased density and microcalcific-ations in the right breast. Surgical histology: extensive right multifocal infiltrating ductal carcinoma requiring a total mastectomy. (b) A 50-year old patient. *Infrared imaging* (A): Significant vascular asymmetry with a near global ΔT of 2.35°C in the left breast (IR-5). *Mammography* (not available) diffuse density. *Surgical histology*: Left multi-focal infiltrating ductal carcinoma requiring a total mastectomy.

new modalities that have recently appeared. While progress in imaging and better training have resulted in the gradual decrease in the average size of breast tumors over the previous decade, the continued search for improved imaging must continue to further reduce the false negative rate and promote earlier detection.

Digital mammography is already recognized as a major imaging facilitator with the capability to do tomosynthesis and substraction, along with state of the art 3D and 4D ultrasound . However, there is now new emphasis on developing functional imaging that can exploit early vascular and metabolic changes associated with tumor initiation that often predate morphological changes that most of our current structural imaging modalities still depend on; thus, the enthusiasm in the development of sestamibi scanning, doppler ultrasound, and MRI of the breast [42,43]. Unfortunately, as promising as these modalities are, they are often too cumbersome, costly, inaccessible, or require intravenous access to be used as first-line detection modalities alongside clinical exam and mammography.

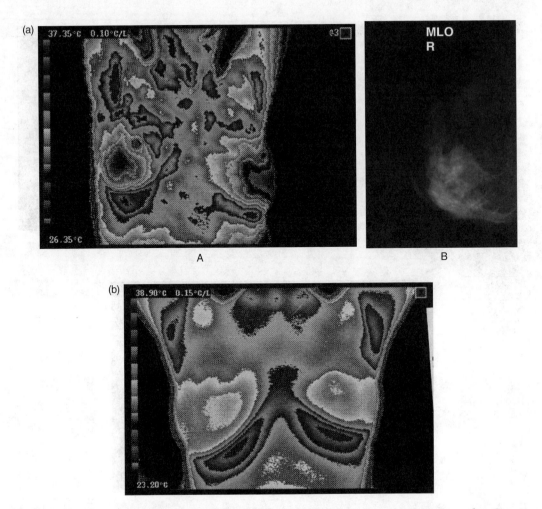

FIGURE 26.11 (See color insert.) (a) Four years post right partial mastectomy, the patient is recurrence free. Current *Infrared imaging* (A): shows no activity and *Mammography* (B): shows scar tissue. (b) *Infrared image*, 5 years following a left partial mastectomy and radiotherapy for carcinoma revealing slight asymmetry of volume, but no abnormal vascular abnormality and resolution of radiation-induced changes. The patient is disease free.

On the other hand, integrating IR imaging, a safe and practical modality into the first-line strategy, can increase the sensitivity at this crucial stage by also providing an early warning signal of an abnormality that in some cases is not evident in the other components. Combining IR imaging and mammography in an "IR-Assisted Mammography Strategy" is particularly appealing in the current era of increased emphasis on detection by imaging with less reliance on palpation as tumor size further decreases.

Intercenter standardization of a protocol concerning patient preparation, temperature controlled environment, digital image production, enhanced grading, and archiving, as well as data collection and sharing are all important factors that are beginning to be addressed. New technology could permit real-time image acquisition that could be submitted to computerized assisted image reading which will further enhance the physician's ability to detect subtle abnormalities.

Physician training is an essential quality control component for this imaging modality to contribute its full potential. A thorough knowledge of all aspects of benign and malignant breast pathology and concomitant access to prior IR imaging that should normally remain stable (Figure 26.9) are all contributory features. This modality needs to benefit from the same quality control previously applied to mammography and should not, at this time, be used as stand alone. It should benefit from the same interaction between clinical knowledge and other imaging tools as is the case in current breast cancer detection in the clinical environment. This is especially important since there are no current IR regulations, as it poses no health threat and does not use radiation, and could thus fall victim to untrained personnel who could misuse it on unsuspecting patients as was previously the case.

Its future promise, however, resides primarily in its ability to qualify and quantify vascular and metabolic changes related to early tumor genesis. The proposals that a higher temperature difference (ΔT) and increased vascular asymmetry are prognostic factors of tumor aggressivity need to be validated by further research (Figure 26.10). The same applies to the probability that the reduction of IR changes seen with pre-operative chemohormonotherapy reflect reduction in neo-angiogenesis and thus treatment efficacy. These remain, at the very least, extremely interesting and promising areas for future research, particularly

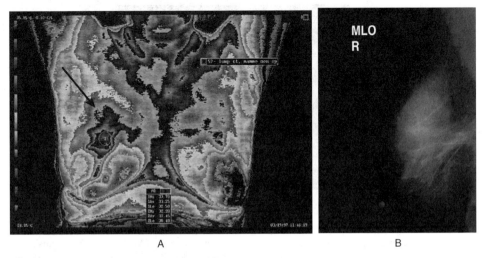

FIGURE 26.12 (See color insert.) A 52-year old patient, 5 years following right partial mastectomy, radiation, and chemotherapy for right breast cancer. Recent follow-up Infrared Imaging (A) now reveals significant vascular asymmetry (SVA) in the right breast with a ΔT of 1.5°C in the area of the previous surgery (IR-4). *Corresponding mammography* (B): Density and scar issue vs. possible recurrence. *Surgical histology:* 4 cm, recurrent right carcinoma in the area of the previous resection.

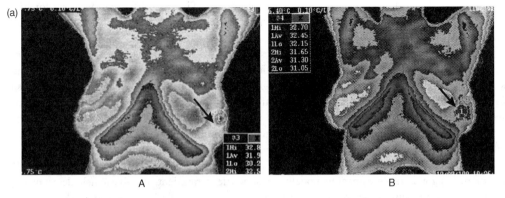

FIGURE 26.13 (See color insert.) (a) A 45-year old patient with small nodular process just inferior and medial to the left nipple areolar complex. *Infrared imaging* (A), without digital enhancement, was carried out and circles were placed on the nipple area rather than just below and medial to it. The nonenhanced IR image was thus initially misinterpreted as normal with a ΔT of 0.25°C. The same image was recalled and *repeated* (B), now with appropriate digital enhancement and once again, documented the presence of increased vascular activity just inferior and medial to the left nipple areolar complex with a ΔT of 1.15°C (IR-4.15). A 1.5 cm. cancer was found just below the left nipple.

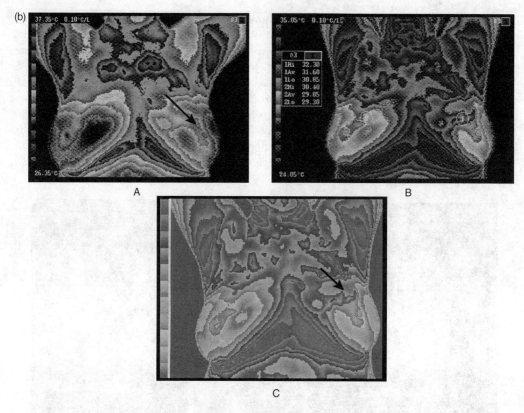

FIGURE 26.13 (Continued.) (See color insert.) (b) A 37-year old patient with lump in the upper inner quadrant of the left breast. Mammography confirms spiculated mass. *Infrared imaging* (A): Reported as "normal." Infrared imaging was repeated after appropriate *digital adjustment* (B): Now reveals obvious significant vascular asymmetry in the same area and a ΔT of 1.75°C (Ir-4) (mod IR-4.75). Using a different IR camera on the *same patient* (C) confirms same finding. *Surgical histology*: 1.5 cm infiltrating ductal CA.

in view of the current interest in new angiogenesis-related therapeutic strategies. Its contribution to monitoring post-operative patients (Figure 26.11) which is problematic with both mammography and ultrasound [44] and its ability to recognize recurrent cancer (Figure 26.12) are other areas for further clinical trials. Adequate physician training and strict attention to image acquisition are essential to avoid false negative interpretation (Figure 26.13).

As is the case for all current imaging modalities, the fact that this modality does not detect all tumors should not detract from its contribution as a functional adjuvant addition to our current first-line imaging strategy that is still based essentially on mammography alone, a structural modality that has reached its full potential. There is already sufficient data regarding IR's sensitivity and specificity that has been more recently validated and on going data collection will be important to justify its continued use in the ever evolving breast imaging field. Infrared imaging will soon replace current imaging modalities as an alternative, which would be both uninvasive and yet more informative first-line tool. In the meantime, to ignore its contribution to the very complex process of promoting earlier breast cancer detection could be questioned. A good first-line imaging modality must be safe, convenient, and able to help detect primarily the more aggressive tumors where early intervention can have a greater impact on survival.

References

[1] Lloyd-Williams K. and Handley R.S. Infra-red thermometry in the diagnosis of breast disease. *Lancet* 2, 1371–1381, 1961.

[2] Handley R.S. The temperature of breast tumors as a possible guide to prognosis. *Acta Unio. Int. Contra. Cancrum.* 18, 822, 1962.

[3] Lawson R.N. and Chughtai M.S. Breast cancer and body temperatures. *Can. Med. Assoc. J.* 88, 68–70, 1963.

[4] Gershen-Cohen J., Haberman J., and Brueschke E.E. Medical thermography: a summary of current status. *Radiol. Clin. North. Am.* 3, 403–431, 1965.

[5] Haberman J. The present status of mammary thermography. *Ca — Can. J. Clin.* 18, 314–321, 1968.

[6] Jones C.H. Thermography of the female breast. In Parsons C.A. (ed.), *Diagnosis of Breast Disease*, University Park Press, Baltimore, pp. 214–234, 1983.

[7] Isard H.J., Becker W., Shilo R. et al. Breast thermography after four years and 10,000 studies. *Am. J. Roentgenol.* 115, 811–821, 1972.

[8] Dodd G.D. Thermography in breast cancer diagnosis. In *Proceedings of the 7th National Cancer Conference*. Los Angeles, CA, September 27–29, Lippincott, Philadelphia, Toronto, p. 267, 1972.

[9] Feig S.A., Shaber G.S., Schwartz G.F. et al. Thermography, mammography, and clinical examination in breast cancer screening. *Radiology* 122, 123–127, 1977.

[10] Wallace J.D. Thermographic examination of the breast: an assessment of its present capabilities. In Gallagher H.S. (ed.), *Early Breast Cancer: Detection and Treatment*. American College of Radiology, Wiley, New York, pp. 13–19, 1975.

[11] Report of the working group to review the national cancer institute breast cancer detection demonstration projects. *J. Natl Cancer Inst.* 62, 641–709, 1979.

[12] Haberman J. An overview of breast thermography in the United States. In Margaret Abernathy and Sumio Uematsu (eds), *Medical Thermography*. American Academy of Thermology, Washington, pp. 218–223, 1986.

[13] Moskowitz M., Milbrath J., Gartside P. et al. Lack of efficacy of thermography as a screening tool for minimal and stage I breast cancer. *N. Engl. J. Med.* 295, 249–252, 1976.

[14] Threatt B., Norbeck J.M., Ullman N.S. et al. Thermography and breast cancer: an analysis of a blind reading. *Ann. N.Y. Acad. Sci.* 335, 501–519, 1980.

[15] Stark A. The use of thermovision in the detection of early breast cancer. *Cancer* 33, 1664–1670, 1964.

[16] Sterns E. and Cardis C. Thermography in breast diagnosis. *Cancer* 50, 323–325, 1982.

[17] Moskowitz M. Breast imaging. In Donegan W.L. and Spratt J.S. (eds), *Cancer of the Breast*. Saunders, New York, pp. 206–239, 1995.

[18] Gautherie M. and Gros C.M. Breast thermography and cancer risk prediction. *Cancer* 45, 51–56, 1980.

[19] Amalric R., Gautherie M., Hobbins W.B. et al. Avenir des femmes à thermogramme infra-rouge mammaire anormal isolé. *La. Nouvelle. Presse Médicale.* 38, 3153–3155, 1981.

[20] Mariel L., Sarrazin D., Daban A. et al. The value of mammary thermography. A report on 655 cases. *Sem. Hop.* 57, 699–701, 1981.

[21] Isard H.J. Other imaging techniques. *Cancer* 53, 658–664, 1984.

[22] Nyirjesy I. and Billingsley F.S. Detection of breast carcinoma in a gynecological practice. *Obstet. Gynecol.* 64, 747–751, 1984.

[23] Bothmann G.A. and Kubli F. Plate thermography in the assessment of changes in the female breast. 2. Clinical and thermographic results. *Fortschr. Med.* 102, 390–393, 1984.

[24] Useki H. Evaluation of the thermographic diagnosis of breast disease: relation of thermographic findings and pathologic findings of cancer growth. *Nippon. Gan. Chiryo. Gakkai. Shi.* 23, 2687–2695, 1988.

[25] Head J.F., Wang F., and Elliott R.L. Breast thermography is a noninvasive prognostic procedure that predicts tumor growth rate in breast cancer patients. *Ann. N.Y. Acad. Sci.* 698, 153–158, 1993.

[26] Head J.F. and Elliott R.L. Breast thermography. *Cancer* 79, 186–188, 1995.

[27] Gamagami P. Indirect signs of breast cancer: angiogreneis study. In *Atlas of Mammography*. Blackwell Science, Cambridge, MA, pp. 231–226, 1996.

[28] Guidi A.J. and Schnitt S.J. Angiogenesis in preinvasive lesions of the breast. *Breast J.* 2, 364–369, 1996.

[29] Anbar M. Hyperthermia of the cancerous breast: analysis of mechanism. *Cancer Lett.* 84, 23–29, 1994.

[30] Anbar M. Breast cancer. In *Quantitative Dynamic Telethermometry in Medical Diagnosis and Management*. CRC Press, Ann Arbor, MI, pp. 84–94, 1994.

[31] Parisky H.R., Sard A. et al. Efficacy of computerized infrared imagng analysis to evaluate mammographically suspicious lesions. *Am. J. Radiol.* 180, 263–272, 2003.

[32] Sickles E.A. Mammographic features of "early" breast cancer. *Am. J. Roentgenol.* 143, 461, 1984.

[33] Thomas D.B., Gao D.L., Self S.G. et al. Randomized trial of breast self-examination in Shanghai: methodology and preliminary results. *J. Natl Cancer Inst.* 5, 355–365, 1997.

[34] Elmore J.G., Wells C.F., Carol M.P.H. et al. Variability in radiologists interpretation of mammograms. *N. Engl. J. Med.* 331, 99–104, 1993.

[35] Boyd N.F., Byng J.W., Jong R.A. et al. Quantitative classification of mammographic densities and breast cancer risk. *J. Natl Cancer Inst.* 87, 670–675, 1995.

[36] Laya M.B. Effect on estrogen replacement therapy on the specificity and sensibility of screening mammography. *J. Natl Cancer Inst.* 88, 643–649, 1996.

[37] Singletary S.E., McNeese M.D., and Hortobagyi G.N. Feasibility of breast-conservation surgery after induction chemotherapy for locally advanced breast carcinoma. *Cancer* 69, 2849–2852, 1992.

[38] Jansson T., Westlin J.E., Ahlstrom H. et al. Position emission tomography studies in patients with locally advanced and/or metastatic breast cancer: a method for early therapy evaluation? *J. Clin. Oncol.* 13, 1470–1477, 1995.

[39] Hendry J. Combined positron emission tomography and computerized tomography. Whole body imaging superior to MRI in most tumor staging. *JAMA* 290, 3199–3206, 2003.

[40] Keyserlingk J.R., Ahlgren P.D., Yu E., and Belliveau N. Infrared imaging of the breast: initial reappraisal using high-resolution digital technology in 100 successive cases of stage I and II breast cancer. *Breast J.* 4, 245–251, 1998.

[41] Keyserlingk J.R., Yassa, M., Ahlgren, P., and Belliveau N. Tozzi. Ville Marie Oncology Center and St. Mary's Hospital, Montreal, Canada D. *Preliminary Evaluation of Digital Functional Infrared Imaging to Reflect Preoperative Chemohormonotherapy-Induced Changes in Neoangiogenesis in Patients with Locally Advanced Breast Cancer*. European Oncology Society, Milan, Italy, September 2001.

[42] Berg et al. Tumor type and breast profile determine value of mammography, ultrasound and MR. *Radiology* 233, 830–849, 2004.

[43] Oestreicher et al. Breast exam and mammography. *Am. J. Radiol.* 151, 87–96, 2004.

[44] Mendelson, Berg et al. Ultrasound in the operated breast; presented at the *2004 RSNA*. Chicago, November 2005.

27

Detecting Breast Cancer from Thermal Infrared Images by Asymmetry Analysis

Hairong Qi
The University of Tennessee

Phani Teja Kuruganti
Oak Ridge National Laboratory

Wesley E. Snyder
North Carolina State University

27.1 Introduction... 27-1
    Measuring the Temperature of Human Body • Metabolic
    Activity of Human Body and Cancer Cells • Early Detection
    of Breast Cancer
27.2 Asymmetric Analysis in Breast Cancer Detection 27-4
    Automatic Segmentation • Asymmetry Identification by
    Unsupervised Learning • Asymmetry Identification Using
    Supervised Learning Based on Feature Extraction
27.3 Conclusions 27-12
References 27-13

One of the popular methods for breast cancer detection is to make comparisons between contralateral images. When the images are relatively symmetrical, small asymmetries may indicate a suspicious region. In thermal infrared (IR) imaging, asymmetry analysis normally needs human intervention because of the difficulties in automatic segmentation. In order to provide a more objective diagnostic result, we describe an automatic approach to asymmetry analysis in thermograms. It includes automatic segmentation and supervised pattern classification. Experiments have been conducted based on images provided by Elliott Mastology Center (Inframetrics 600M camera) and Bioyear, Inc. (Microbolometer uncooled camera).

27.1 Introduction

The application of IR imaging in breast cancer study starts as early as 1961 when Williams and Handley first published their results in the *Lancet* [1]. However, the premature use of the technology and its poorly controlled introduction into breast cancer detection in the 1970s have led to its early demise [2]. IR-based diagnosis was criticized as generating a higher false-positive rate than mammography, and thus was not recommended as a standard modality for breast cancer detection. Therefore, despite its deployment in many areas of industry and military, IR usage in medicine has declined [3]. Three decades later, several papers and studies have been published to reappraise the use of IR in medicine [2,3] for the following three reasons (1) We have greatly improved IR technology. New generations of IR cameras have been developed with much enhanced accuracy; (2) We have much better capabilities in image processing. Advanced techniques including image enhancement, restoration, and segmentation have been effectively used in processing IR images; and (3) We have a deeper understanding of the patho-physiology of heat generation.

The main objective of this work is to evaluate the viability of IR imaging as a noninvasive imaging modality for early detection of breast cancer so that it can be performed both on the symptomatic and the asymptomatic patient and can thus be used as a complement to traditional mammography. This report summarizes how the identification of the asymmetry can be automated using image segmentation, feature extraction, and pattern recognition techniques. We investigate different features that contribute the most toward the detection of asymmetry. This kind of approach helps reduce the false-positive rate of the diagnosis and increase chances of disease cure and survival.

27.1.1   Measuring the Temperature of Human Body

Temperature is a long established indicator of health. The Greek physician, Hippocrates, wrote in 400 B.C. "In whatever part of the body excess of heat or cold is felt, the disease is there to be discovered" [4]. The ancient Greeks immersed the body in wet mud and the area that dried more quickly, indicating a warmer region, was considered the diseased tissue. The use of hands to measure the heat emanating from the body remained well into the 16th and the 17th centuries. It wasn't until Galileo, who made a thermoscope from a glass tube, that some form of temperature sensing device was developed, but it did not have a scale. It is Fahrenheit and later Celsius who have fixed the temperature scale and proposed the present day clinical thermometer. The use of liquid crystals is another method of displaying skin temperature. Cholesteric esters can have the property of changing colors with temperature and this was established by Lehmann in 1877. It was involved in use of elaborative panels that encapsulated the crystals and were applied to the surface of the skin, but due to large area of contact, they affected the temperature of the skin. All the methods discussed above are contact based.

Major advances over the past 30 years have been with IR thermal imaging. The astronomer, Sir William Herschel, in Bath, England discovered the existence of IR radiation by trying to measure the heat of the separate colors of the rainbow spectrum cast on a table in the darkened room. He found that the highest temperature was found beyond the red end of the spectrum. He reported this to the Royal society as Dark Heat in 1800, which eventually has been turned the IR portion of the spectrum. IR radiation occupies the region between visible and microwaves. All objects in the universe emit radiations in the IR region of the spectra as a function of their temperature. As an object gets hotter, it gives off more intense IR radiation, and it radiates at a shorter wavelength [3]. At moderate temperatures (above 200°F), the intensity of the radiation gets high enough that the human body can detect that radiation as heat. At sufficiently high temperatures (above 1200°F), the intensity gets high enough and the wavelength gets short enough that the radiation crosses over the threshold to the red end of the visible light spectrum. The human eye cannot detect IR rays, but they can be detected by using the thermal IR cameras and detectors.

27.1.2   Metabolic Activity of Human Body and Cancer Cells

Metabolic process in a cell can be briefly defined as the sum total of all the enzymatic reactions occurring in the cell. It can be further elaborated as a highly coordinated, purposeful activity in which many sets of interrelated multienzyme systems participate, exchanging both matter and energy between the cell and its environment. Metabolism has four specific functions (1) To obtain chemical energy from the fuel molecules; (2) To convert exogenous nutrients into the building blocks or precursor of macromolecular cell components; (3) To assemble such building blocks into proteins, nucleic acids, lipids, and other cell components; and (4) To form and degrade biomolecules required in specialized functions of the cell.

Metabolism can be divided into two major phases, Catabolism and Anabolism. Catabolism is the degradative phase of metabolism in which relatively large and complex nutrient molecules (carbohydrates, lipids, and proteins) are degraded to yield smaller, simpler molecules such as lactic acid, acetic acid, CO_2, ammonia, or urea. Catabolism is accompanied by conservation of some of the energy of the nutrient in the form of phosphate bond energy of adenosine triphosphate (ATP). Conversely, anabolism is the building up phase of metabolism, the enzymatic biosynthesis of such molecular components of cells as the nucleic acids, proteins, lipids, and carbohydrates from their simple building block precursors. Biosynthesis of organic molecules from simple precursors requires input of chemical energy, which is furnished by ATP generated during catabolism. Each of these pathways is promoted by a sequence of specific enzymes catalyzing consecutive reactions. The energy produced by the metabolic pathways is utilized by the cell for its division. Cells undergo mitotic cell division, a process in which a single cell divides into many cells and forms tissues, leading further into the development and growth of the multicellular organs. When cells divide, each resultant part is a complete relatively small cell. Immediately after division the newly formed cells grow rapidly soon reaching the size of the original cell. In humans, growth occurs through mitotic cell division with subsequent enlargement and differentiation of the reproduced cells into organs. Cancer cells also grow similarly but lose the ability to differentiate into organs. So, a cancer may be defined as an actively dividing undifferentiated mass of cells called the "tumor."

Cancer cells result from permanent genetic change in a normal cell triggered by some external physical agents such as chemical agents, x-rays, UV rays, etc. They tend to grow aggressively and do not obey normal pattern of tissue formation. Cancer cells have a distinctive type of metabolism. Although they possess all the enzymes required for most of the central pathways of metabolism, cancer cells of nearly all types show an anomaly in the glucose degradation pathway (viz. Glycolysis). The rate of oxygen consumption is somewhat below the values given by normal cells. However the malignant cells tend to utilize anywhere from 5 to 10 times as much glucose as normal tissue and convert most of it into lactate instead of pyruvate (lactate is a low energy compound whereas pyruvate is a high energy compound). The net effect is that in addition to the generation of ATP in mitochondria from respiration, there is a very large formation of ATP in extramitochondrial compartment from glycolysis. The most important effect of this metabolic imbalance in cancer cells is the utilization of a large amount of blood glucose and release of large amounts of lactate into blood. The lactate so formed is recycled in the liver to produce blood glucose again. Since the formation of blood glucose by the liver requires 6 molecules of ATP whereas breakdown of glucose to lactate produces only 2 ATP molecules, the cancer cells are looked upon as metabolic parasites dependent on the liver for a substantial part of their energy. Large masses of cancer cells thus can be a considerable metabolic drain on the host organism. In addition to this, the high metabolic rate of cancer cells causes an increase in local temperature as compared to normal cells. Local metabolic activity ceases when blood supply is stopped since glycolysis is an oxygen dependent pathway and oxygen is transported to the tissues by the hemoglobin present in the blood; thus, blood supply to these cells is important for them to proliferate. The growth of a solid tumor is limited by the blood supply. If it were not invaded by capillaries a tumor would be dependent on the diffusion of nutrients from its surroundings and could not enlarge beyond a diameter of a few millimeters. Thus, in order to grow further the tumor cells stimulate the blood vessels to form a capillary network that invades the tumor mass. This phenomenon is popularly called "angiogenesis," which is a process of vascularization of a tissue involving the development of new capillary blood vessels.

Vascularization is a growth of blood vessels into a tissue with the result that the oxygen and nutrient supply is improved. Vascularization of tumors is usually a prelude to more rapid growth and often to metastasis (advanced stage of cancer). Vascularization seems to be triggered by angiogenesis factors that stimulate endothelial cell proliferation and migration. In the context of this paper the high metabolic rate in the cancer cells and the high density of packaging makes them a key source of heat concentration (since the heat dissipation is low) thus enabling thermal IR imaging as a viable technique to visualize the abnormality.

27.1.3 Early Detection of Breast Cancer

There is a crucial need for early breast cancer detection. Research has shown that if detected earlier (tumor size less than 10 mm), the breast cancer patient has an 85% chance of cure as opposed to 10% if the cancer is detected late [5].

Different kinds of diagnostic imaging techniques exist in the field of breast cancer detection. The most popularly used method presently is x-ray mammography. The drawback of this technique is that it is invasive and experts believe that electromagnetic radiation can also be a triggering factor for cancerous growth. Because of this, periodic inspection might have a negative effect on the patient's health. Research shows that the mammogram sensitivity is higher for older women (age group 60 to 69 years) at 85% compared with younger women (<50 years) at 64% [5]. A new study in a British medical journal (The LANCET [6]) has asserted that there is no reliable evidence that screening with mammography for breast cancer reduces mortality. They show that screening actually leads to more aggressive treatment, increasing the number of mastectomies by about 20%, and the number of mastectomies and tumorectomies by about 30%.

In contrast to this IR imaging uses a noninvasive imaging technique as the diagnostic tool. The main source of IR rays is heat emitted from different bodies whose temperature is above absolute zero. Thus a thermogram of a patient provides the heat distribution in the body. The cancerous cells, due to high metabolic rates and angiogenesis, are at a higher temperature than the normal cells around it. Thus the cancer cells can be imaged as hotspots in the IR images. The thermogram provides more dynamic information of the tumor since the tumor can be small in size but can be fast growing making it appear as a high temperature spot in the thermogram [7,8]. However, this is not the case in mammography, in which unless the tumor is beyond certain size, it cannot be imaged as x-rays essentially pass through it unaffected. This qualifies IR imaging as an effective diagnostic tool for early detection of breast cancer. Keyserlingk et al. [2] reported that the average tumor size undetected by thermal imaging is 1.28 cm and 1.66 cm by mammography. It is also reported that thermography can provide results that can be correct even 8 to 10 years before mammography can detect a mass in the patient's body [9,10].

27.2 Asymmetric Analysis in Breast Cancer Detection

Radiologists routinely make comparisons between contralateral images. When the images are relatively symmetrical, small asymmetries may indicate a suspicious region. This is the underlying philosophy in the use of asymmetry analysis for mass detection in breast cancer study [11]. Unfortunately, due to various reasons like fatigue, carelessness, or simply because of the limitation of human visual system, these small asymmetries might not be easy to detect. Therefore, it is important to design an automatic approach to eliminate human factors.

There have been a few papers addressing techniques for asymmetry analysis of mammograms [11–16]. Head et al. [17,18] recently analyzed the asymmetric abnormalities in infrared images. In their approach, the thermograms are segmented first by an operator. Then breast quadrants are derived automatically based on unique point of reference, that is, the chin, the lowest, rightmost, and leftmost points of the breast.

This chapter describes an automatic approach to asymmetry analysis in thermograms. It includes automatic segmentation and pattern classification. Hough transform is used to extract the four feature curves that can uniquely segment the left and right breasts. The feature curves include the left and the right body boundary curves, and the two parabolic curves indicating the lower boundaries of the breasts. Upon segmentation, different pattern recognition techniques are applied to identify the asymmetry.

Both segmentation and classification results are shown on images provided by Elliott Mastology Center (Inframetrics 600M camera) and Bioyear, Inc. (Microbolometer uncooled camera).

27.2.1 Automatic Segmentation

There are several ways to perform segmentation, including *threshold-based* techniques, *edge-based* techniques, and *region-based* techniques. Threshold-based techniques assign pixels above (or below) a specified threshold to be in the same region. Edge-based techniques assume that the boundary formed by adjacent regions (or segments) has high edge strength. Through edge detection, we can identify the boundary that surrounds a region. Region-based methods start with elemental regions and split or merge them [19].

27.2.1.1 Edge Image Generation

In this research work, we choose to use the edge-based segmentation technique as we have identified four dominant curves in the edge image, which we call "feature curves," including the left and right body boundaries, and the two lower boundaries of the breasts (Figure 27.3) or the two shadow boundaries that are below the breasts (Figure 27.2) whichever is stronger.

Edges are areas in the image where the brightness changes suddenly. One way to find edges is to calculate the amplitude of the first derivative (Equation 27.1) that generates the so-called gradient magnitude image where $\partial f / \partial x$ is the derivative of the image f along the x direction, and $\partial f / \partial y$ is the derivative along the y direction (the x and y directions are orthogonal to each other) and to threshold the amplitude image.

$$\text{Gradient magnitude} = \sqrt{\left(\frac{\partial f}{\partial x}\right)^2 + \left(\frac{\partial f}{\partial y}\right)^2} \tag{27.1}$$

Another way is to calculate the second derivative and to locate the zero-crossing points, as the second derivative at edge pixels would appear as a point where the derivatives of its left and right pixels change signs.

Although effective, both derivative images are very sensitive to noise. In order to eliminate or reduce the effect of noise, a Gaussian smoothing low-pass filter is applied before taking the derivatives. The smoothing process, on the other hand, also results in thicker edges. The Canny edge detector [20] solves this problem by taking two extra steps, the *nonmaximum suppression* (NMS) step and the *hysteresis thresholding* step, in order to locate the true edge pixels (only one pixel wide along the gradient direction).

For each edge pixel in the gradient magnitude image, the NMS step looks one pixel in the direction of the gradient, and another pixel in the reverse direction. If the magnitude of the current pixel is not the maximum of the three, then this pixel is not a true edge pixel. NMS helps locate the true edge pixels properly. However, the new edges still suffer from extra edge points problem due to noise and missing edge points.

The hysteresis thresholding improves the quality of edge image by using a dual-threshold approach, in which two thresholds, τ_1 and τ_2 (τ_2 is significantly larger than τ_1), are applied on the NMS-processed edge image to produce two binary edge images, denoted as T_1 and T_2, respectively. Since T_1 was created using a lower threshold, it will contain more extra edge pixels than T_2. Edge pixels in T_2 are therefore considered to be parts of true edges. When some discontinuities in edges occur in the T_2 image, the pixels at the same location of the T_1 image is looked up that could be continuations of the edge. If such pixels are found, they are included in the true edge image. This process continues until the continuation of pixels in T_1 connects with an edge pixel in T_2 or no connected T_1 points are found. (See Figure 27.2 and Figure 27.3 for examples of the edge image derived from Canny edge detector.)

27.2.1.2 Hough Transform for Edge Linking

From Figure 27.2 and Figure 27.3, we find that the edge images still cannot be used directly for segmentation as the edge detector picks up all the intensity changes, which would complicate the segmentation. On the other hand, many edges show gaps among edge pixels that would result in segments that are not closed. We have identified four feature boundaries that could enclose the breast. The body boundaries are easy to detect. Difficulties lie in the detection of the lower boundaries of the breasts or the shadow. We observe that the breast boundaries are generally parabolic in shape. Therefore, the Hough transform [21] is used to detect the parabola.

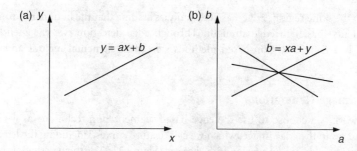

FIGURE 27.1   Illustration of the Hough transform. (a) The original image domain and (b) The parametric domain.

The Hough transform is one type of parametric transforms, in which the object in an image is expressed as a mathematical function of some parameters and the object can be represented in another transformation domain by these parameters. Take a straight edge in an image as an example, in the original image representation domain (or the $x - y$ domain), we can use $y = ax + b$ to describe this edge with a slope of a and an intercept of b, as shown in Figure 27.1a. In order to derive the two parameters, a and b, we can convert the problem to a parametric domain (or the a–b domain) from the original x–y space, and treat x and y as parameters. We find that for each point (x, y) on the edge, there are infinite number of possible corresponding (a, b)s and they form a line in the a–b space, $b = xa + y$. We can imagine that for all the points on the edge, if each of which corresponds to a straight line in the a–b space, then in theory, these lines must intersect at one and only one point (Figure 27.1b), which indicates the true slope and intercept of the edge.

Similarly, the problem of deriving the parameters that describe the parabola can be formulated in a three-dimensional (3D) parametric space of x_0–y_0–p as there are three unknown parameters:

$$y - y_0 = p(x - x_0)^2 \tag{27.2}$$

Each point on the parabola in the x–y space corresponds to a parabola in the x_0–y_0–p space. All the points on the parabola in the x–y space intersect at one point in the x_0–y_0–p space. In order to locate this intersection point in the parametric space, the idea of *accumulator array* is used in which the number of times that a certain pixel in the parametric space is "hit" by a transformed curve (line, parabola, etc.) is treated as the intensity of the pixel. Therefore, the value of the parameters can be derived based on the coordinates of the brightest pixel in the parametric space. The readers are referred to Reference 19 for details on how to implement this accumulator array.

The coordinates of the two brightest spot in the parametric space are used to describe the parabolic functions that form the lower boundaries of the breasts, as shown in Figure 27.2 and Figure 27.3.

27.2.1.3   Segmentation Based on Feature Boundaries

Segmentation is based on three key points, the two armpits (P_L, P_R) derived from the left and right body boundaries by picking up the point where the largest curvature occurs and the intersection (O) of the two parabolic curves derived from the lower boundaries of the breasts/shadow of the breasts. The vertical line that goes through point O and is perpendicular to line $P_L P_R$ is the one used to separate the left and right breasts.

27.2.1.4   Experimental Results

The first set of testing images are obtained using the Inframetrics 600M camera, with a thermal sensitivity of 0.05°K. The images are collected at Elliott Mastology Center. Results from two testing images (*lr*, *nb*) are shown in Figure 27.2, that includes the intermediate results from edge detection, feature curve

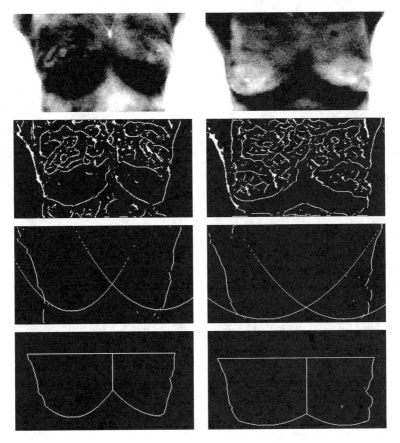

FIGURE 27.2 Segmentation results of two images. Left: results from *lr*. Right: results from *nb*. From top to bottom: original image, edge image, four feature curves, and segments (©2005 IEEE).

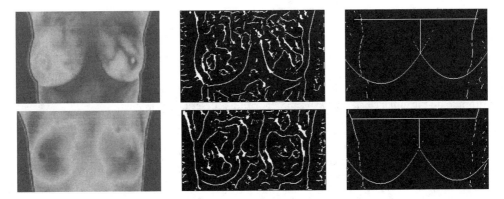

FIGURE 27.3 Hough transform based image segmentation. Top: image of a patient with cancer. Bottom: image of a patient without cancer. From left to right: the original TIR image, the edge image using Canny edge detector, and the segmentation based on Hough transform (©2005 IEEE).

extraction, and segmentation. From the figure, we can see that Hough transform can derive the parabola at the accurate location.

Another set of images are obtained using Microbolometer uncooled camera, with a thermal sensitivity of 0.05°K. Some examples of the segmented images are shown in Figure 27.3.

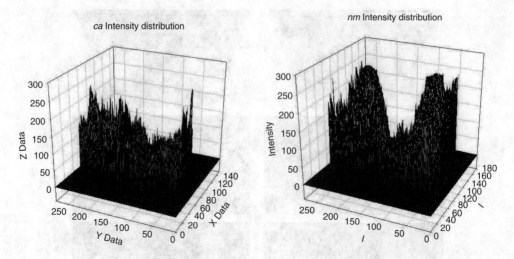

FIGURE 27.4 The left figure show the intensity distribution of a cancerous image and the right figure shows the same for a noncancerous image. The cancerous image is more asymmetrical than the noncancerous one.

Figure 27.4 shows the 3D histogram of the thermal distribution described in the intensity component of the cancerous (*ca*) and noncancerous (*nm*) images. From the graphs, we observe that the *ca* image is more asymmetrical than the *nm* image.

27.2.2 Asymmetry Identification by Unsupervised Learning

Pixel values in a thermogram represent the thermal radiation resulting from the heat emanating from the human body. Different tissues, organs, and vessels have different amount of radiation. Therefore, by observing the heat pattern, or in another word, the pattern of the pixel value, we should be able to discover the abnormalities if there are any.

Usually, in pattern classification algorithms, a set of training data are given to derive the decision rule. All the samples in the training set have been correctly classified. The decision rule is then applied to the testing data set where samples have not been classified yet. This classification technique is also called supervised learning. In unsupervised learning, however, data sets are not divided into training sets or testing sets. No a priori knowledge is known about which class each sample belongs to.

In asymmetry analysis, none of the pixels in the segment knows its class in advance, thus there will be no training set or testing set. Therefore, this is an unsupervised learning problem. We use k-means algorithm to do the initial clustering. k-means algorithm is described as follows:

1. Begin with an arbitrary set of cluster centers and assign samples to nearest clusters
2. Compute the sample mean of each cluster
3. Reassign each sample to the cluster with the nearest mean
4. If the classification of all samples has not changed, then stop, else go to step 2

After each sample is relabeled to a certain cluster, the cluster mean can then be calculated. The segmented image can also be displayed in labeled format. From the difference of mean distribution, we can tell if there is any asymmetric abnormalities.

Figure 27.5 provides the histogram of pixel value from each segment that generated in Figure 27.2 with 10-bin setup. We can tell just from the shape of the histogram that *lr* is more asymmetric than *nb*. However, the histogram only reveals global information. Figure 27.6 displays the classification results for each segment in its labeled format. Here, we choose to use four clusters. The figure also shows the mean difference of each cluster in each segmented image. From Figure 27.6, we can clearly see the much bigger difference shown in the mean distribution or image *lr*, which can also be observed from the labeled image.

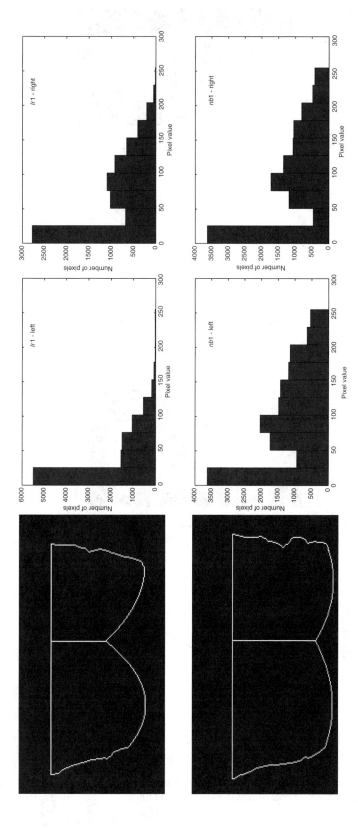

FIGURE 27.5   Histogram of the left and right segments. Top: results from *lr*. Bottom: results from *nb*. From left to right: the segments, histogram of the left segment, histogram of the right segment (©2005 IEEE).

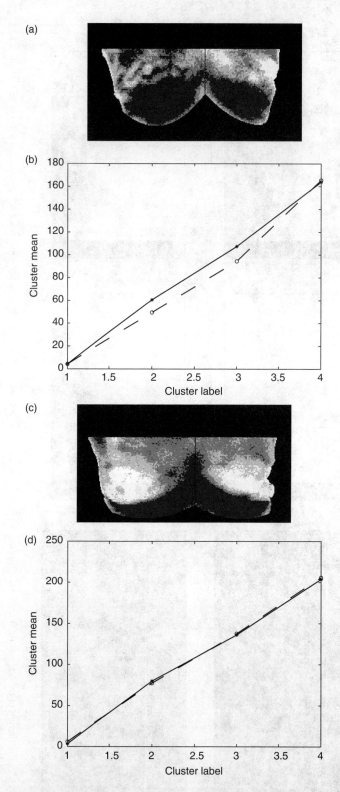

FIGURE 27.6 Labeled image and the profile of mean for each cluster. (a) Results from *lr*, (b) labeled image, (c) results from *nb*, and (d) average pixel value profile of each cluster (©2005 IEEE).

27.2.3 Asymmetry Identification Using Supervised Learning Based on Feature Extraction

Feature extraction is performed on the segmented images. The aim of this research is to identify the effectiveness of the features in contributing toward the asymmetry analysis.

As discussed earlier, TIR imaging is a functional imaging technique representing thermal information as a function of intensity. The TIR image is a pseudo-colored image with different colors assigned to different temperature ranges.

The distribution of different intensities can now be quantified by calculating some high-order statistics as feature elements. We design the following features to form the feature space:

- *Moments of the intensity image*: The intensity component of the image directly corresponds to the thermal energy distribution in the respective areas. The histogram describing the intensity distributions essentially describes the texture of the image. The moments of the histogram give statistical information about the texture of the image. Figure 27.5 shows the intensity distribution of images of a cancerous patient and non-cancerous patient. The four moments, mean, variance, skewness, and kurtosis are taken as

$$\text{Mean } \mu = \frac{1}{N} \sum_{j=1}^{N} p_j \tag{27.3}$$

$$\text{Variance } \sigma^2 = \frac{1}{N-1} \sum_{j=1}^{N} (p_j - \mu)^2 \tag{27.4}$$

$$\text{Skewness } = \frac{1}{N} \sum_{j=1}^{N} \left[\frac{p_j - \mu}{\sigma} \right]^3 \tag{27.5}$$

$$\text{Kurtosis } = \frac{1}{N} \sum_{j=1}^{N} \left(\frac{p_j - \mu}{\sigma} \right)^4 \tag{27.6}$$

where p_j is the probability density of the jth bin in the histogram, and N is the total number of bins.
- *The peak pixel intensity of the correlated image*: The correlated image between the left and right (reflected) breasts is also a good indication of asymmetry. We use the peak intensity of the correlated image as a feature element since the higher the correlation value, the more symmetric the two breast segments.
- *Entropy*: Entropy measures the uncertainty of the information contained in the segmented images. The more equal the intensity distribution, the less information. Therefore, the segment with hot spots should have a lower Entropy.

$$\text{Entropy } H(X) = - \sum_{j=1}^{N} p_j \log p_j \tag{27.7}$$

- *Joint Entropy*: The higher the joint entropy between the left and right breast segments, the more symmetric they are supposedly to be, and the less possible of the existence of tumor.

$$\text{Joint Entropy } H(X, Y) = \sum_{i=1}^{N_X} \sum_{j=1}^{N_Y} p_{ij} \log(p_{ij}) \tag{27.8}$$

TABLE 27.1 Moments of the Histogram

Moments	Cancerous		Noncancerous	
	Left	Right	Left	Right
Mean	0.0010	0.0008	0.0012	0.0010
Variance (10^{-6})	2.0808	1.1487	3.3771	2.7640
Skewness (10^{-6})	2.6821	1.1507	4.8489	4.5321
Kurtosis (10^{-8})	1.0481	0.3459	2.1655	2.3641

TABLE 27.2 Entropy and Correlation Values

Feature	Cancerous	Noncancerous
Correlation	$\times 10^8$	2.35719×10^8
Joint Entropy	9.0100	17.5136
Entropy		
Left	1.52956	1.70684
Right	1.3033	1.4428

where p_{ij} is the joint probability density, N_X and N_Y are the number of bins of the intensity histogram of images X and Y respectively.

From the set of features derived from the testing images, the existence of asymmetry is decided by calculating the ratio of the feature from the left segment to the feature from the right segment. The closer the value to one, the more correlated the features or the less asymmetric the segments. Classic pattern classification techniques like the maximum posterior probability and the kNN classification [22] can be used for the automatic classification of the images. Table 27.1 describes the typical moments for the cancerous and noncancerous images.

The typical values of the cancerous images and noncancerous images are tabulated in Table 27.2. The asymmetry can be clearly stated with a close observation of the given feature values. We used 6 normal patient thermograms and 18 cancer patient thermograms. With a larger database, a training feature set can be derived and supervised learning algorithms like discriminant function or kNN classification can be implemented for a fast, effective, and automated classification.

Figure 27.7 evaluates the effectiveness of the features used. The first data point along the x-axis indicates *entropy*, the second to the fifth points indicate the four statistical moments (*means, variance, skewness, and kurtosis*). The y-axis shows the *closeness* metric we defined as

$$\text{Bilateral ratio closeness to } 1 = \left| \frac{\text{feature value from left segment}}{\text{feature value from right segment}} - 1 \right| \tag{27.9}$$

From the figure, we observe that the high-order statistics are the most effective features to measure the asymmetry, while low-order statistics (*mean*) and *entropy* do not assist asymmetry detection.

27.3 Conclusions

This paper develops a computer-aided approach for automating asymmetry analysis of thermograms. This kind of approach will help the diagnostics as a useful second opinion. The use of TIR images for breast cancer detection and the advantages of thermograms over traditional mammograms are studied. From the experimental results, it can be observed that the Hough transform can be effectively used for breast segmentation. We propose two pattern classification algorithms, the unsupervised learning

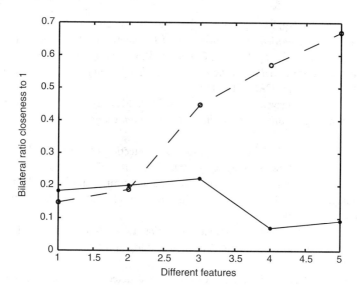

FIGURE 27.7   Performance evaluation of different feature elements. Solid line: non-cancerous image; Dash line: cancerous image. The five data points along the *x*-axis indicate (from left to right): entropy, mean, variance, skewness, and kurtosis (©2005 IEEE).

using k-means and the supervised learning using kNN based on feature extraction. Experimental results show that feature extraction is a valuable approach to extract the signatures of asymmetry, especially the joint entropy. With a larger database, supervised pattern classification techniques can be used to attain more accurate classification. These kind of diagnostic aids, especially in a disease like breast cancer where the reason for the occurrence is not totally known, will reduce the false-positive diagnosis rate and increase the survival rate among the patients since the early diagnosis of the disease is more curable than in a later stage.

References

[1] Llyod-Williams, K. and Handley, R.S., Infrared thermometry in the diagnosis of breast disease. *Lancet*, 2, 1378–1381, 1961.

[2] Keyserlingk, J.R., Ahlgren, P.D., Yu, E., Belliveau, N., and Yassa, M., Functional infrared imaging of the breast, *IEEE Engineering in Medicine and Biology*, 19, 30–41, 2000.

[3] Jones B.F., A reappraisal of the use of infrared thermal image analysis in medicine. *IEEE Transactions on Medical Imaging*, 17, 1019–1027, 1998.

[4] Thermology, http://www.thermology.com/history.htm

[5] Ng, E.Y.K. and Sudarshan, N.M., Numerical computation as a tool to aid thermographic interpretation. *Journal of Medical Engineering and Technology*, 25, 53–60, 2001.

[6] Oslen, O. and Gotzsche, P.C., Cochrane review on screening for breast cancer with mammography. *Lancet*, 9290, 1340–1342, 2001.

[7] Hay, G.A., *Medical Image: Formation, Perception and Measurement*. The Institute of Physics, John Wiley & Sons, 1976.

[8] Watmough, D.J., The role of thermographic imaging in breast screening, discussion by C.R. Hill. In *Medical Images: Formation, Perception and Measurement, 7th L H Gray Conference: Medical Images*, pp. 142–158, 1976.

[9] Gautheire, M., *Atlas of Breast Thermography with Specific Guidelines for Examination and Interpretation*. Milan, Italy: PAPUSA, 1989.

[10] Ng, E.Y.K., Ung, L.N., Ng, F.C., and Sim, L.S.J., Statistical analysis of healthy and malignant breast thermography, *Journal of Medical Engineering and Technology*, 25, 253–263, 2001.

[11] Good, W.F., Zheng, B., Chang, Y. et al., Generalized procrustean image deformation for subtractiuon of mammograms. In *Proceeding of SPIE Medical Imaging — Image Processing*, Vol. 3661, pp. 1562–1573, San Diego, CA, SPIE, 1999.

[12] Shen, L., Shen, Y.P., Rangayyan, R.M., and Desautels J., Measures of asymmetry in mammograms based upon shape spectrum. In *Proceedings of the Annual Conference on EMB*, Vol. 15, pp. 48–49, San Diego, CA, 1993.

[13] Yin, F.F., Giger, M.L., Doi, K. et al., Computerized detection of masses in digital mammograms: analysis of bilateral subtraction images. *Medical Physics*, 18, 955–963, 1991.

[14] Yin, F.F., Giger, M.L., Doi, K. et al., Computerized detection of masses in digital mammograms: automated alignment of breast images and its effect on bilateral-substraction technique. *Medical Physics*, 21, 445–452, 1994.

[15] Yin, F.F., Giger, Vyborny C.J. et al., Comparison of bilateral-subtraction and single-image processing techniques in the computerized detection of mammographic masses. *Investigative Radiology*, 6, 473–481, 1993.

[16] Zheng, B., Chang, Y.H., and Gur, D., Computerized detection of masses from digitized mammograms: comparison of single-image segmentation and bilateral image subtraction. *Academic Radiology*, 2, 1056–1061, 1995.

[17] Head J.F., Lipari, C.C., and Elliott R.L., Computerized image analysis of digitized infrared images of the breasts from a scanning infrared imaging system. In *Proceedings of the 1998 Conference on Infrared Technology and Applications XXIV, Part I*, Vol. 3436, pp. 290–294, San Diego, CA, SPIE, 1998.

[18] Lipari C.A. and Head J.F., Advanced infrared image processing for breast cancer risk assessment. In *Proceedings for 19th International Conference of IEEE/EMBS*, pp. 673–676, Chicago, IL, Oct. 30–Nov. 2. IEEE, 1997.

[19] Snyder, W.E. and Qi, H., *Machine Vision*, Cambridge University Press, 2004.

[20] Canny, J., A computational approach to edge detection. *IEEE Transactions on Pattern Analysis and Machine Intelligence*, 6, 679–698, 1995.

[21] Jafri M.Z. and Deravi, F., Efficient algorithm for the detection of parabolic curves. In *Vision Geometry III*, Vol. 2356, pp. 53–62, SPIE, 1998.

[22] Duda, R.O., Hart, P.E., and Strok, D.G., *Pattern Classification*. John Wiley & Sons, 2nd ed., 2001.

28
Advanced Thermal Image Processing

B. Wiecek
M. Strzelecki
T. Jakubowska
M. Wysocki
C. Drews-Peszynski
Technical University of Lodz

28.1 Histogram-Based First Order Thermal Signatures **28**-3
28.2 Second Order Statistical Parameters.................... **28**-5
28.3 Wavelet Transformation **28**-8
28.4 Classification **28**-9
28.5 Conclusion **28**-12
References **28**-12

Thermal imaging can be useful as an early diagnostic technique that can detect many diseases, such as for example, breast cancer, malignant tumors, etc. There are many different methods that describe image features. A large group of methods is based on statistical parameters calculations. Parameters like mean value, standard deviation, skewness, kurtosis, etc. can be used to compare thermal images. We consider both the first and second order statistical parameters [1,2]. The first order statistical parameters methods use image's histogram (Figure 28.1) to compute signatures, while the second order statistical parameters are defined for so-called co-occurrence matrix of the image [2,11].

In medical applications, one of the principal features of the thermal image is its symmetry of temperature patterns. Thermal images are usually asymmetrical in pathological cases. Any significant asymmetry can indicate a physiologic abnormality (Figure 28.2). This may be pathological (including cancer, fibrocystic disease, an infection, or a vascular disease) or it might indicate an anatomical variant [4–6].

The next group of methods is based on image transformations, such as linear filtering, Fourier or wavelet analysis. All these methods allow to regenerate an image which is processed or converted, and signatures are defined in different domain, for example, frequency or scale domains. Well-known Karhunen-Loeve transform is implemented in form of principle component analysis (PCA). PCA is a technique that is usually used for reducing the dimensionality of multivariate data, preserving most of the variance [7–9].

Thermal image classification is a powerful tool for many medical diagnostic protocols, for example, during breast cancer screening [3,10,11]. Figure 28.3 and Figure 28.4 show thermal images of a healthy breast and that with malignant tumor, respectively. Among the variety of different image features, statistical thermal signatures (first and second order) have been already effectively used for classification of images represented by raw data [1,2,10,12]. In another approach, the features obtained from wavelet transformation can also be used for successful classification.

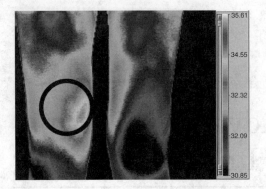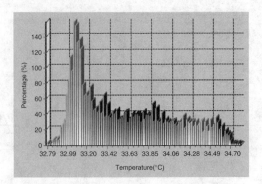

FIGURE 28.1   (See color insert following page 29-16.) ROI of thermal image and its histogram.

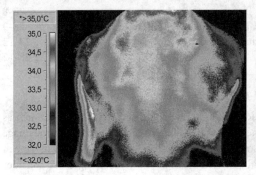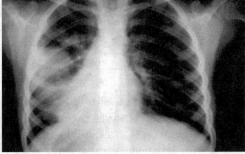

FIGURE 28.2   (See color insert.) Nonsymmetrical temperature distribution for pneumonia with corresponding X-ray image.

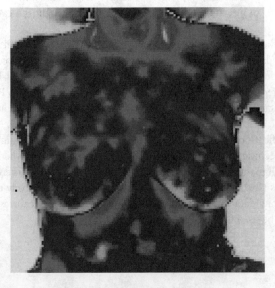

FIGURE 28.3   (See color insert.) Thermal image of the healthy breast.

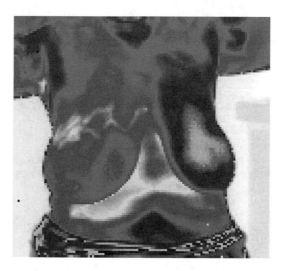

FIGURE 28.4 (See color insert.) Thermal image of the breast with malignant tumor (left side).

It is possible to define many features for an image, and obviously, the selection and reduction are needed. Two approaches are applied, based on Fischer coefficient as well as by using minimization of classification error probability (POE) and average correlation coefficients (ACC), calculated for chosen features [13]. It can reduce the number of features to a few ones. Features preprocessing which generates new parameters after linear or nonlinear transformations can be the next step in the procedure. It allows to get less correlated and of the lower order data. Two approaches are used, that is, PCA and linear discriminant analysis (LDA) [1,3,8]. Finally, classification can be performed using different artificial neural network (ANN), with or without additional hidden layers, and with different number of neurons. Alternatively, nearest neighbor classification (NNC) can also be employed for such image processing.

28.1 Histogram-Based First Order Thermal Signatures

An image is assumed to be a rectangular matrix of discretised data (pixels) pix $[m, n]$, where $m = 0, 1, \ldots, M$, $n = 0, 1, \ldots, N$. Each pixel takes a value from the range $i \in \langle 0, L - 1 \rangle$. The histogram describes the frequency of existence of pixels of the same intensity in whole image or in the region of interest (ROI). Formally, the histogram represents the distribution of the probability function of the existence of the given intensity in an image and it is expressed using Kronecker delta function as:

$$H(i) = \sum_{n}^{N-1} \sum_{m}^{M-1} \delta(p[m, x], i) \qquad \text{for } i = 0, 1, \ldots, L - 1 \tag{28.1}$$

where

$$\delta(p[m, n], i) = \begin{cases} 1, & \text{for } p[m, n] = i \\ 0, & \text{for } p[m, n] \neq i \end{cases} \tag{28.2}$$

Histogram is used for defining first order statistical features of the image, such as mean value μ_H, variance σ_H, skewness, kurtosis, energy, and entropy. The definitions of these parameters are given below.

$$\mu_H = \sum_{i=0}^{L-1} ip(i)$$

$$\sigma_H = \sum_{i=0}^{L-1} (i - \mu_H)^2 p(i)$$

$$skewness = \frac{\sum_{i=0}^{L-1} (i - \mu_H)^3 p(i)}{\sigma_H^3}$$

$$kurtosis = \frac{\sum_{i=0}^{L-1} (i - \mu_H)^4 p(i)}{\sigma_H^4} - 3$$ (28.3)

$$energy = \sum_{i=0}^{L-1} p^2(i)$$

$$entropy = -\sum_{i=0}^{L-1} \log_2(p(i))p(i)$$

Histogram gives global information on an image. By converting histogram we can obtain some very useful image improvement, such as contrast enhancement [1,14]. The first order statistical parameters can be used to separate physiological and pathological breast thermal images. The results for breast cancer screening are presented below.

Thirty-two healthy patients and ten patients with malignant tumors were analyzed using thermography. There were four images registered for every patient that represented each breast in direct and lateral direction to the camera. Histograms were created for these images and on the basis of statistical parameters, the following features were calculated: mean temperature, standard deviation, variance, skewness, and kurtosis. Afterward, differences of parameter values for left and right breast were calculated. The degree of symmetry on the basis of these differences was then estimated (see Figure 28.5 and Figure 28.6).

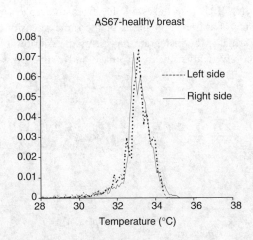

FIGURE 28.5   Histograms of healthy breast thermographs.

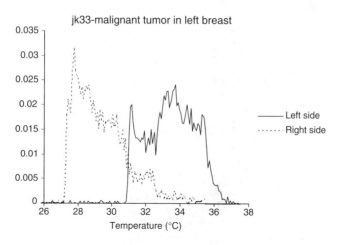

FIGURE 28.6   Histograms of breast thermographs with malignant tumor.

The mean temperature in the healthy group was estimated at the level $30.2 \pm 1.8°C$ in the direct position and $29.7 \pm 1.9°C$ in the lateral one. The mean temperature was higher in 8 cases out of 10 in malignant tumor group. Moreover, 6 cases out of 32 in the healthy group with mean temperatures exceeded normal level. Therefore, we have found that it is necessary to analyze symmetry between left and right breast. Comparison of mean temperature was not sufficient to separate physiological and pathological images. Among analyzed parameters, skewness was the most promising for successful classification of thermal images. Absolute differences of skewness for left and right side was equal to $0.4 \pm 0.3°C$ in frontal position and $0.6 \pm 0.4°C$ in lateral one for the healthy group. These differences were higher for images in lateral position in all cases in the pathological group in comparison to the healthy patients' images.

The image in Figure 28.4 confirm the evidence of asymmetry between left and right side for healthy and malignant tumor cases.

Analyzing the first order statistical parameter let us conclude that it is quite hard to use them for the image classification and detecting tumors. In some cases, only mean temperature and the skewness let us to separate and classify thermal images of breasts with and without malignant tumors. Frontal and lateral positions were used during this investigation, but no significant difference of the obtained result was noticed.

It is concluded that the first order parameters do not give the satisfactory results, and due to some physiological changes of the breast, we could observe that these parameters do not allow separating patients with and without tumors. That was the main reason, that the second order statistical parameters are used for the further investigations.

28.2   Second Order Statistical Parameters

More advanced statistical information on thermal images can be derived from second order parameters. They are defined on so-called co-occurrence matrix. Such a matrix represents the joint probability of two pixels having i-th and j-th intensity at the different distances d, in the different directions. Co-occurrence matrix gives more information on intensity distribution over the whole image, and in this sense, it can effectively be used to separate and classify thermal images.

Let us assume that each pixel has eight neighbors lying in four directions: horizontal, vertical, diagonal and antidiagonal. Let us consider only the nearest neighbors, so the distance $d = 1$ (see Figure 28.7).

As an example let us take an image 4×4 with 4 intensity levels given as (see Figure 28.8).

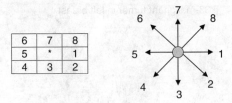

FIGURE 28.7   Eight neighboring pixels in four direct horizontal, vertical, diagonal, and antidiagonal.

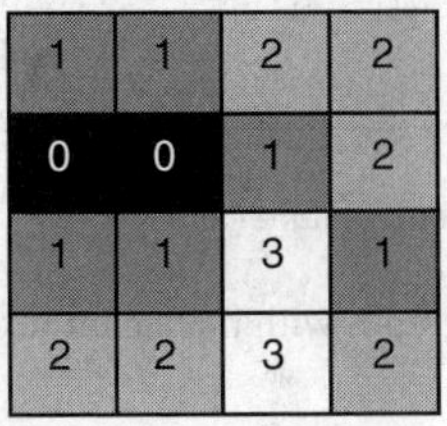

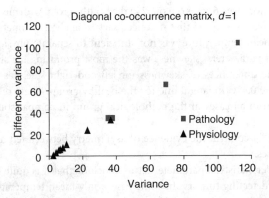

FIGURE 28.8   Example of 4 × 4 image with 4 discrete intensity levels.

Diagonal co-occurrence matrix, $d=1$

FIGURE 28.9   Difference variance vs. variance obtained from co-occurrence matrix for horizontal direction.

For horizontal direction the co-occurrence matrix takes a form:

$$m_{\text{horizontal}} = \begin{bmatrix} 2 & 1 & 0 & 0 \\ 1 & 4 & 2 & 2 \\ 0 & 2 & 4 & 2 \\ 0 & 2 & 2 & 0 \end{bmatrix} \tag{28.4}$$

The co-occurrence matrix is always square and diagonal with the dimension equal to the number of intensity levels in the image. After normalization, we get the matrix of the probabilities $p(i, j)$. Normalization is done by dividing the all elements by number of possible couple pixels for a given direction of analysis. For horizontal and vertical directions this number is equal to $2N(M - 1)$ and $2M(N - 1)$, while for diagonal directions it is $2(M - 1)(N - 1)$, respectively.

Second order parameters are presented by Equation 28.4 and Equation 28.6. As an example of comparing thermal images μ_x, μ_y, σ_x, σ_y are mean values and standard deviations for the elements of co-occurrence matrices that were calculated for horizontal and vertical directions, respectively, and the results are presented in Figure 28.9 and Figure 28.10.

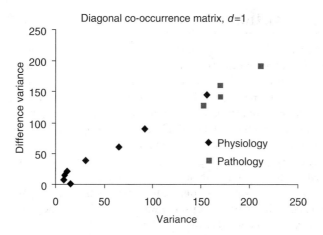

FIGURE 28.10 Difference variance vs. variance obtained from co-occurrence matrix for diagonal direction.

Second order statistical parameters can be used to discriminate the physiological and pathological cases, for example, breast cancers. Most of them successfully discriminate healthy and malignant tumor cases. The protocol of the investigation assumes the symmetry analysis in the following way. At first, the square ROI were chosen for analysis. Then, co-occurrence matrixes were calculated for left and right breasts to evaluate second order statistical parameters for different directions. Only the neighboring pixels are considered in these investigations ($d = 1$). Finally, the differences of the values of these parameters for left and right sides were used for the image classification. Figure 28.9 and Figure 28.10 illustrate that the differences of second order parameters for left and right sides are typically greater for pathological cases. Taking two parameters such as difference variance and variance allows successfully separating almost all healthy and malignant tumor cases.

$$\text{Energy} = \sum_{i=0}^{L-1}\sum_{j=0}^{L-1} p^2(i,j)$$

$$\text{Variance} = \sum_{i=0}^{L-1}\sum_{j=0}^{L-1} (i-j)^2 p(i,j)$$

$$\text{Difference variance} = \text{Var}(p_{x-y})$$

$$(28.5)$$

where

$$p_{x-y}(l) = \sum_{i=0}^{L-1}\sum_{j=0}^{L-1} p(i,j), \quad \text{for } |i-j| = l, \ l = 0,1,\dots,G-2$$

$$\text{Correlation} = \frac{\sum_{i=0}^{L-1}\sum_{j=0}^{L-1}(ij)p(i,j) - \mu_x\mu_y}{\sigma_x\sigma_y}$$

$$(28.6)$$

$$\text{Inverse difference} = \sum_{i=0}^{L-1}\sum_{j=0}^{L-1} \frac{p(i,j)}{1+(i-j)^2}$$

$$\text{Entropy} = -\sum_{i=0}^{L-1}\sum_{j=0}^{L-1} p(i,j)\log_2[p(i,j)]$$

28.3 Wavelet Transformation

Wavelet transformation is actually used in many domains, such as telecommunication and signal processing for compression and to extract quantitative features from the signal. In image processing it can be employed to get new features, representing both global and detail information. Wavelet transformation is based on image filtering represented by rows and columns using low and high pass linear filters (Figure 28.11). After filtering, decimation is used to reduce the number of pixels. The procedure can be repeated until 1×1 images are obtained. Practically, the processing is stopped earlier, after 2 to 4 steps, and then the features are derived from the filtered subimages.

As an example, the investigations of 10 patients with recognized breast tumors, as well as 30 healthy patients are presented. All healthy and pathological cases were confirmed by other diagnostic methods, such as mammography, USG, biopsy, and so on. We have used thermographic camera to take two images for each breast: frontal and side ones. Each patient was relaxing before the experiment for 15 min in a room where temperature were stabilized at 20°C.

Then the numerical procedure was used to calculate features of the images. Figure 28.12 presents the pathological case where left breast has evidently higher temperature and the temperature distribution is very asymmetric.

One of the possible transformations uses wavelets realized by filtering as it has already been mentioned. The result of such processing is presented in Figure 28.13. As it is seen, the different filters are showing different details of the image, that is, high pass filters allows to present gradient of the temperature, while

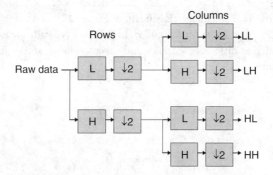

FIGURE 28.11 Wavelet transformation of an image.

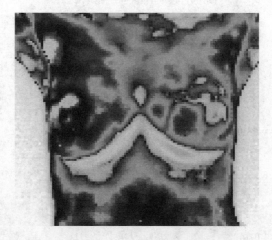

FIGURE 28.12 (See color insert.) Example of thermal image with the tumor.

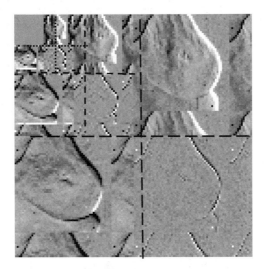

FIGURE 28.13   Result of wavelet transformation.

the low pass ones display the global temperature distribution and the energy of the signal understood as the level of temperature.

As a powerful tool, wavelet transformation gives the possibility of generating new features from different subimages, in different scales and subbands. Filtering can be easily parameterized in the sense of varying cutoff frequency, what provides the additional flexibility in the algorithm. It denotes, that a lot of different features can be produced by this method. Obviously, the selection of these features is necessary to obtain only these ones, which are the most discriminative and weakly correlated [11].

28.4 Classification

Artificial neural network are typically used for classification. The selected image features are used as inputs. It means that the number of input nodes is equal to number of the features. The number of neurons in the first hidden layer can be equal or lower than the number of features in the classification, as shown in Figure 28.14. ANN can have user-defined next hidden layers, which allow additional nonlinear processing of the input features. As ANN is the nonlinear system, such technique allows to additional decorrelating and data reduction, what in consequence improves the classification. Such approach is known as nonlinear discriminant analysis (NDA) [3,11].

It is well known that the training of ANN is the very important step in the entire protocol. It is an multivariable optimization problem typically based on back-propagation technique. In general case it can lead to wrong solutions if the there is no single minimum of the error function. That is why we need enough data during learning phase, and sometimes it is better or necessary to repeat training of ANN with different initial values of the neuron weight coefficients.

Classification can start from the raw data analysis. As seen in Figure 28.15, two classes of images containing (1) nonhealthy and (2) healthy cases are chosen. In this example, selection of features reduces the number of features to two, derived from the co-occurrence matrix (sum of squares and inverse difference moment) [1,10,12]. The third one is based on wavelet transformation — energy E_{HL} for the scale no.1 and high and low frequency subbands. Raw data analysis (Figure 28.15) does not give satisfactory feature separation and classification. It is hard to separate clusters of features corresponding to physiological and pathological images. The distance in between them in the multivariate space is not large enough, which means that the probability of erroneous classification is still quite high.

The next results were obtained by LDA (Figure 28.16), in which the most discriminative features (MDF) are generated [10,13]. LDA creates typically new set with smaller number of features. LDA is the linear

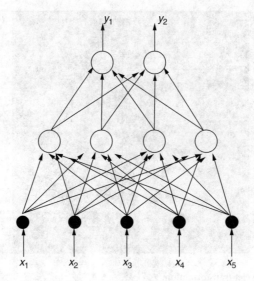

FIGURE 28.14 Neural network example with input, single hidden, and output layers.

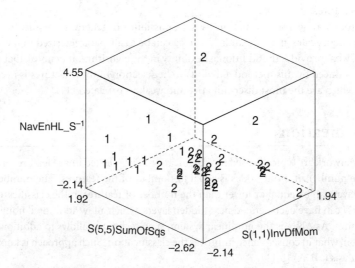

FIGURE 28.15 Raw data analysis result.

transformation, and produces linearly separated features, which means that in general case it is also not possible to separate them fully. This case is illustrated in Figure 28.16.

Nonlinear transformation of the features obtained by ANN with additional hidden layer is the most promising technique. The output of this additional hidden layer creates the new smaller set of features, which are typically much better separable. It can be simple verified by the larger value of Fisher coefficient. In our investigation, seven original features were selected using POE and ACC selection criteria. The first and second hidden layers contained only one and two neurons, respectively. It denotes that the original features were reduced to two new ones. The expectation that this approach allows better separation and classification is now confirmed [2].

The results of NDA are presented in Figure 28.17 and Figure 28.18. Two new features are far away from each other on the feature space, both for frontal and side images. It is even not very surprising that the value of Fisher coefficient $F = 2.7$ for original features is now increased to $F = 443.4$. ANN together with

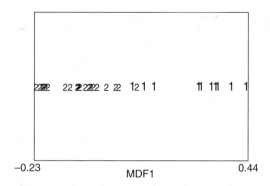

FIGURE 28.16 Nonacceptable separation of cluster using LDA.

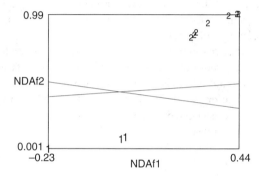

FIGURE 28.17 NDA classification results for side thermal images of the breast.

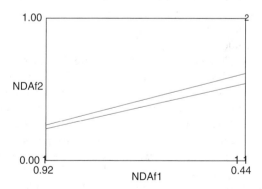

FIGURE 28.18 NDA classification results for frontal thermal images of the breast.

NDA have one more advantage. Besides data reduction and decorrelating, it also allows implementing classification realized by the last output layer of ANN.

We faced one problem in the presented research. The number of pathological cases was small, only ten. As it has been already mentioned it is difficult to get well diagnosed patients, especially in the young age [4–6]. The research is still in progress, and we actually enlarging our image database day-by-day. This research is a preliminary one, and shows the possibility of using advanced image processing tools. The effectiveness of the screening procedure can be verified later, when we will have enough input data.

Because of the above limits, the classification was carried out in the following simplified way: First we have chosen equal number of physiological and pathological images, that is, 10 + 10. Every image from

TABLE 28.1 Errors of Classification

	Frontal positions		Side positions	
	False negative	False positive	False negative	False positive
Raw data	2/10	3/30	1/10	2/30
PCA	2/10	3/30	1/10	2/30
LDA	1/10	2/30	1/10	1/30
NDA	2/10	2/30	0/10	2/30

each class (healthy and nonhealthy) was extracted, and the training of ANN was performed for all the rest. Then this one not being used before during learning was employed now for classification.

The results are presented in Table 28.1. First three rows in this table present nearest neighbor (NN) classification of the image features. The first results were obtained by using feature calculated on a image and NN classification after feature selection. In the subsequent experiments, preprocessing of original features using PCA and LDA was employed.

Finally, calculation using NDA was performed with an additional hidden layer that consisted of two neurons for generating two new more discriminative features. The results in Table 28.1 confirm the effectiveness of using both NN and ANN classifiers. Although it was not evidently proved that NDA results are better in the classification, we definitely conclude that ANN is a powerful tool for thermal image processing during breast cancer screening. Reducing false/positive errors of classification is the most important task for the future research.

28.5 Conclusion

This chapter presents the preliminary results of the feature analysis for thermal images for different medical applications, mainly used in breast oncology. Thermography as the additional and adjacent method can be very helpful for early screening that helps to recognize tumors. At first, we consider first and second order statistical parameters. Although we do not have many pathological cases for investigations yet, the first results are very promising. The second order parameters are more sensitive to the overall structure of an image. Actually, the study is being extended by choosing second order parameters for multivariate data classification. The presented approach includes the PCA to reduce the dimensionality of the problem and by selecting the eigen vectors it is possible to generate data, which represents the tumors more evidently.

Breast cancer screening is a challenge today for medical engineering. Breast temperature depends not only due to some pathological changes, but it also varies in normal physiological situations, it is even a consequence of emotional state of a patient. It was a main reason that we are looking for more advanced methods of thermal image processing, that could give satisfactory results.

One of the possible alternative for such processing is ANN classification based on multidimensional feature domain, with use of modern transformations, such as wavelets. The preliminary investigations are quite successful, and can be improved by increasing the number of samples taken for processing.

Future research will concentrate around selection of features and adjusting wavelet transformation parameters to get the best classification. We assume that the more satisfactory results can be obtained by using features based on asymmetry between left and right sides of a patient. It could help for one-side cancerous lesion classification, what is the most typical pathological case and frequently happens today.

References

[1] P. Cichy, "Texture analysis of digital images, doctoral thesis, *Technical University of Lodz, Institute of Electronics*, Lodz, 2000, in Polish.

[2] A. Materka, M. Strzelecki, R. Lerski, and L. Schad, "Evaluation of texture features of test objects for magnetic resonance imaging," *Infotech Oulu Workshop on Texture Analysis in Machine Vision,* June 1999, Oulu, Finland.

[3] P. Debiec, M. Strzelecki, and A. Materka, "Evaluation of texture generation methods based on CNN and GMRF image texture models," *Proceedings of the International Conference on Signals and Electronic Systems,* 17–20 October 2000, Ustron, pp. 187–192.

[4] E.Y.K. Ng, L.N. Ung, F.C. Ng, and L.S.J. Sim "Statistical analysis of healthy and malignant breast thermography," *Journal of Medical Engineering and Technology,* 25, 253–263, 2001.

[5] B.F.J. Manly, *Multivariate Statistical Method: A Primer.* London, Chapman & Hall, 1994.

[6] Michael Bennett, "Breast cancer screening using high-resolution digital thermography," *Total Health,* 22, 44, 1985.

[7] I.T. Jolliffe, *Principal Component Analysis.* New York, Springer-Verlag, 1986.

[8] B.F.J. Manly, *Multivariate Statistical Method: A Primer.* New York, London, Chapman & Hall, 1994.

[9] D.R. Causton, *A Biologist's Advanced Mathematics,* London, Allen and Unwin, 1987.

[10] Schürman J. *Pattern Classification,* New York, John Wiley & Sons, 1996.

[11] M. Kociolek, A. Materka, M. Strzelecki, and P. Szczypinski, "Discrete wavelet transform-derived features for digital image texture analysis," *Proceedings of the International Conference on Signals and Electronic Systems ICSES'2001,* Lodz, 18–21 September 2001, pp. 111–116.

[12] T. Jakubowska, B. Wiecek, M. Wysocki, and C. Drews-Peszynski, "Thermal signatures for breast cancer screening comparative study," *Proceedings of the IEEE EMBS Conference,* Cancun, Mexico, 17–21 September, 2003.

[13] P. Debiec, M. Strzelecki, and A. Materka, "Evaluation of texture generation methods based on CNN and GMRF image texture models," *International Conference on Signals and Electronic Systems ICSES'2000,* Ustron, October 2000, pp. 187–192.

[14] B. Wiecek and S. Zwolenik, "Thermal wave method — limits and potentialities of active thermography in biology and medicine," *2nd Joint EMBS-BMES Conference, 24th Annual International Conference of the IEEE Engineering in Medicine and Biology Society,* BMES-EMS 2002, Houston, 23–26 October, 2002.

29

Biometrics: Face Recognition in Thermal Infrared

I. Pavlidis
University of Houston

P. Tsiamyrtzis
Athens University of Economics and Business

P. Buddharaju
C. Manohar
University of Houston

29.1 Introduction... **29**-1
29.2 Face Detection in Thermal Infrared **29**-2
      Facial Tissue Delineation Using a Bayesian Approach
29.3 Facial Feature Extraction in Thermal Infrared......... **29**-6
      Morphological Reconstruction of Superficial Blood Vessels
29.4 Conclusion **29**-13
Acknowledgments... **29**-14
References **29**-15

29.1 Introduction

Biometrics has received a lot of attention in the last few years both from the academic and business communities. It has emerged as a preferred alternative to traditional forms of identification, like card IDs, which are not emedded into one's physical characteristics. Research into several biometric modalities including face, fingerprint, iris, and retina recognition has produced varying degrees of success [1]. Face recognition stands as the most appealing modality, since it is the natural mode of identification among humans and totally unobtrusive. At the same time, however, it is one of the most challenging modalities [2]. Faces are 3D objects with rich details that vary with orientation, illumination, age, and artifacts (e.g., glasses).

Research into face recognition has been biased towards the visible spectrum for a variety of reasons. Among those is the availability and low cost of visible band cameras and the undeniable fact that face recognition is one of the primary activities of the human visual system. Machine recognition of human faces, however, has proved more problematic than the seemingly effortless face recognition performed by humans. The major culprit is light variability, which is prevalent in the visible spectrum due to the reflective nature of incident light in this band. Secondary problems are associated to the difficulty of detecting facial disguises [3].

As a cure to the aforementioned problems, researchers have started investigating the use of thermal infrared for face recognition purposes [4,5]. Efforts were directed into solving three complementary problems: face detection, feature extraction, and classification (see Figure 29.1) [6,7]. Face detection is a prerequisite step, since a face cannot be recognized unless first it is detected in the scene. Feature extraction follows face detection and reduces the face to a succinct mathematical description — the feature vector. Classification operates upon the feature vector and matches the incoming face to one of the records kept in the database.

Many of the research efforts in thermal face recognition use the thermal infrared band as a way to see in the dark or reduce the deleterious effect of light variability [8]. Methodologically, they do not differ very much from face recognition algorithms in the visible band [9]. In this chapter, we will present a novel approach to the problem of thermal facial recognition that realizes the full potential of the thermal infrared band. It consists of a statistical face detection and physiological feature extraction algorithm tailored to thermal phenomenology. We will not elaborate on classification, since we do not have to add anything new in this part of the face recognition process. Our goal is to promote a different way of thinking in areas where thermal infrared should be approached in a distinct manner with respect to other modalities.

29.2   Face Detection in Thermal Infrared

We approach the face detection problem in thermal infrared from a statistical point of view. Due to its physiology, a typical human face consists of *hot* and *cold* parts. Hot parts correspond to tissue areas that are rich in vasculature (e.g., periorbital and forehead). Cold parts correspond to tissue areas that feature either sparse vasculature or multi-sided exposure to the environment (e.g., cheeks and nose). This casts the human face as a bimodal distribution entity. The background can also be described by a bimodal distribution. It typically consists of walls (*cold* objects) and the upper part of the subject's body dressed in clothes (*hot* objects). The bimodal distributions of the face and background vary over time, due to thermophysiological processes and environmental noise respectively. Therefore, the problem renders itself naturally to the Bayesian framework, since we have a priori knowledge of the bimodal nature of the scene, which can be updated over time by the incoming evidence (new thermal frames from the camera).

29.2.1   Facial Tissue Delineation Using a Bayesian Approach

We consider an indoor area that is being monitored with a thermal infrared camera. The objective is to detect and delineate a human face should this become available in the scene. The segmented face data feed the feature extraction and classification modules, which complete the face recognition process (see Figure 29.1). Initially, we consider the face detection problem at the pixel level and label every pixel as either facial skin *s* or background *b* pixel.

In more detail, we use a mixture of two Normal distributions to model facial skin temperature. The dominant mode is in the upper band of the values where usually about 60 to 70% of the probability mass

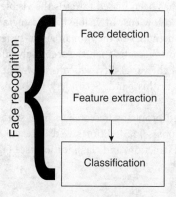

FIGURE 29.1   Architecture of a face recognition system. We will focus on face detection and feature extraction, where thermal infrared warrants a totally different approach from the one usually undertaken in the literature.

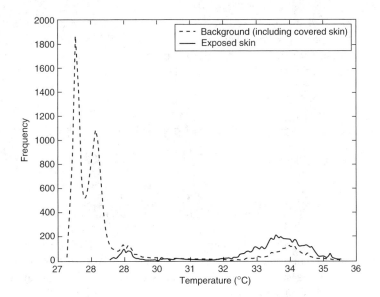

FIGURE 29.2 Temperature distributions of exposed skin and background from a set of facial thermal images in the University of Houston database. The bimodal nature of the distributions is evident.

resides. The secondary mode is in the lower band of the values. For subjects in climate controlled rooms a typical temperature range for the dominant skin mode is $\sim(32–35)°C$, while for the secondary mode is $\sim(28–30)°C$. The latter may overlap with the background distribution since areas of the face like the nose and ears have temperatures similar to the environment (see Figure 29.2).

Similarly, we use a mixture of two Normal distributions to model background temperature. The dominant mode is in the lower band of the values where about 80% of the background probability mass resides (typically, in the range $\sim[27$ to $29]°C$). The secondary background mode has its mean somewhere between the two modes of the skin distribution and variance large enough to cover almost the entire band. Therefore, the secondary background distribution includes some relatively high temperature values. These are due to the fact that light clothes offer spots of high temperature (e.g., places where the clothes touch the skin), which mimic the skin distribution but are not skin (see Figure 29.2).

For each pixel we have some prior distribution (information) available of whether this particular pixel represents skin ($\pi(s)$) or background ($\pi(b) = 1 - \pi(s)$). Then, the incoming pixel value represents the data (likelihood) that will be used to update the prior to posterior distribution via the Bayes theorem. Based on the posterior distribution we will draw our inference of whether the specific pixel represents s or b. At the end, this posterior distribution will be used as the prior for the next incoming data point.

We call θ the parameter of interest, which takes two possible values (s and b) with some probability. The prior distribution at time t consists of the probabilities of the two complementary events, s and b. Thus, we have:

$$\pi^{(t)}(\theta) = \begin{cases} \pi^{(t)}(s), & \text{when } \theta = s \\ \pi^{(t)}(b) = 1 - \pi^{(t)}(s), & \text{when } \theta = b \end{cases} \tag{29.1}$$

The incoming pixel value x_t has a conditional distribution $f(x_t|\theta)$, which depends on whether the particular pixel is skin (i.e., $\theta = s$) or background (i.e., $\theta = b$). Based on our bimodal view of the skin and background distributions we will have for the likelihood:

$$f(x_t|\theta) = \begin{cases} f(x_t|s): \omega_s^{(t)} N(\mu_{s_1}^{(t)}, \sigma_{s_1}^{2(t)}) + (1 - \omega_s^{(t)}) N(\mu_{s_2}^{(t)}, \sigma_{s_2}^{2(t)}), & \text{when } \theta = s \\ f(x_t|b): \omega_b^{(t)} N(\mu_{b_1}^{(t)}, \sigma_{b_1}^{2(t)}) + (1 - \omega_b^{(t)}) N(\mu_{b_2}^{(t)}, \sigma_{b_2}^{2(t)}), & \text{when } \theta = b \end{cases} \tag{29.2}$$

There are ten parameters that are involved in the conditional distribution of Equation 29.2, namely, 2 weights, 4 means, and 4 variances. We will discuss later on, how to initialize and update these parameters.

The prior distribution, $\pi^{(t)}(\theta)$, will be combined with the likelihood, $f(x_t \mid \theta)$, to provide (via the Bayes theorem) the posterior distribution $p^{(t)}(\theta \mid x_t)$. Thus, we will have:

$$p^{(t)}(\theta \mid x_t) = \begin{cases} p^{(t)}(s \mid x_t), & \text{when } \theta = s \\ p^{(t)}(b \mid x_t) = 1 - p^{(t)}(s \mid x_t), & \text{when } \theta = b \end{cases} \tag{29.3}$$

where according to the Bayes theorem:

$$p^{(t)}(s \mid x_t) = \frac{\pi^{(t)}(s)f(x_t \mid s)}{\pi^{(t)}(s)f(x_t \mid s) + \pi^{(t)}(b)f(x_t \mid b)} \tag{29.4}$$

In the Bayesian philosophy the posterior distribution of the parameter of interest represents how the prior information (distribution) is updated in light of new evidence (data). At every time point t our inference (on whether the particular pixel represents s or b) will be based on the posterior distribution, $p^{(t)}(\theta \mid x_t)$.

This posterior distribution will also be used to provide the prior distribution for the next stage. More precisely:

$$\pi^{(t+1)}(\theta) = \begin{cases} \pi^{(t+1)}(s) = p^{(t)}(s \mid x_t), & \text{when } \theta = s \\ \pi^{(t+1)}(b) = p^{(t)}(b \mid x_t) = 1 - \pi^{(t+1)}(s), & \text{when } \theta = b \end{cases} \tag{29.5}$$

29.2.1.1 Initialization

As part of the initialization, we need to specify two things: the prior distribution, $\pi^{(1)}(\theta)$ and the likelihood $f(x_1 \mid \theta)$. Absence of information on whether a pixel is skin or background, leads us to adopt a noninformative prior distribution where a priori each pixel is equally likely to be s or b. Thus, we have:

$$\pi^{(1)}(s) = \frac{1}{2} = \pi^{(1)}(b) \tag{29.6}$$

Regarding the likelihood, we need to calculate the initial values of the ten parameters involved in the likelihood Equation 29.2. For that, we select N facial frames (off-line) from a variety of subjects. This is the so-called training set. It is important for this set to be representative, that is, to include people of both sexes, different ages, and with different physical characteristics. We manually segment on all the N frames, skin and, background areas (see Figure 29.3). The segmentation needs to be representative. For example,

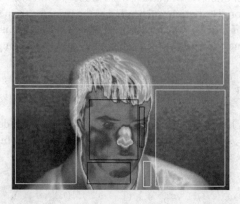

FIGURE 29.3 (See color insert following page **29**-16.) Manual segmentation of skin (black rectangles) and background (white rectangles) areas for initialization purposes.

in the case of skin areas, we need to include eyes, ears, nose and the other facial areas, not parts thereof. Out of the N frames the segmentation will yield N_s skin and N_b background pixels.

For the skin distribution we have available at the initial state the pixels $x_1, x_2, \ldots, x_{N_s}$, which are assumed to be sampled from a mixture of two Normal distributions:

$$f(x_j \mid s) = \sum_{i=1}^{2} \omega_{s_i} N(\mu_{s_i}, \sigma_{s_i}^2) \tag{29.7}$$

where $\omega_{s_2} = 1 - \omega_{s_1}$. We estimate the mixture parameters ω_{s_i}, μ_{s_i}, and $\sigma_{s_i}^2$ using the N_s skin pixels of the training set via the EM algorithm. Initially, we provide the EM algorithm with some crude estimates of the parameters of interest: $\omega_{s_i}^{(0)}$, $\mu_{s_i}^{(0)}$, and $(\sigma_{s_i}^{(0)})^2$. Then, we apply the following loop: For $k = 0, 1, \ldots$, we calculate:

$$z_{ij}^{(k)} = \frac{\omega_{s_i}^{(k)} (\sigma_{s_i}^{(k)})^{-1} \exp \left\{ -\frac{1}{2(\sigma_{s_i}^{(k)})^2} (x_j - \mu_{s_i}^{(k)})^2 \right\}}{\sum_{t=1}^{2} \omega_{s_t}^{(k)} (\sigma_{s_t}^{(k)})^{-1} \exp \left\{ -\frac{1}{2(\sigma_{s_t}^{(k)})^2} (x_j - \mu_{s_t}^{(k)})^2 \right\}} \tag{29.8}$$

$$\omega_{s_i}^{(k+1)} = \frac{\sum_{j=1}^{N_s} z_{ij}^{(k)}}{N_s} \tag{29.9}$$

$$\mu_{s_i}^{(k+1)} = \frac{\sum_{j=1}^{N_s} z_{ij}^{(k)} x_j}{N_s \omega_{s_i}^{(k+1)}} \tag{29.10}$$

$$(\sigma_{s_i}^{(k+1)})^2 = \frac{\sum_{j=1}^{N_s} z_{ij}^{(k)} (x_j - \mu_{s_i}^{(k+1)})^2}{N_s \omega_{s_i}^{(k+1)}} \tag{29.11}$$

for $i = 1, 2$ and $j = 1, \ldots, N_s$. Then, we set $k = k + 1$ and repeat the loop. The condition for terminating the loop is:

$$|\omega_{s_i}^{(k+1)} - \omega_{s_i}^{(k)}| < \varepsilon \quad i = 1, 2 \tag{29.12}$$

where ε is a small positive number $(10^{-3}, 10^{-4}, \ldots)$. We apply a similar EM process for determining the initial parameters of the background distributions.

29.2.1.2 Inference

Once a data point x_t becomes available we are faced with the decision of whether the particular pixel represents skin or background. In a decision theory framework this can be cast as testing the statistical hypotheses for the parameter of interest θ:

$$\left\{ \begin{array}{l} H_0\colon \theta = s \text{ (i.e., the pixel represents skin)} \\ H_1\colon \theta = b \text{ (i.e., the pixel represents background)} \end{array} \right\}$$

Using Equation 29.2 and Equation 29.4 we combine the data with the prior distributions to obtain the posterior distributions. Our inference will be based on these posterior distributions. We need to decide whether we will accept H_0 or H_1. The easiest way to do this within the Bayesian framework is to favor the hypothesis that has the highest a posteriori coverage. That simply means:

$$\left\{ \begin{array}{l} \text{Accept } H_0 \text{ if: } p^{(t)}(s \mid x_t) > p^{(t)}(b \mid x_t) \Leftrightarrow p^{(t)}(s \mid x_t) > 0.5 \\ \text{Accept } H_1 \text{ if: } p^{(t)}(s \mid x_t) < p^{(t)}(b \mid x_t) \Leftrightarrow p^{(t)}(s \mid x_t) < 0.5 \end{array} \right\}$$

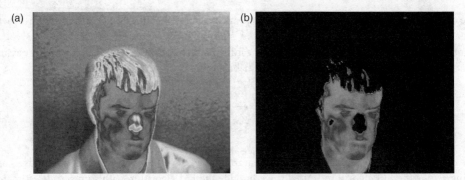

FIGURE 29.4   (See color insert.) Visualization of Bayesian segmentation on a subject: (a) original image; (b) segmented image. The nose has been erroneously segmented as background and a couple of hair patches have been erroneously marked as facial skin. This is due to occasional overlapping between portions of the skin and background distributions. The isolated nature of these mislabeled patches makes them easily correctable through post-processing.

Figure 29.4 visualizes the results of Bayesian segmentation on a typical facial thermal image from the University of Houston database.

29.3   Facial Feature Extraction in Thermal Infrared

Once the face is delineated from the rest of the scene, one can extract the features necessary for classification. In contrast to the visible band, thermal infrared provides the capability to extract physiological features. In particular, blood that flows in the major superficial vessels creates a substantial convective heat effect that is manifested in thermal imagery. Segmentation of the vascular network can provide the basis of a unique feature vector. The topology and extent of the recovered vascular network depend on the genetic traits and physical characteristics of the individual (e.g., facial skin fat deposits). Therefore, facial vasculature is an identifying entity that endures through aging and superficial changes of appearance.

The problem for vessel segmentation has been solved in other imaging modalities using a variety of methods. To the best of our knowledge, it is the first time that vessel segmentation is reported in the thermal imaging modality. In our effort, we took into account methodologies used for vessel segmentation in modalities other than thermal imaging (e.g., ultrasound and MRI). We can broadly categorize these methodologies as follows:

- Center line detection approaches
- Ridge-based approaches
- Region growing approaches
- Differential geometry-based approaches
- Matched filter approaches
- Mathematical morphology approaches

In the center line extraction scheme, the vasculature is developed by traversing the vessels' center lines. The method employs thresholding and thinning of the image, followed by connected component analysis. Center line extraction techniques are used by References 10 and 11. They use graph search theory to find out vessel center lines and then curvature features to reconstruct the vasculature. In Reference 12, the authors detect center lines from images acquired from different angles. As a result, they are able to represent the 3D shape of the vessels.

Ridge-based approaches convert a 2D gray scale image into a 3D surface by mapping the intensity values along the z-axis. Once the surface is generated, the local ridge points are those where the directional gradient is the steepest. The ridges are invariant to affine transforms and this property is exploited in medical registration [13,14]. The method of segmentation of vessels using the ridge-based approach is discussed in Reference 15 and more extensive details are available in its references.

One of the most widely used methods of vessel segmentation is the region growing method. Traditionally, the parameters used for growing the vessel region are pixel intensity and proximity. Recent improvements in this method include gradient and texture [16,17]. Such methods, although they give good results, depend upon initialization. In Reference 18, based on the starting seed provided by the user the region grows upon similar spatial, temporal, and structural features. A similar method is also used in Reference 19.

If a 2D image is mapped into a 3D surface, then the crest lines are the most salient features of that surface. This gives rise to the differential geometry based methods for vessel segmentation. The crest lines are obtained by linking the crest points in the image, which are the local maxima of the surface curvature. A prominent differential geometry-based method is the directional anisotropic diffusion (DAD), which is discussed in Reference 20. It uses Gaussian convolution to remove the image noise. This method is a generalized form of the method reported in Reference 21 and uses the gradient as well as the minimum and maximum curvature information to differentiate the diffusion equation. The method removes the noise without blurring and is thus, very useful in edge enhancement procedures.

The matched filtering approach uses a series of Gaussian kernels of different sizes and orientations. In Reference 22 the orientation of the Gaussian filters is chosen using the Hessian matrix. A similar approach is used in Reference 23 to enhance and detect vessels in real time. These methods are similar to the Gabor filters, which are extensively used in texture analysis.

29.3.1 Morphological Reconstruction of Superficial Blood Vessels

In our method, first, we smooth the image to remove the unwanted noise and then, we apply the morphological operators. In thermal imagery of human tissue the major blood vessels do not have strong edges. Due to the thermal diffusion process the edges that we get have a sigmoid temperature profile. A sigmoid function can be written as $y = 1/(1 + e^{-x})$ (see Figure 29.5).

The method of anisotropic diffusion has proved very effective in handling sigmoid edges [24,25]. Nonlinear anisotropic diffusion filters are iterative filters introduced by Perona et al. [21]. Greig et al. [26] used such filters to enhance MR images. Sapiro et al. [27] used a similar technique to perform edge preserving smoothing of MR images. Others have shown that diffusion filters can be used to enhance and detect object edges within images [21,28].

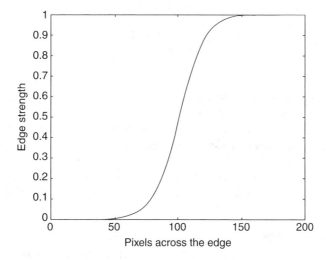

FIGURE 29.5 Sigmoid function plot.

The anisotropic diffusion filter is formulated as a process that enhances object boundaries by performing intra-region as opposed to inter-region smoothing. The mathematical equation for the process is:

$$\frac{\partial I(\bar{x}, t)}{\partial t} = \nabla(c(\bar{x}, t)\nabla I(\bar{x}, t)) \tag{29.13}$$

In our case $I(\bar{x}, t)$ is the thermal image, $\bar{x}$ refers to the spatial dimensions, and t to time. The function $c(\bar{x}, t)$ is a monotonically decreasing function of the image gradient magnitude and is called the *diffusion function*

$$c(\bar{x}, t) = f(|\nabla I(\bar{x}, t)|) \tag{29.14}$$

This allows locally adaptive diffusion strengths. Edges are thus, selectively smoothed or enhanced on the basis of the evaluated diffusion function.

Perona and Malik have suggested the following two formulations for the diffusion function:

$$c_1(\bar{x}, t) = \exp\left(-\left(\frac{|\nabla I(\bar{x}, t)|}{k}\right)^2\right) \tag{29.15}$$

$$c_2(\bar{x}, t) = \exp\left(\frac{1}{1 + \left(\frac{|\nabla I(\bar{x}, t)|}{k}\right)^{1+\alpha}}\right) \tag{29.16}$$

Typical responses of the thermal image of the wrist to the Perona–Malik filters with diffusion functions c_1 and c_2 respectively are shown in Figure 29.6. One can observe that for the same image gradient and value of the k parameter a steeper slope is obtained for c_1 as compared to c_2.

The discrete version of the anisotropic diffusion filter of Equation 29.13 is as follows:

$$I_{t+1}(x, y) = I_t + \frac{1}{4} \times [c_{N,t}(x, y)\nabla I_{N,t}(x, y) + c_{S,t}(x, y)\nabla I_{S,t}(x, y)$$
$$+ c_{E,t}(x, y)\nabla I_{E,t}(x, y) + c_{W,t}\nabla I_{W,t}(x, y)] \tag{29.17}$$

The four diffusion coefficients and gradients in Equation 29.17 correspond to four directions (i.e., North, South, East, and West) with respect to location (x, y). Each diffusion coefficient and the corresponding gradient are calculated in a similar manner. For example, the coefficient along the north direction is calculated as:

$$c_{N,t}(x, y) = \exp\left(\frac{-\nabla I_{N,t}^2(x, y)}{k^2}\right) \tag{29.18}$$

where $\nabla I_{N,t} = I_t(x, y + 1) - I_t(x, y)$.

Figure 29.7a,b show the original thermal image of skin tissue (wrist in this case) and its temperature surface plot respectively. One can observe in the surface plot the noisy ridges formed due to the hair. Figure 29.7c shows the filtered skin image. The hair has been removed from the surface, resulting into smoother ridges and heightened peaks in the temperature surface plot (Figure 29.7d).

As these figures testify anisotropic diffusion is highly beneficial in improving the contrast in the image and removing the noise. This is in preparation of vessel segmentation through morphological methods.

29.3.1.1 Image Morphology

Image morphology is a way of analyzing imagery based on shapes. It is rooted on set theory, the Minkowski operators, and DeMorgan's Laws. The Minkowski operators are usually applied to binary images where it

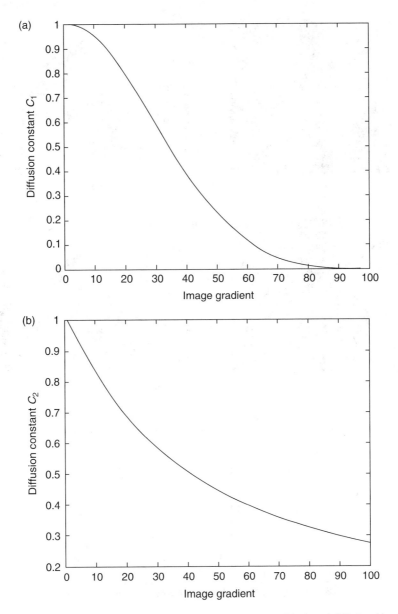

FIGURE 29.6 (a) Plot of diffusion function c_1 against the image gradient. (b) Plot of diffusion function c_2 against the image gradient.

is easy to perform OR and AND operations. The same operators can be applied to gray scale images with small modifications.

Image morphology is a simple but effective tool for shape analysis and segmentation. In retinotherapy it has shown great results in localization of blood vessels in the retina. Leandro et al. [29] have used morphological operators for vessel delineation in the retina where the background intensity was very close to that of the blood vessels. In our case, we have the blood vessels, which have a relatively low contrast compared to that of the surrounding tissue. As per our hypothesis the blood vessel is a tubule like structure running either along the length of the forearm or the face. Thus, our problem is to segment tubule structures from the image. We employ for this purpose a top-hat segmentation method, which is a combination of erosion and dilation operations.

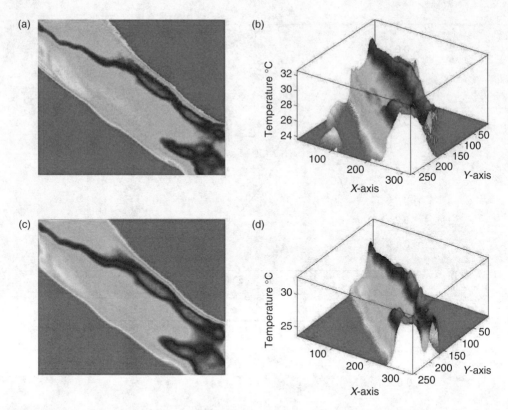

FIGURE 29.7 (See color insert.) (a) Original thermal image of a wrist. (b) Temperature surface plot of the original image. (c) Diffused thermal image of the wrist. (d) Temperature surface plot of the diffused image.

1	1	1
1	1	1
1	1	1

A 3×3 structuring element

0	0	1	0	0
0	1	1	1	0
1	1	1	1	1
0	1	1	1	0
0	0	1	0	0

A 5×5 structuring element

FIGURE 29.8 Structuring elements.

Erosion and dilation are the two most basic operations in mathematical morphology. Both of these operations take two pieces of data as input: an image to be eroded or dilated and a structuring element. The structuring element is similar to what we know as a kernel in the convolution operation. There are a variety of structuring elements available but a simple 3 × 3 square matrix is used more often. Figure 29.8 shows some commonly used structuring elements.

The combination of erosion and dilation results into more advanced morphological operations such as:

- Opening
- Closing
- Skeletonization

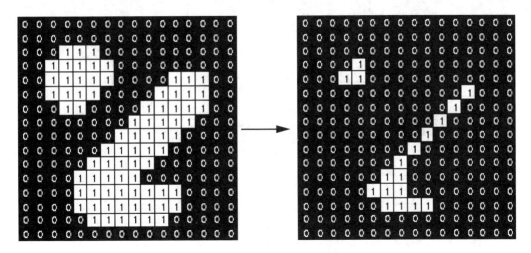

FIGURE 29.9 Binary erosion by a 3 × 3 flat structuring element.

- White top hat segmentation
- Black top hat segmentation

In our application, we are interested only in image opening and top hat segmentation.

1. *Erosion:* The name suggests that this operation erodes the boundary pixels of an image and thus, the resultant image has a shrunk boundary. Mathematically, it is defined as follows:

$$A \oplus B = \{z \mid (A \cap B)_z \subseteq B\} \tag{29.19}$$

Therefore, erosion removes elements smaller than the structuring element. Figure 29.9 shows a simple erosion operation performed on a binary image. Gray scale erosion with a flat structuring element generally darkens the image. Bright regions surrounded by dark regions shrink in size and dark regions surrounded by bright regions grow in size. Small bright spots in images disappear, as they are eroded away down to the surrounding intensity value. In contrast, small dark spots grow. The effect is most pronounced at places in the image where the intensity changes rapidly. Regions of fairly uniform intensity are left more or less unchanged except at their edges.

2. *Dilation:* The name suggests that this operation gradually expands the boundary pixels of an image and thus, the resultant image will have an enlarged boundary. Dilation results in fusing small holes in the boundary area, by enlarging the boundary pixels. This is the equivalent of a smoothing function. Mathematically, it is defined as follows:

$$A \oplus B = \{z \mid (\cap B)_z \cap A \neq \emptyset\} \tag{29.20}$$

Therefore, dilation fills in gaps smaller than the structuring element. Figure 29.10 shows a simple dilation operation performed on a binary image. Gray scale dilation with a flat structuring element generally brightens the image. Bright regions surrounded by dark regions grow in size and dark regions surrounded by bright regions shrink in size. Small dark spots in images disappear as they are "filled in" to the surrounding intensity values. In contrast, small bright spots will grow in size. The effect is most pronounced at places in the image where the intensity changes rapidly. Regions of fairly uniform intensity will be largely unchanged except at their edges.

3. *Opening:* The basic effect of an opening operation is reminiscent of erosion, since it tends to remove some of the foreground (bright) pixels at the edges. However, it is less destructive than erosion. The size and shape of the structuring element plays an important role in performing opening. The operation

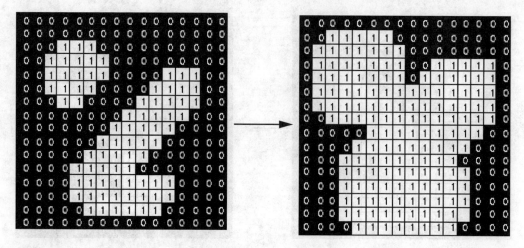

FIGURE 29.10 Binary dilation by a 3 × 3 flat structuring element.

preserves foreground regions that have a shape similar to its structuring element while erodes all other regions of foreground pixels. In mathematical terms opening can be written as:

$$A \circ B = (A \ominus B) \oplus B \quad \text{or} \quad A \circ B = \cup[(B)_z \mid (B)_z \subseteq A] \tag{29.21}$$

While erosion can be used to eliminate small clumps of undesirable foreground pixels (e.g., "salt noise") quite effectively, it has the disadvantage that it affects all foreground regions indiscriminately. Opening gets around this by performing both erosion and dilation on the image. The effect of opening can be visualized quite easily. Imagine taking the structuring element and sliding it inside each foreground region without changing its orientation. All foreground pixels that can be covered by the structuring element with the structuring element being entirely within the foreground region will be preserved. However, all foreground pixels which cannot be reached by the structuring element without parts of it moving out of the foreground region will be eroded away. After the opening has been carried out, the new boundaries of foreground regions will all be such that the structuring element fits inside them. Therefore, further openings with the same element have no effect, a property known as idempotence. The effect of an opening on a binary image using a 3 × 3 flat structuring element is illustrated in Figure 29.11.

4. *White Top Hat Segmentation:* Many times gray scale images feature poor contrast. For example, in our case thermal imagery of human tissue has poor contrast around the vessels due to the thermal diffusion process. As a result, image thresholding yields very poor results. Top-hat segmentation is a morphological operation that corrects this problem. Top hat segmentation has two forms:

- White top hat segmentation
- Black top hat segmentation

The white top-hat segmentation process enhances the bright objects in the image, while the black top-hat segmentation enhances the dark objects. In our case, we are interested in enhancing the bright (hot) ridge like structures corresponding to the blood vessels. Therefore, we are interested only in the white top-hat segmentation process. Two methods have been introduced for performing the white top hat segmentation. The first one proposed in Reference 30 is based on image opening using a flat structuring element, while the second one proposed in Reference 31 uses H-dome transformation. We have adopted the first method where the image is first opened and then this opened image is subtracted from the original image. This gives only the peaks in the image and thus enhances the maxima. The step by step evolution of the original image toward the top-hat segmented image is shown in Figure 29.12. The simple functioning of top-hat transformation can be understood from the line profile plots in Figure 29.13.

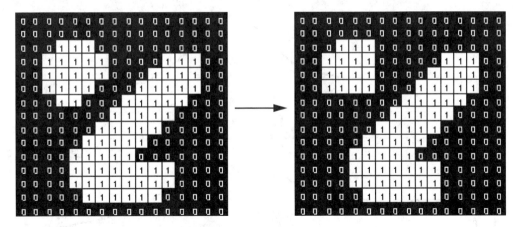

FIGURE 29.11   Binary opening by a 3 × 3 flat structuring element.

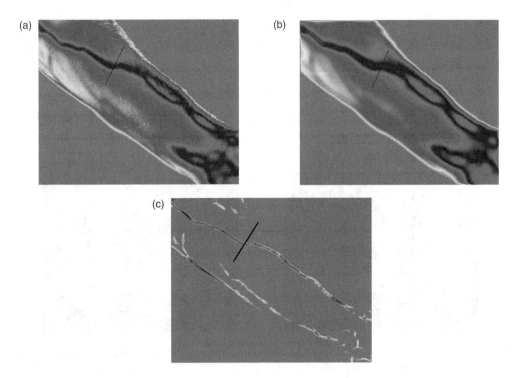

FIGURE 29.12   (See color insert.) Thermal image of a wrist: (a) original, (b) opened, and (c) top hat segmented.

29.4   Conclusion

We have outlined a novel approach to the problem of face recognition in thermal infrared. The cornerstones of the approach are a Bayesian face detection method followed by a physiological feature extractor. The face detector capitalizes upon the bimodal temperature distribution of human skin and typical indoor backgrounds. The physiological feature extractor delineates the facial vascular network based on a white top hat segmentation preceded by anisotropic diffusion (see Figure 29.14). These novel tools can be used

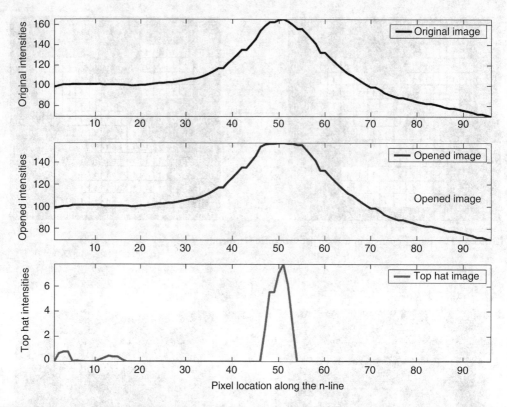

FIGURE 29.13   Image line profiles for (a) original, (b) opened, and (c) top-hat segmented image. The profiles were taken along the line shown in Figure 29.8.

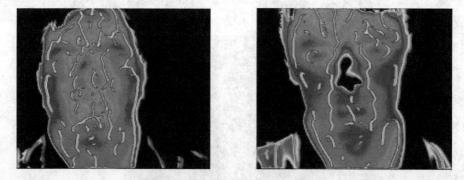

FIGURE 29.14   (See color insert.) Segmented facial images annotated with the facial vascular network (yellow lines) as per the approach detailed in this chapter.

in combination with traditional classification methods to exploit the full potential of thermal infrared for face recognition — one of the fastest growing biometrics.

Acknowledgments

Research related to the content of this chapter was supported by NSF grant #0313880 and ONR/DARPA grant #N00014-03-1-0622. The views expressed in this chapter do not necessarily represent the views of the funding Agencies.

References

[1] Jain, A., Bolle, R., Pankanti, S., and Jain, A.K., *Biometrics: Personal Identification in Networked Society*, 1st ed., Kluwer Academic Publishers, 1999.

[2] Zhao, W., Chellapa, R., Phillips, P.J., and Rosenfeld, A., Face recognition: a literature survey, *ACM Computing Surveys (CSUR)*, 35, 399, 2003.

[3] Pavlidis, I. and Symosek, P., The imaging issue in an automatic face/disguise detection system, in *Proceedings of the IEEE Workshop on Computer Vision Beyond the Visible Spectrum: Methods and Applications*, Hilton Head Island, South Carolina, 2000, p. 15.

[4] Wilder, J., Phillips, P., Jiang, C., and Wiener, S., Comparison of visible and infrared imagery for face recognition, in *Proceedings of the Second International Conference on Automatic Face and Gesture Recognition*, Killington, Vermont, 1996, p. 182.

[5] Socolinsky, D. and Selinger, A., A comparative analysis of face recognition performance with visible and thermal infrared imagery, in *Proceedings of the 16th International Conference on Pattern Recognition*, Vol. 4, Quebec, Canada, 2002, p. 217.

[6] Srivastava, A., Liu, X., Thomasson, B., and Hesher, C., Spectral probability models for IR images with applications to IR face recognition, in *Proceedings of the IEEE Workshop on Computer Vision Beyond the Visible Spectrum: Methods and Applications*, Kauai, Hawaii, 2001.

[7] Buddharaju, P., Pavlidis, I., and Kakadiaris, I., Face recognition in the thermal infrared spectrum, in *Proceedings of the Joint IEEE Workshop on Object Tracking and Classification Beyond the Visible Spectrum*, Washington D.C., 2004.

[8] Socolinsky, D., Wolff, L., Neuheiser, J., and Evelenad, C., Illumination invariant face recognition using thermal infrared imagery, in *Proceedings of the IEEE Computer Society Conference on Computer Vision and Pattern Recognition*, Vol. 1, Kauai, Hawaii, 2001, p. 527.

[9] Cutler, R., Face recognition using infrared images and eigenfaces, http://www.cs.umd.edu/rgc/face/face.htm, 1996.

[10] Niki, N., Kawata, Y., Satoh, H., and Kumazaki, T., 3D imaging of blood vessels using x-ray rotational angiographic system, in *Proceedings of the IEEE Nuclear Science Symposium and Medical Imaging Conference*, Vol. 3, San Francisco, California, 1993, p. 1873.

[11] Kawata, Y., Niki, N., and Kumazaki, T., Characteristics measurement for blood vessels diseases detection based on cone-beam CT images, in *Proceedings of the IEEE Nuclear Science Symposium and Medical Imaging Conference*, Vol. 3, 1995, p. 1660.

[12] Parker, D.L., Wu, J., and van Bree, R.E., Three-dimensional vascular reconstruction from projections: a theoretical review, in *Proceedings of the IEEE Engineering in Medicine and Biology Society Conference*, Vol. 1, New Orleans, 1998, p. 399.

[13] Aylward, S., Pizer, S., Bullit, E., and Eberl, D., Intensity ridge and widths for tubular object segmentation and registration, in *Proceedings of the Workshop on Mathematical Methods in Biomedical Image Analysis*, 1996, p. 131.

[14] Aylward, S. and Bullitt, E., Analysis of parameter space of a metric for registering 3D vascular images, *MICCAI*, 2001.

[15] Bullitt, E. and Aylward, S.R., Analysis of time-varying images using 3D vascular models, *Applied Imagery Pattern Recognition Works*, 2001, p. 9.

[16] Jones, T. and Metaxas, D., Image segmentation based on the integration of pixel affinity and deformable models, in *Proceedings of the IEEE Computer Society Conference on Computer Vision and Pattern Recognition*, Santa Barbara, California, 1998, p. 330.

[17] Pednekar, A.S. and Kakadiaris, I.A., Applications of virtual reality in surgery, in *Proceedings of the Indian Conference on Computer Vision, Graphics, and Image Processing*, Bangalore, India, 2000, p. 215.

[18] O'Brien, J.F. and Exquerra, N.F., Automated segmentation of coronary vessels in angiographic image sequences utilizing temporal, spatial, and structural constraints, in *Proceedings of the SPIE Visualisation Conference in Biomedical Computing*, 1994.

[19] Schmitt, H., Grass, M., Rasche, V., Schramm, O., Haehnel, S., and Sartor, K., An x-ray based method for determination of the contrast agent propagation ub in 3D vessel structures, *IEEE Transactions on Medical Imaging*, 21, 251, 2002.

[20] Krissian, K., Malandain, G., and Ayache, N., Directional Anisotropic Diffusion Applied to Segmentation of Vessels in 3D Images, Technical Report 3064, INRIA, 1996.

[21] Perona, P. and Malik, J., Scale-space and edge detection using anisotropic diffusion, *IEEE Transactions on Pattern Analysis and Machine Intelligence*, 12, 629, 2003.

[22] Sato, Y., Nakjima, S., Shiraga, N., Atsumi, H., Yoshida, S., Kikker, T., Greig, G., and Kikinis, R., 3D multiscale line filter for segmentation and visualization of curvilinear structures in medical images, *IEEE Medical Image Analysis*, 2, 143, 1998.

[23] Poli, R. and Valli, G., An algorithm for real-time vessel enhancement and detection, *Computer Methods and Programming in Biomedicine*, 52, 1, 1997.

[24] Acton, S.T., Bovik, A.C., and Crawford, M.M., Anisotropic diffusion pyramids for image segmentation, in *Proceedings of the IEEE International Conference on Image Processing*, Vol. 3, Austin, Texas, 1994, p. 478.

[25] Acton, S.T., Edge enhancement of infrared imagery by way of the anisotropic diffusion pyramid, in *Proceedings of the IEEE International Conference on Image Processing*, Vol. 1, Laussane, Switzerland, 1996, p. 865.

[26] Gerig, G., Kubler, O., Kikinis, R., and Jolesz, F.A., Nonlinear anisotropic filtering of MRI data, *IEEE Transactions on Medical Imaging*, 11, 221, 1992.

[27] Sapiro, G. and Tannenbaum, A., Edge Preserving Geometric Smoothing of MRI Data, Technical Report, University of Minnesota, Department of Electrical Engineering, April 1994.

[28] Nordstrom, N., Biased anisotropic diffusion — a unified generalization and diffusion approach to edge detection, *Image and Vision Computing*, 8, 318, 1990.

[29] Leandro, J., Cesar, R.M. Jr., and Jelinek, H., Blood vessel segmentation in retina: preliminary assessment of the mathematical morphology and wavelet transform techniques, *14th Brazilian Symposium on Computer Graphics and Image Processing*, 2001, p. 84.

[30] Dougherty, E.R., Euclidean gray-scale granulometries: representation and umbra inducement, *Journal of Mathematical Imaging and Vision*, 1, 7, 1992.

[31] Vincent, L., Morphological grayscale reconstruction in image analysis: application and efficient algorithms, *IEEE Transactions on Image Processing*, 2, 176, 1993.

(a)

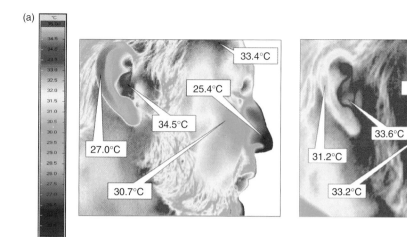

(b)

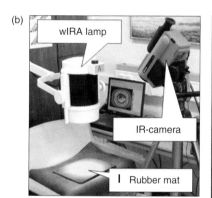

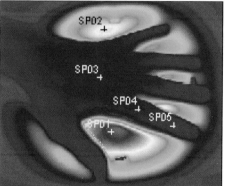

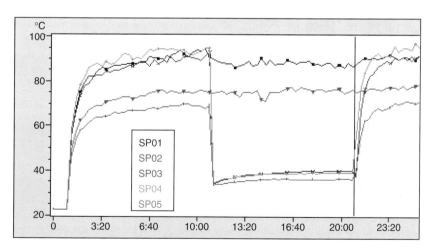

FIGURE 21.1 (a) A Thermogram of a healthy 52-year-old male subject in a cold environment (ca. 15°C; left panel) and in a warm environment (ca. 25°C; right panel). In the cold environment arteriovenous anastomoses in the nose and the auricle region of the ears are closed, resulting in low skin temperatures at these sites. Also note reduced blood flow in the cheeks but not on the forehead, where the blood vessels in the skin are unable to vasoconstrict. (b) Efficiency of skin blood flow as a heat transporter. The photograph in the upper left panel shows a rubber mat being heated with a water-filtered infrared-A irradiator at high intensity (400 mW/cm^2) for a period of 20 min. In the lower panel the time course of surface temperature of the mat at five selected spots as measured by an IR-camera is given. During the last 10 min of the 20-min heating period the left hand of a healthy 54-year-old male subject was placed on the mat. Note that skin surface temperature of the hand remains below 39°C.

(a) 30 min equilibration in cool environment (20°C, 30% rh)

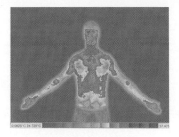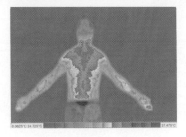

30 min equilibration in warm environment (41°C, 30% rh)

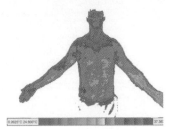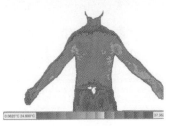

Range of temperature (°C) within regions at two climatic conditions.

	Anterior torso	Posterior torso	Anterior arms	Posterior arms	Palmer hands	Dorsal hands
Cool 20°C	5.0	5.1	6.3	4.5	5.2	4.0
Warm 41°C	3.0	3.2	3.2	3.6	4.0	3.5

(b)

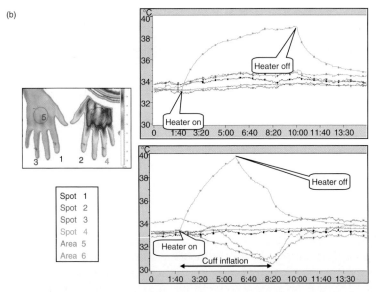

FIGURE 21.2 (a) A The thermoregulatory response of the torso when exposed to a cool or warm environment. Note the heterogeneous temperature distribution in the cool environment as opposed to the more homogeneous temperature distribution in the warm environment. Different colors represent different temperatures. One might recognize the difficulty related to choosing one point (thermocouple data) as the reference value in a region. (b) Skin heating with and without intact circulation in a 65-year-old healthy male subject. The two panels on the right show the time course of 6 selected measuring sites (4 spot measurements and 2 area measurements) of skin temperatures as determined by IR-thermography before, during, and after a period in which the skin surface on the back of the left hand was heated with a water-filtered infrared-A irradiator at high intensity (400 mW/cm^2) in two separate experiments. The results shown in the upper right panel were performed under a situation with a normal intact blood circulation, while the results shown in the lower left panel were made during total occlusion of circulation in the right arm by means of an inflated pressure cuff placed around the upper arm. The time of occlusion is indicated. The IR-thermogram on the left was taken just prior to the end of the heating period in the experiment described in the upper panel. The location of the temperature measurement sites on the hand (4 spot measurements [Spot 1–Spot 4] and the average temperature within a circle [Area 5 and Area 6]) are indicated in on the thermogram.

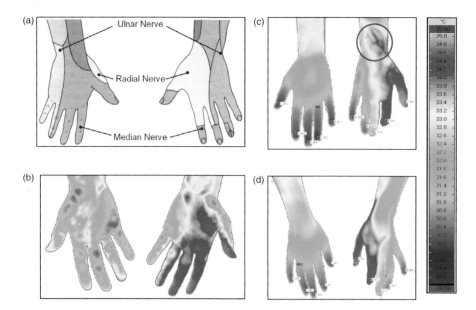

FIGURE 21.3 (a) The distribution of cutaneous nerves to the hand. (b) IR-thermogram of a 40-year-old female patient following a successful nerve block of the left median nerve. (c and d) IR-thermograms of the hands of a 36-year-old female patient whose left wrist (middle of the red circle) was punctured with a sharp object resulting in partial nerve damage (motor and sensory loss). The strong vasodilatory response resulting from partially severed nerves can be easily seen.

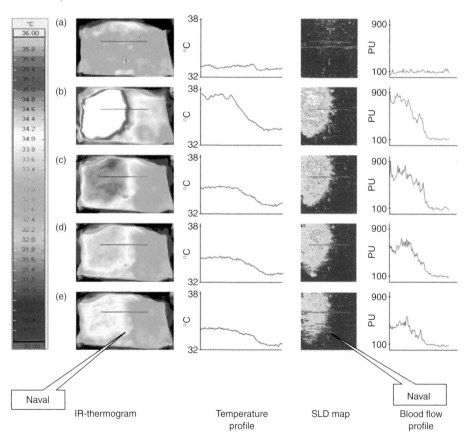

FIGURE 21.4 IR-thermograms, temperature profiles, scanning laser Doppler scans (SLD), and blood flow profiles (perfusion units PU) of the abdominal area of a 44-year-old healthy female subject before (a), immediately after (b), and 5 min (c), 10 min (d) and 20 min (e) after a 20 min heating of the right side of the abdomen with a water-filtered infrared-A irradiation lamp. The blue horizontal lines in the IR-thermograms indicate the position of the temperature profiles. The red horizontal lines in the SLD scans indicate the position of the blood flow profiles. In IR-thermogram (b) the white color indicates skin temperatures greater than 36°C.

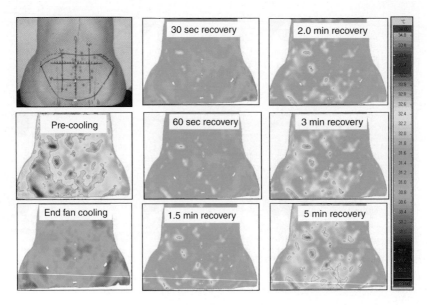

FIGURE 21.5 Abdominal cooling in a 32-year-old female patient prior to breast reconstruction surgery. In this procedure skin and fat tissue from the abdominal area was used to reconstruct a new breast. The localization of suitable perforating vessels for reconnection to the mammary artery is an important part of the surgical procedure. In this sequence of thermograms the patient was first subjected to a mild cooling of the abdominal skin (2 min fan cooling). IR-thermograms of the skin over the entire abdominal area were taken prior to, immediately after, and at various time intervals during the recovery period following the cooling period. To help highlight the perforating vessels an outline function has been employed in which all skin areas having a temperature greater than 32.5°C are enclosed in solid lines.

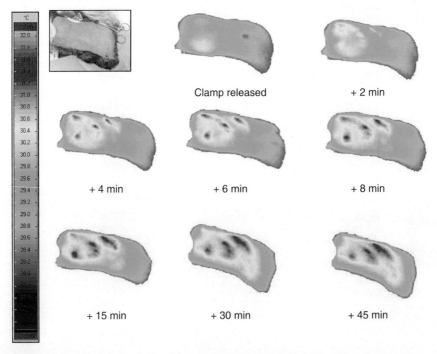

FIGURE 21.6 Infrared thermal images of an abdominal skin flap during breast reconstruction surgery. The sequence of IR-thermal images demonstrates the return of heat to the excised skin flap following reestablishing its blood supply (anastomizing of a mammary artery and vein to a single branch of the deep inferior epigastric artery and a concomitant vein). Prior to this procedure the excised skin flap had been without a blood supply for about 50 min and consequently cooled down. The photograph in the upper left panel shows the skin flap in position on the chest wall prior to being shaped into a new breast.

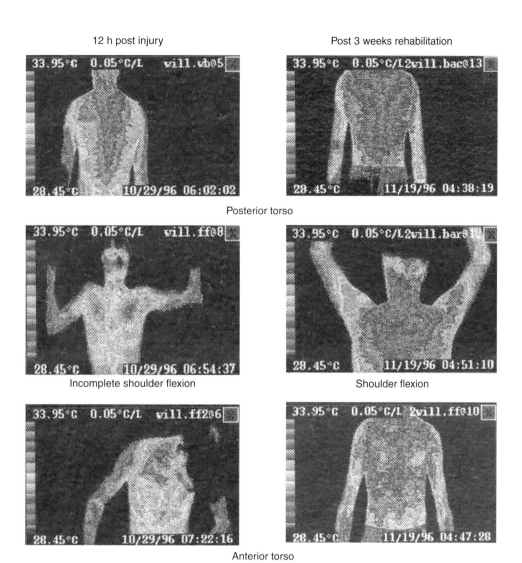

FIGURE 21.7 An American football player who suffered a helmet impact to the right shoulder (left side of image). The athlete was unable to flex his arm above shoulder level. Note the asymmetrical torso pattern in the posterior torso.

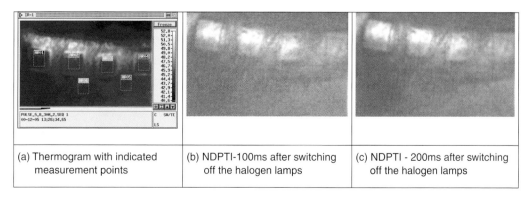

FIGURE 22.13 Classical thermogram (a) and PT normalized differential thermography index pictures of burns (b) and (c).

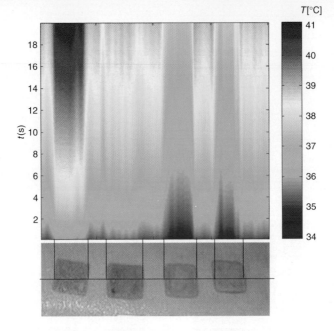

FIGURE 22.16 Thermal transients of burn fields of degree: I, IIa, IIb, IIb.

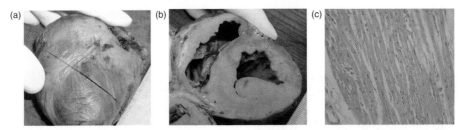

FIGURE 22.18 Pig's heart after heart infarct evoked by the indicated clamp (a), the cross section of the heart with visible area of the stroke (the necrosis of the left ventricle wall — under the finger — is evidenced by darker shadow) (b) and the micro-histopathologic picture showing the cell necrosis (c).

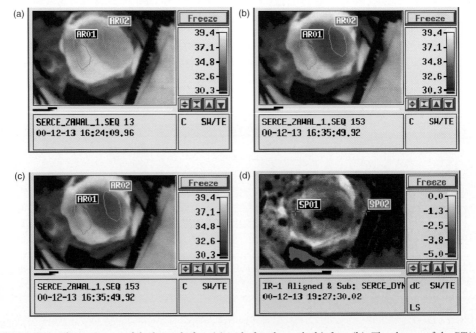

FIGURE 22.19 Thermograms of the heart: before (a) and after the evoked infarct (b). The change of the PT/ADT pictures in time (indicated in the subscript of the thermogram) 0.5 h after the LAD clamping (the tissue is still alive) (c) and 3 h later (the necrosis is evidenced by the change of thermal properties of the tissue) (d).

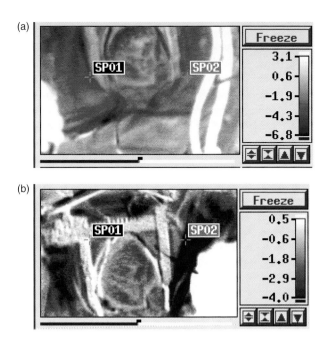

FIGURE 22.21 ADT picture of clinical intervention — before the CABG (a) and after the operation (b). Important is more uniform temperature distribution after the operation proving that intervention was fully successful.

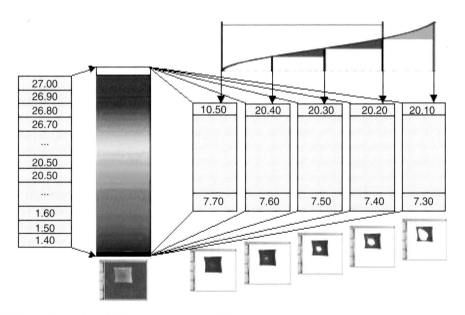

FIGURE 23.3 Simulation of slicing operation on pork fat.

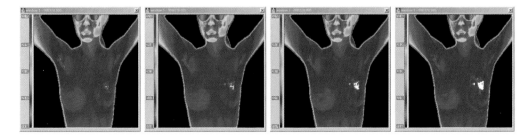

FIGURE 23.4 Slicing of patient with lobular carcinoma in the left breast.

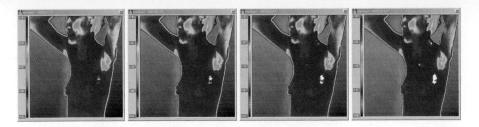

FIGURE 23.5 Slicing of patient with ductal carcinoma in the left breast.

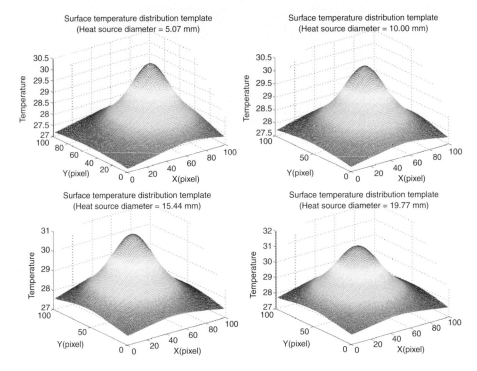

FIGURE 23.9 Surface temperature distribution templates.

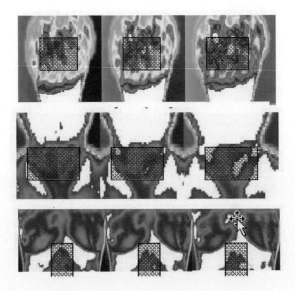

FIGURE 23.10 Endocrine logical triple images of breast. From top to bottom, three signatures of the endocrine logical triple.

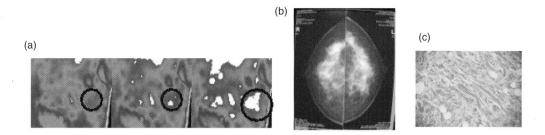

FIGURE 23.11 Benign bumps compared between TTM and MMT, confirmed by pathology. (a) TTM image of January 16, 2004 indicates the slices of abnormal thermo-source in the out-upper quadrant on left breast. These slices of thermo-source show the regular morphology and less vascular. (b) MMT image of January 16, 2004 shows a 0.6 × 0.5 cm, clear-edged lump in the outboard on the left breast. (c) Pathology diagnosis of fatty tumor.

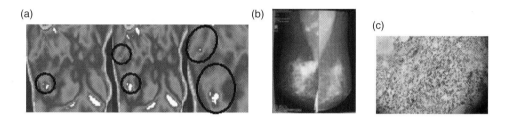

FIGURE 23.12 Malignant bumps compared between TTM and MMT, confirmed by pathology. (a) TTM image of February 4, 2004 indicates the slices of abnormal breast thermo-source that were of irregular morphology, more vascular and higher heat values accompanied with swollen auxiliary lymph node. (b) MMT image taken on February 4, 2004 shows a blurred boundary mass with sand-grained calcification in the outboard on the right breast. (c) Pathology is infiltrated duct carcinoma.

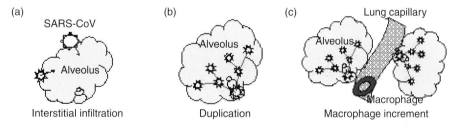

FIGURE 23.13 SARS-CoV infection stages.

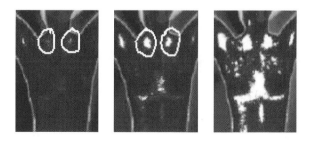

FIGURE 23.14 TTM slicing of normal case.

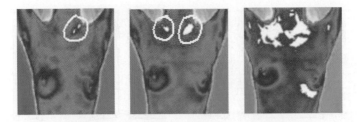

FIGURE 23.15   TTM slicing of lung TB condition.

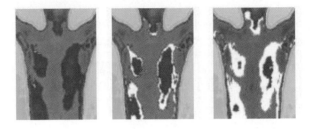

FIGURE 23.16   TTM slicing of SARS patient 1.

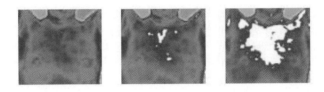

FIGURE 23.17   TTM slicing of SARS patient 2.

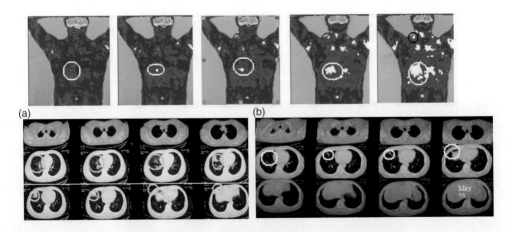

FIGURE 23.18   Comparison between CT and TTM in SARS diagnosis — TTM image of May 23, 2003 indicates the abnormal heat pattern of lower right lung lesion which is confirmed by the CT image of the same date. First row: TTM slicing shows the abnormal heat pattern with the depth of heat source 6 cm from skin surface; in addition, the subclavian area has a lower temperature than that of the right lung. Second row: (a) CT image of April 26, 2003 showed right lung lesion of SARS progress stage; (b) CT image of May 23, 2003 showed right lung lesion of SARS recovery stage.

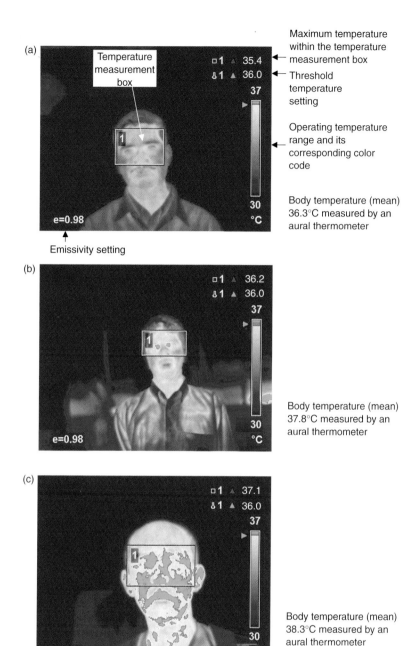

FIGURE 24.1   Examples of temperature profiles using thermal imager with temperature readings.

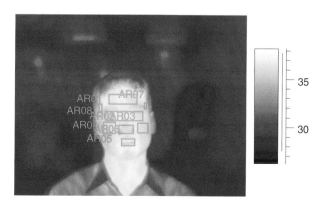

FIGURE 24.5   Processed thermal image of the frontal profile.

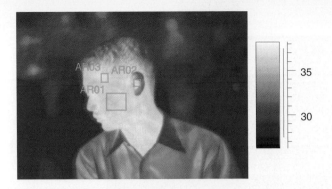

FIGURE 24.6 Processed thermal images of the side profile.

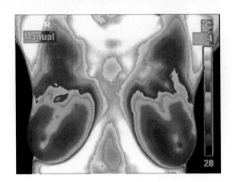

FIGURE 25.1 Bilateral frontal.

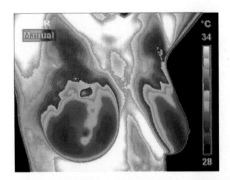

FIGURE 25.2 Right oblique.

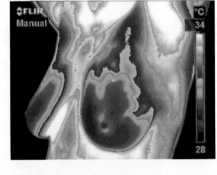

FIGURE 25.3 Left oblique.

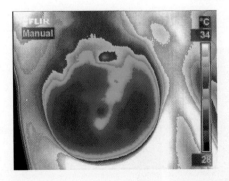

FIGURE 25.4 Right close-up.

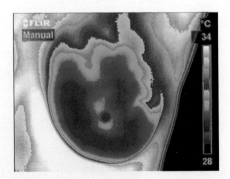

FIGURE 25.5 Left close-up.

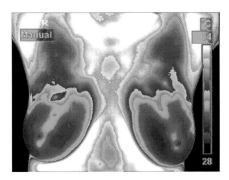

FIGURE 25.6 TH1 (Normal non-vascular).

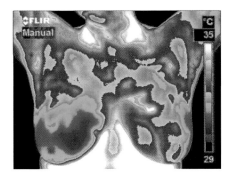

FIGURE 25.7 Left TH5 (Severely Abnormal).

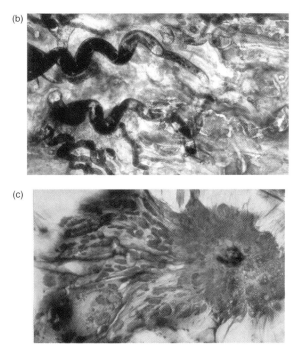

FIGURE 26.2 (b) High nuclear grade ductal carcinoma *in situ* with numerous blood vessels (angiogenesis) (Tabar).
(c) Invasive ductal carcinoma with central necrosis and angiogenesis (Tabar).

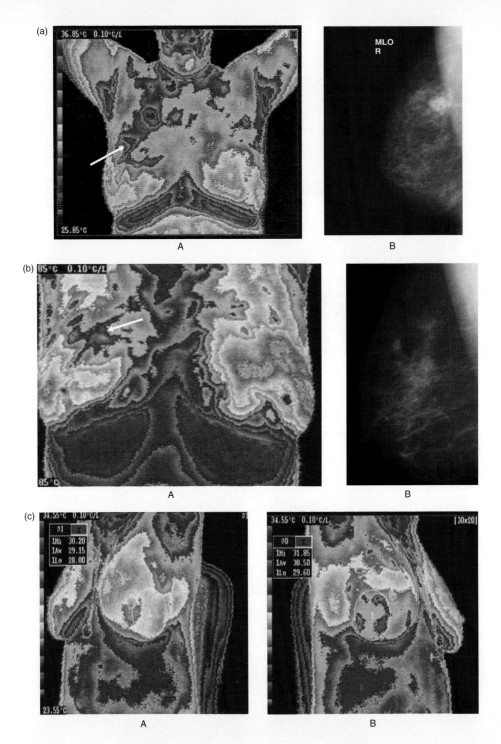

FIGURE 26.4 (a) A 46-year old patient: Lump in the upper central area of the right breast. *Infrared imaging* (A): Significant vascular asymmetry (SVA) in the upper central area of the right breast (IR-3). *Mammography* (B): Corresponding speculated opacity. *Surgical histology*: 2 cm infiltrating ductal carcinoma with negative sentinel nodes. (b) A 44-year old patient. *Infrared imaging* (A): Revealed a significant vascular asymmetry in the upper central and inner quadrants of the right breast with a ΔT of 1.8°C (IR-4.8). *Corresponding mammography* (B): Reveals a spiculated lesion in the upper central portion of the right breast. *Surgical histology*: 0.7 cm infiltrating ductal carcinoma. Patient underwent adjuvant brachytherapy. (c) A 52-year old patient presented with a mild fullness in the lower outer quadrant of the right breast. *Infrared imaging* (A): Left breast (B): right breast reveals extensive significant vascular asymmetry with a ΔT of 1.35°C (IR-5.3). A 2 cm cancer was found in the lower outer area of the right breast.

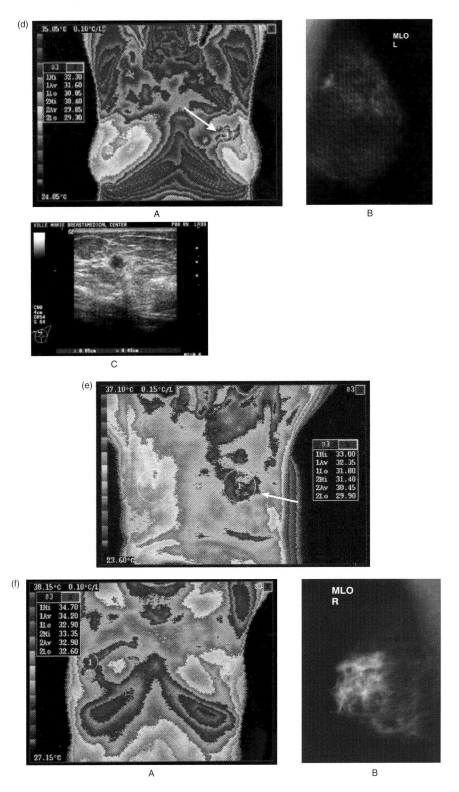

FIGURE 26.4 (d) A 37-year old patient. *Infrared image* (A): Significant vascular asymmetry in the upper inner quadrant of the left breast with a ΔT of 1.75°C (IR-4) (mod IR-4.75). *Mammography* (B): Corresponding spiculated lesion. *Ultrasound* (C): 6 mm lesion. *Surgical histology*: 0.7 cm infiltrating ductal carcinoma. (e) An 82-year old patient. *Infrared imaging anterior view*: Significant vascular asymmetry and a ΔT of 1.90°C (IR-4) in the left subareolar area. *Corresponding mammography*: (not included) asymmetrical density in the left areolar area. *Surgical histology*: Left subareolar 1 cm infiltrating ductal carcinoma. (f) A 34-year old patient with a palpable fullness in the supra-areolar area of the right breast. *Infrared imaging* (A): Extensive significant vascular asymmetry and a ΔT of 1.3°C in the right supra areolar area (IR-4) (mod IR-5.3). *Mammography* (B): Scattered and clustered central microcalcifications. *Surgical histology*: After total right mastectomy and TRAM flap: multifocal DCIS and infiltrating ductal CA centered over a 3 cm area of the supra areolar area.

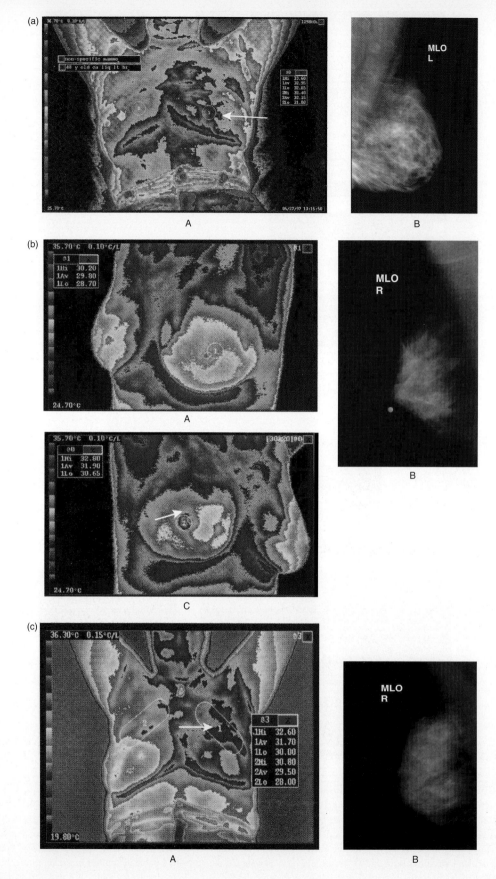

FIGURE 26.5

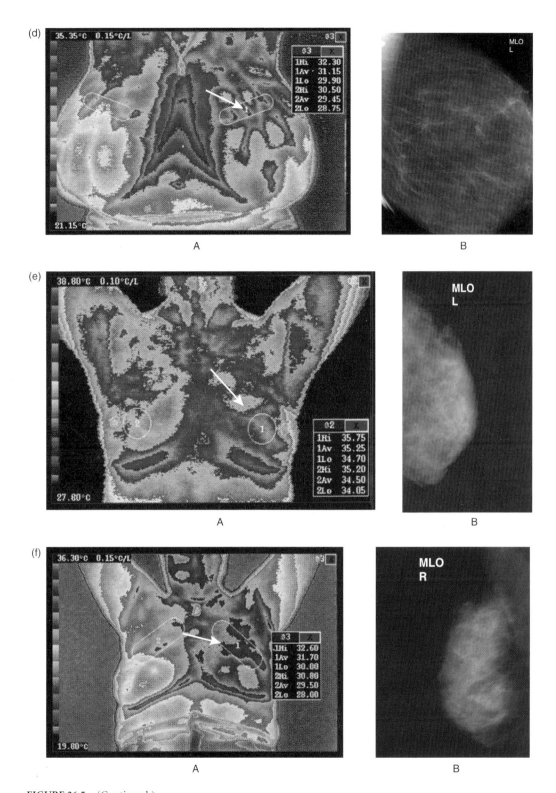

(d)

θ3	X
1Hi	32.30
1Av	31.15
1Lo	29.90
2Hi	30.50
2Av	29.45
2Lo	28.75

35.35°C 0.15°C/L

21.15°C

MLO
L

A   B

(e)

θ2	X
1Hi	35.75
1Av	35.25
1Lo	34.70
2Hi	35.20
2Av	34.50
2Lo	34.05

38.80°C 0.10°C/L

27.80°C

MLO
L

A   B

(f)

θ3	X
1Hi	32.60
1Av	31.70
1Lo	30.00
2Hi	30.80
2Av	29.50
2Lo	28.00

36.30°C 0.15°C/L

19.80°C

MLO
R

A   B

FIGURE 26.5 (Continued.)

(g)

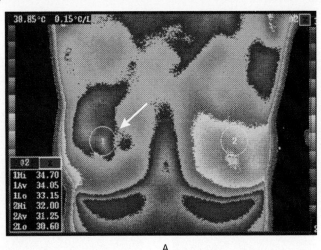

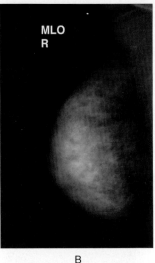

A

B

FIGURE 26.5 (a) A 48-year old patient *Infrared imaging* (A): Significant vascular asymmetry and a ΔT of 0.8°C (IR-3) in the lower inner quadrant of the left breast. *Corresponding mammography* (B): A nonspecific density. *Surgical histology:* 1.6 cm left lower inner quadrant infiltrating ductal carcinoma. (b) A 40-year old patient. *Infrared imaging* (A): left breast (B) right breast: focal hot spot in the right subareolar area on a background of increased vascular activity with a ΔT of 1.1°C (IR-4). *Corresponding mammography* (C): Reveals dense tissue bilaterally. *Surgical histology:* reveals a 1 cm right infiltrating ductal carcinoma and positive lymph nodes. (c) A 51-year old patient. *Infrared imaging* (A): Significant vascular asymmetry and a ΔT of 2.2°C (IR-5) in the upper central area of the left breast. *Corresponding mammography* (B): Mild scattered densities. *Surgical histology:* 2.5 cm infiltrating ductal carcinoma in the upper central area of the left breast. (d) A 44-year old patient. *Infrared imaging* (A): Significant vascular asymmetry and a ΔT of 1.58°C (IR-4) in the upper inner quadrant of the left breast. *Corresponding mammography* (B): A nonspecific corresponding density. *Surgical histology:* A 0.9 cm left upper inner quadrant infiltrating ductal carcinoma. (e) A 45-year old patient with a nodule in central area of left breast. *Infrared imaging* (A): Extensive significant vascular asymmetry (SVA) in the central inner area of the left breast with a ΔT of 0.75°C (IR-3) (mod IR-4.75). *Mammography* (B): Non-contributory. *Surgical histology:* 1.5 cm infiltrating ductal carcinoma with necrosis in the central inner area and 3 + axillary nodes. (f) A 51-year old patient. *Infrared imaging* (A): Extensive significant vascular asymmetry and a ΔT of 2.2° (IR-5) (mod IR-6.2) in the upper central area of the left breast. *Corresponding mammography* (B) scattered densities. *Surgical histology:* 2.5 cm infiltrating ductal carcinoma in the upper central area of the left breast. (g) A 74-year old patient. *Infrared imaging* (A): significant vascular asymmetry in the upper central portion of the right breast with a ΔT of 2.8°C (IR-5) (Mod VM IR: 6.8). *Corresponding mammography* (B): Bilateral extensive density. *Surgical histology:* 1 cm right central quadrant infiltrating ductal carcinoma.

(a)

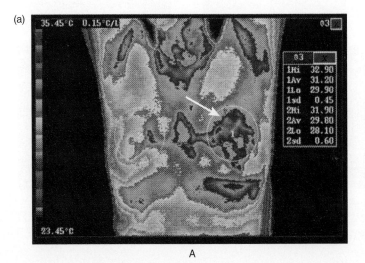

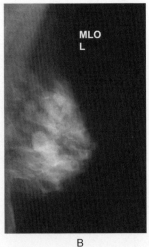

A

B

FIGURE 26.6 (Continued.)

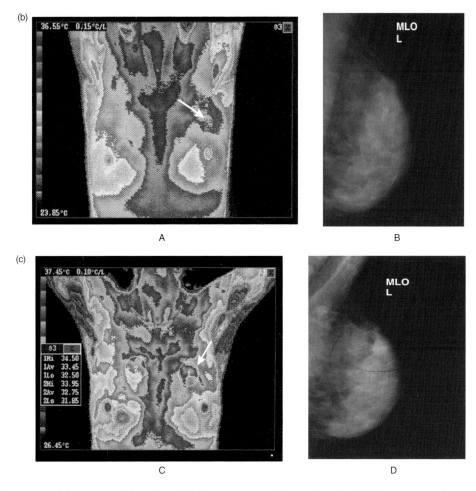

FIGURE 26.6 (a) A 66-year old patient. Initially seen 2 years prior to diagnosis of left breast cancer for probable fibrocystic disorder (FCD) and scattered cysts, mostly on the left side. *Initial infrared imaging* (A): Extensive significant vascular asymmetry left breast and a near global ΔT of 1.4°C (IR-4) (Mod IR: 5.4). *Initial mammography* (B): Scattered opacities and ultrasound and cytologies were consistent with FCD. Two years later a 1.7 cm cancer was found in the central portion of the left breast. (b) A 49-year old patient. *Infrared imaging* 1997 (A): Significant vascular asymmetry in the upper central aspect of the left breast (IR-3) *Corresponding mammography* 1997 (B): Dense tissue (contd. 6B2) (c) Patient presents 2 years later with a lump in the upper central portion of the left breast. *Corresponding infrared imaging* (C): Still reveals significant vascular asymmetry and a ΔT of 0.7°C (IR-3) (Mod VM IR″: 3.7). *Corresponding mammography* (D): Now reveals an opacity in the upper aspect of the left breast. *Surgical histology*: 1 cm infiltrating ductal carcinoma.

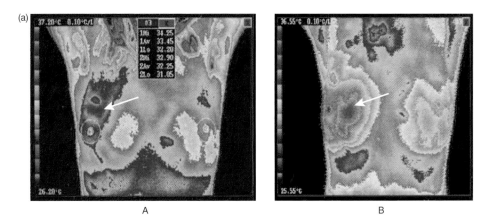

FIGURE 26.7 (Continued.)

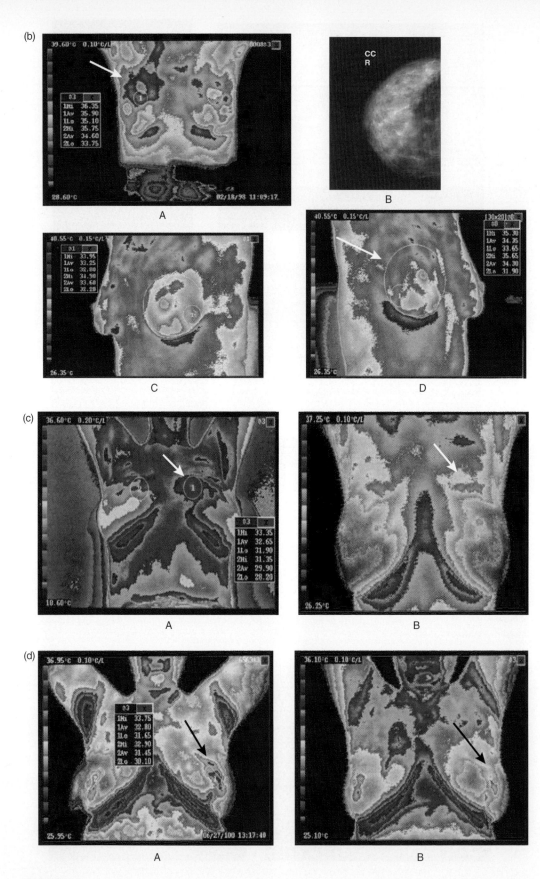

FIGURE 26.7

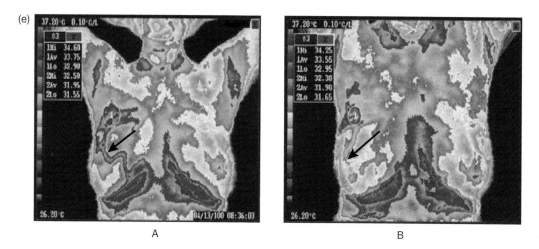

(e)

FIGURE 26.7 (a) A 52-year old patient. *Infrared imaging* (A): Extensive vascular asymmetry (SVA) in the right breast with a ΔT of 1.2°C (IR-5.2). The patient was started on pre-operative chemotherapy (PCT). *Post-PCT infrared imaging* (B): Resolution of previously noted SVA (IR-2). *Surgical histology:* no residual carcinoma in the resected right breast specimen. (b) A 32-year old patient. *Infrared imaging* (A): Extensive significant vascular asymmetry and tortuous vascular pattern and a ΔT of 1.3°C (IR-5.3) in the right breast. *Corresponding mammography* (B): Scattered densities. Patient was started on pre-operative chemotherapy (PCT). *Post-PCT infrared image* (C — left breast; D — right breast): Notable resolution of SVA, with a whole breast ΔT of 0.7°C (IR-2). *Surgical histology:* No residual right carcinoma and chemotherapy induced changes. (c) A 47-year old patient. *Infrared imaging* (A): Extensive significant vascular asymmetry in the inner half of the left breast with a ΔT of 2°C (IR-6.0). The patient was started on pre-operative chemotherapy (PCT). *Post-PCT infrared imaging* (B): no residual asymmetry (IR-1). *Surgical histology:* No viable residual carcinoma, with chemotherapy induced dense fibrosis surrounding nonviable tumor cells. (d) A 56-year old patient. *Pre-chemotherapy infrared imaging* (A): Significant vascular asymmetry overlying the central portion of the left breast with a ΔT of 1.35°C (IR-4.35). The patient was given pre-operative chemotherapy (PCT). *Post-PCT infrared* (C): mild bilateral vascular symmetry (IR-). *Surgical histology:* no residual tumor. (e) A 54-year old patient. *Infrared image* (A): extensive significant vascular asymmetry right breast with a rT of 2.8°C (IR-6.8). Received pre-operative chemotherapy (PCT). *Post-PCT infrared* (B): Mild local residual vascular asymmetry with a rT of 1.65°C (IR-3.65). *Surgical pathology:* No residual viable carcinoma.

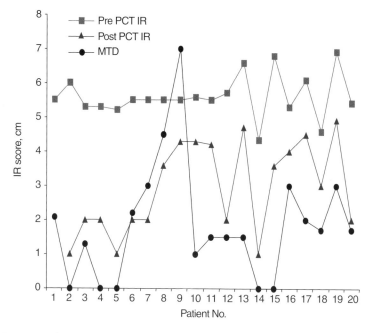

FIGURE 26.8 Pre-PCT and Post-PCT IR Score and Histological Maximum tumor dimension (MTD).

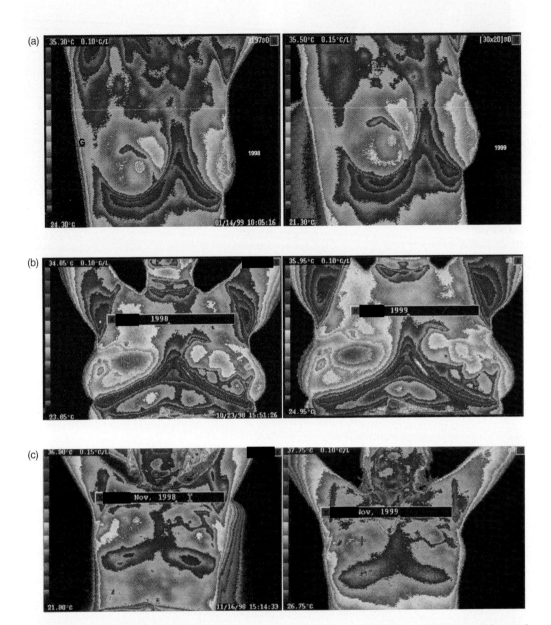

FIGURE 26.9 (a) A stable vascular distribution in the lower inner quadrant of the left breast over a 12-month period. *Infrared imaging* of the breast usually remains remarkably stable in the absence of any on going developing significant pathology. It is important in grading these images to determine if the findings are to be considered evolving and important or stable and possibly relating to the patient's vascular anatomy. (b) An identical vascular distribution of the left breast over a 12-month period. (c) A stable vascular distribution in both breasts over a 12-month period.

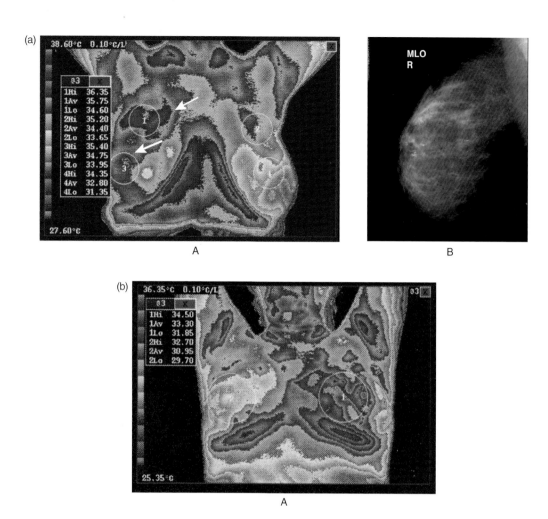

FIGURE 26.10 (a) A 50-year old patient. *Infrared imaging* (A): Significant vascular asymmetry and a ΔT of 3.4°C (IR-5) in the right breast. *Corresponding mammography* (B): Increased density and microcalcifications in the right breast. Surgical histology: extensive right multifocal infiltrating ductal carcinoma requiring a total mastectomy. (b) A 50-year old patient. *Infrared imaging* (A): Significant vascular asymmetry with a near global ΔT of 2.35°C in the left breast (IR-5). *Mammography* (not available) diffuse density. *Surgical histology*: Left multi-focal infiltrating ductal carcinoma requiring a total mastectomy.

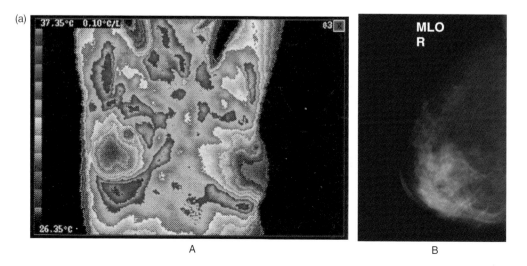

FIGURE 26.11 (Continued.)

(b)

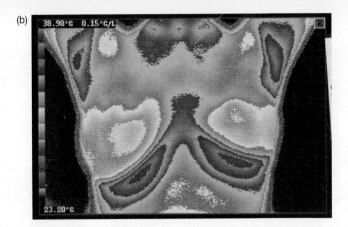

FIGURE 26.11 (a) Four years post right partial mastectomy, the patient is recurrence free. Current *Infrared imaging* (A): shows no activity and *Mammography* (B): shows scar tissue. (b) *Infrared image*, 5 years following a left partial mastectomy and radiotherapy for carcinoma revealing slight asymmetry of volume, but no abnormal vascular abnormality and resolution of radiation-induced changes. The patient is disease free.

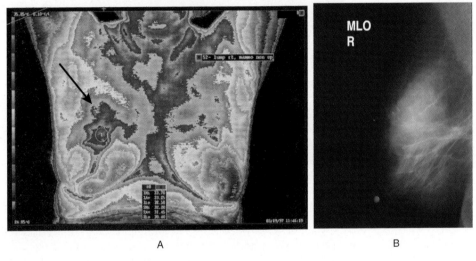

A   B

FIGURE 26.12 A 52-year old patient, 5 years following right partial mastectomy, radiation, and chemotherapy for right breast cancer. Recent follow-up Infrared Imaging (A) now reveals significant vascular asymmetry (SVA) in the right breast with a ΔT of 1.5°C in the area of the previous surgery (IR-4). *Corresponding mammography* (B): Density and scar issue vs. possible recurrence. *Surgical histology*: 4 cm, recurrent right carcinoma in the area of the previous resection.

(a)

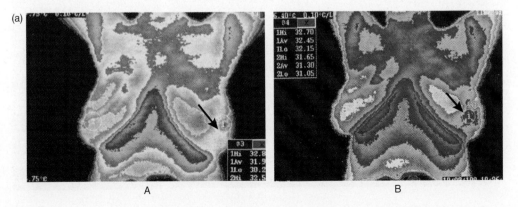

A   B

FIGURE 26.13 (Continued.)

(b)

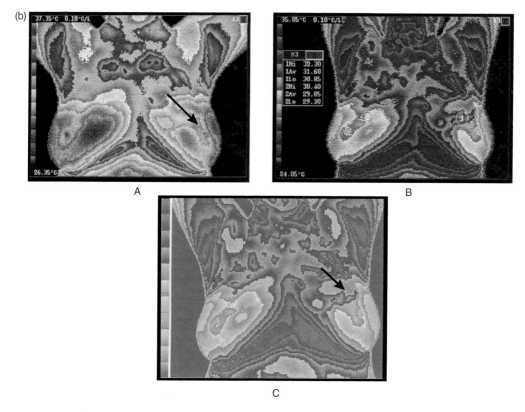

A

B

C

FIGURE 26.13 (a) A 45-year old patient with small nodular process just inferior and medial to the left nipple areolar complex. *Infrared imaging* (A), without digital enhancement, was carried out and circles were placed on the nipple area rather than just below and medial to it. The nonenhanced IR image was thus initially misinterpreted as normal with a ΔT of 0.25°C. The same image was recalled and *repeated* (B), now with appropriate digital enhancement and once again, documented the presence of increased vascular activity just inferior and medial to the left nipple areolar complex with a ΔT of 1.15°C (IR-4.15). A 1.5 cm. cancer was found just below the left nipple. (b) A 37-year old patient with lump in the upper inner quadrant of the left breast. Mammography confirms spiculated mass. *Infrared imaging* (A): Reported as "normal." Infrared imaging was repeated after appropriate *digital adjustment* (B): Now reveals obvious significant vascular asymmetry in the same area and a ΔT of 1.75°C (Ir-4) (mod IR-4.75). Using a different IR camera on the *same patient* (C) confirms same finding. *Surgical histology*: 1.5 cm infiltrating ductal CA.

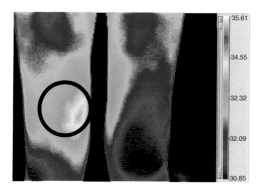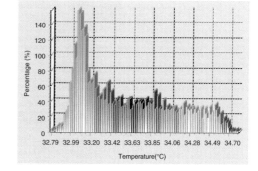

FIGURE 28.1 ROI of thermal image and its histogram.

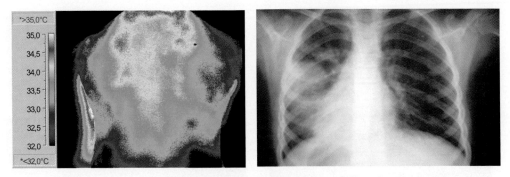

FIGURE 28.2 Nonsymmetrical temperature distribution for pneumonia with corresponding X-ray image.

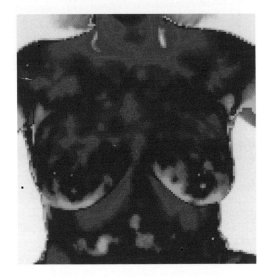

FIGURE 28.3 Thermal image of the healthy breast.

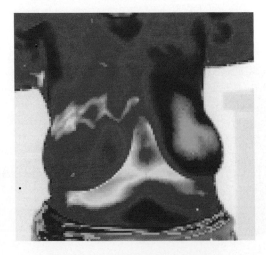

FIGURE 28.4 Thermal image of the breast with malignant tumor (left side).

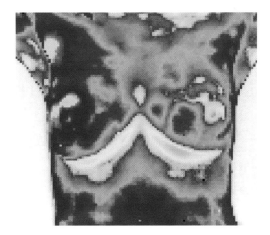

FIGURE 28.12 Example of thermal image with the tumor.

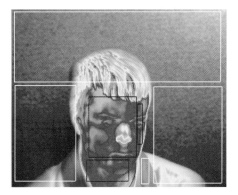

FIGURE 29.3 Manual segmentation of skin (black rectangles) and background (white rectangles) areas for initialization purposes.

(a) (b)

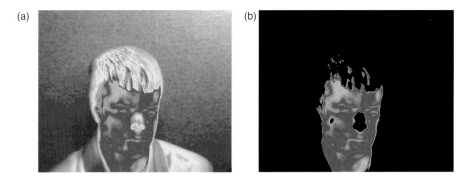

FIGURE 29.4 Visualization of Bayesian segmentation on a subject: (a) original image; (b) segmented image. The nose has been erroneously segmented as background and a couple of hair patches have been erroneously marked as facial skin. This is due to occasional overlapping between portions of the skin and background distributions. The isolated nature of these mislabeled patches makes them easily correctable through post-processing.

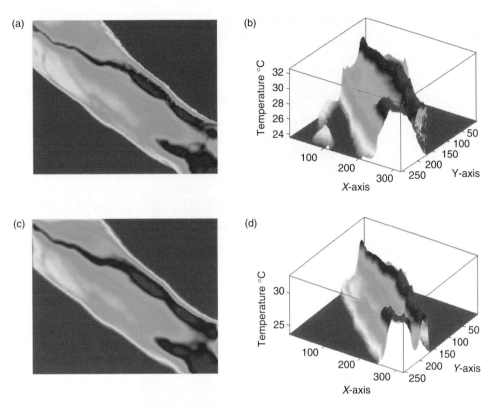

FIGURE 29.7 (a) Original thermal image of a wrist. (b) Temperature surface plot of the original image. (c) Diffused thermal image of the wrist. (d) Temperature surface plot of the diffused image.

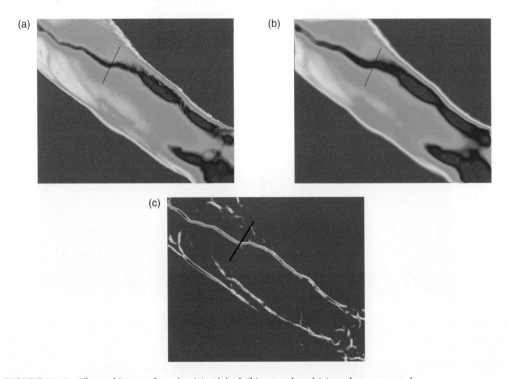

FIGURE 29.12 Thermal image of a wrist: (a) original, (b) opened, and (c) top hat segmented.

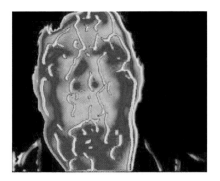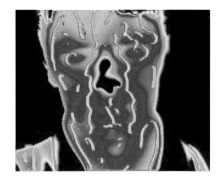

FIGURE 29.14 Segmented facial images annotated with the facial vascular network (yellow lines) per the approach detailed in chapter 29.

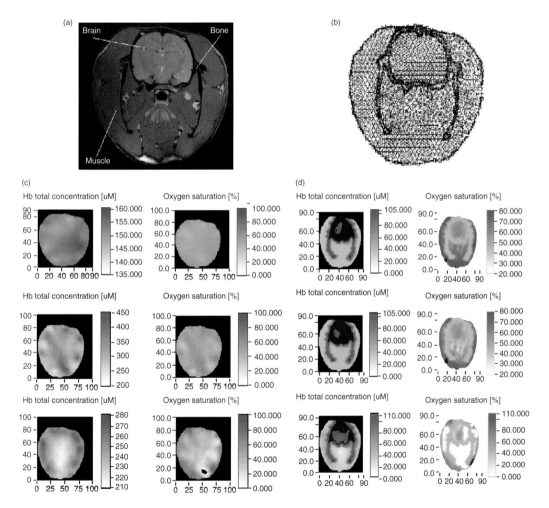

FIGURE 30.2 Functional imaging of rat cranium during changes in inhaled oxygen concentration: (a) MRI image; (b) creation of the mesh to distinguish different compartments in the brain; (c) Map of hemoglobin concentration and oxygen saturation of the rat brain without structural constraints from MRI; (d) Same as (c) with structural constraints including tissue heterogeneity. In (c) and (d) the rows from top correspond to 13, 8, and 0% (after death) oxygen inhaled.

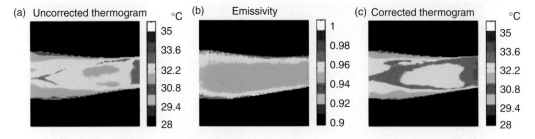

FIGURE 30.8 An example of images obtained from the forearm of a normal healthy male subject. (1) Original thermogram; (b) emissivity image; (c) thermogram corrected by emissivity.

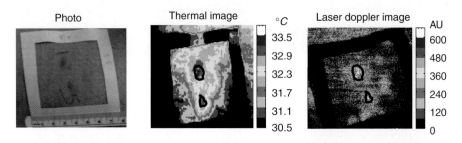

FIGURE 30.10 Typical multi-modality images obtained from a patient with KS lesion. The number "1" and "5" in the visual image were written on the skin to identify the lesions for tumor measurement. The solid line in the thermal and LDI demarks the border of the visible KS lesion.

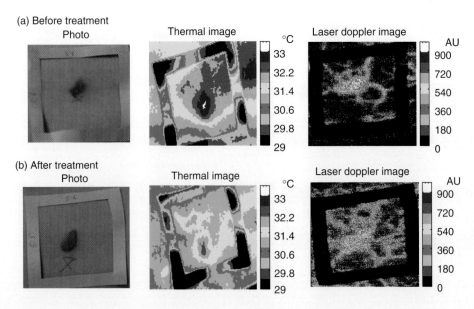

FIGURE 30.12 Typical example of lesion obtained from a subject with KS (a) before, and (b) after the treatment. Improvement after the treatment can be assessed by the thermal or LDI images after 18 weeks.

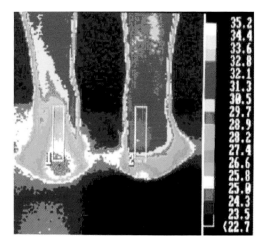

FIGURE 31.1 Acute tendonitis of the right Achilles tendon in a patient suffering from inflammatory spondylarthropathy.

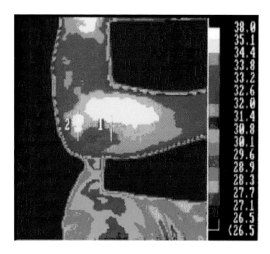

FIGURE 31.2 Tennis elbow with a typical hot spot in the region of tendon insertion.

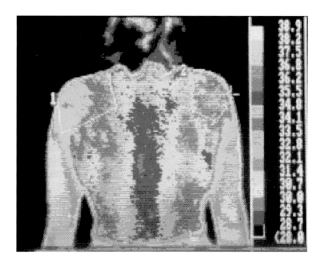

FIGURE 31.3 Decreased temperature in patient with a frozen shoulder on the left hand side.

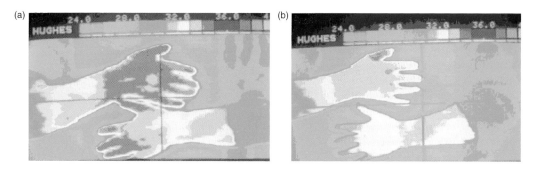

FIGURE 31.5 Early CRPS after radius fracture. Left: 2 h after cast removal; Right: 1 week later.

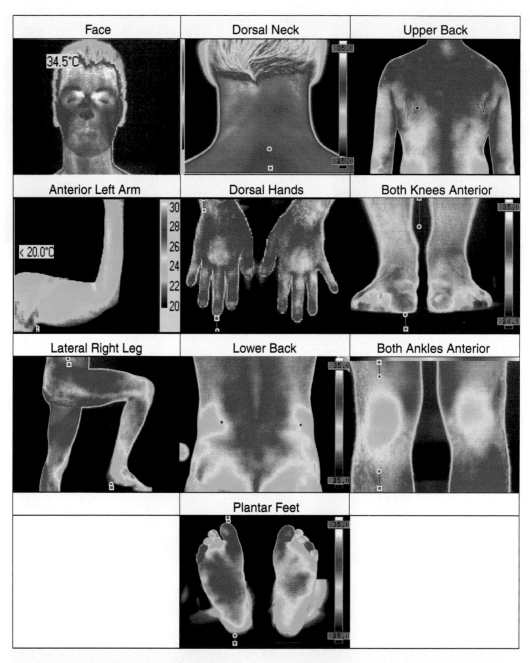

FIGURE 36.1 Body views investigated.

30

Infrared Imaging for Tissue Characterization and Function

Moinuddin Hassan
Victor Chernomordik
Abby Vogel
David Hattery
Israel Gannot
Richard F. Little
Robert Yarchoan
Amir H. Gandjbakhche
National Institutes of Health

30.1 Near-Infrared Quantitative Imaging of Deep Tissue
Structure.. 30-2
Optical Properties of Biological Tissue • Measurable
Quantities and Experimental Techniques • Models of
Photon Migration in Tissue • RWT Applied to Quantitative
Spectroscopy of the Breast • Quantitative Fluorescence
Imaging and Spectroscopy • Future Directions
30.2 Infrared Thermal Monitoring of Disease Processes:
Clinical Study 30-15
Emissivity Corrected Temperature • Temperature
Calibration • Clinical Study: Kaposi's Sarcoma
Acknowledgments... 30-20
References 30-21

Noninvasive imaging techniques are emerging into the forefront of medical diagnostics and treatment monitoring. Both near- and mid-infrared imaging techniques have provided invaluable information in the clinical setting.

Near-infrared imaging in the spectrum of 700 to 1100 nm has been used to functionally monitor diseases processes including cancer and lymph node detection and optical biopsies. Spectroscopic imaging modalities have been shown to improve the diagnosis of tumors and add new knowledge about the physiological properties of the tumor and surrounding tissues. Particular emphasis should be placed on identifying markers that predict the risk of precancerous lesions progressing to invasive cancers, thereby providing new opportunities for cancer prevention. This might be accomplished through the use of markers as contrast agents for imaging using conventional techniques or through refinements of newer technologies such as MRI or PET scanning. The spectroscopic power of light, along with the revolution in molecular characterization of disease processes has created a huge potential for *in vivo* optical imaging and spectroscopy.

In the infrared thermal waveband, information about blood circulation, local metabolism, sweat gland malfunction, inflammation, and healing can be extracted. Infrared thermal imaging has been increasingly used for detection of cancers. As this field evolves, abnormalities or changes in infrared images could be able to provide invaluable information to physicians caring for patients with a variety of disorders. The current status of modern infrared imaging is that of a first line supplement to both clinical exams and current imaging methods. Using infrared imaging to detect breast pathology is based on the principle that both metabolic and vascular activity in the tissue surrounding a new and developing tumor is usually higher than in normal tissue. Early cancer growth is dependent on increasing blood circulation by creating new blood vessels (angiogenesis). This process results in regional variations that can often be detected by infrared imaging.

Section 30.1 discusses near-infrared (NIR) imaging and its applications in imaging biological tissues. Infrared thermal imaging techniques, calibration and a current clinical trial of Kaposi's sarcoma are described in Section 30.2.

30.1 Near-Infrared Quantitative Imaging of Deep Tissue Structure

In vivo optical imaging has traditionally been limited to superficial tissue surfaces, directly or endoscopically accessible, and to tissues with a biological window (e.g., along the optical axis of the eye). These methods are based on geometric optics. Most tissues scatter light so strongly, however, that for geometric optics-based equipment to work, special techniques are needed to remove multiply scattered light (such as pinholes in confocal imaging or interferometry in optical coherence microscopies). Even with these special designs, high resolution optical imaging fails at depths of more than 1 mm below the tissue surface.

Collimated visible or infrared (IR) light impinging upon thick tissue is scattered many times in a distance of ~1 mm, so the analysis of light-tissue interactions requires theories based on the diffusive nature of light propagation. In contrast to x-ray and Positron Emission Tomography (PET), a complex underlying theoretical picture is needed to describe photon paths as a function of scattering and absorption properties of the tissue.

Approximately a decade ago, a new field called "Photon Migration" was born that seeks to characterize the statistical physics of photon motion through turbid tissues. The goal has been to image macroscopic structures in 3D at greater depths within tissues and to provide reliable pathlength estimations for noninvasive spectral analysis of tissue changes. Although geometrical optics fails to describe light propagation under these conditions, the statistical physics of strong, multiply scattered light provides powerful approaches to macroscopic imaging and subsurface detection and characterization. Techniques using visible and NIR light offer a variety of functional imaging modalities, in addition to density imaging, while avoiding ionizing radiation hazards.

In Section 30.1.1, optical properties of biological tissue will be discussed. Section 30.1.2 is devoted to differing methods of measurements. Theoretical models for spectroscopy and imaging are discussed in Section 30.1.3. In Sections 30.1.4 and 30.1.5, two studies on breast imaging and the use of exogenous fluorescent markers will be presented as examples of NIR spectroscopy. Finally, the future direction of the field will be discussed in Section 30.1.6.

30.1.1 Optical Properties of Biological Tissue

The difficulty of tissue optics is to define optical coefficients of tissue physiology and quantify their changes to differentiate structures and functional status *in vivo*. Light-tissue interactions dictate the way that these parameters are defined. The two main approaches are the wave and particle descriptions of light propagation. The first leads to the use of Maxwell's equations, and therefore quantifies the spatially varying permittivity as a measurable quantity. For simplistic and historic reasons, the particle interpretation of light has been mostly used (see section on models of photon migration). In photon transport theory, one considers the behavior of discrete photons as they move through the tissue. This motion is characterized by absorption and scattering, and when interfaces (e.g., layers) are involved, refraction. The absorption

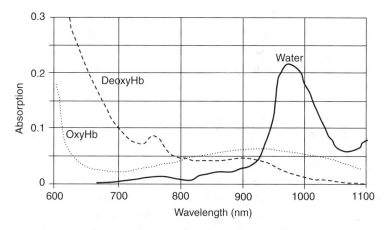

FIGURE 30.1 Absorption spectra of the three major components of tissue in the NIR region; oxy-hemoglobin, deoxy-hemoglobin and water.

coefficient, μ_a(mm^{-1}), represents the inverse mean pathlength of a photon before absorption. $1/\mu_a$ is the distance in a medium where intensity is attenuated by a factor of $1/e$ (Beer's Lambert Law). Absorption in tissue is strongly wavelength dependent and is due to chromophores and water. Among the chromophores in tissue, the dominant component is the hemoglobin in blood. In Figure 30.1, hemoglobin absorption is devided in to oxy- and deoxy-hemoglobin. As seen in this figure, in the visible range (600–700 nm), the blood absorption is relatively high compared to absorption in the NIR. By contrast, water absorption is low in the visible and NIR regions and increases rapidly above approximately 950 nm. Thus, for greatest penetration of light in tissue, wavelengths in the 650–950 nm spectrum are used most often. This region of the light spectrum is called "the therapeutic window." One should note that different spectra of chromophores allow one to separate the contribution of varying functional species in tissue (e.g., quantification of oxy- and deoxy-hemoglobin to study tissue oxygenation).

Similarly, scattering is characterized by a coefficient, μ_s, which is the inverse mean free path of photons between scattering events. The average size of the scattered photons in tissue, in proportion to the wavelength of the light, places the scattering in the Mie region. In the Mie region, a scattering event does not result in isotropic scattering angles [1,2]. Instead, the scattering in tissue is biased in the forward direction.

For example, by studying the development of neonatal skin, Saidi et al. [3] were able to show that the principal sources of anisotropic scattering in muscle are collagen fibers. The fibers were determined to have a mean diameter of 2.2 μm. In addition to the Mie scattering from the fibers, there is isotropic Rayleigh scattering due to the presence of much smaller scatterers such as organelles in cells.

Anisotropic scattering is quantified in a coefficient, g, which is defined as the mean cosine of the scattering angle, where $p(\theta)$ is the probability of a particular scattering angle,

$$g = \langle \cos(\theta) \rangle = \frac{\int_0^\pi p(\theta)\cos(\theta)\sin(\theta)\mathrm{d}\theta}{\int_0^\pi p(\theta)\sin(\theta)\mathrm{d}\theta} \tag{30.1}$$

For isotropic scattering, $g = 0$. For complete forward scattering, $g = 1$, and for complete back scattering, $g = -1$. In tissue, g is typically 0.7 to 0.98 [3–5].

Likewise, different tissue types have differing scattering properties which are also wavelength dependent. The scattering coefficients of many soft tissues have been measured at a variety of optical wavelengths, and are within the range 10 to 100 mm^{-1}. In comparison to absorption, however, scattering changes, as a function of wavelength, are more gradual and have smaller extremes. Abnormal tissues such as tumors, fibro-adenomas, and cysts all have scattering properties that are different from normal tissue [6,7]. Thus, the scattering coefficient of an inclusion may also be an important clue to disease diagnoses.

Theories of photon migration are often based on isotropic scattering. Therefore, one must find the appropriate scaling relationships that will allow use of an isotropic scattering model. For the case of diffusion-like models (e.g., see Reference 8), it has been shown that one may use an isotropic scattering model with a corrected scattering coefficient, μ'_s, and obtain equivalent results where:

$$\mu'_s = \mu_s(1 - g) \tag{30.2}$$

The corrected scattering coefficient is smaller than the actual scattering which corresponds to a greater distance between isotropic scattering events than would occur with anisotropic scattering. For this reason, μ'_s is typically called the transport-corrected scattering coefficient.

There are instances in which the spectroscopic signatures will not be sufficient for detection of disease. This can occur when the specific disease results in only very small changes to the tissue's scattering and absorption properties, or when the scattering and absorption properties are not unique to the disease. Although it is not clear what the limits of detectability are in relationship to diseased tissue properties, it is clear that there will be cases for which optical techniques based on elastic absorption are inadequate. In such cases, another source of optical contrast, such as fluorescence, will be required to detect and locate the disease. Presence of fluorescent molecules in tissues can provide useful contrast mechanisms. Concentration of these endogenous fluorophores in the body can be related to functional and metabolic activities, and therefore to the disease processes. For example, the concentrations of fluorescent molecules such as collagen and NADH have been used to differentiate between normal and abnormal tissue [9].

Advances in the molecular biology of disease processes, new immunohistopathological techniques, and the development of fluorescently-labeled cell surface markers have led to a revolution in specific molecular diagnosis of disease by histopathology, as well as in research on molecular origins of disease processes (e.g., using fluorescence microscopy in cell biology). As a result, an exceptional level of specificity is now possible due to the advances in the design of exogenous markers. Molecules can now be tailor-made to bind only to specific receptor sites in the body. These receptor sites may be antibodies or other biologically interesting molecules. Fluorophores may be bound to these engineered molecules and injected into the body, where they will preferentially concentrate at specific sites of interest [10,11].

Furthermore, fluorescence may be used as a probe to measure environmental conditions in a particular locality by capitalizing on changes in fluorophore lifetimes [12,13]. Each fluorophore has a characteristic lifetime that quantifies the probability of a specific time delay between fluorophore excitation and emission. In practice, this lifetime may be modified by specific environmental factors such as temperature, pH, and concentrations of substances such as oxygen. In these cases, it is possible to quantify local concentrations of specific substances or specific environmental conditions by measuring the lifetime of fluorophores at the site. Whereas conventional fluorescence imaging is very sensitive to non-uniform fluorophore transport and distribution (e.g., blood does not transport molecules equally to all parts of the body), fluorescence lifetime imaging is insensitive to transport non-uniformity as long as a detectable quantity of fluorophores is present in the site of interest. Throughout the following sections, experimental techniques and differing models used to quantify these sources of optical contrast will be presented.

30.1.2 Measurable Quantities and Experimental Techniques

Three classes of measurable quantities prove to be of interest in transforming results of remote sensing measurements in tissue into useful physical information. The first is the spatial distribution of light or the intensity profile generated by photons re-emitted through a surface and measured as a function of the radial distance from the source and the detector when the medium is continually irradiated by a point source (often a laser). This type of measurement is called continuous wave (CW). The intensity, nominally, does not vary in time. The second class is the temporal response to a very short pulse (~picosecond) of photons impinging on the surface of the tissue. This technique is called time-resolved and the temporal response is known as the time-of-flight (TOF). The third class is the frequency-domain technique in which an intensity-modulated laser beam illuminates the tissue. In this case, the measured outputs are the AC modulation amplitude and the phase shift of the detected signal. These techniques could be implemented in geometries with different arrangements of source(s) and detector(s); (a) in the reflection mode, source(s) and detector(s) are placed at the same side of the tissue; (b) in the transmission mode, source(s) and detector(s) are located on opposite sides of the tissue. In the latter, the source(s) and detector(s) can move in tandem while scanning the tissue surface and detectors with lateral offsets also can be used; and (c) tomographic sampling often uses multiple sources and detectors placed around the circumference of the target tissue.

For CW measurements, the instrumentation is simple and requires only a set of light sources and detectors. In this technique, the only measurable quantity is the intensity of light, and, due to multiple scattering, strong pathlength dispersion occurs which results in a loss of localization and resolution. Hence, this technique is widely used for spectroscopic measurements of bulk tissue properties in which the tissue is considered to be homogeneous [14,15]. However, CW techniques for imaging abnormal targets that use only the coherent portion of light, and thereby reject photons with long paths, have also been investigated. Using the transillumination geometry, collimated detection is used to isolate un-scattered photons [16–18]. Spatial filtering has been proposed which employs a lens to produce the Fourier spectrum of the spatial distribution of light from which the high-order frequencies are removed. The resulting image is formed using only the photons with angles close to normal [19]. Polarization discrimination has been used to select those photons which undergo few scattering events and therefore preserve a fraction of their initial polarization state, as opposed to those photons which experience multiple scattering resulting in complete randomization of their initial polarization state [20]. Several investigators have used heterodyne detection which involves measuring the beat frequency generated by the spatial and temporal combination of a light beam and a frequency modulated reference beam. Constructive interference occurs only for the coherent portion of the light [20–22]. However, the potential of direct imaging using CW techniques in very thick tissue (e.g., breast) has not been established. On the other hand, use of models of photon migration implemented in inverse method based on backprojection techniques has shown promising results. For example, Phillips Medical has used 256 optical fibers placed at the periphery of a white conical shaped vessel. The area of interest, in this case the breast, is suspended in the vessel, and surrounded by a matching fluid. Three CW laser diodes sequentially illuminate the breast using one fiber. The detection is done simultaneously by 255 fibers. It is now clear that CW imaging cannot provide direct images with clinically acceptable resolution in thick tissue. Attempts are underway to devise inverse algorithms to separate the effects of scattering and absorption and therefore use this technique for quantitative spectroscopy as proposed by Phillips [23]. However, until now, clinical application of CW techniques in imaging has been limited by the mixture of scattering and absorption of light in the detected signal. To overcome this problem, time-dependent measurement techniques have been investigated.

Time-domain techniques involve the temporal resolution of photons traveling inside the tissue. The basic idea is that photons with smaller pathlengths are those that arrive earlier to the detector. In order to discriminate between un-scattered or less scattered light and the majority of the photons, which experience a large number of multiple scattering, subnanosecond resolution is needed. This short time gating of an imaging system requires the use of a variety of techniques involving ultra-fast phenomena and/or fast detection systems. Ultra-fast shuttering is performed using the Kerr effect. The birefringence in the Kerr cell, placed between two crossed polarizers, is induced using very short pulses. Transmitted light through the Kerr cell is recorded, and temporal resolution of a few picoseconds is achieved [19]. When an impulse of light (~picoseconds or hundreds of femtoseconds) is launched at the tissue surface, the whole temporal distribution of photon intensity can be recorded by a streak camera. The streak camera can achieve temporal resolution on the order of few picoseconds up to several nanoseconds detection time. This detection system has been widely used to assess the performance of breast imaging and neonatal brain activity [24,25]. The time of flight recorded by the streak camera is the convolution of the pulsed laser source (in practice with a finite width) and the actual Temporal Point Spread Function (TPSF) of the diffuse photons. Instead of using very short pulse lasers (e.g., Ti–Sapphire lasers), the advent of pulse diode lasers with relatively larger pulse widths (100 to 400 psec) have reduced the cost of time-domain imaging. However, deconvolution of the incoming pulse and the detected TPSF have been a greater issue. Along with diode laser sources, several groups have also used time-correlated single photon counting with photomultipliers for recording the TPSF [26,27]. Fast time gating is also obtained by using Stimulated Raman Scattering. This phenomenon is a nonlinear Raman interaction in some materials such as hydrogen gas involving the amplification of photons with Stokes shift by a higher energy pump beam. The system operates by amplifying only the earliest arriving photons [28]. Less widely used techniques such as second-harmonic generation [29], parametric amplification [30] and a variety of others have been proposed for time-domain (see an excellent review in Reference 31).

For frequency-domain measurements, the requirement is to measure the DC amplitude, the AC amplitude, and the phase shift of the photon density wave. For this purpose a CW light source is modulated with a given frequency (~100 MHz). Lock-in Amplifiers and phase sensitive CCD camera have been used to record the amplitude and phase [32,33]. Multiple sources at different wavelengths can be modulated with a single frequency or multiple frequencies [6,34]. In the latter case a network analyzer is used to produce modulation swept from several hundreds of MHz to up to 1 GHz.

30.1.3 Models of Photon Migration in Tissue

Photon Migration theories in biomedical optics have been borrowed from other fields such as astrophysics, atmospheric science, and specifically from nuclear reactor engineering [35,36]. The common properties of these physical media and biological tissues are their characterization by elements of randomness in both space and time. Because of many difficulties surrounding the development of a theory based on a detailed picture of the microscopic processes involved in the interaction of light and matter, investigations are often based on statistical theories. These can take a variety of forms, ranging from quite detailed multiple-scattering theories [36] to transport theory [37]. However, the most widely used theory is the time-dependent diffusion approximation to the transport equation:

$$\vec{\nabla} \cdot (D\vec{\nabla}\Phi(\vec{r}, t)) - \mu_a \Phi(\vec{r}, t) = \frac{1}{c}\frac{\partial \Phi(\vec{r}, t)}{\partial t} - S(\vec{r}, t) \tag{30.3}$$

where $\vec{r}$ and t are spatial and temporal variables, c is the speed of light in tissue, and D is the diffusion coefficient related to the absorption and scattering coefficients as follows:

$$D = \frac{1}{3[\mu_a + \mu_s']} \tag{30.4}$$

The quantity $\Phi(\vec{r}, t)$ is called the fluence, defined as the power incident on an infinitesimal volume element divided by its area. Note that the equation does not incorporate any angular dependence, therefore assuming an isotropic scattering. However, for the use of the diffusion theory for anisotropic scattering, the diffusion coefficient is expressed in terms of the transport-corrected scattering coefficient. $S(\vec{r}, t)$ is the source term. The gradient of fluence, $J(\vec{r}, t)$, at the tissue surface is the measured flux of photons by the detector:

$$J(\vec{r}, t) = -D\vec{\nabla}\Phi(\vec{r}, t) \tag{30.5}$$

For CW measurements, the time-dependence of the flux vanishes, and the source term can be seen as the power impinging in its area. For time-resolved measurements, the source term is a Dirac delta function describing a very short photon impulse. Equation 30.3 has been solved analytically for different types of measurements such as reflection and transmission modes assuming that the optical properties remain invariant through the tissue. To incorporate the finite boundaries, the method of images has been used. In the simplest case, the boundary has been assumed to be perfectly absorbing which does not take into account the difference between indices of refraction at the tissue–air interface. For semi-infinite and transillumination geometries, a set of theoretical expressions has been obtained for time-resolved measurements [38].

The diffusion approximation equation in the frequency-domain is the Fourier transformation of the time-domain with respect to time. Fourier transformation applied to the time-dependent diffusion equation leads to a new equation:

$$\vec{\nabla} \cdot (D\vec{\nabla}\Phi(\vec{r}, \omega)) - \left[\mu_a + \frac{i\omega}{c}\right]\Phi(\vec{r}, \omega) + S(\vec{r}, \omega) = 0 \tag{30.6}$$

Here the time variable is replaced by the frequency ω. This frequency is the modulation angular frequency of the source. In this model, the fluence can be seen as a complex number describing the amplitude and phase of the photon density wave, dumped with a DC component:

$$\Phi(\vec{r}, \omega) = \Phi_{AC}(\vec{r}, \omega) + \Phi_{DC}(\vec{r}, 0) = I_{AC}\exp(i\theta) + \Phi_{DC}(\vec{r}, 0) \tag{30.7}$$

In the RHS of Equation 30.7, the quantity θ is the phase shift of the diffusing wave. For a nonabsorbing medium, its wavelength is:

$$\lambda = 2\pi\sqrt{\frac{2c}{3\mu'_s\omega}} \tag{30.8}$$

Likewise in the time-domain, Equation 30.3 has an analytical solution for the case that the tissue is considered homogeneous. The analytical solution permits one to deduce the optical properties in a spectroscopic setting.

For imaging, where the goal is to distinguish between structures in tissue, the diffusion coefficient and the absorption coefficient in Equation 30.3 and Equation 30.6 become spatial-dependent and are replaced by $D(r)$ and $\mu_a(r)$. For the cases that an abnormal region is embedded in otherwise homogeneous tissue, perturbation methods based on Born approximation or Rytov approximation have been used (see excellent review in Reference 39). However, for the cases that the goal is to reconstruct the spectroscopic signatures inside the tissue, no analytical solution exists. For these cases, inverse algorithms are devised to map the spatially varying optical properties. Numerical methods such as finite-element or finite-difference methods have been used to reconstruct images of breast, brain, and muscle [40–42]. Furthermore, in those cases that structural heterogeneity exists, a priori information from other image modalities such as MRI can be used. An example is given in Figure 30.2. Combining MRI and NIR imaging, rat cranium functional imaging during changes in inhaled oxygen concentration was studied [43]. Figure 30.2a,b correspond to the MRI image and the corresponding constructed finite-element mesh. Figure 30.2c,d correspond to the oxygen map of the brain with and without incorporation of MRI geometry and constraints.

The use of MRI images has improved dramatically the resolution of the oxygen map. The use of optical functional imaging in conjunction with other imaging modalities has opened new possibilities in imaging and treating diseases at the bedside.

The second theoretical framework used in tissue optics is the random walk theory (RWT) on a lattice developed at the National Institutes of Health [44,45] and historically precedes the use of the diffusion approximation theory. It has been shown that RWT may be used to derive an analytical solution for the distribution of photon path-lengths in turbid media such as tissue [44]. RWT models the diffusion-like motion of photons in turbid media in a probabilistic manner. Using RWT, an expression may be derived for the probability of a photon arriving at any point and time given a specific starting point and time.

Tissue may be modeled as a 3D cubic lattice containing a finite inclusion, or region of interest, as shown in Figure 30.3. The medium has an absorbing boundary corresponding to the tissue surface, and the lattice spacing is proportional to the mean photon scattering distance, $1/\mu'_s$. The behavior of photons in the RWT model is described by three dimensionless parameters, ρ, n, μ, which are respectively the radial distance, the number of steps, and the probability of absorption per lattice step. In the RWT model, photons may move to one of the six nearest neighboring lattice points, each with probability 1/6. If the number of steps, n, taken by a photon traveling between two points on the lattice is known, then the length of the photon's path is also known.

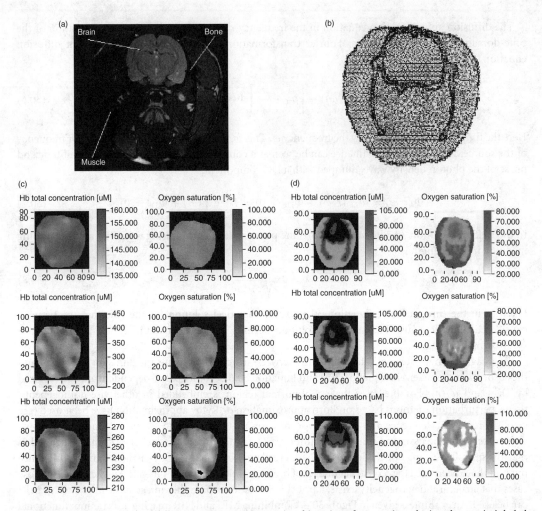

FIGURE 30.2   (See color inset following page **29**-16.) Functional imaging of rat cranium during changes in inhaled oxygen concentration: (a) MRI image; (b) creation of the mesh to distinguish different compartments in the brain; (c) map of hemoglobin concentration and oxygen saturation of the rat brain without structural constraints from MRI; (d) same as (c) with structural constraints including tissue heterogeneity. In (c) and (d) the rows from top correspond to 13, 8, and 0% (after death) oxygen inhaled. (Courtesy of Dartmouth College.)

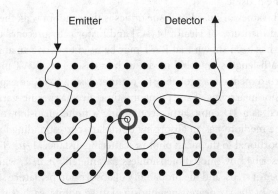

FIGURE 30.3   2D random walk lattice showing representative photon paths from an emitter to a specific site and then to a detector.

Random walk theory is useful in predicting the probability distribution of photon path lengths over distances of at least five mean photon scattering distances. The derivation of these probability distributions is described in papers [44,45]. For simplicity in this derivation, the tissue–air interface is considered to be perfectly absorbing; a photon arriving at this interface is counted as arriving at a detector on the tissue surface. The derivation uses the Central Limit Theorem and a Gaussian distribution around lattice points to obtain a closed-form solution that is independent of the lattice structure.

The dimensionless RWT parameters, ρ, n, and μ, described above, may be transformed to actual parameters, in part, by using time, t, the speed of light in tissue, c, and distance traveled, r, as follows:

$$\rho \to \frac{r\mu_s'}{\sqrt{2}}, \qquad n \to \mu_s'ct, \qquad \mu \to \frac{\mu_a}{\mu_s'} \tag{30.9}$$

As stated previously, scattering in tissue is highly anisotropic. Therefore, one must find the appropriate scaling relationships that will allow the use of an isotropic scattering model such as RWT. Like diffusion theory, for RWT [46], it has been shown that one may use an isotropic scattering model with a corrected scattering coefficient, μ_s', and obtain equivalent results. The corrected scattering coefficient is smaller than the actual scattering that corresponds to a greater distance between isotropic scattering events than would occur with anisotropic scattering. RWT has been used to show how one would transition from the use of μ_s to μ_s' as the distance under considerable increases [47].

As an example, for a homogeneous slab into which a photon has been inserted, the probability, P, of a photon arriving at a point ρ after n steps is [48]:

$$P(n, \rho) = \frac{\sqrt{3}}{2} \left[\frac{1}{2\pi(n-2)} \right]^{3/2} e^{-3\rho^2/2(n-2)} \sum_{k=-\infty}^{\infty} \left[e^{-3[(2k+1)L-2]^2/2(n-2)} - e^{-3[(2k+1)L]^2/2(n-2)} \right] e^{-n\mu}$$

$$\tag{30.10}$$

where L is the thickness of the slab. The method of images has been used to take into account the two boundaries of the slab. Plotting Equation 30.10 yields a photon arrival curve as shown in Figure 30.4; Monte Carlo simulation data are overlaid. In the next two sections the use of RWT for imaging will be presented.

30.1.4 RWT Applied to Quantitative Spectroscopy of the Breast

One important and yet extremely challenging areas to apply diffuse optical imaging of deep tissues is the human breast (see review article of Hawrysz and Sevick-Muraca [49]). It is clear that any new imaging

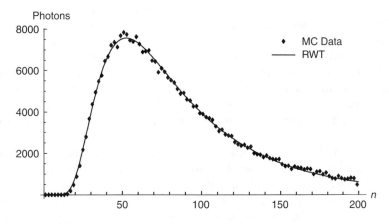

FIGURE 30.4 RWT prediction and Monte Carlo simulation results for transillumination of a 15-mm thick slab with scattering 1/mm and 109 photons.

or spectroscopic modalities that can improve the diagnosis of breast tumors or can add new knowledge about the physiological properties of the breast and surrounding tissues will have a great significance in medicine.

Conventional transillumination using continuous wave (CW) light was used for breast screening several decades ago [50]. However, because of the high scattering properties of tissue, this method resulted in poor resolution. In the late 1980s, time-resolved imaging techniques were proposed to enhance spatial resolution by detecting photons with very short time-of-flight within the tissue. In this technique, a very short pulse, of ~picosecond duration, impinges upon the tissue. Photons experience dispersion in their pathlengths, resulting in temporal dispersion in their time-of-flight (TOF).

To evaluate the performance of time-resolved transillumination techniques, RWT on a lattice was used. The analysis of breast transillumination was based on the calculation of the point spread function (PSF) of time resolved photons as they visit differing sites at different planes inside a finite slab of thickness L. The PSF [51], is defined as the probability that a photon inserted into the tissue visits a given site, is detected at the nth step (i.e., a given time), and has the following rather complicated analytical expression:

$$W_n(\mathbf{s}, \mathbf{r}, \mathbf{r}_0) = \sum_{l=0}^{n} p_l(\mathbf{r}, \mathbf{s}) p_{n-l}(\mathbf{s}, \mathbf{r}_0) = \frac{9}{16\pi^{5/2} n^{3/2}} \sum_{k=-\infty}^{\infty} \sum_{m=-\infty}^{\infty} \{F_n[\alpha_+(k), \beta_+(m,p)] \tag{30.11}$$

$$+ F_n[\alpha_-(k), \beta_-(m,p)] - F_n[\alpha_+(k), \beta_-(m,p)] - F_n[\alpha_-(k), \beta_+(m,p)]\}$$

$$F_n(a,b) = \left(\frac{1}{a} + \frac{1}{b}\right) \exp\left[-\frac{(a+b)^2}{n}\right] \tag{30.12}$$

$$\alpha_\pm(k) = \left\{\frac{3}{2}\left[s_1^2 + (s_3 + 2kN \pm 1)^2\right]\right\}^{\frac{1}{2}} \tag{30.13}$$

$$\beta_\pm(k,\rho) = \left\{\frac{3}{2}\left[(\rho - s_1)^2 + (N - s_3 + 2kN \pm 1)^2\right]\right\}^{\frac{1}{2}} \tag{30.14}$$

where $N = (\mu_s'/\sqrt{2}) + 1$ is dimensionless RWT thickness of the slabs, $\bar{s}(s_1, s_2, s_3)$ are the dimensionless coordinates (see Equation 30.9) of any location for which the PSF is calculated. Evaluation of time-resolved imaging showed that strong scattering properties of tissues prevent direct imaging of abnormalities [52]. Hence, devising theoretical constructs to separate the effects of the scattering from the absorption was proposed, thus allowing one to map the optical coefficients as spectroscopic signatures of an abnormal tissue embedded in thick, otherwise normal tissue. In this method, accurate quantification of the size and optical properties of the target becomes a critical requirement for the use of optical imaging at the bedside. RWT on a lattice has been used to analyze the time-dependent contrast observed in time-resolved transillumination experiments and deduce the size and optical properties of the target and the surrounding tissue from these contrasts. For the theoretical construction of contrast functions, two quantities are needed. First, the set of functions [51] defined previously. Second, the set of functions [53] defined as the probability that a photon is detected at the nth step (i.e., time) in a homogeneous medium (Equation 30.10)[48].

To relate the contrast of the light intensity to the optical properties and location of abnormal targets in the tissue, one can take advantage of some features of the theoretical framework. One feature is that the early time response is most dependent on scattering perturbations, whereas the late time behavior is most dependent on absorptive perturbations, thus allowing one to separate the influence of scattering and absorption perturbations on the observed image contrast. Increased scattering in the abnormal target is modeled as a time delay. Moreover, it was shown that the scattering contrast is proportional to the time-derivative of the PSF, $\mathrm{d}W_n/\mathrm{d}n$, divided by P_n [53]. The second interesting feature in RWT methodology assumes that the contrast from scattering inside the inclusion is proportional to the cross-section of the target (in the z direction) [51,53], instead of depending on its volume as modeled in the perturbation analysis [54].

Several research groups intend to implement their theoretical expressions into general inverse algorithms for optical tomography, that is, to reconstruct three-dimensional maps of spatial distributions of tissue optical characteristics [49], and thereby quantify optical characteristics, positions and sizes of abnormalities. Unlike these approaches, method is a multi-step analysis of the collected data. From images observed at differing flight times, we construct the time-dependent contrast functions, fit our theoretical expressions, and compute the optical properties of the background, and those of the abnormality along with its size. The outline of data analysis is given in Reference 55.

By utilizing the method for different wavelengths, one can obtain diagnostic information (e.g., estimates of blood oxygenation of the tumor) for corresponding absorption coefficients that no other imaging modality can provide directly. Several research groups have already successfully used multi-wavelength measurements using frequency-domain techniques, to calculate physiological parameters (oxygenation, lipid, water) of breast tumors (diagnosed with other modalities) and normal tissue [56].

Researchers at Physikalisch-Technische-Bundesanstalt (PTB) of Berlin have designed a clinically practical optical imaging system, capable of implementing time-resolved *in vivo* measurements on the human breast [27]. The breast is slightly compressed between two plates. A scan of the whole breast takes but a few minutes and can be done in mediolateral and craniocaudal geometries. The first goal is to quantify the optical parameters at several wavelengths and thereby estimate blood oxygen saturation of the tumor and surrounding tissue under the usual assumption that the chromophores contributing to absorption are oxy- and deoxy-hemoglobin and water. As an example, two sets of data, obtained at two wavelengths ($\lambda = 670$ and 785 nm), for a patient (84-year-old) with invasive ductal carcinoma, were analyzed. Though the images exhibit poor resolution, the tumor can be easily seen in the optical image shown in Figure 30.5a. In this figure, the image is obtained from reciprocal values of the total integrals of the distributions of times of flight of photons, normalized to a selected "bulk" area. The tumor center is located at $x = -5$, $y = 0.25$ mm.

The best spatial resolution is observed, as expected, for shorter time-delays allowing one to determine the position of the tumor center on the 2-D image (transverse coordinates) with accuracy $\sim$2.5 mm. After preliminary data processing that includes filtering and deconvolution of the raw time-resolved data, we created linear contrast scans passing through the tumor center and analyzed these scans, using our algorithm. It is striking that one observes similar linear dependence of the contrast amplitude on the derivative of PSF ($\lambda = 670$ nm), as expected in the model (see Figure 30.5b). The slope of this linear dependence was used, to estimate the amplitude of the scattering perturbation [55].

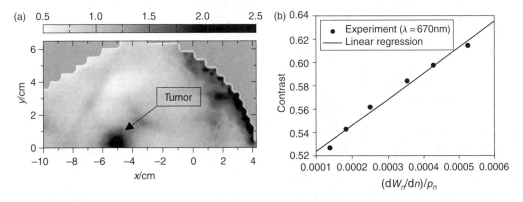

FIGURE 30.5 (a) 2-D optical image of the breast with the tumor. (Courtesy of Physikalisch-Technische-Bundesanstalt, Berlin.) (b) Contrast obtained from linear scan through the tumor plotted vs. the derivative of PSF. From the linear regression the scattering coefficient of the tumor is deduced.

TABLE 30.1   Optical Parameters of Tumor and
Background Breast Tissue

Unknown coefficients	Reconstructed values (mm^{-1})	
	$\lambda = 670$ nm	$\lambda = 785$ nm
Absorption (background)	0.0029^{-1}	0.0024^{-1}
Scattering (background)	1.20^{-1}	1.10^{-1}
Absorption (tumor)	0.0071^{-1}	0.0042^{-1}
Scattering (tumor)	1.76^{-1}	1.6^{-1}

Dimensions and values of optical characteristics of the tumor and surrounding tissues were then reconstructed for both wavelengths. Results show that the tumor had larger absorption and scattering than the background. Estimated parameters are presented in Table 30.1.

Both absorption and scattering coefficients of the tumor and background all proved to be larger at the red wavelength (670 nm). Comparison of the absorption in the red and near infrared range is used to estimate blood oxygen saturation of the tumor and background tissue. Preliminary results of the analysis gave evidence that the tumor tissue is in a slightly deoxygenated state with higher blood volume, compared to surrounding tissue.

The spectroscopic power of optical imaging, along with the ability to quantify physiological parameters of human breast, have opened a new opportunity for assessing metabolic and physiological activities of the human breast during treatment.

30.1.5   Quantitative Fluorescence Imaging and Spectroscopy

As mentioned in Section 30.1.1, advances in the molecular biology of disease processes, new immunohis-topathological techniques, and the development of specific fluorescently-labeled cell surface markers have led a revolution in research on the molecular origins of disease processes. On the other hand, reliable, sensitive, and specific, non-invasive techniques are needed for *in vivo* determinations of abnormalities within tissue. If successfully developed, noninvasive "optical biopsies" may replace conventional surgical biopsies and provide the advantages of smaller sampling errors, reduction in cost and time for diagnosis resulting in easier integration of diagnosis and therapy by following the progression of disease or regression in response to therapy. Clinically practical fluorescence imaging techniques must meet several requirements. First, the pathology under investigation must lie above a depth where the attenuation of the signal results in a poor signal-to-noise ratio and resolvability. Second, the specificity of the marker must be high enough that one can clearly distinguish between normal and abnormal lesions. Finally, one must have a robust image reconstruction algorithm which enables one to quantify the fluorophore concentration at a given depth.

The choices of projects in this area of research are dictated by the importance of the problem, and the impact of the solution on health care. Below, the rationale of two projects, are described that National Institutes of Health are pursuing.

Sjogren's Syndrome (SS) has been chosen as an appropriate test case for developing a noninvasive optical biopsy based on 3-D localization of exogenous specific fluorescent labels. SS is an autoimmune disease affecting minor salivary glands which are near (0.5 to 3.0 mm below) the oral mucosal surface [57]. Therefore the target pathology is relatively accessible to noninvasive optical imaging. The hydraulic conductivity of the oral mucosa is relatively high, which along with the relatively superficial location of the minor salivary glands, makes topical application and significant labeling of diseased glands with large fluorescent molecules easy to accomplish. Fluorescence ligands (e.g., fluorescent antibodies specific to CD4$^+$ T cell-activated lymphocytes infiltrating the salivary glands) are expected to bind specifically to the atypical cells in the tissue, providing high contrast and a quantitative relationship to their concentration (and therefore to the stage of the disease process). The major symptoms (dry eyes and dry mouth due to decreased tear and saliva secretion) are the result of progressive immune-mediated dysfunction of the lacrimal and salivary glands. Currently, diagnosis is made by excisional biopsies of the minor salivary glands in the lower lip. This exam, though considered the best criterion for diagnosis, involves a surgical procedure under local anesthesia followed by postoperative discomfort (swelling, pain) and frequently a temporary loss of sensation at the lower lip biopsy site. Additionally, biopsy is inherently subject to sampling errors and the preparation of histopathological slides is time consuming, complicated, expensive, and requires the skills of several professionals (dentist, pathologist, and laboratory technician). Thus, there is a clear need for a noninvasive diagnostic procedure which reflects the underlying gland pathology and has good specificity. A quantitative, noninvasive assay would also allow repetition of the test to monitor disease progression and the effect of treatment. However, the quantification of fluorophore concentration within the tissue from surface images requires determining the intensities of different fluorophore sources, as a function of depth and transverse distance and predicting the 3-D distribution of fluorophores within the tissue from a series of images [58].

The second project involves the lymphatic imaging-sentinel node detection. The stage of cancer at initial diagnosis often defines prognosis and determines treatment options. As part of the staging procedure of melanoma and breast cancer, multiple lymph nodes are surgically removed from the primary lymphatic draining site and examined histologically for the presence of malignant cells. Because it is not obvious which nodes to remove at the time of resection of the primary tumor, standard practice involves dissection of as many lymph nodes as feasible. Since such extensive removal of lymphatic tissue frequently results in compromised lymphatic drainage in the examined axilla, alternatives have been sought to define the stage at the time of primary resection. A recent advance in lymph node interrogation has been the localization and removal of the "sentinel" node. Although there are multiple lymphatic channels available for trafficking from the primary tumor, the assumption was made that the anatomic location of the primary tumor in a given individual drains into lymphatic channels in an orderly and reproducible fashion. If that is in fact the case, then there is a pattern by which lymphatic drainage occurs. Thus, it would be expected that malignant cells from a primary tumor site would course from the nearest and possibly most superficial node into deeper and more distant lymphatic channels to ultimately arrive in the thoracic duct, whereupon malignant cells would gain access to venous circulation. The sentinel node is defined as the first drainage node in a network of nodes that drain the primary cancer. Considerable evidence has accrued validating the clinical utility of staging breast cancer by locating and removing the sentinel node at the time of resection of the primary tumor. Currently, the primary tumor is injected with a radionucleotide one day prior to removal of the primary tumor. Then, just before surgery, it is injected with visible dye. The surgeon localizes crudely the location of the sentinel node using a hand-held radionucleotide detector, followed by a search for visible concentrations of the injected dye. The method requires expensive equipment and also presents the patient and hospital personnel with the risk of exposure to ionizing radiation. As an alternative to the radionucleotide, we are investigating the use of IR-dependent fluorescent detection methods to determine the location of sentinel node(s).

For *in vivo* fluorescent imaging, a complicating factor is the strong attenuation of light as it passes through tissue. This attenuation deteriorates the signal-to-noise ratio of detected photons. Fortunately, development of fluorescent dyes (such as porphyrin and cyanine) that excite and re-emit in the "biological window" at NIR wavelengths, where scattering and absorption coefficients are relatively low, have provided new possibilities for deep fluorescence imaging in tissue. The theoretical complication occurs at depths greater than 1 mm where photons in most tissues enter a diffusion-like state with a large dispersion in their path-lengths. Indeed, the fluorescent intensity of light detected from deep tissue structures depends not only on the location, size, concentration, and intrinsic characteristics (e.g., lifetime, quantum efficiency) of the fluorophores, but also on the scattering and absorption coefficients of the tissue at both the excitation and emission wavelengths. Hence, in order to extract intrinsic characteristics of fluorophores within tissue, it is necessary to describe the statistics of photon pathlengths which depend on all these differing parameters.

Obviously, the modeling of fluorescent light propagation depends on the kinds of experiments that one plans to perform. For example, for frequency-domain measurements, Patterson and Pogue [59] used the diffusion approximation of the transport equation to express their results in terms of a product of two Green's function propagators multiplied by a term that describes the probability of emission of a fluorescent photon at the site. One Green's function describes the movement of an incident photon to the fluorophore, and the other describes movement of the emitted photon to the detector. In this representation, the amount of light emitted at the site of the fluorophore is directly proportional to the total amount of light impinging on the fluorophore, with no account for the variability in the number of visits by a photon before an exciting transformation. Since a transformation on an early visit to the site precludes a transformation on all later visits, this results in an overestimation of the number of photons which have a fluorescence transformation at a particular site. This overestimation is important when fluorescent absorption properties are spatially inhomogeneous and largest at later arrival times. RWT has been used to allow for this spatial inhomogeneity by introducing the multiple-passage probabilities concept, thus rendering the model more physically plausible [60]. Another incentive to devise a general theory of diffuse fluorescence photon migration is the capability to quantify local changes in fluorescence lifetime. By selecting fluorophore probes with known lifetime dependence on specific environmental variables, lifetime imaging enables one to localize and quantify such metabolic parameters as temperature and pH, as well as changes in local molecular concentrations *in vivo*.

In the probabilistic RWT model, the description of a photon path may be divided into three parts: the path from the photon source to a localized, fluorescing target; the interaction of the photon with the fluorophore; and finally, the path of the fluorescently emitted photon to a detector. Each part of the photon path may be described by a probability: first, the probability that an incident photon will arrive at the fluorophore site; second, the probability that the photon has a reactive encounter with the fluorophore and the corresponding photon transit delay, which is dependent on the lifetime of the fluorophore and the probability of the fluorophore emitting a photon; and third, the probability that the photon emitted by the fluorophore travels from the reaction site to the detector. Each of these three sequences is governed by a stochastic process. The mathematical description of the three processes is extremely complicated. The complete solution for the probability of fluorescence photon arrival at the detector is [61]:

$$\hat{\gamma}(r, s, r_0) = [\eta \Phi \hat{p}'_\xi(r \mid s) \hat{p}_\xi(s \mid r_0)] \times \left[\langle \Delta n \rangle (1 - \eta)[\exp(\xi) - 1] \right.$$

$$\left. + \{\eta \langle \Delta n \rangle [\exp(\xi) - 1] + 1\} \left\{ 1 + \left[(1/8)(3/\pi)^{3/2} \sum_{j=1}^{\infty} \exp(-2j\xi)/j^{3/2} \right] \right\} \right]^{-1} \quad (30.15)$$

where η is the probability of fluorescent absorption of an excitation wavelength photon, Φ is the quantum efficiency of the fluorophore which is the probability that an excited fluorophore will emit a photon at the emission wavelength, $\langle \Delta n \rangle$ is the mean number of steps the photon would have taken had the photon not been exciting the fluorophore (which corresponds to the fluorophore lifetime in random walk parameters) and ξ is a transform variable corresponding to the discrete analog of the Laplace transform and may be considered analogous to frequency. The probability of a photon going from the excitation source to the fluorophore site is $\hat{p}_\xi(s \mid r_0)$, and the probability of a fluorescent photon going from the fluorophore site to the detector is $\hat{p}'_\xi(r \mid s)$; the prime indicates that the wavelength of the photon has changed and therefore the optical properties of the tissue may be different. In practice, this solution is difficult to work with, so some simplifying assumptions are desired. With some simplification the result in the frequency domain is:

$$\hat{\gamma}(r, s, r_0) = \eta \Phi \{\hat{p}'_\xi(r \mid s) \hat{p}_\xi(s \mid r_0) - \xi \langle \Delta n \rangle \hat{p}'_\xi(r \mid s) \hat{p}_\xi(s \mid r_0)\} \quad (30.16)$$

The inverse Laplace transform of this equation gives the diffuse fluorescent intensity in the time-domain, and the integral of the latter over time leads to CW measurements. The accuracy of such cumbersome equations is tested in well-defined phantoms and fluorophores embedded in *ex vivo* tissue. In Figure 30.6, a line scan of fluorescent intensity collected from 500 μm^3 fluorescent dye (Molecular Probe, far red microspheres: 690 nm excitation; 720 nm emission), embedded in 10.4 mm porcine tissue

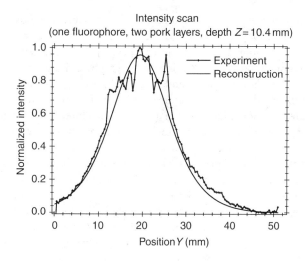

FIGURE 30.6   Intensity scan of a fluorophore 10.4 mm below the tissue surface.

with a lot of heterogeneity (e.g., fat), are presented. The dashed line is the corresponding RWT fit. The inverse algorithm written in C++ was able to construct the depth of the fluorophore with 100% accuracy. Knowing the heterogeneity of the tissue (seen in the intensity profile) this method presents huge potential to interrogate tissue structures deeply embedded in tissue for which specific fluorescent labeling such as antibodies for cell surfaces exists.

30.1.6   Future Directions

A clinically useful optical imaging device requires multidisciplinary and multi-step approaches. At the desk, one devises quantitative theories, and develop methodologies applicable to *in vivo* quantitative tissue spectroscopy and tomographic imaging in different imaging geometries (i.e., transmission or reflection), different types of measurements (e.g., steady-state or time-resolved). Effects of different optical sources of contrast such as endogenous or exogenous fluorescent labels, variations in absorption (e.g., hemoglobin or chromophore concentration) and scattering should be incorporated in the model. At the bench, one designs and conducts experiments on tissue-like phantoms and runs computer simulations to validate the theoretical findings. If successful, one tries to bring the imaging or spectroscopic device to the bedside. For this task, one must foster strong collaborations with physicians who can help to identify physiological sites where optical techniques may be clinically practical and can offer new diagnostic knowledge and less morbidity over existing methods. An important intermediate step is the use of animal models for preclinical studies. Overall, this is a complicated path. However, the spectroscopic power of light, along with the revolution in molecular characterization of disease processes has created a huge potential for *in vivo* optical imaging and spectroscopy. Maybe the twenty-first century will be the second "*siècle des lumieres.*"

30.2   Infrared Thermal Monitoring of Disease Processes: Clinical Study

The relationship between a change in body temperature and health status has been of interest to physicians since Hippocrates stated "should one part of the body be hotter or colder than the rest, then disease is present in that part." Thermography provides a visual display of the surface temperature of the skin. Skin temperature recorded by an infrared scanner is the resultant balance of thermal transport within the tissues and transport to the environment. In medical applications, thermal images of human skin contain a large amount of clinical information that can help to detect numerous pathological conditions ranging from cancer to emotional disorders. For the clinical assessment of cancer, physicians need to determine the activity of the tumor and its location, extent, and its response to therapy. All of these factors make it possible for tumors to be examined using thermography. Advantages to using this method are that it is completely nonionizing, safe, and can be repeated as often as required without exposing the patient to risk. Unfortunately, the skin temperature distribution is misinterpreted in many cases, because a high skin temperature does not always indicate a tumor. Therefore, thermography requires extensive education about how to interpret the temperature distribution patterns as well as additional research to clarify various diseases based on skin temperature.

Before applying the thermal technique in the clinical setting, it is important to consider how to avoid possible error in the results. Before the examination, the body should attain thermal equilibrium with its environment. A patient should be unclothed for at least 20 min in a controlled environment at a temperature of approximately 22°C. Under such clinical conditions, thermograms will show only average temperature patterns over an interval of time. The evaluation of surface temperature by infrared techniques requires wavelength and emissive properties of the surface (emissivity) to be examined over the range of wavelengths to which the detector is sensitive. In addition, a thermal camera should be calibrated with a known temperature reference source to standardize clinical data.

Before discussing a specific clinical application of thermography, an accurate technique for measuring emissivity is presented in Section 30.2.1. In Section 30.2.2, a procedure for temperature calibration of an infrared detector is discussed. The clinical applications of thermography with Kaposi's sarcoma are detailed in Section 30.2.3.

30.2.1 Emissivity Corrected Temperature

Emissivity is described as a radiative property of the skin. It is a measure of how well a body can radiate energy compared to a black body. Knowledge of emissivity is important when measuring skin temperature with an infrared detector system at different ambient radiation temperatures. Currently, different spectral band infrared detector systems are used in clinical studies such as 3–5 and 8–14 μm. It is well known that the emissivity of the skin varies according to the spectral range. The skin emits infrared radiation mainly between 2–20 μm with maximum emission at a wavelength around 10 μm [62]. Jones [63] showed with an InSb detector that only 2% of the radiation emitted from a thermal black body at 30°C was within the 3–5 μm spectral range; the wider spectral response of HgCdTe detector (8–14 μm) corresponded to 40–50% of this black body radiation.

Many investigators have reported on the values for emissivity of skin *in vivo*, measured in different spectral bands with different techniques. Hardy [64] and Stekettee [65] showed that the spectral emissivity of skin was independent of wavelength (λ) when $\lambda > 2$ μm. These results contradicted those obtained by Elam et al. [66]. Watmough and Oliver [67] pointed out that emissivity lies within 0.98–1 and was not less than 0.95 for a wavelength range of 2–5 μm. Patil and Williams [68] reported that the average emissivity of normal breast skin was 0.99 ± 0.045, 0.972 ± 0.041, and 0.975 ± 0.043 within the ranges 4–6, 6–18, and 4–18 μm respectively. Steketee [65] indicated that the average emissivity value of skin was 0.98 ± 0.01 within the range 3–14 μm. It is important to know the precise value of emissivity because an emissivity difference of 0.945–0.98 may cause an error of skin temperature of 0.6°C [64].

There is considerable diversity in the reported values of skin emissivity even in the same spectral band. The inconsistencies among reported values could be due to unreliable and inadequate theories and techniques employed for measuring skin emissivity. Togawa [69] proposed a technique in which the emissivity was calculated by measuring the temperature upon a transient stepwise change in ambient radiation temperature [69,70] surrounding an object surface as shown in Figure 30.7.

The average emissivity for the 12 normal subjects measured by a radiometer and infrared camera are presented in Table 30.2. The emissivity values were found to be significantly different between the 3–5 and 8–14 μm spectral bands ($p < .001$). An example of a set of images obtained during measurement using an infrared camera (3–5 μm band) on the forearm of a healthy male subject is shown in Figure 30.8.

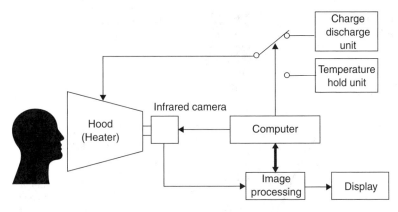

FIGURE 30.7 Schematic diagram of the emissivity measurement system [70].

TABLE 30.2 Emissivity Values

Average normal forearm skin of 12 subjects	
Infrared camera (3–5 μm)	0.958 ± 0.002
Radiometer (8–14 μm)	0.973 ± 0.0003

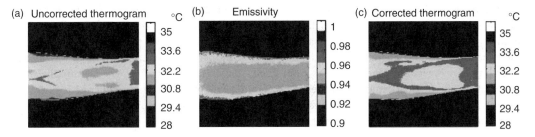

FIGURE 30.8 (See color insert.) An example of images obtained from the forearm of a normal healthy male subject. (a) Original thermogram; (b) emissivity image; (c) thermogram corrected by emissivity.

An accurate value of emissivity is important, because an incorrect value of emissivity can lead to a temperature error in radiometric thermometry especially when the ambient radiation temperature varies widely. The extent to which skin emissivity depends on the spectral range of the infrared detectors is demonstrated in Table 30.2, which shows emissivity values measured at 0.958 ± 0.002 and 0.973 ± 0.003 by an infrared detector with spectral bands of 3–5 and 8–14 μm respectively. These results can give skin temperatures that differ by 0.2°C at a room temperature of 22°C. Therefore, it is necessary to consider the wavelength dependence of emissivity, when high precision temperature measurements are required.

Emissivity not only depends on wavelength but is also influenced by surface quality, moisture on the skin surface, etc. In the infrared region of 3 to 50 μm, the emissivity of most nonmetallic substances is higher for a rough surface than a smooth one [71]. The presence of water also increases the value of emissivity [72]. These influences may account for the variation in results.

30.2.2 Temperature Calibration

In infrared thermography, any radiator is suitable as a temperature reference if its emissivity is known and constant within a given range of wavelengths. Currently, many different commercial blackbody calibrators are available to be used as temperature reference sources. A practical and simple blackbody radiator with a

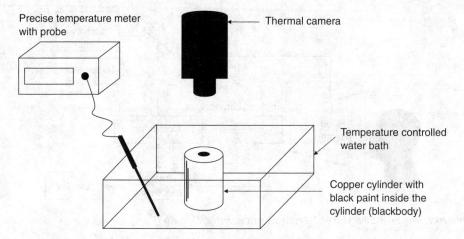

FIGURE 30.9   Schematic diagram of temperature calibration system.

known temperature and measurement system is illustrated in Figure 30.9. The system consists of a hollow copper cylinder, a temperature controlled water bath and a precise temperature meter with probe. The height of the cylinder is 15 cm and the diameter is 7.5 cm. The cylinder is closed except for a hole in the center of the upper end which is 2 cm in diameter. To make the blackbody radiator, the inner surface of the cylinder is coated with black paint (3M Velvet Coating no. 2010) with emissivity of 0.93. Before the calibration, $\frac{3}{4}$ of the cylinder is placed vertically in the water and the thermal camera is placed on the top of the cylinder in a vertical direction with a distance of focus length between the surface of the hole and the camera. The water temperature ranges from 18 to 45°C by increments of 2°C. This range was selected since human temperature generally varies from 22 to 42°C in clinical studies. After setting the water temperature, the thermal camera measures the surface temperature of the hole while the temperature meter with probe measures the water temperature. The temperature of the camera is calibrated according to the temperature reading of the temperature meter.

30.2.3   Clinical Study: Kaposi's Sarcoma

The oncology community is testing a number of novel targeted approaches such as antiangiogenic, anti-vascular, immuno- and gene therapies for use against a variety of cancers. To monitor such therapies, it is desirable to establish techniques to assess tumor vasculature and changes with therapy [73]. Currently, several imaging techniques such as dynamic contrast-enhanced magnetic resonance (MR) imaging [74–76], positron emission tomography (PET) [77–79], computed tomography (CT) [80–83], color Doppler ultrasound (US) [84,85], and fluorescence imaging [86,87] have been used in angiogenesis-related research. With regard to monitoring vasculature, it is desirable to develop and assess noninvasive and quantitative techniques that can not only monitor structural changes, but can also assess the functional characteristics or the metabolic status of the tumor. There are currently no standard noninvasive techniques to assess parameters of angiogenesis in lesions of interest and to monitor changes in these parameters with therapy. For antiangiogenic therapies, factors associated with blood flow are of particular interest.

Kaposi's sarcoma (KS) is a highly vascular tumor that occurs frequently among people infected with acquired immunodeficiency syndrome (AIDS). During the first decade of the AIDS epidemic, 15 to 20% of AIDS patients developed this type of tumor [88]. Patients with KS often display skin and oral lesions. In addition, KS frequently involves lymph nodes and visceral organs [89]. KS is an angio-proliferative disease characterized by angiogenesis, endothelial spindle-cell growth (KS cell growth), inflammatory-cell infiltration and edema [90]. A gamma herpesvirus called Kaposi's sarcoma associated herpesvirus (KSHV) or human herpesvirus type 8 (HHV-8) is an essential factor in the pathogenesis of KS [91]. Cutaneous

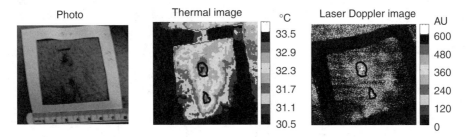

FIGURE 30.10 (See color insert.) Typical multi-modality images obtained from a patient with KS lesion. The number "1" and "5" in the visual image were written on the skin to identify the lesions for tumor measurement. The solid line in the thermal and LDI demarks the border of the visible KS lesion. Shown is a representative patient from the study reported in Reference 95.

KS lesions are easily accessible for noninvasive techniques that involve imaging of tumor vasculature, and they may thus represent a tumor model in which to assess certain parameters of angiogenesis [92,93].

Recently, two such potential noninvasive imaging techniques, infrared thermal imaging (thermography) and laser Doppler imaging (LDI) have been used to monitor patients undergoing an experimental anti-KS therapy [94,95]. Thermography graphically depicts temperature gradients over a given body surface area at a given time. It is used to study biological thermoregulatory abnormalities that directly or indirectly influence skin temperature [96–100]. However, skin temperature is only an indirect measure of skin blood flow, and the superficial thermal signature of skin is also related to local metabolism. Thus, this approach is best used in conjunction with other techniques. LDI can more directly measure the net blood velocity of small blood vessels in tissue, which generally increases as blood supply increases during angiogenesis [101,102]. Thermal patterns were recorded using an infrared camera with a uniform sensitivity in the wavelength range of 8 to 12 μm and LDI images were acquired by scanning the lesion area of the KS patients at two wavelengths, 690 and 780 nm.

An example of the images obtained from a typical KS lesion using different modalities is shown in Figure 30.10 [95]. As can be seen in the thermal image, the temperature of the lesion was approximately 2°C higher than that of the normal tissue adjacent to the lesion. Interestingly, in a number of lesions, the area of increased temperature extended beyond the lesion edges as assessed by visual inspection or palpation [95]. This may reflect relatively deep involvement of the tumor in areas underlying normal skin. However, the thermal signature of the skin not only reflects superficial vascularity, but also deep tissue metabolic activity. In the LDI image of the same lesion, there was increased blood flow in the area of the lesion as compared to the surrounding tissue, with a maximum increase of over 600 AU (arbitrary units). Unlike the thermal image, the increased blood velocity extended only slightly beyond the area of this visible lesion, possibly because the tumor process leading to the increased temperature was too deep to be detected by LDI. Both of these techniques were used successfully to visualize KS lesions [95], and although each measures an independent parameter (temperature or blood velocity), there was a strong correlation in a group of 16 patients studied by both techniques (Figure 30.11) [95]. However, there were some differences in individual lesions since LDI measured blood flow distribution in the superficial layer of the skin of the lesion, whereas the thermal signature provided a combined response of superficial vascularity and metabolic activities of deep tissue.

In patients treated with an anti-KS therapy, there was a substantial decrease in temperature and blood velocity during the initial 18-week treatment period as shown in Figure 30.12 [95]. The changes in these two parameters were generally greater than those assessed by either measurement of tumor size or palpation. In fact, there was no statistically significant decrease in tumor size overall. These results suggest that thermography and LDI may be relatively more sensitive in assessing the response of therapy in KS than conventional approaches. Assessing responses to KS therapy is now generally performed by visual measuring and palpating the numerous lesions and using rather complex response criteria. However, the current tools are rather cumbersome and often subject to observer variation, complicating the assessment

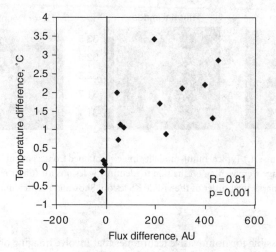

FIGURE 30.11 Relationship between the difference in temperature and flux of the lesion and surrounding area of the lesion of each subject. A positive correlation was observed between these two methods ($R = 0.8$, $p < .001$). (Taken from Hassan et al., TCRT, 3, 451–457, 2004. With permission.)

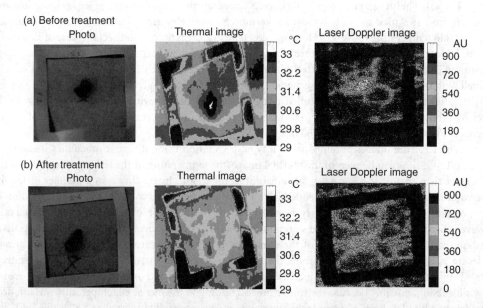

FIGURE 30.12 (See color insert.) Typical example of lesion obtained from a subject with KS (a) before, and (b) after the treatment. Improvement after the treatment can be assessed by the thermal or LDI images after 18 weeks. Shown is a patient from the clinical trial reported in Reference 95.

of new therapies. The techniques described here, possibly combined with other techniques to assess vasculature and vessel function, have the potential of being more quantitative, sensitive, and reproducible than established techniques. Moreover, it is possible that they may show a response to therapy sooner than conventional than conventional means of tumor assessment.

Acknowledgments

Special thanks go to Dr. Herbert Rinneberg (Physikalisch-Technische-Bundesanstalt, Berlin) and Dr. Brian Pogue (Dartmouth College) for providing the optical images. The authors also wish to express their thanks to Dr. Tatsuo Togawa, a former professor of the Institutes of Biomaterials and Bioengineering,

Tokyo Medical and Dental University, Tokyo, Japan for his valuable suggestions and allowing emissivity measurements to be performed in his lab. The authors also like to thanks Kathleen Wyvill and Karen Aleman for their help.

References

[1] M. Born and E. Wolf, *Principles in Optics*, 7th ed. Cambridge: Cambridge University Press, 1999.

[2] A.T. Young, "Rayleigh scattering," *Phys. Today*, 42, 1982.

[3] I.S. Saidi, S.L. Jacques, and F.K. Tittel, "Mie and Rayleigh modeling of visible-light scattering in neonatal skin," *Appl. Opt.*, 34, 7410, 1995.

[4] M.J.C. Van Gemert, S.L. Jacques, H.J.C.M. Sterenberg, and W.M. Star, "Skin optics," *IEEE Trans.*, 36, 1146, 1989.

[5] R. Marchesini, A. Bertoni, S. Andreola, E. Melloni, and A. Sicherolli, "Extinction and absorption coefficients and scattering phase functions of human tissues *in vitro*," *Appl. Opt.*, 28, 2318, 1989.

[6] J. Fishkin, O. Coquoz, E. Anderson, M. Brenner, and B. Tromberg, "Frequency-domain photon migration measurements of normal and malignant tissue optical properties in a human subject," *Appl. Opt.*, 36, 10, 1997.

[7] T.L. Troy, D.L. Page, and E.M. Sevick-Muraca, "Optical properties or normal and diseased breast tissues: prognosis for optical mammography," *J. Biomed. Opt.*, 1, 342, 1996.

[8] A.H. Gandjbakhche, R.F. Bonner, and R. Nossal, "Scaling relationships for anisotropic random walks," *J. Stat. Phys.*, 69, 35, 1992.

[9] G.A. Wagnieres, W.M. Star, and B.C. Wilson, "*In vivo* fluorescence spectroscopy and imaging for oncological applications," *Photochem. Photobiol.*, 68, 603, 1998.

[10] R. Weissleder, "A clearer vision for *in vivo* imaging," *Nat. Biotechnol.*, 19, 316, 2001.

[11] V.F. Kamalov, I.A. Struganova, and K. Yoshihara, "Temperature dependent radiative lifetime of J-aggregates," *J. Phys. Chem.*, 100, 8640, 1996.

[12] S. Mordon, J.M. Devoisselle, and V. Maunoury, "*In vivo* pH measurement and imaging of a pH-sensitive fluorescent probe (5–6 carboxyfluorescein): instrumental and experimental studies," *Photochem. Photobiol.*, 60, 274, 1994.

[13] C.L. Hutchinson, J.R. Lakowicz, and E.M. Sevick-Muraca, "Fluorescence lifetime-based sensing in tissues: a computational study," *Biophys. J.*, 68, 1574, 1995.

[14] F.F. Jobsis, "Noninvasive infrared monitoring of cerebral and myocardial oxygen sufficiency and circulatory parameters," *Science*, 198, 1264, 1977.

[15] T.J. Farrell, M.S. Patterson, and B. Wilson, "A diffusion theory model of spatially resolved, steady-state diffuse reflectance for the noninvasive determination of tissue optical properties *in vivo*," *Med. Phys.*, 9, 879, 1992.

[16] P.C. Jackson, P.H. Stevens, J.H. Smith, D. Kear, H. Key, and P. N. T. Wells, "Imaging mammalian tissues and organs using laser collimated transillumination," *J. Biomed. Eng.*, 6, 70, 1987.

[17] G. Jarry, S. Ghesquiere, J.M. Maarek, F. Fraysse, S. Debray, M.-H. Bui, and D. Laurent, "Imaging mammalian tissues and organs using laser collimated transillumination," *J. Biomed. Eng.*, 6, 70, 1984.

[18] M. Kaneko, M. Hatakeyama, P. He, Y. Nakajima, H. Isoda, M. Takai, T. Okawada, M. Asumi, T. Kato, S. Goto "Construction of a laser transmission photo-scanner: pre-clinical investigation," *Radiat. Med.*, 7, 129, 1989.

[19] L. Wang, P.P. Ho, C. Liu, G. Zhang, and R.R. Alfano, "Ballistic 2-D imaging through scattering walls using an ultrafast optical Kerr gate," *Science*, 253, 769, 1991.

[20] A. Schmitt, R. Corey, and P. Saulnier, "Imaging through random media by use of low-coherence optical heterodyning," *Opt. Lett.*, 20, 404, 1995.

[21] H. Inaba, M. Toida, and T. Ichmua, "Optical computer-assisted tomography realized by coherent detection imaging incorporating laser heterodyne method for biomedical applications," *SPIE Proc.*, 1399, 108, 1990.

[22] H. Inaba, "Coherent detection imaging for medical laser tomography," In *Medical Optical Tomography: Functional Imaging and Monitoring*, Muller, G., ed. p. 317, 1993.

[23] S.B. Colak, D.G. Papaioannou, G.W. T'Hoooft, M.B. van der Mark, H. Schomberg, J.C.J. Paasschens, J.B.M. Melissen, and N.A.A.J. van Austen, "Tomographic image reconstruction from optical projections in light diffusing media," *Appl. Opt.*, 36, 180, 1997.

[24] J.C. Hebden, D.J. Hall, M. Firbank, and D.T. Delpry, "Time-resolved optical imaging of a solid tissue-equivalent phantom," *Appl. Opt.*, 34, 8038, 1995.

[25] J.C. Hebden, "Evaluating the spatial resolution performance of a time-resolved optical imaging system," *Med. Phys.*, 19, 1081, 1992.

[26] R. Cubeddu, A. Pifferi, P. Taroni, A. Torriceli, and G. Valentini, "Time-resolved imaging on a realistic tissue phantom: us' and ua images versus time-integrated images," *Appl. Opt.*, 35, 4533, 1996.

[27] D. Grosenick, H. Wabnitz, H. Rinneberg, K.T. Moesta, and P. Schleg, "Development of a time-domain optical mammograph and first *in-vivo* application," *Appl. Opt.*, 38, 2927, 1999.

[28] M. Bashkansky, C. Adler, and J. Reinties, "Coherently amplified Raman polarization gate for imaging through scattering media," *Opt. Lett.*, 19, 350, 1994.

[29] K.M. Yoo, Q. Xing, and R.R. Alfano, "Imaging objects hidden in highly scattering media using femtosecond second-harmonic-generation cross-correlation time gating," *Opt. Lett.*, 16, 1019, 1991.

[30] G.W. Faris and M. Banks, "Upconverting time gate for imaging through highly scattering media," *Opt. Lett.*, 19, 1813, 1994.

[31] J.C. Hebden, S.R. Arridge, and D.T. Delpry, "Optical imaging in medicine I: experimental techniques," *Phys. Med. Biol.*, 42, 825, 1997.

[32] J.R. Lakowitz and K. Brendt, "Frequency domain measurements of photon migration in tissues," *Chem. Phys. Lett.*, 166, 246, 1990.

[33] M.A. Franceschini, K.T. Moesta, S. Fantini, G. Gaida, E. Gratton, H. Jess, W.W. Mantulin, M. Seeber, P.M. Schlag, and M. Kaschke, "Frequency-domain techniques enhance optical mammography: initial clinical results," *Proc. Natl Acad. Sci., Med. Sci.*, 94, 6468, 1997.

[34] B. Tromberg, O. Coquoz, J.B. Fishkin, T. Pham, E. Anderson, J. Butler, M. Cahn, J.D. Gross, V. Venugopalan, and D. Pham, "Non-invasive measurements of breast tissue optical properties using frequency-domain photon migration," *Philos. Trans. R. Soc. Lond. Ser. B*, 352, 661, 1997.

[35] J.J. Duderstadt and L.J. Hamilton, *Nuclear Reactor Analysis*. New York: Wiley, 1976.

[36] K.M. Case and P.F. Zweifel, *Linear Transport Theory*. Reading: Addison Wesley, 1967.

[37] A. Ishimaru, *Wave Propogation and Scattering in Random Media*. New York: Academic Press, 1978.

[38] M.S. Patterson, B. Chance, and B. Wilson, "Time resolved reflectance and transmittance for the non-invasive measurement of tissue optical properties," *Appl. Opt.*, 28, 2331, 1989.

[39] S.R. Arridge and J.C. Hebden, "Optical imaging in medicine: II. Modelling and reconstruction," *Phys. Med. Biol.*, 42, 841, 1997.

[40] S.R. Nioka, M. Miwa, S. Orel, M. Schnall, M. Haida, S. Zhao, and B. Chance, "Optical imaging of human breast cancer," *Adv. Exp. Med. Biol.*, 361, 171, 1994.

[41] S. Fantini, S.A. Walker, M.A. Franceschini, M. Kaschke, P.M. Schlag, and K.T. Moesta, "Assessment of the size, position, and optical properties of breast tumors *in vivo* by noninvasive optical methods," *Appl. Opt.*, 37, 1982, 1998.

[42] M. Maris, E. Gratton, J. Maier, W. Mantulin, and B. Chance, "Functional near-infrared imaging of deoxygenated haemoglobin during exercise of the finger extensor muscles using the frequency-domain techniques," *Bioimaging*, 2, 174, 1994.

[43] B.W. Pogue and K.D. Paulsen, "High-resolution near-infrared tomographic imaging simulations of the rat cranium by use of a priori magnetic resonance imaging structural information," *Opt. Lett.*, 23, 1716, 1998.

[44] R.F. Bonner, R. Nossal, S. Havlin, and G.H. Weiss, "Model for photon migration in turbid biological media," *J. Opt. Soc. Am. A*, 4, 423, 1987.

[45] A.H. Gandjbakhche and G.H. Weiss, "Random walk and diffusion-like models of photon migration in turbid media," *Progress in Optics*, Wolf, E., ed. Elsevier Science B.V., vol. XXXIV, p. 333, 1995.

[46] A.H. Gandjbakhche, R. Nossal, and R.F. Bonner, "Scaling relationships for theories of anisotropic random walks applied to tissue optics," *Appl. Opt.*, 32, 504, 1993.

[47] V. Chernomordik, R. Nossal, and A.H. Gandjbakhche, "Point spread functions of photons in time-resolved transillumination experiments using simple scaling arguments," *Med. Phys.*, 23, 1857, 1996.

[48] A.H. Gandjbakhche, G.H. Weiss, R.F. Bonner, and R. Nossal, "Photon path-length distributions for transmission through optically turbid slabs," *Phys. Rev. E*, 48, 810, 1993.

[49] D.J. Hawrysz and E.M. Sevick-Muraca, "Developments toward diagnostic breast cancer imaging using near-infrared optical measurements and fluorescent contract agents," *Neoplasia*, 2, 388, 2000.

[50] M. Cutler, "Transillumination as an aid in the diagnosis of breast lesions," *Surg. Gynecol. Obstet.*, 48, 721, 1929.

[51] A. H. Gandjbakhche, V. Chernomordik et al., "Time-dependent contract functions for quantitative imaging in time-resolved transillumination experiments," *Appl. Opt.*, 37, 1973, 1998.

[52] A.H. Gandjbakhche, R. Nossal, and R.F. Bonner, "Resolution limits for optical transillumination of abnormalities deeply embedded in tissues," *Med. Phys.*, 21, 185, 1994.

[53] V. Chernomordik, D. Hattery, A. Pifferi, P. Taroni, A. Torricelli, G. Valentini, R. Cubeddu, and A.H. Gandjbakhche, "A random walk methodology for quantification of the optical characteristics of abnormalities embedded within tissue-like phantoms," *Opt. Lett.*, 25, 951, 2000.

[54] M. Morin, S. Verreault, A. Mailloux, J. Frechette, S. Chatigny, Y. Painchaud, and P. Beaudry, "Inclusion characterization in a scattering slab with time-resolved transmittance measurements: perturbation analysis," *Appl. Opt.*, 39, 2840–2852, 2000.

[55] V. Chernomordik, D.W. Hattery, D. Grosenick, H. Wabnitz, H. Rinneberg, K.T. Moesta, P.M. Schlag, and A.H. Gandjbakhche, "Quantification of optical properties of a breast tumor using random walk theory," *J. Biomed. Opt.*, 7, 80–87, 2002.

[56] A.P. Gibson, J.C. Hebden, and S.R. Arridge, "Recent advances in diffuse optical imaging," *Phys. Med. Biol.*, 50, R1–R43, 2005.

[57] R.I. Fox, "Treatment of patient with Sjogren syndrome," *Rhem. Dis. Clin. North Amer.*, 18, 699–709, 1992.

[58] V. Chernomordik, D. Hattery, I. Gannot, and A.H. Gandjbakhche, "Inverse method 3D recon-struction of localized in-vivo fluorescence. Application to Sjogren syndrome," *IEEE J. Select Topics in Quant. Elec.*, 5, 930, 1999.

[59] M.S. Patterson and B.W. Pogue, "Mathematical model for time-resolved and frequency-domain fluorescence spectroscopy in biological tissue," *Appl. Opt.*, 33, 1963, 1994.

[60] A.H. Gandjbakhche, R.F. Bonner, R. Nossal, and G.H. Weiss, "Effects on multiple passage probabilities on fluorescence signals from biological media," *Appl. Opt.*, 36, 4613, 1997.

[61] D. Hattery, V. Chernomordik, M. Loew, I. Gannot, and A.H. Gandjbakhche, "Analytical solutions for time-resolved fluorescence lifetime imaging in a turbid medium such as tissue," *JOSA(A)*, 18, 1523, 2001.

[62] E. Samuel, "Thermography — some clinical applications," *Biomed. Eng.*, 4, 15–19, 1969.

[63] C.H. Jones, "Physical aspects of thermography in relation to clinical techniques," *Bibl. Radiol.*, 6, 1–8, 1975.

[64] J. Hardy, "The radiation power of human skin in the infrared," *Am. J. Physiol.*, 127, 454–462, 1939.

[65] J. Steketee, "Spectral emissivity of skin and pericardium," *Phys. Med. Biol.*, 18, 686–694, 1973.

[66] R. Elam, D. Goodwin, and K. Williams, "Optical properties of human epidermics," *Nature*, 198, 1001–1002, 1963.

[67] D.J. Watmough and R. Oliver, "Emissivity of human skin in the waveband between 2micra and 6micra," *Nature*, 219, 622–624, 1968.

[68] K.D. Patil and K.L. Willaiam, "Spectral study of human radiation. Non-ionizing radiation," *Non-Ionizing Radiation*, 1, 39–44, 1969.

[69] T. Togawa, "Non-contact skin emissivity: measurement from reflectance using step change in ambient radiation temperature," *Clin. Phys. Physiol. Meas.*, 10, 39–48, 1989.

[70] M. Hassan and T. Togawa, "Observation of skin thermal inertia distribution during reactive hyperaemia using a single-hood measurement system," *Physiol. Meas.*, 22, 187–200, 2001.

[71] W.H. McAdams, *Heat Transmission*. New York: McGraw Hill, p. 472, 1954.

[72] H.T. Hammel, J.D. Hardy, and D. Murgatroyd, "Spectral transmittance and reflectance of excised human skin," *J. Appl. Physiol.*, 9, 257–264, 1956.

[73] D.M. McDonald and P.L. Choyke, "Imaging of angiogenesis: from microscope to clinic," *Nat. Med.*, 9, 713–725, 2003.

[74] J.S. Taylor, P.S. Tofts, R. Port, J.L. Evelhoch, M. Knopp, W.E. Reddick, V.M. Runge, and N. Mayr, "MR imaging of tumor microcirculation: promise for the new millennium," *J. Magn. Reson. Imaging*, 10, 903–907, 1999.

[75] K.L. Verstraete, Y. De Deene, H. Roels, A. Dierick, D. Uyttendaele, and M. Kunnen, "Benign and malignant musculoskeletal lesions: dynamic contrast-enhanced MR imaging—parametric 'first-pass' images depict tissue vascularization and perfusion," *Radiology*, 192, 835–843, 1994.

[76] L.D. Buadu, J. Murakami, S. Murayama, N. Hashiguchi, S. Sakai, K. Masuda, S. Toyoshima, S. Kuroki, and S. Ohno, "Breast lesions: correlation of contrast medium enhancement patterns on MR images with histopathologic findings and tumor angiogenesis," *Radiology*, 200, 639–649, 1996.

[77] A. Fredriksson and S. Stone-Elander, "PET screening of anticancer drugs. A faster route to drug/target evaluations *in vivo*," *Meth. Mol. Med.*, 85, 279–294, 2003.

[78] G. Jerusalem, R. Hustinx, Y. Beguin, and G. Fillet, "The value of positron emission tomography (PET) imaging in disease staging and therapy assessment," *Ann. Oncol.*, 13, 227–234, 2002.

[79] H.C. Steinert, M. Hauser, F. Allemann, H. Engel, T. Berthold, G.K. von Schulthess, and W. Weder, "Non-small cell lung cancer: nodal staging with FDG PET versus CT with correlative lymph node mapping and sampling," *Radiology*, 202, 441–446, 1997.

[80] S. D. Rockoff, "The evolving role of computerized tomography in radiation oncology," *Cancer*, 39, 694–696, 1977.

[81] K.D. Hopper, K. Singapuri, and A. Finkel, "Body CT and oncologic imaging," *Radiology*, 215, 27–40, 2000.

[82] K.A. Miles, M. Hayball, and A.K. Dixon, "Colour perfusion imaging: a new application of computed tomography," *Lancet*, 337, 643–645, 1991.

[83] K.A. Miles, C. Charnsangavej, F.T. Lee, E.K. Fishman, K. Horton, and T.Y. Lee, "Application of CT in the investigation of angiogenesis in oncology," *Acad. Radiol.*, 7, 840–850, 2000.

[84] N. Ferrara, "Role of vascular endothelial growth factor in physiologic and pathologic angiogenesis: therapeutic implications," *Semin. Oncol.*, 29, 10–14, 2002.

[85] D.E. Goertz, D.A. Christopher, J.L. Yu, R.S. Kerbel, P.N. Burns, and F.S. Foster, "High-frequency color flow imaging of the microcirculation," *Ultrasound Med. Biol.*, 26, 63–71, 2000.

[86] E.M. Gill, G.M. Palmer, and N. Ramanujam, "Steady-state fluorescence imaging of neoplasia," *Meth. Enzymol.*, 361, 452–481, 2003.

[87] K. Svanberg, I. Wang, S. Colleen, I. Idvall, C. Ingvar, R. Rydell, D. Jocham, H. Diddens, S. Bown, G. Gregory, S. Montan, S. Andersson-Engels, and S. Svanberg, "Clinical multi-colour fluorescence imaging of malignant tumours — initial experience," *Acta Radiol.*, 39, 2–9, 1998.

[88] V. Beral, T.A. Peterman, R.L. Berkelman, and H.W. Jaffe, "Kaposi's sarcoma among persons with AIDS: a sexually transmitted infection?" *Lancet*, 335, 123–128, 1990.

[89] B.A. Biggs, S.M. Crowe, C.R. Lucas, M. Ralston, I.L. Thompson, and K. J. Hardy, "AIDS related Kaposi's sarcoma presenting as ulcerative colitis and complicated by toxic megacolon," *Gut*, 28, 1302–1306, 1987.

[90] E. Cornali, C. Zietz, R. Benelli, W. Weninger, L. Masiello, G. Breier, E. Tschachler, A. Albini, and
M. Sturzl, "Vascular endothelial growth factor regulates angiogenesis and vascular permeability in
Kaposi's sarcoma," *Am. J. Pathol.*, 149, 1851–1869, 1996.

[91] Y. Chang, E. Cesarman, M.S. Pessin, F. Lee, J. Culpepper, D.M. Knowles, and P.S. Moore, "Identification of herpesvirus-like DNA sequences in AIDS-associated Kaposi's sarcoma," *Science*, 266,
1865–1869, 1994.

[92] R. Yarchoan, "Therapy for Kaposi's sarcoma: recent advances and experimental approaches,"
J. Acquir. Immune Defic. Syndr., 21, S66–73, 1999.

[93] R.F. Little, K.M. Wyvill, J.M. Pluda, L. Welles, V. Marshall, W.D. Figg, F.M. Newcomb, G. Tosato,
E. Feigal, S.M. Steinberg, D. Whitby, J.J. Goedert, and R. Yarchoan, "Activity of thalidomide in
AIDS-related Kaposi's sarcoma," *J. Clin. Oncol.*, 18, 2593–2602, 2000.

[94] M. Hassan, D. Hattery, V. Chernomordik, K. Aleman, K. Wyvill, F. Merced, R.F. Little, R. Yarchoan,
and A. Gandjbakhche, "Non-invasive multi-modality technique to study angiogenesis associated
with Kaposi's sarcoma," *Proceedings of EMBS BMES*, pp. 1139–1140, 2002.

[95] M. Hassan, R.F. Little, A. Vogel, K. Aleman, K. Wyvill, R. Yarchoan, and A. Gandjbakhche, "Quantitative assessment of tumor vasculature and response to therapy in Kaposi's sarcoma using functional
noninvasive imaging," *TCRT*, 3, 451–458, 2004.

[96] C. Maxwell-Cade, "Principles and practice of clinical thermography," *Radiography*, 34, 23–34,
1968.

[97] J.F. Head and R.L. Elliott, "Infrared imaging: making progress in fulfilling its medical promise,"
IEEE Eng. Med. Biol. Mag., 21, 80–85, 2002.

[98] S. Bornmyr and H. Svensson, "Thermography and laser-Doppler flowmetry for monitoring
changes in finger skin blood flow upon cigarette smoking," *Clin. Physiol.*, 11, 135–141, 1991.

[99] K. Usuki, T. Kanekura, K. Aradono, and T. Kanzaki, "Effects of nicotine on peripheral cutaneous
blood flow and skin temperature," *J. Dermatol. Sci.*, 16, 173–181, 1998.

[100] M. Anbar, "Clinical thermal imaging today," *IEEE Eng. Med. Biol. Mag.*, 17, 25–33, 1998.

[101] J. Sorensen, M. Bengtsson, E.L. Malmqvist, G. Nilsson, and F. Sjoberg, "Laser Doppler perfusion
imager (LDPI) — for the assessment of skin blood flow changes following sympathetic blocks,"
Acta Anaesthesiol. Scand., 40, 1145–1148, 1996.

[102] A. Rivard, J.E. Fabre, M. Silver, D. Chen, T. Murohara, M. Kearney, M. Magner, T. Asahara, and
J.M. Isner, "Age-dependent impairment of angiogenesis," *Circulation*, 99, 111–120, 1999.

31

Thermal Imaging in Diseases of the Skeletal and Neuromuscular Systems

31.1 Introduction... **31**-1
31.2 Inflammation **31**-2
31.3 Paget's Disease of Bone **31**-3
31.4 Soft Tissue Rheumatism............................... **31**-4
Muscle Spasm and Injury • Sprains and Strains • Enthesopathies • Fibromyalgia

E. Francis Ring
University of Glamorgan

Kurt Ammer
Ludwig Boltzmann Research Institute for Physical Diagnostics and University of Glamorgan

31.5 Peripheral Nerves **31**-6
Nerve Entrapment • Peripheral Nerve Paresis
31.6 Complex Regional Pain Syndrome **31**-9
31.7 Thermal Imaging Technique **31**-11
Room Temperature • Clinical Examination
References **31**-11

31.1 Introduction

Clinical medicine has made considerable advances over the last century. The introduction of imaging modalities has widened the ability of physicians to locate and understand the extent and activity of a disease. Conventional radiography has dramatically improved, beyond the mere demonstration of bone and calcified tissue. Computed tomography ultrasound, positron emission tomography, and magnetic resonance imaging are now available for medical diagnostics.

Infrared imaging has also added to this range of imaging procedures. It is often misunderstood, or not been used due to lack of knowledge of thermal physiology and the relationship between temperature and disease.

In Rheumatology, disease assessment remains complex. There are a number of indices used, which testify to the absence of any single parameter for routine investigation. Most indices used are subjective.

Objective assessments are of special value, but may be more limited due to their invasive nature. Infrared imaging is noninvasive, and with modern technology has proved to be reliable and useful in rheumatology.

From early times physicians have used the cardinal signs of inflammation, that is, pain, swelling, heat, redness, and loss of function. When a joint is acutely inflamed, the increase in heat can be readily detected by touch. However, subtle changes in joint surface temperature occur and increase and decrease in temperature can have a direct expression of reduction or exacerbation of inflammation.

31.2 Inflammation

Inflammation is a complex phenomenon, which may be triggered by various forms of tissue injury. A series of cellular and chemical changes take place that are initially destructive to the surrounding tissue. Under normal circumstances the process terminates when healing takes place, and scar tissue may then be formed.

A classical series of events take place in the affected tissues. First, a brief arteriolar constriction occurs, followed by a prolonged dilatation of arterioles, capillaries, and venules. The initial increased blood flow caused by the blood vessel dilation becomes sluggish and leucocytes gather at the vascular endothelium. Increased permeability to plasma proteins causes exudates to form, which is slowly absorbed by the lymphatic system. Fibrinogen, left from the reabsorption partly polymerizes to fibrin. The increased permeability in inflammation is attributed to the action of a number of mediators, including histamines, kinins, and prostaglandins. The final process is manifest as swelling caused by the exudates, redness, and increased heat in the affected area resulting from the vasodilation, and increased blood flow. Loss of function and pain accompany these visible signs.

Increase in temperature and local vascularity can be demonstrated by some radionuclide procedures. In most cases, the isotope is administered intravenously and the resulting uptake is imaged or counted with a gamma camera. Superficial increases in blood flow can also be shown by laser doppler imaging although the response time may be slow. Thermal imaging, based on infrared emission from the skin is both fast and noninvasive.

This means that it is a technique that is suitable for repeated assessment, and especially useful in clinical trials of treatment whether by drugs, physical therapy, or surgery.

Intra-articular injection, particularly to administer corticosteroids came into use in the middle of the last century. Horvath and Hollander in 1949 [1] used intra-articular thermocouples to monitor the reduction in joint inflammation and synovitis following treatment. This method of assessment while useful to provide objective evidence of anti-inflammatory treatment was not universally used for obvious ethical reasons.

The availability of noncontact temperature measurement for infrared radiometry was a logical progression. Studies in a number of centers were made throughout the 1960s to establish the best analogs of corticosteroids and their effective dose. Work by Collins and Cosh in 1970 [2] and Ring and Collins 1970 [3] showed that the surface temperature of an arthritic joint was related to the intra-articular joint, and to other biochemical markers of inflammation obtained from the exudates. In a series of experiments with different analogues of prednisolone (all corticosteroids), the temperature measured by thermal imaging in groups of patients can be used to determine the duration and degree of reduction in inflammation [4,5].

At this time, a thermal challenge test for inflamed knees was being used in Bath, based on the application of a standard ice pack to the joint. This form of treatment is still used, and results in a marked decrease of joint temperature, although the effect may be transient.

The speed of temperature recovery after an ice pack of 1 kg of crushed ice to the knee for 10 min, was shown to be directly related to the synovial blood flow and inflammatory state of the joint. The mean temperature of the anterior surface of the knee joint could be measured either by infrared radiometry or by quantitative thermal imaging [6].

A number of new nonsteroid anti-inflammatory agents were introduced into rheumatology in the 1970s and 1980s. Infrared imaging was shown to be a powerful tool for the clinical testing of these drugs, using temperature changes in the affected joints as an objective marker. The technique had been successfully used on animal models of inflammation, and effectively showed that optimal dose response curves could be obtained from temperature changes at the experimental animal joints. The process with human patients suffering from acute Rheumatoid Arthritis was adapted to include a washout period for previous medication. This should be capable of relieving pain but no direct anti-inflammatory action per se. The compound used by all the pharmaceutical companies was paracetamol. It was shown by Bacon et al. [7] that small joints such as fingers and metacarpal joints increased in temperature quite rapidly while paracetamol treatment was given, even if pain was still suppressed. Larger joints, such as knees and ankles required more than one week of active anti-inflammatory treatment to register the same effect. Nevertheless, the commonly accepted protocol was to switch to the new test anti-inflammatory treatment after one week of washout with the analgesic therapy. In every case if the dose was ineffective the joint temperature was not reduced. At an effective dose, a fall in temperature was observed, first in the small joints, then later in the larger joints. Statistical studies were able to show an objective decrease in joint temperature by infrared imaging as a result of a new and successful treatment. Not all the new compounds found their way into routine medicine; a few were withdrawn as a result of undesirable side effects. The model of infrared imaging to measure the effects of a new treatment for arthritis was accepted by all the pharmaceutical companies involved and the results were published in the standard peer reviewed medical journals. More recently attention has been focused on a range of new biological agents for reducing inflammation. These also are being tested in trials that incorporate quantitative thermal imaging.

To facilitate the use and understanding of joint temperature changes, Ring and Collins [3], Collins et al. [8] devised a system for quantitation. This was based on the distribution of isotherms from a standard region of interest. The Thermal Index was calculated as the mean temperature difference from a reference temperature. The latter was determined from a large study of 600 normal subjects where the average temperature threshold for ankles, knees, hands, elbows, and shoulder were calculated. Many of the clinical trials involved the monitoring of hands, elbows, knees, and ankle joints. Normal index figure obtained from controls under the conditions described was from 1 to 2.5 on this scale. In inflammatory arthritis this figure was increased to 4–5, while in osteoarthritic joints, the increase in temperature was usually less, 3–4. In gout and infection higher values around 6–7 on this scale were recorded.

However, to determine normal values of finger joints is a very difficult task. This difficulty arises partly from the fact, that cold fingers are not necessarily a pathological finding. Tender joints showed higher temperatures than nontender joints, but a wide overlap of readings from nonsymptomatic and symptomatic joints was observed [9]. Evaluation of finger temperatures from the reference database of normal thermograms [10] of the human body might ultimately solve the problem of being able to establish a normal range for finger joint temperatures in the near future.

31.3 Paget's Disease of Bone

The early descriptions of Osteitis Deformans by Czerny [11] and Paget [12] refer to "chronic inflammation of bone." An increased skin temperature over an active site of this disease has been a frequent observation and that the increase may be around 4°C. Others have shown an increase in peripheral blood flow in almost all areas examined. Increased periosteal vascularity has been found during the active stages of the disease. The vascular bed is thought to act as an arterio-venous shunt, which may lead to high output cardiac failure. A number of studies, initially to monitor the effects of calcitonin, and later bisphosphonate therapy have been made at Bath (UK). As with the clinical trials previously mentioned, a rigorous technique is required to obtain meaningful scientific data. It was shown that the fall in temperature during calcitonin treatment was also indicated more slowly, by a fall in alkaline phosphatase, the common biochemical marker. Relapse and the need for retreatment was clearly indicated by thermal imaging. Changes in the thermal index often preceded the onset of pain and other symptoms by 2 to 3 weeks. It was also shown that the level of increased temperature over the bone was related to the degree of bone pain. Those patients who had maximal temperatures recorded at the affected bone experienced severe bone pain. Moderate pain was found in those with raised temperature, and no pain in those patients with normal temperatures. The most dramatic temperature changes were observed at the tibia, where the bone is very close to the skin surface. In a mathematical model, Ring and Davies [13] showed that the increased temperature measured over the tibia was primarily derived from osseous blood flow and not from metabolic heat. This disease is often categorized as a metabolic bone disease.

31.4   Soft Tissue Rheumatism

31.4.1   Muscle Spasm and Injury

Muscle work is the most important source for metabolic heat. Therefore, contracting muscles contribute to the temperature distribution at the body's surface of athletes [14,15]. Pathological conditions such as muscle spasms or myofascial trigger points may become visible at regions of increased temperature [16]. An anatomic study from Israel proposes in the case of the levator scapulae muscle that the frequently seen hot spot on thermograms of the tender tendon insertion on the medial angle of the scapula might be caused by an inflamed bursae and not by a taut band of muscle fibers [17].

Acute muscle injuries may also be recognized by areas of increased temperature [18] due to inflammation in the early state of trauma. However, long lasting injuries and also scars appear at hypothermic areas caused by reduced muscle contraction and therefore reduced heat production. Similar areas of decreased temperature have been found adjacent to peripheral joints with reduced range of motion due to inflammation or pain [19]. Reduced skin temperatures have been related to osteoarthritis of the hip [20] or to frozen shoulders [21,22]. The impact of muscle weakness on hypothermia in patients suffering from paresis was discussed elsewhere [23].

31.4.2   Sprains and Strains

Ligamentous injuries of the ankle [24] and meniscal tears of the knee [25] can be diagnosed by infrared thermal imaging. Stress fractures of bone may become visible in thermal images prior to typical changes in x-rays [26] Thermography provides the same diagnostic prediction as bone scans in this condition.

31.4.3   Enthesopathies

Muscle overuse or repetitive strain may lead to painful tendon insertions or where tendons are shielded by tendon sheaths or adjacent to bursae, to painful swellings. Tendovaginitis in the hand was successfully diagnosed by skin temperature measurement [27]. The acute bursitis at the tip of the elbow can be detected through an intensive hot spot adjacent to the olecranon [28]. Figure 31.1 shows an acute tendonitis of the Achilles tendon in a patient suffering from inflammatory spondylarthropathy.

31.4.3.1   Tennis Elbow

Painful muscle insertion of the extensor muscles at the elbow is associated with hot areas on a thermogram [29]. Thermal imaging can detect persistent tendon insertion problems of the elbow region in a similar way as isotope bone scanning [30]. Hot spots at the elbow have also been described as having a high association with a low threshold for pain on pressure [31]. Such hot areas have been successfully used as outcome measure for monitoring treatment [32,33]. In patients suffering from fibromyalgia, bilateral hot spots at the elbows is a common finding [34]. Figure 31.2 is the image of a patient suffering from tennis elbow with a typical hot spot in the region of tendon insertion.

31.4.3.2   Golfer Elbow

Pain due to altered tendon insertions of flexor muscles on the medial side of the elbow is usually named Golfer's elbow. Although nearly identical in pathogenesis as the tennis elbow, temperature symptoms in this condition were rarely found [35].

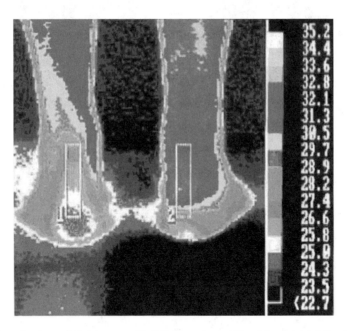

FIGURE 31.1 (See color insert following page **29**-16.) Acute tendonitis of the right Achilles tendon in a patient suffering from inflammatory spondylarthropathy.

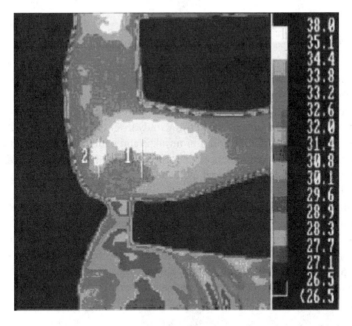

FIGURE 31.2 (See color insert.) Tennis elbow with a typical hot spot in the region of tendon insertion.

31.4.3.3 Periarthropathia of the Shoulder

The term periarthropathia includes a number of combined alterations of the periarticular tissue of the humero-scapular joint. The most frequent problems are pathologies at the insertion of the supraspinous and infraspinous muscles, often combined with impingement symptoms in the subacromial space. Long lasting insertion alteration can lead to typical changes seen on radiographs or ultrasound images, but

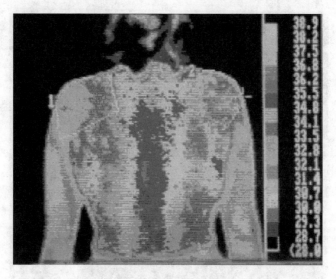

FIGURE 31.3   (See color insert.) Decreased temperature in patient with a frozen shoulder on the left-hand side.

unfortunately there are no typical temperature changes caused by the disease [22,36]. However, persistent loss in range of motion will result in hypothermia of the shoulder region [21,22,36,37]. Figure 31.3 gives an example of an area of decreased temperature over the left shoulder region in patient with restricted range of motion.

31.4.4 Fibromyalgia

The terms tender points (important for the diagnosis of fibromyalgia) and trigger points (main feature of the myofascial pain syndrome) must not be confused. Tender points and trigger points may give a similar image on the thermogram. If this is true, patients suffering from fibromyalgia may present with a high number of hot spots in typical regions of the body. A study from Italy could not find different patterns of heat distribution in patients suffering from fibromyalgia and patients with osteoarthritis of the spine [38]. However, they reported a correspondence of nonspecific hyperthermic patterns with painful muscle areas in both groups of patients. Our thermographic investigations in fibromyalgia revealed a diagnostic accuracy of 60% of hot spots for tender points [34]. The number of hot spot was greatest in fibromyalgia patients and the smallest in healthy subjects. More than 7 hot spots seem to be predictive for tenderness of more than 11 out of 18 specific sites [39]. Based on the count of hot spots, 74.2% of 252 subjects (161 fibromyalgia, 71 with widespread pain but less than 11 tender sites out of 18, and 20 healthy controls) have been correctly diagnosed. However, the intra- and inter-observer reproducibility of hot spot count is rather poor [40]. Software assisted identification of hot or cold spots based on the angular distribution around a thermal irregularity [41] might overcome that problem of poor repeatability.

31.5   Peripheral Nerves

31.5.1 Nerve Entrapment

Nerve entrapment syndromes are compression neuropathies at specific sites in human body. These sites are narrow anatomic passages where nerves are situated. The nerves are particularly prone to extrinsic or intrinsic pressure. This can result in paraesthesias such as tingling or numb feelings, pain, and ultimately in muscular weakness and atrophy.

Uematsu [42] has shown in patients with partial and full lesion of peripheral nerves that both conditions can be differentiated by their temperature reaction to the injury. The innervated area of partially lesioned nerve appears hypothermic caused by activation of sympathetic nerve fibers. Fully dissected nerves result in a total loss of sympathetic vascular control and therefore in hyperthermic skin areas.

The spinal nerves, the brachial nerve plexus, and the median nerve at the carpal tunnel are the most frequently affected nerves with compression neuropathy.

31.5.1.1 Radiculopathy

A slipped nucleus of an intervertebral disk may compress the adjacent spinal nerve or better the sensory and motor fibers of the dorsal root of the spinal nerve. This may or must not result in symptoms of compression neuropathy in the body area innervated by these fibers.

The diagnostic value of infrared thermal imaging in radiculopathies is still under debate. A review by Hoffman et al. [43] from 1991 concluded that thermal imaging should be used only for research and not in clinical routine. This statement was based on the evaluation of 28 papers selected from a total of 81 references.

The study of McCulloch et al. [44] planned and conducted at a high level of methodology, found thermography not valid. However, the applied method of recording and interpretation of thermal images was not sufficient. The chosen room temperature of 20 to 22°C might have been too low for the identification of hypothermic areas. Evaluation of thermal images was based on the criterion that at least 25% of a dermatome present with hypothermia of 1°C compared to the contralateral side. This way of interpretation might be feasible for contact thermography, but does not meet the requirements of quantitative infrared imaging.

The paper of Takahashi et al. [45] showed that the temperature deficit identified by infrared imaging is an additional sign in patients with radiculoapathy. Hypothermic areas did not correlate with sensory dermatomes and only slightly with the underlying muscles of the hypothermic area. The diagnostic sensitivity (22.9–36.1%) and the positive predictive value (25.2–37.0%) were low for both, muscular symptoms such as tenderness or weakness and for spontaneous pain and sensory loss. In contrast, high specificity (78.8–81.7%), high negative predictive values (68.5–86.2%), and a high diagnostic accuracy were obtained.

Only the papers by Kim and Cho [46] and Zhang et al. [47] found thermography of high value for the diagnosis of both lumbosacral and cervical radiculopathies. However, these studies have several methodological flaws. Although a high number of patients were reported, healthy control subjects were not mentioned in the study on lumbosacral radiculopathy. The clinical symptoms are not described and the reliability of the used thermographic diagnostic criteria remains questionable.

31.5.1.2 Thoracic Outlet Syndrome

Similar to fibromyalgia, the disease entity of the thoracic outlet syndrome (TOS) is under continuous debate [48]. Consensus exists, that various subforms related to the severity of symptoms must be differentiated. Recording thermal images during diagnostic body positions can reproducibly provoke typical temperature asymmetries in the hands of patients with suspected thoracic outlet syndrome [49,50]. Temperature readings from thermal images from patients passing that test can be reproduced by the same and by different readers with high precision [51]. The original protocol included a maneuver in which the fist was opened and closed 30 times before an image of the hand was recorded. As this test did not increase the temperature difference between index and little finger, the fist maneuver was removed from the protocol [52]. Thermal imaging can be regarded as the only technique that can objectively confirm the subjective symptoms of mild thoracic outlet syndrome. It was successfully used as outcome measure for the evaluation of treatment for this pain syndrome [53]. However, in a patient with several causes for the symptoms paraestesias and coldness of the ulnar fingers, thermography could show only a marked cooling of the little finger, but could not identify all reasons for that temperature deficit [54]. It was also difficult to differentiate between subjects whether they suffer from TOS or carpal tunnel syndrome. Only

66.3% of patients were correctly allocated to three diagnostic groups, while none of the carpal tunnel syndromes have been identified [55].

31.5.1.3   Carpal Tunnel Syndrome

Entrapment of the median nerve at the carpal tunnel is the most common compression neuropathy. A study conducted in Sweden revealed a prevalence of 14.4%; for pain, numbness, and tingling in the median nerve distribution in the hands. Prevalence of clinically diagnosed carpal tunnel syndrome (CTS) was 3.8 and 4.9% for pathological results of nerve conduction of the median nerve. Clinically and electrophysiologically confirmed CTS showed a prevalence of 2.7% [56].

The typical distribution of symptoms leads to the clinical suspect of CTS [57], which must be confirmed by nerve conduction studies. The typical electroneurographic measurements in patients with CTS show a high intra- and inter-rater reproducibility [58]. The course of nerve conduction measures for a period of 13 years in patients with and without decompression surgery was investigated and it was shown that most of the operated patients presented with less pathological conduction studies within 12 months after operation [59]. Only 2 of 61 patients who underwent a simple nerve decompression by division of the carpal ligament as therapy for CTS had pathological findings in nerve conduction studies 2 to 3 years after surgery [60].

However, nerve conduction studies are unpleasant for the patient and alternative diagnostic procedures are welcome. Liquid crystal thermography was originally used for the assessment of patients with suspected CTS [61–64]. So et al. [65] used infrared imaging for the evaluation of entrapment syndromes of the median and ulnar nerves. Based on their definition of abnormal temperature difference to the contralateral side, they found thermography without any value for assisting diagnosis and inferior to electrodiagnostic testing. Tchou reported infrared thermography of high diagnostic sensitivity and specificity in patients with unilateral CTS. He has defined various regions of interest representing mainly the innervation area of the median nerve. Abnormality was defined if more than 25% of the measured area displayed a temperature increase of at least 1°C when compared with the asymptomatic hand [66].

Ammer has compared nerve conduction studies with thermal images in patients with suspected CTS. Maximum specificity for both nerve conduction and clinical symptoms was obtained for the temperature difference between the 3rd and 4th finger at a threshold of 1°C. The best sensitivity of 69% was found if the temperature of the tip of the middle finger was by 1.2°C less than temperature of the metacarpus [67].

Hobbins [68] combined the thermal pattern with the time course of nerve injuries. He suggested the occurrence of a hypothermic dermatome in the early phase of nerve entrapment and hyperthermic dermatomes in the late phase of nerve compression. Ammer et al. [69] investigated how many patients with a distal latency of the median nerve greater than 6 msec present with a hyperthermic pattern. They reported a slight increase of the frequency of hyperthermic patterns in patients with severe CTS indicating that the entrapment of the median nerve is followed by a loss of the autonomic function in these patients.

Ammer [70] has also correlated the temperature of the index finger with the temperature of the sensory distribution of the median nerve on the dorsum of the hand and found nearly identical readings for both areas. A similar relationship was obtained for the ulnar nerve. The author concluded from these data that the temperature of the index or the little finger is highly representative for the temperature of the sensory area of the median or ulnar nerve, respectively.

Many studies on CTS have used a cold challenge to enhance the thermal contrast between affected fingers. A slow recovery rate after cold exposure is diagnostic for Raynaud's Phenomenon [71]. The coincidence of CTS and Raynaud's phenomenon was reported in the literature [72,73].

31.5.1.4   Other entrapment syndromes

No clear thermal pattern was reported for the entrapment of the ulnar nerve [65]. A pilot study for the comparison of hands from patients with TOS or entrapment of the ulnar nerve at the elbow found only 1 out of 7 patients with ulnar entrapment who presented with temperature asymmetry of the affected extremity [74]. All patients with TOS who performed provocation test during image recording showed at least in one thermogram an asymmetric temperature pattern.

31.5.2 Peripheral Nerve Paresis

Paresis is an impairment of the motor function of the nervous system. Loss of function of the sensory fibers may be associated with motor deficit, but sensory impairment is not included in the term paresis. Therefore, most of the temperature signs in paresis are related to impaired motor function.

31.5.2.1 Brachial Plexus Paresis

Injury of the brachial plexus is a severe consequence of traffic accidents and motor cyclers are most frequently affected. The loss of motor activity in the affected extremity results in paralysis, muscle atrophy, and decreased skin temperature. Nearly 0.5 to 0.9% of newborns acquire brachial plexus paresis during delivery [75]. Early recovery of the skin temperature in babies with plexus paresis precede the recovery of motor function as shown in a study from Japan [76].

31.5.2.2 Facial Nerve

The seventh cranial nerve supplies the mimic muscles of the face and an acquired deficit is often named Bell's palsy. This paresis has normally a good prognosis for full recovery. Thermal imaging was used as outcome measure in acupuncture trials for facial paresis [77,78]. Ammer et al. [79] found slight asymmetries in patients with facial paresis, in which hyperthermia of the affected side occurred more frequently than hypothermia. However, patients with apparent herpes zoster causing facial palsy presented with higher temperature differences to the contralateral side than patients with nonherpetic facial paresis [80].

31.5.2.3 Peroneal Nerve

The peroneal nerve may be affected by metabolic neuropathy in patients with metabolic disease or by compression neuropathy due to intensive pressure applied at the site of fibula head. This can result in "foot drop," an impairment in which the patient cannot raise his forefoot. The thermal image is characterized by decreased temperatures on the anterior lower leg, which might become more visible after the patient has performed some exercises [81].

31.6 Complex Regional Pain Syndrome

A temperature difference between the affected and the nonaffected limb equal or greater than 1°C is one of the diagnostic criteria of the complex regional pain syndrome (CRPS) [82]. Ammer conducted a study in patients after radius fracture treated conservatively with a plaster cast [83]. Within 2 h after plaster removal and 1 week later thermal images were recorded. After the second thermogram an x-ray image of both hands was taken. The mean temperature difference between the affected and unaffected hand was 0.6 after plaster removal and 0.63 one week later. In 21 out of 41 radiographs slight bone changes suspected of algodystropy have been found. Figure 31.4 summarizes the results with respect to the outcome of x-ray images. Figure 31.5 shows the time course of an individual patient.

It was also shown, that the temperature difference decrease during successful therapeutic intervention and temperature effect was paralleled by reduction of pain and swelling and resolution of radiologic changes [84].

Disturbance of vascular adaptation mechanism and delayed response to temperature stimuli was obtained in patients suffering from CRPS [85,86]. These alterations have been interpreted as being caused by abnormalities of the autonomic nerve system. It was suggested to use a cold challenge on the contralateral side of the injured limb for prediction and early diagnosis of CRPS. Gulevich et al. [87] confirmed the high diagnostic sensitivity and specificity of cold challenge for the CRPS. Wasner et al. [88] achieved similar results by whole body cooling or whole body warming. Most recently a Dutch study found that the asymmetry factor, which was based on histograms of temperatures from the affected and nonaffected

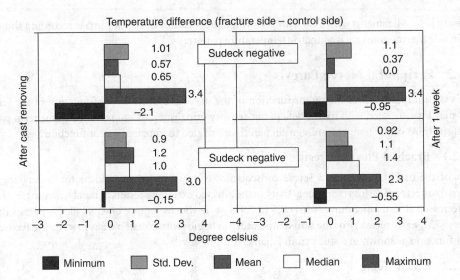

FIGURE 31.4 Diagram of temperatures obtained in patients with positive or negative x-ray images. (From Ammer, K. *Thermol. Österr.*, 1, 4, 1991. With permission.)

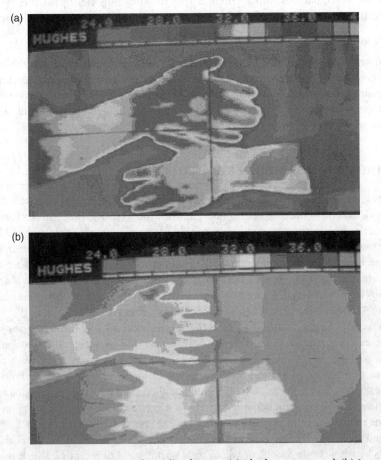

FIGURE 31.5 (See color insert.) Early CRPS after radius fracture. (a) 2 h after cast removal; (b) 1 week later.

hand had the highest diagnostic power for CRPS, while the difference of mean temperatures did not discriminate between disease and health [89].

31.7   Thermal Imaging Technique

The parameters for a reliable technique have been described in the past. Engel et al. [90] is a report published in 1978 by a European working group on Thermography in Locomotor Diseases. This paper discusses aspects of standardization including the need for adequate temperature control of the examination room and the importance of standard views used for image capture. More recently Ring and Ammer [91] described an outline of necessary considerations for good thermal imaging technique in clinical medicine. This outline has been subsequently expanded to encompass a revised set of standard views, and associated regions of interest for analysis. The latter is especially important for standardization, since the normal approach used is to select a region of interest subjectively. This means that without a defined set of reference points it is difficult for the investigator to reproduce the same region of interest on subsequent occasions. It is also even more difficult for another investigator to achieve the same, leading to unacceptable variables in the derived data. The aspects for standardization of the technique and the standard views and regions of interest recently defined are the product of a multicentered Anglo-Polish study who are pursuing the concept of a database of normal reference thermograms. The protocol can be found on a British University Research Group's website from University of Glamorgan [10].

31.7.1   Room Temperature

Room temperature is an important issue when investigating this group of diseases. Inflammatory conditions such as arthritis, are better revealed in a room temperature of 20°C, for the extremities, and may need to be at 18°C for examining the trunk. This presumes that the relative humidity will not exceed 45%, and a very low airspeed is required. At no time during preparatory cooling or during the examination should the patient be placed in a position where they can feel a draught from moving air. However in other clinical conditions where an effect from neuromuscular changes is being examined, a higher room temperature is needed to avoid forced vasoconstriction. This is usually performed at 22 to 24°C ambient. At higher temperatures, the subject may begin to sweat, and below 17°C shivering may be induced. Both of these thermoregulatory responses by the human body are undesirable for routine thermal imaging.

31.7.2   Clinical Examination

In this group of diseases, it can be particularly important that the patient receives a clinical examination in association with thermal imaging. Observations on medication, range of movement, experience of pain related to movement, or positioning may have a significant effect on the interpretation of the thermal images. Documentation of all such clinical findings should be kept on record with the images for future reference.

References

[1] Horvath, S.M. and Hollander, J.L. Intra-articular temperature as a measure of joint reaction. *J. Clin. Invest.*, 13, 615, 1949.

[2] Collins, A.J. and Cosh, J.A. Temperature and biochemical studies of joint inflammation. *Ann. Rheum. Dis.*, 29, 386, 1970.

[3] Ring, E.F.J. and Collins, A.J. Quantitative thermography. *Rheumatol. Phys. Med.*, 10, 337, 1970.

[4] Esselinckx, W. et al. Thermographic assessment of three intra-articular prednisolone analogues given in rheumatoid arthritis. *Br. J. Clin. Pharm.*, 5, 447, 1978.

[5] Bird, H.A., Ring, E.F.J., and Bacon, P.A. A thermographic and clinical comparison of three intra-articular steroid preparations in rheumatoid arthritis. *Ann. Rheum. Dis.*, 38, 36, 1979.

[6] Collins, A.J. and Ring, E.F.J. Measurement of inflammation in man and animals. *Br. J. Pharm.*, 44, 145, 1972.

[7] Bacon, P.A., Ring, E.F.J., and Collins, A.J. Thermography in the assessment of anti rheumatic agents, in *Rheumatoid Arthritis*. Gordon, J.L. and Hazleman, B.L., Eds., Elsevier/North Holland Biomedical Press, Amsterdam, 1977, p. 105.

[8] Collins, A.J. et al. Quantitation of thermography in arthritis using multi-isothermal analysis. I. The thermographic index. *Ann. Rheum. Dis.*, 33, 113, 1974.

[9] Ammer, K., Engelbert, B., and Kern, E. The determination of normal temperature values of finger joints. *Thermol. Int.*, 12, 23, 2002.

[10] Website address, Standard protocol for image capture and analysis, www.medimaging.org

[11] Czerny, V. Eine fokale Malazie des Unterschenkels. *Wien. Med. Wochenschr.*, 23, 895, 1873.

[12] Paget, J. On a form of chronic inflammation of bones. *Med. Chir. Transact.*, 60, 37, 1877.

[13] Ring, E.F.J. and Davies, J. Thermal monitoring of Paget's disease of bone. *Thermology*, 3, 167, 1990.

[14] Tauchmannova, H., Gabrhel, J., and Cibak, M. Thermographic findings in different sports, their value in the prevention of soft tissue injuries. *Thermol. Österr.* 3, 91–95, 1993.

[15] Smith, B.L, Bandler, M.K, and Goodman, P.H. Dominant forearm hyperthermia, a study of fifteen athletes. *Thermology*, 2, 25–28, 1986.

[16] Fischer, A.A. and Chang, C.H. Temperature and pressure threshold measurements in trigger points. *Thermology*, 1, 212, 1986.

[17] Menachem, A., Kaplan, O., and Dekel, S. Levator scapulae syndrome: an anatomic–clinical study. *Bull. Hosp. Jt. Dis.*, 53, 21, 1993.

[18] Schmitt, M. and Guillot, Y. Thermography and muscle injuries in sports medicine, in *Recent Advances in; Medical Thermography*, Ring, E.F.J. and Philips, J., Eds., Plenum Press, London, 1984, p. 439.

[19] Ammer, K. Low muscular activity of the lower leg in patients with a painful ankle. *Thermol. Österr.*, 5, 103, 1995.

[20] Kanie, R. Thermographic evaluation of osteoarthritis of the hip. *Biomed. Thermol.*, 15, 72, 1995.

[21] Vecchio, P.C. et al. Thermography of frozen shoulder and rotator cuff tendinitis. *Clin. Rheumatol.*, 11, 382, 1992.

[22] Ammer, K. et al. Thermography of the painful shoulder. *Eur. J. Thermol.*, 8, 93, 1998.

[23] Hobbins, W.B. and Ammer, K. Controversy: why is a paretic limb cold, high activity of the sympathetic nerve system or weakness of the muscles? *Thermol. Österr.*, 6, 42, 1996.

[24] Ring, E.F.J. and Ammer, K. Thermal imaging in sports medicine. *Sports Med. Today*, 1, 108, 1998.

[25] Gabrhel, J. and Tauchmannova, H. Wärmebilder der Kniegelenke bei jugendlichen Sportlern. *Thermol. Österr.*, 5, 92, 1995.

[26] Devereaux, M.D. et al. The diagnosis of stress fractures in athletes. *JAMA*, 252, 531, 1984.

[27] Graber, J. Tendosynovitis detection in the hand. *Verh. Dtsch. Ges. Rheumatol.*, 6, 57, 1980.

[28] Mayr, H. Thermografische Befunde bei Schmerzen am Ellbogen. *Thermol. Österr.*, 7, 5–10, 1997.

[29] Binder, A.I. et al. Thermography of tennis elbow, in *Recent Advances in Medical Thermography*. Ring, E.F.J. and Philips, J., Eds., Plenum Press, London, 1984, p. 513.

[30] Thomas, D. and Savage, J.P. Persistent tennis elbow: evaluation by infrared thermography and nuclear medicine isotope scanning. *Thermology*, 3, 132; 1989.

[31] Ammer, K. Thermal evaluation of tennis elbow, in *The Thermal Image in Medicine and Biology*. Ammer, K. and Ring, E.F.J., Eds., Uhlen Verlag, Wien, 1995, p. 214.

[32] Devereaux, M.D., Hazleman, B.L., and Thomas, P.P. Chronic lateral humeral epicondylitis — a double-blind controlled assessment of pulsed electromagnetic field therapy. *Clin. Exp. Rheumatol.* 3, 333, 1985.

[33] Ammer, K. et al. Thermographische und algometrische Kontrolle der physikalischen Therapie bei Patienten mit Epicondylopathia humeri radialis. *ThermoMed*, 11, 55–67, 1995.

[34] Ammer, K., Schartelmüller, T., and Melnizky, P. Thermography in fibromyalgia. *Biomed. Thermol.* 15, 77, 1995.

[35] Ammer, K. Only lateral, but not medial epicondylitis can be detected by thermography. *Thermol. Österr.*, 6, 105, 1996.

[36] Hirano, T. et al. Clinical study of shoulder surface temperature in patients with periarthritis scapulohumeralis (abstract). *Biomed. Thermol.*, 11, 303, 1991.

[37] Jeracitano, D. et al. Abnormal temperature control suggesting sympathetic dysfunction in the shoulder skin of patients with frozen shoulder. *Br. J. Rheumatol.*, 31, 539, 1992.

[38] Biasi, G. et al. The role computerized telethermography in the diagnosis of fibromyalgia syndrome. *Minerva Medica*, 85, 451, 1994.

[39] Ammer, K. Thermographic diagnosis of fibromyalgia. *Ann Rheum Dis. XIV European League Against Rheumatism Congress, Abstracts*, 135, 1999.

[40] Ammer, K., Engelbert, B., and Kern, E. Reproducibility of the hot spot count in patients with fibromyalgia, an intra- and inter-observer comparison. *Thermol. Int.*, 11, 143, 2001.

[41] Anbar, M. Recent technological developments in thermology and their impact on clinical applications. *Biomed. Thermol.*, 10, 270, 1990.

[42] Uematsu, S. Thermographic imaging of cutaneous sensory segment in patients with peripheral nerve injury. *J. Neurosurg.*, 62, 716–720, 1985.

[43] Hoffman, R.M., Kent, D.L., and. Deyo, R.A. Diagnostic accuracy and clinical utility of thermography for lumbar radiculopathy. A meta-analysis. *Spine*, 16, 623, 1991.

[44] McCulloch, J. et al. Thermography as a diagnostic aid in sciatica. *J. Spinal Disord.*, 6, 427, 1993.

[45] Takahashi, Y., Takahashi, K., and Moriya, H. Thermal deficit in lumbar radiculopathy. *Spine*, 19, 2443, 1994.

[46] Kim, Y.S. and Cho, Y.E. Pre- and postoperative thermographic imaging of lumbar disk herniations. *Biomed. Thermol.*, 13, 265, 1993.

[47] Zhang, H.Y., Kim, Y.S., and Cho, Y.E. Thermatomal changes in cervical disc herniations. *Yonsei Med. J.*, 40, 401, 1999.

[48] Cuetter, A.C. and Bartoszek, D.M. The thoracic outlet syndrome: controversies, overdiagnosism overtreatment and recommendations for management. *Muscle Nerve*, 12, 419, 1989.

[49] Schartelmüller, T. and Ammer, K. Thoracic outlet syndrome, in *The Thermal Image in Medicine and Biology*. Ammer, K. and Ring, E.F.J., Eds., Uhlen Verlag, Wien, 1995, p. 201.

[50] Schartelmüller, T. and Ammer, K. Infrared thermography for the diagnosis of thoracic outlet syndrome. *Thermol. Österr.*, 6, 130, 1996.

[51] Melnizky, P, Schartelmüller, T., and Ammer, K. Prüfung der intra-und interindividuellen Verläßlichkeit der Auswertung von Infrarot-Thermogrammen. *Eur. J. Thermol.*, 7, 224, 1997.

[52] Ammer, K. Thermographie der Finger nach mechanischem Provokationstest. *ThermoMed*, 17/18, 9, 2003.

[53] Schartelmüller, T., Melnizky, P., and Engelbert, B. Infrarotthermographie zur Evaluierung des Erfolges physikalischer Therapie bei Patenten mit klinischem Verdacht auf Thoracic Outlet Syndrome. *Thermol. Int.*, 9, 20, 1999.

[54] Schartelmüller, T. and Ammer, K. Zervikaler Diskusprolaps, Thoracic Outlet Syndrom oder periphere arterielle Verschlußkrankheit-ein Fallbericht. *Eur. J. Thermol.*, 7, 146, 1997.

[55] Ammer, K. Diagnosis of nerve entrapment syndromes by thermal imaging, in *Proceedings of The First Joint BMES/EMBS Conference. Serving Humanity, Advancing Technology*, October 13–16, 1999, Atlanta, GA, USA, p. 1117.

[56] Atroshi, I. et al. Prevalence of carpal tunnel syndrome in a general population. *JAMA*, 282, 153, 1999.

[57] Ammer, K., Mayr, H., and Thür, H. Self-administered diagram for diagnosing carpal tunnel syndrome. *Eur. J. Phys. Med. Rehab.*, 3, 43, 1993.

[58] Melnizky, P., Ammer, K., and Schartelmüller, T. Intra- und interindividuelle Verläßlichkeit der elektroneurographischen Untersuchung des Nervus medianus. *Österr. Z. Phys. Med. Rehab.*, 7, S83, 1996.

[59] Schartelmüller, T., Ammer, K., and Melnizky, P. Natürliche und postoperative Entwicklung elektroneurographischer Untersuchungsergebnisse des N. medianus von Patienten mit Carpaltunnelsyndrom (CTS). *Österr. Z. Phys. Med.*, 7, 183, 1997.

[60] Rosen, H.R. et al. Is surgical division of the carpal ligament sufficient in the treatment of carpal tunnel syndrome? *Chirurg*, 61, 130, 1990.

[61] Herrick, R.T. et al. Thermography as a diagnostic tool for carpal tunnel syndrome, in *Medical Thermology*, Abernathy, M. and Uematsu, S., Eds., American Academy of Thermology, 1986, p. 124.

[62] Herrick, R.T. and Herrick, S.K., Thermography in the detection of carpal tunnel syndrome and other compressive neuropathies. *J. Hand Surg.*, 12A, 943–949, 1987.

[63] Gateless, D., Gilroy, J., and Nefey, P. Thermographic evaluation of carpal tunnel syndrome during pregnancy. *Thermology*, 3, 21, 1988.

[64] Meyers, S. et al. Liquid crystal thermography, quantitative studies of abnormalities in carpal tunnel syndrome. *Neurology*, 39, 1465, 1989.

[65] So, Y.T., Olney, R.K., and Aminoff, M.J. Evaluation of thermography in the diagnosis of selected entrapment neuropathies. *Neurology*, 39, 1, 1989.

[66] Tchou, S. and Costich, J.F. Thermographic study of acute unilateral carpal tunnel syndromes. *Thermology*, 3, 249–252, 1991.

[67] Ammer, K. Thermographische Diagnose von peripheren Nervenkompressionssyndromen. *ThermoMed*, 7, 15, 1991.

[68] Hobbins, W.B. Autonomic vasomotor skin changes in pain states: significant or insignificant? *Thermol. Österr.*, 5, 5, 1995.

[69] Ammer, K. et al. The thermal image of patients suffering from carpal tunnel syndrome with a distal latency higher than 6.0 msec. *Thermol. Int.*, 9, 15, 1999.

[70] Ammer, K. and Melnizky, P. Determination of regions of interest on thermal images of the hands of patients suffering from carpal tunnel syndrome. *Thermol. Int.*, 9, 56, 1999.

[71] Ammer, K. Thermographic diagnosis of Raynaud's Phenomenon. *Skin Res. Technol.*, 2, 182, 1996.

[72] Neundörfer, B., Dietrich, B., and Braun, B. Raynaud–Phänomen beim Carpaltunnelsyndrom. *Wien. Klin. Wochenschr.*, 89, 131–133, 1977.

[73] Grassi, W. et al. Clinical diagnosis found in patients with Raynaud's phenomenon: a multicentre study. *Rheumatol. Int.*, 18, 17, 1998.

[74] Mayr, H. and Ammer, K. Thermographische Diagnose von Nervenkompressionssyndromen der oberen Extremität mit Ausnahme des Karpaltunnelsyndroms (abstract). *Thermol. Österr.*, 4, 82, 1994.

[75] Mumenthaler, M. and Schliack, H. *Läsionen periphere Nerven*. Georg Thieme Verlag, Stuttgart-New York, Auflage, 1982, p. 4.

[76] Ikegawa, S. et al. Use of thermography in the diagnosis of obstetric palsy (abstract). *Thermol. Österr.*, 7, 31, 1997.

[77] Zhang, D. et al. Preliminary observation of imaging of facial temperature along meridians. *Chen Tzu Yen Chiu*, 17, 71, 1992.

[78] Zhang, D. et al. Clinical observations on acupuncture treatment of peripheral facial paralysis aided by infra-red thermography — a preliminary report. *J. Tradit. Chin. Med.*, 11, 139, 1991.

[79] Ammer, K., Melnizky, P. and Schartelmüller, T. Thermographie bei Fazialisparese. *ThermoMed*, 13, 6–11, 1997.

[80] Schartelmüller, T., Melnizky, P., and Ammer, K. Gesichtsthermographie, Vergleich von Patienten mit Fazialisparese und akutem Herpes zoster ophthalmicus. *Eur. J. Thermol.*, 8, 65, 1998.

[81] Melnizky, P., Ammer, K., and Schartelmüller, T. Thermographische Überprüfung der Heilgymnastik bei Patienten mit Peroneusparese. *Thermol. Österr.*, 5, 97, 1995.

[82] Wilson, P.R. et al. Diagnostic algorithm for complex regional pain syndromes, in *Reflex Sympathetic Dystrophy, A Re-appraisal*. Jänig, W. and Stanton-Hicks, M., Eds., Seattle, IASP Press, 1996, p. 93.

[83] Ammer, K. Thermographie nach gipsfixierter Radiusfraktur. *Thermol. Österr.*, 1, 4, 1991.

[84] Ammer, K. Thermographische Therapieüberwachung bei M.Sudeck. *ThermoMed*, 7, 112–115, 1991.

[85] Cooke, E.D. et al. Reflex sympathetic dystrophy (algoneurodystrophy): temperature studies in the upper limb. *Br. J. Rheumatol.*, 8, 399, 1989.

[86] Herrick, A. et al. Abnormal thermoregulatory responses in patients with reflex sympathetic dystrophy syndrome. *J. Rheumatol.*, 21, 1319, 1994.

[87] Gulevich, S.J. et al. Stress infrared telethermography is useful in the diagnosis of complex regional pain syndrome, type I (formerly reflex sympathetic dystrophy). *Clin. J. Pain*, 13, 50, 1997.

[88] Wasner, G., Schattschneider, J., and Baron, R. Skin temperature side differences — a diagnostic tool for CRPS? *Pain*, 98, 19, 2002.

[89] Huygen, F.J.P.M. et al. Computer-assisted skin videothermography is a highly sensitive quality tool in the diagnosis and monitoring of complex regional pain syndrome type I. *Eur. J. Appl. Physiol.*, 91, 516, 2004.

[90] Engel, J.M. et al. Thermography in locomotor diseases, recommended procedure. Anglo-dutch thermographic society group report. *Eur. J. Rheumatol. Inflam.*, 2, 299–306, 1979.

[91] Ring, E.F.J. and Ammer, K. The technique of infra red imaging in medicine. *Thermol. Int.*, 10, 7, 2000.

32

Functional Infrared Imaging in Clinical Applications

32.1	Introduction...	**32**-1
32.2	Quantifying the Relevance and Stage of Disease with the τ Image Technique	**32**-2
32.3	Raynaud's Phenomenon.................................	**32**-5
32.4	Diagnosis of Varicocele and Follow-Up of the Treatment	**32**-8
32.5	Analysis of Skin Temperature During Exercise	**32**-11
32.6	Discussion and Conclusion	**32**-13
References	....	**32**-13

Arcangelo Merla
Gian Luca Romani
University "G. d'Annunzio"

32.1 Introduction

Infrared imaging allows the representation of the surface thermal distribution of the human body. Several studies have been performed so far to assess the contribution that such information may provide to the clinicians. The skin temperature distribution of the human body depends on the complex relationships defining the heat exchange processes between skin tissue, inner tissue, local vasculature, and metabolic activity. All of these processes are mediated and regulated by the sympathetic and parasympathetic activity to maintain the thermal homeostasis. The presence of a disease can locally affect the heat balance or exchange processes resulting in an increase or in a decrease of the skin temperature. Such a temperature change can be better estimated with respect to the surrounding regions or the unaffected contra lateral region. But then, the disease should also effect the local control of the skin temperature. Therefore, the characteristic parameters modeling the activity of the skin thermoregulatory system can be used as diagnostic parameters. The functional infrared (fIR) Imaging — also named infrared functional imaging (fIR imaging) — is the study for diagnostic purposes, based on the modeling of the bio-heat exchange processes, of the functional properties and alterations of the human thermoregulatory system. In this chapter, we will review some of the most important recent clinical applications of the functional infrared imaging of our group.

32.2 Quantifying the Relevance and Stage of Disease with the τ Image Technique

Infrared imaging can provide diagnostic information according different possible approaches. The approach generally followed consists of the detection of significant differences between the skin thermal distributions of the two hemisoma or in the pattern recognition of specific features with respect to average healthy population [1]. The underlying hypothesis is that the skin temperature distribution, at a given time, is considered at a steady state. Of course this is a rough approximation of the reality because of the homeostasis. More valuable and quantitative information can be obtained from the study of the skin temperature dynamics in the unsteady state, where the processes involved and controlled by the thermoregulatory system can be modeled and described through their characteristic parameters [2–7]. The presence of diseases interfering with the skin thermoregulatory system can be then inferred by the analysis of its functional alterations [8–18]. To enhance the functional content of the thermoregulatory response, one needs to pass through modeling of the thermal properties and dynamics of the skin thermoregulatory system. Such a modeling can bring more quantitative and detailed diagnostic parameters with respect to the particular disease being analyzed. Merla et al. [7,17,19,20] proposed a new imaging technique, based on this approach, for the clinical study of a variety of diseases. The theory behind the technique is based on the fact that the human thermoregulatory system maintains a reasonably constant body temperature against a wide range of environmental conditions. The body uses several physiological processes to control the heat exchange with the environment. The mechanism controlling thermal emission and dermal microcirculation is driven by the sympathetic nervous system. A disease locally affecting the thermoregulatory system (i.e., traumas, lesions, vein thrombosis, varicocele, dermatitis, Raynaud's phenomenon, and scleroderma, etc.) may produce an altered sympathetic function and a change in the local metabolic rate. Local vasculature and microvasculature may be rearranged resulting in a modification of the skin temperature distribution.

Starting from a general energy balance equation, it is straightforward to demonstrate that the recovery time from any kind of thermal stress for a given region of interest depends on the region thermal parameters. A given disease may alter the normal heat capacity and the tissue/blood ratio mass density of a region. An example is given in Figure 32.1 that shows the different thermoregulatory behaviors exhibited by two

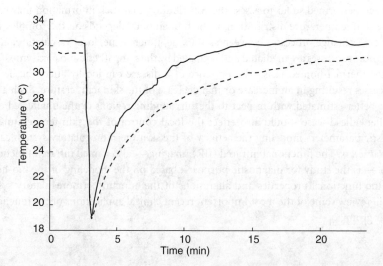

FIGURE 32.1 Muscular lesion on the left thigh abductor with hemorrhage shedding: thermal recovery curves following a cold thermal stress. The dotted line represents the recovery of a healthy area close to the damaged one. The continuous line represents the curve related to a muscular lesion region. Both recoveries exhibit exponential feature; the injured area exhibits a faster rewarming with a shorter time constant.

adjacent regions — one healthy and one affected by a muscular lesion — after local cooling applied to the skin. A controlled thermal stress applied to the region of interest and the surrounding tissue permits to study and to model the response of the region itself. The most important terms involved in the energy balance during the recovery are the heat storage in the tissue, heat clearance by blood perfusion, and convective heat exchange with the environment, as described by the following equation:

$$\frac{\partial T}{\partial t} \rho \cdot c \cdot V = hA\,(T_o - T) + \rho_{bl} \cdot c_{bl} \cdot w_{bl}(t) \cdot (T_{bl} - T) \tag{32.1}$$

where subscripts o and bl designate the properties of the environment and blood, respectively, while ρ is the density, c is the specific heat, V is the volume, T is the temperature, t is the time, h is the combined heat transfer coefficient between the skin and the environment, A is the surface area, and w is the blood perfusion rate.

The initial condition for (32.1) is

$$T = T_i \quad \text{for } t = 0 \tag{32.2}$$

where T_i is the skin temperature and $t = 0$ is the time at the recovery starting.

Equation 32.1 can be easily integrated under the assumption of constant blood perfusion rate w_{bl} and blood temperature T_{bl}, yielding:

$$T(t) = \frac{W \cdot (T_{bl} - T_o)}{W + H} + \left(T_i - T_o - \frac{W \cdot (T_{bl} - T_o)}{W + H} \right) \cdot e^{-(W+H)\cdot t} + T_o \tag{32.3}$$

where

$$H = \frac{h \cdot A}{\rho \cdot c \cdot V} \qquad W = \frac{\rho_{bl} \cdot c_{bl} \cdot w_{bl}}{\rho \cdot c \cdot V} \tag{32.4}$$

The time t_f to reach a certain preset (final) temperature T_f is then given by:

$$t_f = -\frac{1}{W + H} \ln \left(\frac{(1 + (H/W)) \cdot (T_f - T_o) - W(T_{bl} - T_o)}{(1 + (H/W)) \cdot (T_i - T_o) - W(T_{bl} - T_o)} \right) \tag{32.5}$$

Equation 32.5, with the assumption of constant blood perfusion, relates the time to reach a preset temperature to the local thermal properties and to local blood perfusion.

The exponential solution described in (32.3) suggests to use the time constant τ as a characterizing parameter for the description of the recovery process after any kind of controlled thermal stress, with τ mainly determined by the local blood flow and thermal capacity of the tissue.

The fIR imaging permits an easy evaluation of τ, which can be regarded as a parameter able to discriminate areas interested by the specific disease from healthy ones.

Rather than a static imaging of the skin thermal distribution to pictorially describe the effect of the given disease, an image reporting the τ recovery time pixel to pixel can be used to characterize that disease [7,17,19,20]. Areas featuring an associated blood shedding, or an inflammatory state, or an increased blood reflux, often exhibit a faster recovery time with respect to the surroundings. Those areas then exhibit a smaller τ value. In contrast, in presence of localized calcifications, early ulcers or scleroderma, and impaired microvascular control, the involved areas show a slower recovery than the healthy surrounding areas and are therefore characterized by a longer τ time.

The reliability and value of the τ image technique rely on the good quality of the data and on their appropriate processing. While the interested reader can find a detailed description for proper materials and method for the τ image technique in Reference 17, it is worthwhile to report hereby the general algorithm for the method:

1. Subject marking (to permit movement correction of the thermal image series) and acclimation to the measurement room kept at controlled environmental conditions

2. Adequate calibration of the thermal imaging device
3. Recording of the baseline temperature dynamics for the region of interest
4. Execution of the thermal stress (usually performed through a cold or warm dry patch at controlled temperature and temperature exchange rate)
5. Recording of the thermal recovery until the complete restoration of the baseline features
6. Postprocessing movement correction of the thermal image series
7. Fitting of the pixel by pixel experimental recovery data to an exponential curve and extraction of the time constant τ for each pixel of the region of interest
8. Pixel by pixel color coding and mapping of the time constant τ values

The τ image technique has been first proposed as complementary diagnostic tool for the diagnosis of muscular lesions, Raynaud's phenomenon, and deep vein thrombosis [7,17,19,20]. In those studies, the technique correctly depicted the stages of the diseases accordingly with the gold standard evaluation techniques. A mild cold stress has been used as a thermal stress. For the muscular lesions, according to the importance of the lesion, the lower values (2–4 min) of the recovery time τ were found in agreement with the location and the severity of the trauma (Figure 32.2). The dimensions of the lesions as estimated by ultrasonography were proportionally related to those of their tracks on the τ image. In the diagnosis of Raynaud's phenomenon secondary to scleroderma greater values (18–20 min) of the recovery time τ corresponded to finger districts more affected by the disease (Figure 32.3). Clinical investigation and capillaroscopy confirmed the presence of scleroderma and the microvascular damage.

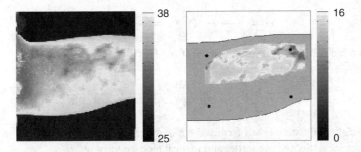

FIGURE 32.2 Second-class muscular lesion on the left leg abductor — Medial view. Left: Static thermography image. The bar shows the pixel temperature. The light gray spots indicate the presence of the trauma. Right: Time constant τ image after mild cold stress. The bar illustrates the recovery time, in minutes, for each pixel. The black spots are the markers used as position references. (From Merla et al., *IEEE Eng. Med. Biol. Magn.*, 21, 86, 2002. With permission.)

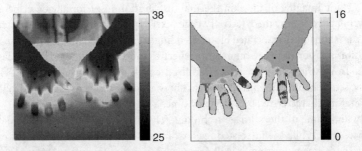

FIGURE 32.3 Raynaud's Phenomenon Secondary to Scleroderma. Left: Static thermography image. The bar shows the pixel temperature. Right: Time constant τ image after mild cold stress. The bar illustrates the recovery time, in minutes, for each pixel. The regions associated with longer recovery times identify the main damaged finger regions. (From Merla et al., *IEEE Eng. Med. Biol. Magn.*, 21, 86, 2002. With permission.)

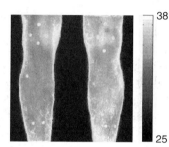 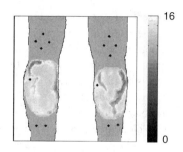

FIGURE 32.4 Bi-lateral vein thrombosis. Left: Static thermography image. The bar shows the pixel temperature. Right: Time constant τ image after mild cold stress. The bar illustrates the recovery time, in minutes, for each pixel. The areas associated with shorter recovery times identify the regions interested by the thrombosis. (From Merla et al., *IEEE Eng. Med. Biol. Magn.*, 21, 86, 2002. With permission.)

In the reported deep vein thrombosis cases, the authors found the lower values (1–3 min) of the recovery time τ in agreement with the location and the severity of the blood flow reflux according to the Echo Color Doppler findings (Figure 32.4).

The τ image technique provides useful diagnostic information and can be applied also as a follow-up tool. It is an easy and not invasive diagnostic procedure that can be successfully used in the diagnosis and monitoring of several diseases affecting the local thermoregulatory properties, both in a direct and an indirect way. The τ image technique opens new possibilities for the applications of IR imaging in the clinical field. It is worth noting that a certain amount of information is already present — but embedded — in the traditional static image (see Figure 32.2), but the interpretation is difficult and relies on the ability of the clinicians. The method is based on the assumptions of a time constant blood perfusion and blood temperature. While such assumptions are not completely correct from the physiological point of view, the experimental exponential-shaped recovery function allows such a simplification. With respect to some diseases, such as the Raynaud's phenomenon, the τ image technique may provide useful information to image the damage and quantitatively follow its time evolution.

32.3 Raynaud's Phenomenon

Raynaud's phenomenon (RP) is defined as a painful vasoconstriction — that may follow cold or emotional stress — of small arteries and arterioles of extremities, like fingers and toes. RP can be primary (PRP) or secondary Systemic Sclerosis (SSc) to scleroderma. The latter is usually associated with a connective tissues disease. RP precedes the systemic autoimmune disorders development, particularly scleroderma, by many years and it can evolve into secondary RP. The evaluation of vascular disease is crucial in order to distinguish between PRP and SSc. In PRP, episodic ischemia in response to cold exposure or to emotional stimuli is usually completely reversible: absence of tissue damage is the typical feature [21], but also mild structural changes are demonstrated [22]. In contrast, scleroderma RP shows irreversible tissue damage and severe structural changes in the finger vascular organization [2]. None of the physiological measurement techniques currently in use, but infrared imaging, is completely satisfactory in focusing primary or secondary RP [3]. The main limit of such techniques (nail fold capillary microscopy, cutaneous laser-Doppler flowmetry, and plethysmography) is the fact that they can proceed just into a partial investigation, usually assessing only one finger once. The measurement of skin temperature is an indirect method to estimate change in skin thermal properties and blood flow. Thermography, protocols [3–5, 23–27] usually include cold patch testing to evaluate the capability of the patients hands to rewarm. The pattern of the rewarming curves is usually used to depict the underlying structural diseases. Analysis of rewarming curves has been used in several studies to differentiate healthy subjects from PRP or SSc Raynaud's patients. Parameters usually considered so far are: the lag time preceding the onset of rewarming

[3–5] or to reach a preset final temperature [26]; the rate of the rewarming and the maximum temperature of recovery [27]; and the degree of temperature variation between different areas of the hands [25].

Merla et al. [14,16] proposed to model the natural response of the fingertips to exposure to a cold environment to get a diagnostic parameter derived by the physiology of such a response. The thermal recovery following a cold stress is driven by thermal exchange with the environment, transport by the incoming blood flow, conduction from adjacent tissue layers, and metabolic processes. The finger temperature is determined by the net balance of the energy input/output. The more significant contribution come from the input power due to blood perfusion and the power lost to the environment [28]:

$$\frac{dQ}{dt} = -\frac{dQ_{env}}{dt} + \frac{dQ_{ctr}}{dt} \tag{32.6}$$

Normal finger recovery after a cold stress is reported in Figure 32.5. In absence of thermoregulatory control, fingers exchange heat only with the environment: in this case, their temperature T_{exp} follows an exponential pattern with time constant τ given by:

$$\tau = \frac{\rho \cdot c \cdot V}{h \cdot A} \tag{32.7}$$

where ρ is the mass density, c the specific heat, V the finger volume, h is the combined heat transfer coefficient between the finger and the environment, and A is the finger surface area. Thanks to the thermoregulatory control, the finger maintains its temperature T greater than T_{exp}. For a Δt time, the area of the trapezoid $ABCF$ times $h \cdot A$ in Figure 32.5 computes the heat provided by the thermoregulatory system, namely ΔQ_{ctrl}. This amount summed to ΔQ_{env} yields Q, the global amount of heat stored in the finger.

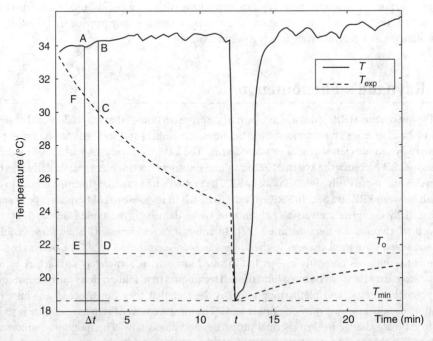

FIGURE 32.5 Experimental rewarming curves after cold stress in normal subjects. The continuous curve represents the recorded temperature finger. The outlined curve represents the exponential temperature pattern exhibited by the finger in absence of thermoregulatory control. In this case, the only heat source for the finger is the environment. (From Merla et al., *IEEE Eng. Med. Biol. Mag.*, 21, 73, 2002. With permission.)

Then, the area of the trapezoid *ABDE* is proportional to the amount Q of heat stored in the finger during a Δt interval. Therefore, Q can be computed integrating the area surrounded by the temperature curve T and the constant straight line T_0:

$$Q = -h \cdot A \cdot \int_{t_1}^{t_2} (T_0 - T(\varsigma)) \, d\varsigma \tag{32.8}$$

where the minus sign takes into account that the heat stored by the finger is counted as positive. Q is intrinsically related to the finger thermal capacity, according to the expression

$$\Delta Q = \rho \cdot c \cdot V \cdot \Delta T \tag{32.9}$$

Under the hypothesis of constant T_0, the numerical integration in (32.8) can be used to characterize the rewarming exhibited by a healthy or a suffering finger.

The Q parameter has been used in References 14 and 16 to discriminate and classify PRP, SSc, and healthy subjects on a set of 40 (20 PRP, 20 SSc), and 18 healthy volunteers, respectively. For each subject, the response to a mild cold challenge of hands in water was assessed by fIR imaging. Rewarming curves were recorded for each of the five fingers of both hands; the temperature integral Q was calculated along the 20 min following the cold stress. Ten subjects, randomly selected within the 18 normal ones, repeated two times and in different days the test to evaluate the repeatability of the fIR imaging findings. The repeatability test confirmed that fIR imaging and Q computation is a robust tool to characterize the thermal recovery of the fingers.

The grand average Q values provided by the first measurement was $(1060.0 \pm 130.5)°C$ min, while for the second assessment it was $(1012 \pm 135.1)°C$ min ($p > .05$, one-way ANOVA test). The grand average Q values for PRP, SSc, and healthy subjects' groups are shown in Figure 32.6, whereas single values obtained for each finger of all of the subjects are reported in Figure 32.7.

The results in References 14 and 16 highlight that the PRP group features low intra- and inter-individual variability whereas the SSc group displays a large variability between healthy and unhealthy fingers. Q values for SSc finger are generally greater than PRP ones.

The temperature integral at different finger regions yields very similar results for all fingers of the PRP group, suggesting common thermal and BF properties. SSc patients showed different thermoregulatory

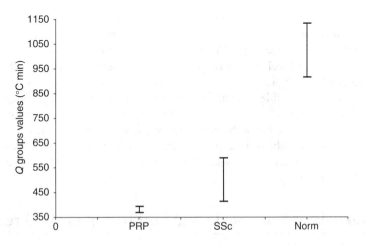

FIGURE 32.6 One-way ANOVA test applied to the Q parameter calculated for each group (PRP, SSc, and healthy). The Q parameter clearly discriminates among the three groups. (From Merla et al., *IEEE Eng. Med. Biol. Magn.*, 21, 73, 2002. With permission.)

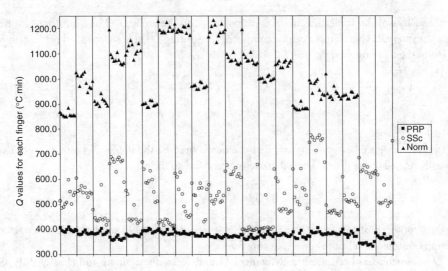

FIGURE 32.7   *Q* values calculated for each finger of each subjects. Vertical grid lines are placed to discriminate the ten fingers. PRP fingers are characterized by a strong intra- and inter-individual homogeneity. Greater mean *Q* values and greater intra- and inter-individual variations characterizes the SSc fingers. (From Merla et al., *IEEE Eng. Med. Biol. Magn.*, 21, 73, 2002. With permission.)

responses in the different segments of finger. This feature is probably due to the local modification in the tissue induced by the scleroderma. Scleroderma patients also featured a significantly different behavior across the five fingers depending on the disease involvement.

In normal and PRP groups all fingers show a homogeneous behavior and PRP fingers always exhibit a poorer recovery than normal ones. Additionally, in both groups, the rewarming always starts from the finger distal area differently from what happens in SSc patients. The sensitivity of the method in order to distinguish patients from normal is 100%. The specificity in distinguishing SSc from PRP is 95%.

The grand average *Q* clearly highlights the difference between PRP, SSc, and between normal subjects. It provides useful information about the abnormalities of their thermoregulatory finger properties. The PRP patients exhibited common features in terms of rewarming. Such behavior can be explained in terms of an equally low and constant BF in all fingers and to differences in the amount of heat exchanged with the environment [2].

Conversely, no common behavior was found for the SSc patients, since their disease determines — for each finger — very different thermal and blood perfusion properties. Scleroderma seems to increase the tissue thermal capacity with a reduced ability to exchange. As calculated from the rewarming curves, *Q* parameter seems to be particularly effective to describe the thermal recovery capabilities of the finger. The method clearly highlighted the difference between PRP and SSc patients and provides useful information about the abnormalities of their thermal and thermoregulatory finger properties.

In consideration of the generally accepted theory that the different recovery curves of the patients are a reflection of the slow deterioration of the microcirculation, so that over time in the same patients it is possible to observe changes in the thermal recovery curves, the method described earlier could be used to monitor the clinical evolution of the disease. In addition, pharmacological treatment effects could be advantageously followed up.

32.4   Diagnosis of Varicocele and Follow-Up of the Treatment

Varicocele is a widely spread male disease consisting of a dilatation of the pampiniform venous plexus and of the internal spermatic vein. Consequences of such a dilatation are an increase of the scrotal temperature and a possible impairment of the potential fertility [29,30]. In normal men, testicular temperature is

3 to 4°C lower than core body temperature [29]. Two thermoregulatory processes maintain this lower temperature: heat exchange with the environment through the scrotal skin and heat clearance by blood flow through the pampiniform plexus. Venous stasis due to the varicocele may increase the temperature of the affected testicle or pampiniform plexus. Thus, an abnormal temperature difference between the two hemiscrota may suggest the presence of varicocele [6,29–31] (see Figure 32.8). Telethermography can reveal abnormal temperature differences between the two testicles and altered testicular thermal recovery after an induced cold stress. Affected testicles return to prestress equilibrium temperatures faster than do normal testicles [6]. The fIR imaging has been used to determine whether altered scrotal thermoregulation is related to subclinical varicocele [15]. In a study conducted in 2001, Merla and Romani enrolled 60 volunteers, 18 to 27 years of age (average age, 21 ± 2 years), with no symptoms or clinical history of varicocele. After clinical examination, echo color Doppler imaging (the gold standard) and fIR imaging were performed. The fIR imaging evaluation consisted of obtaining scrotal images, measuring the basal temperature at the level of the pampiniform plexus (T_p) and the testicles (T_t), and determining thermal recovery of the scrotum after cold thermal stress. The temperature curve of the hemiscrotum during rewarming showed an exponential pattern and was, therefore, fitted to an exponential curve. The time constant τ of the best exponential fit depends on the thermal properties of the scrotum and its blood perfusion [15]. Therefore τ provides a quantitative parameter assessing how much the scrotal thermoregulation is affected by varicocele. Cooling was achieved by applying a dry patch to the scrotum that was 10°C colder than the basal scrotal temperature. The fIR measurements were performed according to usual standardization procedures [15]. The basal prestress temperature and the recovery time constant τ_p at the level of the pampiniform plexus and of the testicles (τ_t) were evaluated on each hemiscrotum. A basal testicular temperature greater than 32°C and basal pampiniform plexus temperature greater than 34°C were considered warning thresholds. Temperature differences among testicles (ΔT_t) or pampiniform plexus ΔT_p and temperature greater than 1.0°C were also considered warning values, as were τ_p and $\Delta \tau_t$ values longer than 1.5 min. The fIR imaging evaluation classified properly the stages of disease, as confirmed by the echo color Doppler imaging and clinical examination in a blinded manner. In 38 subjects, no warning basal temperatures or differences in rewarming temperatures were observed. These subjects were considered to be normal according to fIR imaging. Clinical examination and echo color Doppler imaging confirmed the absence of varicocele ($p < .01$, one-way ANOVA test).

In 22 subjects, one or more values were greater than the warning threshold for basal temperatures or differences in rewarming temperatures. Values for ΔT_p and the $\Delta \tau_p$ were higher than the warning thresholds in 8 of the 22 subjects, who were classified as having grade 1 varicocele. Five subjects had ΔT_t and $\Delta \tau_t$ values higher than the threshold. In 9 subjects, 3 or more infrared functional imaging values were greater than the warning threshold values. The fIR imaging classification was grade 3 varicocele. Clinical examination and echo color Doppler imaging closely confirmed the fIR imaging evaluation of the stage of the varicocele. The fIR imaging yielded no false-positive or false-negative results. All participants with positive results on fIR imaging also had positive results on clinical examination and echo color Doppler imaging. The sensitivity and specificity of fIR test were 100 and 93%, respectively. An abnormal change in the temperature of the testicles and pampiniform plexus may indicate varicocele, but the study demonstrated that impaired thermoregulation is associated with varicocele-induced alteration of blood flow. Time of recovery of prestress temperature in the testicles and pampiniform plexus appears to assist in classification of the disease. The fIR imaging accurately detected 22 nonsymptomatic varicocele.

The control of the scrotum temperature should improve after varicocelectomy as a complementary effect of the reduction of the blood reflux. Moreover, follow-up of the changes in scrotum thermoregulation after varicocelectomy may provide early indications on possible relapses of the disease.

To answer these questions, Merla et al. [9] used fIR imaging to study changes in the scrotum thermoregulation of 20 patients (average age, 27 ± 5 years) that were judged eligible for varicocelectomy on the basis of the combined results of the clinical examination, Echo color Doppler imaging, and spermiogram. No bilateral varicoceles were included in the study.

Patients underwent clinical examination, echo color Doppler imaging and instrument varicocele grading, and infrared functional evaluation before varicocelectomy and every 2 weeks thereafter, up to the

24th week. Out of 20, 14 patients suffered from grade 2 left varicocele. All of them were characterized by basal temperatures and recovery time after cold stress according to Reference 15. Varicoceles were surgically treated via interruption of the internal spermatic vein using modified Palomo's technique. The fIR imaging documented changes in the thermoregulatory control of the scrotum after the treatment as following: 13 out of the 14 grade 2 varicocele patients exhibited normal basal T_t, T_p on the varicocele side of the scrotum, and normal temperature differences ΔT_t and ΔT_p starting from the 4th week after varicocelectomy. Their $\Delta\tau_t$ and $\Delta\tau_p$ values returned to normal range from the 4th to the 6th week. Four out of the Six grade 3 varicocele patients exhibited normal basal T_t, T_p on the varicocele side of the scrotum, and normal temperature differences ΔT_t and ΔT_p starting from the 6th week after varicocelectomy. Their $\Delta\tau_t$ and $\Delta\tau_p$ values returned to normal range from the 6th to the 8th week. The other three patients did not return to normal values of the above-specified parameters. In particular, $\Delta\tau_t$ and $\Delta\tau_p$ remained much longer than the threshold warming values [6,15] up to the last control (Figure 32.8). Echo color Doppler imaging and clinical examination assessed relapses of the disease. The study proved that the surgical treatment of the varicocele induces modification in the thermoregulatory properties of the scrotum, reducing the basal temperature of the affected testicle and pampiniform plexus, and slowing down its recovery time after thermal stress. Among the 17 with no relapse, 4 exhibited return to normal T_t, T_p, ΔT_t, and ΔT_p for the latero-anterior side of the scrotum, while the posterior side of the scrotum remained hyperthermal or characterized by ΔT_t and ΔT_p higher than the threshold warning value. This fact suggested that the surgical treatment via interruption of the internal spermatic vein using Palomo's technique may not be the most suitable method for those varicoceles. The time requested by the scrotum to restore normal temperature distribution and control seems to be positively correlated to the volume and duration of the blood reflux lasting: the greater the blood reflux, the longer the time. The study

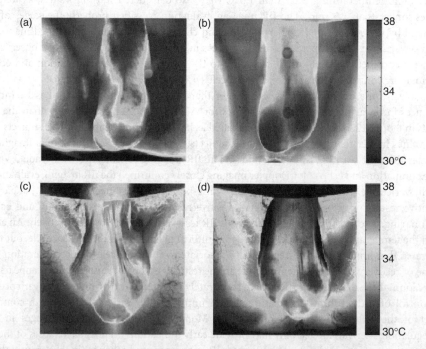

FIGURE 32.8   (a) Second grade right varicocele. The temperature distribution all over the scrotum clearly highlights significant differences between affected and unaffected testicles. (b) The same scrotum after varicocelectomy. The surgical treatment reduced the increased temperature on the affected hemiscrotum and restored the symmetry in the scrotal temperature distribution. (c) Third grade left varicocele. (d) The same scrotum after varicocelectomy. The treatment was unsuccessful into repairing the venous reflux, as documented by the persisting asymmetric scrotal distribution.

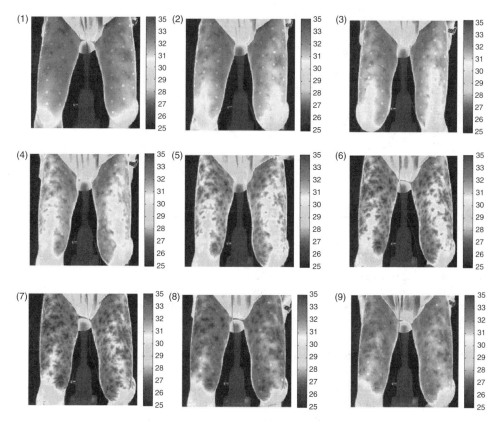

FIGURE 32.9 From top right to bottom left, fIR image sequence recorded along the exercise for a fit level subject. Images 1 and 2 were recorded during the warm up. Images 3 to 5 were recorded during the load phase of the exercise, with constant increasing working load. Image 6 corresponds to the maximum load and the beginning of the recovery phase. Note the arterovenous shunts opening to improve the core muscle layer cooling. (From Merla et al. in *Proceedings of the 24th IEEE Engineering in Medicine and Biology Society Conference*, Houston, October 23–25, 2002. With permission.)

demonstrated that IR imaging may provide early indication on the possible relapsing of the disease and may be used as a suitable complementary follow-up tool.

32.5 Analysis of Skin Temperature During Exercise

Skin temperature depends on complex thermal exchanges between skin tissue, skin blood, the environment, and the inner warmer tissue layers [31]. Johnson [32], Kenney and Johnson [33], and Zontak et al. [34] documented modifications in blood flow of the skin during: a reduction of the skin blood flow characterizes the initial phase of the exercise; while increase in skin blood flow accompanies increased working load. Zontak et al. [34] showed — by means of thermography — that dynamics of hand skin temperature response during leg exercise depends on the type of the exercise (graded vs. constant load): graded load exercise results in a constant decrease of finger temperature reflecting a constantly dominating vasoconstrictor response; steady state exercise causes a similar initial temperature decrease followed by rewarming of hands reflecting dominance of the thermoregulatory reflexes at a later stage of the exercise.

Merla et al. [18] studied directly the effects of graded load exercise on the thigh skin temperature, by means of fIR imaging. The study was aimed to assess possible relationship between the dynamics of the skin temperature along the exercise, the way the exercise is executed, and the fitness level of the subject.

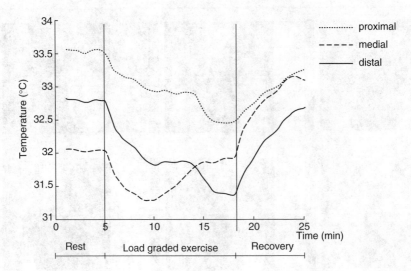

FIGURE 32.10 T_{ts} vs. time curves of each third of the left thigh for the subject in Figure 32.9. The distal third exhibits a different behavior with respect to the more proximal ones, probably because of a different involving in the execution of the exercise. (From Merla et al., in *Proceedings of the 24th IEEE Engineering in Medicine and Biology Society Conference*. With permission.)

In their study, the authors recruited 35 volunteers (24 M/11 F; age $= 22 \pm 1.5$ yr; height $= 173 \pm 2.8$ cm; body weight $= 68 \pm 4.2$ kg), with normal response to cardiac effort test. The thigh skin temperature (T_{ts}) of the subject was continuously recorded under conditions of rest, increasing physical load, and recovery from exercise. Three different regions T_{ts} (proximal, medial, and distal third of thigh length, frontal view) were studied. After 2.5-min rest fIR recording, exercise testing was performed using a calibrated bicycle ergometer. The ergometer was controlled by a special software, that after measurement of Body Mass Index, total body fat percentage, arterial pressure, biceps strength, and back flexibility, extrapolates VO_2 (oxygen consumption) values during the several steps of the exercise test, and the fitness level monitoring the heartbeat rate (HR). The subjects underwent a load graded exercise test — 25 W every 3 min increasing workloads, 50 rpm — up to reaching the submaximal HR condition. The recovery phase was defined as the time necessary to restore the rest HR by means of recovery exercise and rest. T_{ts} distribution was continuously monitored, while fIR images were recorded every 1-min along the exercise and the recovery phases (Figure 32.9). For all of the subjects, the temperature featured an exponential pattern, decreasing in the warming up and increasing during the recovery. Time constants of the T_{ts} vs. time curves were calculated for the graded exercise (τ_{ex}) and the recovery (τ_{rec}) phases, respectively (Figure 32.10).

Artery–venous shunt openings were noticed during the restoring phase to improve the cooling of the core of the muscle. Different T_{ts} vs. time curves were observed for the three chosen recording regions according to the specific involvement of the underlying muscular structures (Figure 32.10). Each subject produced different T_{ts} vs. time curves, according to the fitness level and VO_2 consumption: the greater VO_2 consumption and better fitness, the faster τ_{ex} and τ_{rec} (see Table 32.1).

The results obtained by Merla et al. are consistent with previous observations [32–34]: the muscles demand increased blood flow at the beginning of the exercise that results in skin vasoconstriction. Prolonged work causes body temperature increase that invokes thermal regulatory processes with heat conduction to the skin. Therefore, skin thermoregulatory processes are also invoked by the exercise and can be recorded by fIR imaging. Executing of graded exercise determines a decreasing of the skin temperature throughout the exercise period, in association with increasing demand of blood from the working muscles. As the muscles stop working and the recovery and the restoration phase start, thermoregulatory control is invoked to limit body temperature increase and the skin vessels dilate to increase heat conduction to the skin and, then, to the environment [34]. One remarkable result is the fact that different T_{ls} vs. time curves for contralateral-homologous regions or different thirds have been found in some of the

TABLE 32.1 VO$_2$ Consumption and Average Constant Time on the Whole Thigh Length

Fitness level	Number of subjects	VO$_2$ (ml/kg min)	τ_{ex} (min)	τ_{rec} (min)
Excellent	12	56.7 ± 2.5	8.5 ± 2.2	2.4 ± 1.5
Fit	9	30.4 ± 3.8	10.1 ± 2.5	4.8 ± 2.0
Fair	8	25.9 ± 3.4	12.5 ± 2.6	7.3 ± 1.8
Needs work	6	18.3 ± 2.9	15.3 ± 2.3	10.3 ± 1.9

Source: Taken from Merla et al. in *Proceedings of the 24th IEEE Engineering in medicine and Biology Society Conference,* Houston, October 23–25, 2002.

subjects. This fact may be likely explained as a different involvement of the several parts of the muscles used or as expression of different work capabilities of the lower arms in the exercise. The fIR recording of skin temperature during exercise may be therefore regarded as a tool to get information about the quality of the execution of the exercise and the fitness level state of the subjects.

32.6 Discussion and Conclusion

The fIR imaging is a biomedical imaging technique that relies on high-resolution IR imaging and on the modeling of the heat exchange and control processes at the skin layer. The fIR imaging is aimed to provide quantitative diagnostic parameters through the functional investigation of the thermoregulatory processes. It is also aimed to provide further information about the studied disease to the physicians, like explanation of the possible physics reasons of some thermal behaviors and their relationships with the physiology of the involved processes. One of the great advantages of fIR imaging is the fact that it is not invasive and it is a touchless imaging technique. The fIR is not a static imaging investigation technique. Therefore, data for fIR imaging need to be processed adequately for movement. Adequate bio heat modeling is also required. The medical fields for possible applications of fIR imaging are numerous, ranging from those described in this chapter, to psychometrics, cutaneous blood flow modeling, peripheral nervous system activity, and some angiopathies. The applications described in this chapter show that fIR imaging provides highly effective diagnostic parameters. The method is highly sensitive, and also highly specific to discriminating different conditions of the same disease. For the studies reported hereby, fIR imaging is sensitive and specific as the corresponding golden standard techniques, at least. In some cases, fIR represents a useful follow-up tool (like in varicocelectomy to promptly assess possible relapses) or even an elective diagnostic tool, as in the Raynaud's phenomenon. The τ image technique represents an innovative technique that provides useful and additional information to the golden standard techniques. Thanks to it, the whole functional processes associated to a disease can be depicted and summarized into just a single image.

References

[1] Aweruch, M.S., Thermography: its current diagnostic status in muscular–skeletal medicine, *Med. J. Aust.*, 154, 441, 1991.

[2] Prescott et al., Sequential dermal microvascular and perivascular changes in the development of scleroderma, *J. Pathol.*, 166, 255, 1992.

[3] Herrick, A.L. and Clark, S., Quantifying digital vascular disease in patients with primary Raynaud's phenomenon and systemic sclerosis, *Ann. Rheum. Dis.*, 57, 70, 1998.

[4] Darton, K. and Black, C.M., Pyroelectric vidicon thermography and cold challenge quantify the severity of Raynaud's phenomenon, *Br. J. Rheumatol.*, 30, 190, 1991.

[5] Javanetti, S. et al., Thermography and nailfold capillaroscopy as noninvasive measures of circulation in children with Raynaud's phenomenon, *J. Rheumatol.*, 25, 997, 1998.

[6] Merla, A. et al., Dynamic digital telethermography: a novel approach to the diagnosis of varicocele, *Med. Biol. Eng. Comp.*, 37, 1080, 1999.

[7] Merla, A. et al., Correlation of telethermographic and ultrasonographic reports in the therapeutic monitoring of second-class muscular lesions treated by hyperthermia, *Med. Biol. Eng. Comp.*, 37, 942, 1999.

[8] Merla, A., Biomedical applications of functional infrared imaging, presented at the *21st Annual Meeting of Houston Society of Engineering in Medicine and Biology*, Houston, TX, February 12–13, 2004.

[9] Merla, A. et al., Assessment of the effects of the varicocelectomy on the thermoregulatory control of the scrotum, *Fertil. Steril.*, 81, 471, 2004.

[10] Merla, A. et al., Recording of the sympathetic thermal response by means of infrared functional imaging, in *Proceedings of the 25th Annual International Conference of the IEEE Engineering in Medicine and Biology Society*, Cancun, Mexico, September 17–21, 2003.

[11] Merla, A. et al., Infrared functional imaging applied to the study of emotional reactions: preliminary results, in *Proceedings of the 4th International Non-Invasive Functional Source Imaging*, Chieti, Italy, September 9–13, 2003.

[12] Merla, A. and Romani, G.L., Skin blood flow rate mapping through functional infrared imaging, in *Proceedings of the World Congress of Medical Physics WC2003*, Sidney, August 24–29, 2003.

[13] Merla, A. Cianflone, F., and Romani, G.L., Skin blood flow rate estimation through functional infrared imaging analysis, in *Proceedings of the 5th International Federation of Automatic Control Symposium on Modelling and Control in Biomedical Systems*, Melbourne, August 19–23, 2003.

[14] Merla, A. et al., Raynaud's phenomenon: infrared functional imaging applied to diagnosis and drugs effects, *Int. J. Immun. Pharm.* 15, 41, 2002.

[15] Merla, A. et al., Use of infrared functional imaging to detect impaired thermoregulatory control in men with asymptomatic varicocele, *Fertil. Steril.*, 78, 199, 2002.

[16] Merla, A. et al., Infrared functional imaging applied to Raynaud's phenomenon, *IEEE Eng. Med. Biol. Mag.*, 21, 73, 2002.

[17] Merla, A. et al., Quantifying the relevance and stage of disease with the tau image technique. *IEEE Eng. Med. Biol. Mag.*, 21, 86, 2002.

[18] Merla, A. et al., Infrared functional imaging: analysis of skin temperature during exercise, in *Proceedings of the 24th IEEE Engineering in Medicine and Biology Society Conference*, Houston, October 23–25, 2002.

[19] Merla, A. et al., Time recovery image: a diagnostic image technique based on the dynamic digital telethermography, *Thermol. Int.*, 10, 142, 2000.

[20] Merla, A. et al., Tau image: a diagnostic imaging technique based on the dynamic digital telethermography, *in Proceedings of the WC2000 Chicago World Congress on Medical Physics and Biomedical Engineering and 22nd International Conference of IEEE Engineering in Medicine and Biology Society*, Digest of Papers CD, track 1,TU-FXH, July 2000, Chicago.

[21] Allen, E.V. and Brown, G.E., Raynaud's disease: a critical review of minimal requisites for diagnosis, *Am. J. Med. Sci.*, 183, 187, 1932.

[22] Subcommittee for Scleroderma Criteria of the American Rheumatism Association Diagnostic and Therapeutic Criteria Committee, Preliminary criteria for the classification of systemic sclerosis (scleroderma), *Arthr. Rheum.*, 23, 581, 1980.

[23] O'Reilly, D. et al., Measurement of cold challenge response in primary Raynaud's phenomenon and Raynaud's phenomenon associated with systemic sclerosis, *Ann. Rheum. Dis.*, 51, 1193, 1992.

[24] Clarks, S. et al., The distal–dorsal difference as a possible predictor of secondary Raynaud's phenomenon, *J. Rheumatol.*, 26, 1125, 1999.

[25] Schuhfried, O. et al., Thermographic parameters in the diagnosis of secondary Raynaud's phenomenon, *Arch. Phys. Med. Rehab.,* 81, 495, 2000.

[26] Ring, E.F.J., Ed., Cold stress test for the hands, in *The thermal image in Medicine and Biology,* Uhlen Verlag, Wien, 1995.

[27] Merla, A. et al., Combined approach to the initial stage Raynaud's phenomenon diagnosis by means of dynamic digital telethermography, capilloroscopy and pletismography: preliminary findings, *Med. Biol. Eng. Comp.,* 37, 992, 1999.

[28] Shitzer, A. et al., Lumped parameter tissue temperature–blood perfusion model of a cold stressed finger, *J. Appl. Physiol.,* 80, 1829, 1996.

[29] Mieusset, R. and Bujan, L., Testicular heating and its possible contributions to male infertility: a review, *Int. J. Andr.,* 18, 169, 1995.

[30] Trum, J.W., The value of palpation, varicoscreen contact thermography and colour Doppler ultrasound in the diagnosis of varicocele, *Hum. Reprod.,* 11, 1232, 1996.

[31] Brengelmann, G.L. et al., Altered control of skin blood flow during exercise at high internal temperatures, *J. Appl. Physiol.,* 43, 790, 1977.

[32] Johnson, J.M., Exercise and the cutaneous circulation, *Exerc. Sport Sci. Rev.* 20, 59, 1992.

[33] Kenney, W.L. and Johnson, J.M., Control of skin blood flow during exercise, *Med. Sci. Sports Exerc.,* 24, 303, 1992.

[34] Zontak, A. et al., Dynamic thermography: analysis of hand temperature during exercise, *Ann. Biomed. Eng.,* 26, 988, 1998.

[35] ASHRAE: handbook fundamentals SI edition, ASHRAE, Atlanta, GA, 1985.

[36] Cooke, E.D. et al., Reflex sympathetic dystrophy and repetitive strain injury: temperature and microcirculatory changes following mild cold stress, *J.R. Soc. Med.,* 86, 690, 1993.

[37] Di Benedetto, M., Regional hypothermia in response to minor injury, *Am. J. Phys. Med. Rehab.,* 75, 270, 1996.

[38] Garagiola, U., Use of telethermography in the management of sports injuries, *Sports Med.,* 10, 267, 1990.

[39] Maricq, H.R. et al., Diagnostic potential of in vivo capillary microscopy in scleroderma and related disorders, *Arthr. Rheum.,* 23, 183, 1980.

[40] Rodnan, G.P., Myerowitz, R.I., and Justh, G.O., Morphological changes in the digital arteries of patients with progressive systemic sclerosis and Raynaud phenomenon, *Medicine,* 59, 393, 1980.

[41] Tucker, A., Infrared thermographic assessment of the human scrotum, *Fertil. Steril.,* 74, 802, 2000.

33

Thermal Imaging in Surgery

33.1 Overview 33-1
33.2 Energized Systems 33-2
33.3 Thermal Imaging Systems 33-3
33.4 Calibration 33-3
33.5 Thermal Imaging During Energized Surgery 33-4
RF Electrosurgery • Analysis of Collateral Damage
33.6 Laser Applications in Dermatology.................... 33-6
Overview
33.7 Laser-Tissue Interactions 33-8
33.8 Optimizing Laser Therapies........................... 33-9
33.9 Thermographic Results of Laser Positioning 33-11
33.10 Computerized Laser Scanning 33-11
Case Study 1: Port Wine Stain • Case Study 2: Laser
Depilation
33.11 Conclusions 33-15
References 33-17

Paul Campbell
Ninewells Hospital

Roderick Thomas
Swansea Institute of Technology

33.1 Overview

Advances in miniaturization and microelectronics, coupled with enhanced computing technologies, have combined to see modern infrared imaging systems develop rapidly over the past decade. As a result, the instrumentation has become considerably improved, not only in terms of its inherent resolution (spatial *and* temporal) and detector sensitivity (values ca. 25 mK are typical) but also in terms of its portability: the considerable reduction in bulk has resulted in light, camcorder (or smaller) sized devices. Importantly, cost has also been reduced so that entry to the field is no longer prohibitive. This attractive combination of factors has led to an ever increasing range of applicability across the medical spectrum. Whereas the mainstay application for medical thermography over the past 40 years has been with rheumatological and associated conditions, usually for the detection and diagnosis of peripheral vascular diseases such as Raynaud's phenomenon, the latest generations of thermal imaging systems have seen active service within new surgical realms such as orthopaedics, coronary by-pass operations, and also in urology. The focus of this chapter relates not to a specific area of surgery per se, but rather to a generic and pervasive aspect of all modern surgical approaches: the use of *energized* instrumentation during surgery. In particular, we will concern ourselves with the use of thermal imaging to accurately monitor temperature within the tissue locale surrounding an energy-activated instrument. The rationale behind this is that it facilitates optimization of operation specific protocols that may either relate to thermally based therapies, or else to reduce the extent of collateral damage that may be introduced when inappropriate power levels, or excessive pulse durations, are implemented during surgical procedures.

33.2 Energized Systems

Energy-based instrumentation can considerably expedite fundamental procedures such as vessel sealing and dissection. The instrumentation is most often based around ultrasonic, laser, or radio-frequency (RF)-current based technologies. Heating tissue into distinct temperature regimes is required in order to achieve the desired effect (e.g., vessel sealing, cauterization, or cutting). In the context of electrical current heating, the resultant effect of the current on tissue is dominated by two factors: the temperature attained by the tissue; and the duration of the heating phase, as encapsulated in the following equation:

$$T - T_0 = \frac{1}{\sigma \rho c} J^2 \delta t \tag{33.1}$$

where T and T_0 are the final and initial temperatures (in degrees Kelvin [K]) respectively, σ is the electrical conductivity (in S/m), ρ is the tissue density, c is the tissue specific heat capacity ($J\,kg^{-1}\,K^{-1}$), J is the current density (A/m^2), and δt is the duration of heat application. The resultant high temperatures are not limited solely to the tissue regions in which the electrical current flow is concentrated. Heat will flow away from hotter regions in a time dependence fashion given by the Fourier equation:

$$Q(r, t) = -k\nabla T(r, t) \tag{33.2}$$

where Q is the heat flux vector, the proportionality constant k is a scalar quantity of the material known as the thermal conductivity, and $\nabla T(r, t)$ is the temperature gradient vector. The overall spatio-temporal evolution of the temperature field is embodied within the differential equation of heat flow (alternatively known as the diffusion equation)

$$\frac{1}{\alpha} \frac{\partial T(r, t)}{\partial t} = \nabla^2 T(r, t) \tag{33.3}$$

where α is the thermal diffusivity of the medium defined in terms of the physical constants, k, ρ, and c thus:

$$\alpha = k/\rho c \tag{33.4}$$

and temperature T is a function of both the three dimensions of space (r) and also of time t. In other words, high temperatures are not limited to the region specifically targeted by the surgeon, and this is often the source of an added surgical complication caused by collateral or proximity injury. Electrosurgical damage, for example, is the most common cause of iatrogenic bowel injury during laparoscopic surgery and 60% of mishaps are missed, that is, the injury is not recognized during surgery and declares itself with peritonitis several days after surgery or even after discharge from hospital. This level of morbidity can have serious consequences, in terms of both the expense incurred by re-admission to hospital, or even the death of the patient. By undertaking *in vivo* thermal imaging during energized dissection it becomes possible to determine, in real time, the optimal power conditions for the successful accomplishment of specific tasks, and with minimal collateral damage. As an adjunct imaging modality, thermal imaging may also improve surgical practice by facilitating easier identification and localization of tissues such as arteries, especially by less experienced surgeons. Further, as tumors are more highly vascularized than normal tissue, thermal imaging may facilitate their localization and staging, that is, the identification of the tumor's stage in its growth cycle. Figure 33.1 shows a typical set-up for implementation of thermography during surgery.

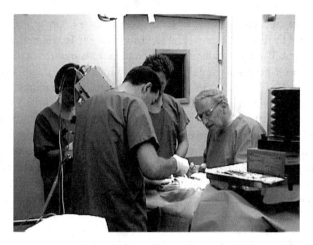

FIGURE 33.1 Typical set-up for a thermal imaging in surgery. The camera is tripod mounted toward the foot of the operating table and aimed at the surgical access site (camera visible over the left shoulder of the nearmost surgeon).

33.3 Thermal Imaging Systems

As skin is a close approximation to an ideal black body (the emissivity, ε, of skin is 0.98, whereas that of an ideal black body has $\varepsilon = 1$), then we can feel reasonably confident in applying the relevant physics directly to the situation of thermography in surgery. One important consideration must be the waveband of detector chosen for thermal observations of the human body. It is known from the thermal physics of black bodies, that the wavelength at which the maximum emissive power occurs, λ_{max} (i.e., the peak in the Planck curve), is related to the body's temperature T through Wien's law:

$$\lambda_{max} T = 0.002898 \qquad (33.5)$$

Thus for bodies at 310 K (normal human body temperature), the peak output is around 10 μm, and the majority of the emitted thermal radiation is limited to the range from 2 to 20 μm. The optimal detectors for passive thermal imaging of normal skin should thus have best sensitivity around the 10 μm range, and this is indeed the case with many of the leading thermal imagers manufactured today, which often rely on GaAs quantum well infrared photodetectors (QWIPs) with a typical waveband of 8–9 μm. A useful alternative to these longwave detectors involves the use of indium–antimonide (InSb) based detectors to detect radiation in the mid-wave infrared (3–5 μm). Both these materials have the benefit of enhanced temperature sensitivity (ca. 0.025 K), and are both wholly appropriate even for quantitative imaging of hotter surfaces, such as may occur in energized surgical instrumentation.

33.4 Calibration

Whilst the latest generation of thermal imaging systems are usually robust instruments exhibiting low drift over extended periods, it is sensible to recalibrate the systems at regular intervals in order to preserve the integrity of captured data. For some camera manufacturers, recalibration can be undertaken under a service agreement and this usually requires shipping of the instrument from the host laboratory. However for other systems, recalibration must be undertaken in-house, and on such occasions, a black body source (BBS) is required.

Most BBS are constructed in the form of a cavity at a known temperature, with an aperture to the cavity that acts as the black body, effectively absorbing all incident radiation upon it. The cavity temperature must be measured using a high accuracy thermometric device, such as a platinum resistance thermometer

(PRT), with performance characteristics traceable to a thermometry standard. Figure 33.2b shows one such system, as developed by the UK National Physical Laboratory at Teddington, and whose architecture relies on a heat-pipe design. The calibration procedure requires measurement of the aperture temperature at a range of temperature set-points that are simultaneously monitored by the PRT (e.g., at intervals of 5° between temperature range of 293 and 353 K). Direct comparison of the radiometric temperature measured by the thermal camera with the standard temperature monitored via the PRT allows a calibration table to be generated across the temperature range of interest. During each measurement, sufficient time must be allowed in order to let the programmed temperature set-point equilibrate, otherwise inaccuracies will result. Further, the calibration procedure should ideally be undertaken under similar ambient conditions to those under which usual imaging is undertaken. This may include aspects such as laminar, or even fan-assisted, flow around the camera body which will affect the heat transfer rate from the camera to the ambient and in turn may affect the performance of the detector (viz Figure 33.2b).

33.5   Thermal Imaging During Energized Surgery

Fully remote-controlled cameras may be ideally suited to overhead bracket mountings above the operating table so that a bird's eye view over the surgical site is afforded. However, without a robotized arm to fully control pitch and location, the view may be restrictive. Tripod mounting, as illustrated in Figure 33.1, and with a steep look-down angle from a distance of about 1 m to the target offers the most versatile viewing without compromising the surgeon's freedom of movement. However, this type of set-up demands that a camera operator be on hand continually in order to move the imaging system to those positions offering best viewing for the type of energized procedure being undertaken.

33.5.1   RF Electrosurgery

As mentioned earlier, the most common energized surgical instrumentation employ a physical system reliant on either (high frequency) electrical current, an ultrasonic mechanism, or else incident laser energy in order to induce tissue heating. Thermal imaging has been used to follow all three of these procedures. There are often similarities in approach between the alternative modalities. For example, vessel sealing often involves placement of elongated forcep-style electrodes across a target vessel followed by ratcheted compression, and then a pulse of either RF current, or alternatively ultrasonic activation of the forceps, is applied through the compressed tissue region. The latest generations of energized instrumentation may have active feedback control over the pulse to facilitate optimal sealing with minimal thermal spread (e.g., the Valleylab *Ligasure* instrument) however under certain circumstances, such as with calcified tissue or in excessively liquid environments the performance may be less predictable.

   Figure 33.3 illustrates how thermal spread may be monitored during the instrument activation period of one such "intelligent" feedback device using RF current. The initial power level for each application is determined through a fast precursor voltage scan that determines the natural impedance of the compressed tissue. Then, by monitoring the temperature dependence of impedance (of the compressed tissue) during current activation, the microprocessor controlled feedback loop automatically maintains an appropriate power level until a target impedance is reached indicating that the seal is complete. This process typically takes between 1 and 6 sec, depending on the nature of the target tissue. Termination of the pulse is indicated by an audible tone burst from the power supply box. The performance of the system has been evaluated in preliminary studies involving gastric, colonic and small bowel resection [1]; hemorraoidectomy [2]; prostatectomy [3]; and cholecystectomy [4].

   Perhaps most strikingly, the facility for real time thermographic monitoring, as illustrated in Figure 33.3, affords the surgeon immediate appreciation of the instrument temperature, providing a visual cue that automatically alerts to the potential for iatrogenic injury should a hot instrument come into close contact with vital structures. By the same token, the *in situ* thermal image also indicates when the tip of the instrument has cooled to ambient temperature. It should be noted that the amount by which the activated

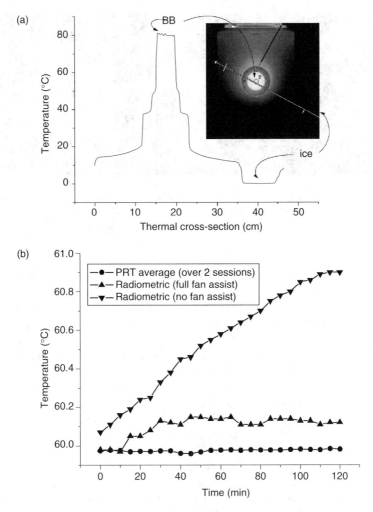

FIGURE 33.2 Thermal cross-section (profile) through the black body calibration source together with equilibrated crushed ice, which acts as a convenient secondary temperature gauge *in situ*. (Insert [left] thermal view with linear region of interest highlighted, and [right] optical view of the black body cavity and beaker of [equilibrated] crushed ice to the lower right.) (b) Radiometric detector drift during start up under two different ambient conditions. The detector readout is centered on the black body cavity source shown in (a), which was itself maintained at a target temperature of 59.97°C throughout the measurements (solid circles). Without fan-assisted cooling of the camera exterior, the measured temperature drifted by 0.8°C over 2 h, hence the importance of calibration under typical operating conditions. With fan-assisted cooling, the camera "settles" within around 30 min of switching on. (Camera: Raytheon Galileo [Raytheon Systems].)

head's temperature rises is largely a function of device dimensions, materials, and the power levels applied together with the pulse duration.

33.5.2 Analysis of Collateral Damage

Whilst thermograms typical of Figure 33.3 offer a visually instructive account of the thermal scene and its temporal evolution, a quantitative analysis of the sequence is more readily achieved through the identification of a linear region of interest (LROI), as illustrated by the line bisecting the device head in Figure 33.4a. The data constituted by the LROI is effectively a snapshot thermal profile across those pixels lying on this designated line (Figure 33.4b). A graph can then be constructed to encapsulate the

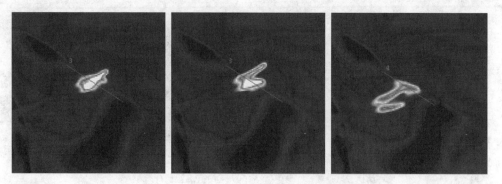

FIGURE 33.3 Thermographic sequence taken with the Dundee thermal imaging system and showing (33.1) ener-gized forceps attached to bowel (white correlates with temperature), (33.2) detachment of the forceps revealing hot tissue beneath, (33.3) remnant hot-spot extending across the tissue and displaying collateral thermal damage covering 4.5 mm either side of the instrument jaws.

time dependent evolution of the LROI. This is displayed as a 3D surface (a function of spatial co-ordinate along the LROI, time, and temperature) upon which color-mapped contours are evoked to represent the different temperature domains across the LROI (Figure 33.4c). In order to facilitate measurement of the thermal spread, the 3D surface, as represented in matrix form, can then be interrogated with a mathematical programming package, or alternatively inspected manually, a process that is most easily undertaken after projecting the data to the 2D coordinate-time plane, as illustrated in Figure 33.4d. The critical temperature beyond which tangible heat damage can occur to tissue is assumed to be 45°C [5]. Thermal spread is then calculated by measuring the maximum distance between the 45°C contours on the planar projection, then subtracting the electrode "footprint" diameter from this to get the total spread. Simply dividing this result by two gives the thermal spread either side of the device electrodes.

The advanced technology used in some of the latest generations of vessel sealing instrumentation can lead to a much reduced thermal spread, compared with the earlier technologies. For example with the Ligasure LS1100 instrument, the heated peripheral region is spatially confined to less than 2 mm, even when used on thicker vessels/structures. A more advanced version of the device (LS1200 [*Precise*]) consistently produces even lower thermal spreads, typically around 1 mm (viz Figure 33.4). This performance is far superior to other commercially available energized devices.

For example, Kinoshita and co-workers [6] have observed (using infrared imaging) that the typical lateral spread of heat into adjacent tissue is sufficient to cause a temperature of over 60°C at radial distances of up to 10 mm from the active electrode when an ultrasonic scalpel is used. Further, when standard bipolar electro-coagulation instrumentation is used, the spread can be as large as 22 mm. Clearly, the potential for severe collateral and iatrogenic injury is high with such systems unless power levels are tailored to the specific procedure in hand and real time thermal imaging evidently represents a powerful adjunct technology to aid this undertaking.

Whilst the applications mentioned thusfar relate to "open" surgical procedures requiring a surgical incision to access the site of interest, thermal imaging can also be applied as a route to protocol optimization for other less invasive procedures also. Perhaps the most important surgical application in this regime involves laser therapy for various skin diseases/conditions. Application of the technique in this area is discussed below.

33.6 Laser Applications in Dermatology

33.6.1 Overview

Infrared thermographic monitoring (ITM) has been successfully used in medicine for a number of years and much of this has been documented by Prof. Francis Ring [http://www.medimaging.org/], who has

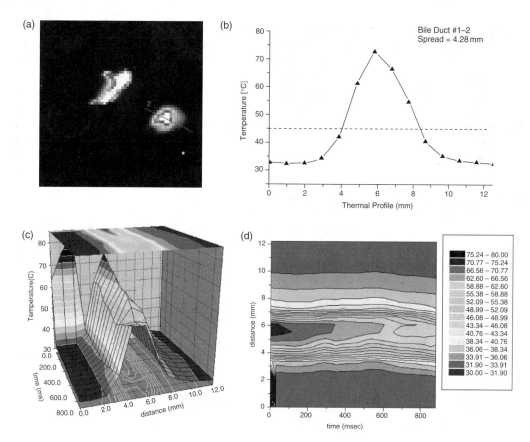

FIGURE 33.4 (a) Mid-infrared thermogram taken at the instant an energized forceps (Ligasure LS1200 "*Precise*") is removed from the surgical scene after having conducted a seal on the bile duct. The hot tips of the forceps are clearly evident in the infrared view (just left of center), as is the remnant hot-spot where the seal has occurred on the vessel. By generating a linear region of interest (LROI) through the hot-spot, as indicated by the highlighted line in the figure, it is possible to monitor the evolution of the hot-spot's temperature in a quantitative fashion. (b) Thermal profile corresponding to the LROI shown in (a). (c) By tracking the temporal evolution of the LROI, it is possible to generate a 3D plot of the thermal profile by simply stacking the individual profiles at each acquisition frame. In this instance the cooling behavior of the hot-spot is clearly identified. Manual estimation of the thermal spread is most easily achieved by resorting to the 2D contour plot of the thermal profile's temporal evolution, as shown in (d). In this instance, the maximal spread of the 45°C contours is measured as 4.28 mm. By subtracting the forcep "footprint" (2.5 mm for the device shown) and dividing the result by 2, we arrive at the thermal spread for the device. The average thermal spread (for 6 bile-duct sealing events) was 0.89 ± 0.35 mm.

established a database and archive within the Department of Computing at the University of Glamorgan, UK, spanning over 30 years of ITM applications. Examples include monitoring abnormalities such as malignancies, inflammation, and infection that cause localized increases in skin temperature, which show as hot spots or as asymmetrical patterns in an infrared thermogram.

A recent medical example that has benefited by the intervention of ITM is the treatment by laser of certain dermatological disorders. Advancements in laser technology have resulted in new portable laser therapies, examples of which include the removal of vascular lesions (in particular Port Wine Stains [PWS]), and also cosmetic enhancement approaches such as hair-(depilation) and wrinkle removal.

In these laser applications it is a common requirement to deliver laser energy uniformly without overlapping of the beam spot to a sub-dermal target region, such as a blood vessel, but with the minimum of collateral damage to the tissue locale. Temperature rise at the skin surface, and with this the threshold to burning/scarring is of critical importance for obvious reasons. Until recently, this type of therapy had not yet benefited significantly from thermographic evaluation. However, with the introduction of the latest generation thermal imaging systems, exhibiting the essential qualities of portability, high resolution, and high sensitivity, significant inroads to laser therapy are beginning to be made.

Historically, lasers have been used in dermatology for some 40 years [25]. In recent years there have been a number of significant developments particularly regarding the improved treatment of various skin disorders most notably the removal of vascular lesions using dye lasers [8,12,15,17,19] and depilation using ruby lasers [9,14,16]. Some of the general indicators as to why lasers are the preferred treatment of choice are summarized in Table 33.1.

33.7 Laser-Tissue Interactions

The mechanisms involved in the interaction between light and tissue depend on the characteristics of the impinging light and the targeted human tissue [24]. To appreciate these mechanisms the optical properties of tissue must be known. It is necessary to determine the tissue reflectance, absorption, and scattering properties as a function of wavelength. A simplified model of laser light interaction with the skin is illustrated in Figure 33.5.

Recent work has shown that laser radiation can penetrate through the epidermis and basal structure to be preferentially absorbed within the blood layers located in the lower dermis and subcutis. The process is termed selective photothermolysis, and is the specific absorption of laser light by a target tissue in order to eliminate that target without damaging surrounding tissue. For example, in the treatment of Port Wine

TABLE 33.1 Characteristics of Laser Therapy during and after Treatment

General indicators	Dye laser vascular lesions	Ruby laser depilation
During treatment	Varying output parameters	Varying output parameters
	Portable	Portable
	Manual and scanned	Manual and scanned
	Selective destruction of target chromophore (Haemoglobin)	Selective destruction of target chromophore (melanin)
After treatment (desired effect)	Slight bruising (purpura)	Skin returns to normal coloring (no bruising)
	Skin retains its elasticity	Skin retains surface markings
	Skin initially needs to be protected from UV and scratching	Skin retains its ability to tan after exposure to ultraviolet light
	Hair follicles are removed	Hair removed

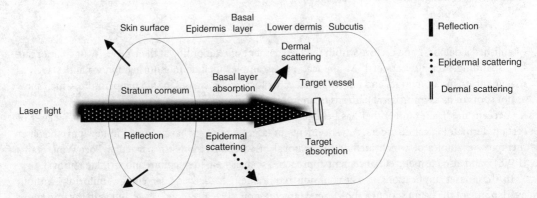

FIGURE 33.5 Passage of laser light within skin layers.

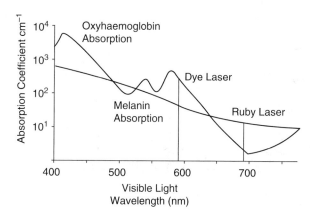

FIGURE 33.6 Spectral absorption curves for human blood and melanin.

TABLE 33.2 Interaction Effects of Laser Light and Tissue

Effect	Interaction
Photothermal	
Photohyperthermia	Reversible damage of normal tissue (37–42°C)
Photothermolysis	Loosening of membranes (odema), tissue welding (45–60°C)
Photocoagulation	Thermal-dynamic effects, micro-scale overheating
Photocarbonization	Coagulation, necrosis (60–100°C)
Photovaporization	Drying out, vaporization of water, carbonization (100–300°C)
	Pyrolysis, vaporization of solid tissue matrix (>300°C)
Photochemical	
Photochemotherapy	Photodynamic therapy, black light therapy
Photoinduction	Biostimulation
Photoionization	
Photoablation	Fast thermal explosion, optical breakdown, mechanical shockwave

Stains (PWS), a dye laser of wavelength 585 nm has been widely used [10] where the profusion of small blood vessels that comprise the PWS are preferentially targeted at this wavelength. The spectral absorption characteristics of light through human skin have been well established [7] and are replicated in Figure 33.6 for the two dominant factors: melanin and oxyhaemoglobin.

There are three types of laser/tissue interaction, namely: photothermal, photochemical, and protoionization (Table 33.2), and the use of lasers on tissue results in a number of differing interactions including photodisruption, photoablation, vaporization, and coagulation, as summarized in Figure 33.7.

The application of appropriate laser technology to medical problems depends on a number of laser operating parameters including matching the optimum laser wavelength for the desired treatment. Some typical applications and the desired wavelengths for usage are highlighted in Table 33.3.

33.8 Optimizing Laser Therapies

There are a number of challenges in optimizing laser therapy, mainly related to the laser parameters of wavelength, energy density, and spot size. Combined with these are difficulties associated with poor positioning of hand-held laser application that may result in uneven treatment [overlapping spots and/or uneven coverage (stippling) of spots], excessive treatment times, and pain. Therefore, for enhanced efficacy an improved understanding of the thermal effects of laser–tissue interaction benefits therapeutic

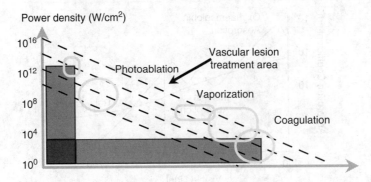

FIGURE 33.7 Physiological characteristics of laser therapy. (From Thomas et al., 2002, *Proceedings of SPIE*, 1–4 April, Orlando, USA. With permission.)

TABLE 33.3 Laser Application in Dermatology

Laser	Wavelength (nm)	Treatment
Flashlamp short-pulsed dye	510	Pigmented lesions, for example, freckles, tattoos
Flashlamp long-pulsed dye	585	PWS in children, warts, hypertrophic scars
Ruby single-pulse or Q-switched	694	Depilation of hair
Alexandrite Q-switched	755	Multicolored tattoos, viral warts, depilation
Diode variable	805	Multicolored tattoos, viral warts
Neodymium yitrium aluminum (Nd-YAG) Q-switched	1064	Pigmented lesions; adult port-wine stains, black/blue tattoos
Carbon dioxide continuous pulsed	10600	Tissue destruction, warts, tumors

approaches. Here, variables for consideration include:

1. Thermal effects of varying spot size.
2. Improved control of hand-held laser minimising overlapping and stippling.
3. Establishment of minimum gaps.
4. Validation of laser computer scanning.

Evaluation (Figure 33.8) was designed to elucidate whether or not measurements of the surface temperature of the skin are reproducible when illuminated by nominally identical laser pulses. In this case a 585 nm dye laser and a 694 nm ruby laser were used to place a number of pulses manually on tissue. The energy emitted by the laser is highly repeatable. Care must be taken to ensure that both the laser and radiometer position are kept constant and that the anatomical location used for the test had uniform tissue pigmentation.

Figure 33.8 shows the maximum temperature for each of twenty shots fired on the forearm of a representative Caucasian male with type 2 skin*. Maximum temperature varies between 48.90 and 48.10°C representing a variance of 1°C ($\pm$0.45°C). This level of reproducibility is pleasing since it shows that, despite the complex scenario, the radiometer is capable of repeatedly and accurately measuring surface tissue temperatures. In practice the radiometer may be used to inform the operator when any accumulated temperature has subsided allowing further treatment without exceeding some damage threshold.

Energy density is also an important laser parameter and can be varied to match the demands of the application. It is normal in the discipline to measure energy density (fluence) in J/cm^2. In treating vascular lesions most utilize an energy density for therapy of 5 to 10 J/cm^2 [13]. The laser operator needs to be sure that the energy density is uniform and does not contain hot-spots that may take the temperature above the damage threshold inadvertently. Preliminary characterization of the spot with thermal imaging can

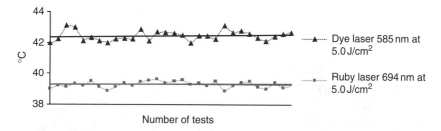

FIGURE 33.8 Repeatability of initial maximum skin temperatures (°C) of two lasers with similar energy density but different wavelengths.

then aid with fine tuning of the laser and reduce the possibility of excessive energy density and with that the possibility of collateral damage.

33.9   Thermographic Results of Laser Positioning

During laser therapy the skin is treated with a number of spots, applied manually depending on the anatomical location and required treatment. It has been found that spot size directly affects efficacy of treatment. The wider the spot size the higher the surface temperature [22]. The type and severity of lesion also determines the treatment required. Its color severity (dark to light) and its position on skin (raised to level). Therefore the necessary treatment may require a number of passes of the laser over the skin. It is therefore essential as part of the treatment that there is a physical separation between individual spots so that:

1. The area is not over treated with overlapping spots that could otherwise result in local heating effects from adjacent spots resulting in skin damage
2. The area is not under treated leaving stippled skin
3. The skin has cooled sufficiently before second or subsequent passes of the laser

Figure 33.9 shows two laser shots placed next to each other some 4 mm apart. The time between the shots is 1 sec. There are no excessive temperatures evident and no apparent temperature build-up in the gap. This result, which concurs with Lanigan [18], suggests a minimum physical separation of 5 mm between all individual spot sizes.

The intention is to optimize the situation leading to a uniform therapeutic and aesthetic result without either striping or thermal build-up. This is achieved by initially determining the skin color (Chromotest) for optimum energy settings, followed by a patch test and subsequent treatment. Increasing the number of spots to 3 with the 4 mm separation reveals a continuing trend, as shown in Figure 33.10. The gap between the first two shots is now beginning to merge in the 2 sec period that has lapsed. The gap between shots 2 and 3 remains clear and distinct and there are clearly visible thermal bands across the skin surface of between 38–39 and 39–40°C. These experimental results supply valuable information to support the development of both free-hand treatment and computer-controlled techniques.

33.10   Computerized Laser Scanning

Having established the parameters relating to laser spot positioning, the possibility of achieving reproducible laser coverage of a lesion by automatic scanning becomes a reality. This has potential advantages, which include:

1. Accurate positioning of the spot with the correct spacing from the adjacent spots
2. Accurate timing allowing the placement at a certain location at the appropriate lapsed time

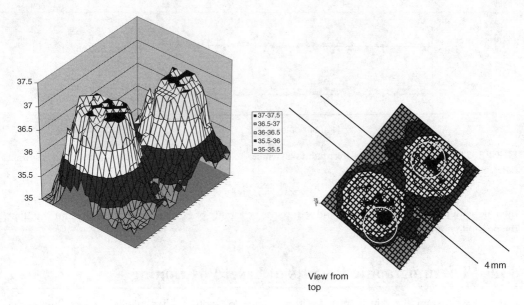

FIGURE 33.9 Two-dye laser spots with a minimum of 4 mm separation (585 nm at 4.5 J/cm^2, 5 mm spot).

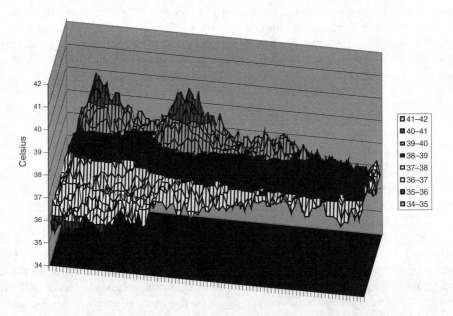

FIGURE 33.10 Three-dye laser spots, 2 sec apart with a 5 mm separation (585 nm at 5 J/cm^2, 5 mm spot).

There are some disadvantages that include the need for additional equipment and regulatory approvals for certain market sectors

A computerized scanning system has been developed [9] that illuminates the tissue in a pre-defined pattern. Sequential pulses are not placed adjacent to an immediately preceding pulse thereby ensuring the minimum of thermal build-up. Clement et al. [9] carried out a trial, illustrating treatment coverage using a hand-held system compared to a controlled computer scanning system. Two adjacent areas (lower arm) were selected and shaved. A marked hexagonal area was subjected to 19 shots using a hand-held system, and an adjacent area of skin was treated with a scanner whose computer control is designed to uniformly fill the area with exactly 19 shots. Such tests were repeated and the analyzed statistics showed that, on

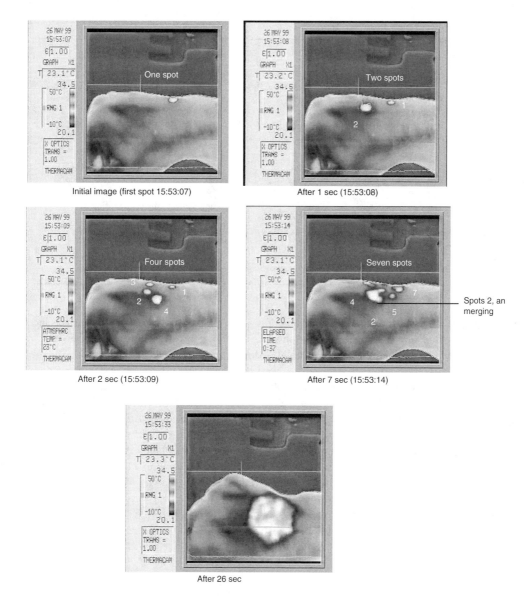

FIGURE 33.11 Sample sequences during computer laser scanning.

average, only 60% of area is covered by laser spots. The use of thermography allowed the validation and optimization of this automated system in a way that was impossible without thermal imaging technology. The following sequence of thermal images, Figure 33.11, captures the various stages of laser scanning of the hand using a dye laser at 5.7 J/cm². Thermography confirms that the spot temperature from individual laser beams will merge and that both the positioning of spots and the time duration between spots dictate the efficacy of treatment.

33.10.1 Case Study 1: Port Wine Stain

Vascular naevi are common and are present at birth or develop soon after. Superficial lesions are due to capillary networks in the upper or mid dermis, but larger angiomas can be located in the lower dermis and subcutis. An example of vascular naevi is the Port-Wine Stain (PWS) often present at birth, is an irregular

TABLE 33.4   Vasculature Treatment Types

Treatment type	Process	Possible concerns
Camouflage	Applying skin colored pigments to the surface of the skin. Enhancement to this technique is to tattoo skin colored inks into the upper layer of the lesion	Only a temporary measure and is very time consuming. Efficacy dependant on flatter lesions
Cryosurgery	Involves applying super-cooled liquid nitrogen to the lesion to destroy abnormal vasculature	May require several treatments
Excision	Common place where the lesion is endangering vital body functions	Not considered appropriate for purely cosmetic reasons. Complex operation resulting in a scar. Therefore, only applicable to the proliferating haemangioma lesion.
Radiation therapy	Bombarding the lesion with radiation to destroy vasculature	Induced number of skin cancer in a small number of cases
Drug therapy	Widely used administering steroids	Risk of secondary complications affecting bodily organs

red or purple macule which often affects one side of the face. Problems can arise if the naevus is located close to the eye and some cases where a PWS involves the trigeminal nerve's ophthalmic division may have an associated intracranial vascular malformation known as Sturge Weber Syndrome. The treatment of vascular naevi can be carried out a number of ways often dependent on the nature, type, anatomical and severity of lesion location, as highlighted in Table 33.4.

A laser wavelength of 585 nm is preferentially absorbed by haemoglobin within the blood, but there is partial absorption in the melanin rich basal layer in the epidermis. The objective is to thermally damage the blood vessel, by elevating its temperature, while ensuring that the skin surface temperature is kept low. For a typical blood vessel, the temperature–time graph appears similar to Figure 33.12. This suggests that it is possible to selectively destroy the PWS blood vessels, by elevating them to a temperature in excess of 100°C, causing disruption to the small blood vessels, whilst maintaining a safe skin surface temperature. This has been proven empirically via thermographic imaging with a laser pulsing protocol that was devised and optimized on the strength of Monte-Carlo based models [26] of the heat dissipation processes [11]. The two-dimensional Cartesian thermal transport equation is:

$$\nabla T^2 + \frac{Q(x,y)}{k} = \frac{1}{\alpha}\frac{\partial T}{\partial t} \tag{33.6}$$

where temperature T has both an implied spatial and temporal dependence and the volumetric source term, $Q(x, y)$, is obtained from the solution of the Monte-Carlo radiation transport problem [27].

33.10.2   Case Study 2: Laser Depilation

The 694 nm wavelength laser radiation is preferentially absorbed by melanin, which occurs in the basal layer and particularly in the hair follicle base, which is the intended target using an oblique angle of laser beam (see Figure 33.13). A Monte-Carlo analysis was performed in a similar manner to *Case Study 1* above, where the target region in the dermis is the melanin rich base of the hair follicle. Figures 33.14a,b show the temperature–time profiles for 10 and 20 J cm^2 laser fluence [23]. These calculations suggest that it is possible to thermally damage the melanin-rich follicle base whilst restricting the skin surface temperature to values that cause no superficial damage. Preliminary clinical trials indicated that there is indeed a beneficial effect, but the choice of laser parameters still required optimizing.

Thermographic analysis has proved indispensable in this work. Detailed thermometric analysis is shown in Figure 33.15a. Analysis of this data shows that in this case, the surface temperature is raised to

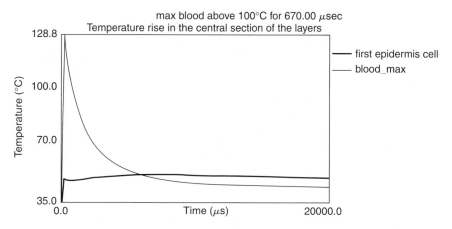

FIGURE 33.12   Typical temperatures for PWS problem, indicating thermal disruption of blood vessel, while skin surface temperature remains low.

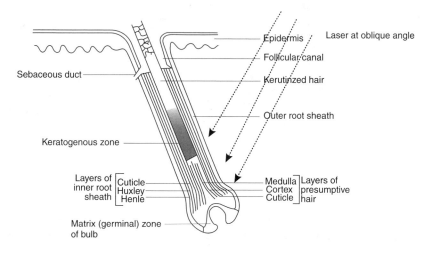

FIGURE 33.13   Oblique laser illumination of hair follicle.

about 50°C. The thermogram also clearly shows the selective absorption in the melanin-dense hair. The temperature of the hair is raised to over 207°C. This thermogram illustrates direct evidence for selective wavelength absorption leading to cell necrosis. Further clinical trials have indicated a maximum fluence of 15 J cm^2 for type III caucasian skin. Figure 33.15b illustrates a typical thermographic image obtained during the real-time monitoring.

33.11   Conclusions

The establishment, development, and consequential success of medical infrared thermographic (MIT) intervention with laser therapy is primarily based on the understanding of the following, that are described in more detail below:

1. Problem/condition to be monitored
2. Set-up and correct operation of infrared system (appropriate and validated training)
3. Appropriate conditions during the monitoring process
4. Evaluation of activity and development of standards and protocol

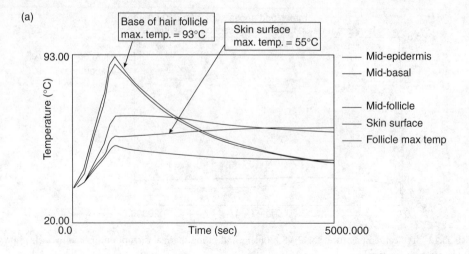

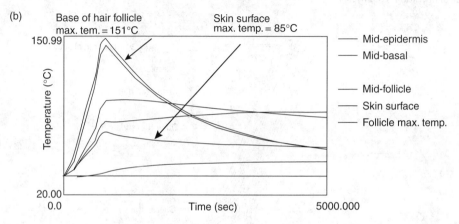

FIGURE 33.14   (a) Temperature–time profiles at 10 J cm^2 ruby (694 nm), 800 μsec laser pulse on caucasian skin type III. (b) Temperature–time profiles for 20 J cm^2 ruby (694 nm), 800 μsec laser pulse on Caucasian skin type III.

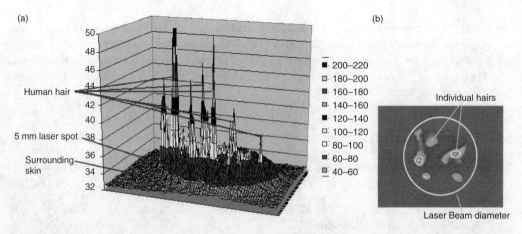

FIGURE 33.15   (a) Post-processed results of 5 mm. (b) Simplified thermogram diameter 694 nm 20 J cm^2 800 μsec ruby pulse of ruby laser pulse, with 5 mm spot at 20 J cm^2.

With reference to (1) above in the conclusions, the condition to be monitored, there needs to be a good knowledge as to the physiological aspects of the desired medical process; in laser therapy an understanding as to the mechanisms involved in laser–tissue interaction. A good reference source of current practice can be found in the Handbook of Optical Biomedical Diagnostics, published by The International Society for Optical Engineering (SPIE).

In this application fast data-capture (>50 Hz), good image quality (256 × 256 pixels), temperature sensitivity, and repeatability were considered important and an Inframetrics SC1000 Focal Plane Array Radiometer (3.4 to 5μm, CMOS PtSi Cooled Detector) with a real-time data acquisition system (Dynamite) was used. There are currently very fast systems available with data acquisition speeds in terms of hundreds of Hertz with detectors that provide excellent image quality. In (2) the critical aspect is training [21]. Currently, infrared equipment manufacturers design systems with multiple applications in mind. This has resulted in many aspects of good practice and quality standards. This is one of the reasons why industrial infrared thermography is so successful. This has not necessarily been the case in medicine. However, it is worth noting that there are a number of good infrared training organizations throughout the world, particularly in the United States. The advantages of adopting training organizations such as these is that they have experience of training with reference to a very wide range and type of infrared thermographic systems, in a number of different applications. This will help in the identification of the optimum infrared technology. In (3) consideration as to the conditions surrounding the patient and the room environment are important for optimum results. In the United Kingdom for example, Prof. Francis Ring, University of Glamorgan has led the way in the development and standardizations of clinical infrared practice [20]. Finally, (4) the evaluation of such practice is crucial if lessons are to be learnt and protocol and standards are to emerge.

Infrared thermal imaging provides an important tool for optimizing energized surgical interventions and facilitates validation of theoretical models of evolving temperature fields.

References

[1] Heniford, B.T., Matthews, B.D., Sing, R.F., Backus, C., Pratt, P., and Greene, F.L. (2001) Initial results with an electrothermal bipolar vessel sealer. *Surg. Endosc.* 15: 799–801.

[2] Palazzo, F.F., Francis, D.L., and Clifton, M.A. (2002) Randomised clinical trial of ligasure versus open haemorrhoidectomy. *Br. J. Surg.* 89, 154–157.

[3] Sengupta, S. and Webb, D.R. (2001) Use of a computer controlled bipolar diathermy system in radical prostatectomies and other open urological surgery. *ANZ J. Surg.* 71: 538–540.

[4] Schulze, S., Krztiansen, V.B., Fischer-Hansen, B., and Rosenberg, J. (2002) Sealing of the cystic duct with bipolar electrocoagulation. *Surg. Endosc.* 16: 342–344.

[5] Reidenbach, H.D. and Buess, G. (1992). Anciliary technology: electrocautery, thermoregulation and laser. In Cuschieri, A., Buess, G., and Perrisat, L. Eds., *Operative Manual of Endoscopic Surgery*. Springer-Verlag, Berlin-Heidelberg-New York, pp. 44–60.

[6] Kinoshita, T., Kanehira, E., Omura, K., Kawakami, K., and Watanabe, Y. (1999) Experimental study on heat production by a 23.5 kHz ultrasonically activated device for endoscopic surgery. *Surg. Endosc.* 13: 621–625.

[7] Andersen, R.R. and Parrish, J.A. (1981) Microvasculature can be selectively damaged using dye lasers. *Lasers Surg. Med.* 1: 263–270.

[8] Barlow, R.J., Walker, N.P.J., and Markey, A.C. (1996) Treatment of proliferative haemangiomas with 585nm pulsed dye laser. *Br. J. Dermatol.* 134: 700–704.

[9] Clement, R.M., Kiernan, M.N., Thomas, R.A., Donne, K.E., and Bjerring, P.J. (1999) The use of thermal imaging to optimise automated laser irradiation of tissue, *Skin Research and Technology*. Vol. 5, No. 2, *6th Congress of the International Society for Skin Imaging*, July 4–6, 1999, Royal Society London.

[10] Clement, R.M., Donne, K.D., Thomas, R.A., and Kiernan, M.N. (2000) Thermographic condition monitoring of human skin during laser therapy, *Quality Reliability Maintenance, 3rd International Conference*, St Edmund Hall, University of Oxford, 30–31 March 2000.

[11] Daniel, G. (2002) An investigation of thermal radiation and thermal transport in laser–tissue interaction, PhD Thesis, Swansea Institute.

[12] Garden, J.M., Polla, L.L., and Tan, O.T. (1988) Treatment of port wine stains by pulsed dye laser — analysis of pulse duration and long term therapy. *Arch. Dermatol.* 124: 889–896.

[13] Garden, J.M. and Bakus, W. (1996) Clinical efficacy of the pulsed dye laser in the treatment of vascular lesions. *J. Dermatol. Surg. Oncol.* 19: 321–326.

[14] Gault, D., Clement, R.M., Trow, R.B., and Kiernan, M.N. (1998) Removing unwanted hairs by laser. *Face* 6: 129–130.

[15] Glassberg, E., Lask, G., Rabinowitz, L.G., and Tunnessen, W.W. (1989) Capillary haemangiomas: case study of a novel laser treatment and a review of therapeutic options. *J. Dermatol. Surg. Oncol.* 15: 1214–1223.

[16] Grossman et al. (1997) Damage to hair follicle by normal mode ruby laser pulse. *J. Amer. Acad. Dermatol.* 889–894.

[17] Kiernan, M.N. (1997) An analysis of the optimal laser parameters necessary for the treatment of vascular lesions, PhD Thesis, The University of West of England.

[18] Lanigan, S.W. (1996) Port wine stains on the lower limb: response to pulsed dye laser therapy. *Clin. Exp. Dermatol.* 21: 88–92.

[19] Motley, R.J., Katugampola, G., and Lanigan, S.W. (1996) Microvascular abnormalities in port wine stains and response to 585 nm pulsed dye laser treatment. *Br. J. Dermatol.* 135: Suppl. 47: 13–14.

[20] Ring, E.F.J. (1995) History of thermography. In Ammer, K. and Ring, E.F.J., Eds., *The Thermal Image in Medicine and Biology*. Uhlen Verlag, Vienna, pp. 13–20.

[21] Thomas, R.A. (1999) *Thermography*. Coxmoor Publishers, Oxford, pp. 79–103.

[22] Thomas, R.A., Donne, K.E., Clement, R.M., and Kiernan, M. (2002) Optimised laser application in dermatology using infrared thermography, *Thermosense XXIV*, *Proceedings of SPIE*, April 1–4, Orlando, USA.

[23] Trow, R. (2001) The design and construction of a ruby laser for laser depilation, PhD Thesis, Swansea Institute.

[24] Welsh, A.J. and van Gemert, M.V.C. (1995) *Optical–Thermal Response of Laser-Irradiated Tissue*. Plenum Press, ISBN 0306449269.

[25] Wheeland, R.G. (1995) Clinical uses of lasers in dermatology. *Lasers Surg. Med.* 16: 2–23.

[26] Wilson, B.C. and Adam, G. (1983) A Monte Carlo model for the absorption and flux distributions of light in tissue. *Med. Phys. Biol.* 1.

[27] Donne, K.E. (1999) Two dimensional computer model of laser tissue interaction. Private communication.

34

Infrared Imaging Applied to Dentistry

34.1 The Importance of Temperature 34-1
34.2 The Skin and Skin-Surface Temperature Measurement 34-2
34.3 Two Common Types of Body Temperature Measurements 34-2
34.4 Diagnostic Applications of Thermography 34-3
34.5 The Normal Infrared Facial Thermography 34-3
34.6 Abnormal Facial Conditions Demonstrated with Infrared Facial Thermography 34-4

Assessing Temporomandibular Joint (TMJ) Disorders with Infrared Thermography • Assessing Inferior Alveolar Nerve (IAN) Deficit with Infrared Thermography • Assessing Carotid Occlusal Disease with Infrared Thermography • Additional Applications of Infrared Thermography • Future Advances in Infrared Imaging

Acknowledgments 34-5
References 34-5

Barton M. Gratt
University of Washington

34.1 The Importance of Temperature

Temperature is very important in all biological systems. Temperature influences the movement of atoms and molecules and their rates of biochemical activity. Active biological life is, in general, restricted to a temperature range of 0 to 45°C [1]. Cold-blooded organisms are generally restricted to habitats in which the ambient temperature remains between 0 and 40°C. However, a variety of temperatures well outside of this occurs on earth, and by developing the ability to maintain a constant body temperature, warm-blooded animals; for example, birds, mammals, including humans have gained access to a greater variety of habitats and environments [1].

With the application of common thermometers, elevation in the core temperature of the body became the primary indicator for the diagnosis of fever. Wunderlich introduced fever measurements as a routine procedure in Germany, in 1872. In 1930, Knaus inaugurated a method of basal temperature measurement, achieving full medical acceptance in 1952. Today, it is customary in hospitals throughout the world to take body temperature measurements on all patients [2].

The scientists of the first part of the 20th century used simple thermometers to study body temperatures. Many of their findings have not been superseded, and are repeatedly confirmed by new investigators using new more advanced thermal measuring devices. In the last part of the 20th century, a new discipline termed "thermology" emerged as the study of surface body temperature in both health and in disease [2].

34.2 The Skin and Skin-Surface Temperature Measurement

The skin is the outer covering of the body and contributes 10% of the body's weight. Over 30% of the body's temperature-receptive elements are located within the skin. Most of the heat produced within the body is dissipated by way of the skin, through radiation, evaporation, and conduction. The range of ambient temperature for thermal comfort is relatively broad (20 to 25°C). Thermal comfort is dependent upon humidity, wind velocity, clothing, and radiant temperature. Under normal conditions there is a steady flow of heat from the inside of a human body to the outside environment. Skin temperature distribution within specific anatomic regions; for example, the head vs. the foot, are diverse, varying by as much as ±15°C. Heat transport by convection to the skin surface depends on the rate of blood flow through the skin, which is also variable. In the trunk region of the body, blood flow varies by a factor of 7; at the foot, blood flow varies by a factor of 30; while at the fingers, it can vary by a factor of 600 [3].

It appears that measurements of body (core) temperatures and skin (surface) temperature may well be strong physiologic markers indicating health or disease. In addition, skin (surface) temperature values appear to be unique for specific anatomic regions of the body.

34.3 Two Common Types of Body Temperature Measurements

There are two common types of body temperature measurements that are made and utilized as diagnostic indicators.

1. *The Measurement of Body Core Temperature.* The normal core temperature of the human body remains within a range of 36.0 to 37.5°C [1]. The constancy of human core temperature is maintained by a large number of complex regulatory mechanisms [3]. Body core temperatures are easily measured orally (or anally) with contacting temperature devices including: manual or digital thermometers, thermistors, thermocouples, and even layers of liquid temperature sensitive crystals, etc. [4–6].
2. *The Measurement of Body Surface Temperature.* While body core temperature is very easy to measure, the body's skin surface temperature is very difficult to measure. Any device that is required to make contact with the skin cannot measure the body's skin surface temperature reliably. Since skin has a relatively low heat capacity and poor lateral heat conductance, skin temperature is likely to change on contact with a cooler or warmer object [2]. Therefore, an indirect method of obtaining skin surface temperature is required, a common thermometer on the skin, for example, will not work.

Probably the first research efforts that pointed out the diagnostic importance of the infrared emission of human skin and thus initiated the modern era of thermometry were the studies of Hardy in 1934 [7,8]. However, it took 30 years for modern thermometry to be applied in laboratories around the world. To conduct noncontact thermography of the human skin in a clinical setting, an advanced computerized infrared imaging system is required. Consequently, clinical thermography required the advent of microcomputers developed in the late 1960s and early 1970s. These sophisticated electronic systems employed advanced microtechnology, requiring large research and development costs.

Current clinical thermography units use single detector infrared cameras. These work as follows: infrared radiation emitted by the skin surface enters the lens of the camera, passes through a number of rapidly spinning prisms (or mirrors), which reflect the infrared radiation emitted from different parts of the field of view onto the infrared sensor. The sensor converts the reflected infrared radiation into electrical signals. An amplifier receives the electric signals from the sensor and boosts them to electric potential signals of a few volts that can be converted into digital values. These values are then fed into a computer. The computer uses this input, together with the timing information from the rotating mirrors, to reconstruct a digitized thermal image from the temperature values of each small area within the field of observation. These digitized images are easily viewed and can be analyzed using computer software and stored on a computer disk for later reference.

34.4   Diagnostic Applications of Thermography

In 1987, the *International Bibliography of Medical Thermology* was published and included more than 3000 cited publications on the medical use of thermography, including applications for anesthesiology, breast disease, cancer, dermatology, gastrointestinal disorders, gynecology, urology, headache, immunology, musculoskeletal disorders, neurology, neurosurgery, ophthalmology, otolaryngology, pediatrics, pharmacology, physiology, pulmonary disorders, rheumatology, sports medicine, general surgery, plastic and reconstructive surgery, thyroid, cardiovascular and cerebrovascular, vascular problems, and veterinary medicine [9]. In addition, changes in human skin temperature has been reported in conditions involving the orofacial complex, as related to dentistry, such as the temporomandibular joint [10–25], and nerve damage and repair following common oral surgery [25–27]. Thermography has been shown not to be useful in the assessment of periapical granuloma [28]. Reports of dedicated controlled facial skin temperature studies of the orofacial complex are limited, but follow findings consistent with other areas of the body [29,30].

34.5   The Normal Infrared Facial Thermography

The pattern of heat dissipation over the skin of the human body is normally symmetrical and this includes the human face. It has been shown that in normal subjects, the difference in skin temperature from side-to-side on the human body is small, about 0.2°C [31]. Heat emission is directly related to cutaneous vascular activity, yielding enhanced heat output on vasodilatation and reduced heat output on vasoconstriction. Infrared thermography of the face has promise, therefore, as a harmless, noninvasive, diagnostic technique that may help to differentiate selected diagnostic problems. The literature reports that during clinical studies of facial skin temperature a significant difference between the absolute facial skin temperatures of men vs. women was observed [32]. Men were found to have higher temperatures over all 25 anatomic areas measured on the face (e.g., the orbit, the upper lip, the lower lip, the chin, the cheek, the TMJ, etc.) than women. The basal metabolic rate for a normal 30-year-old male, 1.7 m tall (5 ft, 7 in.), weighing 64 kg (141 lbs), who has a surface area of approximately 1.6 m^2, is approximately 80 W; therefore, he dissipates about 50 W/m^2 of heat [33]. On the other hand, the basal metabolic rate of a 30-year-old female, 1.6 m tall (5 ft, 3 in.), weighing 54 kg (119 lbs), with a surface area of 1.4 m^2, is about 63 W, so that she dissipates about 41 W/m^2 of heat [33,34]. Assuming that there are no other relevant differences between males and females, women's skin is expected to be cooler, since less heat is lost per unit (per area of body surface). Body heat dissipation through the face follows this prediction. In addition to the effect of gender on facial temperature, there are indications that age and ethnicity may also affect facial temperature [32].

When observing patients undergoing facial thermography, there seems to be a direct correlation between vasoactivity and pain, which might be expected since both are neurogenic processes. Differences in facial skin temperature, for example, asymptomatic adult subjects (low temperatures differences) and adult patients with various facial pain syndromes (high temperature differences) may prove to be a useful criterion for the diagnosis of many conditions [35]. Right- vs. left-side temperature differences (termed: delta T or ΔT) between many specific facial regions in normal subjects were shown to be low (<0.3°C) [40], while similar ΔT values were found to be high (>0.5°C) in a variety of disorders related to dentistry [35].

34.6 Abnormal Facial Conditions Demonstrated with Infrared Facial Thermography

34.6.1 Assessing Temporomandibular Joint (TMJ) Disorders with Infrared Thermography

It has been shown that normal subjects have symmetrical thermal patterns over the TMJ regions of their face. Normal subjects had ΔT values of 0.1°C (±0.1°C) [32,36]. On the other hand, TMJ pain patients were found to have asymmetrical thermal patterns, with increased temperatures over the affected TMJ region, with ΔT values of +0.4°C (±0.2°C) [37]. Specifically, painful TMJ patients with internal derangement and painful TMJ osteoarthritis were both found to have asymmetrical thermal patterns and increased temperatures over the affected TMJ, with mean area TMJ ΔT of +0.4°C (±0.2°C) [22,24]. In other words, the correlation between TMJ pain and hyper perfusion of the region seems to be independent of the etiology of the TMJ disorder (osteoarthritis vs. internal derangement). In addition, a study of mild-to-moderate TMD (temporomandibular joint dysfunction) patients indicated that area ΔT values correlated with the level of the patient's pain symptoms [38]. And a more recent double-blinded clinical study compared active orthodontic patients vs. TMD patients vs. asymptomatic TMJ controls, and showed average ΔT values of +0.2, +0.4, and +0.1°C; for these three groups respectively. This study showed that thermography could distinguish between patients undergoing active orthodontic treatment and patients with TMD [39].

34.6.2 Assessing Inferior Alveolar Nerve (IAN) Deficit with Infrared Thermography

The thermal imaging of the chin has been shown to be an effective method for assessing inferior alveolar nerve deficit [40]. Whereas normal subjects (those without inferior alveolar nerve deficit) show a symmetrical thermal pattern, (ΔT of +0.1°C [±0.1°C]); patients with inferior alveolar nerve deficit had elevated temperature in the mental region of their chin (ΔT of +0.5°C [±0.2°C]) on the affected side [41]. The observed vasodilatation seems to be due to blockage of the vascular neuronal vasoconstrictive messages, since the same effect on the thermological pattern could be invoked in normal subjects by temporary blockage of the inferior alveolar nerve, using a 2% lidocaine nerve block injection [42].

34.6.3 Assessing Carotid Occlusal Disease with Infrared Thermography

The thermal imaging of the face, especially around the orbits, has been shown to be an effective method for assessing carotid occlusal disease. Cerebrovascular accident (CVA), also called stroke, is well known as a major cause of death. The most common cause of stroke is atherosclerosotic plaques forming emboli, which travel within vascular blood channels, lodging in the brain, obstructing the brain's blood supply, resulting in a cerebral vascular accident (or stroke). The most common origin for emboli is located in the lateral region of the neck where the common carotid artery bifurcates into the internal and the external carotid arteries [43,44]. It has been well documented that intraluminal carotid plaques, which both restrict and reduce blood flow, result in decreased facial skin temperature [43–54]. Thermography has demonstrated the ability to detect a reduction of 30% (or more) of blood flow within the carotid arteries [55]. Thermography shows promise as an inexpensive painless screening test of asymptomatic elderly adults at risk for the possibility of stroke. However, more clinical studies are required before thermography may be accepted for routine application in screening toward preventing stroke [55,56].

34.6.4 Additional Applications of Infrared Thermography

Recent clinical studies assessed the application of thermography on patients with chronic facial pain (orofacial pain of greater than 4 month's duration). Thermography classified patients as being "normal" when selected anatomic ΔT values ranged from 0.0 to ±0.25°C, and "hot" when ΔT values were >+0.35°C, and "cold" when area ΔT values were $< -0.35°C$. The study population consisted of 164 dental pain patients and 164 matched (control) subjects. This prospective, matched study determined that subjects classified with "hot" thermographs had the clinical diagnosis of (1) sympathetically maintained pain, (2) peripheral nerve-mediated pain, (3) TMJ arthropathy, or (4) acute maxillary sinusitis. Subjects classified with "cold" areas on their thermographs were found to have the clinical diagnosis of (1) peripheral nerve-mediated pain, or (2) sympathetically independent pain. Subjects classified with "normal" thermographs included patients with the clinical diagnosis of (1) cracked tooth syndrome, (2) trigeminal neuralgia, (3) pretrigeminal neuralgia, or (4) psychogenic facial pain. This new system of thermal classification resulted in 92% (301 or 328) agreement in classifying pain patients vs. their matched controls. In brief, ΔT has been shown to be within $\pm 0.4°C$ in normal subjects, while showing values greater than $+0.7°C$ and less than $-0.6°$ C in abnormal facial pain patients [10], making "ΔT" an important diagnostic parameter in the assessment of orofacial pain [35].

34.6.5 Future Advances in Infrared Imaging

Over the last 20 years there have been additional reports in the dental literature giving promise to new and varied applications of infrared thermography [57–63]. While, infrared thermography is promising, the future holds even greater potential for temperature measurement as a diagnostic tool, the most promising being termed dynamic area telethermometry (DAT) [64,65]. Newly developed DAT promises to become a new more advanced tool providing quantitative information on the thermoregulatory frequencies (TRFs) manifested in the modulation of skin temperature [66]. Whereas the static thermographic studies discussed above demonstrate local vasodilatation or vasoconstriction, DAT can identify the mechanism of thermoregulatory frequencies and thus it is expected, in the future, to significantly improve differential diagnosis [66].

In summary, the science of thermology, including static thermography, and soon to be followed by DAT, appears to have great promise as an important diagnostic tool in the assessment of orofacial health and disease.

Acknowledgments

This chapter is dedicated to Professor Michael Anbar, of Buffalo, New York: A brilliant scientist, my thermal science mentor, and "The Father of Dynamic Area Telethermography."

References

[1] Grobklaus, R. and Bergmann, K.E. Physiology and regulation of body temperature. In *Applied Thermology: Thermologic Methods*. J.-M. Engel, U. Fleresch, and G. Stuttgen, Eds., Federal Republic of Germany: VCH (1985), pp. 11–20.

[2] *Applied Thermology: Thermologic Methods*. J.-M. Engel, U. Fleresch, and G. Stuttgen, Eds., Federal Republic of Germany: VCH (1985), pp. 11–20.

[3] Kirsch, K.A. Physiology of skin-surface temperature. In *Applied Thermology: Thermologic Methods*. J.-M. Engel, U. Fleresch, and G. Stuttgen, Eds., Federal Republic of Germany: VCH (1985), pp. 1–9.

[4] Anbar, M., Gratt, B.M., and Hong, D. Thermology and facial telethermography: part I. History and technical review. *Dentomaxillofac. Radiol.* (1998) 27: 61–67.

[5] Anbar, M. and Gratt, B.M. Role of nitric oxide in the physiopathology of pain. *J. Musc. Skeletal Joint Pain* (1997) 14: 225–254.

[6] Rost, A. Comparative measurements with an infrared and contact thermometer for thermal stress reaction. In *Thermological Methods*. J.-M. Engel, U. Flesch, and G. Stuttgen, Eds., Weinheim: VCH Verlag (1985), pp. 169–170.

[7] Hardy, J.D. The radiation of heat from the human body: I–IV. *J. Clin. Invest.* (1934) 13: 593–620.

[8] Hardy, J.D. The radiation of heat from the human body: I–IV. *J. Clin. Invest.* (1934) 13: 817–883.

[9] Abernathy, M. and Abernathy, T.B. International bibliography of thermology. *Thermology.* (1987) 2: 1–533.

[10] Berry, D.C. and Yemm, R. Variations in skin temperature of the face in normal subjects and in patients with mandibular dysfunction. *Br. J. Oral Maxillofac. Surg.* (1971) 8: 242–247.

[11] Berry, D.C. and Yemm, R. A further study of facial skin temperature in patients with mandibular dysfunction. *J. Oral Rehabil.* (1974) 1: 255–264.

[12] Kopp, S. and Haraldson, T. Normal variations in skin temperature of the face in normal subjects and in patients with mandibular dysfunction. *Br. J. Oral Maxillofac. Surg.* (1983) 8: 242–247.

[13] Johansson, A., Kopp, S., and Haraldson, T. Reproducibility and variation of skin surface temperature over the temporomandibular joint and masseter muscle in normal individuals. *Acta Odontol. Scand.* (1985) 43: 309–313.

[14] Tegelberg, A. and Kopp, S. Skin surface temperature over the temporo-mandibular and metacarpophalangeal joints in individuals with rheumatoid arthritis. *Odontol. Klin.*, Box 33070, 400 33 Goteborg, Sweden (1986) Report No. 31, pp. 1–31.

[15] Akerman, S. et al. Relationship between clinical, radiologic and thermometric findings of the temporomandibular joint in rheumatoid arthritis. *Odontol. Klin.*, Box 33070, 400 33 Goteborg, Sweden (1987) Report No. 41, pp. 1–30.

[16] Finney, J.W., Holt, C.R., and Pearce, K.B. Thermographic diagnosis of TMJ disease and associated neuromuscular disorders. *Special Report: Postgraduate Medicine* (March 1986), pp. 93–95.

[17] Weinstein, S.A. Temporomandibular joint pain syndrome — the whiplash of the 1980s, *Thermography and Personal Injury Litigation, Ch. 7.* S.D. Hodge, Jr., Ed., New York, USA: John Wiley & Sons (1987), pp. 157–164.

[18] Weinstein, S.A., Gelb, M., and Weinstein, E.L. Thermophysiologic anthropometry of the face in home sapiens. *J. Craniomand. Pract.* (1990) 8: 252–257.

[19] Pogrel, M.A., McNeill, C., and Kim, J.M. The assessment of trapezius muscle symptoms of patients with temporomandibular disorders by the use of liquid crystal thermography. *Oral Surg. Oral Med. Oral. Pathol. Oral Radiol. Endod.* (1996) 82: 145–151.

[20] Steed, P.A. The utilization of liquid crystal thermography in the evaluation of temporomandibular dysfunction. *J. Craniomand. Pract.* (1991) 9: 120–128.

[21] Gratt, B.M., Sickles, E.A., Graff-Radford, S.B., and Solberg, W.K. Electronic thermography in the diagnosis of atypical odontalgia: a pilot study. *Oral Surg. Oral Med. Oral Pathol. Oral Radiol. Endod.* (1989) 68: 472–481.

[22] Gratt, B.M. et al. Electronic thermography in the assessment of internal derangement of the TMJ. *J. Orofacial Pain* (1994) 8: 197–206.

[23] Gratt, B.M., Sickles, E.A., Ross, J.B., Wexler, C.E., and Gornbein, J.A. Thermographic assessment of craniomandibular disorders: diagnostic interpretation versus temperature measurement analysis. *J. Orofacial Pain* (1994) 8: 278–288.

[24] Gratt, B.M., Sickles, E.A., and Wexler, C.E. Thermographic characterization of osteoarthrosis of the temporomandibular joint. *J. Orofacial Pain* (1994) 7: 345–353.

[25] Progrell, M. A., Erbez, G., Taylor, R.C., and Dodson, T.B. Liquid crystal thermography as a diagnostic aid and objective monitor for TMJ dysfunction and myogenic facial pain. *J. Craniomand. Disord. Facial Oral Pain* (1989) 3: 65–70.

[26] Dmutpueva, B.C., and Alekceeva, A.H. Applications of thermography in the evaluation of the postoperative patient. *Stomatologiia* (1986) 12: 29–30 (Russian).

[27] Cambell, R.L., Shamaskin, R.G., and Harkins, S.W. Assessment of recovery from injury to inferior alveolar and mental nerves. *Oral Surg. Oral Med. Oral Pathol. Oral Radiol. Endod.* (1987) 64: 519–526.

[28] Crandall, C.E. and Hill, R.P. Thermography in dentistry: a pilot study. *Oral Surg. Oral Med. Oral Pathol. Oral Radiol. Endod.* (1966) 21: 316–320.

[29] Gratt, B.M., Pullinger, A., and Sickles, E.A. Electronic thermography of normal facial structures: A pilot study. *Oral Surg. Oral Med. Oral Pathol. Oral Radiol. Endod.* (1989) 68: 346–351.

[30] Weinstein, S.A., Gelb, M., and Weinstein, E.L. Thermophysiologic anthropometry of the face in homo sapiens. *J. Craniomand. Pract.* (1990) 8: 252–257.

[31] Uematsu, S. Symmetry of skin temperature comparing one side of the body to the other. *Thermology* (1985) 1: 4–7.

[32] Gratt, B.M. and Sickles, E.A. Electronic facial thermography: an analysis of asymptomatic adult subjects. *J. Orofacial Pain* (1995) 9: 222–265.

[33] Blaxter, K. Energy exchange by radiation, convection, conduction and evaporation. In *Energy Metabolism in Animals and Man.* New York: Cambridge University Press (1989), pp. 86–99.

[34] Blaxter, K. The minimal metabolism. In *Energy Metabolism in Animals and Man.* New York: Cambridge University Press (1989) 120–146.

[35] Gratt, B.M, Graff-Radford, S.B., Shetty, V., Solberg, W.K., and Sickles, E.A. A six-year clinical assessment of electronic facial thermography. *Dentomaxillofac. Radiol.* (1996) 25: 247–255.

[36] Gratt, B.M., and Sickles, E.A. Thermographic characterization of the asymptomatic TMJ. *J. Orofacial Pain* (1993) 7: 7–14.

[37] Gratt, B.M., Sickles, E.M., and Ross, J.B. Thermographic assessment of craniomandibular disorders: diagnostic interpretation versus temperature measurement analysis. *J. Orofacial Pain* (1994) 8: 278–288.

[38] Canavan, D. and Gratt, B.M. Electronic thermography for the assessment of mild and moderate TMJ dysfunction. *Oral Surg. Oral Med. Oral Pathol. Oral Radiol. Endod.* (1995) 79: 778–786.

[39] McBeth, S.A., and Gratt, B.M. A cross-sectional thermographic assessment of TMJ problems in orthodontic patients. *Am. J. Orthod. Dentofac. Orthop.* (1996) 109: 481–488.

[40] Gratt, B.M., Shetty, V., Saiar, M., and Sickles, E.A. Electronic thermography for the assessment of inferior alveolar nerve deficit. *Oral Surg. Oral Med. Oral Pathol. Oral Radiol. Endod.* (1995) 80: 153–160.

[41] Gratt, B.M., Sickles, E.A., and Shetty, V. Thermography for the clinical assessment of inferior alveolar nerve deficit: a pilot study. *J. Orofacial Pain* (1994) 80: 153–160.

[42] Shetty, V., Gratt, B.M., and Flack, V. Thermographic assessment of reversible inferior alveolar nerve deficit. *J. Orofacial Pain* (1994) 8: 375–383.

[43] Wood, E.H. Thermography in the diagnosis of cerebrovascular disease: preliminary report. *Radiology* (1964) 83: 540–546.

[44] Wood, E.H. Thermography in the diagnosis of cerebrovascular disease. *Radiology* (1965) 85: 207–215.

[45] Steinke, W., Kloetzsch, C., and Hennerici, M. Carotid artery disease assessed by color Doppler sonography and angiography. *AJR* (1990) 154: 1061–1067.

[46] Hu, H.-H. et al. Color Doppler imaging of orbital arteries for detection of carotid occlusive disease. *Stroke* (1993) 24: 1196–1202.

[47] Carroll, B.A., Graif, M., and Orron, D.E. Vascular ultrasound. In *Peripheral Vascular Imaging and Intervention.* D. Kim and D.E. Orron, Eds., St. Louis, MO, Mosby/Year Book (1992), pp. 211–225.

[48] Mawdsley, C., Samuel, E., Sumerling, M.D., and Young, G.B. Thermography in occlusive cerebrovascular diseases. *Br. Med. J.* (1968) 3: 521–524.

[49] Capistrant, T.D. and Gumnit, R.J. Thermography and extracranial cerebrovascular disease: a new method to predict the stroke-prone individual. *Minn. Med.* (1971) 54: 689–692.

[50] Karpman, H.L., Kalb, I.M., and Sheppard, J.J. The use of thermography in a health care system for stroke. *Geriatrics* (1972) 27: 96–105.

[51] Soria, E. and Paroski, M.W. Thermography as a predictor of the more involved side in bilateral carotid disease: case history. *Angiology* (1987) 38: 151–158.

[52] Capistrat, T.D. and Gumnit, R.J. Detecting carotid occlusive disease by thermography. *Stroke* (1973) 4: 57–65.

[53] Abernathy, M., Brandt, M.M., and Robinson, C. Noninvasive testing of the carotid system. *Am. Fam. Physic.* (1984) 29: 157–164.

[54] Dereymaeker, A., Kams-Cauwe, V., and Fobelets, P. Frontal dynamic thermography: improvement in diagnosis of carotid stenosis. *Eur. Neurol.* (1978) 17: 226–234.

[55] Gratt, B.M., Halse, A., and Hollender, L. A pilot study of facial infrared thermal imaging used as a screening test for detecting elderly individuals at risk for stroke. *Thermol. Int.* (2002) 12: 7–15.

[56] Friedlander A.H. and Gratt B.M. Panoramic dental radiography and thermography as an aid in detecting patients at risk for stroke. *J. Oral Maxillofac. Surg.* (1994) 52: 1257–1262.

[57] Graff-Radford, S.B., Ketalaer, M.-C., Gratt, B.M., and Solberg, W.K. Thermographic assessment of neuropathic facial pain: a pilot study. *J. Orofacial Pain* (1995) 9: 138–146.

[58] Pogrel, M.A., Erbez, G., Taylor, R.C., and Dodson, T.B. Liquid crystal thermography as a diagnostic aid and objective monitor for TMJ dysfunction and myogenic facial pain. *J. Craniobandib. Disord. Facial Oral Pain* (1989) 3: 65–70.

[59] Pogrel, M.A., Yen, C.K., and Taylor, R.C. Infrared thermography in oral and maxillo-facial surgery. *Oral Surg. Oral Med. Oral Pathol. Oral Radiol. Endod.* (1989) 67: 126–131.

[60] Graff-Radford, S.B., Ketlaer, M.C., Gratt, B.M., and Solberg, W.K. Thermographic assessment of neuropathic facial pain. *J. Orofacial Pain* (1995) 9: 138–146.

[61] Biagioni, P.A., Longmore, R.B., McGimpsey, J.G., and Lamey, P.J. Infrared thermography: its role in dental research with particular reference to craniomandibular disorders. *Dentomaxillofac. Radiol.* (1996) 25: 119–124.

[62] Biagioni, P.A., McGimpsey, J.G., and Lamey, P.J. Electronic infrared thermography as a dental research technique. *Br. Dent. J.* (1996) 180: 226–230.

[63] Benington, I.C., Biagioni, P.A., Crossey, P.J., Hussey, D.L., Sheridan, S., and Lamel, P.J. Temperature changes in bovine mandibular bone during implant site preparation: an assessment using infra-red thermography. *J. Dent.* (1996) 24: 263–267.

[64] Anbar, M. Clinical applications of dynamic area telethermography. In *Quantitative Dynamic Telthermography in Medical Diagnosis*. CRC Press: Boca Raton, FL (1994), pp. 147–180.

[65] Anbar, M. Dynamic area telethermography and its clinical applications. *SPIE Proc.* (1995) 2473: 3121–3323.

[66] Anbar M., Grenn, M.W., Marino, M.T., Milescu, L., and Zamani, K. Fast dynamic area telethermography (DAT) of the human forearm with a Ga/As quantum well infrared focal plane array camera. *Eur. J. Therol.* (1997) 7: 105–118.

35

Use of Infrared Imaging in Veterinary Medicine

Ram C. Purohit
Auburn University

Tracy A. Turner
Private Practice

David D. Pascoe
Auburn University

35.1 Historical Perspective 35-1
35.2 Standards for Reliable Thermograms 35-2
35.3 Dermatome Patterns of Horses and Other Animal
Species 35-3
35.4 Peripheral Neurovascular Thermography 35-4
Horner's Syndrome • Neurectomies • Vascular Injuries
35.5 Musculoskeletal Injuries 35-5
35.6 Thermography of the Testes and Scrotum in
Mammalian Species 35-6
35.7 Conclusions 35-6
References 35-7

35.1 Historical Perspective

In the mid-1960s and early 1970s, several studies were published indicating the value of IR (infrared) thermography in veterinary medicine [1–3]. In the 1965 research of Delahanty and George [2], the thermographic images required at least 6 min to produce a thermogram, a lengthy period of time during which the veterinarian had to keep the horse still while the scan was completed. This disadvantage was overcome by the development of high speed scanners using rotating IR prisms which then could produce instantaneous thermograms.

Stromberg [4–6] and Stromberg and Norberg [7] used thermography to diagnose inflammatory changes of the superficial digital flexor tendons in race horses. With thermography, they were able to document and detect early inflammation of the tendon, 1 to 2 weeks prior to the detection of lameness using clinical examination. They suggested that thermography could be used for early signs of pending lameness and it could be used for preventive measures to rest and treat race horses before severe lameness became obvious on physical examination.

In 1970, the Horse Protection Act was passed by the United States Congress to ban the use of chemical or mechanical means of "soring" horses. It was difficult to enforce this act because of the difficulty in obtaining measurable and recordable proof of violations. In 1975, Nelson and Osheim [8] documented that soring caused by chemical or mechanical means on the horse's digit could be diagnosed as having a definite abnormal characteristic IR emission pattern in the affected areas of the limb. Even though thermography at that time became the technique of choice for the detection of soring, normal thermography patterns in horses were not known. This prompted the USDA to fund research for the uses of thermography in veterinary medicine.

Purohit et al. [9] established a protocol for obtaining normal thermographic patterns of the horses' limbs and other parts of the body. This protocol was regularly used for early detection of acute and chronic inflammatory conditions in horses and other animal species. Studies at Auburn University vet school used an AGA 680 liquid cooled thermography system that had a black and white and an accessory color display units that allows the operator to assign the array of ten isotherms to temperature increments from 0.2 to 10.0°C. Images were captured within seconds rather than the 6 min required for earlier machines. In veterinary studies at Auburn University, the thermographic isotherms were imaged with nine colors and white assigned to each isotherm that varied in temperature between either 0.5 or 1.0°C.

In a subsequent study, Purohit and McCoy [10] established normal thermal patterns (temperature and gradients) of the horse, with special attention directed towards thoracic and pelvic limbs. Thermograms of various parts of the body were obtained 30 min before and after the exercise for each horse. Thermographic examination was also repeated for each horse on six different days. Thermal patterns and gradients were similar in all horses studied with a high degree of right to left symmetry in IR emission.

At the same time, Turner et al. [11] investigated the influence of the hair coat and hair clipping. This study demonstrated that the clipped leg was always warmer. After exercise, both clipped and unclipped legs had similar increases in temperature. The thermal patterns and gradients were not altered by clipping and/or exercise [10,11]. This indicated that clipping hair in horses with even hair coats was not necessary for thermographic evaluation. However, in some areas where the hair is long hair and not uniform, clipping may be required. Recently, concerns related to hair coat, thermographic imaging, and temperature regulation were investigated in llamas exposed to the hot humid conditions of the southeast [12]. While much of the veterinary research has focused on the thermographic imaging as a diagnostic tool, this study expanded its use into the problems of thermoregulation in various non endemic species.

Current camera technology has improved scanning capabilities that are combined with computer-assisted software programs. This new technology provides the practitioner with numerous options for image analysis, several hundred isotherms capable of capturing temperature differences in the hundredths of a degree Celsius, and better image quality. Miniaturized electronics have reduced the size of the units, allowing some systems to be housed in portable hand-held units. With lower cost of equipment, more thermographic equipment are being utilized in human and animal veterinary medicine and basic physiology studies.

It was obvious from initial studies by several authors that standards needed to be established for obtaining reliable thermograms in different animal species. The variations in core temperature and differences in the thermoregulatory mechanism responses between species emphasizes the importance of individually established norms for thermographic imagery.

A further challenge in veterinary medicine may occur when animal patient care may necessitate outdoor imaging.

35.2   Standards for Reliable Thermograms

Thermography provides an accurate, quantifiable, noncontact, noninvasive measure and map of skin surface temperatures. Skin surface temperatures are variable and change according to blood flow regulation to the skin surface. As such, IR thermography practitioner must be aware of the internal and external influences that alter this dynamic process of skin blood flow and temperature regulation. While imaging equipment can vary widely in price, these differences are often reflective of the wave-length capturing capability of the detectors and adjunct software that can aid in image analysis. The thermographer needs to understand the limitations of their IR system in order to make appropriate interpretations of their data. There have been some published studies that have not adhered to reliable standards and equipment prerequisites, thereby detracting from the acceptance of thermography as a valuable research and clinical technique. In some cases a simple cause–effect relationship was assumed to demonstrate the diagnosis of a disease or syndrome based on thermal responses as captured by thermographic images.

Internal and external factors have a significant effect on the skin surface temperature. Therefore, the use of thermography to evaluate skin surface thermal patterns and gradient requires an understanding of the dynamic changes which occur in blood flow at systemic, peripheral, regional, and local levels [9,10]. Thus, to enhance the diagnostic value of thermography, we recommend the following standards for veterinary medical imaging:

1. The environmental factors which interfere with the quality of thermography should be minimized. The room temperature should be maintained between 21 and 26°C. Slight variations in some cases may be acceptable, but room temperature should always be cooler than the animal's body temperature and free from air drafts.
2. Thermograms obtained outdoors under conditions of direct air drafts, sunlight, and extreme variations in temperature may provide unreliable thermograms in which thermal patterns are altered. Such observations are meaningless as a diagnostic tool.
3. When an animal is brought into a temperature controlled room, it should be equilibrated at least 20 min or more, depending on the external temperature from which the animal was transported. Animals transported from extreme hot or cold environments may require up to 60 min of equilibration time. Equilibration time is adequate when the thermal temperatures and patterns are consistently maintained over several minutes.
4. Other factors affecting the quality of thermograms are exercise, sweating, body position and angle, body covering, systemic and topical medications, regional and local blocks, sedatives, tranquilizers, anesthetics, vasoactive drugs, skin lesions such as scars, surgically altered areas, etc. As stated prior, the hair coat may be an issue with uneven hair length or a thick coat.
5. It is recommended that the infrared imaging should be performed using an electronic non contact cooled system. The use of long wave detectors is preferable.

The value of thermography is demonstrated by the sensitivity to changes in heat on the skin surface and its ability to detect temporal and spatial changes in thermal skin responses that corresponds to temporal and spatial changes in blood flow. Therefore, it is important to have well documented normal thermal patterns and gradients in all species under controlled environments prior to making any claims or detecting pathological conditions.

35.3 Dermatome Patterns of Horses and Other Animal Species

Certain chronic and acute painful conditions associated with peripheral neurovascular and neuromuscular injuries are easy to confuse with spinal injuries associated with cervical, thoracic, and lumbar-sacral areas [13,14]. Similarly, inflammatory conditions such as osteoarthritis, tendonitis, and other associated conditions may also be confused with other neurovascular conditions. Thus, studies have been done over the last 25 years at Auburn University to map cutaneous and differentiate the sensory-sympathetic dermatome patterns of cervical, thoracic, and lumbosacral regions in horses [13,14]. Infrared thermography was used to map the sensory-sympathetic dermatome in horses. The dorsal or ventral spinal nerve(s) were blocked with 0.5% of mepevacine as a local anesthetic. The sensory sympathetic spinal nerve block produced two effects. First, blocking the sympathetic portion of the spinal nerve caused increased thermal patterns and produced sweating of the affected areas. Second, the areas of insensitivity produced by the sensory portion of the block were mapped and compared with the thermal patterns. The areas of insensitivity were found to correlate with the sympathetic innervations.

Thermography was used to provide thermal patterns of various dermatome areas from cervical areas to epidural areas in horses. Clinical cases of cervical area nerve compression provided cooler thermal patterns, away from the site of injuries. In cases of acute injuries, associated thermal patterns were warmer than normal cases at the site of the injury. Elucidation of dermatomal (thermatom) patterns provided location for spinal injuries for the diagnosis of back injuries in horses. Similarly, in a case of a dog where the neck injury (subluxation of atlanto-axis) the diagnosis was determined by abnormal thermal patterns and gradients.

35.4   Peripheral Neurovascular Thermography

When there are alterations in skin surface temperature, it may be difficult to distinguish and diagnose between nerve and vascular injuries. The cutaneous circulation is under sympathetic vasomotor control. Peripheral nerve injuries and nerve compression can result in skin surface vascular changes that can be detected thermographically. It is well known that inflammation and nerve irritation may result in vasoconstriction causing cooler thermograms in the afflicted areas. Transection of a nerve and/or nerve damage to the extent that there is a loss of nerve conduction results in a loss in sympathetic tone which causes vasodilation indicated by an increase in the thermogram temperature. Of course, this simple rationale is more complicated with different types of nerve injuries (neuropraxia, axonotomesis, and neurotmesis). Furthermore, lack of characterization of the extent and duration of injuries may make thermographic interpretation difficult.

Studies were done on horses and other animal species to show that if thermographic examination is performed properly under controlled conditions, it can provide an accurate diagnosis of neurovascular injuries. The rationale for a neurovascular clinical diagnosis is provided in the following Horner's Syndrome case.

35.4.1   Horner's Syndrome

In four horses, Horner's Syndrome was also induced by transaction of vagosympathetic trunk on either left or right side of the neck [15]. Facial thermograms of a case of Horner's Syndrome were done 15 min before and after the exercise. Sympathetic may cause the affected side to be warm by 2–3°C more than the non-transected side. This increased temperature after denervation is reflective of an increase in blood flow due to vasodilation in the denervated areas [15, 16]. The increased thermal patterns on the affected side were present up to 6–12 weeks. In about 2–4 months, neurotraumatized side blood flow readjusted to the local demand of circulation. Thermography of both non-neuroectomized and neuroectomized sides looked similar and normal [16]. In some cases, this readjustment took place as early as five days and it was difficult to distinguish the affected side. The intravenous injection of 1 mg of epinephrine in a 1000 lb horse caused an increase in thermal patterns on the denervated side, the same as indicating the presence of Horner's Syndrome. Administration of I V acetyl promazine (30 mg/1000 lb horse) showed increased heat (thermal pattern) on the normal non-neuroectomized side, whereas acetylpromazine had no effect on the neurectomized side. Alpha-blocking drug acetylpromazine caused vasodilation and increased blood flow to normal non-neuroectomized side, whereas no effect was seen in the affected neurectomized side due to the lack of sympathetic innervation [16–18].

35.4.2   Neurectomies

Thermographic evaluation of the thoracic (front) and pelvic (back) limbs were done before and after performing digital neurectomies in several horses. After posterior digital neurectomy there were significant increases in heat in the areas supplied by the nerves [17]. Within 3–6 weeks, readjustment of local blood flow occurred in the neurectomized areas, and it was difficult to differentiate between the non-neurectomized and the neurectomized areas. Ten minutes after administration of 0.06 mg/kg I V injection of acetylpromazine, a 2–3°C increase in heat was noted in normal non-neurectomized areas, whereas the neurectomized areas of the opposite limb were not affected.

35.4.3 Vascular Injuries

Thermography has been efficacious in the diagnosis of vascular diseases. It has been shown that the localized reduction of blood flow occurs in the horse with navicular disease [11]. This effect was more obvious on thermograms obtained after exercise than before exercise. Normally, 15–20 min of exercise will increase skin surface temperature by 2–2.5°C in horses [10,11]. In cases of arterial occlusion, the area distal to the occlusion in the horses' limb shows cooler thermograms. The effects of exercise or administration of alpha-blocking drugs like acetylpromazine causes increased blood flow to peripheral circulation in normal areas with intact vascular and sympathetic responses [17,18]. Thus, obtaining thermograms either after exercise or after administration of alpha-blocking drugs like acetylpromazine provides prognostic value for diagnosis of adequate collateral circulation. Therefore, the use of skin temperature as a measure of skin perfusion merits consideration for peripheral vascular flow, perfusion, despite some physical and physiological limitations, which are inherent in methodology [19].

Furthermore, interference with the peripheral vascular blood flow can result from neurogenic inhibition, vascular occlusion, and occlusion as a result of inflammatory vascular compression. Neurogenic inhibition can be diagnosed through the administration of alpha-blocking drugs which provide an increase in blood flow. Vascular impairment may also be associated with local injuries (inflammation, edema, swelling, etc.) which may provide localized cooler or hotter thermograms. Thus, evaluation using thermography should note the physical state and site of the injury.

35.5 Musculoskeletal Injuries

Thermography has been used in the clinical and subclinical cases of osteoarthritis, tendonitis, navicular disease, and other injuries such as sprains, stress fractures, and shin splints [10,11,20,21]. In some cases thermal abnormalities may be detected two weeks prior to the onset of clinical signs of lameness in horses, especially in the case of joint disease [21], tendonitis [10], and navicular problems [11,20].

Osteoarthritis is a severe joint disease in horses. Normally, diagnosis is made by clinical examination and radiographic evaluation. Radiography detects the problem after deterioration of the joint surface has taken place. Clinical evaluation is only done when horses show physical abnormalities in their gait due to pain. An early sign of osteoarthritis is inflammation, which can be detected by thermography prior to it becoming obvious on radiograms [21].

In studies of standard bred race horses, the effected tarsus joint can demonstrate abnormal thermal patterns indicating inflammation in the joint two to three weeks prior to radiographic diagnosis [21]. The abnormal thermograms obtained in this study were more distinct after exercise than before exercise. Thus, thermography provided a subclinical diagnosis of osteoarthritis in this study.

Thermography was used to evaluate the efficacy of corticosteroid therapy in amphotericine-B induced arthritis in ponies [22]. The intra-articular injection of 100 mg of methylprednisolone acetate was effective in alleviating the clinical signs of lameness and pain. It is important to note that when compared with clinical signs of non-treated arthritis, it was difficult to differentiate increased thermal patterns between corticosteroid treated vs. non-treated, arthritis-induced joints. However, corticosteroid therapy did not decrease the healing time of intercarpal arthritis, whereas corticosteroid therapy did decrease the time for return to normal thermographic patterns for tibiotarsal joints. In this study, thermography was useful in detecting inflammation in the absence of clinical signs of pain in corticosteroid treated joints and aiding the evaluation of the healing processes in amphotericin B-induced arthritis [22].

The chronic and acute pain associated with neuromuscular conditions can also be diagnosed by this technique. In cases where no definitive diagnosis can be made using physical examination and x-rays, thermography has been efficacious for early diagnosis of soft tissue injuries [10,23]. The conditions such as subsolar abscesses, laminitis, and other leg lameness can be easily differentiated using thermography [10,11]. We have used thermography for quantitative and qualitative evaluation of anti-inflammatory drugs such as phenylbutazone in the treatment of physical or chemically induced inflammation. The most useful application of thermography in veterinary medicine and surgery has been to aid early detection of an acute and chronic inflammatory process.

35.6 Thermography of the Testes and Scrotum in Mammalian Species

The testicular temperature of most mammalian species must be below body temperature for normal spermatogenesis. The testes of most domestic mammalian species migrates out of the abdomen and are retained in the scrotum, which provides the appropriate thermal environment for normal spermatogenesis [24,25]. The testicular arterial and venous structure is such that arterial coils are enmeshed in the pampiniform plexus of the testicular veins, which provides a counter current heating regulating mechanism by which arterial blood entering the testes is cooled by the venous blood leaving the testes [24,25]. In the ram, the temperature of the blood in the testicular artery decreases by 4°C from the external inguinal ring to the surface of the testes. Thus, to function effectively, the mammalian testes are maintained at a lower temperature.

Purohit [26,27] used thermography to establish normal thermal patterns and gradients of the scrotum in bulls, stallions, bucks, dogs, and llamas. The normal thermal patterns of the scrotum in all species studied is characterized by right to left symmetrical patterns, with a constant decrease in the thermal gradients from the base to the apex. In bulls, bucks, and stallions, a thermal gradient of 4–6°C from the base to apex with concentric hands signifies normal patterns. Inflammation of one testicle increased ipsilateral scrotal temperatures of 2.5–3°C [26,28] If both testes were inflamed, there was an overall increase of 2.5–3°C temperature and a reduction in temperature gradient was noted.

Testicular degeneration could be acute or chronic. In chronic testicular degeneration with fibrosis, there was a loss of temperature gradient, loss of concentric thermal patterns, and some areas were cooler than others with no consistent patterns [26]. Reversibility of degenerative changes depends upon the severity and duration of the trauma. The infrared thermal gradients and patterns in dogs [27] and llamas [27,29] are unique to their own species and the patterns are different from that of the bull and buck.

Thermography has also been used in humans, indicating a normal thermal pattern which is characterized by symmetric and constant temperatures between 32.5 and 34.5°C [30–33]. Increased scrotal infrared emissions were associated with intrascrotal tumor, acute and chronic inflammation, and varicoceles [34,35]. Thermography has been efficacious for early diagnosis of acute and/or chronic testicular degeneration in humans and many animal species. The disruption of the normal thermal patterns of the scrotum is directly related to testicular degeneration. The testicular degeneration may cause transient or permanent infertility in the male. It is well established that increases in scrotal temperature above normal causes disruption of spermatogenesis, affects sperm maturation, and contributes toward subfertile or infertile semen quality. Early diagnosis of pending infertility has a significant impact on economy and reproduction in animals.

35.7 Conclusions

The value of thermography can only be realized if it is used properly. All species studied thus far have provided remarkable bilateral symmetrical patterns of infrared emission. The high degree of right-to-left symmetry provides a valuable asset in diagnosis of unilateral problems associated with various inflammatory disorders. On the other hand, bilateral problems can be diagnosed due to changes in thermal gradient and/or overall increase or decrease of temperature, away from the normal established thermal patterns in a given area of the body. Various areas of the body on the same side have normal patterns and gradients. This can be used to diagnose a change in gradient patterns. Alteration in normal thermal patterns and gradients indicates a thermal pathology. If thermal abnormalities are evaluated carefully, early diagnosis can be made, even prior to the appearance of clinical signs of joint disease, tendonitis, and various musculoskeletal problems in various animal species. Thermography can be used as a screening device for early detection of an impending problem, allowing veterinarian institute treatment before the problem becomes more serious. During the healing process post surgery, animals may appear physically sound. Thermography can be used as a diagnostic aid in assessing the healing processes. In equine sports medicine, thermography can be used on a regular basis for screening to prevent severe injuries to the horse. Early detection and treatment can prevent financial losses associated with delayed diagnosis and treatment.

The efficacy of non contact electronic infrared thermography has been demonstrated in numerous clinical settings and research studies as a diagnostic tool for veterinary medicine. It has had a strong impact on veterinary medical practice and thermal physiology where accurate skin temperatures need to be assessed under normal conditions, disease pathologies, injuries, and thermal stress. The importance of infrared thermography as a research tool cannot be understated for improving the medical care of animals and for the contributions made through animal research models that improve our understanding of human structures and functions.

References

[1] Smith W.M. Application of thermography in veterinary medicine. *Ann. NY Acad. Sci.*, 121, 248, 1964.

[2] Delahanty D.D. and George J.R. Thermography in equine medicine. *J. Am. Vet. Med. Assoc.*, 147, 235, 1965.

[3] Clark J.A. and Cena K. The potential of infrared thermography in veterinary diagnosis. *Vet. Rec.*, 100, 404, 1977.

[4] Stromberg B. The normal and diseased flexor tendon in racehorses. *Acta Radiol.* [Suppl.] 305, 1, 1971.

[5] Stromberg B. Thermography of the superficial flexor tendon in race horses. *Acta Radiol.* [Suppl.] 319, 295, 1972.

[6] Stromberg B. The use of thermograph in equine orthopedics. *J. Am. Vet. Radiol. Soc.*, 15, 94, 1974.

[7] Stromberg B. and Norbert I. Infrared emission and Xe-disappearance rate studies in the horse. *Equine Vet. J.*, 1, 1–94, 1971.

[8] Nelson H.A. and Osheim D.L. Soring in Tennessee walking horses: detection by thermography. *USDA-APHIS, Veterinary Services Laboratories*, Ames, Iowa, pp. 1–14, 1975.

[9] Purohit R.C., Bergfeld II W.A. McCaoy M.D., Thompson W.M., and Sharman R.S. Value of clinical thermography in veterinary medicine. *Auburn Vet.*, 33, 140, 1977.

[10] Purohit R.C. and McCoy M.D. Thermography in the diagnosis of inflammatory processes in the horse. *Am. J. Vet. Res.*, 41, 1167, 1980.

[11] Turner T.A. et al. Thermographic evaluation of podotrochlosis in horses. *Am. J. Vet. Res.*, 44, 535, 1983.

[12] Heath A.M., Navarre C.B., Simpkins A.S., Purohit R.C., and Pugh D.G. A comparison of heat tolerance between sheared and non sheared alpacas (llama pacos). *Small Ruminant Res.*, 39, 19, 2001.

[13] Purohit R.C. and Franco B.D. Infrared thermography for the determination of cervical dermatome patterns in the horse. *Biomed. Thermol.*, 15, 213, 1995.

[14] Purohit R.C., Schumacher J, Molloy J.M., Smith, and Pascoe D.D. Elucidation of thoracic and lumbosacral dermatomal patterns in the horse. *Thermol. Int.*, 13, 79, 2003.

[15] Purohit R.C., McCoy M.D., and Bergfeld W.A. Thermographic diagnosis of Horner's syndrome in the horse. *Am. J. Vet. Res.*, 41, 1180, 1980.

[16] Purohit R.C. The diagnostic value of thermography in equine medicine. *Proc. Am. Assoc. Equine Pract.*, 26, 316–326, 1980.

[17] Purohit R.C. and Pascoe D.D. Thermographic evaluation of peripheral neurovascular systems in animal species. *Thermology*, 7, 83, 1997.

[18] Purohit R.C., Pascoe D.D., Schumacher J, Williams A., and Humburg J.H. Effects of medication on the normal thermal patterns in horses. *Thermol. Osterr.*, 6, 108, 1996.

[19] Purohit R.C. and Pascoe D.D. Peripheral neurovascular thermography in equine medicine. *Thermol. Osterr.*, 5, 161, 1995.

[20] Turner T.A., Purohit R.C., and Fessler J.F. Thermography: a review in equine medicine. *Comp. Cont. Education Pract. Vet.*, 8, 854, 1986.

[21] Vaden M.F., Purohit R.C. Mcoy, and Vaughan J.T. Thermography: a technique for subclinical diagnosis of osteoarthritis. *Am. J. Vet. Res.*, 41, 1175–1179, 1980.

[22] Bowman K.F., Purohit R.C., Ganjan, V.K., Peachman R.D., and Vaughan J.T. Thermographic evaluation of corticosteroids efficacy in amphotericin-B induced arthritis in ponies. *Am. J. Vet. Res.* 44, 51–56, 1983.

[23] Purohit R.C. Use of thermography in the diagnosis of lameness. *Auburn Vet.*, 43, 4, 1987.

[24] Waites G.M.H. and Setchell B.P. Physiology of testes, epididymis, and scrotum. In *Advances in Reproductive Physiology*. McLaren A., Ed., London, Logos, Vol. 4, pp. 1–21, 1969.

[25] Waites G.M.H. Temperature regulation and the testes. In *The Testis*, Johnson A.D., Grones W.R., and Vanderwork N.L., Eds., New York, Academy Press, Inc., Vol. 1, pp. 241–237, 1970.

[26] Purohit R.C., Hudson R.S., Riddell M.G., Carson R.L., Wolfe D.F., and Walker D.F. Thermography of bovine scrotum. *Am. J. Vet. Res.*, 46, 2388–2392, 1985.

[27] Purohit R.C., Pascoe D.D., Heath A.M. Pugh D.G., Carson R.L., Riddell M.G., and Wolfe D.F. Thermography: its role in functional evaluation of mammalian testes and scrotum. *Thermol. Int.*, 12, 125–130, 2002.

[28] Wolfe D.F., Hudson R.S., Carson R.L., and Purohit, R.C. Effect of unilateral orchiectomy on semen quality in bulls. *J. Am. Vet. Med. Assoc.*, 186, 1291, 1985.

[29] Heath A.M., Pugh D.G., Sartin E.A., Navarre B., and Purohit R.C. Evaluation of the safety and efficacy of testicular biopsies in llamas. *Theriogenology*, 58, 1125, 2002.

[30] Amiel J.P., Vignalou L., Tricoire J. et al. Thermography of the testicle: preliminary study. *J. Gynecol. Obstet. Biol. Reprod.*, 5, 917, 1976.

[31] Lazarus B.A. and Zorgiotti A.W. Thermo-regulation of the human testes. *Fertil. Steril.*, 26, 757, 1978.

[32] Lee J.T. and Gold R.H. Localization of occult testicular tumor with scrotal thermography. *J. Am. Med. Assoc.*, 1976, 236, 1976.

[33] Wegner G. and Weissbach Z. Application of palte thermography in the diagnosis of scrotal disease. *MMW*, 120, 61, 1978.

[34] Gold R.H., Ehrlich R.M., Samuels B. et al. Scrotal thermography. *Radiology*, 1221, 129, 1979.

[35] Coznhaire F., Monteyne R., and Hunnen M. The value of scrotal thermography as compared with selective retrograde venography of the internal spermatic vein for the diagnosis of subclinical varicoceles. *Fertil. Steril.*, 27, 694, 1976.

36

Standard Procedures for Infrared Imaging in Medicine

Kurt Ammer
Ludwig Boltzmann Research
Institute for Physical Diagnostics
and University of Glamorgan

E. Francis Ring
University of Glamorgan

36.1 Introduction.. 36-1
36.2 Definition of Thermal Imaging......................... 36-2
   Accuracy • Precision • Responsiveness
36.3 Sources of Variability of Thermal Images.............. 36-3
   Object or Subject • Camera Systems, Standards, and
   Calibration • Patient Position and Image Capture •
   Information Protocols and Resources • Image Processing •
   Image Analysis • Image Exchange • Image Presentation
References 36-9

36.1 Introduction

Infra red thermal imaging has been used in medicine since the early 1960s. Working groups within the European Thermographic Association (now European Association of Thermology) produced the first publications on standardization of thermal imaging in 1978 [1] and 1979 [2]. However, Collins and Ring established already in 1974 a quantitative thermal index [3], which was modified in Germany by J.-M. Engel in 1978 [4]. Both indices opened the field of quantitative evaluation of medical thermography.

Further recommendations for standardization appeared in 1983 [5] and 1984, the later related to essential techniques for the use of thermography in clinical drug trials [6]. J.-M. Engel published a booklet entitled "Standardized thermographic investigations in rheumatology and guideline for evaluation" in 1984 [7]. The author presented his ideas for standardization of image recording and assessment including some normal values for wrist, knee, and ankle joints. Engel's measurements of knee temperatures were first published in 1978 [4]. Normal temperature values of the lateral elbow, dorsal hands, anterior knee, lateral and medial malleolus and the 1st metatarsal joint were published by Collins in 1976 [8].

The American Academy of Thermology published technical guidelines in 1986 including some recommendations for thermographic examinations [9]. However, the American authors concentrated on determining the symmetry of temperature distribution rather than the normal temperature values of particular body regions. Uematsu in 1985 [10] and Goodman, 1986 [11] published the side to side variations of surface temperatures of the human body. These symmetry data were confirmed by E.F. Ring for the lower leg in 1986 [12].

In Japan, medical thermal imaging has been an accepted diagnostic procedure since 1981 [13]. Recommendations for the analysis of neuromuscular thermograms were published by Fujimasa et al. in 1986 [14]. Five years later more detailed proposals for the thermal image based analysis of physiological functions were published in *Biomedical Thermology* [15], the official journal of the Japanese Society of thermology. This paper was the result of a workshop on clinical thermography criteria.

Recently, the thermography societies in Korea have published a book, which summarizes in 270 pages general standards for imaging recording and interpretation of thermal images in various diseases [16].

As the relationship between skin blood flow and body surface temperature has been obvious from the initial use of thermal imaging in medicine, quantitative assessments were developed at an early stage. E.F. Ring developed a thermographic index for the assessment of ischemia in 1980, that was originally used for patients suffering from Raynauds' disease [17]. The European Association of Thermology published a statement in 1988 on the subject of Raynaud's Phenomenon [18]. Normal values for recovering after a cold challenge have been published since 1976 [19,20]. A range of temperatures were applied in this thermal challenge test, the technique was reviewed by E.F. Ring in 1997 [21].

An overview of recommendations gathered from, The Japanese Society of Biomedical Thermology and the European Association of Thermology was collated and published by Clark and Goff in 1997 [22]. This paper is based on the practical implications of the foregoing papers taken from the perspective of the modern thermal imaging systems available to medicine.

Finally, a project at the University of Glamorgan, aims to create an atlas of normal thermal images of healthy subjects [23]. This study, started in 2001, has generated a number of questions related to the influence of body positions on accuracy and precision of measurements from thermal images [24,25].

36.2   Definition of Thermal Imaging

Thermal imaging is regarded as a technique for temperature measurements based on the infrared radiation from objects. Unlike images created by x-rays or proton activation through magnetic resonance, thermal imaging is not related to morphology. The technique provides only a map of the distribution of temperatures on the surface of the object imaged.

Whenever infrared thermal imaging is considered as a method for measurement, the technique must meet all criteria of a measurement. The most basic features of measurement are accuracy (in the medical field also named validity) and precision (in medicine reliability). Anbar [26] has listed five other terms related to the precision of infrared based temperature measurements. When used as an outcome measure, responsiveness or sensitivity to change is an important characteristic.

36.2.1   Accuracy

Measurements are basic procedures of comparison namely to compare a standardized meter with an object to be measured. Any measurement is prone to error, thus a perfect measurement is impossible. However, the smaller the variation of a particular measurement from the standardized meter, the higher is the accuracy of the measurement or in other words, an accurate measurement is as close as possible to the true value of measurement. In medicine, accuracy is often named validity, mainly caused by the fact, that medical measurements are not often performed by the simple comparison of meter and object. For example, assessments from various features of a human being may be combined into a new construct, resulting in a innovative measurement of health.

36.2.2   Precision

A series of measurements can not achieve totally identical results. The smaller the variation between single results, the higher is the precision or repeatability (reliability) of the measurement. However, reliability without accuracy, is useless. For example, a sports archer who always hits the same peripheral sector of the recorded in such a manner. In radiography, standardized positions of the body for image capture have been included in the protocol for quality assurance for a long time. Although thermal imaging does not provide much anatomical information compared to other imaging techniques, variation of body positions and the related fields of view affects the precision of temperature readings from thermograms. However, the intra- and inter-rater repeatability of temperature values from the same thermal image was found to be excellent [56].

36.3.3.1 Location for Thermal Imaging

The size of investigation room does not influence the quality of temperature measurements from thermal images, unless the least distance in one direction is not shorter than the distance between the camera and an object of 1.2 m height [57]. Such a condition will result in thermal images out of focus. Other important features of the examination room are thermal insulation and prevention of any direct or reflected infrared radiation sources. Following this proposal will result in an increase of accuracy and precisison of measurements.

36.3.3.2 Ambient Temperature Control

This is a primary requirement for most clinical applications of thermal imaging. A range of temperatures from 18 to 25°C should be attainable and held for at least 1 h to better than 1°C. Due to the nature of human thermoregulation, stability of the room temperature is a critical feature. It have been shown, that subjects acclimatized for 40–60 min to a room temperature of 22°C showed differences in surface temperature at various measuring sites of the face after lowering the ambient temperature by 2°C [58]. While the nose cooled on average by 4°C, the forehead and the meatus decreased the surface temperature by only by 0.4–0.45%. Similar changes may occur at other acral sites such as tips of fingers or toes, as both regions are highly involved in heat exchange for temperature regulation.

At lower temperatures, the subject is likely to shiver, and over 25°C room temperature will cause sweating, at least in most European countries. Variations may be expected in colder or warmer climates, in the latter case, room temperatures may need to be 1 to 2°C higher [59].

Additonal techniques for cooling particular regions of the body have been developed [60,61]. Immersion of the hands in water at various tempeatures is a common challenge for the assessment of vasospastic disease [21].

Heat generated in the investigation room affects the room temperature. Possible heat sources are electronic equipment such as the scanner and its computer, but also human bodies. For this reason the air-conditioning unit should be capable of compensating for the maximum number of patients and staff likely to be in the room at any one time. These effects will be greater in a small room of 2 × 3 m or less.

Air convection is a very effective method of skin cooling and related to the wind speed. Therefore, air conditioning equipment should be located so that direct draughts are not directed at the patient, and that overall air speed is kept as low as possible. A suspended perforated ceiling with ducts diffusing the air distribution evenly over the room is ideal [62].

A cubicle or cubicles within the temperature controlled area is essential. These should provide privacy for disrobing and a suitable area for resting through the acclimatization period.

36.3.3.3 Pre-Imaging Equilibration

On arrival at the department, the patient should be informed of the examination procedure, instructed to remove appropriate clothing and jewellery, and asked to sit or rest in the preparation cubicle for a fixed time. The time required to achieve adequate stability in blood pressure and skin temperature is generally considered to be 15 min, with 10 min as a minimum [63–65]. After 30 min cooling, oszillations of the skin temperature can be detected, in different regions of the body with different amplitudes resulting in a temperature asymmetry between left and right sides [64].

Contact of body parts with the environment or with other body parts alters the surface temperature due to heat transfer by conduction. Therefore, during the preparation time the patient must avoid folding or crossing arms and legs, or placing bare feet on a cold surface. If the lower extremities are to be examined, a stool or leg rest should be provided to avoid direct contact with the floor [66]. If these requirements are not met, poor precision of measurements may result.

36.3.3.4 Positions for Imaging

As in anatomical imaging studies, it is preferable to standardize on a series of standard views for each body region. The EAT Locomotor Diseases Group recommendations include a triangular marker system to indicate anterior, posterior, lateral, and angled views [2,67]. However, reproduction of positions for angled views may be difficult, even when aids such as rotating platforms are used [68].

Modern image processing software provide comment boxes which can be used to encode the angle of view which will be stored with the image [69]. It should be noted that the position of the patient for scanning and in preparation must be constant. Standing, sitting, or lying down affect the surface area of the body exposed to the ambient, therefore an image recorded with the patient in a sitting position may not be comparable with one recorded on a separate occasion in a standing position. In addition, blood flow against the influence of gravity contributes to the skin temperature of fingers in various limb positions [70].

36.3.3.5 Field of View

Image size is dependent on the distance between the camera and the patient and the focal length of the infrared camera lens. The lens is generally fixed on most medical systems, so it is good practice to maintain a constant distance from the patient for each view, in order to acquire a reproducible field of view for the image. If in different thermograms different fields of the same subject are compared, the variable resolution can lead to false temperature readings [71]. However, maintaining the same distance between object and camera, cannot compensate for individual body dimensions, for example, big subjects will have big knees and therefore maintaining the same distance as for a tiny subjects knee is not applicable.

To overcome this problem, the field of view has been defined in the standard protocol at the University of Glamorgan in a two fold way, that is, body position and alignment of anatomical landmarks to the edge of the image [23]. These definitions enabled us to investigate the reproducibilty of body views using the distance in pixels between anatomical landmarks and the outline of the infrared images [24–72].

Figure 36.1 gives examples of the views, that have been investigated for the reproduciblity of body positions. Table 36.2 shows the mean value, standard deviation, and 95% confidence interval of the variation of body views of the upper and the lower part of the human body. Variations in views of the lower part of the body were bigger than in views of the upper part. The highest degree of variation was found in the view "Both Ankles Anterior," but the smallest variation in the view "Face."

36.3.4 Information Protocols and Resources

Human skin temperature is the product of heat dissipated from the vessels and organs within the body, and the effect of the environmental factors on heat loss or gain. There are a number of further influences which are controllable, such as cosmetics [29], alcohol intake [73–75], and smoking [76–78]. In general terms the patient attending for examination should be advised to avoid all topical applications such as ointments and cosmetics on the day of examination to all the relevant areas of the body [31,47,79,80]. Large meals and above average intake of tea or coffee should also be excluded, although studies supporting this recommendation are hard to find and the results are not conclusive [81,82].

Patients should be asked to avoid tight fitting clothing, and to keep physical exertion to a minimum. This particularly applies to methods of physiotherapy such as electrotherapy [83,85], ultrasound [86,87], heat treatment [88,90], cryotherapy [91–94], massage [95–97], and hydrotherapy [31,32,98,99], because thermal effects from such treatment can last for 4 to 6 h under certain conditions. Heat production by muscular exercise is a well documented phenomenon [65,100–103].

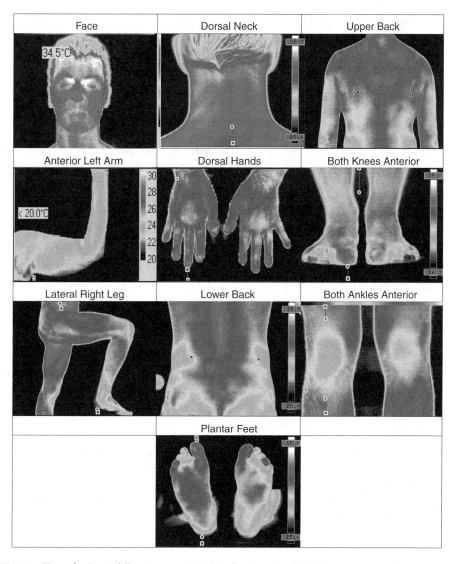

FIGURE 36.1 (See color insert following page **29**-16.) Body views investigated.

TABLE 36.2 Variation of Positions of All the Investigated Views

View	Upper edge (pixel) mean ± SD (95% CI)	Lower edge (pixel) mean ± SD (95% CI)	Left side edge (pixel) mean ± SD (95% CI)
Face	0.5 ± 5.3 (−2.2 to 1.9)	4.0 ± 10.9 (−0.03 to 8.2)	
Dorsal neck	−8.4 ± 36.4 (−18.3 to 1.6)	122.6 ± 146.6 (82.6 to 162.6)	
Upper back	4.5 ± 9.9 (0.8 to 8.2)	28.1 ± 22.0 (19.9 to 36.4)	
Anterior left arm	22.4 ± 33.0 (8.7 to 36.0)	15.8 ± 15.4 (9.5 to 22.2)	12.5 ± 16.0 (5.9 to 19.1)
Dorsal hands	41.8 ± 17.8 (35.5 to 48.2)	33.2 ± 22.3 (25.3 to 41.5)	
Both knees anterior	80.7 ± 47.3 (60.7 to 100.7)	84.3 ± 37.0 (68.6 to 99.9)	
Lateral right leg	16.7 ± 21.0 (5.9 to 27.5)	17.2 ± 15.8 (9.0 to 25.3)	
Lower back	17.1 ± 4.2 (8.6 to 25.6)	16.3 ± 4.6 (16.3 ro 34.9)	
Both ankles anterior	158.8 ± 12.2 (133.6 to 184.1)	54.9 ± 9.1 (36.1 to 37.8)	
Plantar feet	31.0 ± 24.1 (23.2 to 38.7)	25.7 ± 23.1 (18.3 to 33.1)	

Drug treatment can also affect the skin temperature. This phenomenon was used to evaluate the therapeutic effects of medicaments [6]. Drugs affecting the cardiovascular system must be reported to the thermographer, in order that the correct interpretation of thermal images will be given [104–107].

Omiting just one of the above mentioned conditions will result in reduced precision of temperature measurements.

36.3.5 Image Processing

Every image or block of images must carry the indication of temperature range, with color code/temperature scale. The color scale itself should be standardized. Industrial software frequently provides a grey-scale picture and one or more color scales. However, modern image processing software permits to squeeze the color scale in already recorded images in order to increase the image contrast. Such a procedure will affect the temperature readings from thermal images as temperatures outside of the compressed temperature scale will not be included in the statistics of selected regions of interest. This will result in erroneous temperature readings, affecting both accuracy and precision of measurements.

36.3.6 Image Analysis

Almost all systems now use image processing techniques and provide basic quantitation of the image [108–110]. In some cases this may be operated from a chip within the camera, of may be carried out through an on- or off- line computer. For older equipment like the AGA 680 series several hardware adaptations have been reported to achieve quantitation of the thermograms [111–113].

It has to be emphasized that false color coding of infrared images does not provide means for temperature measurement. If colors are separated by a temperature distance of 1°C, the temperature difference between two points situated in adjacent colors may be between 0.1 and 1.9°C. It is obvious, that false colored images provide at its best an estimation of temperature, but not a measurement. The same is true for liquid crystal thermograms.

Nowadays, temperature measurements in thermal images are based on the definition of regions of interest (ROI). However, standards for shape, size and placement of these regions are not available or incomplete. Although a close correlation exists for ROI of different size in the same region [114], the precision of measurement is affected when ROIS of different size and location are used for repeated measurements.

The Glamorgan protocol [23] is the very first attempt to create a complete standard for the definition of regions of interest in thermal images based on anatomical limits. Furthermore, in the view "both knee anterior" the shape with the highest reproducibility was investigated. During one of the Medical Infrared Training-Courses at the University of Glamorgan, three newly trained investigators defined on the same thermal image of both anterior knees twice the region of interest in the shape of a box, an ellipsoid or as an hour-glass shape. Similar to the result of a pilot study that compared these shapes for repeateabilty, the highest reliability was found for temperature readings from the hour-glass shape, followed by readings from ellipsoids and boxes [53]. The repeatabilty of the regions on the view "Left Anterior Arm," "Both Ankles Anterior," "Dorsal Feet," and "Plantar Feet" were also investigated and resulted in reliabilty coefficients between 0.7 (right ankle) and 0.93 (forearm). The intraclass correlation coefficients ranged between 0.48 (upper arm) and 0.87 (forearm). Applying the Glamorgan protocol consequently, will result in precise temperature measurements from thermal images.

36.3.7 Image Exchange

Most of the modern infrared systems store the recorded thermal images in an own image format, which may not compatible with formats of thermal images from other manufacturers. However, most of this images can be transformed into established image formats such as TIF, JPEG, GIF, and others. As a thermal image is the pictographic representation of a temperature map, the sole image is not enough unless the related temperature information is not provided. Consequently, temperature measurements from standard computer images derived from thermograms is not possible.

Providing both temperature scale and a scale of grey shades, allows the exchange of thermal images over long distance and between different, but compatible image processing software [115]. The grey scale must be derived from the original grey shade thermal image. If it has been transformed from a false color image, the resulted black-and-white thermogram may not be representative for the original grey scale gradient as the grey scale of individual colors may deviate from the particular grey shade of the image. This can then result in false temperature readings.

36.3.8 Image Presentation

Image presentation does not influence the result of measurements from thermal images. However, if thermograms are read by eyes, their appearance will affect the credibility of the information in thermal images. This is for instance the case, when thermal images are use as evidence in legal trials [116].

It was stated, that for forensic acceptability of thermography standardization and repeatability of the technique are very important features [117]. This supports the necessity of quantitative evaluation of thermal images and standards strictly applied to the technique of infrared imaging will finally result in high accuracy and precision of this method of temperature measurement. At that stage it can be recommended as responsive outcome measure for clinical trials in rheumatology [6,8], angiopathies [107,118], neuromuscular disorders [119], surgery [120], and paediatrics [121].

References

[1] Aarts, N.J.M. et al. Thermograp. terminology. *Acta Thermograp.*, 1978, Suppl. 2.

[2] Engel, J.M. et al. Thermography in locomotor diseases — recommended procedure. *Eur. J. Rheum. Inflamm.*, 2, 299, 1979.

[3] Collins, A.J. et al. Quantitation of thermography in arthritis using multi-isothermal analysis. *Ann. Rheum. Dis.*, 33, 113, 1974.

[4] Engel, J.-M. Quantitative Thermographie des Kniegelenks. *Z. Rheumatol.*, 37, 242, 1978.

[5] Ring, E.F.J. Standardisation of thermal imaging in medicine: physical and environmental factors, in *Thermal Assessment of Breast Health*, Gautherie, M., Albert, E., and Keith, L., Eds., MTP Press Ltd, Lancaster/Boston/The Hague, 1983, p. 29.

[6] Ring, E.F.J., Engel, J.M., and Page-Thomas, D.P. Thermologic methods in clinical pharmacology — skin temperature measurement in drug trials. *Int. J. Clin. Pharm. Ther. Tox.*, 22, 20, 1984.

[7] Engel, J.-M. and Saier, U. *Thermographische Standarduntersuchungen in der Rheumatologie und Richtlinien zu deren Befundung.* Luitpold, München, 1984.

[8] Collins, A.J. Anti-inflammatory drug assessment by the thermographic index. *Acta Thermograp.*, 1, 73, 1976.

[9] Pochaczevsky, R. et al. *Technical Guidelines*, 2nd ed. *Thermology*, 2, 108, 1986.

[10] Uematsu, S. Symmetry of skin temperatures comparing one side of the body to the other. *Thermology*, 1, 4, 1985.

[11] Goodman, P.H. et al. Normal temperature asymmetry of the back and extremities by computer-assisted infrared imaging. *Thermology*, 1, 195, 1986.

[12] Bliss, P. et al. Investigation of nerve root irritation by infrared thermography, in *Back Pain — Methods for Clinical Investigation and Assessment*, Hukins, D.W.L. and Mulholland, R.C., Eds., University Press, Manchester, 1986, p. 63.

[13] Atsumi, K. High technology applications of medical thermography in Japan. *Thermology*, 1, 79–80, 1985.

[14] Fujimasa, I. et al. A new computer image processing system for the analysis of neuromuscular thermograms: a feasibility study. *Thermology*, 1, 221, 1986.

[15] Fujimasa, I. A proposal for thermographic imaging diagnostic procedures for temperature related physiologic function analysis. *Biomed. Thermol.*, 11, 269, 1991.

[16] Lee, D.-I. (Ed.) *Practical Manual of Clinical Thermology*, ISBN 89-954013-04.

[17] Ring, E.F.J. A thermographic index for the assessment of ischemia. *Acta thermograp.*, 5, 35, 1980.

[18] Aarts, N. P. et al. Raynaud's phenomenon: assessment by thermography. *Thermology*, 3, 69, 1988.

[19] Acciarri, L., Carnevale, F., and Della Selva, A. Thermography in the hand angiopathy from vibrating tools. *Acta thermograp.*, 1, 18, 1976.

[20] Ring, E.F. and Bacon, P.A. Quantitative thermographic assessment of inositol nicotinate therapy in Raynaud's phenomena. *J. Int. Med. Res.*, 5, 217, 1977.

[21] Ring, E.F.J. Cold stress test for the hands, in *The Thermal Image in Medicine and Biology*, Ammer, K. and Ring, E.F.J., Eds., Uhlen-Verlag, Wien, 1995, p. 237.

[22] Clark, R.P. and de Calcina-Goff, M. Guidelines for Standardisation in Medical Thermography Draft International Standard Proposals. *Thermol. Osterr.*, 7, 47, 1997.

[23] Website address, Atlas of Normals, www.medimaging.org.

[24] Ammer, K. et al. Rationale for standardised capture and analysis of infrared thermal images, in *Proceedings Part II, EMBEC'02 2.European Medical & Biological Engineering Conference*. Hutten, H. and Krösel, P., Eds. IFMBE, Graz, 2002, p. 1608.

[25] Ring, E.F.J. et al. Errors and artefacts in thermal imaging, in *Proceedings Part II, EMBEC'02 2.European Medical & Biological Engineering Conference*. Hutten, H. and Krösel, P., Eds., IFMBE, Graz, 2002, p. 1620.

[26] Anbar, M. Recent technological developments in thermology and their impact on clinical applications. *Biomed. Thermol.*, 10, 270, 1990.

[27] Hardy, J.D. The radiation of heat from the human body. III. The human skin as a black body radiator. *J. Clin. Invest.*, 13, 615, 1934.

[28] Togawa, T. and Saito, H. Non-contact imaging of thermal properties of the skin. *Physiol. Meas.*, 15, 291, 1994.

[29] Engel, J.-M. Physical and physiological influence of medical ointments of infrared thermography, in *Recent Advances in Medical Thermology*, Ring, E.F.J. and Phillips, B., Eds., Plenum Press, New York, 1984, p. 177.

[30] Hejazi, S. and Anbar, M. Effects of topical skin treatment and of ambient light in infrared thermal images. *Biomed. Thermol.*, 12, 300, 1992.

[31] Ammer, K. The influence of antirheumatic creams and ointments on the infrared emission of the skin, in *Abstracts of the 10th International Conference on Thermogrammetry and Thermal Engineering in Budapest 18–20, June 1997*, Benkö, I. et al., Eds., MATE, Budapest, 1997, p. 177.

[32] Ammer, K. Einfluss von Badezusätzen auf die Wärmeabstrahlung der Haut. *ThermoMed*, 10, 71, 1994.

[33] Ammer, K. The influence of bathing on the infrared emission of the skin, in *Abstracts of the 9th International Conference on Thermogrammetry and Thermal Engineering in Budapest 14–16, June 1995*, Benkö, I., Lovak., and Kovacsics, I., Eds., MATE, Budapest, 1995, p. 115.

[34] Ammer, K. Thermographie in lymphedema, in *Advanced Techniques and Clinical Application in Biomedical Thermologie*, Mabuchi, K., Mizushina, S., and Harrison, B., Eds., Harwood Academic Publishers, Chur/Schweiz, 1994, p. 213.

[35] Heath, A.M. et al. A comparison of surface and rectal temperatures between sheared and non-sheared alpacas (*Lama pacos*). *Small Rumin. Res.*, 39, 19, 2001.

[36] Purohit, R.C. et al. Thermographic evaluation of animal skin surface temperature with and without haircoat. *Thermol. Int.*, 11, 83, 2001.

[37] Damm, F., Döring, G., and Hildebrandt, G. Untersuchungen über den Tagesgang von Hautdurchblutung und Hauttemperatur unter besonderer Berücksichtigung der physikalischen Temperaturregulation. *Z. Physik. Med. Rehabil.*, 15, 1, 1974.

[38] Reinberg, A. Circadian changes in the temperature of human beings. *Bibl. Radiol.*, 6, 128, 1975.

[39] Schmidt, K.-L., Mäurer, R., and Rusch, D. Zur Wirkung örtlicher Wärme und Kälteanwendungen auf die Hauttemperatur am Kniegelenk. *Z. Rheumatol.*, 38, 213, 1979.

[40] Kanamori, T. et al. Circadian rhythm of body temperature. *Biomed. Thermol.*, 11, 292, 1991.

[41] Friedrich, K.H. Assessment criteria for infrared thermography systems. *Acta thermograp*, 5, 68, 1980.

[42] Alderson, J.K.A. and Ring, E.F.J. "Sprite" high resolution thermal imaging system. *Thermology*, 1, 110, 1985.

[43] Dibley, D.A.G. Opto-mechanical systems for thermal imaging, in *The Thermal Image in Medicine and Biology*, Ammer, K., and Ring, E.F.J., Eds., Uhlen-Verlag, Wien, 1995, p. 33.

[44] Plassmann, P. Advances in image processing for thermology, *Presented at Int. Cong. of Thermology*, Seoul, June 5–6, 2004, p. 3.

[45] Kutas, M. Staring focal plane array for medical thermal imaging, in *The Thermal Image in Medicine and Biology*, Ammer, K., and Ring, E.F.J., Eds., Uhlen-Verlag, Wien, 1995, p. 40.

[46] Ring, E.F.J., Minchinton, M., and Elvins, D.M. A focal plane array system for clinical infrared imaging. *IEEE/EMBS Proceedings*, Atlanta 1999, p. 1120.

[47] Hejazi, S. and Spangler, R.A. A multi-wavelength thermal imaging system, in *Proc. 11th Annual Int. Conf. IEEE Engineering in Medicine and Biology Society*, II, 1989, p. 1153.

[48] Ring, E.F.J. Quality control in infrared thermography, in *Recent Advances in Medical Thermology*, Ring, E.F.J. and Phillips, B., Eds., Plenum Press, New York, 1984, p. 185.

[49] Clark, R.P. et al. Thermography and pedobarography in the assessment of tissue damage in neuropathicand atherosclerotic feet. *Thermology*, 3, 15, 1988.

[50] Clark, J.A. Effects of surface emissivity and viewing angle errors in thermography. *Acta thermograp*, 1, 138, 1976.

[51] Steketee, J. Physical aspects of infrared thermography, in *Recent Advances in Medical Thermology*, Ring, E.F.J. and Phillips, B., Eds., Plenum Press, New York, 1984, p. 167.

[52] Wiecek, B., Jung, A., and Zuber, J. Emissivity-Bottleneck and Challenge for thermography. *Thermol. Int.*, 10, 15, 2000.

[53] Ammer K. Need for standardisation of measurements, in *Thermal Imaging in Thermography and Lasers in Medicine*, Wiecek, B., Ed., Akademickie Centrum Graficzno-Marketigowe Lodart S.A, Lodz, 2003, p. 13.

[54] Anbar, M. Potential artifacts in infrared thermographic measurements. *Thermology*, 3, 273, 1991.

[55] Ring, E.F.J. and Dicks, J.M. Spatial resolution of new thermal imaging systems, *Thermol. Int.*, 9, 7, 1999.

[56] Melnizky, P., Schartelmüller, T., and Ammer, K. Prüfung der intra-und interindividuellen Verlässlichkeit der Auswertung von Infrarot-Thermogrammen. *Eur. J. Thermol.*, 7, 224, 1997.

[57] Ring, E.F.J. and Ammer, K. The technique of thermal imaging in medicine. *Thermol. Int.*, 10, 7, 2000.

[58] Khallaf, A. et al. Thermographic study of heat loss from the face. *Thermol. Österr.*, 4, 49, 1994.

[59] Ishigaki, T. et al. Forehead–back thermal ratio for the interpretation of infrared imaging of spinal cord lesions and other neurological disorders. *Thermology*, 3, 101, 1989.

[60] Schuber, T.R. et al. Directed dynamic cooling,a methodic contribution in telethermography. *Acta thermograp*, 1, 94, 1977.

[61] Di Carlo, A. Thermography in patients with systemic sclerosis. *Thermol. Österr.*, 4, 18, 1994.

[62] Love, T.J. Heat transfer considerations in the design of a thermology clinic. *Thermology*, 1, 88, 1985.

[63] Ring, E.F.J. Computerized thermography for osteo-articular diseases. *Acta thermograp.*, 1, 166, 1976.

[64] Roberts, D.L. and Goodman, P.H. Dynamic thermoregulation of back and upper extremity by computer-aided infrared imaging. *Thermology*, 2, 573, 1987.

[65] Mabuchi, K. et al. Development of a data processing system for a high-speed thermographic camera and its use in analyses of dynamic thermal phenomena of the living body, in *The Thermal Image in Medicine and Biology*, Ammer, K., and Ring, E.F.J., Eds., Uhlen-Verlag, Wien, 1995, p. 56.

[66] Cena, K. Environmental heat loss, in *Recent Advances in Medical Thermology*, Ring, E.F.J. and Phillips, B., Eds., Plenum Press, New York, 1984, p. 81.

[67] Engel, J.-M. Kennzeichnung von Thermogrammen, in *Thermologische Messmethodik*, Engel, J.-M., Flesch, U., and Stüttgen, G., Eds., Notamed, Baden–Baden, 1983, p. 176.

[68] Park, J.-Y. Current development of medical infrared imaging technology, *Presented at Int. Congr. of Thermology*, Seoul, June 5–6, 2004, p. 9.

[69] Plassmann, P. and Ring, E.F.J. An open system for the acquisition and evaluation of medical thermological images. *Eur. J. Thermol.* 7, 216, 1997.

[70] Abramson, D.I. et al. Effect of altering limb position on blood flow, O_2 uptake and skin temperature. *J. Appl. Physiol.*, 17, 191, 1962.

[71] Schartelmüller, T. and Ammer, K. Räumliche Auflösung von Infrarotkameras. *Thermol. Österr.*, 5, 28, 1995.

[72] Ammer, K. Update in standardization and temperature measurement from thermal images, *Presented at Int. Cong. of Thermology*, Seoul, June 5–6, 2004, p. 7.

[73] Mannara, G., Salvatori, G.C., and Pizzuti, G.P. Ethyl alcohol induced skin temperature changes evaluated by thermography. Preliminary results. *Boll. Soc. Ital. Biol. Sper.*, 69, 587, 1993.

[74] Melnizky, P. and Ammer, K. Einfluss von Alkohol und Rauchen auf die Hauttemperatur des Gesichts, der Hände und der Kniegelenke. *Thermol. Int.*, 10, 191, 2000.

[75] Ammer, K., Melnizky, P., and Rathkolb, O. Skin temperature after intake of sparkling wine, still wine or sparkling water. *Thermol. Int.*, 13, 99, 2003.

[76] Gershon-Cohen, J., Borden, A.G., and Hermel, M.B. Thermography of extremities after smoking. *Br. J. Radiol.*, 42, 189, 1969.

[77] Usuki, K. et al. Effects of nicotine on peripheral cutaneous blood flow and skin temperature. *J. Dermatol. Sci.*, 16, 173, 1998.

[78] Di Carlo, A. and Ippolito, F. Early effects of cigarette smoking in hypertensive and normotensive subjects. An ambulatory blood pressure and thermographic study. *Minerva Cardioangiol.*, 51, 387, 2003.

[79] Collins, A.J. et al. Some observations on the pharmacology of "deep-heat," a topical rubifacient. *Ann. Rheum. Dis.*, 43, 411, 1984.

[80] Ring, E.F. Cooling effects of Deep Freeze Cold gel applied to the skin, with and without rubbing, to the lumbar region of the back. *Thermol. Int.*, 14, 64, 2004.

[81] Federspil, G. et al. Study of diet-induced thermogenesis using telethermography in normal and obese subjects. *Recent Prog. Med.*, 80, 455, 1989.

[82] Shlygin, G.K. et al. Radiothermometric research of tissues during the initial reflex period of the specific dynamic action of food. *Med. Radiol. (Mosk)*, 36, 10, 1991.

[83] Danz, J. and Callies, R. Infrarothermometrie bei differenzierten Methoden der Niederfrequenztherapie. *Z. Physiother.*, 31, 35, 1979.

[84] Rusch, F., Neeck, G., and Schmidt, K.L. Über die Hemmung von Erythemen durch Capsaicin. 3.Objektivierung des Capsaicin-Erythems mittels statischer und dynamischer Thermographie, *Z. Phys. Med. Baln. Med. Klim.*, 17, 18, 1988.

[85] Mayr, H., Thür, H., and Ammer, K. Electrical stimulation of the stellate ganglia, in *The Thermal Image in Medicine and Biology*, Ammer, K., and Ring, E.F.J., Eds., Uhlen-Verlag, Wien, 1995, p. 206.

[86] Danz, J. and Callies R. Thermometrische Untersuchungen bei unterschiedlichen Ultraschallintensitäten. *Z. Physiother.*, 30, 235, 1978.

[87] Demmink, J.H., Helders, P.J., Hobaek, H., and Enwemeka, C. The variation of heating depth with therapeutic ultrasound frequency in physiotherapy. *Ultrasound Med. Biol.*, 29, 113–118, 2003.

[88] Rathkolb, O. and Ammer, K. Skin temperature of the fingers after different methods of heating using a wax bath. *Thermol Österr.*, 6, 125, 1996.

[89] Ammer, K. and Schartelmüller, T. Hauttemperatur nach der Anwendung von Wärmepackungen und nach Infrarot-A-Bestrahlung. *Thermol. Österr.*, 3, 51, 1993.

[90] Goodman, P.H., Foote, J.E., and Smith, R.P. Detection of intentionally produced thermal artifacts by repeated thermographic imaging. *Thermology*, 3, 253, 1991.

[91] Dachs, E., Schartelmüller, T., and Ammer, K. Temperatur zur Kryotherapie und Veränderungen der Hauttemperatur am Kniegelenk nach Kaltluftbehandlung. *Thermol. Österr.*, 1, 9, 1991.

[92] Rathkolb, O. et al. Hauttemperatur der Lendenregion nach Anwendung von Kältepackungen unterschiedlicher Größe und Applikationsdauer. *Thermol. Österr.*, 1, 15, 1991.

[93] Ammer, K. Occurrence of hyperthermia after ice massage. *Thermol. Österr.*, 6, 17, 1996.

[94] Cholewka, A. et al. Temperature effects of whole body cryotherapy determined by thermography. *Thermol. Int.*, 14, 57, 2004.

[95] Danz, J., Callies, R., and Hrdina, A. Einfluss einer abgestuften Vakuumsaugmassage auf die Hauttemperatur. *Z. Physiother.*, 33, 85, 1981.

[96] Eisenschenk, A. and Stoboy, H. Thermographische Kontrolle physikalisch-therapeutischer Methoden. *Krankengymnastik*, 37, 294, 1985.

[97] Kainz, A. Quantitative Überprüfung der Massagewirkung mit Hilfe der IR-Thermographie. *Thermol. Österr.*, 3, 79, 1993.

[98] Rusch, D. and Kisselbach, G. Comparative thermographic assessment of lower leg baths in medicinal mineral waters (Nauheim Springs), in *Recent Advances in Medical Thermology*, Ring, E.F.J. and Phillips, B., Eds., Plenum Press, New York, 1984, p. 535.

[99] Ring, E,F.J., Barker, J.R., and Harrison, R.A. Thermal effects of pool therapy on the lower limbs. *Thermology*, 3, 127, 1989.

[100] Konermann, H. and Koob, E. Infrarotthermographische Kontrolle der Effektivität krankengymnastischer Behandlungsmaßnahmen. *Krankengymnastik*, 27, 39, 1975.

[101] Smith, B.L., Bandler, M.K., and Goodman, P.H. Dominant forearm hyperthermia: a study of fifteen athletes. *Thermology*, 2, 25, 1986.

[102] Melnizky, P., Ammer, K., and Schartelmüller, T. Thermographische Überprüfung der Heilgymnastik bei Patienten mit Peroneusparese. *Thermol. Österr.*, 5, 97, 1995.

[103] Ammer, K. Low muscular acitivity of the lower leg in patients with a painful ankle. *Thermol. Österr.*, 5, 103, 1995.

[104] Ring, E.F., Porto, L.O., and Bacon, P.A. Quantitative thermal imaging to assess inositol nicotinate treatment for Raynaud's syndrome. *J. Int. Med. Res.*, 9, 393, 1981.

[105] Lecerof, et al. Acute effects of doxazosin and atenolol on smoking-induced peripheral vasoconstriction in hypertensive habitual smokers. *J. Hypertens.*, 8, S29, 1990.

[106] Tham, T.C., Silke, B., and Taylor, S.H. Comparison of central and peripheral haemodynamic effects of dilevalol and atenolol in essential hypertension. *J. Hum. Hypertens.*, 4, S77, 1990.

[107] Natsuda, H. et al. Nitroglycerin tape for Raynaud's phenomenon of rheumatic disease patients — an evaluation of skin temperature by thermography. *Ryumachi*, 34. 849, 1994.

[108] Engel, J.M. Thermotom- ein Softwarepaket für die thermographische Bildanalyse in der Rheumatologie, in *Thermologische Messmethodik*, Engel, J.-M., Flesch, U., and Stüttgen, G., Eds., Notamed, Baden–Baden, 1983, p. 110.

[109] Bösiger, P. and Scaroni, F. Mikroprozessor-unterstütztes Thermographie-System zur quantitativewn on-line Analyse von statischen und dynamischen Thermogrammen, in *Thermologische Messmethodik*, Engel, J.-M., Flesch, U., and Stüttgen, G., Eds., Notamed, Baden–Baden, 1983, p. 125.

[110] Brandes, P. PIC-Win-Iris Bildverarbeitungssoftware. *Thermol. Österr.*, 4, 33, 1994.

[111] Ring, E.F.J. Quantitative thermography in arthritis using the AGA integrator. *Acta thermograp.*, 2, 172, 1977.

[112] Parr, G. et al. Microcomputer standardization of the AGA 680 M system, in *Recent Advances in Medical Thermology*, Ring, E.F.J. and Phillips, B., Eds., Plenum Press, New York, 1984, pp. 211–214.

[113] Van Hamme, H., De Geest, G., and Cornelis, J. An acquisition and scan conversion unit for the AGA THV680 medical infrared camera. *Thermology*, 3, 205, 1990.

[114] Mayr, H. Korrelation durchschnittlicher und maximaler Temperatur am Kniegelenk bei Auswertung unterschiedlicher Messareale. *Thermol. Österr.*, 5, 89, 1995.

[115] Plassmann, P. On-line Communication for Thermography in Europe, *Presented at Int. Cong. of Thermology*, Seoul, June 5–6, 2004, p. 50.

[116] Ring, E.F.J. Thermal imaging in medico-legal claims. *Thermol. Int.*, 10, 97, 2000.

[117] Sella, G.E. Forensic criteria of acceptability of thermography. *Eur. J. Thermol.*, 7, 205, 1997.

[118] Hirschl, M. et al. Double-blind, randomised, placebo controlled low level laser therapy study in patients with primary Raynaud's phenomenon. *Vasa*, 31, 91, 2002.

[119] Schartelmüller, T., Melnizky, P., and Engelbert, B. Infrarotthermographie zur Evaluierung des Erfolges physikalischer Therapie bei Patienten mit klinischem Verdacht auf Thoracic Outlet Syndrome. *Thermol. Int.*, 9, 20, 1999.

[120] Kim, Y.S. and Cho, Y.E. Pre- and postoperative thermographic imaging in lumbar disc herniations, in *The Thermal Image in Medicine and Biology*, Ammer, K., and Ring, E.F.J., Eds., Uhlen-Verlag, Wien, 1995, p. 168.

[121] Siniewicz, K, et al. Thermal imaging before and after physial exercises in children with orthostatic disorders of the cardiovascular system. *Thermol. Int.*, 12, 139, 2002.

37

Infrared Detectors and Detector Arrays

37.1 Photon Detectors 37-1
    Photoconductive Detectors • Photovoltaic Detectors
37.2 Thermal Detectors 37-6
37.3 Detector Materials 37-7
37.4 Detector Readouts 37-12
    Readouts for Photon Detectors • Thermal Detector Readouts
    • Readout Evolution
37.5 Technical Challenges for Infrared Detectors 37-14
    Uncooled Infrared Detector Challenges • Electronics
    Challenges • Detector Readout Challenges • Optics
    Challenges • Challenges for Third-Generation Cooled
    Imagers
37.6 Summary 37-24
References 37-25

Paul Norton
Stuart Horn
Joseph G. Pellegrino
Philip Perconti
*U.S. Army Communications and
Electronics Research, Development
and Engineering Center (CERDEC)
Night Vision and Electronic Sensors
Directorate*

There are two general classes of detectors: *photon* (or quantum) and *thermal* detectors [1,2]. Photon detectors convert absorbed photon energy into released electrons (from their bound states to conduction states). The material band gap describes the energy necessary to transition a charge carrier from the valence band to the conduction band. The change in charge carrier state changes the electrical properties of the material. These electrical property variations are measured to determine the amount of incident optical power. Thermal detectors absorb energy over a broad band of wavelengths. The energy absorbed by a detector causes the temperature of the material to increase. Thermal detectors have at least one inherent electrical property that changes with temperature. This temperature-related property is measured electrically to determine the power on the detector. Commercial infrared imaging systems suitable for medical applications use both types of detectors. We begin by describing the physical mechanism employed by these two detector types.

37.1 Photon Detectors

Infrared radiation consists of a flux of photons, the quantum-mechanical elements of all electromagnetic radiation. The energy of the photon is given by:

$$E_{ph} = h\nu = hc/\lambda = 1.986 \times 10^{-19}/\lambda \text{ J}/\mu\text{m} \tag{37.1}$$

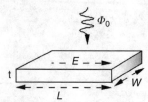

FIGURE 37.1 Photoconductive detector geometery.

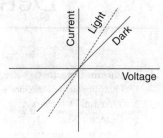

FIGURE 37.2 Current–voltage characteristics of a photoconductive detector.

where h is the Planck's constant, c is the speed of light, and λ is the wavelength of the infrared photon in micrometers (μm).

Photon detectors respond by elevating an bound electron in a material to a free or conductive state. Two types are photon detectors are produced for the commercial market:

- Photoconductive
- Photovoltaic

37.1.1 Photoconductive Detectors

The mechanism of photoconductive detectors is based upon the excitation of bound electrons to a mobile state where they can move freely through the material. The increase in the number of conductive electrons, n, created by the photon flux, Φ_0 allows more current to flow when the detective element is used in a bias circuit having an electric field E. The photoconductive detector element having dimensions of length L, width W, and thickness t is represented in Figure 37.1.

Figure 37.2 illustrates how the current–voltage characteristics of a photoconductor change with incident photon flux (Chapter 4).

The response of a photoconductive detector can be written as:

$$R = \frac{nqRE\tau(\mu_n + \mu_p)}{E_{ph}L}(V/W)$$

(37.2)

where R is the response in volts per Watt, η is the quantum efficiency in electrons per photon, q is the charge of an electron, R is the resistance of the detector element, τ is the lifetime of a photoexcited electron, and μ_n and μ_p are the mobilities of the electrons and holes in the material in volts per square centimeter per second.

Noise in photoconductors is the square root averaged sum of terms from three sources:

- Johnson noise
- Thermal generation-recombination
- Photon generation-recombination

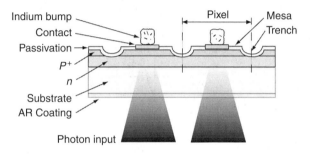

FIGURE 37.3 Photovoltaic detector structure example for mesa diodes.

Expressions for the total noise and each of the noise terms are given in Equation 37.3 to Equation 37.6

$$V_{\text{noise}} = \sqrt{V_{\text{Johnson}}^2 + V_{\text{ph g-r}}^2 + V_{\text{th g-r}}^2} \qquad (37.3)$$

$$V_{\text{Johnson}} = \sqrt{4kTR} \qquad (37.4)$$

$$V_{\text{ph g-r}} = \frac{\sqrt{\eta\phi(WL)}2qRE\tau(\mu_{\text{n}} + \mu_{\text{p}})}{L} \qquad (37.5)$$

$$V_{\text{th g-r}} = \sqrt{\frac{np}{n+p}\tau\left(\frac{Wt}{L}\right)}2qRE(\mu_{\text{n}} + \mu_{\text{p}}) \qquad (37.6)$$

The figure of merit for infrared detectors is called D^*. The units of D^* are cm $(\text{Hz})^{1/2}/\text{W}$, but are most commonly referred to as Jones. D^* is the detector's signal-to-noise (SNR) ratio, normalized to an area of 1 cm^2, to a noise bandwidth of 1 Hz, and to a signal level of 1 W at the peak of the detectors response. The equation for D^* is:

$$D_{\text{peak}}^* = \frac{R}{V_{\text{noise}}}\sqrt{WL}\,(\text{Jones}) \qquad (37.7)$$

where W and L are defined in Figure 37.1.

A special condition of D^* for a photoconductor is noted when the noise is dominated by the photon noise term. This is a condition in which the D^* is maximum.

$$D_{\text{blip}}^* = \frac{\lambda}{2hc}\sqrt{\frac{\eta}{E_{\text{ph}}}} \qquad (37.8)$$

where "blip" notes background-limited photodetector.

37.1.2 Photovoltaic Detectors

The mechanism of photovoltaic detectors is based on the collection of photoexcited carriers by a diode junction. Photovoltaic detectors are the most commonly used photon detectors for imaging arrays in current production. An example of the structure of detectors in such an array is illustrated in Figure 37.3 for a mesa photodiode. Photons are incident from the optically transparent detector substrate side and

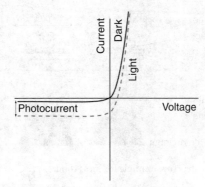

FIGURE 37.4   Current–voltage characteristics of a photovoltaic detector.

are absorbed in the n-type material layer. Absorbed photons create a pair of carriers, an electron and a hole. The hole diffuses to the p-type side of the junction creating a photocurrent. A contact on the p-type side of the junction is connected to an indium bump that mates to an amplifier in a readout circuit where the signal is stored and conveyed to a display during each display frame. A common contact is made to the n-type layer at the edge of the detector array. Adjacent diodes are isolated electrically from each other by a mesa etch cutting the p-type layer into islands.

Figure 37.4 illustrates how the current–voltage characteristics of a photodiode change with incident photon flux (Chapter 4).

The current of the photodiode can be expressed as:

$$I = I_0(e^{qV/kT} - 1) - I_{\text{photo}} \tag{37.9}$$

where I_0 is reverse-bias leakage current and I_{photo} is the photoinduced current. The photocurrent is given by:

$$I = I_0(e^{qV/kT} - 1) - I_{\text{photo}} \tag{37.10}$$

where Φ_0 is the photon flux in photons/cm^2/sec and A is the detector area.

Detector noise in a photodiode includes three terms: Johnson noise, thermal diffusion generation and recombination noise, and photon generation and recombination. The Johnson noise term, written in terms of the detector resistance $dI/dV = R_0$ at zero bias as:

$$i_{\text{Johnson}} = \sqrt{4kT/R_0} \tag{37.11}$$

where k is Boltzmann's constant and T is the detector temperature. The thermal diffusion current is given by:

$$i_{\text{diffusion noise}} = q\sqrt{2I_s \left[\exp\left(\frac{eV}{kT}\right) - 1 \right]} \tag{37.12}$$

where the saturation current, I_s, is given by:

$$I_s = qn_i^2 \left[\frac{1}{N_a}\sqrt{\frac{D_n}{\tau_{n0}}} + \frac{1}{N_d}\sqrt{\frac{D_p}{\tau_{p0}}} \right] \tag{37.13}$$

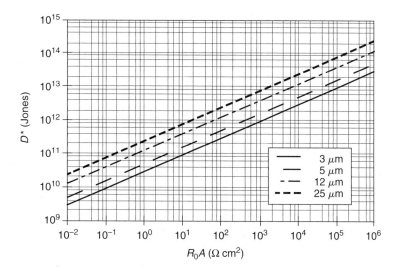

FIGURE 37.5 D^* as a function of the detector resistance-area product, R_0A. This condition applies when detector performance is limited by dark current.

where N_a and N_d are the concentration of p- and n-type dopants on either side of the diode junction, τ_{n0} and τ_{p0} are the carrier lifetimes, and D_n and D_p are the diffusion constants on either side of the junction, respectively.

The photon generation-recombination current noise is given by:

$$i_{\text{photon noise}} = q\sqrt{2\eta\Phi_0} \qquad (37.14)$$

When the junction is at zero bias, the photodiode D^* is given by:

$$D_\lambda^* = \frac{\lambda}{hc}\eta e \frac{1}{\left[(4kT/R_0A) + 2e^2\eta\right]} \qquad (37.15)$$

In the special case of a photodiode that is operated without sufficient cooling, the maximum D^* may be limited by the dark current or leakage current of the junction. The expression for D^* in this case, written in terms of the junction-resistance area product, R_0A, is given by:

$$D_\lambda^* = \frac{\lambda}{hc}\eta e \sqrt{\frac{R_0A}{4kT}} \qquad (37.16)$$

Figure 37.5 illustrates how D^* is limited by the R_0A product for the case of dark-current limited detector conditions.

For the ideal case where the noise is dominated by the photon flux in the background scene, the peak D^* is given by:

$$D_\lambda^* = \frac{\lambda}{hc}\sqrt{\frac{\eta}{2E_{\text{ph}}}} \qquad (37.17)$$

Comparing this limit with that for a photoconductive detector in Equation 37.8, we see that the background-limited D^* for a photodiode is higher by a factor of square root of 2 ($\sqrt{2}$).

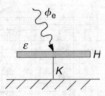

FIGURE 37.6 Abstract bolometer detector structure, where C is the thermal capacitance, G is the thermal conductance, and ε is the emissivity of the surface. Φ_e represents the energy flux in W/cm^2.

37.2 Thermal Detectors

Thermal detectors operate by converting the incoming photon flux to heat [3]. The heat input causes the thermal detector's temperature to rise and this change in temperature is sensed by a bolometer. A bolometer element operates by changing its resistance as its temperature is changed. A bias circuit across the bolometer can be used to convert the changing current to a signal output.

The coefficient α is used to compare the sensitivity of different bolometer materials and is given by:

$$\alpha = \frac{1}{R_d} \frac{dR}{dT} \tag{37.18}$$

where R_d is the resistance of the bolometer element, and dR/dT is the change in resistance per unit change in temperature. Typical values of α are 2 to 3%.

Theoretically, the bolometer structure can be represented as illustrated in Figure 37.6. The rise in temperature due to a heat flux ϕ_e is given by:

$$\Delta T = \frac{\eta P_0}{G(1 + \omega^2 \tau^2)^{1/2}} \tag{37.19}$$

where P_0 is the radiant power of the signal in watts, G is the thermal conductance (K/W), h is the percentage of flux absorbed, and ω is the angular frequency of the signal. The bolometer time constant, τ, is determined by:

$$\tau = \frac{C}{G} \tag{37.20}$$

where C is the heat capacity of detector element.

The sensitivity or D^* of a thermal detector is limited by variations in the detector temperature caused by fluctuations in the absorption and radiation of heat between the detector element and the background. Sensitive thermal detectors must minimize competing mechanisms for heat loss by the element, namely, convection and conduction.

Convection by air is eliminated by isolating the detector in a vacuum. If the conductive heat losses were less than those due to radiation, then the limiting D^* would be given by:

$$D^*(T, f) = 2.8 \times 10^{16} \sqrt{\frac{\varepsilon}{T_2^5 + T_1^5}} \text{Jone} \tag{37.21}$$

where T_1 is the detector temperature, T_2 the background temperature, and ε the value of the detector's emissivity and equally it's absorption. For the usual case of both the detector and background temperature at normal ambient, 300 K, the limiting D^* is 1.8×10^{10} Jones.

Bolometer operation is constrained by the requirement that the response time of the detector be compatible with the frame rate of the imaging system. Most bolometer cameras operate at a 30 Hz frame

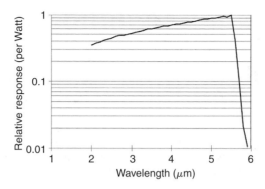

FIGURE 37.7   Spectral response per watt of an InSb detector at 80 K.

rate — 33 msec frame. Response times of the bolometer are usually designed to be on the order of 10 msec. This gives the element a fast enough response to follow scenes with rapidly varying temperatures without objectionable image smearing.

37.3   Detector Materials

The most popular commercial cameras for thermal imaging today use the following detector materials [4]:

- InSb for 5 μm medium wavelength infrared (MWIR) imaging
- $Hg_{1-x}Cd_xTe$ alloys for 5 and 10 μm long wavelength infrared (LWIR) imaging
- Quantum well detectors for 5 and 10 μm imaging
- Uncooled bolometers for 10 μm imaging

We will now review a few of the basic properties of these detector types.

Photovoltaic InSb remains a popular detector for the MWIR spectral band operating at a temperature of 80 K [5,6]. The detector's spectral response at 80 K is shown in Figure 37.7. The spectral response cutoff is about 5.5 μm at 80 K, a good match to the MWIR spectral transmission of the atmosphere. As the operating temperature of InSb is raised, the spectral response extends to longer wavelengths and the dark current increases accordingly. It is thus not normally used above about 100 K. At 80 K the R_0A product of InSb detectors is typically in the range of 10^5 to 10^6 Ω cm^2 — see Equation 37.16 and Figure 37.5 for reference.

Crystals of InSb are grown in bulk boules up to 3 in. in diameter. InSb materials is highly uniform and combined with a planar-implanted process in which the device geometry is precisely controlled, the resulting detector array responsivity is good to excellent. Devices are usually made with a p/n diode polarity using diffusion or ion implantation. Staring arrays of backside illuminated, direct hybrid InSb detectors in 256 × 256, 240 × 320, 480 × 640, 512 × 640, and 1024 × 1024 formats are available from a number of vendors.

HgCdTe detectors are commercially available to cover the spectral range from 1 to 12 μm [7–13]. Figure 37.8 illustrates representative spectral response from photovoltaic devices, the most commonly used type. Crystals of HgCdTe today are mostly grown in thin epitaxial layers on infrared-transparent CdZnTe crystals. SWIR and MWIR material can also be grown on Si substrates with CdZnTe buffer layers. Growth of the epitaxial layers is by liquid phase melts, molecular beams, or by chemical vapor deposition. Substrate dimensions of CdZnTe crystals are in the 25 to 50 cm^2 range and Si wafers up to 5 to 6 in. (12.5 to 15 cm) in diameter have been used for this purpose. The device structure for a typical HgCdTe photodiode is shown in Figure 37.3.

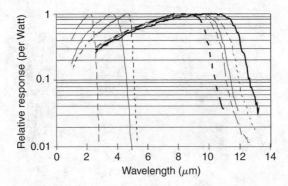

FIGURE 37.8 Representative spectral response curves for a variety of HgCdTe alloy detectors. Spectral cutoff can be varied over the SWIR, MWIR, and LWIR regions.

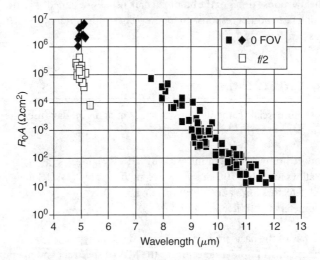

FIGURE 37.9 Values of R_0A product as a function of wavelength for HgCdTe photodiodes. Note that the R_0A product varies slightly with illumination — $0°$ field-of-view compared with $f/2$ — especially for shorter-wavelength devices.

At 80 K the leakage current of HgCdTe is small enough to provide both MWIR and LWIR detectors that can be photon-noise dominated. Figure 37.9 shows the R_0A product of representative diodes for wavelengths ranging from 4 to 12 μm.

The versatility of HgCdTe detector material is directly related to being able to grow a broad range of alloy compositions in order to optimize the response at a particular wavelength. Alloys are usually adjusted to provide response in the 1 to 3 μm short wavelength infrared (SWIR), 3 to 5 μm MWIR, or the 8 to 12 μm LWIR spectral regions. Short wavelength detectors can operate uncooled, or with thermoelectric coolers that have no moving parts. Medium and long wavelength detectors are generally operated at 80 K using a cryogenic cooler engine. HgCdTe detectors in 256 × 256, 240 × 320, 480 × 640, and 512 × 640 formats are available from a number of vendors.

Quantum well infrared photodetectors (QWIPs) consist of alternating layers of semiconductor material with larger and narrower bandgaps [14–20]. This series of alternating semiconductor layers is deposited one layer upon another using an ultrahigh vacuum technique such as molecular beam epitaxy (MBE). Alternating large and narrow bandgap materials give rise to quantum wells that provide bound and quasi-bound states for electrons or holes [1–5].

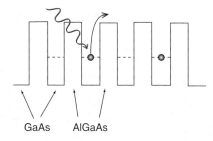

FIGURE 37.10 Quantum wells generate bound states for electrons in the conduction band. The conduction bands for a QWIP structure are shown consisting of $Al_xGa_{1-x}As$ barriers and GaAs wells. For a given pair of materials having a fixed conduction band offset, the binding energy of an electron in the well can be adjusted by varying the width of the well. With an applied bias, photoexcited electrons from the GaAs wells are transported and detected as photocurrent.

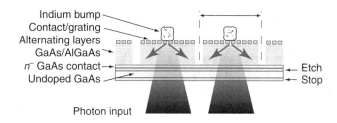

FIGURE 37.11 Backside illuminated QWIP structure with a top side diffraction grating/contact metal. Normally-incident light is coupled horizontally into the quantum wells by scattering off a diffraction grating located at the top of the focal plane array.

Many simple QWIP structures have used GaAs as the narrow bandgap quantum well material and $Al_xGa_{1-x}As$ as the wide bandgap barrier layers as shown in Figure 37.10. The properties of the QWIP are related to the structural design and can be specified by the well width, barrier height, and doping density. In turn, these parameters can be tuned by controlling the cell temperatures of the gallium, aluminum, and arsenic cells as well as the doping cell temperature. The quantum well width (thickness) is governed by the time interval for which the Ga and As cell shutters are left opened. The barrier height is regulated by the composition of the $Al_xGa_{1-x}As$ layers, which are determined by the relative temperature of the Al and Ga cells. QWIP detectors rely on the absorption of incident radiation within the quantum well and typically the well material is doped n-type at an approximate level of 5×10^{17}.

The QWIP detectors require that an electric field component of the incident radiation be perpendicular to the layer planes of the device. Imaging arrays use diffraction gratings as shown in Figure 37.11. In particular, the latter approach is of practical importance in order to realize two-dimensional detector arrays. The QWIP focal plane array is a reticulated structure formed by conventional photolithographic techniques. Part of the processing involves placing a two-dimensional metallic grating over the focal plane pixels. The grating metal is typically angled at 45° patterns to reflect incident light obliquely so as to couple the perpendicular component of the electric field into the quantum wells thus producing the photoexcitation. The substrate material (GaAs) is backside thinned and a chemical/mechanical polish is used to produce a mirrorlike finish on the backside. The front side of the pixels with indium bumps are flip-chip bonded to a readout IC. Light travels through the back side and is unabsorbed during its first pass through the epilayers; upon scattering with a horizontal propagation component from the grating some of it is then absorbed by the quantum wells, photoexciting carriers. An electric field is produced perpendicular to the layers by applying a bias voltage at doped contact layers. The structure then behaves as a photoconductor.

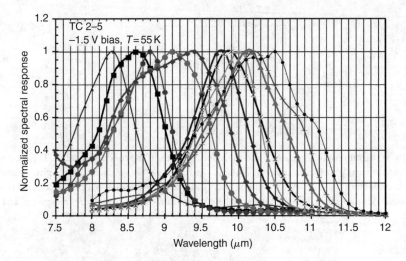

FIGURE 37.12 Representative spectral response of QWIP detectors.

The QWIP detectors require cooling to about 60 K for LWIR operation in order to adequately reduce the dark current. They also have comparatively low quantum efficiency, generally less than 10%. They thus require longer signal integration times than InSb or HgCdTe devices. However, the abundance of radiation in the LWIR band in particular allows QWIP detectors to still achieve excellent performance in infrared cameras.

The maturity of the GaAs-technology makes QWIPs particularly suited for large commercial focal plane arrays with high spatial resolution. Excellent lateral homogeneity is achieved, thus giving rise to a small fixed-pattern noise. QWIPs have an extremely small 1/f noise compared to interband detectors (like HgCdTe or InSb), which is particularly useful if long integration times or image accumulation are required. For these reasons, QWIP is the detector technology of choice for many applications where somewhat smaller quantum efficiencies and lower operation temperatures, compared to interband devices, are tolerable. QWIPs are finding useful applications in surveillance, night vision, quality control, inspection, environmental sciences, and medicine.

Quantum well infrared detectors are available in the 5- and 10-μm spectral region. The spectral response of QWIP detectors can be tuned to a wide range of values by adjusting the width and depth of quantum wells formed in alternating layers of GaAs and GaAlAs. An example of the spectral response from a variety of such structures is shown in Figure 37.12. QWIP spectral response is generally limited to fairly narrow spectral bandwidth — approximately 10 to 20% of the peak response wavelength. QWIP detectors have higher dark currents than InSb or HgCdTe devices and generally must be cooled to about 60 K for LWIR operation.

The quantum efficiencies of InSb, HgCdTe, and QWIP photon detectors are compared in Figure 37.13. With antireflection coating, InSb and HgCdTe are able to convert about 90% of the incoming photon flux to electrons. The QWIP quantum efficiencies are significantly lower, but work at improving them continues to occupy the attention of research teams.

We conclude this section with a description of Type-II superlattice detectors [21–26]. Although Type-II superlattice detectors are not yet used in arrays for in commercial camera system, the technology is briefly reviewed here because of its potential future importance. This material system mimics an intrinsic detector material such as HgCdTe, but is "bandgap engineered." Type-II superlattice structures are fabricated from multilayer stacks of alternating layers of two different semiconductor materials. Figure 37.14 illustrates the structure. The conduction band minimum is in one layer and the valence band minimum is in the adjacent layer (as opposed to both minima being in the same layer as in a Type-I superlattice).

The idea of using type-II superlattices for LWIR detectors was originally proposed in 1977. Recent work on the MBE growth of Type-II systems by [7] has led to the exploitation of these materials for IR

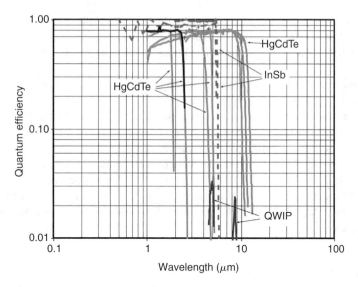

FIGURE 37.13 Comparison of the quantum efficiencies of commercial infrared photon detectors. This figure represents devices that have been antireflection coated.

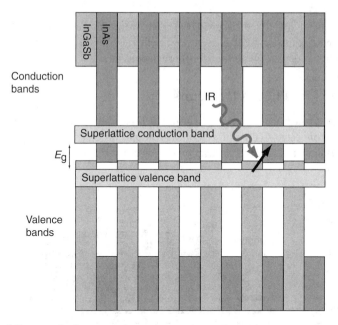

FIGURE 37.14 Band diagram of a short-period InAs/(In,Ga)Sb superlattice showing an infrared transition from the heavy hole (hh) miniband to the electron (e) miniband.

detectors. Short period superlattices of, for example, strain-balanced InAs/(Ga,In)Sb lead to the formation of conduction and valence minibands. In these band states heavy holes are largely confined to the (Ga,In)Sb layers and electrons are primarily confined to the InAs layers. However, because of the relatively low electron mass in InAs, the electron wave functions extend considerably beyond the interfaces and have significant overlap with heavy-hole wave functions. Hence, significant absorption is possible at the minigap energy (which is tunable by changing layer thickness and barrier height).

Cutoff wavelengths from 3 to 20 μm and beyond are potentially possible with this system. Unlike QWIP detectors, the absorption of normally incident flux is permitted by selection rules, obviating the need for grating structures or corrugations that are needed with QWIPs. Finally, Auger transition rates, which place intrinsic limits on the performance of these detectors and severely impact the lifetimes found in bulk, narrow-gap detectors, can be minimized by judicious choices of the structure's geometry and strain profile.

In the future, further advantages may be achievable by using the InAs/Ga(As,Sb) material system where both the InAs and Ga(As,Sb) layers may be lattice matched to InAs substrates. The intrinsic quality obtainable in these structures can be in principle superior to that obtained in InAs/(Ga,In)Sb structures. Since dislocations may be reduced to a minimum in the InAs/Ga(As,Sb) material system, it may be the most suitable Type-II material for making large arrays of photovoltaic detectors.

Development efforts for Type-II superlattice detectors are primarily focused on improving material quality and identifying sources of unwanted leakage currents. The most challenging problem currently is to passivate the exposed sidewalls of the superlattices layers where the pixels are etched in fabrication. Advances in these areas should result in a new class of IR detectors with the potential for high performance at high operating temperatures.

37.4 Detector Readouts

Detectors themselves are isolated arrays of photodiodes, photoconductors, or bolometers. Detectors need a readout to integrate or sample their output and convey the signal in an orderly sequence to a signal processor and display [27].

Almost all readouts are integrated circuits (ICs) made from silicon. They are commonly referred to as readout integrated circuits, or ROICs. Here we briefly describe the functions and features of these readouts, first for photon detectors and then for thermal detectors.

37.4.1 Readouts for Photon Detectors

Photon detectors are typically assembled as a hybrid structure, as illustrated in Figure 37.15. Each pixel of the detector array is connected to the unit cell of the readout through an indium bump. Indium bumps allow for a soft, low-temperature metal connection to convey the signal from the detector to the readout's input circuit.

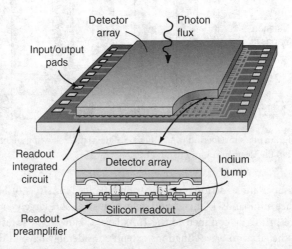

FIGURE 37.15 Hybrid detector array structure consists of a detector array connected to a readout array with indium metal bumps. Detector elements are usually photodiodes or photoconductors, although photocapacitors are sometimes used. Each pixel in the readout contains at least one addressable switch, and more often a preampflifier or buffer together with a charge storage capacitor for integrating the photosignal.

Commercial thermal imagers that operate in the MWIR and LWIR spectral regions generally employ a direct injection circuit to collect the detector signal. This is because this circuit is simple and works well with the relatively high photon currents in these spectral bands. The direct injection transistor feeds the signal onto an integrating capacitor where it stored for a time called the integration time. The integration time is typically around 200 μsec for the LWIR spectral band and 2 msec for the MWIR band, corresponding to the comparative difference in the photon flux available. The integration time is limited by the size of the integration capacitor. Typical capacitors can hold on the order of 3×10^7 electrons.

For cameras operating in the SWIR band, the lower flux levels typically require a more complicated input amplifier. The most common choice employs a capacitive feedback circuit, providing the ability to have significant gain at the pixel level before storage on an integrating capacitor.

Two readout modes are employed, depending upon the readout design:

- Snapshot
- Rolling frame

In the snapshot mode, all pixels integrate simultaneously, are stored, and then read out in sequence, followed by resetting the integration capacitors. In the rolling frame mode the capacitors of each row are reset after each pixel in that row is read. In this case each pixel integrates in different parts of the image frame. A variant of the rolling frame is an interlaced output. In this case the even rows are read out in the first frame and the odd rows in the next. This corresponds to how standard U.S. television displays function.

It is common for each column in the readout to have an amplifier to provide some gain to the signal coming from each row as it is read. The column amplifier outputs are then fed to the output amplifiers. Commercial readouts typically have one, two, or four outputs, depending upon the array size and frame rate. Most commercial cameras operate at 30 or 60 Hz.

Another common feature found on some readouts is the ability to operate at higher frame rates on a subset of the full array. This ability is called windowing. It allows data to be collected more quickly on a limited portion of the image.

37.4.2 Thermal Detector Readouts

Bolometer detectors have comparatively lower resistance than photon detectors and relatively slow inherent response times. This condition allows readouts that do not have to integrate the charge during the frame, but only need to sample it for a brief time. This mode is frequently referred to as pulse-biased.

The unit cell of the bolometer contains only a switch that is pulsed on once per frame to allow current to flow from each row in turn to the column amplifiers. Bias is supplied by the row multiplexer. Sample times for each detector are typically on the order of the frame time divided by the number of rows. Many designs employ differential input column amplifiers that are simultaneously fed an input from a dummy or blind bolometer element in order to subtract a large fraction of the current that flows when the element is biased.

The nature of bolometer operation means that the readout mode is rolling frame. Some designs also provide interlaced outputs for input to TV-like displays.

37.4.3 Readout Evolution

Early readouts required multiple bias supply inputs and multiple clock signals for operation. Today only two clocks and two bias supplies are typically required. The master clock sets the frame rate. The integration clock sets the time that the readout signal is integrated, or that the readout bias pulse is applied. On-chip clock and bias circuits generate the additional clocks and biases required to run the readout. Separate grounds for the analog and digital chip circuitry are usually employed to minimize noise.

Current development efforts are beginning to add on-chip analog-to-digital (A/D) converters to the readout. This feature provides a direct digital output, avoiding significant difficulties in controlling extraneous noise when the sensor is integrated with an imaging or camera system.

37.5   Technical Challenges for Infrared Detectors

Twenty-five years ago, infrared imagining was revolutionized by the introduction of the Probeye Infrared camera. At a modest 8 pounds, Probeye enabled handheld operation, a feature previously unheard of at that time when very large, very expensive IR imaging systems were the rule. Infrared components and technologies have advanced considerably since then. With the introduction of the Indigo Systems Omega camera, one can now acquire a complete infrared camera weighing less than 100 g and occupying 3.5 in.[3].

Many forces are at play enabling this dramatic reduction in camera size. Virtually all of these can be traced to improvements in the silicon IC processing industry. Largely enabled by advancements in photolithography, but additionally aided by improvements in vacuum deposition equipment, device feature sizes have been steadily reduced. It was not too long ago that the minimum device feature size was just pushing to break the 1-μm barrier. Today, foundries are focused on production implementation of 65 to 90 nm feature sizes.

The motivation behind such significant improvements has been the high-dollar/high-volume commercial electronics business. Silicon foundries have expended billions of dollars in capitalization and R&D aimed at increasing the density and speed of the transistors per unit chip area. Cellular telephones, personal data assistants (PDAs), and laptop computers are all applications demanding smaller size, lower power, and more features — performance — from electronic components. Infrared detector arrays and cameras have taken direct advantage of these advancements.

37.5.1   Uncooled Infrared Detector Challenges

The major challenge for all infrared markets is to reduce the pixel size while increasing the sensitivity. Reduction from a 50-μm pixel to a 25-μm pixel, while maintaining or even reducing noise equivalent temperature difference (NETD), is a major goal that is now being widely demonstrated (see Figure 37.16). The trends are illustrated by a simple examination of a highly idealized bolometer: the DC response of a detector in which we neglect all noise terms except temperature fluctuation noise, and the thermal conductance value is not detector area dependent (i.e., we are not at or near the radiation conductance limit). Using these assumptions, reducing the pixel area by a factor of four will reduce the SNR by a factor

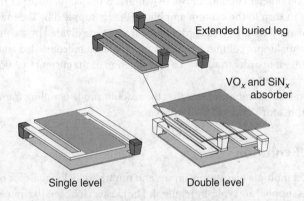

FIGURE 37.16   Uncooled microbolometer pixel structures having noise-equivalent temperature difference (NEΔT) values <50 mK: single level for 2 mil (50 μm) pixels in a 240 × 320 format and double level for 1 mil (25 μm) pixels in a 480 × 640 format (courtesy of Raytheon Vision Systems).

of eight as shown below:

$$\Delta T_{\text{signal}|\text{DCresponse}} = \frac{P_{\text{signalDC}}}{G_{\text{th}}} = \frac{\gamma A_{\text{D}} I_{\text{light}}}{G_{\text{th}}} \tag{37.22}$$

where P_{signalDC} is the DC signal from IR radiation (absorbed power) [W], A_{D} is the detector area [m^2], I_{light} is the light intensity [W/m^2], G_{th} is the thermal conductance [W/K], and γ is a constant that accounts for reflectivity and other factors not relevant to this analysis.

For a detector in the thermal fluctuation limit, the root mean square temperature fluctuation noise is a function of the incident radiation and the thermal conductance of the bolometer bridge.

$$\Delta T_{\text{noise}} \sqrt{\langle \Delta T^2 \rangle} = \sqrt{\frac{kT^2}{C_{\text{th}}}} \tag{37.23}$$

where T is the operating temperature in Kelvin, k is Boltzman's constant, and C_{th} is the total heat capacity of the detector in Joules per Kelvin [J/K].

The total heat capacity can be written as $C_{\text{th}} = c_{\text{p}} A_{\text{d}} Z_{\text{bridge}}$, where Z_{bridge} is the bolometer bridge thickness in meters and c_{p} is the specific heat of the detector in J/K-m^3.

The signal to noise (SNR) is then

$$\frac{\Delta T_{\text{signal}}}{\Delta T_{\text{noise}}} = \frac{\gamma A_{\text{D}} I_{\text{light}}}{G_{\text{th}}} \sqrt{\frac{c_{\text{p}} A_{\text{D}} Z_{\text{bridge}}}{kT^2}} = \frac{\gamma A_{\text{D}} I_{\text{light}}}{G_{\text{th}}} A_{\text{D}}^{3/2} \sqrt{\frac{c_{\text{p}} Z_{\text{bridge}}}{kT^2}} \tag{37.24}$$

It can be seen that the SNR goes as the area to the three halves. Therefore, a 4× reduction in detector area reduces the SNR by a factor of eight for this ideal bolometer case. Thermal conductance is assumed constant, that is, the ratio of leg length to thickness remains constant as the detector area is reduced. In practical constructions, reducing the pixel linear dimensions by 2× also reduces the leg length by 2×, thus the thermal conductance increases and aggravates the problem. In order to improve the SNR caused by the 4× loss in area, one may be tempted to reduce the thermal conductance G_{th} by 8×. To accomplish this, the length of the legs must be increased and their thickness reduced. By folding the legs under the detector, as seen in Figure 37.10, one can achieve this result. However, an 8× reduction in thermal conductance would result in a detrimental increase in the thermal time constant.

The thermal time constant is given by $\tau_{\text{thermal}} = C_{\text{th}}/G_{\text{th}}$. The heat capacity is reduced by 4× because of the area loss. If G_{th} is reduced by a factor of 8×, then $\tau_{\text{thermal}} = 2C_{\text{th}}/G_{\text{th}}$ is increased by a factor of two. This image smear associated with this increased time constant would prove problematic for practical military applications.

In order to maintain the same time constant, the total heat capacity must be reduced accordingly. Making the detector thinner may achieve this result except that it also increases the temperature fluctuation noise. From this simple example one can readily see the inherent relationship between SNR and the thermal time constant.

We would like to maintain both an equivalent SNR and thermal time constant as the detector cell size is decreased. This can be achieved by maintaining the relationships between the thermal conductance, detector area, and bridge thickness as shown in the following.

The thermal time constant is given by the following:

$$\tau_{\text{thermal}} = \frac{C_{\text{th}}}{G_{\text{th}}} = \frac{c_{\text{p}} A_{\text{D}} Z_{\text{bridge}}}{G_{\text{th}}} \tag{37.25}$$

Equating the thermal time constant of the large and small pixels equal and doing the same with the SNR leads to the following relationships, where the primed variables are the parameters required for the new detector cell:

$$\tau_{\text{thermal}} = \frac{c_p A_D Z_{\text{bridge}}}{G_{\text{th}}} = \frac{c_p A_D' Z_{\text{bridge}}'}{G_{\text{th}}'} \qquad (37.26)$$

$$\frac{\Delta T_{\text{signal}}}{\Delta T_{\text{noise}}} = \frac{\gamma A_D I_{\text{light}}}{G_{\text{th}}} \sqrt{\frac{c_p A_D Z_{\text{bridge}}}{kT^2}} = \frac{\gamma A_D' I_{\text{light}}}{G_{\text{th}}'} \sqrt{\frac{c_p A_D' Z_{\text{bridge}}'}{kT^2}} \qquad (37.27)$$

Rearranging τ_{thermal} to find the ratio $G_{\text{th}}/G_{\text{th}}'$ and substituting into the SNR, we obtain:

$$\frac{Z_{\text{bridge}}'}{Z_{\text{bridge}}} = \frac{A_D'}{A_D}, \quad \text{and it follows that} \quad \frac{G_{\text{th}}'}{G_{\text{th}}} = \left(\frac{Z_{\text{bridge}}'}{Z_{\text{bridge}}}\right)^2 \qquad (37.28)$$

So, it becomes evident that a $4\times$ reduction in pixel cell area requires a $16\times$, and not an $8\times$, reduction in thermal conductance to maintain equivalent SNR and thermal time constant. This gives some insight into the problems of designing small pixel bolometers for high sensitivity. It should be noted that in current implementations, the state-of-the-art sensitivity is about $10\times$ from the thermal limits.

37.5.2 Electronics Challenges

Specific technology improvements spawned by the commercial electronics business that have enabled size reductions in IR camera signal processing electronics include:

- Faster digital signal processors (DSPs) with internal memory ≥1 MB
- Higher-density field-programmable gate arrays (FPGAs) (>200 K gates and with an embedded processor core
- Higher-density static (synchronous?) random access memory >4 MB
- Low-power, 14-bit differential A/D converters

Another enabler, also attributable to the silicon industry, is reduction in the required core voltage of these devices (see Figure 37.17). Five years ago, the input voltage for virtually all-electronic components was 5 V. Today, one can buy a DSP with a core voltage as low as 1.2 V. Power consumption of the device is proportional to the square of the voltage. So a reduction from 5- to 1.2-V core represents more than an order of magnitude power reduction.

The input voltage ranges for most components (e.g., FPGAs, memories, etc.) are following the same trends. These reductions are not only a boon for reduced power consumption, but also these lower power devices typically come in much smaller footprints. IC packaging advancements have kept up with the

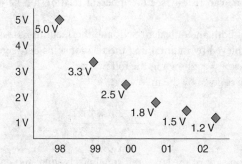

FIGURE 37.17 IC device core voltage vs. time

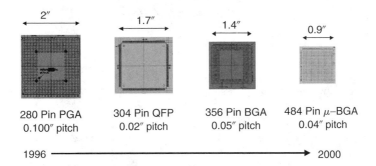

FIGURE 37.18 Advancements in component packaging miniaturization together with increasing pin count that enables reduced camera volume.

higher-density, lower-power devices. One can now obtain a device with almost twice the number of I/Os in 25% of the required area (see Figure 37.18).

All of these lower power, smaller footprint components exist by virtue of the significant demand created by the commercial electronics industry. These trends will continue. Moore's law (logic density in bits/in.[2] will double every 18 months) nicely describes the degree by which we can expect further advancements.

37.5.3 Detector Readout Challenges

The realization of tighter design rules positively affects reduction in camera size in yet another way. Multiplexers, or ROICs, directly benefit from the increased density. Now, without enlarging the size of the ROIC die, more functions can be contained in the device. On-ROIC A/D conversion eliminates the need for a dedicated, discrete A/D converter. On-ROIC clock and bias generation reduces the number of vacuum Dewar feedthroughs to yield a smaller package as well as reducing the complexity and size of the camera power supply. Putting the nonuniformity correction circuitry on the ROIC reduces the magnitude of the detector output signal swing and minimizes the required input dynamic range of the A/D converter. All of these increases in ROIC functionality come with the increased density of the silicon fabrication process.

37.5.4 Optics Challenges

Another continuing advancement that has helped reduced the size of IR cameras is the progress made at increasing the performance of the uncooled detectors themselves. The gains made at increasing the sensitivity of the detectors has directly translated to reduction in the size of the optics. With a sensitivity goal of 100 mK, an $F/1$ optic has traditionally been required to collect enough energy. Given the recent sensitivity improvements in detectors, achievement of 100 mK can be attained with an $F/2$ optic. This reduction in required aperture size greatly reduces the camera size and weight. These improvements in detector sensitivity can also be directly traceable to improvements in the silicon industry. The same photolithography and vacuum deposition equipments used to fabricate commercial ICs are used to make bolometers. The finer geometry line widths translate directly to increased thermal isolation and increased fill factor, both of which are factors in increased responsivity.

Reduction in optics' size was based on a sequence of NEDT performance improvements in uncooled VO_x microbolometer detectors so that faster optics $F/1.4$ to $F/2$ could be utilized in the camera and still maintain a moderate performance level. As indicated by Equation 37.29 to Equation 37.33, the size of the optics is based on the required field-of-view (FOV), number of detectors (format of the detector array), area of the detector, and F# of the optics (see Figure 37.19). The volume of the optics is considered to be approximately a cylinder with a volume of $\pi r^2 L$. In Equation 37.29 to Equation 37.33, FL is the optics focal length equivalent to L, D_o is the optics diameter and $D_o/2$ is equivalent to r, A_{det} is the area of the

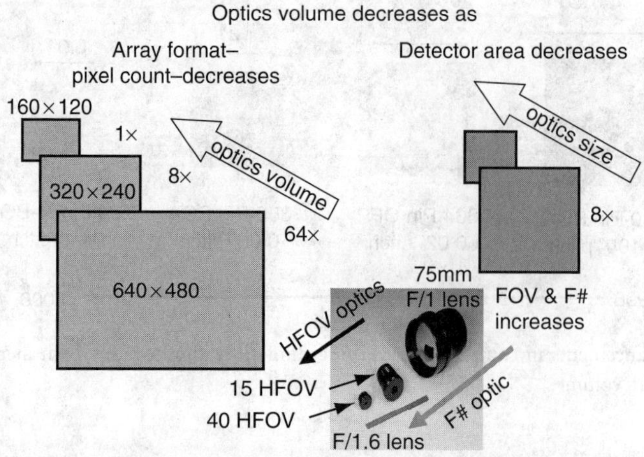

FIGURE 37.19 Trade-off between optics size and volume and $f/\#$, array format, and pixel size.

detector, $F\#$ is the f-number of the optics and HFOV is the horizontal field-of-view.

$$FL = \frac{\#\text{ horizontal detectors}}{\text{Tan(HFOV/2)}} = \frac{\sqrt{A_{\text{det}}}}{2} \tag{37.29}$$

$$D_0 = \frac{\#\text{ horizontal detectors}}{\text{Tan(HFOV/2)}} = \frac{\sqrt{A_{\text{det}}}}{2F\#} \tag{37.30}$$

$$F\# = \frac{FL}{D_0} \tag{37.31}$$

$$\text{Volume}_{\text{optics}} = \pi \left[\frac{D_0}{2}\right]^2 = FL$$

$$= \pi \left[\frac{(\#\text{ horizontal detectors}/(\tan(\text{HFOV}/2))) = (\sqrt{A_{\text{det}}}/2F\#)}{2}\right]^2 = FL \tag{37.32}$$

$$\text{Volume}_{\text{optics}} = \pi \left[\frac{(\#\text{ horizontal detectors}/(\tan(\text{HFOV}/2))) = \sqrt{A_{\text{det}}}}{32F\#^2}\right]^3 \tag{37.33}$$

Uncooled cameras have utilized the above enhancements and are now only a few ounces in weight and require only about 1 W of input power.

37.5.5 Challenges for Third-Generation Cooled Imagers

Third-generation cooled imagers are being developed to greatly extend the range at which targets can be detected and identified [28–30]. U.S. Army rules of engagement now require identification prior to attack. Since deployment of first- and second-generation sensors there has been a gradual proliferation of thermal imaging technology worldwide. Third-generation sensors are intended to ensure that U.S. Army forces maintain a technological advantage in night operations over any opposing force.

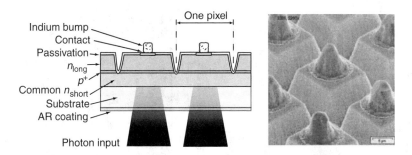

FIGURE 37.20 Illustration of a simultaneous two-color pixel structure — cross section and SEM. Simultaneous two-color FPAs have two indium bumps per pixel. A 50-μm simultaneous two-color pixel is shown.

Thermal imaging equipment is used to first detect an object, and then to identify it. In the detection mode, the optical system provides a wide field-of-view (WFOV — $f/2.5$) to maintain robust situational awareness [31]. For detection, LWIR provides superior range under most Army fighting conditions. Medium wavelength infrared offers higher spatial resolution sensing, and a significant advantage for long-range identification when used with telephoto optics (NFOV — $f/6$).

37.5.5.1 Cost Challenges — Chip Size

Cost is a direct function of the chip size since the number of detector and readout die per wafer is inversely proportion to the chip area. Chip size in turn is set by the array format and pixel size. Third-generation imager formats are anticipated to be in a high-definition 16 × 9 layout, compatible with future display standards, and reflecting the soldier's preference for a wide field-of-view. An example of such a format is 1280 × 720 pixels. For a 30 μm pixel this format yields a die size greater than 1.5 × 0.85 in. (22 × 38 mm). This will yield only a few die per wafer, and will also require the development of a new generation of dewar-cooler assemblies to accommodate these large dimensions. A pixel size of 20 μm results in a cost saving of more than 2×, and allows the use of existing dewar designs.

37.5.5.1.1 Two-Color Pixel Designs

Pixel size is the most important factor for achieving affordable third-generation systems. Two types of two-color pixels have been demonstrated. Simultaneous two-color pixels have two indium–bump connections per pixel to allow readout of both color bands at the same time. Figure 37.20 shows an example of a simultaneous two-color pixel structure. The sequential two-color approach requires only one indium bump per pixel, but requires the readout circuit to alternate bias polarities multiple times during each frame. An example of this structure is illustrated in Figure 37.21. Both approaches leave very little area available for the indium bump(s) as the pixel size is made smaller. Advanced etching technology is being developed in order to meet the challenge of shrinking the pixel size to 20 μm.

37.5.5.2 Sensor Format and Packaging Issues

The sensor format was selected to provide a wide field-of-view and high spatial resolution. Target detection in many Army battlefield situations is most favorable in LWIR. Searching for targets is more efficient in a wider field-of-view, in this case $F/2.5$. Target identification relies on having 12 or more pixels across the target to adequately distinguish its shape and features. Higher magnification, $F/6$ optics combined with MWIR optical resolution enhances this task.

Consideration was also given to compatibility with future standards for display formats. Army soldiers are generally more concerned with the width of the display than the height, so the emerging 16 : 9 width to height format that is planned for high-definition TV was chosen.

A major consideration in selecting a format was the packaging requirements. Infrared sensors must be packaged in a vacuum enclosure and mated with a mechanical cooler for operation. Overall array size was therefore limited to approximately 1 in. so that it would fit in an existing standard advanced dewar

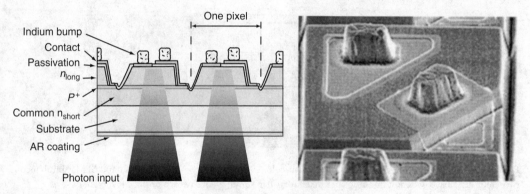

FIGURE 37.21 Illustration of a sequential two-color pixel structure — cross section and SEM. Sequential two-color FPAs have only one indium bump per pixel, helping to reduce pixel size. A 20 μm sequential two-color pixel is shown.

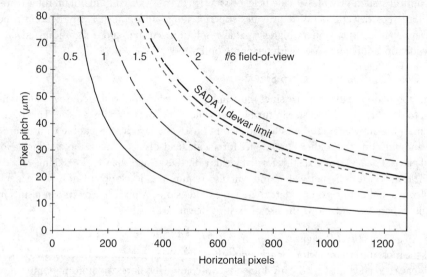

FIGURE 37.22 Maximum array horizontal format is determined by the pixel size and the chip size limit that will fit in an existing SADA dewar design for production commonality. For a 20-μm pixel and a 1.6° FOV, the horizontal pixel count limit is 1280. A costly development program would be necessary to develop a new, larger dewar.

assembly (SADA) dewar design. Figure 37.22 illustrates the pixel size/format/field-of-view trade within the design size constraints of the SADA dewar.

37.5.5.3 Temperature Cycling Fatigue

Modern cooled infrared focal plane arrays are hybrid structures comprising a detector array mated to a silicon readout array with indium bumps (see Figure 37.15).

Very large focal plane arrays may exceed the limits of hybrid reliability engineered into these structures. The problem stems from the differential rates of expansion between HgCdTe and Si, which results in large stress as a device is cooled from 300 K ambient to an operating temperature in the range of 77 to 200 K. Hybrids currently use mechanical constraints to force the contraction of the two components to closely match each other. This approach may have limits — when the stress reaches a point where the chip fractures.

Two new approaches exist that can extend the maximum array size considerably. One is the use of silicon as the substrate for growing the HgCdTe detector layer using MBE. This approach has shown excellent

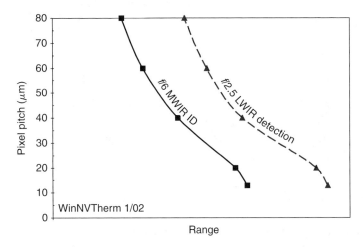

FIGURE 37.23 Range improves as the pixel size is reduced until a limit in optical blur is reached. In the examples above, the blur circle for the MWIR and LWIR cases are comparable since the f/number has been adjusted accordingly. D^* and integration time have been held constant in this example.

results for MWIR detectors, but not yet for LWIR devices. Further improvement in this approach would be needed to use it for Third-Generation MWIR/LWIR two-color arrays.

A second approach that has proven successful for InSb hybrids is thinning the detector structure. HgCdTe hybrids currently retain their thick, 500 μm, CdZnTe epitaxial substrate in the hybridized structure. InSb hybrids must remove the substrate because it is not transparent, leaving only a 10-μm thick detector layer. The thinness of this layer allows it to readily expand and contract with the readout. InSb hybrids with detector arrays over 2 in. (5 cm) on a side have been successfully demonstrated to be reliable.

Hybrid reliability issues will be monitored as a third-generation sensor manufacturing technology and is developed to determine whether new approaches are needed.

In addition to cost issues, significant performance issues must also be addressed for third-generation imagers. These are now discussed in the following section.

37.5.5.4 Performance Challenges

37.5.5.4.1 Dynamic Range and Sensitivity Constraints

A goal of third-generation imagers is to achieve a significant improvement in detection and ID range over Second-Generation systems. Range improvement comes from higher pixel count, and to a lesser extent from improved sensitivity. Figure 37.23 shows relative ID and detection range vs. pixel size in the MWIR and LWIR, respectively. Sensitivity (D^* and integration time) have been held constant, and the format was varied to keep the field-of-view constant.

Sensitivity has less effect than pixel size for clear atmospheric conditions, as illustrated by the clear atmosphere curve in Figure 37.24. Note that here the sensitivity is varied by an order of magnitude, corresponding to two orders of magnitude increase in integration time. Only a modest increase in range is seen for this dramatic change in SNR ratio. In degraded atmospheric conditions, however, improved sensitivity plays a larger role because the signal is weaker. This is illustrated in Figure 37.24 by the curve showing range under conditions of reduced atmospheric transmission.

Dynamic range of the imager output must be considered from the perspective of the quantum efficiency and the effective charge storage capacity in the pixel unit cell of the readout. Quantum efficiency and charge storage capacity determine the integration time for a particular flux rate. As increasing number of quanta are averaged, the SNR ratio improves as the square root of the count. Higher accuracy A/D converters are therefore required to cope with the increased dynamic range between the noise and signal levels. Figure 37.25 illustrates the interaction of these specifications.

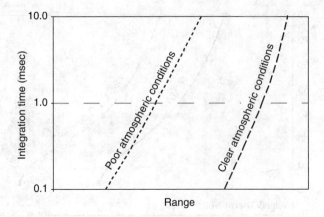

FIGURE 37.24   Range in a clear atmosphere improves only modestly with increased sensitivity. The case modeled here has a 20 μm pixel, a fixed D^*, and variable integration time. The 100× range of integration time corresponds to a 10× range in SNR. Improvement is more dramatic in the case of lower-atmospheric transmission that results in a reduced target signal.

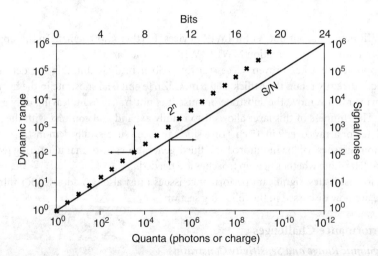

FIGURE 37.25   Dynamic range (2^n) corresponding to the number of digital bits (n) is plotted as a discrete point corresponding to each bit and referenced to the left and top scales. SNR ratio, corresponding to the number of quanta collected (either photons or charge) is illustrated by the solid line in reference to the bottom- and right-hand scales.

System interface considerations lead to some interesting challenges and dilemmas. Imaging systems typically specify a noise floor from the readout on the order of 300 μV. This is because system users do not want to encounter sensor signal levels below the system noise level. With readouts built at commercial silicon foundries now having submicrometer design rules, the maximum bias voltage applied to the readout is limited to a few volts — this trend has been downward from 5 V in the past decade as design rules have shrunk, as illustrated in Figure 37.26. Output swing voltages can only be a fraction of the maximum applied voltage, on the order of 3 V or less.

This means that the dynamic range limit of a readout is about 10,000 — 80 db in power — or less. Present readouts almost approach this constraining factor with 70 to 75 db achieved in good designs. In order to significantly improve sensitivity, the noise floor will have to be reduced.

If sufficiently low readout noise could be achieved, and the readout could digitize on chip to a level of 15 to 16 bits, the data could come off digitally and the system noise floor would not be an issue. Such developments may allow incremental improvement in third-generation imagers in the

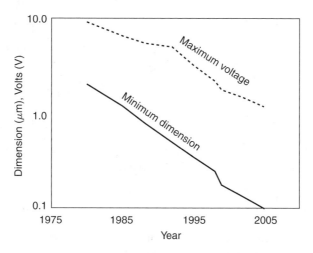

FIGURE 37.26 Trends for design rule minimum dimensions and maximum bias voltage of silicon foundry requirements.

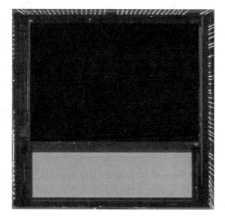

FIGURE 37.27 Focal planes with on-chip A/D converters have been demonstrated. This example shows a 900 × 120 TDI scanning format array. Photo supplied by Lester Kozlowski of Rockwell Scientific, Camarillo, CA.

future. Figure 37.27 illustrates an example of an on-chip A/D converter that has demonstrated 12 bits on chip.

A final issue here concerns the ability to provide high charge storage density within the small pixel dimensions envisioned for third-generation imagers. This may be difficult with standard CMOS capacitors. Reduced oxide thickness of submicrometer design rules does give larger capacitance per unit area, but the reduced bias voltage largely cancels any improvement in charge storage density. Promising technology in the form of ferroelectric capacitors may provide much greater charge storage densities than the oxide-on-silicon capacitors now used. Such technology is not yet incorporated into standard CMOS foundries. Stacked hybrid structures[1] [32] may be needed as at least an interim solution to incorporate the desired charge storage density in detector-readout-capacitor structures.

37.5.5.4.2 High Frame Rate Operation

Frame rates of 30 to 60 fps are adequate for visual display. In third-generation systems we plan to deploy high frame rate capabilities to provide more data throughput for advanced signal processing functions

---

[1]It should be noted that the third-generation imager will operate as an on-the-move wide area step-scanner wit automated ATR versus second-generation systems that rely on manual target searching. This allows the overall narrower field of view for the third-generation imager.

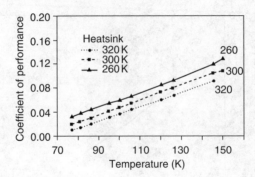

FIGURE 37.28   Javelin cooler coefficient of performance vs. temperature.

such as automatic target recognition (ATR), and missile and projectile tracking. An additional benefit is
the opportunity to collect a higher percentage of available signal. Higher frame rates pose two significant
issues. First, output drive power is proportional to the frame rate and at rates of 480 Hz or higher, this
could be the most significant source of power dissipation on the readout. Increased power consumption
on chip will also require more power consumption by the cryogenic cooler. These considerations lead
us to conclude that high frame rate capabilities need to be limited to a small but arbitrarily positioned
window of 64 × 64 pixels, for which a high frame rate of 480 Hz can be supported. This allows for ATR
functions to be exercised on possible target locations within the full field-of-view.

37.5.5.4.3 *Higher Operating Temperature*

Current tactical infrared imagers operate at 77 K with few exceptions — notably MWIR HgCdTe, which
can use solid-state thermoelectric (TE) cooling. Power can be saved, and cooler efficiency and cooler
lifetime improved if focal planes operate at temperatures above 77 K.

Increasing the operating temperature results in a major reduction of input cryogenic cooler power. As
can be seen from Figure 37.28 the coefficient of performance (COP) increases by a factor of 2.4 from 2.5
to 6% as the operating temperature is raised from 80 to 120 K with a 320 K heat sink. If the operating
temperature can be increased to 150 K, the COP increases fourfold. This can have a major impact on input
power, weight, and size.

Research is underway on an artificial narrow bandgap intrinsic-like material — strained-layer superlattices of InGaAsSb — which have the potential to increase operating temperatures to even higher levels
[33]. Results from this research may be more than a decade away, but the potential benefits are significant
in terms of reduced cooler operating power and maintenance.

The above discussion illustrates some of the challenges facing the development of third-generation
cooled imagers. In addition to these are the required advances in signal processing and display technologies
to translate the focal plane enhancements into outputs for the user. These advances can be anticipated
to not only help to increase the range at which targets can be identified, but also to increase the rate
of detection and identification through the use of two-color cues. Image fusion of the two colors in
some cases is anticipated to help find camouflaged targets in clutter. Improved sensitivity and two-color
response is further anticipated to minimize the loss of target contrast now encountered because of diurnal
crossover. Future two-color imagers together with novel signal processing methods may further enhance
the ability to detect land mines and find obscured targets.

37.6 Summary

Infrared sensors have made major performance strides in the last few years, especially in the uncooled
sensors area. Cost, weight, and size of the uncooled have dramatically been reduced allowing a greater proliferation into the commercial market. Uncooled sensors will find greater use in the medical community

as a result. High-performance cooled sensors have also been dramatically improved including the development of multicolor arrays. The high-performance sensors will find new medical applications because of the color discrimination and sensitivity attributes now available.

References

[1] D.G. Crowe, P.R. Norton, T. Limperis, and J. Mudar, Detectors, in *Electro-Optical Components*, W.D. Rogatto, Ed., Vol. 3, ERIM, Ann Arbor, MI; *Infrared & Electro-Optical Systems Handbook*, J.S. Accetta and D.L. Schumaker, Executive Eds., SPIE, Bellingham, WA, 1993, revised 1996, Chapter 4, pp. 175–283.

[2] P.R. Norton, Detector focal plane array technology, in *Encyclopedia of Optical Engineering*, Vol. 1, R.G. Driggers, Ed., Marcel Dekker, New York, 2003, pp. 320–348.

[3] P.W. Kruse and D.D. Skatrud, Eds., Uncooled infrared imaging arrays and systems in *Semiconductors and Semimetals*, R.K. Willardson and E.R. Weber, Eds., Academic Press, New York, 1997.

[4] P. Norton, Infrared image sensors, *Opt. Eng.*, 30, 1649–1663, 1991.

[5] T. Ashley, I.M. Baker, T.M. Burke, D.T. Dutton, J.A. Haigh, L.G. Hipwood, R. Jefferies, A.D. Johnson, P. Knowles, and J.C. Little, *Proc. SPIE*, 4028, 2000, pp. 398–403

[6] P.J. Love, K.J. Ando, R.E. Bornfreund, E. Corrales, R.E. Mills, J.R. Cripe, N.A. Lum, J.P. Rosbeck, and M.S. Smith, Large-format infrared arrays for future space and ground-based astronomy applications, *Proceedings of SPIE; Infrared Spaceborne Remote Sensing IX*, vol. 4486–38; pp. 373–384, 29 July–3 August, 2001; San Diego, USA.

[7] The photoconductive and photovoltaic detector technology of HgCdTe is summarized in the following references: D. Long and J.L. Schmidt, Mercury-cadmium telluride and closely related alloys, in *Semiconductors and Semimetals* 5, R.K. Willardson and A.C. Beer, Eds., Academic Press, New York, pp. 175–255, 1970; R.A. Reynolds, C.G. Roberts, R.A. Chapman, and H.B. Bebb, Photo-conductivity processes in 0.09 eV bandgap HgCdTe, in *Proceedings of the 3rd International Conference on Photoconductivity*, E.M. Pell, Ed., Pergamon Press, New York, p. 217, 1971; P.W. Kruse, D. Long, and O.N. Tufte, Photoeffects and material parameters in HgCdTe alloys, in *Proceedings of the 3rd International Conference on Photoconductivity*, E.M. Pell, Ed., Pergamon Press, New York, p. 233, 1971; R.M. Broudy and V.J. Mazurczyk (HgCd) Te photoconductive detectors, in *Semiconductors and Semimetals*, 18, R.K. Willardson and A.C. Beer, Eds., chapter 5, Academic Press, New York, pp. 157–199, 1981; M.B. Reine, A.K. Sood, and T.J. Tredwell, Photovoltaic infrared detectors, in *Semiconductors and Semimetals*, 18, R.K. Willardson and A.C. Beer, Eds., chapter 6, pp. 201–311; D. Long, Photovoltaic and photoconductive infrared detectors, in *Topics in Applied Physics* 19, *Optical and Infrared Detectors*, R.J. Keyes, Ed., Springer-Verlag, Heidelberg, pp.101–147, 1970; C.T. Elliot, infrared detectors, in *Handbook on Semiconductors* 4, C. Hilsum, Ed., chapter 6B, North Holland, New York, pp. 727–798, 1981.

[8] P. Norton, Status of infrared detectors, *Proc. SPIE*, 2274, 82–92, 1994.

[9] I.M., Baker, Photovoltaic IR detectors in *Narrow-gap II–VI Compounds for Optoelectronic and Electromagnetic Applications*, P. Capper, Ed., Chapman and Hall, London, pp. 450–73, 1997.

[10] P. Norton, Status of infrared detectors, *Proc. SPIE*, 3379, 102–114, 1998.

[11] M. Kinch., HDVIP® FPA technology at DRS, *Proc. SPIE*, 4369, pp. 566–578, 1999.

[12] M.B. Reine., Semiconductor fundamentals — materials: fundamental properties of mercury cadmium telluride, in *Encyclopedia of Modern Optics*, Academic Press, London, 2004.

[13] A. Rogalski., HgCdTe infrared detector material: history, status and outlook, *Rep. Prog. Phys.* 68, 2267–2336, 2005.

[14] S.D. Guanapala, B.F. Levine, and N. Chand, *J. Appl. Phys.*, 70, 305, 1991.

[15] B.F. Levine, *J. Appl. Phys.*, 47, R1–R81, 1993.

[16] K.K. Choi., *The Physics of Quantum Well Infrared Photodetectors*, World Scientific, River Edge, New Jersey, 1997.

[17] S.D. Gunapala, J.K. Liu, J.S. Park, M. Sundaram, C.A. Shott, T. Hoelter, T.-L. Lin, S.T. Massie, P.D. Maker, R.E. Muller, and G. Sarusi, 9 μm Cutoff 256×256 GaAs/AlGaAs quantum well infrared photodetector hand-held camera, *IEEE Trans. Elect. Dev.*, 45, 1890, 1998.

[18] S.D. Gunapala, S.V. Bandara, J.K. Liu, W. Hong, M. Sundaram, P.D. Maker, R.E. Muller, C.A. Shott, and R. Carralejo, Long-wavelength 640×480 GaAs/AlGaAs quantum well infrared photodetector snap-shot camera, *IEEE Trans. Elect. Dev.*, 44, 51–57, 1997.

[19] M.Z. Tidrow et al., Device physics and focal plane applications of QWIP and MCT, *Opto-Elect. Rev.*, 7, 283–296, 1999.

[20] S.D. Gunapala and S.V. Bandara, Quantum well infrared photodetector (QWIP) focal plane arrays, in *Semiconductors and Semimetals*, R.K. Willardson and E.R. Weber, Eds., 62, Academic Press, New York, 1999.

[21] G.A. Sai-Halasz, R. Tsu, and L. Esaki, *Appl. Phys. Lett.* 30, 651, 1977.

[22] D.L. Smith and C. Mailhiot, Proposal for strained type II superlattice infrared detectors, *J. Appl. Phys.*, 62, 2545–2548, 1987.

[23] S.R. Kurtz, L.R. Dawson, T.E. Zipperian, and S.R. Lee, Demonstration of an InAsSb strained-layer superlattice photodiode, *Appl. Phys. Lett.*, 52, 1581–1583, 1988.

[24] R.H. Miles, D.H. Chow, J.N. Schulman, and T.C. McGill, Infrared optical characterization of InAs/GaInSb superlattices, *Appl. Phys. Lett.* 57, 801–803, 1990.

[25] F. Fuchs, U.Weimar, W. Pletschen, J. Schmitz, E. Ahlswede, M. Walther, J. Wagner, and P. Koidl, *J. Appl. Phys. Lett.*, 71, 3251, 1997.

[26] Gail J. Brown, Type-II InAs/GaInSb superlattices for infrared detection: an overview, *Proceedings of SPIE*, 5783, pp. 65–77, 2005.

[27] J.L. Vampola, Readout electronics for infrared sensors, in *electro-optical components*, chapter 5, vol. 3, W.D. Rogatto, Ed., *Infrared & Electro-Optical Systems Handbook,* J.S. Accetta and D.L. Schumaker, Executive Eds., *ERIM*, Ann Arbor, MI and *SPIE*, Bellingham, WA, pp. 285–342, 1993, revised 1996.

[28] D. Reago, S. Horn, J. Campbell, and R. Vollmerhausen, Third generation imaging sensor system concepts, *SPIE*, 3701, 108–117, 1999.

[29] P. Norton*, J. Campbell III, S. Horn, and D. Reago, Third-generation infrared imagers, *Proc. SPIE*, 4130, 226–236, 2000.

[30] S. Horn, P. Norton, T. Cincotta, A. Stoltz, D. Benson, P. Perconti, and J. Campbell, Challenges for third-generation cooled imagers, *Proc. SPIE*, 5074, 44–51, 2003.

[31] S. Horn, D. Lohrman, P. Norton, K. McCormack, and A. Hutchinson, Reaching for the sensitivity limits of uncooled and minimally cooled thermal and photon infrared detectors, *Proc. SPIE*, 5783, 401–411, 2005.

[32] W. Cabanskia, K. Eberhardta, W. Rodea, J. Wendlera, J. Zieglera, J.Fleißnerb, F. Fuchsb, R. Rehmb, J. Schmitzb, H. Schneiderb, and M. Walther, 3rd gen focal plane array IR detection modules and applications, *Proc. SPIE*, 5406, 184–192, 2004.

[33] S. Horn, P. Norton, K. Carson#, R. Eden, and R. Clement, Vertically-integrated sensor arrays — VISA, *Proc. SPIE*, 5406, 332–340, 2004.

[34] R. Balcerak and S. Horn, Progress in the development of vertically-integrated sensor arrays, *Proc. SPIE*, 5783, 384–391, 2005.

38

Infrared Camera Characterization

Joseph G. Pellegrino
Jason Zeibel
Ronald G. Driggers
Philip Perconti
U.S. Army Communications and Electronics Research, Development and Engineering Center (CERDEC) Night Vision and Electronic Sensors Directorate

38.1 Dimensional Noise **38**-3
38.2 Noise Equivalent Temperature Difference **38**-5
38.3 Dynamic Range **38**-6
38.4 Modulation Transfer Function **38**-8
38.5 Minimum Resolvable Temperature **38**-8
38.6 Spatial Resolution **38**-9
     Pixel Size
References **38**-10

Many different types of infrared (IR) detector technology are now commercially available and the physics of their operation has been described in an earlier chapter. IR imagers are classified by different characteristics such as scan type, detector material, cooling requirements, and detector physics. Thermal imaging cameras prior to the 1990s typically contained a relatively small number of IR photosensitive detectors. These imagers were known as *cooled scanning systems* because they required cooling to cryogenic temperatures and a mechanical scan mirror to construct a two-dimensional (2D) image of the scene. Large 2D arrays of IR detectors, or staring arrays, have enabled the development of *cooled staring systems* that maintain sensitivity over a wide range of scene flux conditions, spectral bandwidths, and frame rates. Staring arrays consisting of small bolometric detector elements, or microbolometers, have enabled the development of *uncooled staring systems* that are compact, lightweight, and low power (see Figure 38.1).

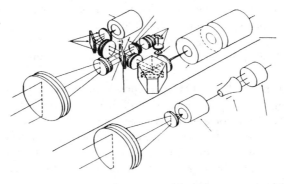

FIGURE 38.1   Scanning and staring system designs.

The sensitivity, or thermal resolution, of uncooled microbolometer focal plane arrays has improved dramatically over the past decade, resulting in IR video cameras that can resolve temperature differences under nominal imaging conditions as small as twenty millidegrees Kelvin using f/1.0 optics. Advancements in the manufacturing processes used by the commercial silicon industry have been instrumental in this progress. Uncooled microbolometer structures are typically fabricated on top of silicon integrated circuitry (IC) designed to readout the changes in resistance for each pixel in the array. The silicon-based IC serves as an electrical and mechanical interface for the IR microbolometer.

The primary measures of IR sensor performance are sensitivity and resolution. When measurements of end-to-end or human-in-the-loop (HITL) performance are required, the visual acuity of an observer through a sensor is included. The sensitivity and resolution are both related to the hardware and software that comprises the system, while the HITL includes both the sensor and the observer. Sensitivity is determined through radiometric analysis of the scene environment and the quantum electronic properties of the detectors. Resolution is determined by analysis of the physical optical properties, the detector array geometry, and other degrading components of the system in much the same manner as complex electronic circuit/signals analysis. The sensitivity of cooled and uncooled staring IR video cameras has improved by more than a factor of ten compared to scanning systems commercially available in the 1980s and early 1990s.[11,12]

Sensitivity describes how the sensor performs with respect to input signal level. It relates noise characteristics, responsivity of the detector, light gathering of the optics, and the dynamic range of the sensor. Radiometry describes how much light leaves the object and background and is collected by the detector. Optical design and detector characteristics are of considerable importance in sensor sensitivity analysis. In IR systems, noise equivalent temperature difference (NETD) is often a first order description of the system sensitivity. The three-dimensional (3D) noise model [1] describes more detailed representations of sensitivity parameters. The sensitivity of scanned long-wave infrared (LWIR) cameras operating at video frame rates is typically limited by very short detector integration times on the order of tens or hundreds of microseconds. The sensitivity of staring IR systems with high quantum efficiency detectors is often limited by the charge integration capacity, or well capacity, of the readout integrated circuit (ROIC). The detector integration time of staring IR cameras can be tailored to optimize sensitivity for a given application and may range from microseconds to tens of milliseconds.

The second type of measure is resolution. Resolution is the ability of the sensor to image small targets and to resolve fine detail in large targets. Modulation transfer function (MTF) is the most widely used resolution descriptor in IR systems. Alternatively, it may be specified by a number of descriptive metrics such as the optical Rayleigh Criterion or the instantaneous field-of-view of the detector. Where these metrics are component-level descriptions, the system MTF is an all-encompassing function that describes the system resolution. Sensitivity and resolution can be competing system characteristics and they are the most important issues in initial studies for a design. For example, given a fixed sensor aperture diameter, an increase in focal length can provide an increase in resolution, but may decrease sensitivity [2]. A more detailed consideration of the optical design parameters is included in the next chapter.

Quite often metrics, such as NETD and MTF, are considered separable. However, in an actual sensor, sensitivity and resolution performance are interrelated. As a result, minimum resolvable temperature difference (MRT or MRTD) has become a primary performance metric for IR systems.

This chapter addresses the parameters that characterize a camera's performance. A website advertising IR camera would in general contain a specification sheet that contains some variation of the terms that follow. A goal of this section is to give the reader working knowledge of these terms so as to better enable them to obtain the correct camera for their application:

- Three-dimensional noise
- NETD (Noise equivalent temperature difference)
- Dynamic range
- MTF

- MRT (minimum resolvable temperature) and MDT (minimum detectable temperature)
- Spatial resolution
- Pixel size

38.1 Dimensional Noise

The 3D noise model is essential for describing the sensitivity of an optical sensor system. Modern imaging sensors incorporate complex focal plane architectures and sophisticated postdetector processing and electronics. These advanced technical characteristics create the potential for the generation of complex noise patterns in the output imagery of the system. These noise patterns are deleterious and therefore need to be analyzed to better understand their effects upon performance. Unlike classical systems where "well behaved" detector noise predominates, current sensor systems have the ability to generate a wide variety of noise types, each with distinctive characteristics temporally, as well as along the vertical and horizontal image directions. Earlier methods for noise measurements at the detector preamplifier port that ignored other system noise sources are no longer satisfactory. System components following the stage that include processing may generate additional noise and even dominate total system noise.

Efforts at the Night Vision and Electronic Sensor Directorate to measure 2nd generation IR sensors uncovered the need for a more comprehensive method to characterize noise parameters. It was observed that the noise patterns produced by these systems exhibited a high degree of directionality. The data set is 3D with the temporal dimension representing the frame sequencing and the two spatial dimensions representing the vertical and horizontal directions within the image (see Figure 38.2).

To acquire this data cube, the field of view of a camera to be measured is flooded with a uniform temperature reference. A set number n (typically around 100) of successive frames of video data are then collected. Each frame of data consists of the measured response (in volts) to the uniform temperature source from each individual detector in the 2D focal plane array (FPA). When many successive frames of data are "stacked" together, a uniform source data cube is constructed. The measured response may be either analog (RS-170) or digital (RS-422, Camera Link, Hot Link, etc.) in nature depending on the camera interface being studied.

To recover the overall temporal noise, first the temporal noise is calculated for each detector in the array. A standard deviation of the n measured voltage responses for each detector is calculated. For an h by v array, there are hv separate values where each value is the standard deviation of n voltage measurements. The median temporal noise among these hv values is stated as the overall temporal noise in volts.

Following the calculation of temporal noise, the uniform source data cube is reduced along each axis according to the 3D noise procedure. There are seven noise terms as part of the 3D noise definition. Three components measure the average noise present along on each axis (horizontal, vertical, and temporal) of the data cube (σ_h, σ_v, and σ_t). Three terms measure the noise common to any given pair of axes in the data cube (σ_{tv}, σ_{th}, and σ_{vh}). The final term measures the uncorrelated random noise (σ_{tvh}). To calculate

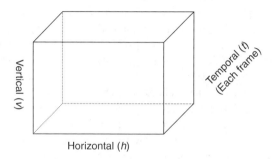

FIGURE 38.2   An example of a uniform source data cube for 3D noise measurements. The first step in the calculation of 3D noise parameters is the acquisition of a uniform source data cube.

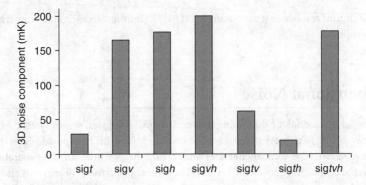

FIGURE 38.3   The 3D noise values for a typical data cube. The spatial nonuniformity can be seen in the elevated values of the spatial only 3D noise components σ_h, σ_v, and σ_{vh}. The white noise present in the system (σ_{tvh}) is roughly the same magnitude as the spatial 3D noise components.

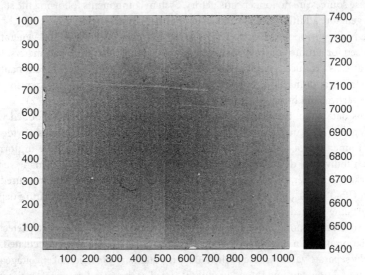

FIGURE 38.4   An example of a camera system with high spatial noise components and very low temporal noise components.

the spatial noise for the camera, each of the 3D noise components that are independent of time (σ_v, σ_h, and σ_{vh}) are added in quadrature. The result is quoted as the spatial noise of the camera in volts.

In order to represent a data cube in a 2D format, the cube is averaged along one of the axes. For example, if a data cube is averaged along the temporal axis, then a time averaged array is created. This format is useful for visualizing purely spatial noise effects as three of the components are calculated after temporal averaging (σ_h, σ_v, and σ_{vh}). These are the time independent components of 3D Noise. The data cube can also be averaged along both spatial dimensions. The full 3D Noise calculation for a typical data cube is shown in Figure 38.3.

Figure 38.4 shows an example of a data cube that has been temporally averaged. In this case, many spatial noise features are present. Column noise is clearly visible in Figure 38.4, however the dominant spatial noise component appears to be the "salt and pepper" fixed pattern noise. The seven 3D Noise components are shown in Figure 38.5. σ_{vh} is clearly the dominant noise term, as was expected due to the high fixed pattern noise. The column noise σ_h and the row noise σ_v are the next dominant. In this example, the overall bulls-eye variation in the average frame dominates the σ_v and σ_h terms. Vertical stripes present in the figure add to σ_v, but this effect is small in comparison, leading to similar values for

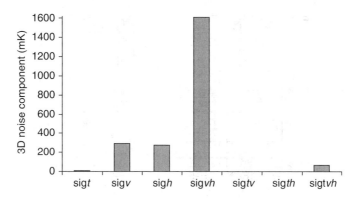

FIGURE 38.5 The 3D noise components for the data cube used to generate. Note that the amount of row and column noise is significantly smaller than the fixed pattern noise. All the 3D noise values with a temporal component are significantly smaller than the purely spatial values.

σ_v and σ_h. In this example, the temporal components of the 3D noise are two orders of magnitude lower than σ_{vh}. If this data cube were to be plotted as individual frames, we would see that successive frames would hardly change and the dominant spatial noise would be present (and constant) in each frame.

38.2 Noise Equivalent Temperature Difference

In general, imager sensitivity is a measure of the smallest signal that is detectable by a sensor. For IR imaging systems, noise equivalent temperature difference (NETD) is a measure of sensitivity. Sensitivity is determined using the principles of radiometry and the characteristics of the detector. The system intensity transfer function (SITF) can be used to estimate the noise equivalent temperature difference. NEDT is the system noise rms voltage over the noise differential output. It is the smallest measurable signal produced by a large target (extended source), in other words the minimum measurable signal.

Equation below describes NETD as a function of noise voltage and the system intensity transfer function. The measured NETD values are determined from a line of video stripped from the image of a test target, as depicted in Figure 38.10. A square test target is placed before a blackbody source. The delta T is the difference between the blackbody temperature and the mask. This target is then placed at the focal point of an off axis parabolic mirror. The mirror serves the purpose of a long optical path length to the target, yet relieves the tester from concerns over atmospheric losses to the temperature difference. The image of the target is shown in Figure 38.6. The SITF slope for the scan line in Figure 38.6 is the $\Delta\Sigma/\Delta T$, where $\Delta\Sigma$ is the signal measured for a given ΔT. The N_{rms} is the background signal on the same line.

$$\text{NETD} = \frac{N_{rms} \, [\text{volts}]}{\text{SITF\_Slope} \, [\text{volts/K}]}$$

After calculating both the temporal and spatial noise, a signal transfer function (SiTF) is measured. The field of view of the camera is again flooded with a uniform temperature source. The temperature of the source is varied over the dynamic range of the camera's output while the mean array voltage response is recorded. The slope of the resulting curve yields the SiTF responsivity in volts per degree Kelvin change in the scene temperature. Once both the SiTF curve and the temporal and spatial noise in volts are known, the NETD can be calculated. This is accomplished by dividing the temporal and spatial noise in volts by the responsivity in volts per degree Kelvin. The resulting NETD values represent the minimum discernable change in scene temperature for both spatial and temporal observation.

The SiTF of an electro-optical (EO) or IR system is determined by the signal response once the dark offset signal has been subtracted off. After subtracting off the offset due to non flux effects, the SiTF

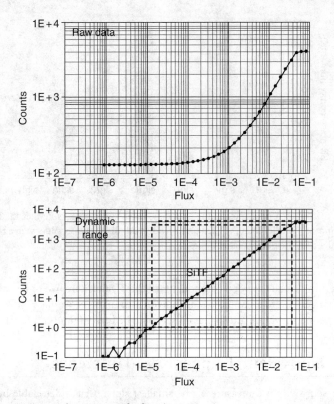

FIGURE 38.6   Dynamic range and system transfer function.

plots the counts output relative to the input photon flux. The SiTF is typically represented in response units of voltage, signal electrons, digital counts, etc. vs. units of the source: blackbody temperature, flux, photons, and so on. If the system behaves linearly within the dynamic range then the slope of the SiTF is constant. The dynamic range of the system, which may be defined by various criteria, is determined by the minimum (i.e., signal to noise ratio = 1) and maximum levels of operation.

38.3   Dynamic Range

The responsivity function also provides dynamic range and linearity information. The camera dynamic range is the maximum measurable input signal divided by the minimum measurable signal. The NEDT is assumed to be the minimum measurable signal. For AC systems, the maximum output depends on the target size and therefore the target size must be specified if dynamic range is a specification. Depending upon the application, the maximum input value may be defined by one of several methods. One method for specifying the dynamic range of a system involves having the ΔV_{sys} signal reach some specified level, say 90% of the saturation level as shown in Figure 38.7. Another method to assess the maximum input value is based on the signal's deviation from linearity. The range of data points that fall within a specified band is designated as the dynamic range. A third approach involves specifying the minimum SiTF of the system.

For most systems, the detector output signal is adjusted both in gain and offset so that the dynamic range of the A/D converter is maximized. Figure 38.8 shows a generic detector system that contains an 8-bit A/D converter. The converter can handle an input signal between 0 and 1 volt and an output between 0 and 255 counts. By selecting the gain and offset, any detector voltage range can be mapped into the digital output. Figure 38.9 shows 3 different system gains and offsets. When the source flux level is less

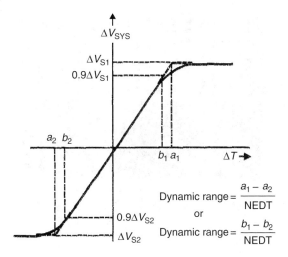

FIGURE 38.7 Dynamic range defined by linearity.

$$\text{Dynamic range} = \frac{a_1 - a_2}{\text{NEDT}}$$

or

$$\text{Dynamic range} = \frac{b_1 - b_2}{\text{NEDT}}$$

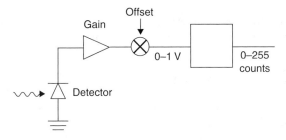

FIGURE 38.8 System with 8-bit A/D converter.

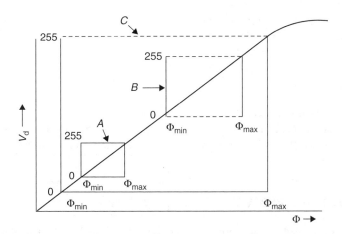

FIGURE 38.9 Different gains and voltage offsets affect the input-to-output transition.

than Φ_{min}, the source will not be seen (i.e. it will appear as 0 counts). When the flux level is greater than Φ_{max}, the source will appear as 255 counts, and the system is said to be saturated. The gain parameters, Φ_{min} and Φ_{max} are redefined for each gain and offset level setting.

Output A below occurs with maximum gain. Point B occurs with moderate gain and C with minimum gain. For the various gains, the detector output gets mapped into the full dynamic range of the A/D converter.

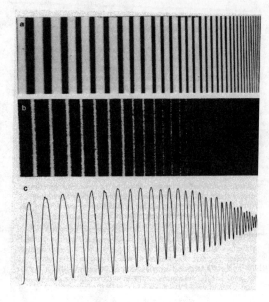

FIGURE 38.10   This figure shows the falloff in MTF as spatial frequency increases. Panel a is a sinusoidal test pattern, panel b is the optical system's (negative) response, and panel c shows the contrast as a function of spatial frequency.

38.4   Modulation Transfer Function

The modulation transfer function (MTF) of an optical system measures a system's ability to faithfully image a given object. Consider for example the bar pattern shown in Figure 38.10, with the cross section of each bar being a sine wave. Since the image of a sine wave light distribution is always a sine wave, no matter how bad the aberrations may be, the image is always a sine wave. The image will therefore have a sine wave distribution with intensity shown in Figure 38.10.

When the bars are coarsely spaced, the optical system has no difficulty faithfully reproducing them. However, when the bars are more tightly spaced, the contrast,

$$\text{Contrast} = \frac{\text{bright} - \text{dark}}{\text{bright} + \text{dark}}$$

begins to fall off as shown in panel c. If the dark lines have intensity = 0, the contrast = 1, and if the bright and dark lines are equally intense, contrast = 0. The contrast is equal to the MTF at a specified spatial frequency. Furthermore, it is evident that the MTF is a function of spatial frequency and position within the field.

38.5   Minimum Resolvable Temperature

Each time a camera is turned on, the observer subconsciously makes a judgement about image quality. The IR community uses the MRT and the MDT as standard measures of image quality. The MRT and MDT depend upon the IR imaging system's resolution and sensitivity. MRT is a measure of the ability to resolve detail and is inversely related to the MTF, whereas the MDT is a measure to detect something. The MRT and MDT deal with an observer's ability to perceive low contrast targets which are embeddedd in noise.

MRT and MDT are not absolute values rather they are temperature differentials relative to a given background. They are sometimes referred to as the minimum resolvable temperature difference (MRTD) and the minimum detectable temperature difference (MDTD).

The theoretical MRT is

$$\mathrm{MRT}(f_x) = \frac{k \cdot (\mathrm{NEDT})}{\mathrm{MTF}_{\mathrm{perceived}}(f_x)} \cdot \sqrt{\{\beta_1 + \cdots + \beta_n\}}$$

where $\mathrm{MTF}_{\mathrm{perceived}} = \mathrm{MTF}_{\mathrm{SYS}}\, \mathrm{MTF}_{\mathrm{MONITOR}}\, \mathrm{MTF}_{\mathrm{EYE}}$. The $\mathrm{MTF}_{\mathrm{system}}$ is defined by the product $\mathrm{MTF}_{\mathrm{sensor}}$ $\mathrm{MTF}_{\mathrm{optics}}\, \mathrm{MTF}_{\mathrm{electronics}}$. Each β_i in the equation is an eye filter that is used to interpret the various components of noise. As certain noise sources increase, the MRT also increases. MRT has the same ambient temperature dependence as the NEDT; as the ambient temperature increases, MRT decreases. Because the MTF decreases as spatial frequency increases, the MRT increases with increasing spatial frequency. Overall system response depends on both sensitivity and resolution. The MRT parameter is bounded by sensitivity and resolution. Figure shows that different systems may have different MRTs. System A has a better sensitivity because it has a lower MRT at low spatial frequencies. At mid-range spatial frequencies, the systems are approximately equivalent and it can be said that they provide equivalent performance. At higher frequencies, System B has better resolution and can display finer detail than system A. In general, neither sensitivity, resolution, nor any other single parameter can be used to compare systems; many quantities must be specified for complete system-to-system comparison.

38.6   Spatial Resolution

The term resolution applies to two different concepts with regard to vision systems. Spatial resolution refers to the image size in pixels — for a given scene, more pixels means higher resolution. The spatial resolution is a fixed characteristic of the camera and cannot be increased by the frame grabber of post-processing techniques. Zooming techniques, for example, merely interpolate between pixels to expand an image without adding any new information to what the camera provided. It is easy to decrease the resolution, however, by simply ignoring part of the data. National Instruments frame grabbers provide for this with a "scaling" feature that instructs the frame grabber to sample the image to return a 1/2, 1/4, 1/8, and so on, scaled image. This is convenient when system bandwidth is limited and you don't require any precision measurements of the image.

The other use of the term "resolution" is commonly found in data acquisition applications and refers to the number of quantization levels used in A/D conversions. Higher resolution in this sense means that you would have improved capability of analyzing low-contrast images. This resolution is specified by the A/D converter; the frame grabber determines the resolution for analog signals, whereas the camera determines it for digital signals (the frame grabber must have the capability of supporting whatever resolution the camera provides, though).

38.6.1   Pixel Size

Camera pixel size consists of the tiny dots that make up a digital image. So let us say that a camera is capable of taking images at 640×480 pixels. A little math shows us that such an image would contain 307,200 pixels or 0.3 megapixels. Now let's say the camera takes 1024×768 images. That gives us 0.8 megapixels. So the larger the number of megapixels, the more image detail you get. Each pixel can be one of 16.7 million colors.

The detector pixel size refers to the size of the individual sensor elements that make up the detector part of the camera. If we had two charge-coupled devices (CCDs) detectors with equal Quantum Efficiency (QEs) but one has 9 μm pixels and the other has 18 μm pixels (i.e., the pixels on CCD#2 are twice the linear size of those on CCD #1) and we put both of these CCDs into cameras that operate identically, then the image taken with CCD#1 will require 4X the exposure of the image taken with CCD#2. This seeming discrepancy is due in its entirety to the area of the pixels in the two CCDs and could be compared to the effectiveness of rain gathering gauges with different rain collection areas: A rain gauge with a 2-in. diameter throat will collect 4X as much rain water as a rain gauge with a 1-in. diameter throat.

References

[1] J. D'Agostino and C. Webb, 3-D analysis framework and measurement methodology for imaging system noise. *Proc. SPIE*, 1488, 110–121 (1991).

[2] R.G. Driggers, P. Cox, and T. Edwards, *Introduction to Infrared and Electro-Optical Systems*, Artech House, Boston, MA, 1998, p. 8.

39

Infrared Camera and Optics for Medical Applications

39.1 Infrared Sensor Calibration **39**-4
39.2 Gain Detector **39**-6
   Nonuniformity Calibration
39.3 Operational Considerations........................... **39**-7
39.4 Infrared Optical Considerations **39**-8
   Resolution
39.5 Spectral Requirement.................................. **39**-10
   Depth of Field
39.6 Selecting Optical Materials **39**-11
   Special Considerations • Coatings • Reflective Optics
Acknowledgments... **39**-14
References **39**-14
Further Information **39**-14

Michael W. Grenn
Jay Vizgaitis
Joseph G. Pellegrino
Philip Perconti
*U.S. Army Communications and
Electronics Research, Development
and Engineering Center (CERDEC)
Night Vision and Electronic Sensors
Directorate*

The infrared radiation emitted by an object above 0 K is passively detected by infrared imaging cameras without any contact with the object and is nonionizing. The characteristics of the infrared radiation emitted by an object are described by Planck's blackbody law in terms of spectral radiant emittance.

$$M_\lambda = \varepsilon(\lambda) \frac{c_1}{\lambda^5 (e^{c_2/\lambda T} - 1)} \ \text{W/cm}^2 \, \mu\text{m}$$

where c_1 and c_2 are constants of 3.7418×10^4 W μm^4/cm^2 and 1.4388×10^4 μm K. The wavelength, λ, is provided in micrometers and $\varepsilon(\lambda)$ is the emissivity of the surface. A blackbody source is defined as an object with an emissivity of 1.0, so that it is a perfect emitter. Source emissions of blackbodies at nominal terrestrial temperatures are shown in Figure 39.1. The radiant exitance of a blackbody at a 310 K, corresponding to a nominal core body temperature of 98.6°F, peaks at approximately 9.5 μm in the LWIR. The selection of an infrared camera for a specific application requires consideration of many factors including sensitivity, resolution, uniformity, stability, calibratability, user controllability, reliability, object of interest phenomenology, video interface, packaging, and power consumption.

Planck's equation describes the spectral shape of the source as a function of wavelength. It is readily apparent that the peak shifts to shorter wavelengths as the temperature of the object of interest increases.

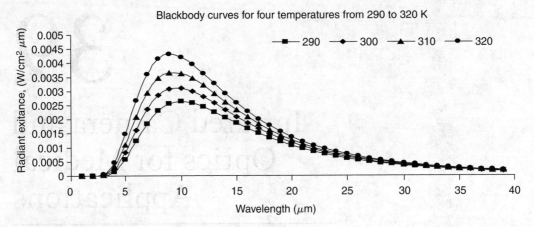

FIGURE 39.1   Planck's blackbody radiation curves.

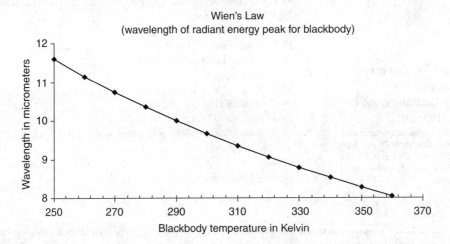

FIGURE 39.2   Location of peak of blackbody radiation, Wien's Law.

If the temperature of a blackbody approaches that of the sun, or 5900 K, the peak of the spectral shape would shift to 0.55 μm or green light. This peak wavelength is described by Wien's displacement law

$$\lambda_{\max} = 2898/T \ \mu\text{m}$$

Figure 39.2 shows the radiant energy peak as a function of temperature in the LWIR. It is important to note that the difference between the blackbody curves is the "signal" in the infrared bands. For an infrared sensor, if the background temperature is 300 K and the object of interest temperature is 302 K, the signal is the 2 K difference in flux between these curves. Signals in the infrared ride on very large amounts of background flux. This is not the case in the visible. For example, consider the case of a white object on a black background. The black background is generating no signal, while the white object is generating a maximum signal assuming the sensor gain is properly adjusted. The dynamic range may be fully utilized in a visible sensor. For the case of an IR sensor, a portion of the dynamic range is used by the large background flux radiated by everything in the scene. This flux is never a small value, hence sensitivity and dynamic range requirements are much more difficult to satisfy in IR sensors than in visible sensors.

A typical infrared imaging scenario consists of two major components, the object of interest and the background. In an IR scene, the majority of the energy is emitted from the constituents of the scene. This emitted energy is transmitted through the atmosphere to the sensor. As it propagates through the atmosphere it is degraded by absorption and scattering. Obscuration by intervening objects and additional energy emitted by the path also affect the target energy. This effect may be very small in short range imaging applications under controlled conditions. All these contributors, which are not the object of interest, essentially reduce one's ability to discriminate the object. The signal is further degraded by the optics of the sensor. The energy is then sampled by the detector array and converted to electrical signals. Various electronics amplify and condition this signal before it is presented to either a display for human interpretation or an algorithm like an automatic target recognizer for machine interpretation. A linear systems approach to modeling allows the components' transfer functions to be treated separately as contributors to the overall system performance. This approach allows for straightforward modifications to a performance model for changes in the sensor or environment when performing tradeoff analyses.

The photon flux levels (photons per square centimeter per second) on Earth is 1.5×10^{17} in the daytime and around 1×10^{10} at night in the visible. In the MWIR, the daytime and nighttime flux levels are 4×10^{15} and 2×10^{15}, respectively, where the flux is a combination of emitted and solar reflected flux. In the LWIR, the flux is primarily emitted where both day and night yield a 2×10^{17} level. At first look, it appears that the LWIR flux characteristics are as good as a daytime visible system, however, there are two other factors limiting performance. First, the energy bandgaps of infrared sensitive devices are much smaller than in the visible, resulting in significantly higher detector dark current. The detectors are typically cooled to reduce this effect. Second, the reflected light in the visible is modulated with target and background reflectivities that typically range from 7 to 20%.

In the infrared, where all terrestrial objects emit, a two-degree equivalent blackbody difference in photon flux between object and background is considered high contrast. The flux difference between two blackbodies of 302 K compared to 300 K can be calculated in a manner similar to that shown in Figure 39.1. The flux difference is the signal that provides an image, hence the difference in signal compared to the ambient background flux should be noted. In the LWIR, the signal is 3% of the mean flux and in the MWIR it is 6% of the mean flux. This means that there is a large flux pedestal associated with imaging in the infrared.

There are two major challenges accompanying the large background pedestal in the infrared. First, the performance of a typical infrared detector is limited by the background photon noise and this noise term is determined by the mean of the pedestal. This value may be relatively large compared to the small signal differences. Second, the charge storage capacity of the silicon input circuit mated to each infrared detector in a staring array limits the amount of integrated charge per frame, typically around 10^7 charge carriers. An LWIR system in a hot desert background would generate 10^{10} charge carriers in a 33 msec integration time. The optical f-number, spectral bandwidth, and integration time of the detector are typically tailored to reach half well for a given imaging scenario for dynamic range purposes. This well capacity limited condition results in a sensitivity, or noise equivalent temperature difference (NETD) of 10 to 30 times below the photon limited condition. Figure 39.3 shows calculations of NETD as a function of background temperature for MWIR and LWIR staring detectors dominated by the photon noise of the incident IR radiation. At 310 K, the NETD of high quantum efficiency MWIR and LWIR focal plane arrays (FPAs) is nearly the same, or about 3 millidegrees K, when the detectors are permitted to integrate charge up to the frame time, or in this case about 33 msec. The calculations show the sensitivity limits from the background photon shot noise only and does not include the contribution of detector and system temporal and spatial noise terms. The effects of residual spatial noise on NETD are described later in the chapter. The well capacity assumed here is 10^9 charge carriers to demonstrate sensitivity that could be achieved under large well conditions. The MWIR device is photon limited over the temperature range and begins to reach the well capacity limit near 340 K. The 24 μm pitch 9.5 μm cutoff LWIR device is well capacity limited over the entire temperature range. The 18 μm pitch 9.5 μm cutoff LWIR device becomes photon limited around 250 K. Various on-chip signal processing techniques, such as charge skimming and

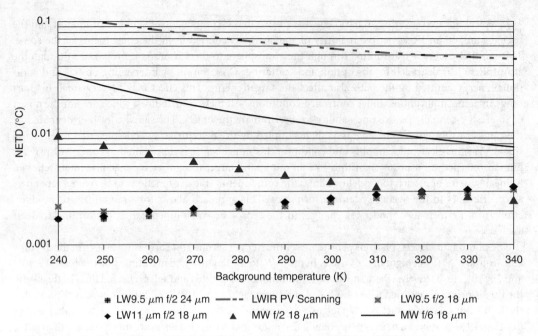

FIGURE 39.3   Background limited NETD for high quantum efficiency MWIR and LWIR detectors.

charge partitioning, have been investigated to increase the charge capacity of these devices. In addition, as the minimum feature sizes of the input circuitry decreases, more real estate in the unit cell can be allocated to charge storage.

Another major difference between infrared and visible systems is the size of the detector and diffraction blur. Typical sizes for MWIR and LWIR detectors, or pixels, range from 20 to 50 μm. Visible detectors less than 6 μm are commercially available today. The diffraction blur for the LWIR is more than ten times larger than the visible blur and MWIR blur is eight times larger than visible blur. Therefore, the image blur due to diffraction and detector size is much larger in an infrared system than a visible system. It is very common for infrared staring arrays to be sampling limited where the sample spacing is larger than the diffraction blur and the detector size. Dither and microscanning are frequently used to enhance performance. A more detailed discussion of the optical considerations of infrared sensors is provided later in the chapter.

Finally, infrared staring arrays consisting of cooled photon detectors or uncooled thermal detectors may have responsivities that vary dramatically from pixel to pixel. It is common practice to correct for the resulting nonuniformity using a combination of factory preset tables and user inputs. The nonuniformity can cause fixed pattern noise in the image that can limit the performance of the system even more than temporal noise and these effects are demonstrated in the next section.

39.1 Infrared Sensor Calibration

Significant advancement in the manufacturing of high-quality FPAs operating in the SWIR, MWIR, and LWIR has enabled industry to offer a wide range of affordable camera products to the consumer. Commercial applications of infrared camera technology are often driven by the value of the information it provides and price points set by the marketplace. The emergence of uncooled microbolometer FPA cameras with sensitivity less than 0.030°C at standard video rates has opened many new applications of the technology. In addition to the dramatic improvement in sensitivity over the past several years, uncooled microbolometer FPA cameras are characteristically compact, lightweight, and low power. Uncooled cameras are commercially available from a variety of domestic and foreign vendors including Agema, BAE Systems, CANTRONIC Systems, Inc., DRS and DRS Nytech, FLIR Systems, Inc., Indigo Systems, Inc.,

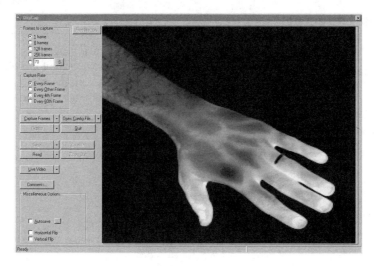

FIGURE 39.4   Windows-based GUI developed at NVESD for an uncooled medical imaging system.

Electrophysics Corp., Inc., Infrared Components Corp., IR Solutions, Inc., Raytheon, Thermoteknix Systems Ltd., ompact, low power The linearity, stability, and repeatability of the SiTF may be measured to determine the suitability of an infrared camera for accurate determination of the apparent temperature of an object of interest. LWIR cameras are typically preferred for imaging applications that require absolute or relative measurements of object irradiance or radiance because emitted energy dominates the total signal in the LWIR. In the MWIR, extreme care is required to ensure the radiometric accuracy of data. Thermal references may be used in the scene to provide a known temperature reference point or points to compensate for detector-to-detector variations in response and improve measurement accuracy. Thermal references may take many forms and often include temperature controlled extended area sources or uniformly coated metal plates with contact temperature sensors. Depending on the stability of the sensor, reference frames may be required in intervals from minutes to hours depending on the environmental conditions and the factory presets. Many sensors require an initial turn-on period to stabilize before accurate radiometric data can be collected. An example of a windows-based graphical user interface (GUI) developed at NVESD for an uncooled imaging system for medical studies is shown in Figure 39.4. The system allows the user to operate in a calibrated mode and display apparent temperature in regions of interest or at any specified pixel location including the pixel defined by the cursor. Single frames and multiple frames at specified time intervals may be selected for storage. Stability of commercially available uncooled cameras is provided earlier.

The LTC 500 thermal imager had been selected as a sensor to be used in a medical imaging application. Our primary goal was to obtain from the imagery calibrated temperature values within an accuracy of approximately a tenth of a degree Celsius. The main impediments to this goal consisted of several sources of spatial nonuniformity in the imagery produced by this sensor, primarily the spatial variation of radiance across the detector FPA due to self heating and radiation of the internal camera components, and to a lesser extent the variation of detector characteristics within the FPA. Fortunately, the sensor provides a calibration capability to mitigate the effects of the spatial nonuniformities.

We modeled the sensor FPA as a 2D array of detectors, each having a gain G and offset K, both of which are assumed to vary from detector to detector. In addition we assumed an internally generated radiance Y for each detector due to the self-heating of the internal sensor components (also varying from detector to detector, as well as slowly with time). Lastly, there is an internally programmable offset C for each detector which the sensor controls as part of its calibration function. Therefore, given a radiance X incident on some detector of the FPA from the external scene, the output Z for that detector is given by:

$$Z = GX + GY + K + C$$

39.2   Gain Detector

Individual detector gains were calculated by making two measurements. First, the sensor was allowed to run for several hours in order for the internal temperatures to stabilize. A uniform blackbody source at temperature T_1 (20°C) was used to fill the field of view (FOV) of the sensor and an output image Z_1 was collected. Next the blackbody temperature was set to T_2 (40°C) and a second output image Z_2 was collected. Since the measurement interval was small (<1 to 2 min) we assume the Y values remain constant, we have (for each detector):

$$Z_1 = GX_1 + GY + K + C$$

$$Z_2 = GX_2 + GY + K + C$$

where X_1 and X_2 refer to the external scene radiance corresponding to temperatures T_1 and T_2 incident on the detector and were calculated by integrating Planck's blackbody function over the 8 to 12 μm spectral band of the sensor. Taking the difference, we have (for each detector):

$$G = \frac{Z_2 - Z_1}{X_2 - X_1}$$

where the numbers here refer to measurements at different temperatures and, again, the value G (as well as Z and X) are assumed to vary from detector to detector (detector subscripts were omitted for clarity).

39.2.1   Nonuniformity Calibration

The LTC 500 provides the capability for nonuniformity calibration that allows the user to remove nonuniformities across the FPA assuming they do not change too rapidly with time. The procedure involves placing a uniform blackbody source across the FOV of the sensor and pressing the calibrate button. At this point, the sensor internally adjusts the value of a programmable offset for each detector so that the output Z of each detector is equal to a constant that we will denote Z_{CAL} (which the sensor sets to the midpoint of the digital pixel range, i.e., 16384).

Let D_1 and D_2 be two detectors selected from the 2D FPA, the outputs Z_1, Z_2 are then given by:

$$Z_1 = G_1 X_1 + G_1 Y_1 + K_1 + C_1$$

$$Z_2 = G_2 X_2 + G_2 Y_2 + K_2 + C_2$$

where now the numbers refer to different detectors, and as before G is gain, X is the incident radiance from the external scene, Y is the internal self heating radiance on the detectors, K is a possible offset variation from detector to detector, and C represents the programmable calibration offset for each detector. If we fill the FOV with a uniform blackbody at some temperature (T_{CAL}) producing a uniform radiance X_{CAL} on the FPA and activate the calibration function, we have:

$$Z_1 = Z_{CAL} = G_1 X_{CAL} + G_1 Y_1 + K_1 + C_1$$

$$Z_2 = Z_{CAL} = G_2 X_{CAL} + G_2 Y_2 + K_2 + C_2$$

so

$$C_1 = Z_{CAL} - G_1 X_{CAL} - G_1 Y_1 - K_1$$

$$C_2 = Z_{CAL} - G_2 X_{CAL} - G_2 Y_2 - K_2$$

where X_{CAL} is calculated by spectrally integrating Planck's function from 8 to 12μm at $T = T_{CAL}$. C_1 and C_2 will now retain these values until the sensor is either recalibrated or powered down. Now, for some arbitrary externally supplied radiance X_1, X_2 on the FPA we have:

$$Z_1 = G_1 X_1 + G_1 Y_1 + K_1 + C_1$$

$$Z_1 = G_1 X_1 + G_1 Y_1 + K_1 + Z_{CAL} - G_1 X_{CAL} - G_1 Y_1 - K_1$$

$$Z_1 = G_1 X_1 + Z_{CAL} - G_1 X_{CAL}$$

$$Z_1 = G_1 (X_1 - X_{CAL}) + Z_{CAL}$$

and, similarly

$$Z_2 = G_2 (X_2 - X_{CAL}) + Z_{CAL}$$

therefore, the output of each detector depends only on the individual detector gain (which we know) and the external radiance incident on the detector. The spatially varying components (Y and K) have been removed.

Rearranging to solve for radiance input X as a function of the output intensity Z we have:

$$X = \frac{(Z - Z_{CAL})}{G} + X_{CAL}$$

Given a precomputed look up table RAD2TEMP of T, X pairs we can take the radiance value X and look up the corresponding temperature T for any pixel in the image. Hence we have computed temperature T_C as a function of radiance X on any detector:

$$T_C = \text{RAD2TEMP}[X]$$

39.3   Operational Considerations

Upon testing the system in a scenario that more accurately reflected the operational usage anticipated (i.e., with up to 10 ft between the sensor and the measured object), we encountered an unexpected discrepancy between the computed temperature values and the actual values as reported by the blackbody temperature display. We decided to assume that actual temperature values would vary linearly with the values computed by the above method. Therefore, we added a second step to the calibration procedure that requires the user to collect an image at a higher temperature than the calibration temperature T_{CAL}. Also, this second measurement would be made at a sensor to blackbody distance of approximately 10 ft. So now, we have two computed temperatures and two actual corresponding temperatures. Then we compute a slope and y-intercept describing the (assumed) linear relationship between the computed and actual temperatures.

$$T_A = M T_C + B$$

where

$$M = \frac{T_{A_2} - T_{A_1}}{T_{C_2} - T_{C_1}}$$

and

$$B = T_{A_1} - M T_{C_1}$$

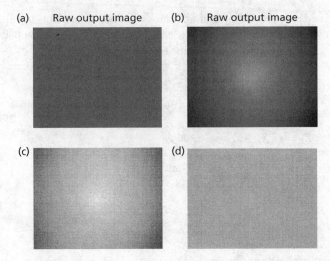

(a) Raw output image   (b) Raw output image

(c)   (d)

FIGURE 39.5 Gain calculation, (a) *low temperature*: uniform 30°C black body source, calibrated at 30°, $\mu = 16381$, $\sigma = 1.9$ (raw counts). (b) *High temperature*: uniform 40°C black body source, calibrated at 30°, $\mu = 16842$, $\sigma = 11.3$ (raw counts). (c) *Processed using uniform gain*: uniform 35°C black body source, calibrated at 30°, $\mu = 34.74$, $\sigma = 0.12$ (°C). (d) *Processed using computed gain*: uniform 35°C black body source, calibrated at 30°, $\mu = 34.74$, $\sigma = 0.04$ (°C).

where T_A is the adjusted temperature, T_C is the computed temperature from the previously described methodology. M and B are recomputed during each nonuniformity calibration.

From a camera perspective, the system intensity transfer function (SiTF) in digital counts for a DC = $A + BeT^4$

$$T = \left(\frac{DN - A}{B\varepsilon} \right)^{1/4}$$

By adding this second step to the calibration process, we were able to improve the accuracy of the computed temperature to within a tenth of a degree for the test data set (Figure 39.5).

39.4   Infrared Optical Considerations

This section focuses mainly on the MWIR and LWIR since optics in the NIR and SWIR and very similar to that of the visible. This area assumes a basic knowledge of optics, and applies that knowledge to the application of infrared systems.

39.4.1   Resolution

Designing an IR optical system is first initiated by developing a set of requirements that are needed. These requirements will be used to determine the focal plane parameters and desired spectral band. These parameters in turn drive the first order design, evolving into the focal length, entrance pupil diameter, FOV, and f/number.

If we start with the user inputs of target distance, size, cycle criteria (or pixel criteria), and spectral band, we can begin designing our sensor. First we calculate the minimum resolution angle (α, in radians). This parameter is also known as the instantaneous field of view (IFOV), and can be calculated by

$$\alpha = \frac{\text{Size}_{\text{tar}}}{(\text{Range})(2 \times \text{Cyles})}$$

or

$$\alpha = \frac{\text{Size}_{\text{tar}}}{(\text{Range})(\text{Pixels})}$$

Based on the wavelength, we can determine the minimum entrance pupil diameter that is necessary to distinguish between the two blur spots.

$$\text{EPD} = \frac{1.22\lambda}{\alpha}$$

Knowing the detector size and pixel pitch we can then determine the minimum focal length based on our IFOV that is required to meet our resolution requirements. Longer focal lengths will provide better spatial resolution.

$$\text{EFL} = \frac{\text{Pitch}}{\alpha}$$

Once we know our focal length, we can determine our FOV based on the height of the detector and the focal length. The vertical and horizontal fields of view are calculated separately based on their respective dimensions.

$$\theta = 2\tan\left[\frac{0.5h}{\text{EFL}}\right]$$

where h is the full detector height (or width). Depending on the system requirements, the size of the FPA may want to be scaled to match the desired FOV. Arrays with more pixels provide for greater resolution for a given FOV. However, smaller arrays cost less. Scaling an optical system to match the FOV for a different array format results in the scaling of the focal length, and thus the resolution.

The f/number is then calculated as the ratio of the focal length to the entrance pupil diameter.

$$f/\text{number} = \frac{\text{EFL}}{\text{EPD}}$$

The f/number of the system can be further optimized based on two parameters: the sensitivity and the blur circle. The minimum f/number is already set based on the calculated minimum entrance pupil diameter and focal length. The f/number can be adjusted to improve sensitivity by trying to optimize the blur circle to match the diagonal dimension of the detector pixel. This method provides a way to maximize the amount of energy on the pixel while minimizing aliasing.

$$f/\text{number} = \frac{\text{Pixel}_{\text{diagonal}}}{2.44\lambda}$$

A faster f/number is good in many ways as it can improve the resolution by reducing the blur spot and increasing the optics cutoff frequency. It also allows more signal to the detector and gives a boost in the signal to noise ratio. A fast f/number is absolutely necessary for uncooled systems because they have to overcome the noise introduced from operation at warmer temperatures. Faster f/numbers also help in environments with poor thermal contrast. However, a faster f/number also means that the optics will be larger, and the optical designs will be more difficult. Faster f/numbers introduce more aberrations into each lens making all aberrations more difficult to correct, and a diffraction limited system harder to achieve. A cost increase may also occur due to larger optics and tighter tolerances. A tradeoff has to occur to find the optimal f/number for the system. The table below shows the tradeoffs between optics diameter, focal length, resolution and FOV.

39.5   Spectral Requirement

The spatial resolution is heavily dependent on the wavelength of light and the f/number. Diffraction limits the minimum blur size based on these two parameters.

$$d_{spot} = 2.44\lambda(f/number)$$

The table compares blur sizes for various wavelengths and f/numbers.

	Spot size (μm)			
f/number	$\lambda = 0.6$	$\lambda = 2$	$\lambda = 4$	$\lambda = 10$
1	1.5	4.9	9.8	24.4
2.5	3.7	12.2	24.4	61.0
4	5.9	19.5	39.0	97.6
5.5	8.1	26.8	53.7	134.2
7	10.2	34.2	68.3	170.8

First Order Parameters Resolution

	f/number	Focal length	Field of view	Entrance pupil diameter
Impact resolution	A faster f/number results in a smaller optics blur due to diffraction. The result is an improved diffraction limit, and thus better spatial resolution. However, two things can adversely impact this improvement. Aberrations increase with faster f/number, potentially moving a system out of being diffraction limited, in which case the faster f/number can potentially hurt you. Also, a fixed front aperture system will have to reduce its focal length to accommodate the faster f/number, thus reducing spatial resolution through a change in focal length	Increasing the focal length will increase spatial resolution. However, the amount of improvement may be limited by the size of the allowed aperture, as having to go to a slower f/number can reduce some of the gains. Longer focal lengths also result in narrower FOVs, which can be limited by stabilization issues	Narrower FOVs are the direct result of longer focal lengths. Longer focal lengths result in improved spatial resolution. The Field of view can also vary by changing the size of the FPA. If all other parameters are maintained, and the FPA size is increased merely through the addition of more pixels, then the FOV increases without impacting resolution. If the number of pixels stay the same, but the pixel size is increased. then resolution is decreased. If pixel size is constant, number of pixels is increased, and focal length is scaled to maintain a constant FOV, then the resolution scales with the focal length	The entrance pupil diameter (EPD) can impact the resolution in three ways. Increasing the EPD while maintaining focal length improves resolution by utilizing a faster f/number. Increasing the EPD while maintaining a constant f/number results in a longer focal length, and thus increase spatial resolution. Maintaining a constant EPD while increasing focal length results in an improved spatial resolution due to the focal length, but a reduced resolution due to diffraction. The point where there is no longer significant improvement is dependent on the pixel size

39.5.1   Depth of Field

It is often desired to image targets that are located at different distances in object space. Two targets that are separated by a distance will both appear to be equally in focus if they fall within the depth of field

(DOF) of the optics. A target that is closer to the optics than the DOF will appear defocused. In order to bring the out-of-focus target back in focus, it is required to refocus the optics so that the image plane shifts back to the location of the detector. Far targets focus shorter than near targets. If it is assumed that the optics are focused for an infinite target distance, the near DOF, known as the hyperfocal distance (HFD), can be found by

$$\text{HFD} = \frac{D^2}{2\lambda}$$

where D is the entrance pupil diameter, and λ is the wavelength in the same units as the diameter. This approximation can be made in the infrared because we can assume that we are utilizing a diffraction limited system.

This formula is dependent only on the aperture diameter and wavelength. It is easily seen that shorter wavelengths and larger apertures have larger HFDs. This relationship is based on the Rayleigh limit which states that as long as the wavefront error is within a $\frac{1}{4}$ wavelength of a true spherical surface, it is essentially diffraction limited. The depth of field can then be improved by focusing the optics to be optimally focused at the HFD. The optics are then in focus from that point to infinity based on the $\frac{1}{4}$ wave criteria, but also for a $\frac{1}{4}$ wave near that target distance. The full DOF of the system then becomes half the HFD to infinity. This is approximated by

$$\text{DOF} = \frac{D^2}{4\lambda}$$

If the region of interest is not within these bounds, it is possible to approximate the near and far focus points for a given object distance with

$$Z_{\text{near}} = \frac{\text{HFD} \times Z_o}{\text{HFD} + (Z_o - f)}$$

$$Z_{\text{far}} = \frac{\text{HFD} \times Z_o}{\text{HFD} - (Z_o - f)}$$

where X is the object distance that the objects are focused for and f is the focal length of the optics.

Work has been done with digital image processing techniques to improve the DOF by applying a method known as Wavefront Coding, developed by Cathey and Dowksi at the University of Colorado. This effectiveness of this technique has been well documented and demonstrated for the visible spectral band. Efforts are underway to demonstrate the effectiveness with LWIR uncooled cameras.

39.6 Selecting Optical Materials

The list of optical materials that transmit in the MWIR and LWIR spectrum is very short compared to that found in the visible spectrum. There are 21 crystalline materials and a handful chalcogenide glasses that transmit radiation at these wavelengths. Of the 21 crystalline materials, only six are practical to use in the LWIR, and nine are usable in the MWIR. The remaining possess poor characteristics such as being hygroscopic, toxic to the touch, etc., making them impractical for use in a real system. The list grows shorter for multi-spectral applications as only four transmit in the visible, MWIR, and LWIR. The chalcogenide glasses are an amorphous conglomerate of two or three infrared transmitting materials. A table of the practical infrared materials is listed along with a chart of their spectral bands. Transmission losses due to absorption can be calculated from the absorption coefficient of the material at the specified wavelength.

$$T_{\text{abs}} = e^{-at}$$

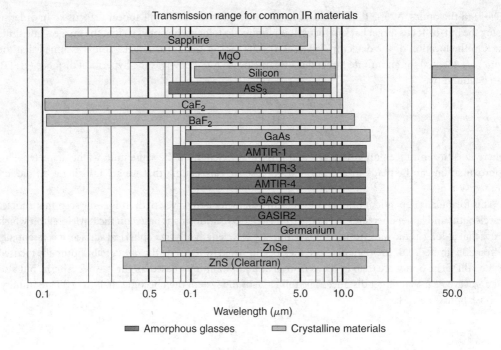

Table of Infrared Optical Materials

Material	Refractive Index		dn/dT (K^{-1})	Spectral range (μm)
	4 μm	=10 μ		
Germanium	4.0243	4.0032	0.000396	2.0–17.0
Gallium arsenide	3.3069	3.2778	0.000148	0.9–16.0
ZnSe	2.4331	2.4065	0.000060	0.55–20.0
ZnS (cleartran)	2.2523	2.2008	0.000054	0.37–14.0
AMTIR-1	2.2514	2.4976	0.000072	0.7–14.0
AMTIR-3	2.6200	2.6002	0.000091	1.0–14.0
AMTIR-4	2.6487	2.6353	−0.000030	1.0–14.0
GASIR 1	2.5100	2.4944	0.000055	1.0–14.0
GASIR 2	2.6038	2.5841	0.000058	1.0–14.0
Silicon	3.4255	N/A	0.000160	1.2–9.0
Sapphire	1.6753	N/A	0.000013	0.17–5.5
BaF$_2$	1.4580	1.4014	−0.000015	0.15–12.5
CaF$_2$	1.4097	1.3002	−0.000011	0.13–10.0
As$_2$S$_3$	2.4112	2.3816	−0.0000086	0.65–8.0
MgO	1.6679	N/A	0.000011	0.4–8.0

39.6.1 Special Considerations

In the LWIR, germanium is by far the best material to use for color correction and simplicity of design due to its high index of refraction and low dispersion. It is possible to design entire systems with germanium, but there are some caveats to this choice. Temperature plays havoc on germanium in two ways. It has a very high dn/dT (0.000396 K^{-1}), defocusing a lens that changes temperature of only a few degrees. It also has an absorption property in the LWIR for temperatures greater than 57°C. As the optic temperature rises above this point, the absorption coefficent increases, reducing the transmission. The high cost of germanium can also be a factor. It is not always good choice for a low-cost sensor, as the lens may end up costing more than the FPA. A good thermal match to compensate for the dn/dT of germanium is AMTIR-4. Its negative dn/dT provides for an excellent compensator for the germanium. It is possible to design a two lens germanium/AMTIR-4 lens system that does not require refocusing for over a 60°C temperature range.

The low-cost optics are silicon, ZnS, and the chalcogenide glasses. Silicon is only usable in the MWIR, and although the material is very inexpensive, its hardness can make it very difficult to diamond turn, and thus expensive. Although it does not diamond turn well, it does grind and polish easily, providing a very inexpensive solution when complex surfaces such as aspheres and diffractives are not used. ZnS is relatively inexpensive to germanium and ZnSe, but is relatively expensive to silicon and the chalcogenide glasses. The chalcogenide glasses are by far the least expensive to make and manufacture making them an excellent solution for low-cost system design. There are three types of the chalcogenide glasses that are moldable. AMTIR-4, a product of Amorphous Materials, Inc., has a lower melting point that the other chalcogenides making it the easiest to mold. Another material GASIR1 and GASIR2, products of Umicore, have also been demonstrated as being moldable. They have similar optical properties to that of AMTIR-1 and AMTIR-3.

39.6.2 Coatings

The high indices of refraction of most infrared materials lead to large fresnel losses, and thus require AR coatings. The transmission for a plane uncoated surface is shown below. In air, $n_1 = 1$.

$$T = 1 - \left(\frac{n_1 - n_2}{n_1 + n_2} \right)^2$$

The total reflectance off both sides of an uncoated plate is the multiplication of the two surfaces. This is in turn multiplied by the transmission of the material due to absorption. An example is given below:

Example
Uncoated Zinc Selenide flat, $n = 2.4$ in air, $t = 1.5$ cm thickness, absorption $= 0.0005$.

Total transmission through both sides $= (0.83)(0.999)(0.83) = 0.688$

Standard AR coatings are readily available for all of the materials previously listed. Generally, better than 99% can be expected for an AR-coated lens for either the MWIR or LWIR. If dual band operation is required, expect this performance to drop to 96%, and for the price to go up. The multispectral coatings are more difficult to design, and result in having many more layers. Infrared beamsplitter coatings can be difficult and expensive to manufacture. Care should be taken in specifying both the transmission and reflection properties of the beamsplitter. Specifications that are too stringent often lead to huge costs and schedule delays. Also, it is very important to note that the choice of which wavelength passes through and which wavelength is reflected can make a significant impact on the performance of a beamsplitter. In general, transmitting the longer wavelength and reflecting the shorter wavelength will boost performance and reduce cost.

39.6.3 Reflective Optics

Reflective optics can be a very useful and effective design too in the infrared. Reflective optics have no chromatic aberrations, and allow for diffraction limited solutions for very wide spectral bands. However, the use of reflective optics is somewhat limited to narrow FOVs and have difficulty with fast f/numbers. In addition, the type of reflective system can impact the performance fairly significantly for longer wavelengths. The most common type of design, the Cassegrain, two mirrors that are aligned on the same optical axis. The secondary mirror acts as an obscuration to the primary, which results in a degraded MTF due to diffraction around the obscuration. This effect is not apparent in most wavebands because the MTF loss occurs after the Nyquist frequency of the detector. However, this is not the case for the LWIR where the MTF drop occurs before Nyquist. To overcome this effect, most reflective systems used in the LWIR are off-axis reflective optics. These optics will provide diffraction limited MTF as long as the f/numbers do not get too fast, and the FOVs do not get too large. The off-axis nature makes these reflective systems hard to align, and expensive to manufacture.

Acknowledgments

Thanks to John O'Neill, Jason Zeibel, Tim Mikulski, Kent McCormack for data. EO-IR Measurements, Inc. for developing the graphical user interface for the medical infrared imaging camera. Leonard Bonnell, Vipera Systems, Inc., for development of the infrared endoscope.

References

[1] J. D'Agostino and C. Webb, 3-D analysis framework and measurement methodology for imaging system noise. *Proc. SPIE*, 1488, 110–121 (1991).

[2] R.G. Driggers, P. Cox, and T. Edwards, *Introduction to Infrared and Electro-Optical Systems*. Artech House, Boston, MA, 1998, p. 8.

[3] G.C. Holst, *Electro-Optical Imaging System Performance*. JCD Publishing, Winter Park, FL, 1995, p. 347.

[4] M.W. Grenn, Recent advances in portable infrared imaging cameras. *Proc. IEEE-EMBS*, 1996, Amsterdam.

[5] M.W. Grenn, Performance of portable staring infrared cameras. *Proc. IEEE/EMBS* Oct.30–Nov. 2, 1997 Chicago, IL, USA.

Further Information

D'Agostino, J. and Webb, C. "3-D Analysis Framework and Measurement Methodology for Imaging System Noise," *Proc. SPIE*, 1488, 110–121 (1991).

Holst, G.C. *Electro-Optical Imaging System Performance*. JCD Publishing, Winter Park, FL, 1995, p. 432.

Johnson, J. "Analysis of Image Forming Systems," *Proceedings of IIS*, 249–273 (1958).

O.H. Schade, "Electro-optical Characteristics of Television Systems," *RCA Review*, IX(1–4) (1948).

Ratches, J.A. "NVL Static Performance Model for Thermal Viewing Systems," USA Electronics Command Report ECOM 7043, AD-A011212 (1973).

Sendall, R. and Lloyd, J.M. "Improved Specifications for Infrared Imaging Systems," *Proceedings of IRIS*, 14, 109–129 (1970).

Vollmerhausen, R.H. and Driggers, R.G. "NVTHERM: Next Generation Night Vision Thermal Model," *Proceedings of IRIS Passive Sensors*, 1 (1999).

IV

Medical Informatics

Luis G. Kun
IRMC/National Defense University

40 Hospital Information Systems: Their Function and State
T. Allan Pryor **40**-1

41 Computer-Based Patient Records
J. Michael Fitzmaurice **41**-1

42 Overview of Standards Related to the Emerging Health Care
Information Infrastructure
Jeffrey S. Blair **42**-1

43 Introduction to Informatics and Nursing
Kathleen A. McCormick, Joyce Sensmeier, Connie White Delaney,
Carol J. Bickford **43**-1

44 Non-AI Decision Making
Ron Summers, Derek G. Cramp, Ewart R. Carson **44**-1

45 Medical Informatics and Biomedical Emergencies: New Training and
Simulation Technologies for First Responders
Joseph M. Rosen, Christopher Swift, Eliot B. Grigg, Matthew F. McKnight,
Susan McGrath, Dennis McGrath, Peter Robbie, C. Everett Koop **45**-1

W HAT IS IT? In the summer of 2004 I was invited to lecture at Dartmouth. Dr. Rosen, my host, asked me if I could address my interpretation of Medical Informatics during my lecture. This presentation made me review and reflect on some old and new concepts that have appeared in the literature, in some cases. I have observed, for example, that the definition varies greatly depending on the profession of the person who answers this question. A few years earlier, while at the CDC, I had the opportunity to participate in a lecture by Ted Shortliffe, in which he explained a model of Medical Informatics that appears in his book (*Handbook of Medical Informatics*). I also like portions of the content that appears at the Vanderbilt University website in its program of medical informatics (MI) and finally the work of Musen/Von Bemmel reflected on their *Handbook of Medical Informatics*.

Healthcare informatics has been defined by these authors, respectively as:

- "A field of study concerned with the broad range of issues in the management and use of biomedical information, including medical computing and the study of the nature of medical information itself." Shortliffe E.H., Perreault L.E., Eds. *Medical Informatics: Computer Applications in Health Care and Biomedicine.* New York: Springer, 2001.
- "The science that studies the use and processing of data, information, and knowledge applied to medicine, health care and public health." Von Bemmel J.H., Musen M.A., Eds. *Handbook of Medical Informatics.* AW Houten, Netherlands: Bohn Stafleu Van Loghum; Heidelberg, Germany: Springer Verlag, 1997.

Vanderbilt's MI program uses a *"simplistic definition"*: *Computer applications in medical care* and a *"better definition"*: *Biomedical Informatics is an emerging discipline that has been defined as the study, invention, and implementation of structures and algorithms to improve communication, understanding, and management of medical information. The end objective of biomedical informatics is the coalescing of data, knowledge, and the tools necessary to apply that data and knowledge in the decision making process, at the time and place that a decision needs to be made. The focus on the structures and algorithms necessary to manipulate the information separates Biomedical Informatics from other medical disciplines where information content is the focus.*

The Vanderbilt model shows Medical Informatics as the intersection of three different domains: Biological Science, Information Analysis and Presentation (i.e., informatics, computation, statistics) and Clinical Health Services Research (i.e., Policy, Outcomes). The first two at the intersection create Bioinformatics, while the second and third create health informatics [through the translation from bench to bedside]. Some more definitions:

The noun informatics has one meaning; the sciences concerned with gathering and manipulating and storing and retrieving, and classifying recorded information [1]. in.for.mat.ics n. *Chiefly British.* Information science, and bi.o.in.for.mat.ics n. Information technology as applied to the life sciences, especially the technology used for the collection, storage, and retrieval of genomic data [2].

In the *Handbook of Medical Informatics* (Musen/VonBemmel et al.) medical informatics is located at the intersection of information technology and the different disciplines of medicine and health care. These authors decided not to enter into a fundamental discussion of the possible differences between medical informatics and health informatics, however several definitions of medical informatics (medical information science, health informatics) were given. Some of these take into account both the scientific and the applied sides of the field. They cited two definitions:

1. *Medical information science is the science of using system-analytic tools. . .to develop procedures (algorithms) for management, process control, decision making, and scientific analysis of medical knowledge* [3].
2. *Medical informatics comprises the theoretical and practical aspects of information processing and communication, based on knowledge and experience derived from processes in medicine and health care* [4].

According to Wikipedia: Medical informatics is the name given to the application of information technology to healthcare. It is the: "understanding, skills, and tools that enable the sharing and use of information to deliver healthcare and promote health" *(British Medical Informatics Society).*

Medical informatics is often called *healthcare informatics* or *biomedical informatics,* and forms part of the wider domain of *eHealth*. These later-generation terms reflect the substantive contribution of the citizen

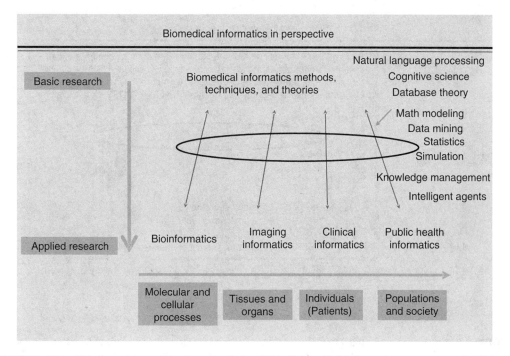

FIGURE IV.1 This figure is a modification of Ted Shortliffe's: "biomedical informatics in perspective." (Adapted from T. Shortliffe: Editorial, *Journal of Biomedical Informatics* 35 (2002) 279–280; republished with permission of the author).

and non-medical professions to the generation and usage of healthcare data and related information. Additionally, medical informaticians are active in bioinformatics and other fields not strictly defined as health care.

Biomedical Informatics: An Evolving Perspective

Some view medical informatics as a basic medical science with a wide variety of potential areas of applications. At the same time, the development and evaluation of new methods and theories are a primary focus of activities in this field. Using the results of experiences, allows, for example, the understanding, structuring, and encoding of knowledge, thus allowing its use in information processing by others, in the same field of specialty (i.e., within the field of clinical informatics) or in other areas (i.e., nursing informatics, dental informatics, and veterinary informatics). In Shortliffe's "biomedical informatics in perspective," his fundamental diagram shows how a clinician or researcher could "move" from basic research to applied research looking at molecular and cellular processes (bioinformatics), tissues and organs (imaging informatics), individual patients (clinical informatics) and populations and society (public health informatics). The important concept is, that a core series of informatics methods, tools and techniques, are the same regardless of the applied research area chosen.

This core includes: natural language processing, cognitive science, mathematical modeling and simulation, database theory, statistics, data mining, knowledge management, and intelligent agents. Many of these information technologies were developed in other fields and later applied by the "medical/health" community. In other cases the reverse has occurred. For example, the skeleton of an expert system developed for a medical diagnosis and treatment application, could be used by others to diagnose and correct problems in a computer system.

The basic core mentioned in the previous paragraph, then requires expertise in many different fields that include: biology, biomathematics, medicine, nursing, dentistry, veterinary, computer science–electrical

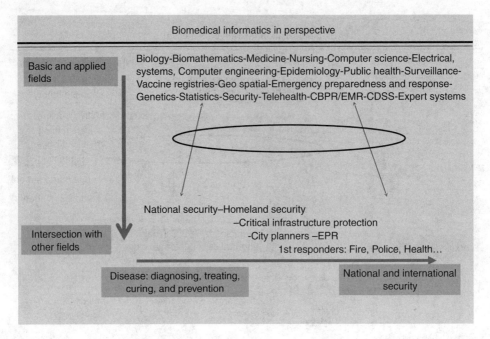

FIGURE IV.2 This is an example of applying the model shown in Figure IV.1, to other disciplines. It depicts biomedical informatics: tools, methods, techniques, and theories applied to individuals interested in the use of medical and public health informatics from a national security perspective. It also shows at the top, some of the different areas of expertise that may be touched by this field.

systems, computer engineering, epidemiology, public health, surveillance, geo-spatial information systems, emergency preparedness and response, genetics, statistics, security, telehealth, computer-based patient records, clinical decision support systems, expert systems, data mining/warehousing, etc. Figure IV.2, shows how if we start with the basic sciences and applied fields, we can develop a model that allows, through the use of medical and public health informatics, deal with issues such as national and international security and the critical infrastructure protection (CIP) of the public health infrastructure. This figure also shows many of the different professions or areas of expertise involved on the field of medical informatics.

Societal changes have occurred, in particular during the past four decades to information processing. In the last decade, for those that have observed the Internet and World Wide Web (WWW) evolution, many of these changes come as part of a new resulting culture. The convergence of computers and communications have played a key role in this evolving field of medical informatics. The way physicians, nurses, biomedical engineers, veterinarians, dentists, laboratory technicians, public health specialists, and other healthcare professionals do their "business" regardless if it is clinical, administrative, research and development or academic, requires and demands not only a clear understanding of these terms, but what their "business process" is all about.

For example, around the 1986 timeframe as technical manager for the requirements definition of the nursing point of care system for IBM Federal Systems in Gaithersburg, I had the opportunity to better understand the nursing process of information. Let us assume that a patient fall to the ground as he was having a heart attack. He cut his forehead, his left hand, arm, knee, and twisted his left ankle. When brought into an emergency room in a hospital the medical diagnosis given is: myocardial infarction. Yet from a nursing point of view, the patient diagnosis is different. He is assessed and evaluated, classified and care plans are developed for each of the diagnosis (for each of the injuries) according to a list that would include not only the heart attack (and the follow-up ordered by the physician), but the forehead, left hand, left arm, left knee, and left ankle. Following the NANDA diagnosis there will be a process to be followed for each wound or injury and that would facilitate the patient's discharge.

Each of the professionals mentioned above, that is, healthcare providers, etc. may have a piece of the patient's health puzzle which may need to be included in their record. In my professional life I have been involved in different activities that involved the utilization of different pieces of computer hardware, systems and application software and other devices that acquire, transmit, process, and store information, and in different forms (i.e., signals, voice, images from different modalities: CT, MRI, ultrasound, nuclear, x-ray, scanned/document images, etc.). In my early years at IBM in the late 70s, the concepts of "patient-centered" information was one of the leading concepts helping us drive towards the implementation of electronic health records. But in this day and age, we have a significant number of new devices, which were not made for that particular purpose and yet they are being used to collect, transmit, process, or store patient-related information. Biomedical engineers are and will be faced with these new challenges, where patient information may not be flowing from conventional data collection devices. Information now could come from sensing devices, RFID tags and through a myriad of wireless devices and networks. An RFID tag was approved in the 4Q 2004, by the FDA, that could be implanted into a patient. Aside from the issues of privacy and security of that information, the repercussions of such actions can be magnificent. It may improve the life of some or even save lives. Imagine, for example, patients suffering from either Alzheimer's or Parkinson's disease being admitted into an emergency room after an accident and not being able to convey any personal or medical-related information. Having available some basic but critical medical information can identify who the patient is, what medications they may be allergic, etc.

In the last 30 years, the field of medical informatics has grown tremendously both in its complexity and in content. As a result, two sections will be written in this handbook. The first one, represented in the chapters, will be devoted to areas that form a key "core" of computer technologies. These include: hospital information systems (HIS), computer-based patient records (CBPR or CPR), imaging, communications, standards, and other related areas. The second section includes the following topics: artificial intelligence, expert systems, knowledge-based systems neural networks, and robotics. Most of the techniques describe in the second section will require the implementation of systems explained in this first section. We could call most of these chapters the information infrastructure required to apply medical informatics techniques to medical data. These topics are crucial because they not only lay the foundation required to treat a patient within the walls of an institution but they also provide the roadmap required to deal with the patient's lifetime record while allowing selected groups of researchers and clinicians to analyze the information and generate outcomes research and practice guidelines information.

As an example, a network of associated hospitals in the East Coast (a health care provider network) may want to utilize an expert system that was created and maintained at Stanford University. This group of hospitals, HMOs, clinics, physician's offices, and the like would need a "standard" computer-based patient record (CPR) that can be used by the clinicians from any of the physical locations. In addition in order to access the information, all these institutions require telecommunications and networks that will allow for the electronic "dialogue." The different forms of the data, particularly clinical images, will require devices for displaying purposes, and the information stored in the different HIS, Clinical Information Systems (CIS), and departmental systems needs to be integrated. The multimedia type of record would become the data input for the expert system which could be accessed remotely (or locally) from any of the enterprise's locations. On the application side, the expert system could provide these institutions which techniques that can help in areas such as diagnosis and patient treatment. However, several new trends such as: total quality management (TQM), outcome research, and practice guidelines could be followed. It should be obvious to the reader that to have the ability to compare information obtained in different parts of the world by dissimilar and heterogeneous systems, certain standards need to be followed (or created) so that when analyzing the data, the information obtained will make sense.

Many information systems issues described in this introduction will be addressed in this section. The artificial intelligence chapters which follow should be synergistic with these concepts. A good understanding of the issues in this section is required prior to the utilization of the actual expert system. These issues are part of this section of medical informatics, other ones, however, for example, systems integration and process reengineering, will not be addressed here in detail but will be mentioned by the different authors. I encourage the reader to follow up on the referenced material at the end of each chapter, since the citations contain very valuable information.

Several perspectives in information technologies need to be taken in consideration when reading this section. One of them is described very accurately in the book entitled Globalization, Technology and Competition [5]. The first chapter of this book talks about new services being demanded by end users which include the integration of computers and telecommunications. From their stages theory point of view, the authors described very appropriately, that "we are currently" nearing the end of the micro era and the beginning of the network era. From an economy point of view, the industrial economy (1960s and 1970s) and the transitional economy (1970s and 1980s) moved into an information economy (1990s and beyond).

In the prior editions I mentioned that: "*Many other questions and answers reflected some of the current technological barriers and users needs. Because of these trends it was essential to include in this Handbook technologies that today may be considered state of the art but when read about 10 years from now will appear to be transitional only. Information technologies are moving into a multimedia environment which will require special techniques for acquiring, displaying, storing, retrieving, and communicating the information. We are in the process of defining some of these mechanisms.*" This is precisely what has occurred. In some instances such as imaging, this Handbook contains a full section dedicated to the subject. That section contains the principles, the associated math algorithms, and the physics related to all medical imaging modalities. The intention in this section was to address issues related to imagining as a form of medical information. These concepts include issues related then to acquisition, storage and retrieval, display and communications of document and clinical images, for example, picture archival and communications systems (PACS). From a CPR point of view, clinical and document images will become part of this electronic chart, therefore many of the associated issues will be discussed in this section more extensively. The state of the telecommunications has been described as a revolution; data and voice communications as well s full-motion video have come together as a new dynamic field. Much of what is happening today is a result of technology evolution and need. The connecting thread between evolutionary needs and revolutionary ideas is an integrated perspective of both sides of multiple industries. This topic will also be described in more detail in this section.

A Personal (Historical) Perspective on Information Technology in Healthcare: During my first 14 "professional years" I worked with IBM (1978–1992) across the country: Los Angeles, Dallas, Gaithersburg, Dallas and Houston. As I moved from city to city I noticed that while financial transactions would simply follow me (from place-to-place), that is, with the use of the same credit cards; this was not the case with my medical records. In fact, there wasn't an "electronic" version available. In today's terms my "paper-trail record" was a "cut and paste" document that I had to create and take with me wherever I went.

At work, I was engaged since 1983, on the development of concepts of the "All Digital Medical Record" (ADMR), bedside terminals, PACS, Integrated Diagnostics Systems, and other related topics such as Telemedicine. In the 1986 timeframe and while at IBM, Al Potvin (former IEEE-EMBS President) asked me to become part of the IEEE-USA Health Care Engineering Policy Committee, (HCEPC), and I did. I formed and chaired then, the Electronic Medical Record/High Performance Computers and Communications (EMR/HPCC) working group. Many of these concepts were presented at EMBS [6] and AAMI [7, 8] annual meetings, in Biomedical Engineering classes [9, 10], and even at National [11–13] and International Conferences/Meetings [14–19]. Nine and ten years ago respectively, we (the HCEPC) had 2 meetings where the Role of Technology in the Cost of Health Care were explored [20, 21]. At that time, (in the early 1990s.), and given the rate at which the American Health Care system was growing, the HCEPC asked me to organize a special Technology Policy session during the 1993 EMBS meeting in San Diego [22]. (After the formal presentations, the participants, who represented the United States, Canada and Europe had a terrific discussion that lasted well over 3 h from the allotted time for the session.) Costs were the fundamental and center piece of these discussions. The Clinton-Gore administration encouraged the use of information technology for health care reform and as a consequence we organized a meeting in 1995 [23] to address these needs.

Near seven years later the book entitled: To Err is Human[24] changed the focal point from "costs" to "human lives taken by medical errors". Experts estimated that as many as 98,000 people die (in the United States) in any given year from medical errors that occur in hospitals. That's more than die from motor vehicle accidents, breast cancer, or AIDS — three causes that receive far more public attention. Indeed, more people die annually from medication errors than from workplace injuries. Add the financial cost to the human tragedy, and medical error easily rose to the top ranks of urgent, widespread public problems. This book broke the silence that has surrounded medical errors and their consequence — but not by pointing fingers at caring health care professionals who make honest mistakes. After all, to err is human. Instead, it set forth a national agenda — with state and local implications — for reducing medical errors and improving patient safety through the design of a safer health system. It revealed the often startling statistics of medical error and the disparity between the incidence of error and public perception of it, given many patients' expectations that the medical profession always performs perfectly. A careful examination was made of how the surrounding forces of legislation, regulation, and market activity influenced the quality of care provided by health care organizations and then looked at their handling of medical mistakes. (Using a detailed case study, the book reviews the current understanding of why these mistakes happen. A key theme is that legitimate liability concerns discourage reporting of errors — which begs the question, "How can we learn from our mistakes?") Balancing regulatory versus market-based initiatives and public versus private efforts, the Institute of Medicine presented wide-ranging recommendations for improving patient safety, in the areas of leadership, improved data collection and analysis, and development of effective systems at the level of direct patient care. The bottom line was that it asserted that the problem is not bad people in health care — it is that good people are working in bad systems that need to be made safer.

A series of efforts, including both private and public sectors that is, e-Health Initiative [25], occurred which prompted a series of actions, documents and even proposed legislation in 2003, that is, HR 2915 The National Health Information Infrastructure (NHII); and also a National meeting where the requirements for such an infrastructure were agreed upon. A follow-up meeting took place on July 20–23, 2004 here in Washington, D.C.

The Secretarial Summit on Health Information Technology launching the National Health Information Infrastructure 2004: Cornerstones for Electronic Healthcare was well attended by over 1500 people representing the private and public healthcare industry. In challenging both sectors of the healthcare industry, Secretary Tommy G. Thompson stated, "Health information technology can improve quality of care and reduce medical errors, even as it lowers administrative costs. It has the potential to produce savings of 10% of our total annual spending on health care, even as it improves care for patients and provides new support for health care professionals." A report, titled "The Decade of Health Information Technology: Delivering Consumer-centric and Information-rich Health Care," ordered by President George W. Bush in April, was presented on July 21st by David Brailer, the National Coordinator for Health Information Technology, whom the president appointed to the new position in May. The report lays out the broad steps needed to achieve always-current, always-available electronic health records (EHR) for Americans. This responds to the call by President Bush to achieve EHRs for most Americans within a decade. The report identifies goals and action areas, as well as a broad sequence needed to achieve the goals, with joint private or public cooperation and leadership. The heads of every agency within DHHS (i.e., AHRQ, NIH, CDC, FDA, CMS, HRSA, etc.) were present and each made a presentation on how the NHII would affect their own area of service (e.g., research and development, education, reimbursement, etc.)

For more details about the news coverage on the NHII conference, please link to the following sites:

1. HHS Fact Sheet-HIT Report at-a-glance 7/21/04:
   http://www.hhs.gov/news/press/2004pres/20040721.html
2. NY Times 7/21/04:
   http://www.nytimes.com/2004/07/21/technology/21record.html

3. GovExec.com 7/21/04:
   http://www.governmentexecutive.com/dailyfed/0704/072104dk1.htm
4. Center for Health Transformation 7/21/04:
   http://www.healthtransformation.net/news/chtnews.asp
5. iHealthbeat 7/26/04:
   http://www.ihealthbeat.org/index.cfm?Action=dspItem&itemid=104473
6. USNews.com 8/2/04:
   http://www.usnews.com/usnews/tech/articles/040802/2wired.htm

New issues of the Information Age

As time passes by, we ("the educated world population") are becoming more accustomed to see how the Internet for example is being used to manage the health of the elderly and for homecare purposes. People living in urban, suburban, and rural areas are using telehealth as one of several mechanisms to deal with their personal health. This is one of the many ways that in my opinion healthcare costs have the potential to be reduced [26]. The Balanced Budget Act of 1997 was in fact the first time that the U.S. government decided to measure cost and medical effectiveness through telemedicine, involving elderly patients with diabetes. (A grant of about $28 million was given to Columbia University Medical Center in March 2000 and was renewed in 2004.)

In the United States the constant rising prices of medications however, are also making the elderly (in particular) look for alternative mechanisms to purchase them, that is, the Internet. The new questions that should be raised are: How can we ensure the quality of those drugs ordered through this mechanism? (i.e., Who is accountable? Who is the producer of such medications? etc.) How many people may be dying (or affected negatively) by those that are self-prescribing medications?

Several bills in the U.S. Congress are trying to deal, with some of these issues. The language has the potential to affect prescribing medications during interactive video consultations. The intent of this legislation, to ensure patients have access to safe and appropriate medicine, is a good one; however it may limit what we will be able to do through this type of technology. Some Internet Rx Legislation Under Consideration. (Bills can be accessed online at http://Thomas.loc.gov.):

- S 2464: Internet Pharmacy Consumer Protection Act aka Ryan Haight Act. *Sen. Coleman (MN). Co-sponsor: Feinstein.* Requires an in-person medical evaluation in order for a practitioner to dispense a prescription to a patient.
- HR 3880: Internet Pharmacy Consumer Protection Act. *Rep. Davis (VA) Cosponsors: Waxman.* Requires an in-person medical evaluation in order for a practitioner to dispense a prescription to a patient.
- S 2493: Safe Importation of Medical Products and Other Rx Therapies Act of 2004. *Sen. Gregg (NH). Co-sponsors: Smith.* Requires a treating provider to perform a documented patient evaluation (including a patient history and physical examination) of an individual to establish the diagnosis for which a prescription drug is prescribed.
- HR 3870: Prescription Drug Abuse Elimination Act of 2004. *Rep. Norwood (GA). Co-sponsor: Strickland.* Defines treating provider as a health care provider who has performed a documented patient evaluation of the individual involved (including a patient history and physical examination) to establish the diagnosis for which a prescription drug involved is prescribed.
- HR 2652: Internet Pharmacy Consumer Protection Act. *Rep. Stupak (MI).*States that a person may not introduce a prescription drug into interstate commerce or deliver the prescription drug for introduction into such commerce pursuant to a sale state requires an in-person medical evaluation in order for a practitioner to dispense a prescription to a patient.

In some cases, the defined requirements or the language used (i.e., in person patient evaluation) may act precisely against the use of that technology (i.e., tele-consultation). It is in the best interest of society, that biomedical engineers, among others get involved in "educating" the law-makers regarding the intrinsic value that the technology may bring into the system.

Summary of the Medical Informatics Section Covered in the Prior Edition(s)

In the first chapter Allan Pryor provided us with a tutorial on hospital information systems (HIS). He described not only the evolution of HIS and departmental systems and clinical information systems (CIS), but also their differences. Within the evolution he followed these concepts with the need for the longitudinal patient record and the integration of patient data. This chapter included patient database strategies for the HIS, data acquisition, patient admission, transfer and discharge functions. Also discussed were patient evaluation and patient management issues. From an end-user point of view, a terrific description on the evolution of data-driven and time-driven systems was included, culminating with some critical concepts on HIS requirements for decision support and knowledge base functionality. His conclusions were good indication of his vision.

Michael Fitzmaurice followed with "Computer-Based Patient Records" (CBPR or CPR). In the introduction, it was explained what is the CPR and why it is a necessary tool for supporting clinical decision making and how it is enhanced when it interacts with medial knowledge sources. This was followed by clinical decision support systems (CDSS): knowledge server, knowledge sources, medical logic modules (MLM), and nomenclature. This last issue in particular was one which needed to be well understood. The nomenclature used by physicians and by the CPRs differ among institutions. Applying logic to the wrong concepts can produce misinterpretations. The scientific evidence in this chapter included: patient care process, CDSS hurdles, CPR implementation, research data bases, telemedicine, hospital, and ambulatory care systems. A table of hospital and ambulatory care computer-based patient records systems concluded this chapter.

Because of the fast convergence of computers, telecommunications, and healthcare applications; already in the last edition it was impossible to separate these elements (i.e., communications and networks). Both are part of information systems. Soumitra Sengupta provided us in this chapter with a tutorial-like presentation which included an introduction and history, impact of clinical data, information types, and platforms. The importance of this section was reflected both in the contents reviewed under current technologies — LANs, WANs, middleware, medical domain middleware; integrated patient data base, and medical vocabulary — as well as in the directions and challenges section which included improved bandwidth, telemedicine, and security management. In the conclusions the clear vision is that networks will become the de facto fourth utility after electricity, water, and heat. Since the publishing of the last edition, both the Internet and the World Wide Web (WWW) had taken off in multiple directions, creating a societal-vision, which is much different than the one that most people expected then. For example, the use of telemedicine was seen as a tool for rural medicine and for emergency medicine and not an accepted one for Home care for the elderly and for persons suffering from a large number Chronic Diseases, both here in the United States and in the rest of the world.

"Non-AI Decision Making" was covered by Ron Summers and Ewart Carson. This chapter included an introduction which explained the techniques of procedural or declarative knowledge. The topics covered in this section included: analytical models, and decision theoretic models, including clinical algorithms, and decision trees. The section that followed covered a number of key topics which appear while querying large clinical databases to yield evidence of either diagnostic or treatment or research value; statistical models, database search, regression analysis, statistical pattern analysis, bayesian analysis, Depster-Shafer theory, syntactic pattern analysis, causal modeling, artificial neural networks. In the summary the authors clearly advised the reader to read this section in conjunction with the expert systems chapters that followed.

The standards section was closely associated with the CPR chapter of this section. Jeff Blair did a terrific job with his overview of standards related to the emerging health care information infrastructure. This chapter gave the reader not only an overview of the major existing and emerging health care information standards but an understanding of all (the "then," current) efforts, national and international, to coordinate, harmonize, and accelerate these activities. The introduction summarized how this section was organized. It included identifier standards (patient's, site of care, product, and supply labeling), communications (message format) standards, content, and structure standards. This section was followed by a summary of clinical data representations, guidelines for confidentiality, data, security, and authentication. After that quality indicators and data sets were described along with international standards. Coordinating and promotion organizations were listed at the end of this chapter including points of contact which proved to be very beneficial for those who needed to follow up.

Design issues in developing clinical decision support and monitoring systems by John Goethe and Joseph Bronzino provided insight for the development of clinical decision support systems. In their introduction and throughout this chapter, the authors provided a step-by-step tutorial with practical advice and make recommendations on design of the systems to achieve end-user acceptance. After that a description of a clinical monitoring system, developed and implemented by them for a psychiatric practice, was presented in detail. In their conclusions, the human engineering issue was discussed.

What is New in This Edition

There are two new chapters. One is an Introduction to Nursing Informatics by Kathleen McCormick et al. and one is on Medical Informatics and Biomedical Emergencies: New Training and Simulation Technologies for First Responders, by Joseph Rosen et al. Since nurses work side by side with physicians, biomedical engineers, information technologists, and others, the understanding becomes crucial of this profession and what they do in their daily hospital activities becomes crucial.

Delivering detection, diagnostic, and treatment information to first responders remains a central challenge in disaster management. This is particularly true in biomedical emergencies involving highly infectious agents. Adding inexpensive, established information technologies to existing response system will produce beneficial outcomes. In some instances, however, emerging technologies will be necessary to enable an immediate, continuous response. This article identifies and describes new training, education and simulation technologies that will help first responders cope with bioterrorist events.

Two revisions from the prior edition, were made by Summers and Carson and Michael Fitzmaurice respectively.

The authors of this section represented industry, academia, and government. Their expertise in many instances is multiple from developing to actual implementing these technical ideas. I am very grateful for all our discussions and their contributions.

References

[1] WordNet 1.7.1 Copyright© 2001 by Princeton University. All rights reserved.
[2] The American Heritage® Dictionary of the English Language, 4th ed. Copyright© 2004, 2000 by Houghton Mifflin Company. Published by Houghton Mifflin Company. All rights reserved.
[3] Shortliffe E.H. The science of biomedical computing. *Med. Inform.* 1984; 9: 185–93.
[4] Von Bemmel J.H. The structure of medical informatics. *Med. Inform.* 1984; 9: 175–80.
[5] (The Fusion of Computers and Telecommunications in the 1990s) by Bradley, Hausman and Nolan (1993).
[6] Invited Lecturer for the IEEE-EMBS, Dallas/Fort Worth Section. Session Topic — "Paperless Hospital" University of Texas, Arlington, TX; October 1989.
[7] Kun, L., Chairman during the *24th Annual AAMI-Association for the Advancement of Medical Instrumentation-Conference*, Session Topic — "The paperless hospital." Presentation: "Trends for the creation of an All Digital Medical Record," St. Louis, Missouri; May 1989.

[8] Kun, L., Guest Speaker to the *Association for the Advancement of Medical Instrumentation*. Session: Technology Management in 21st Century Health Care. Topic: "Electronic Community Medical Records." Anaheim, CA; May 1995.

[9] Kun, L., Invited lecturer Trinity College/*The Hartford Graduate Center Biomedical Engineering Seminar Series Fall 1990*. Session Topic — "The Digital Medical Record" Hartford, CT.

[10] Kun, L., UTA Biomedical Engineering Dept. Graduate Seminar. Topic —"All Digital Medical Record". Arlington, TX; October 1988.

[11] Kun, L., Guest lecturer for the *Emergency Physicians Training Conference*. Session Topic — "All Digital Medical Record at the ER", Infomart, Dallas, TX; June 1990.

[12] Kun, L., Guest Speaker to the *1st National Symposium on Coupling Technology to National Need*. Topic: "Impact of the Electronic Medical Record and the High Performance Computing and Communications in Health Care. Albuquerque, New Mexico; August 1993.

[13] Kun, L., Distinguished Lecturer and part of a debate panel on the topic: "The Vision of the Future of Health Care Technology and Health Care Reform." Presentation topic: "The Role of the EMR and the HPCC in Controlling the Cost of Health Care." *Sigma-Xi Distinguished Lectureship Program at the University of Connecticut*, April 1994.

[14] Kun, L., Applications of Microcomputers in Government, Industry and University. Centro Internacional de Fisica y la Universidad Nacional Quito, Ecuador , Course 4 Topic: "*The All Digital Medical Record. Image, Voice, Signals, Text and Graphics used for Patient Care*"; July 1987.

[15] Kun, L., Universidad Nacional, Santo Domingo, Dominican Republic. Course 4 Topic: "The All Digital Medical Record. Image, Voice, Signals, Text and Graphics used for Patient Care"; July 1987.

[16] Kun, L., *Seminar Manager for the 1 week IBM Europe Institute: "Medical Computing: The Next Decade."* Presentation — "All Digital Medical Record", Garmisch-Partenkirchen, Germany. August 1989.

[17] Kun, L., *Seminar Technical Chairman IBM Research/IBM France*. Topic - "Medical Imaging Computing: The Next Decade." Presentation — "The Paperless Hospital", Lyon, France; June 1990.

[18] Kun, L., Guest Speaker and Session Chairman to the 1994 *2nd International Symposium Biomedical Engineering in the 21st Century*. Topics: "Telemedicine" and "The Computer Based Patient Record." Center for Biomedical Engineering, College of Medicine, National Taiwan University, Taipei Convention Center, Taipei, Taiwan, R.O.C. September 1994.

[19] Kun, L., Invited lecturer to the Director of Health Industry Marketing Asia/Pacific. Session Topic - "The All Digital Medical Record", Tokyo, Japan. Sponsor IBM Japan/Asia Pacific HQ; April 1991.

[20] Kun, L., Guest Speaker to the Role of Technology in the Cost of Health Care Conference. Session: "The Role of Information Systems in Controlling Costs". Topic: "The Electronic Medical Record and the High Performance Computing and Communications Controlling Costs of Health Care." Washington, DC; April 1994.

[21] Kun, L., Guest Speaker to the Role of Technology in the Cost of Health Care: Providing the Solutions Conference. Health Care Technology Policy II Topic: " Transfer & Utilization of Government Technology Assets to the Private Sector in the Fields of Health Care and Information Technologies". Moderator Session: "Use of Information Systems as a Management Tool". Washington, DC; May 1995.

[22] Kun, L., Session Chairman of a Special Mini-Symposia on: "Engineering Solutions to Healthcare Problems: Policy Issues", during the *15th annual International Conference IEEE-EMBS*. Also presenter of the lecture: "Health Care Reform Addressed by Technology Transfer: The Electronic Medical Record & the High Performance Computers & Communications Efforts. San Diego, California; October 1993.

[23] Kun, L., Conference Chairman — Health Care Information Infrastructure, Part of *SPIE's 1995 Symposium on Information, Communications and Computer Technology, Applications and Systems*. Philadelphia, Pennsylvania; October 1995

[24] Kohn, L., Janet M. Corrigan, and Molla S. Donaldson, Editors; Committee on Quality of Health Care in America, Institute of Medicine, "To Err is Human: Building a Safer Health System", (2000) Institute of Medicine.

[25] Foundation for eHealth Initiative: http://www.ncpdp.org/pdf/eHIOverview.pdf

[26] Kun, L., Guest lecture: "Healthcare of the elderly in the 21st century. Can we afford not to use telemedicine?" CIMIC, Rutgers University, NJ; December 12, 1996: http://cimic.rutgers.edu/seminars/kun.html

40

Hospital Information Systems: Their Function and State

40.1 Patient Database Strategies for the HIS **40**-2
40.2 Data Acquisition **40**-3
40.3 Patient Admission, Transfer, and
     Discharge Functions **40**-4
40.4 Patient Evaluation **40**-4
40.5 Patient Management..................................... **40**-5
40.6 Conclusion **40**-7
References **40**-7

T. Allan Pryor
University of Utah

The definition of a hospital information system (HIS) is unfortunately not unique. The literature of both the informatics community and health care data processing world is filled with descriptions of many differing computer systems defined as an HIS. In this literature, the systems are sometimes characterized into varying level of HISs according to the functionally present within the system. With this confusion from the literature, it is necessary to begin this chapter with a definition of an HIS. To begin this definition, I must first describe what it is not. The HIS will incorporate information from the several departments within the hospital, but an HIS is not a departmental system. Departmental systems such as a pharmacy or a radiology system are limited in their scope. They are designed to manage only the department that they serve and rarely contain patient data captured from other departments. Their function should be to interface with the HIS and provide portions of the patient medical/administrative record that the HIS uses to manage the global needs of the hospital and patient.

A clinical information system is likewise not an HIS. Again, although the HIS needs clinical information to meets its complete functionality, it is not exclusively restricted to the clinical information supported by the clinical information systems. Examples of clinical information systems are ICU systems, respiratory care systems, nursing systems. Similar to the departmental systems, these clinical systems tend to be one-dimensional with a total focus on one aspect of the clinical needs of the patient. They provide little support for the administrative requirements of the hospital.

If we look at the functional capabilities of both the clinical and departmental systems, we see many common features of the HIS. They all require a database for recording patient information. Both types of systems must be able to support data acquisition and reporting of patient data. Communication of information to other clinical or administrative departments is required. Some form of management support can be found in all the systems. Thus, again looking at the basic functions of the system one cannot differentiate the clinical/departmental systems from the HIS. It is this confusion that makes defining the HIS difficult and explains why the literature is ambiguous in this matter.

The concept of the HIS appears to be, therefore, one of integration and breadth across the patient or hospital information needs. That is, to be called an HIS the system must meet the global needs of those it is to serve. In the context, if we look at the hospital as the customer of the HIS, then the HIS must be able to provide global and departmental information on the state of the hospital. For example, if we consider the capturing of charges within the hospital to be an HIS function, then the system must capture all patient charges no matter which departmental originated those charges. Likewise all clinical information about the patient must reside within the database of the HIS and make possible the reporting and management of patient data across all clinical departments and data sources. It is totality of function that differentiates the HIS from the departmental or restricted clinical system, not the functions provided to a department or clinical support incorporated within the system.

The development of an HIS can take many architectural forms. It can be accomplished through interfacing of a central system to multiple departmental or clinical information systems. A second approach which has been developed is to have, in addition to a set of global applications, departmental or clinical system applications. Because of the limitation of all existing systems, any existing comprehensive HIS will in fact be a combination of interfaces to departmental/clinical systems and the applications/database of the HIS purchased by the hospital.

The remainder of this chapter will describe key features that must be included in today's HIS. The features discussed below are patient databases, patient data acquisition, patient admission/bed control, patient management and evaluation applications, and computer-assisted decision support. This chapter will not discuss the financial/administrative applications of an HIS, since those applications for the purposes of this chapter are seen as applications existing on a financial system that may not be integral application of the HIS.

40.1 Patient Database Strategies for the HIS

The first HISs were considered only an extension of the financial and administrative systems in place in the hospital. With this simplistic view many early systems developed database strategies that were limited in their growth potential. Their databases mimicked closely the design of the financial systems that presented a structure that was basically a "flat file" with well-defined fields. Although those fields were adequate for capturing the financial information used by administration to track the patient's charges, they were unable to adapt easily to the requirement to capture the clinical information being requested by health care providers. Today's HIS database should be designed to support a longitudinal patient record (the entire clinical record of the patient spanning multiple inpatient, outpatient encounters), integration of all clinical and financial data, and support of decision support functions.

The creation of a longitudinal patient record is now a requirement of the HIS. Traditionally the databases of the HISs were encounter-based. That is, they were designed to manage a single patient visit to the hospital to create a financial record of the visit and make available to the care provider data recorded during the visit. Unfortunately, with those systems the care providers were unable to view the progress of the patient across encounters, even to the point that in some HISs critical information such as patient allergies needed to be entered with each new encounter. From the clinical perspective, the management of a patient must at least be considered in the context of a single episode of care. This episode might include one or more visits to the hospital's outpatient clinics, the emergency department, and multiple inpatient stays. The care provider to manage properly the patient, must have access to all the information recorded from those multiple encounters. The need for a longitudinal view dictates that the HIS database structure must both allow for access to the patient's data independent of an encounter and still provide for encounter-based access to adapt to the financial and billing requirements of the hospital.

The need for integration of the patient data is as important as the longitudinal requirement. Traditionally the clinical information tended to be stored in separate departmental files. With this structure it was easy to report from each department, but the creation of reports combining data from the different proved difficult if not impossible. In particular in those systems where access to the departmental data was provided only though interfaces with no central database, it was impossible to create an integrated patient evaluation report. Using those systems the care providers would view data from different screens at their terminal and extract with pencil onto paper the results from each departmental (clinical laboratory, radiology, pharmacy, and so on) the information they needed to properly evaluate the patient. With the integrated clinical database the care provider can view directly on a single screen the information from all departments formatted in ways that facilitate the evaluation of the patient.

Today's HIS is no longer merely a database and communication system but is an assistant in the management of the patient. That is, clinical knowledge bases are an integral part of the HIS. These knowledge bases contain rules and/or statistics with which the system can provide alerts or reminders or implement clinical protocols. The execution of the knowledge is highly dependent on the structure of the clinical database. For example, a rule might be present in the knowledge base to evaluate the use of narcotics by the patient. Depending on the structure of the database, this may require a complex set of rules looking at every possible narcotic available in the hospital's formulary or a single rule that checks the presence of the class narcotics in the patient's medical record. If the search requires multiple rules, it is probably because the medical vocabulary has been coded without any structure. With this lack of structure there needs to be a specific rule to evaluate every possible narcotic code in the hospital's formulary against the patient's computer medication record. With a more structured data model a single rule could suffice. With this model the drug codes have been assigned to include a hierarchical structure where all narcotics would fall into the same hierarchical class. Thus, a single rule specific only to the class "narcotics" is all that is needed to compare against the patient's record.

These enhanced features of the HIS database are necessary if the HIS is going to serve the needs of today's modern hospital. Beyond these inpatient needs, the database of the HIS will become part of an enterprise clinical database that will include not only the clinical information for the inpatient encounters but also the clinical information recorded in the physician's office or the patient's home during outpatient encounters. Subsets of these records will become part of state and national health care databases. In selecting, therefore, and HIS, the most critical factor is understanding the structure and functionality of its database.

40.2 Data Acquisition

The acquisition of clinical data is key to the other functions of the HIS. If the HIS is to support an integrated patient record, then its ability to acquire clinical data from a variety of sources directly affect its ability to support the patient evaluation and management functions described below. All HIS systems provide for direct terminal entry of data. Depending on the system this entry may use only the keyboard or other "point and click" devices together with the keyboard.

Interfaces to other systems will be necessary to compute a complete patient record. The physical interface to those systems is straightforward with today's technology. The difficulty comes in understanding the data that are being transmitted between systems. It is easy to communicate and understand ASCII textual information, but coded information from different systems is generally difficult for sharing between systems. This difficulty results because there are no medical standards for either medical vocabulary or the coding systems. Thus, each system may have chose an entirely different terminology or coding system to describe similar medical concepts. In building the interface, therefore, it may be necessary to build unique translation tables to store the information from one system into the databases of the HIS. This requirement has limited the building of truly integrated patient records.

Acquisition of data from patient monitors used in the hospital can either be directly interfaced to the HIS or captured through an interface to an ICU system. Without these interfaces the acquisition of the monitoring data must be entered manually by the nursing personnel. It should be noted that whenever possible automated acquisition of data is preferable to manual entry. The automated acquisition is more accurate and reliable and less resource intensive. With those HISs which do not have interfaces to patient monitors, the frequency of data entry into the system is much less. The frequency of data acquisition affects the ability of the HIS to implement real-time medical decision logic to monitor the status of the patient. That is, in the ICU where decisions need to be made on a very timely manner, the information on which the decision is based must be entered as the critical event is taking place. If there is no automatic entry of the data, then the critical data needed for decision making may not be present, thus preventing the computer from assisting in the management of the patient.

40.3 Patient Admission, Transfer, and Discharge Functions

The admission application has three primary functions. The first is to capture for the patient's computer record pertinent demographic and financial/insurance information. A second function is to communicate that information to all systems existing on the hospital network. The third is to link the patient to previous encounters to ensure that the patient's longitudinal record is not compromised. This linkage also assists in capturing the demographic and financial data needed for the current encounter, since that information captured during a previous encounter may need not to be reentered as part of this admission. Unfortunately in many HISs the linkage process is not as accurate as needed. Several reasons explain this inaccuracy. The first is the motivation of the admitting personnel. In some hospitals they perceive their task as a business function responsible only for ensuring that the patient will be properly billed for his or her hospital stay. Therefore, since the admission program always allows them to create a new record and enter the necessary insurance/billing information, their effort to link the patient to his previous record may not be as exhaustive as needed.

Although the admitting program may interact with many financial and insurance files, there normally exists two key patient files that allow the HIS to meet its critical clinical functions. One is a master patient index (MPI) and the second is the longitudinal clinical file. The MPI contains the unique identifier for the patient. The other fields of this file are those necessary for the admitting clerk to identify the patient. During the admitting process the admitting clerk will enter identifying information such as name, sex, birth date, social security number. This information will be used by the program to select potential patient matches in the MPI from which the admitting clerk can link to the current admission. If no matches are detected by the program, the clerk creates a new record in the MPI. It is this process that all too frequently fails. That is, the clerk either enters erroneous data and finds no match or for some reason does not select as a match one of the records displayed. Occasionally the clerk selects the wrong match causing the data from this admission to be posted to the wrong patient. In the earlier HISs where no longitudinal record existed, this problem was not critical, but in today's system, errors in matching can have serious clinical consequences. Many techniques are being implemented to eliminate this problem including probabilistic matching, auditing processes, postadmission consolidation.

The longitudinal record may contain either a complete clinical record of the patient or only those variables that are most critical in subsequent admissions. Among the data that have been determined as most critical are key demographic data, allergies, surgical procedures, discharge diagnoses, and radiology reports. Beyond these key data elements more systems are beginning to store the complete clinical record. In those systems the structure of the records of the longitudinal file contain information regarding the encounter, admitting physician, and any other information that may be necessary to view the record from an encounter view or as a complete clinical history of the patient.

40.4 Patient Evaluation

The second major focus of application development for the HIS is creation of patient evaluation applications. The purpose of these evaluation programs is to provide to the care giver information about the patient which assists in evaluating the medical status of the patient. Depending on the level of data integration in the HIS, the evaluation applications will be either quite rudimentary or highly complex. In the simplest form these applications are departmentally oriented. With this departmental orientation the care giver can access through terminals in the hospital departmental reports. Thus, laboratory reports, radiology reports, pharmacy reports, nursing records, and the like can be displayed or printed at the hospital terminals. This form of evaluation functionality is commonly called results review, since it only allows the results of tests from the departments to be displayed with no attempt to integrate the data from those departments into an integrated patient evaluation report.

The more clinical HISs as mentioned above include a central integrated patient database. With those systems patient reports can be much more sophisticated. A simple example of an integrated patient evaluation report is a diabetic flowsheet. In this flowsheet the caregiver can view the time and amount of insulin given, which may have been recorded by the pharmacy or nursing application, the patient's blood glucose level recorded in the clinical laboratory or again by the nursing application. In this form the caregiver has within single report, correlated by the computer, the clinical information necessary to evaluate the patient's diabetic status rather than looking for data on reports from the laboratory system, the pharmacy system, and the nursing application. As the amount and type of data captured by the HIS increases, the system can produce ever-more-useful patient evaluation reports. There exist HISs which provide complete rounds reports the summarize on one to two screens all the patient's clinical record captured by the system. These reports not only shorten the time need by the caregiver to locate the information, but because of the format of the report, can present the data in a more intuitive and clinically useful form.

40.5 Patient Management

Once the caregiver has properly evaluated the state of the patient, the next task is to initiate therapy that ensures an optimal outcome for the patient. The sophistication of the management applications is again a key differentiation of HISs. At the simplest level management applications consist of order-entry applications. The order-entry application is normally executed by a paramedical personnel. That is, the physician writes the order in the patient's chart, and another person reviews from the chart the written order and enters it into the computer. For example, if the order is for a medication, then it will probably be a pharmacist who actually enters the order into the computer. For most of the other orders a nurse or ward clerk is normally assigned this task. The HIS records the order in the patient's computerized medical record and transmits the order to the appropriate department for execution. In those hospitals where the departmental systems are interfaced to the HIS, the electronic transmission of the order to the departmental system is a natural part of the order entry system. In many systems the transmission of the order is merely a printout of the order in the appropriate department.

The goal of most HISs is to have the physician responsible for management of the patient enter the orders into the computer. The problem that has troubled most of the HISs in achieving this goal has been the inefficiency of the current order-entry programs. For these programs to be successful they have to complete favorably with the traditional manner in which the physician writes the order. Unfortunately, most of the current order-entry applications are too cumbersome to be readily accepted by the physician. Generally they have been written to assist the paramedic in entering the order resulting with far too many screens or fields that need to be reviewed by the physician to complete the order. One approach that has been tried with limited success is the use of order sets. The order sets have been designed to allow the physician to easily from a single screen enter multiple orders. The use of order sets has improved the acceptability of the order-entry application to the physician, but several problems remain preventing universal acceptance by the physicians. One problem is that the order set will never be sufficiently complete to contain all orders that the physician would want to order. Therefore, there is some subset of patients orders that will have to be entered using the general ordering mechanisms of the program. Depending on the frequency of those orders, the acceptability of the program changes. Maintenance issues also arise with order sets, since it may be necessary to formulate order sets for each of the active physicians. Maintaining of the physician-specific order sets soon becomes a major problem for the data processing department.

It becomes more problematic if the HIS to increase the frequency of a given order being present on an order set allows the order sets to be not only physician-defined but problem-oriented as well. Here it is necessary to again increase the number of order sets or have the physicians all agree on those orders to be included in an order set for a given problem.

Another problem, which makes use of order entry by the physician difficult, is the lack of integration of the application into the intellectual tasks of the physician. That is, in most of the systems the physicians are asked to do all the intellectual work in evaluating and managing the care of the patient in the traditional manner and then, as an added task, enter the results of that intellectual effort into the computer. It is at this last step that is perceived by the physician as a clerical task at which the physician rebels. Newer systems are beginning to incorporate more efficiently the ordering task into other applications. These applications assist the physical throughout the entire intellectual effort of patient evaluation and management of the patient. An example of such integration would be the building of evaluation and order sets in the problem list management application. Here when the care provider looks at the patient problem list he or she accesses problem-specific evaluation and ordering screens built into the application, perhaps shortening the time necessary for the physician to make rounds on the patient.

Beyond simple test ordering, many newer HISs are implementing decision support packages. With these packages the system can incorporate medical knowledge usually as rule sets to assist the care provider in the management of patients. Execution of the rule sets can be performed in the foreground through direct calls from an executing application or in the background with the storing of clinical data in the patient's computerized medical record. This latter mode is called data-driven execution and provides an extremely powerful method of knowledge execution and alerting. that is, after execution of the rule sets, the HIS will "alert" the care provider of any outstanding information that may be important regarding the status of the patient or suggestions on the management of the patient. Several mechanisms have been implemented to direct the alerts to the care provider. In the simplest form notification is merely a process of storing the alert in the patient's medical record to be reviewed the next time the care provider accesses that patient's record. More sophisticated notification methods have included directed printouts to individuals whose job it is to monitor the alerts, electronic messages sent directly to terminals notifying the users that there are alerts which need to be viewed, and interfacing to the paging system of the hospital to direct alert pages to the appropriate personnel.

Execution of the rule sets are sometimes, time-driven. This mode results in sets of rules being executed at a particular point in time. The typical scenario for time-driven execution is to set a time of day for selected rule set execution. At that time each day the system executes the given set of rules for a selected population in the hospital. Time drive has proven to be a particularly useful mechanism of decision support for those applications that require hospitalwide patient monitoring.

The use of decision support has ranged from simple laboratory alerts to complex patient protocols. The responsibility of the HIS is to provide the tools for creation and execution of the knowledge base. The hospitals and their designated "experts" are responsible for the actual logic that is entered into the rule sets. Many studies are appearing in the literature suggesting that the addition of knowledge base execution to the HIS is the next major advancement to be delivered with the HIS. This addition will become a tool to better manage the hospital in the world of managed care.

The inclusion of decision support functionality in the HIS requires that the HIS be designed to support a set of knowledge tools. In general a knowledge bases system will consist of a knowledge base and an inference engine. The knowledge base will contain the rules, frames, and statistics that are used by the inference applications to substantiate a decision. We have found that in the health care area the knowledge base should be sufficiently flexible to support multiple forms of knowledge. That is, no single knowledge representation sufficiently powerful to provide a method to cover all decisions necessary in the hospital setting. For example, some diagnostic decisions may well be best suited for bayesian methods, whereas other management decisions may follow simple rules. In the context of the HIS, I prefer the term application manager to inference engine. The former is intended to imply that different applications may require different knowledge representations as well as different inferencing strategies to traverse the knowledge base. Thus, when the user selects the application, he or she is selecting a particular inference engine that may be unique to that application. The tasks, therefore, of the application manager are to provide the "look and feel" of the application, control the functional capabilities of the application, and invoke the appropriate inference engine for support of any "artificial intelligence" functionality.

40.6 Conclusion

Today's HIS is no longer the financial/administrative system that first appeared in the hospital. It has extended beyond that role to become an adjunct to the care of the patient. With this extension into clinical care the HIS has not only added new functionality to its design but has enhanced its ability to serve the traditional administrative and financial needs of the hospital as well. The creation of these global applications which go well beyond those of the departmental/clinical systems is now making the HIS the patient-focused system. With this global information the administrators and clinical staff together can accurately access where there are inefficiencies in the operation of the hospital from the delivery of both the administrative and medical care. This knowledge allows changes in the operation of the hospital that will ensure that optimal care continues to be provided to the patient at the least cost to the hospital. These studies and operation changes will continue to grow as the use of an integrated database and implementation of medical knowledge bases become increasingly routine in the functionality of the HIS.

References

[1] Pryor T.A., Gardner R.M., Clayton P.D. et al. (1983) The HELP system. *J. Med. Syst.* 7: 213.
[2] Pryor T.A., Clayton P.D., Haug P.J. et al. (1987) Design of a knowledge driven HIS. *Proc. 11th SCAMC*, 60.
[3] Bakker A.R. (1984) The development of an integrated and co-operative hospital information system. *Med. Inf.* 9: 135.
[4] Barnett G.O. (1984) The application of computer-based medical record systems in ambulatory practice. *N. Engl. J. Med.* 310: 1643.
[5] Bleich H.L., Beckley R.F., Horowitz G.L. et al. (1985) Clinical computing in a teaching hospital. *N. Engl. J. Med* 312: 756.
[6] Whiting-O'Keefe Q.E., Whiting A., and Henke J. (1988) The STOR clinical information system. *MD Comput.* 5: 8.
[7] Hendrickson G., Anderson R.K., Clayton P.D. et al. (1992). The integrated academic information system at Columbia-Presbyterian Medical Center. *MD Comput.* 9: 35.
[8] Safran C., Slack W.V., and Bleich H.L. (1989) Role of computing in patient care in two hospitals. *MD Comput.* 6: 141.
[9] Bleich H.L., Safran C., and Slack W.V. (1989) Departmental and laboratory computing in two hospitals. *MD Comput.* 6: 149.
[10] ASTM E1238-91 (1992) Specifications for transferring clinical observations between independent computer systems. Philadelphia, American Society for Testing and Materials.
[11] Tierney W.M., Miller M.E., and Donald C.J. (1990) The effect on test ordering of informing physicians of the charges for outpatient diagnostic tests. *N. Engl. J. Med.* 322: 1499.
[12] Stead W.W. and Hammond W.E. (1983) Functions required to allow TMR to support the information requirements of a hospital. *Proc. 7th SCAMC*, 106.
[13] Safran C., Herrmann F., Rind D. et al. (1990) Computer-based support for clinical decision making. *MD Comput.* 7: 319.
[14] Tate K.E., Gardner R.M., and Pryor T.A. (1989) Development of a computerized laboratory alerting system. *Comp. Biomed. Res.* 22: 575.
[15] Orthner H.F. and Blum B.I. (Eds.) (1989) *Implementing Health Care Information Systems*, Springer-Verlag.
[16] Dick R.S. and Steen E.B. (Eds.) (1991) *The Computer-Based Patient Record*, National Academy Press.

41

Computer-Based Patient Records

41.1	Computer-Based Patient Record.......................	**41**-2
41.2	Clinical Decision Support Systems	**41**-3
	Knowledge Server • Knowledge Sources • Medical Logic Modules • Nomenclature	
41.3	Scientific Evidence	**41**-5
	Patient Care Processes • Incentives • Evaluation • CDSS Hurdles • Research Databases • Telemedicine	
41.4	Federal Initiatives for Health Information System Interoperability and Connectivity	**41**-7
	PITAC	
41.5	Private Sector Initiatives...............................	**41**-9
41.6	Driving Forces for CPRS	**41**-9
	Patient Safety • Quality of Care	
41.7	Extended Uses of CPR Data...........................	**41**-11
41.8	Federal Programs	**41**-11
41.9	Selected Issues..	**41**-12
	Standards • Security • Data Quality • Varying State Requirements	
41.10	Summary	**41**-15
	Acknowledgment...	**41**-15
	References	**41**-16

J. Michael Fitzmaurice
Agency for Healthcare Research and Quality

The objective of this section is to present the computer-based patient record (CPR) as a powerful tool for organizing patient care data to improve patient care and strengthen communication of patient care data among healthcare providers. The CPR is even more powerful when used in a system that retrieves applicable medical knowledge to support clinical decision making, improving patient safety, and promoting quality improvement. Evidence exists that the use of CPR systems (CPRS) can change both physician behavior and patient outcomes of care. As the speed and cost efficiency of computers rise, the cost of information storage and retrieval falls, and the breadth of ubiquitous networks becomes broader, it is essential that CPRs and systems that use them be evaluated for the improvements in health care that they can bring, and for their protection of the confidentiality of individually identifiable patient information.

Any opinions expressed in this chapter are those solely of the author and not of the U.S. Department of Health and Human Services or of the Agency for Healthcare Research and Quality.

The primary role of the CPR is to support the delivery of medical care to a particular patient. Serving this purpose, ideally the CPR brings past and current information about a particular patient to the physician, promotes communication among healthcare givers about that patient's care, and documents the process of care and the reasoning behind the choices that are made. Thus, the data in a CPR should be acquired as part of the normal process of healthcare delivery, by the providers of care and their institutions to improve data accuracy and timeliness of decision support. And these data should be shared for the benefit of the patient's care, perhaps with the permission or direction of the patient to safeguard confidentiality.

The CPR can also be an instrument for building a clinical data repository that is useful for collecting information about which medical treatments are effective in the practice of medicine in the community and for improving population-based health care. A clinical data repository may be provider-based or patient-based; it may be disease specific and geographically specific. Additional applications of CPR data beyond direct patient care can improve population-based care. These applications bring personal and public benefits, but also raise issues that must be addressed by healthcare policy makers.

Because patient information is likely to be located in the medical records of several of the patient's providers, providing high quality of care often requires exchanges of this information among providers. The vision of health information technology applications to improving the quality of health care contains a role for a national health information infrastructure. This infrastructure could take many forms but the most likely form is a combination of local or regional networks through which the required exchanges of patient information could take place. Currently most of these exchanges are done using faxed messages or phone calls. Sometimes the patient is just given the information to carry to the next provider. The CPR can be an even more powerful tool when it is connected to an electronic network and interoperable with other CPRs. Like the use of CPR applications, the use of health information networks also brings issues to be addressed by healthcare policy makers.

Clinical data standards, personal health identification, and communication networks, all critical factors for using CPRs effectively, are also addressed separately in other sections of this book.

41.1 Computer-Based Patient Record

A CPR is a collection of data about a patient's health care in electronic form. The CPR, also called an electronic health record (EHR) is part of a system (a CPRS, usually maintained in a hospital, physician's office, or an Internet or application service provider if it is web-based) that encompasses data entry and presentation, storage, and access to the clinical decision maker — usually a physician or nurse. The data are entered by keyboard, dictation and transcription, voice recognition and interpretation, light pen, touch screen, hand-held computerized notepad or a hand-held personal digital assistant (perhaps wireless) with gesture, and character recognition and grouping capabilities. Entry may also be by other means, for example, by direct instrumentation from electronic patient monitors and bedside terminals, nursing stations, bar code readers, radio-frequency identification (RFID), analyses by other linked computer systems such as laboratory autoanalyzers, and intensive care unit monitors, or even another provider's CPRS via a secure network. While the CPR could include patient-entered data, some medical providers may question the validity of such information for making their decisions; others may rely on such data for diagnosis and treatment.

Patient care data collected by a CPRS may be stored centrally or they may be stored in many places (e.g., distributed among the patient's providers) for retrieval at the request of an authorized user (most likely with the patient's authorization) through a database management system. The CPR may present data to the physician as text, tables, graphs, sound, images, full-motion video, and signals on an electronic screen, cell phones, pagers, or even paper. The CPR may also point to the location of additional patient data that cannot be easily incorporated into the CPR.

In too many current clinical settings (hospitals, physicians' offices, and ambulatory care centers), data pertaining to a patient's medical care are recorded and stored in a paper medical record. If the paper record is out of its normal location, or accompanying the patient during a procedure or an off-site study, it is

TABLE 41.1 Core Functions of an Electronic Health Record System

Health information and data
Results management
Order entry/management
Decision support
Electronic communication and connectivity
Patient support
Administrative processes
Reporting and population health management

Source: Institute of Medicine [2003]. *Patient Safety: Achieving a New Standard for Care.* Aspden P., Corrigan J.M., Wolcott J., and Erickson S.M. (eds). National Academic Press, Washington, D.C.

not available to the nurse, the attending physician, or the expert consultant. In paper form, data entries are often illegible and not easily retrieved and read by multiple users one at a time. On the other hand, an electronic form provides legible, clinical information which can be available to all users simultaneously, thus improving timely access to patient care data and communication among care providers.

Individual hospital departments (e.g., laboratory or pharmacy) often lose the advantages of automated data when their own computer systems print the computerized results onto paper. The pages are then sent to the patient's hospital floor and assembled into a paper record. The lack of standards for the electronic exchange of this data and the lack of implementation of existing standards, such as using the Logical Observation Identifiers, Names and Codes (LOINC) standard for reporting laboratory results, hinders the integration of computerized departmental systems. Searching electronic files is often more efficient than searching through paper. Weaknesses of paper medical record systems for supporting patient care and health care providers have long been known [Korpman, 1990, 1991].

Many of the functions of a CPR and how it operates within a healthcare information system to satisfy user demands are explained in the Institute of Medicine's (IOM) report, The Computer-Based Patient Record: An Essential Technology for Health Care [1991, 1997]. In response to a request by the Agency for Healthcare Research and Quality, IOM provided guidance to DHHS in 2003 on a set of "basic functionalities" that an electronic health record system should possess to promote patient safety [IOM, 2003], shown in Table 41.1.

This guidance is the basis for a new Health Level Seven (HL7, a standard developing organization) standard that specifies the functions of an EHR that will be useful for EHR purchasers to specify what functions they want and for vendors of EHR systems to describe the functions they offer [HL7, 2004].

41.2 Clinical Decision Support Systems

One of the roles of the CPR is to enable a clinical decision support system (CDSS) — computer software designed to aid clinical decision making — to provide the physician with medical knowledge that is pertinent to the care of the patient. Diagnostic suggestions, testing prompts, therapeutic protocols, practice guidelines, alerts of potential drug–drug and drug–food reactions, evidence-based treatment suggestions, and other decision support services can be obtained through the interaction of the CPR with a CDSS.

41.2.1 Knowledge Server

Existing knowledge about potential diagnoses and treatments, practice guidelines, and complicating factors pertinent to the patient's diagnosis and care is needed at the time treatment decisions are made. The go-between that makes this link is a "knowledge server," which acquires the necessary information for the decision maker from the knowledge server's information sources. The knowledge server can assist the clinical decision maker to put this information, that is, specific data and information about the patient's identification and condition(s) and medical knowledge, into the proper context for treating the patient [Tuttle et al., 1994].

41.2.2 Knowledge Sources

Knowledge sources include a range of options, from internal development and approval by a hospital's staff, for example, to sources outside the hospital, such as the National Guidelines Clearinghouse, see www.guideline.gov, initiated by the Agency for Healthcare Research and Quality (AHRQ), the American Medical Association, and the Association of American Health Plans; the Physicians Data Query program at the National Cancer Institute at http://www.nci.nih.gov/cancertopics/pdq; other consensus panel guidelines sponsored by the National Institutes of Health; guidelines developed by medical and other specialty societies and others; and specialized information from private-sector knowledge vendors. Additional sources of knowledge include the medical literature, which can be searched for high quality, comprehensive review articles, and for particular subjects using the "PubMed" program to explore the MEDLINE literature database available through the National Library of Medicine at http://www.ncbi.nlm.nih.gov/entrez/query.fcgi?db=PubMed&itool=toolbar. AHRQ-supported Evidence-based Practice Center reports summarizing scientific evidence on specific topics of medical interest are available to support guideline development, see http://www.guideline.gov/resources/epc_reports.aspx.

41.2.3 Medical Logic Modules

If medical knowledge needs are anticipated, acquired beforehand, and put into a medical logic module (MLM), software can provide rule-based alerts, reminders and suggestions for the care provider at the point (time and place) of health service delivery. One format for MLMs is the Arden Syntax, which standardizes the logical statements [ASTM, 1992]. For example, an MLM might be interpreted as, "If sex is female, and age is greater than 50 years, and no Pap smear test result appears in the CPR, then recommend a Pap smear test to the patient." If MLMs are to have a positive impact on physician behavior and the patient-care process, then physicians using MLMs must agree on the rules in the logical statements or conditions and recommended actions that are based on interactions with patient-care data in the CPR. Another format is GLIF (the Guideline Interchange Format), a computer-interpretable language framework for modeling and executing clinical practice guidelines. GLIF uses GELLO, a guideline expression language that is better suited for GLIF's object-oriented data model, is extensible, and allows implementation of expressions that are not supported by the Arden Syntax [Wang 2004; also see http://www.openclinical.org/gmm_glif.html].

Because MLMs are usually independent, the presence or absence of one MLM does not affect the operation of other MLMs in the system. If done carefully and well, MLMs developed in one healthcare organization can be incorporated in the CPRSs of other healthcare organizations. However, this requires much more than using accepted medical content and logical structure. If the medical concept terminology (the nomenclature and code sets used by physicians and by the CPR) differs among organizations, the knowledge server may misinterpret what is in the CPR, apply logic to the wrong concept, or select the wrong MLM. Further, the physician receiving its message may misinterpret the MLM [Pryor and Hripcsak, 1994].

41.2.4 Nomenclature

For widespread use of CDSSs, a uniform medical nomenclature, consistent with the scientific literature is necessary. Medical knowledge is information that has been evaluated by experts and converted into useful medical concepts, options, and rules for decisions. For CDSSs to search through a patient's CPR, identify the medical concepts, retrieve appropriate patient data and information, and provide a link to the relevant knowledge, the CDSS has to recognize the names used in the CPR for the concepts [Cimino, 1993]. Providing direction for coupling terms and codes found in patient records to medical knowledge is the goal of the Unified Medical Language System (UMLS) project of the National Library of Medicine [NLM, 2005a]. "The UMLS Metathesaurus supplies information that computer programs can use to create standard data, interpret user inquiries, interact with users to refine their questions, and convert the users' terms into the vocabulary used in relevant information sources" [IOM, 2005b].

The developers of medical informatics applications need a controlled medical terminology so that their applications will work across various sites of care and medical decision making. The desiderata, or requirements, of a controlled medical terminology as described by Cimino [1998] include: "vocabulary content, concept orientation, concept permanence, nonsemantic concept identifiers, polyhierarchy, formal definitions, rejection of 'not elsewhere classified' terms, multiple granularities, multiple consistent views, context representation, graceful evolution, and recognized redundancy."

The National Committee on Vital and Health Statistics (NCVHS) is an 18-private-sector member, federal advisory committee with a 50-year history of advising the Secretary of Health and Human Services (HHS) on issues relating to health data, statistics, privacy, and national health information policy [http://aspe.dhhs.gov/ncvhs/]. Recognizing that "[w]ithout national standard vocabularies, precise clinical data collection and accurate interpretation of such data is difficult to achieve," NCVHS recommended in 2000 that the Secretary of HHS "should provide immediate funding to accelerate the development and promote early adoption of PMRI standards." This recommendation included clinical terminology activities of the National Library of Medicine, the Agency for Healthcare Research and Quality, and the Food and Drug administration to augment, develop and test clinical vocabularies, and to make them available publicly at low cost [NCVHS, PMRI, 2000]. The Consolidated Health Informatics work group, a White House, Office of Management and Budget, interagency, eGovernment Initiative dominated by HHS, Department of Veterans Affairs (VA), and Department of Defense (DoD) staff, made similar recommendations over the next 3 years. This encouragement led HHS to negotiate a national license for free use of SNOMED-CT (Systematized Nomenclature for Medicine — Clinical Terms), adopt 20 clinical data standards, and begin developing drug terminology and structured drug information, mapping vocabularies to SNOMED-CT, and investigating the standardization of data elements used for reporting patient safety adverse events.

41.3 Scientific Evidence

41.3.1 Patient Care Processes

Controlled trials have shown the effectiveness of CDSS for modifying physician behavior using preventive care reminders. In an early review of the scientific literature up, Johnston et al. [1994] reported that controlled trials of CDSSs have shown significant, favorable effects on care processes from (1) providing preventive care information to physicians and patients [McDonald et al., 1984; Tierney et al., 1986], (2) supporting diagnosis of high-risk patients [Chase et al., 1983], (3) determining the toxic drug dose for obtaining the desired therapeutic levels [White et al., 1987], and (4) aiding active medical care decisions [Tierney, 1988]. Johnston found clinician performance was generally improved when a CDSS was used and, in a small number of cases (3 of 10 trials), significant improvements in patient outcomes.

In a randomized, controlled clinical trial, one that randomly assigned some teams of physicians to computer workstations with screens designed to promote cost-effective ordering (e.g., of drugs and laboratory tests), Tierney et al. [1993] reported patient lengths of stay were 0.89 days shorter, and charges generated by the intervention teams were $887 lower, than for the control teams of physicians. These gains were not without an offset. Time and motion studies showed that intervention physician teams spent 5.5 min longer per patient during 10-h observation periods. This study is a rare controlled trial that sheds light on the resource impact and the effectiveness of using a CDSS.

In this setting, physician behavior was changed and resources were reduced by the application of logical algorithms to computer-based patient record information. Nevertheless, a different hospital striving to attain the same results would have to factor in the cost of the equipment, installation, maintenance, and software development plus the need to provide staff training in the use of a CDSS.

Additional evidence, rigorously obtained, shows beneficial effects of the use of EHRs within a CDSS on medical practices. As reported in the response of the Department of Health and Human Services to the GAO report, *Health and Human Services' Estimate of Health Care Cost Savings Resulting from the Use of Information Technology,* many studies published in peer-reviewed journals show "substantial improvement in clinical processes" when physicians use EHRs:

> The effects of EHRs include reducing laboratory and radiology test ordering by 9 to 14% [Bates, 1999; Tierney, 1990; Tierney, 1987], lowering ancillary test charges by up to 8% [Tierney, 1988], reducing hospital admissions, costing an average of $17,000 each, by 2 to 3% [Jha, 2001], and reducing excess medication usage by 11% [Wang, 2003; Teich, 2000] [GAO, 2005].

41.3.2 Incentives

As can be seen from the literature, CDSS can improve quality and in many cases reduce resources needed for treatment. The benefit of this resource reduction, however, goes most frequently to health plans under cost-based reimbursement of providers. The provider of care may need additional incentives to adopt CDSS as part of the regular work process. Otherwise, any added time needed to access and respond to the CDSS prompts and alerts may reduce the provider's personal productivity (see the extra 5.5 min per patient noted earlier) without offsetting compensation. These additional incentives may be funds for purchase of the hardware and software needed for CDSS, payment for using CDSS, or payment for reporting evidence of improved quality of care or cost reduction.

41.3.3 Evaluation

Clinical decision support systems should be evaluated according to how well they enhance performance in the user's environment [Nykanen et al., 1992]. If CDSS use is to become widespread and supported, society should judge CDSSs not only on enhanced provider performance, but also on whether patient outcomes are improved and system-wide healthcare costs are contained. Evaluation of information systems is extremely difficult because so many changes occur when they are introduced into an existing work flow. Attributing changes in productivity, costs of care, and patient outcomes to the introduction and use of a CDSS or a CPRS is difficult when the work patterns and the culture of the workplace are also changing. Many clinical information system applications have been self-evaluated in their original development site. While impressive findings have been published, the generalizability of those findings needs verification.

41.3.4 CDSS Hurdles

In a review of medical diagnostic decision support systems, Miller [1994] examines the development of CDSSs over the past 40 years, and identifies several hurdles to be overcome before large-scale, generic CDSSs grow to widespread use. These hurdles include determining (1) how to support medical knowledge base construction and maintenance over time, (2) the amount of reasoning power and detailed representation of medical knowledge required (e.g., how strong a match of medical terms is needed to join medical concepts with appropriate information), (3) how to integrate CDSSs into the clinical environment to reduce the costs of patient data capture, and (4) how to provide flexible user interfaces and environments that adjust to the abilities and desires of the user (e.g., with regard to typing expertise and pointing devices).

41.3.5 Research Databases

Computer-based patient records can have great value for developing research databases, medical knowledge, and quality assurance information that would otherwise require an inordinate amount of manual resources to obtain in their absence. An example of CPR use in research is found in a study undertaken at Latter Day Saints (LDS) Hospital. Using the HELP CPR system to gather data on 2847 surgical patients, this study found that administering antibiotics prophylactically during the 2-h window before surgery (as opposed to earlier or later within a 48-h window) minimized the chance of surgical-wound infection. It also reduced the surgical infection rate for this time category to 0.59%, compared to the 1.5% overall infection rate for all the surgical patients under study [Classen et al., 1992].

The same system was used at LDS Hospital to link the clinical information system data (including a measure of nursing acuity) with the financial systems' data. Using clinical data to adjust for the severity of patient illness, Evans et al. [1994] measured the effect of adverse drug events due to hospital drug administration on hospital length of stay and cost. The difference attributable to adverse drug events among similar patients was estimated to be an extra 1.94 patient days and $1939 in costs.

41.3.6 Telemedicine

A CPR may hold and exchange radiological and pathological images of the patient taken or scanned in digital form. The advantage is that digital images may be transferred long distances without a reduction in quality of appearance. This allows patients to receive proficient medical advice even when they and their local family practitioners are far from the consulting physicians. It also allows health managers to move such clinical work to take advantage of excess radiology and pathology capacity elsewhere in the system. Further, joint telemedicine consults in real time can also add to the ability of local physicians to become better at diagnosing and treating some conditions (such as those requiring expertise in dermatology) by learning from the long-distance specialist as he or she treats their patients. Nevertheless, while telemedicine has been shown to work in actual practice, the scientific literature does not present definitive findings of cost effectiveness or efficacy [Hersch, 2001a,b].

When personally identifiable healthcare data are transported electronically across state borders for telemedicine uses, the applicability of state laws and policies regarding the confidentiality and privacy of this data is not often obvious to the sender or receiver. This uncertainty raises legal questions for organizations that wish to move this data over national networks for patient management, business, or analytical reasons. When vendors of CPRS plan nationwide distribution of their products, they must consider among other things variation in state laws regarding the validity of electronic information for use in official medical records, the length of time for retention of medical record information, and liability for the consequences of EHR failure. The users of systems that exchange patient information across state borders for treatment must also consider the appropriate state licensing requirements.

41.4 Federal Initiatives for Health Information System Interoperability and Connectivity

For years, the Department of Veterans Affairs (VISTA — Veterans Health Information Systems and Technology Architecture) and the Department of Defense (CHCS-II — Composite Health Care System) have invested in the development of CPRS to improve care for veterans and active servicemen. The Indian Health Service has adopted and modified the VA's VISTA system for its own CPRS use. HHS has a history of undertaking national terminology development [Humphreys et al., 1998] and medical informatics research [Fitzmaurice et al., 2002]. In 2004, however, the federal government began to take the initiative to lay the foundation for improving the coordination of these efforts and promoting the interoperability and connectivity of health information systems across the country.

During the 2004–2005 period, the President placed a greater federal emphasis on using health information technology to improve patient safety and the quality of health care. President George Bush in his 2004 State of the Union message said, "By computerizing health records, we can avoid dangerous medical mistakes, reduce costs, and improve care." And on April 26, 2004, "Within ten years, every American must have a personal electronic medical record. That's a good goal for the country to achieve" [Bush, 2004].

As recommended by NCVHS [2001] and others, the President created the Office of the National Coordinator for Health Information Technology [Bush, 2004], and on May 6, 2004, the Secretary of

Health and Human Services (1) appointed David Brailer, M.D, Ph.D., as the first National Coordinator, and (2) announced that the medical vocabulary known as SNOMED CT (Systematized Nomenclature for Medicine — Clinical Terms, a clinical reference language standard created by the College of American Pathologists) could be downloaded free for use in the United States through HHS' National Library of Medicine [US DHHS, 2004]. By July 21, 2004, the National Coordinator produced a strategic framework to guide the nationwide implementation of health information technology in both the public and private sectors. This plan has four major goals to be pursued for the vision of improved health care. They are to build an interoperable national health information system that will:

1. Inform clinical practice
2. Interconnect clinicians
3. Personalize care
4. Improve population health [ONCHIT, 2004]

Through its Transforming Healthcare Quality Through Health Information Technology Program, the AHRQ in September 2004 awarded 100 grants ($139 Million over 3 years), 5 state demonstration contracts ($25 million over 5 years), a National Health Information Technology Resource Center contract ($18.4 million over 5 years), and initiated a data standards program ($10 million in 1 year). AHRQ's research program embodies the vision of the federal strategic framework for promoting and invests federal research funds to build a knowledge base of how regional and local information technology networks and applications can improve quality of care and patient safety [AHRQ, 2004].

Recognizing the benefits of CPRS and the exchange of clinical information, the President in his State of the Union message to the American people on February 3, 2005, called for additional investment, saying, "I ask Congress to move forward on ... improved information technology to prevent medical error and needless costs ..." The federal government has begun to devote resources to support its vision of national networks for the exchange of clinical information to benefit patient care. The vision is one of interoperable clinical applications of health information technology applications over a national set of regional networks and of connectivity to all health providers to these networks.

Health information systems are beginning to rely on intranet networks within the health enterprise to link the information created by disparate applications currently in use (e.g., to link existing [legacy] applications such as laboratory, radiology, and pharmacy information systems), and on private networks to exchange patient information among health providers. These systems use web browsers, object-oriented technology, and document formatting languages, including hypertext markup language (HTML) and extensible markup language (XML). Indeed, the structure of HL7's Version 3 of its suite of clinical message standards for health institutions' electronic clinical messages employs this technology [HL7, 2001], as does ASTM's proposed Continuity of Care Record standard [ASTM, 2005].

Currently, the health industry does not have acceptable standards for encrypting clinical message exchanges and for electronic signatures that are in widespread use. Although the confidentiality of subjects of personal health information is considered sufficiently protected and the authentication of the sender and receiver sufficiently assured for those providers who currently exchange clinical information through fax and telephone, pilot tests of electronic prescribing conducted by the Medicare Program should provide additional information on ways to improve protection and authentication for clinical exchanges through electronic networks. These 2006 pilots are mandated by the Medicare Prescription Drug, Improvement, and Modernization Act of 2003 (MMA) [Public Law, 2003].

41.4.1 PITAC

The President's Information Technology Advisory Committee (PITAC) is a private-sector member committee chartered originally in 1998 to provide the president with independent expert advice on maintaining America's preeminence in advanced information technology. In its 2004 report, *Revolutionizing Health Care Through Information Technology*, PITAC recommended Federal leadership in developing a national framework containing four essential elements. These elements are: electronic health records, computer-assisted clinical decision support, computerized provider order entry, and "secure, private, interoperable, electronic health information exchange, including both highly specific standards for capturing new data and tools for capturing non-standards-compliant electronic information from legacy systems" [PITAC, 2004]. In 2005, the President folded PITAC into the President's Council of Advisors on Science and Technology (PCAST).

41.5 Private Sector Initiatives

The Markle Foundation with support from The Robert Wood Johnson Foundation under its Connecting for Health program and in collaboration with the eHealth Initiative organizes working groups representing the public and private sectors to tackle the barriers to the development of an interconnected health information infrastructure. These working groups have produced papers On Linking Health Care Information (February 2005), Achieving Electronic Connectivity in Health Care (July 2004), Connecting Americans to Their Healthcare (July 2004), and Financial, Legal and Organizational Approaches to Achieving Electronic Connectivity in Healthcare (October 2004) and Connecting Healthcare in the Information Age (June 5, 2003). The Markle Foundation [Markle Foundation, 2005] convenes recognized experts and health sector stakeholders to reach consensus on how specific barriers should be tackled and preparing roadmaps for action.

The Healthcare Information and Management Systems Society (HIMSS) is a membership organization that focuses on providing leadership for the optimal use of healthcare information technology and management systems to better human health. One of its projects, Integrating the Healthcare Enterprise (IHE), is a multi-year initiative that has as its goal to create "the framework for passing vital health information seamlessly — from application to application, system to system, and setting to setting — across the entire healthcare enterprise." HIMSS, the Radiological Society of North America (RSNA), and the American College of Cardiology (ACC) work collaboratively with the aim "to improve the way computer systems in healthcare share critical information." In 2005, at the HIMSS Annual Conference, the IHE Connect-a-thon and Interoperability Showcase demonstrated the communication of documents containing patient care information found in ASTM's. Continuity of Care Record standard across the products of 32 health information system and application vendors using existing health data standards [HIMSS, IHE, 2005, http://www.himss.org/ASP/topics_ihe.asp.]. Public demonstrations of the applications of health data standards are invaluable for learning what works in the electronic exchange of patient care data and how it works. Essentially, what is learned is how to make health data standards work for specific health care applications and how to make them better.

41.6 Driving Forces for CPRS

41.6.1 Patient Safety

Patient safety is a real concern in the U.S. healthcare system but is not well understood. The publication of the IOM study *To Err is Human* in 1999, informed the American public that between 44,000 and 98,000 people died of medical errors in hospitals [IOM, 1999]. In 2003, Zhan and Miller estimated that complications of often preventable injuries and complications in hospitals in the United States lead to more than 32,000 deaths, 2.4 million extra days of care, and costs exceeding $9B annually [Zahn and Miller, 2003]. Among the conditions studied were accidental puncture and laceration, anesthesia complications, postoperative infections and bedsores, surgical wounds reopening, and obstetric traumas during childbirth. Health information technology is clearly part of the remedy. In a study of 36 hospitals, Barker et al., found that 19% of the doses were in error and that "the percentage of [drug] errors rated potentially harmful was 7%, or more than 40 per day in a typical 300-patient facility" [Barker, 2003]. Bates et al., found that the rate of serious medication errors dropped by more than half after a large tertiary teaching hospital implemented a computerized physician order entry system [Bates et al., 1998]. IOM recommends that "[t]o reduce the number of medical errors, the nation's health care system must harness available technologies and build an infrastructure for national health information" [IOM, 2003b Patient Safety: Achieving a New Standard for Care, IOM, 2003b].

IOM, which is a foremost advisor to the nation in evaluating scientific evidence and obtaining professional opinion pertaining to patient safety and quality of care, recommends that: "[t]o reduce the number of medical errors, the nation's healthcare system must harness available technologies and build an infrastructure for national health information." More specifically, IOM recommends a seamless national network that requires EHRs, secure platforms for exchange of info among providers and patients, and data standards that would make health information understandable by the information systems of different providers. Further, healthcare organizations must adopt information technology systems that are able to collect and share essential health information on patients and their care [IOM, 2003b].

41.6.2 Quality of Care

In *Crossing the Quality Chasm: A New Health System for the 21st Century*, [IOM, 2001], IOM noted that a chasm exists between current practice and the best we can do and urged the United States (1) to adopt six attributes of quality care: safe, effective, patient-centered, timely, efficient, and equitable and (2) to use information technology to improve the quality of care.

Quality of care deficiencies are widespread in the United States and, judging from one study, evenly distributed across metropolitan areas [McGlynn et al., 2003], from a random sample of health care experiences of adults living in 12 metropolitan areas in the United States over a 2-year period found that study participants received 54.9% of recommended care. They evaluated health system performance on 439 indicators of quality of care for 30 acute and chronic conditions as well as preventive care, with the participants receiving 53.5, 56.1, and 54.9% of the recommended care, respectively for the three categories. In the 12 metropolitan areas studied, Seattle, Washington, received the recommended care 59% of the time (the highest), Little Rock, Arkansas, 51% (the lowest) [Kerr, 2004].

The contribution of CPRSs for improving quality of care is to deliver medical knowledge and appropriate patient information to the healthcare decision makers — especially the physician and patient — at the time such information is needed and to aggregate clinical entries to obtain quality measures more efficiently than by combing through paper medical records. Once in place, CPRS can also reduce the cost of obtaining standardized quality measures, compared with manual abstractions of paper medical records.

41.6.2.1 Rising Healthcare Spending

Healthcare expenditures in the United States totaled $1.7 trillion in 2003 ($5,670 per capita) and 15.3% of our gross domestic product. This increase was a 7.7% increase over 2002 expenditures and exceeded the rate of inflation of the Consumers Price Index (2.3%) threefold [Smith, 2005; and Bureau of Labor Statistics, 2005]. Two major concerns over rising health spending are matters of (1) obtaining value for the dollar spent on health care and (2) achieving productive competitiveness in the U.S. A study by Hussey et al., showed that the United States spends more per capita on health care than four other comparable countries: Australia, Canada, New Zealand, and England. However, the United States underperforms on such measures as: breast cancer deaths, leukemia deaths, asthma deaths, suicide rates, and cancer screening. The implication is that even though the United States spends more, outcomes are not necessarily better.

41.6.2.2 Competition in the U.S. Economy

Firms in the United States are concerned that many goods produced in the United States are more expensive than in other parts of the world in part because of the higher costs of health care in the United States, and the larger portion of healthcare costs they incur as part of their labor costs. Also, if the U.S. healthcare system itself is not as productive as are the healthcare systems of other countries, our workers will spend more time obtaining health care and recovering from illness, and less time working. As a result, U.S. companies are encouraging health plans to improve the quality of care provided to their employees and to contract with lower cost providers. The Leapfrog Group and other employer groups are promoting a better health system by encouraging employer purchasers to buy healthcare services from providers using:

- Computer physician order entry to permit computer-generated prompts, alerts, and reminders to inform treatment decisions.
- ICU physician staffing — the use of board-certified hospital intensivists, hospital-based physicians that would take over a patient's care in the hospital intensive care unit.
- Evidence-based hospital referral — particularly for high-risk surgery and high-risk neonatal intensive care [Birkmeyer, 2001].

41.7 Extended Uses of CPR Data

Data produced by such systems have additional value beyond supporting the care of specific patients. For example, subsets of individual patient care data from CPRs can be used for research purposes, quality assurance purposes, developing and assessing patient care treatment paths (planned sequences of medical services to be implemented after the diagnoses and treatment choices have been made), assessments of treatment strategies across a range of choices, and postmarketing surveillance of drugs and medical device technologies in use in the community after their approval by the Food and Drug Administration. When linked with data measuring patient outcomes, CPR data may be used to help model the results achieved by different treatments, sites of care, and organizations of care.

If patient care data were uniformly defined and recorded, accurately linked, and collected into databases pertaining to particular geographical areas, they would be useful for research into the patient outcomes of alternative medical treatments for specific conditions and for developing information to assist consumers, healthcare providers, health plans, payers, public health officials, and others in making choices about treatments, technologies, sites and providers of care, health plans, and community health needs. This is currently an ambitious vision for research considering the presently limited use of CPRs. There are insufficient incentives for validating, storing, and sharing electronic patient record data, plus improvements are needed that push forward the state of the art in measuring the severity of patient illness so that the outcomes of like patients can be compared. Many healthcare decisions are now based on data of inferior quality or no data at all. The importance of these decisions, however, to the healthcare market is driving higher the demand for uniform, accurate clinical data.

41.8 Federal Programs

Uniform, electronic clinical patient data could be useful to many Federal programs that have responsibility for improving, safeguarding, and financing America's health. For example, the AHRQ is charged "to enhance the quality, appropriateness, and effectiveness of health services, and access to such services, through the establishment of a broad base of scientific research and through the promotion of improvements in clinical and health system practices, including the prevention of diseases and other health conditions" [PL, 1999].

The findings that result from such research should improve patient outcomes of care, quality measurement, and cost and access problems. To examine the influence on patient outcomes of alternative treatments for specific conditions, research needs to account for the simultaneous effects of many patient risk factors, such as diabetes and hypertension. Health insurance claims for payment data do not have sufficient clinical detail for many research, quality assurance, and evaluation purposes. Often, administrative data (such as claims data) must be supplemented with data abstracted from the patients' medical records to be useful. In many cases, the data must be identified and collected prospectively from patients (with their permission) and their providers to ensure availability and uniformity. The use of a CPR could reduce the burden of this data collection, support practice guideline development in the private sector, and support the development, testing, and use of quality improvement measures. Having uniform, computerized patient care data in CPRs would allow disease registries to be developed for many more patient conditions.

Other federal, state, and local health agencies also could benefit from CPR-based data collections. For example, the Food and Drug Administration, which conducts postmarketing monitoring to learn the incidence of unwanted effects of drugs after they are approved, could benefit from analyses of the next 20,000 cases, in which a particular pharmaceutical is prescribed, using data collected in a CPR. Greater confidence in postmarket surveillance could speed approval of new drug applications. The Centers for Medicare and Medicaid Services (CMS) is providing guidance and information to its Quality Improvement Organizations (QIOs) about local and nationwide medical practice patterns founded on analyses of national and regional clinical data about Medicare beneficiaries. Medicare QIOs could analyze more data from provider's CPRs in their own states to provide constructive, quality-enhancing feedback providers of care at less expense. As a further example, the Centers for Disease Control and Prevention with access to locally available (and perhaps anonymized) CPR data on patient care could more quickly and completely monitor the incidence and prevalence of communicable diseases, and engage in real-time surveillance for monitoring bioterrorism threats. State and local public health departments could allocate resources more quickly to address changing health needs with early recognition of community health problems.

Many of these uses require linked data networks and data repositories that communities and patients trust with their health data, or a filter of data flows that searches for events that would trigger a health alert. A national health information network could provide guidance, governance, and principles for the sharing of electronic patient information. Of paramount importance is the protection of the confidentiality of patient information. This may require an approach that gives patients a choice to opt in to such systems of sharing their information to obtain the benefits or to opt out of having the system use their own information.

41.9   Selected Issues

While there are personal and public benefits to be gained from extended use of CPR data beyond direct patient care, the use of personal medical information for these uses, particularly if it contains personal identification, brings with it some requirements and issues that must be faced. Some of the issues that must be addressed by health care policy makers, as well as by private markets, are as follows.

41.9.1   Standards

Standards are needed for the nomenclature, coding, and structure of clinical patient care data; the content of data sets for specific purposes; and the electronic transmission of such data to integrate data efficiently across departmental systems within a hospital and data from the systems of other hospitals and healthcare providers. If benefits are to be realized from rapidly accessing and transmitting patient care data for managing patient care, consulting with experts across long distances, linking physician offices and hospitals, undertaking research, and other applications, data standards are essential [Fitzmaurice, 1994].

The United States has the framework for coordination of U.S. standards developing organizations, development and coordination of the U.S. position on international standards issues, and representation at the technical committee that develops and approves international health data standards. The Healthcare Informatics Standards Board of the American National Standards Institute coordinates the standard developing organizations that work on such standards in the United States, and produces special summary reports on administrative and clinical health data standards [ANSI HISB, 1997, 1998]. The U.S. Technical Advisory Group to the Organization of International Standards (ISO) Technical Committee (TC) 215, Health Informatics, develops and represents U.S. positions on international health data standards issues, new work items, and recommends the U.S. vote on international standards ballots. The ISO TC 215, Health Informatics, was formed in 1998 by over 30 countries to provide a forum for international coordination of health informatics standards.

TABLE 41.2   HIPAA Administrative Simplification Standards

Transactions and Code Sets (TCS) Rule — October 16, 2002/2003
    Claims Attachments — Proposed rule 2005
    TCS Revisions — Expected 2005
Identifiers
    Employer ID — July 30, 2004
    National Provider ID — May 23, 2007
    Health Plan ID — Expected 2005
    Individual ID — Put on hold by Congress
Security Rule — April 21, 2005
Privacy Rule — April 14, 2003

Note: Small health plans have an additional year before their use of HIPAA standards is mandatory.

Within the United States, administrative health data standards are mandated in the Health Insurance Portability and Accountability Act (HIPAA) of 1996 [Public Law, 1996]. In this law, the Secretary of Health and Human Services (HHS) is directed to adopt standards for nine common health transactions (enrollment, claims, payment, and others) that must be used if those transactions are conducted electronically. Penalties are capped at $100 per violation and a maximum of $25,000 per year for each provision violated. Digital signatures, when adopted by the Secretary, may be deemed to satisfy federal and state statutory requirements for written signatures for HIPAA transactions but there is no industry standard to date. The four categories of HIPAA standards with the dates on which specific standards are mandatory, or the year in which they are expected to be published, are shown in Table 41.2. Published standards are expected to be mandatory about 2 years and 60 days after they are published in final form.

41.9.2 Security

Confidentiality and privacy of individually identifiable patient care and provider data are the most important issues. For most purposes, the HIPAA Privacy Rule [U.S. Department of Health and Human Services, Office of Civil Rights, 2003] is quite stringent with respect to establishing a privacy floor across all states. It creates a fence around the individually identifiable health information it protects, that is, such information that is in the hands of health plans, clearinghouses, and providers who undertake HIPAA transactions (covered entities). Covered entities may use protected health information only for purposes of treatment, payment, or health operations. Without an individual's authorization, there are only 12 ways for a covered entity to legally disclose or use protected health information. Each of these exceptions has requirements of its own.

The HIPAA Privacy Rule is an essential cornerstone for building a national health information infrastructure that eases the way for personal health information to be shared. It gives patients new rights and controls nationwide, including the right to see, obtain a copy of, and add amendments to their health information. For uses and disclosures not permitted by the Privacy Rule, HIPAA-covered entities must obtain the individual's authorization. The penalties for violating the Privacy Rule can be expensive and include imprisonment.

System security and integrity become important as more and more information for patient treatment and other uses is exchanged through national networks. Not only does this issue relate to purposeful violations of privacy, but also to the accuracy of medical knowledge for patient benefit. If the system fails to transmit accurately what was sent to a physician — for example, an MRI, patient history, a practice guideline, or a clinical research finding — and if a physician's judgment and recommendation is based on a flawed image or other misreported medical knowledge — who bears the legal responsibility for a resulting inappropriate patient outcome due to system failure?

TABLE 41.3   Exceptions to the HIPAA Privacy Rule

As required by law
For public health
Victims of abuse
For health oversight activities
For judicial and administrative proceedings
For law enforcement
Disclosures about decedents (coroner, medical examiner)
To facilitate organ transplantation
For research
To avert serious threats to health or safety
For specialized government functions
For workers' compensation

Note: Individual authorization is not required for disclosures and uses of protected health information.

National HIPAA security standards for assuring the confidentiality of electronic protected health information are mandatory as of April 20, 2005. The HIPAA Security Rule addresses the administrative, technical, and physical security procedures that HIPAA-covered entity must use. Some procedure specifications are required; others must be addressed following a risk analysis by the HIPAA-covered entity [Health Insurance Reform, 2003]. This rule supports the Privacy Rule in that it establishes what security protections are reasonable to safeguard electronic health information from impermissible uses and disclosures.

41.9.3 Data Quality

The quality of stored and exchanged clinical data may be questioned in the absence of organized programs and criteria to assess the reliability, validity, and sufficiency of this data. There should be a natural reluctance to use questionable data for making treatment decisions, undertaking research, and for providing useful information to consumers, medical care organizers, and payers. For proper use and analysis, the user should take special care in judging that the information is of sufficient quality to measure and assess the relevant risk factors influencing patient conditions and outcomes. Providers of care may have reluctance even in relying on data supplied by their own patients without some assurance that it is valid.

41.9.4 Varying State Requirements

Electronically stored records in one state may be considered to be legally the same as paper records, but not in another state. In law, regulation, and practice, many states require pen and ink recording and signatures, apparently ruling out electronic records and signatures. To reduce this inconsistency and uncertainty and to provide national guidance, the Electronic Signatures in Global and National Commerce Act was enacted by the U.S. government effective on October 1, 2000. This law gives electronic signatures the same legality as hand-written ones where all parties agree for transactions that are commercial, consumer, or business in nature [Public Law, 2000]. To add to the variability, State privacy laws that (1) conflict with the HIPAA Privacy Rule and (2) are more stringent override the federal Privacy Rule:

Standard unique identifiers for patients, health care providers, institutions and payers are needed to obtain economies and accuracy when linking patient care data at different locations, and patient care data with other relevant data. Under HIPAA, the Secretary of HHS must adopt standards for uniquely identifying providers, health plans, employers, and individuals. Because of national concerns about the confidentiality of personal health information that may be linked using the unique individual health identifier, final implementation of that identifier must await explicit approval by Congress.

Malpractice liability concerns arise as telemedicine and information technology allow physician specialists to give medical advice across state borders electronically to other physicians, other healthcare providers, and patients. Physicians are normally licensed by a state to practice within its own state borders. Does a physician who is active in telemedicine need to obtain a license from each state in which he or she practices medicine from outside the state? If the expert physician outside the patient's state gives bad advice, which state's legal system has jurisdiction for liability considerations?

Benefit–cost analysis methods must be developed and applied to inform investment decision makers about the most productive applications of CPR systems. There is a need for a common approach to measuring the benefits and the costs for comparing alternative information technology applications. Certainly this is difficult since so many things change with the introduction of CPRS. As hard as they are to do well, valid business risk and benefit assessments can advance the development and implementation of commercial CPR applications.

Regional health data repositories and information exchange networks for the benefit of patients, providers, employers, hospital groups, consumers, and state health and service delivery programs raise issues about the ownership of patient care data, the use of identifiable patient care data, and the governance of health data repositories. A study by the IOM [1994] examined the power of regional health data repositories for improving public health, supporting better private health decisions, recognizing medically and cost-effective healthcare providers and health plans, and generally providing the information necessary to improve the quality of healthcare delivery in all settings. Because these data may include personally identifiable data and move outside the environment in which they were created, resolving these issues is of paramount importance for the development of regional health networks.

41.10 Summary

In summary, the benefits of CPRS are becoming better known and accepted. What is unknown are the costs of achieving these benefits in sites other than where the CPRSs were developed and how to successfully overcome institutional obstacles to their implementation. The widespread use of systems that provide clinical decision support depends in good part on the development and use of a common medical terminology or, at least, a reference terminology that contains all the relevant concepts to which different medical terminologies can map. This would enable interoperable electronic health information systems to accurately exchange information about those concepts. Although the HIPAA Privacy Rule gives patients the right to obtain a copy of their health information, research findings are lacking on the benefits of sharing CPR information with the patients themselves.

Strong initiatives by the federal government are leading the private and the government sectors to consider what infrastructure is needed to support patient information exchanges by clinical systems for the care of a patient. Indeed, a patient's CPR may not be a real data repository but a set of links to a patient's data that resides in many diverse electronic medical records — a virtual CPR. In addition, the federal government is making substantial investments in regional, often statewide, health information network demonstrations, and in research that studies local health information technology applications. The purpose of these investments is to learn how these networks can resolve important issues regarding the connectivity of providers to the network, the interoperability of their systems, and how successful they can be for improving patient safety and the quality of care. Many issues have been presented that must be resolved if the vision of a national health information infrastructure to be even partially achieved. The good news is that there is a national will to tackle them.

Acknowledgment

The author is Senior Science Advisor for Information Technology, Agency for Healthcare Research and Quality in the U.S. Department of Health and Human Services.

References

American National Standards Institute, Healthcare Informatics Standards Board (1997). HISB Inventory of Health Care Information Standards Pertaining to the Health Insurance Portability and Accountability Act of 1996, P.L. 104–191. New York.

American National Standards Institute, Healthcare Informatics Standards Board (1998). Inventory of Clinical Information Standards, New York. http://web.ansi.org/rooms/room_41/public/docs.html

Agency for Healthcare Research and Quality (2004). Fact Sheet: The Agency for Healthcare Research and Quality Health Information Technology Programs. Accessed on March 5, 2005, at http://www.ahrq.gov/research/hitfact.htm.

ASTM International (1992). E1460-92: Standard Specifications for Defining and Sharing Modular Health Knowledge Bases (Arden Syntax for Medical Logic Modules). ASTM, Philadelphia, PA.

ASTM International (2005). WK4363 Standard Specification for the Continuity of Care Record (CCR). Accessed on April 8, 2005, at http://www.astm.org/cgi-bin/SoftCart.exe/DATABASE.CART/WORKITEMS/WK4363.htmL+mystore+lghb8081

Barker K.N., Flynn E.A., Pepper G.A., Bates D.W., and Mikeal R.L. Medication errors observed in 36 healthcare facilities. *Arch. Intern. Med.* 2002; 162: 1897–1903.

Bates D.W., Leape L.L., Cullen D.J., Laird N., Petersen L.A., Teich J.M., Burdick E., Hickey M., Kleefield S., Shea B., VanderVliet M., and Seger D.L. Effect of computerized physician order entry and a team intervention on prevention of serious medication errors. *JAMA*, 1998; 280: 1311–1316.

Bates D.W., Kuperman G.J., Rittenberg E., Teich J.M., Fiskio J., Ma'luf N., Onderonk A., Wybenga D., Winkelman J., Brennan T.A., Komeroff A.L., and Tanasijevic M. A randomized trial of a computer-based intervention to reduce utilization of redundant laboratory tests. *Am. J. Med.* 1999; 106: 144–150.

Birkmeyer J.D., Birkmeyer C.M., Wennberg D.E., and Young M. (2000). Leapfrog patient safety standards: the potential benefit of universal adoption. Washington, D.C.: The Leapfrog Group for Patient Safety Accessed on April 8, 2005, at http://www.leapfroggroup.org/media/file/Leapfrog-Launch-Executive_Summary.pdf

Bureau of Labor Statistics (2005) "Table 1A. Consumer Price Index for All Urban Consumers (CPI-U): U.S. city average, by expenditure category and commodity and service group. Accessed on October 11, 2005 at http://www.bls.gov/cpi/cpid03av.pdf.

Bush G.W. (2004a). Incentives for the Use of Health Information Technology and Establishing the Position of the National Health Information Technology Coordinator. Executive Order (April 27, 2004). Accessed at http://www.whitehouse.gov/news/releases/2004/04/20040427-4.html on February 21, 2005.

Bush G.W. (2004b). President Unveils Tech Initiatives for Energy, Health Care, Internet. Remarks by the President at American Association of Community Colleges Annual Convention, Minneapolis Convention Center, Minneapolis, Minnesota (April 26, 2004). Accessed at http://www.whitehouse.gov/news/releases/2004/04/20040426-6.html on February 28, 2005.

Chase C.R., Vacek P.M., Shinozaki T., Giard A.M., and Ashikaga T. Medical information management: Improving the transfer of research results to presurgical evaluation. *Med. Care.* 1983; 21: 410–424.

Cimino, J.J. Saying what you mean and meaning what you say: coupling biomedical terminology and knowledge. *Acad. Med.* 1993; 68: 257–260.

Cimino J.J. Desiderata for controlled medical vocabularies in the twenty-first century. *Meth. Inf. Med.* 1998; 37: 394–403.

Classen D.C., Evans R.S., Pestotnik S.L., Horn S.D., Menlove R. L., and Burke J.P. The timing of prophylactic administration of antibiotics and the risk of surgical wound infection. *NEJM* 1992; 326: 281–285.

Cynthia Smith, Cathy Cowan, Art Sensenig, Aaron Catlin and the Health Accounts Team. Health spending growth slows in 2003. *Health Affairs.* 2005; 24(1): 185–194.

Donaldson M.S. and Lohr K.N. (Eds.) (1994). *Health Data in the Information Age: Use, Disclosure, and Privacy.* National Academy Press, Washington, D.C.

Evans R.S., Pestotnik S.L., Classen D.C., and Burke J.R. Development of an automated antibiotic consultant. *MD Comput.* 1993; 10: 17–22.

Evans R.S., Classen D.C., Stevens M.S., Pestotnik S.L., Gardner R.M., Lloyd J.F., and Burke J.P. Using a health information system to assess the effects of adverse drug events. In *AMIA Proceedings of the 17th Annual Symposium on Computer Applications in Medical Care*, McGraw-Hill, Inc., New York, pp. 161–165.

Fitzmaurice J.M. (1994b). Health Care and the NII. In: Putting the Information Infrastructure to Work: Report of the Information Infrastructure Task Force Committee on Applications and Technology, pp. 41–56. National Institute of Standards and Technology, Gaithersburg, MD.

Fitzmaurice J.M., Adams K., and Eisenberg, J.M. Three decades of research on computer applications in health care. *J. Am. Med. Inform. Assoc.* 2002; 9: 144–160.

General Accounting Office, Health and Human Services' Estimate of Health Care Cost Savings Resulting from the Use of Information Technology. GAO-05-309R (February 17, 2005), pp. 1–9. Accessed on February 20, 2005 at http://www.gao.gov/new.items/d05309r.pdf.

Health Insurance Reform: Security Standards; Final Rule (2003). Federal Register. Rules and Regulations. 45 CFR Parts 160, 162, and 164.68(34); (Feb. 20, 2003): 8334–8381.

Hersh W.R., Wallace J.A., Patterson P.K., Shapiro S.E., Kraemer D.F., Eilers G.M., Chan B.K.S., Greenlick M.R., and Helfand M. (2001a). *Telemedicine for the Medicare Population.* Evidence Report/Technology Assessment No. 24 (Prepared by Oregon Health Sciences University, Portland, OR under Contract No. 290-97-0018). AHRQ Publication No. 01-E012. Rockville (MD): Agency for Healthcare Research and Quality. July 2001. Accessed on April 10, 2005 at http://www.ahrq.gov/clinic/evrptfiles.htm

Hersh W.R., Wallace J.A., Patterson P.K., Kraemer D.F., Nichol W.P., Greenlick M.R., Krages K.P., Helfand M. (2001b). Telemedicine for the Medicare Population: Pediatric, obstetric, and clinician-indirect home interventions. Evidence Report/Technology Assessment No. 24S, Supplement (Prepared by Oregon Health Sciences University, Portland, OR under Contract No. 290-97-0018). AHRQ Publication No. 01-E060. Rockville (MD): Agency for Healthcare Research and Quality. August 2001. Accessed on April 10, 2005 at http://www.ahrq.gov/clinic/evrptfiles.htm

HL7 EHR System Functional Model Draft Standard for Trial Use, July, 2004. Eds: Dickinson G., Fischetti L., and Heard S. Ann Arbor, Michigan: Health Level Seven, Inc., 2004. Accessed on April 7, 2005, at http://www.hl7.org/ehr/downloads/index.asp

HL7 Version 3.0 (Draft), Ann Arbor, Michigan: Health Level Seven. 2001. Accessed on April 8, 2005 at http://www.hl7.org/library/standards.cfm

Humphreys B.L., Lindberg D.A., Schoolman H.M., and Barnett G.O. The Unified Medical Language System: an informatics research collaboration. *J. Am. Med. Inform. Assoc.* 1998; 5: 1–11.

Hussey P.S., Anderson G.F., Osborn R., Feek C., McLaughlin V., Millar J., and Epstein A. How does the quality of care compare in five countries? *Health Affairs* 2004; 23: 89–99.

Institute of Medicine (1991). Revised edition 1997. The Computer-Based Patient Record: An Essential Technology for Health Care, Detmer D.E., Dick R.S., and Steen E.B. (Eds.). *Committee on Improving the Patient Record*, National Academy Press, Washington, D.C.

Institute of Medicine, Committee on Data Standards for Patient Safety. 2003a. *Key Capabilities of an Electronic Health Record System. Letter Report.* 2003. Washington, D.C.:The National Academies Press. Accessed at http://books.nap.edu/html/ehr/NI000427.pdf on February 20, 2005.

Institute of Medicine (1994). *Health Data In the Information Age: Use, Disclosure, and Privacy.* Donaldson M.S. and Lohr K.N. (Eds.), National Academy Press, Washington, D.C.

Institute of Medicine (1999). *To Err Is Human: Building a Safer Health System.* Kohn L.T., Corrigan J., and Donaldson M.S. (Eds.). Committee on Quality of Health Care in America. National Academy Press, Washington, D.C.

Institute of Medicine (2001). *Crossing the Quality Chasm: A New Health System for the 21st Century.* National Academy Press, Washington, D.C.

Institute of Medicine (2003b). *Patient Safety: Achieving a New Standard for Care.* Aspden P., Corrigan J.M., Wolcott J., and Erickson S.M. (Eds.). Committee on Data Standards for Patient Safety. National Academies Press, Washington, D.C.

Jha A.K., Kuperman G.J., Rittenberg E., Teich J.M., and Bates D.W. Identifying hospital admissions due to adverse drug events using a computer-based monitor. *Pharmacoepidemiol. Drug Safety*, 2001; 10: 113–119.

Johnston M.E., Langton K.B., Haynes R.B., and Mathieu A. Effects of computer-based clinical decision support systems on clinician performance and patient outcome. *Ann. Int. Med.* 1994; 120: 135–142.

Kerr E.A., McGlynn E.A., Adams J., Keesey J., and Asch S.M. Profiling the quality of care in twelve communities: results from the CQI study. *Health Affairs* 2004; 23: 247–256.

Korpman R.A. Patient care automation; the future is now. Part 2. The current paper system — can it be made to work? *Nurs. Econ.* 1990; 8: 263–267.

Korpman, R.A. Patient care automation; the future is now, Part 8. Does reality live up to the promise? *Nurs. Econ.* 1991; 9: 175–179.

Markle Foundation, Connecting for Health, General Resources (2005). Accessed on April 7, 2005 at http://www.connectingforhealth.org/resources/generalresources.html

McDonald C.J., Hui S.J., Smith D.M., Tierney W.M., Cohen S.J., Weinberger M., et al. Reminders to physicians from an introspective computer medical record. A two-year randomized trial. *Ann. Int. Med.* 1984; 100: 130–138.

McGlynn E.A., Asch S.M., Adams J., Keesey J., Hicks J., DeCristofaro A., and Kerr E.A. The Quality of Health Care Delivered to Adults in the United States, *N. Engl. J. Med.* 2003; 348: 2635–2645.

Miller, R.A. Medical diagnostic decision support systems — past, present, and future. *J. Am. Med. Inform. Assoc.* 1994; 1: 8–27.

National Committee On Vital and Health Statistics (2000). Report to the Secretary of the U.S. Department of Health and Human Services on Uniform Data Standards for Patient Medical Record Information. Department of HHS: July 6, 2000, Accessed at http://www.ncvhs.hhs.gov/hipaa000706.pdf on February 28, 2005.

National Committee on Vital and Health Statistics. Information for Health — A Strategy for Building the National Health Information Infrastructure: Report and Recommendations From the NCVHS. Washington, D.C., Department of Health and Human Services, November 15, 2001. Accessed on April 9, 2005, at http://www.ncvhs.hhs.gov/nhiilayo.pdf.

National Coordination Office for High Performance Computing and Communication (1994). HPCC FY 1995 Implementation Plan. Executive Office of The President, Washington, D.C.

National Library of Medicine (2005a). Unified Medical Language System, Section 2, Metathesaurus. Accessed on April 9, 2005 at http://www.nlm.nih.gov/research/umls/meta2.html

National Library of Medicine (2005b). Unified Medical Language System, Metathesaurus. Accessed on April 9, 2005 at http://www.nlm.nih.gov/pubs/factsheets/umlsmeta.html

Nykanen, P., Chowdhury, S., and Wiegertz, O. Evaluation of decision support systems in medicine. *Comput Methods Programs Biomed*; 1991; 34(2-3): 229–238.

Office of the National Coordinator for Health Information Technology (ONCHIT) (2004). *Strategic Framework: The Decade of Health Information Technology: Delivering Consumer-centric and Information-rich Health Care.* July 21, 2004, Washington, D.C., Dept. of Health and Human Services. Accessed at http://www.hhs.gov/healthit/frameworkchapters.html on February 21, 2005.

President's Information Technology Advisory Committee (2004). Revolutionizing health care through information technology. Arlington, VA. NCO for ITRD National Coordinating Office for Information Technology Research and Development, June 2004.

Pryor, T. Allan and Hripcsak, George. (1994). Sharing MLMs: An Experiment Between Columbia-Presbyterian and LDS Hospital. In *AMIA Proceedings of the 17th Annual Symposium on Computer Applications in Medical Care*, McGraw-Hill, Inc., New York, pp. 399–403.

Public Law 104–191, 1996. The Health Insurance Portability and Accountability Act of 1996, August 21, 1996.

Public Law 105–277, Department of Transportation and Related Agencies Appropriations Act, October 21, 1998.

Public Law 106–129, Healthcare Research and Quality Act of 1999, December 6, 1999. Accessed on April 8, 2005, at http://www.ahrq.gov/ hrqa99a.htm

Public Law 106–229. June 30, 2000. Electronic signatures in global and National commerce act. Accessed on March 5, 2005, at http://frwebgate.access.gpo.gov/cgi-bin/getdoc.cgi?dbname=106_cong_public_laws&docid=f:publ229.106.pdf

Public Law 108–173, Medicare Prescription Drug, Improvement, and Modernization Act of 2003, December 8, 2003. Accessed on April 8, 2005, at http://www.cms.hhs.gov/medicarereform/MMAactFullText.pdf

Teich J.M, Merchia P.R., Schmiz J.L., Kuperman G.J., Spurr C.D., and Bates D.W. Effects of computerized physician order entry on prescribing practices. *Arch. Intern. Med.* 2000; 160: 2741–2747.

Tierney W.M., McDonald C.J., Martin D.K, and Rogers M.P. Computerized display of past test results. Effect on outpatient testing. *Ann. Intern. Med.* 1987; 107: 569–574.

Tierney, W.M., McDonald, C.J., Hui S.J., and Martin, D.K. Computer predictions of abnormal test results. Effects on outpatient testing. *JAMA* 1988; 259: 1194–11988.

Tierney W.M., Miller M.E., and McDonald C.J. The effect on test ordering of informing physicians of the charges for outpatient diagnostic tests. *NEJM* 1990; 322: 1499–1504.

Tierney W.N. and McDonald C.M. Practice Databases and their uses in clinical research. *Statist. Med.* 1991; 10: 541–557.

Tierney W.M., Miller M.E., Overhage J.M., and McDonald C.J. Physician inpatient order writing on microcomputer workstations. *JAMA* 1993; 269: 379–383.

Tuttle M.S., Sherertz D.D., Fagan L.M., Carlson R.W., Cole W.G., Shipma P.B., and Nelson S.J. 1994. Toward an interim standard for patient-centered knowledge-access. In *AMIA Proceedings of the 17th Annual Symposium on Computer Applications in Medical Care*, McGraw-Hill, Inc., New York, pp. 564–568.

U.S. Department of Health and Human Services, Office of Civil Rights (2003). Standards for Privacy of Individually Identifiable Health Information; Security Standards for the Protection of Electronic Protected Health Information; General Administrative Requirements Including, Civil Money Penalties: Procedures for Investigations, Imposition of Penalties, and Hearings. Regulation Text (Unofficial Version) (45 CFR Parts 160 and 164); December 28, 2000 as amended: May 31, 2002, August 14, 2002, February 20, 2003, and April 17, 2003. (August 2003). Accessed on April 9, 2005, at http://www.hhs.gov/ocr/combinedregtext.pdf

U.S. Department of Health and Human Services Press Release. May 6, 2004. Secretary Thompson, Seeking Fastest Possible Results, Names First Health Information Technology Coordinator. Accessed on March 5, 2005, at http://www.hhs.gov/news/press/2004pres/20040506.html.

U.S. Senate (1999). Healthcare Research and Quality Act of 1999, Senate Bill.580. Introduced January 6, 1999, signed into law on December 6, 1999. Accessed on March 5, 2005, at http://www.ahrq.gov/hrqa99a.htm.

Wang S.J., Middleton B., Prosser L.A., Bardon C.G., Spurr C.D., Carchidi P.J., Kittler A.F., Goldzer R.C., Fairchild D.G., Sussman A.J., Kuperman G.J., and Bates D.W. A cost–benefit analysis of electronic medical records in primary care. *Am. J. Med.* 2003; 114: 397–403.

Wang D., Peleg M., Tu S.W., Boxwala A.A., Ogunyemi O., Zeng Q., Greenes R.A., Patel V.L., and Shortliffe E.H. Design and implementation of the GLIF3 guideline execution engine. *Biomed. Inform.* 2004; 37: 305–18.

Zhan C. and Miller M.R. Excess length of stay, charges, mortality are attributable to medical injuries during hospitalization. *JAMA* 2003; 290: 1868–1874

42

Overview of Standards Related to the Emerging Health Care Information Infrastructure

42.1 Identifier Standards **42**-2
   Patient Identifiers • Provider Identifiers • Site-of-Care
   Identifiers • Product and Supply Labeling Identifiers
42.2 Communications (Message Format) Standards **42**-3
   ASC X12N • American Society for Testing and Materials •
   Digital Imaging and Communications • Health Level Seven
   (HL7) • Institute of Electrical and Electronics Engineers, Inc.
   P1157
42.3 Content and Structure Standards **42**-5
42.4 Clinical Data Representations (Codes) **42**-5
42.5 Confidentiality, Data Security, and Authentication ... **42**-6
42.6 Quality Indicators and Data Sets **42**-7
42.7 International Standards **42**-7
42.8 Standards Coordination and Promotion
   Organizations **42**-7
42.9 Summary **42**-8
References **42**-8
Further Reading **42**-10

Jeffrey S. Blair
IBM Health Care Solutions

As the cost of health care has become a larger percentage of the gross domestic product of many developed nations, the focus on methods to improve health care productivity and quality has increased. To address this need, the concept of a health care information infrastructure has emerged. Major elements of this concept include patient-centered care facilitated by computer-based patient record systems, continuity of care enabled by the sharing of patient information across information networks, and outcomes measurement aided by greater availability and specificity of health care information.

   The creation of this health care information infrastructure will require the integration of existing and new architectures, products, and services. To make these diverse components work together, health care information standards (classifications, guides, practices, terminology) will be required [ASTM, 1994]. This chapter will give you an overview of the major existing and emerging health care information standards, and the efforts to coordinate, harmonize, and accelerate these activities. It is organized into the major topic areas of:

- Identifier standards
- Communications (message format) standards
- Content and structure standards
- Clinical data representations (codes)
- Confidentiality, data security, and authentication
- Quality indicators and data sets
- International Standards
- Coordinating and promotion organizations
- Summary

42.1 Identifier Standards

There is a universal need for health care identifiers to uniquely specify each patient, provider, site of care, and product; however, there is no universal acceptance or satisfaction with these systems.

42.1.1 Patient Identifiers

The social security number (SSN) is widely used as a patient identifier in the United States today. However, critics point out that it is not an ideal identifier. They say that not everyone has an SSN; several individuals may use the same SSN; and the SSN is so widely used for other purposes that it presents an exposure to violations of confidentiality. These criticisms raise issues that are not unique to the SSN. A draft document has been developed by the American Society for Testing and Materials (ASTM) E31.12. Subcommittee to address these issues. It is called the "Guide for the Properties of a Universal Health Care Identifier" (UHID). It presents a set of requirements outlining the properties of a national system creating a UHIC, includes critiques of the SSN, and creates a sample UHD [ASTM E31.12, 1994]. Despite the advantages of a modified/new patient identifier, there is not yet a consensus as to who would bear the cost of adopting a new patient identifier system.

42.1.2 Provider Identifiers

The Health Care Financing Administration (HCFA) has created a widely used provider identifier known as the Universal Physician Identifier Number (UPIN) [Terrell et al., 1991]. The UPIN is assigned to physicians who handle Medicare patients, but it does not include nonphysician caregivers. The National Council of Prescription Drug Programs (NCPDP) has developed the standard prescriber identification number (SPIN) to be used by pharmacists in retail settings. A proposal to develop a new national provider identifier number has been set forth by HCFA [1994]. If this proposal is accepted, then HCFA would develop a national provider identifier number which would cover all caregivers and sites of care, including Medicare, Medicaid, and private care. This proposal is being reviewed by various state and federal agencies. It has also been sent to the American National Standards, Institute's Health Care Informatics Standards Planning Panel (ANSI HISPP) Task Force on Provider Identifiers for review.

42.1.3 Site-of-Care Identifiers

Two site-of-care identifier systems are widely used. One is the health industry number (HIN) issued by the Health Industry Business Communications Council (HIBCC). The HIN is an identifier for health care facilities, practitioners, and retail pharmacies. HCFA has also defined provider of service identifiers for Medicare usage.

42.1.4 Product and Supply Labeling Identifiers

Three identifiers are widely accepted. The labeler identification code (LIC) identifies the manufacturer or distributor and is issued by HIBCC [1994]. The LIC is used both with and without bar codes for products and supplies distributed within a health care facility. The universal product code (UPC) is maintained by the Uniform Code Council and is typically used to label products that are sold in retail settings. The national drug code is maintained by the Food and Drug Administration and is required for reimbursement by Medicare, Medicaid, and insurance companies. It is sometimes included within the UPC format.

42.2 Communications (Message Format) Standards

Although the standards in this topic area are still in various stages of development, they are generally more mature than those in most of the other topic areas. They are typically developed by committees within standards organizations and have generally been accepted by users and vendors. The overviews of these standards given below were derived from many sources, but considerable content came from the Computer-based Patient Record Institute's (CPRI) "Position Paper on Computer-based Patient Record Standards" [CPRI, 1994] and the Agency for Health Care Policy and Research's (AHCPR) "Current Activities of Selected Health Care Informatics Standards Organizations" [Moshman Associates, 1994].

42.2.1 ASC X12N

This committee is developing message format standards for transactions between payers and providers. It is rapidly being accepted by both users and vendors. It defines the message formats for the following transaction types [Moshman Associates, 1994]:

- 834 — enrollment
- 270 — eligibility request
- 271 — eligibility response
- 837 — health care claim submission
- 835 — health care claim payment remittance
- 276 — claims status request
- 277 — claims status response
- 148 — report of injury or illness

ASC X12N is also working on the following standards to be published in the near future:

- 257, 258 — Interactive eligibility response and request. These transactions are an abbreviated form of the 270/271.
- 274, 275 — patient record data response and request. These transactions will be used to request and send patient data (tests, procedures, surgeries, allergies, etc.) between a requesting party and the party maintaining the database.
- 278, 279 — health care services (utilization review) response and request. These transactions will be used to initiate and respond to a utilization review request.

ASC X12N is recognized as an accredited standards committee (ASC) by the American National Standards Institute (ANSI).

42.2.2 American Society for Testing and Materials

42.2.2.1 Message Format Standards

The following standards were developed within American Society for Testing and Materials (ASTM) Committee E31. This committee has applied for recognition as an ASC by ANSI:

1. ASTM E1238 standard specification for transferring clinical observations between independent systems. E1238 was developed by ASTM Subcommittee E31.11. This standard is being used by most of

the largest commercial laboratory vendors in the United States to transmit laboratory results. It has also been adopted by a consortium of 25 French laboratory system vendors. Health level seven (HL7), which is described later in this topic area, has incorporated E1238 as a subset within its laboratory results message format [CPRI, 1994].

2. ASTM E1394 standard specification for transferring information between clinical instruments. E1394 was developed by ASTM Subcommittee E31.14. This standard is being used for communication of information from laboratory instruments to computer systems. This standard has been developed by a consortium consisting of most U.S. manufacturers of clinical laboratory instruments [CPRI, 1994].

3. ASTM 1460 specification for defining and sharing modular health knowledge bases (Arden Syntax). E1460 was developed by ASTM Subcommittee E31.15. The Arden Syntax provides a standard format and syntax for representing medical logic and for writing rules and guidelines that can be automatically executed by computer systems. Medical logic modules produced in one site-of-care system can be sent to a different system within another site of care and then customized to reflect local usage [CPRI, 1994].

4. ASTM E1467 specification for transferring digital neurophysical data between independent computer systems. E1467 was developed by ASTM Subcommittee E31.17. This standard defines codes and structures needed to transmit electrophysiologic signals and results produced by electroencephalograms and electromyograms. The standard is similar in structure to ASTM E1238 and HL7; and it is being adopted by all the EEG systems manufacturers [CPRI, 1994].

42.2.3 Digital Imaging and Communications

This standard is developed by the American College of Radiology — National Electronic Manufacturers' Association (ACR-NEMA). It defines the message formats and communications standards for radiologic images. Digital imaging and communications (DICOM) is supported by most radiology picture archiving and communications systems (PACS) vendors and has been incorporated into the Japanese Image Store and Carry (ISAC) optical disk system as well as Kodak's PhotoCD. ACR-NEMA is applying to be recognized as an accredited organization by ANSI [CPRI, 1994].

42.2.4 Health Level Seven (HL7)

HL7 is used for intra-institution transmission of orders; clinical observations and clinical data, including test results; admission, transfer, and discharge records; and charge and billing information. HL7 is being used in more than 300 U.S. health care institutions including most leading university hospitals and has been adopted by Australia and New Zealand as their national standard. HL7 is recognized as an accredited organization by ANSI [Hammond, 1993; CPRI, 1994].

42.2.5 Institute of Electrical and Electronics Engineers, Inc. P1157

42.2.5.1 Medical Data Interchange Standard

Institute of Electrical and Electronics Engineers, Inc. (IEEE) Engineering in Medicine and Biology Society (EMB) is developing the medical data interchange standard (MEDIX) standards for the exchange of data between hospital computer systems [Harrington, 1993; CPRI, 1994]. Based on the International Standards Organization (ISO) standards for all seven layers of the OSI reference model, MEDIX is working on a framework model to guide the development and evolution of a compatible set of standards. This activity is being carried forward as a joint working group under ANSI HISPP's Message Standards Developers Subcommittee (MSDS). IEEE is recognized as an accredited organization by ANSI.

IEEE P1073 Medical Information Bus (MIB): This standard defines the linkages of medical instrumentation (e.g., critical care instruments) to point-of-care information systems [CPRI, 1994].

National Council for Prescription Drug Programs (NCPDP): These standards developed by NCPDP are used for communication of billing and eligibility information between community pharmacies and third-party payers. They have been in use since 1985 and now serve almost 60% of the nation's community pharmacies. NCPDP has applied for recognition as an accredited organization by ANSI [CPRI, 1994].

42.3   Content and Structure Standards

Guidelines and standards for the content and structure of computer-based patient record (CPR) systems are being developed within ASTM Subcommittees E31.12 and E31.19. They have been recognized by other standards organizations (e.g., HL7); however, they have not matured to the point where they are generally accepted or implemented by users and vendors.

A major revision to E1384, now called a standard description for content and structure of the computer-based patient record, has been made within Subcommittee E31.19 [ASTM, 1994]. This revision includes work from HISPP on data modeling and an expanded framework that includes master tables and data views by user.

Companion standards have been developed within E31.19. They are E1633, A Standard Specification for the Coded Values Used in the Automated Primary Record of Care [ASTM, 1994], and E1239–94, A Standard Guide for Description of Reservation/Registration-A/D/T Systems for Automated Patient Care Information Systems [ASTM, 1994]. A draft standard is also being developed for object-oriented models for R-A/D/T functions in CPR systems. Within the E31.12 Subcommittee, domain specific guidelines for nursing, anesthesiology, and emergency room data within the CPR are being developed [Moshman Associates, 1994; Waegemann, 1994].

42.4   Clinical Data Representations (Codes)

Clinical data representations have been widely used to document diagnoses and procedures. There are over 150 known code systems. The codes with the widest acceptance in the United States include:

1. International Classification of Diseases (ICD) codes, now in the ninth edition (ICD-9), are maintained by the World Health Organization (WHO) and are accepted worldwide. In the United States, HCFA and the National Center for Health Statistics (NCHS) have supported the development of a clinical modification of the ICD codes (ICD-9-CM). WHO has been developing ICD-10; however, HCFA projects that it will not be available for use within the United States for several years. Payers require the use of ICD-9-CM codes for reimbursement purposes, but they have limited value for clinical and research purposes due to their lack of clinical specificity [Chute, 1991].

2. Current Procedural Terminology (CPT) codes are maintained by the American Medical Association (AMA) and are widely used in the United States for reimbursement and utilization review purposes. The codes are derived from medical specialty nomenclatures and are updated annually [Chute, 1991].

3. The systematized nomenclature of medicine (SNOMED) is maintained by the College of American Pathologists and is widely accepted for describing pathologic test results. It has a multiaxial (11 fields) coding structure that gives it greater clinical specificity than the ICD and CPT codes, and it has considerable value for clinical purposes. SNOMED has been proposed as a candidate to become the standardized vocabulary for computer-based patient record systems [Rothwell et al., 1993].

4. Digital imaging and communications (DICOM) is maintained by the American College of Radiology — National Electronic Manufacturers' Association (ACR-NEMA). It sets forth standards for indices of radiologic diagnoses as well as for image storage and communications [Cannavo, 1993].

5. Diagnostic and Statistical Manual of Mental Disorders (DSM), now in its fourth edition (DSM-IV), is maintained by the American Psychiatric Association. It sets forth a standard set of codes and descriptions for use in diagnoses, prescriptions, research, education, and administration [Chute, 1991].

6. Diagnostic Related Groups (DRGs) are maintained by HCFA. They are derivatives of ICD-9-CM codes and are used to facilitate reimbursement and case-mix analysis. They lack the clinical specificity to be of value in direct patient care or clinical research [Chute, 1991].

7. Unified Medical Language System (UMLS) is maintained by the National Library of Medicine (NLM). It contains a metathesaurus that links clinical terminology, semantics, and formats of the major clinical coding and reference systems. It links medical terms (e.g., ICD, CPT, SNOMED, DSM, CO-STAR, and D-XPLAIN) to the NLM's medical index subject headings (MeSH codes) and to each other [Humphreys, 1991; Cimino et al., 1993].

8. The Canon Group has not developed a clinical data representation, but it is addressing two important problems: clinical data representations typically lack clinical specificity and are incapable of being generalized or extended beyond a specific application. "The Group proposes to focus on the design of a general schema for medical-language representation including the specification of the resources and associated procedures required to map language (including standard terminologies) into representations that make all implicit relations "visible," reveal "hidden attributes," and generally resolve "ambiguous references" [Evans et al., 1994].

42.5   Confidentiality, Data Security, and Authentication

The development of computer-based patient record systems and health care information networks have created the opportunity to address the need for more definitive confidentiality, data security, and authentication guidelines and standards. The following activities address this need:

1. During 1994, several bills were drafted in Congress to address health care privacy and confidentiality. They included the Fair Health Information Practices Act of 1994 (H.R. 4077), the Health Care Privacy Protection Act (S. 2129), and others. Although these bills were not passed as drafted, their essential content is expected to be included as part of subsequent health care reform legislation. They address the need for uniform comprehensive federal rules governing the use and disclosure of identifiable health and information about individuals. They specify the responsibilities of those who collect, use, and maintain health information about patients. They also define the rights of patients and provide a variety of mechanisms that will allow patients to enforce their rights.

2. ASTM Subcommittee E31.12 on Computer-based Patient Records is developing Guidelines for Minimal Data Security Measures for the Protection of Computer-based patient Records [Moshman Associates, 1994].

3. ASTM Subcommittee E31.17 on Access, Privacy, and Confidentiality of Medical Records is working on standards to address these issues [Moshman Associates, 1994].

4. ASTM Subcommittee E31.20 is developing standard specifications for authentication of health information [Moshman Associates, 1994].

5. The Committee on Regional Health Data Networks convened by the Institute of Medicine (IOM) has completed a definitive study and published its findings in a book entitled Health Data in the Information Age: Use, Disclosure, and Privacy [Donaldson and Lohr, 1994].

6. The Computer-based Patient Record Institute's (CPRI) Work Group on Confidentiality, Privacy, and Legislation has completed white papers on "Access to Patient Data" and on "Authentication," and a publication entitled "Guidelines for Establishing Information Security: Policies at Organizations using Computer-based Patient Records" [CPRI, 1994].

7. The Office of Technology Assessment has completed a two-year study resulting in a document entitled "Protecting Privacy in Computerized Medical Information." It includes a comprehensive review of system/data security issues, privacy information, current laws, technologies used for protection, and models.

8. The U.S. Food and Drug Administration (FDA) has created a task force on Electronic/Identification Signatures to study authentication issues as they relate to the pharmaceutical industry.

42.6   Quality Indicators and Data Sets

The Joint Commission on Accreditation of Health Care Organizations (JCAHO) has been developing and testing obstetrics, oncology, trauma, and cardiovascular clinical indicators. These indicators are intended to facilitate provider performance measurement. Several vendors are planning to include JCAHO clinical indicators in their performance measurement systems [JCAHO, 1994].

The health employers data and information set (HEDIS) version 2.0 has been developed with the support of the National Committee for Quality Assurance (NCQA). It identifies data to support performance measurement in the areas of quality (e.g., preventive medicine, prenatal care, acute and chronic disease, and mental health), access and patient satisfaction, membership and utilization, and finance. The development of HEDIS has been supported by several large employers and managed care organizations [NCQA, 1993].

42.7   International Standards

The ISO is a worldwide federation of national standards organizations. It has 90 member countries. The purpose of ISO is to promote the development of standardization and related activities in the world. ANSI was one of the founding members of ISO and is representative for the United States [Waegemann, 1994].

ISO has established a communications model for open systems interconnection (OSI). IEEE/MEDIX and HL7 have recognized and built upon the ISO/OSI framework. Further, ANSI HISPP has a stated objective of encouraging compatibility of U.S. health care standards with ISO/OSI. The ISO activities related to information technology take place within the Joint Technical Committee (JTC) 1.

The Comite Europeen de Noramalisation (CEN) is a European standards organization with 16 technical committees (TCs). Two TCs are specifically involved in health care: TC 251 (Medical Informatics) and TC 224 WG12 (Patient Data Cards) [Waegemann, 1994].

The CEN TC 251 on Medical Informatics includes work groups on: Modeling of Medical Records; Terminology, Coding, Semantics, and Knowledge Bases; Communications and Messages; Imaging and Multimedia; Medical Devices; and Security, Privacy, Quality, and Safety. The CEN TC 251 has established coordination with health care standards development in the United States through ANSI/HISPP.

In addition to standards developed by ISO and CEN, there are two other standards of importance. United Nations (U.N.) EDIFACT is a generic messaging-based communications standard with health-specific subsets. It parallels X12 and HL7, which are transaction-based standards. It is widely used in Europe and in several Latin American countries. The READ Classification System (RCS) is a multiaxial medical nomenclature used in the United Kingdom. It is sponsored by the National Health Service and has been integrated into computer-based ambulatory patient record systems in the United Kingdom [CAMS, 1994].

42.8   Standards Coordination and Promotion Organizations

In the United States, two organizations have emerged to assume responsibility for the coordination and promotion of health care standards development: the ANSI Health Care Informatics Standards Planning Panel (HISPP) and the Computer-based Patient Record Institute (CPRI). The major missions of an ANSI HISPP are:

1. To coordinate the work of the standards groups for health care data interchange and health care informatics (e.g., ACR/NEMA, ASTM, HL7, IEEE/MEDIX) and other relevant standards groups (e.g., X3, X12) toward achieving the evolution of a unified set of nonredundant, nonconflicting standards.
2. To interact with and provide input to CEN TC 251 (Medical Informatics) in a coordinated fashion and explore avenues of international standards development. The first mission of coordinating

standards is performed by the Message Standards Developers Subcommittee (MSDS). The second mission is performed by the International and Regional Standards Subcommittee. HISPP also has four task groups (1) Codes and Vocabulary, (2) Privacy, Security, and Confidentiality, (3) Provider Identification Numbering Systems, and (4) Operations. Its principal membership is composed of representatives of the major health care standards development organizations (SDOs), government agencies, vendors, and other interested parties. ANSI HISPP is by definition a planning panel, not an SDO [Hammond, 1994; ANSI HISPP, 1994].

The CPRI's mission is to promote acceptance of the vision set forth in the Institute of Medicine Study report "The Computer-based Patient Record: An Essential Technology for Health Care." CRPI is a nonprofit organization committed to initiating and coordinating activities to facilitate and promote the routine use of computer-based patient records. The CPRI takes initiatives to promote the development of CPR standards, but it is not an SDO itself. CPRI members represent the entire range of stakeholders in the health care delivery system. Its major work groups are the: (1) Codes and Structures Work Group; (2) CPR Description Work Group; (3) CPR Systems Evaluation Work Group; (4) Confidentiality, Privacy, and Legislation Work Group; and (5) Professional and Public Education Work Group [CPRI, 1994].

Two work efforts have been initiated to establish models for principal components of the emerging health care information infrastructure. The CPR Description Work Group of the CPRI is defining a consensus-based model of the computer-based patient record system. A joint working group to create a common data description has been formed by the MSDS Subcommittee of ANSI HISPP and IEEE/MEDIX. The joint working group is an open standards effort to support the development of a common data model that can be shared by developers of health care informatics standards [IEEE, 1994].

The CPRI has introduced a proposal defining a public/private effort to accelerate standards development for computer-based patient record systems [CPRI, 1994]. If funding becomes available, the project will focus on obtaining consensus for a conceptual description of a computer-based patient record system; addressing the need for universal patient identifiers; developing standard provider and sites-of-care identifiers; developing confidentiality and security standards; establishing a structure for and developing key vocabulary and code standards; completing health data interchange standards; developing implementation tools; and demonstrating adoptability of standards in actual settings. This project proposes that the CPRI and ANSI HISPP work together to lead, promote, coordinate, and accelerate the work of SDOs to develop health care information standards.

The Workgroup on Electronic Data Interchange (WEDI) is a voluntary, public/private task force which was formed in 1991 as a result of the call for health care administrative simplification by the director of the Department of Health and Human Services, Dr. Louis Sullivan. They have developed an action plan to promote health care EDI which includes: promotion of EDI standards, architectures, confidentiality, identifiers, health cards, legislation, and publicity [WEDI, 1993].

42.9 Summary

This chapter has presented an overview of major existing and emerging health care information infrastructure standards and the efforts to coordinate, harmonize, and accelerate these activities. Health care informatics is a dynamic area characterized by changing business and clinical processes, functions, and technologies. The effort to create health care informatics standards is therefore also dynamic. For the most current information on standards, refer to the "For More Information" section at the end of this chapter.

References

American National Standards Institute's Health Care Informatics Standards Planning Panel (1994). Charter statement. New York.

American Society for Testing and Materials (ASTM) (1994). Guide for the properties of a universal health care identifier. ASTM Subcommittee E31.12, Philadelphia.

American Society for Testing and Materials (ASTM) (1994). Membership information packet: ASTM Committee E31 on computerized systems, Philadelphia.

American Society for Testing and Materials (ASTM) (1994). A standard description for content and structure of the computer-based patient record, E1384–91/1994 revision. ASTM Subcommittee E31.19, Philadelphia.

American Society for Testing and Materials (ASTM) (1994). Standard guide for description of reservation registration-admission, discharge, transfer (R-ADT) systems for automated patient care information systems, E1239–94. ASTM Subcommittee E31.19, Philadelphia.

American Society for Testing and Materials (ASTM) (1994). A standard specification for the coded values used in the automated primary record of care, E1633. ASTM Subcommittee E31.19, Philadelphia.

Cannavo M.J. (1993). The last word regarding DEFF & DICOM. Healthcare Informatics 32.

Chute C.G. (1991). Tutorial 19: Clinical data representations. Washington, DC, Symposium on Computer Applications in Medical Care.

Cimino J.J., Johnson S.B., Peng P. et al. (1993). *From ICD9-CM to MeSH Using the UMLS: A How-to-Guide*, SCAMC, Washington, DC.

Computer Aided Medical Systems Limited (CAMS) (1994). CAMS News 4: 1.

Computer-based Patient Record Institute (CPRI) (1994). CPRI-Mail 3: 1.

Computer-based Patient Record Institute (CPRI) (1994). Position paper computer-based patient record standards. Chicago.

Computer-based Patient Record Institute (CPRI) (1994). Proposal to accelerate standards development for computer-based patient record systems. Version 3.0, Chicago.

Donaldson M.S. and Lohr K.N. (Eds.) (1994). *Health Data in the Information Age: Use, Disclosure, and Privacy*. Washington, DC, Institute of Medicine, National Academy Press.

Evans D.A., Cimino J.J., Hersh W.R. et al. (1994). Toward a medical-concept representation language. *J. Am. Med. Inform. Assoc.* 1: 207.

Hammond W.E. (1993). Overview of health care standards and understanding what they all accomplish. *HIMSS Proceedings*, Chicago, American Hospital Association.

Hammond W.E., McDonld C., Beeler G. et al. (1994). Computer standards: Their future within health care reform. *HIMSS Proceedings*, Chicago, Health Care Information and Management Systems Society.

Harrington J.J. (1993). *IEEE P1157 MEDIX: A Standard for Open Systems Medical Data Interchange*. New York, Institute of Electrical and Electronic Engineers.

Health Care Financing Administration (HCFA) (1994). Draft issue papers developed by HCFA's national provider identifier/national provider file workgroups. Baltimore.

Health Industry Business Communications Council (HIBCC) (1994). Description of present program standards activity. Phoenix.

Humphreys B. (1991). Tutorial 20: Using and assessing the UMLS knowledge sources. Symposium on Computer Applications in Medical Care, Washington, DC.

Institute of Electrical and Electronics Engineers (IEEE) (1994). Trial-use standard for health care data interchange — Information model methods: Data model framework. IEEE Standards Department, New York.

Joint Commission on Accreditation of Health Organizations (JCAHO) (1994). The Joint Commission Journal on Quality Improvement. Oakbrook Terrace, IL.

Moshman Associates, Inc. (1994). Current activities of selected health care informatics standards organizations. Bethesda, MD. Office of Science and Data Development, Agency for Health Care Policy and Research.

National Committee for Quality Assurance (1993). Hedis 2.0: Executive summary. Washington, DC.

Rothwell D.J., Cote R.A., Cordeau J.P. et al. (1993). Developing a standard data structure for medical language — The SNOMED proposal. Washington, DC, SCAMC.

Terell S.A., Dutton B.L., Porter L. et al. (1991). In search of the denominator: Medicare physicians — How many are there? Baltimore, Health Care Financing Administration.

Waegemann C.P. (1994). Draft — 1994 resource guide: Organizations involved in standards and development work for electronic health record systems. Newton, Mass, Medical Records Institute.

Workgroup for Electronic Data Interchange (WEDI) (1993). WEDI report: October 1993. Convened by the Department of Health and Human Services, Washington, DC.

Further Reading

For copies of standards accredited by ANSI, you can contact the American National Standards Institute, 11 West 42d St., NY, NY 10036 (212), 642–4900. For information on ANSI Health Care Informatics Standards Planning Panel (HISPP), contact Steven Cornish (212) 642–4900.

For copies of individual ASTM standards, you can contact the American Society for Testing and Materials, 1916 Race Street, Philadelphia, PA 19103–1187 (215), 299–5400.

For copies of the "Proposal to Accelerate Standards Development for Computer-based Patient Record Systems," contact the Computer-based Patient Record Institute (CPRI), Margaret Amatayakul, 1000 E. Woodfield Road, Suite 102, Schaumburg, IL 60173 (708) 706–6746.

For information on provider identifier standards and proposals, contact the Health Care Financing Administration (HCFA), Bureau Program Operations, 6325 Security Blvd., Baltimore, MD 21207 (410), 966–5798. For information on ICD-9-CM codes, contact HCFA, Medical Coding, 401 East Highrise Bldg. 6325 Security Blvd., Baltimore, MD 21207 (410), 966–5318.

For information on site-of-care and supplier labeling identifiers, contact the Health Industry Business Communications Council (HIBCC), 5110 N. 40th Street, Suite 250, Phoenix, AZ 85018 (602), 381–1091.

For copies of standards developed by Health Level 7, you can contact HL7, 3300 Washtenaw Avenue, Suite 227, Ann Arbor, MI 48104 (313), 665–0007.

For copies of standards developed by the Institute of Electrical and Electronic Engineers/Engineering in Medicine and Biology Society, in New York City, call (212) 705–7900. For information on IEEE/MEDIX meetings, contact Jack Harrington, Hewlett-Packard, 3000 Minuteman Rd., Andover, MA 01810 (508), 681–3517.

For more information on clinical indicators, contact the Joint Commission on Accreditation of Health Care Organizations (JCAHO), Department of Indicator Measurement, One Renaissance Blvd., Oakbrook Terrace, IL 60181 (708), 916–5600.

For information on pharmaceutical billing transactions, contact the National Council for Prescription Drug Programs (NCPDP), 2401 N. 24th Street, Suite 365, Phoenix, AZ 85016 (602), 957–9105.

For information on HEDIS, contact the National Committee for Quality Assurance (NCQA), Planning and Development, 1350 New York Avenue, Suite 700, Washington, D.C. 20005 (202), 628–5788.

For copies of ACR/NEMA DICOM standards, contact David Snavely, National Equipment Manufacturers Association (NEMA), 2101 L. Street N.W., Suite 300, Washington, D.C. 20037 (202), 457–8400.

For information on standards development in the areas of computer-based patient record concept models, confidentiality, data security, authentication, and patient cards, and for information on standards activities in Europe, contact Peter Waegemann, Medical Records Institute (MRI), 567 Walnut, P.O. Box 289, Newton, MA 02160 (617), 964–3923.

43

Introduction to Informatics and Nursing

43.1	Introduction...	**43**-1
43.2	Demography	**43**-2
43.3	Nurses — Largest Group Using Computers and Implementing Information Systems....................	**43**-2
	Expanding Nursing Informatics Roles	
43.4	Definition of "Nursing Informatics"....................	**43**-3
	Informatics Nurses Have a United Voice	
43.5	Nursing Process	**43**-4
	Ethics and Regulation	
43.6	Standards in Vocabularies and Data Sets	**43**-5
43.7	Clinical Information Systems	**43**-6
43.8	Bridging Nursing and Engineering Specialties: The Bioinformatics Partnership of Nurses and Engineers	**43**-7
	Benefits of Using Information Systems in Patient Care	
43.9	Barriers to Creating an Effective Healthcare Information Infrastructure............................	**43**-9
	Opportunities to Create an Effective Healthcare Information Infrastructure	
43.10	Research and Development Needs......................	**43**-11
43.11	Summary	**43**-13
	References	**43**-13

Kathleen A. McCormick
SAIC

Joyce Sensmeier
HIMSS

Connie White Delaney
The University of Minnesota

Carol J. Bickford
American Nurses Association

43.1 Introduction

Everyday in hospitals, critical care environments, ambulatory clinics, academic environments, and vendor corporations, nurses are working side-by-side with colleagues in engineering to develop, evaluate, and maintain information systems and other technology solutions in healthcare. Together these professional teams have evolved from a domain specific focus to the development and implementation of integrated systems with decision support that enhance patient care, verify if outcomes are met, assure quality safe care, and document resource consumption. This chapter provides an overview of the demography of the profession, definitions of nursing informatics, current nursing informatics activities, and examples of bridging healthcare informatics and nursing.

43.2   Demography

Registered nurses comprise the largest healthcare provider group in the United States. Their work environments include traditional healthcare settings such as hospitals, ambulatory care clinics, private practice settings, schools, correctional facilities, home health, community health, and public health environments. Nurses are the most frequent providers of healthcare services to homeless populations, faith communities, and other disenfranchised, underserved, and uninsured populations in the less traditional health related settings. In each setting, the registered nurse serves as the unrecognized knowledge worker, addressing the data, information, and knowledge needs of both patients and healthcare providers. Nurses' record keeping and written documentation provide integral support for the necessary communication activities between nurses and other healthcare providers and therefore must reflect the chronology of findings, decision-making processes, activities, evaluations, and outcomes.

The definition of nursing has evolved over the years. In 2003 the American Nurses Association published this contemporary definition that reflects the holistic and health focus of registered nurses in the United States:

> Nursing is the protection, promotion, and optimization of health and abilities, prevention of illness and injury, alleviation of suffering through the diagnosis and treatment of human response, and advocacy in the care of individuals, families, communities, and populations [ANA, 2003].

Like other professions, after initial educational preparation and licensure, the registered nurse may continue studying for preparation in a specialty practice, such as pediatrics, gerontology, cardiology, women's health, oncology, and perioperative nursing. Graduate preparation in clinical specialties may lead to designation as an advanced practice registered nurse or APRN, nurse anesthetist, or midwife. Others may be interested in preparing for a role specialty, such as administration, education, case management, or informatics.

In studies since the 1980s, nurses have been identified as the largest users of information systems in healthcare and play a critical role in creating an effective healthcare information infrastructure.

43.3   Nurses — Largest Group Using Computers and Implementing Information Systems

The 2000 National Sample Survey of Registered Nurses projects that 8406 or 0.4% of the approximately 2.7 million registered nurses in the United States identify nursing informatics as their nursing specialty (http://bhpr.hrsa.gov/healthworkforce/). Because of the increased national interest in healthcare informatics and implementation of healthcare information systems, coupled with the increased numbers of graduate nursing informatics educational programs, the 2004 National Sample Survey of Registered Nurses is expected to report a greater prevalence of informatics nurses.

Nearly three-quarters of nurse informaticists are currently developing or implementing clinical documentation systems according to a first-of-its-kind survey performed by the Healthcare Information and Management Systems Society (HIMSS) and sponsored by Omnicell, Inc. [HIMSS, 2004a]. A total of 537 responses were received to the web-based survey, which was performed to gain a better understanding of the background of nurse informaticists, the issues they address and the tools they use to perform their jobs. Two-thirds of respondents reported that systems implementation is their top job responsibility.

Drawing on their extensive clinical background, another three-quarters are involved with their organization's clinical information systems implementation. Over half are involved in the development or implementation of computerized provider order entry (CPOE), and 48% are developing or implementing an electronic medical record (EMR). Nurse informaticists are also actively involved in developing or implementing Bar Coded Medication Management, ICU, Master Patient Index (MPI) and Picture Archival and Communication Systems (PACS).

Approximately half of the respondents indicated that they were involved with five or fewer areas of development or implementation. Conversely, 12% of respondents are involved in ten or more areas. Many of the nurses (46%) indicated that they have been involved with the removal/replacement of at least one system.

43.3.1 Expanding Nursing Informatics Roles

Like the expanding roles of other registered nurses, the role of the informatics nurse reflects significant diversity and expertise. Consider the listing provided in the Scope and Standards of Nursing Informatics Practice [ANA, 2001b]: project manager, consultant, educator, researcher, product developer, decision support/outcomes manager, advocate/policy developer, entrepreneur, chief information officer, and business owner. Some of these experts are purchasers of information systems in hospitals, outpatient settings, community and home care nursing environments. Information system vendors have begun designating a senior executive level nurse, Chief Nursing Officer (CNO) to direct the informatics nurse contingent and patient care software development components of the organization, quite like the CNO role in a hospital or multifacility healthcare enterprise. Recent job announcements posted at the HIMSS, the American Medical Informatics Association (AMIA), and the Capitol Area Roundtable in Nursing Informatics (CARING) Web sites sought individuals for systems analyst, database administrator, and implementation specialist positions.

43.4 Definition of "Nursing Informatics"

Health informatics comprises multiple discipline-specific informatics practices; nursing informatics is one of these specialties. Nursing informatics, an applied science, is defined by the American Nurses Association [2001] as a specialty that:

> integrates nursing science, computer science, and information science to manage and communicate data, information, and knowledge in nursing practice. Nursing informatics facilitates the integration of data, information, and knowledge to support patients, nurses, and other providers in their decision-making in all roles, and settings. This support is accomplished through the use of information structures, information processes, and information technology (p. 17).

43.4.1 Informatics Nurses Have a United Voice

Increasing numbers of local and regional networking groups of informatics nurses prompted the Nursing Informatics Working Group of the American Medical Informatics Association (AMIA), the professional nurses represented by the Healthcare Information and Management Systems Society (HIMSS), and the American Nurses Association (ANA) to foster and support the recent development of the Alliance for Nursing Informatics (ANI). This new entity represents more than 2000 nurses and brings together 18 distinct nursing informatics groups (see Table 43.1) in the United States that function separately at local, regional, national, and international levels and have established programs, publications, and organizational structures for their members [HIMSS, 2004c]. The basic objectives of the Alliance are to:

1. Provide a consolidated forum for the informatics community
2. Provide input to a national nursing informatics research agenda
3. Facilitate the dissemination of nursing informatics best practices
4. Present the collective voice of the nursing informatics specialty in national public policy initiatives and standards activities

TABLE 43.1 Eighteen Distinct Nurses Informatics Groups in the U.S. That Have Come Together as an Alliance for Nursing Informatics (ANI) 2004

AMIA	American Medical Informatics Association Nursing Informatics Working Group
ANA	American Nurses Association (Liaison)
ANIA	American Nursing Informatics Association
BANIC	Boston Area Nursing Informatics Consortium
CARING	Capital Area Roundtable on Informatics in Nursing
CSRA-CIN	Central Savannah River Area Clinical Informatics Network
CHIN	Connecticut Healthcare Informatics Network
DVNCN	Delaware Valley Nursing Computer Network
HINJ	Health Informatics of New Jersey
HIMSS	Healthcare Information and Management Systems Society
	Nursing Informatics Community
	Iowa HIMSS Nursing Informatics Committee
INFO	Informatics Nurses From Ohio
MNIN	Michigan Nursing Informatics Network
MINING	Minnesota Nursing Informatics Group
CONI	North Carolina State Nurses Association Council on NI
NISCNE	Nursing Information Systems Council of New England
PISUG	Perinatal Information Systems User Group
PSNI	Puget Sound Nursing Informatics
SCINN	South Carolina Informatics Nursing Network
UNIN	Utah Nursing Informatics Network

In one of its first joint efforts, the nurses represented by the ANI provided testimony to the President's Information Technology Advisory Committee (PITAC) during an open meeting on April 13, 2004. In part, this testimony focused on the benefits of creating an effective health care information infrastructure in all settings for all healthcare providers.

43.5 Nursing Process

Most nurses have been prepared in their educational programs to use the nursing process as a framework to guide thinking and professional practice. Assessment, diagnosis or problem/issue definition, planning, implementation, and evaluation comprise the steps in the nursing process. Employers value the demonstrated expertise and critical thinking skills of the informatics nurse who uses the nursing process. The nursing process serves as the foundation for the *Scope and Standards of Nursing Informatics Practice* [ANA, 2001b], which provides specific standards of practice and standards of professional performance statements that assist the informatics nurse in practice. The content can be used when developing position descriptions and performance appraisals, and also provides a structure for informatics curriculum development for educators and a research agenda for nursing and interdisciplinary groups such as bioengineers and nurses.

43.5.1 Ethics and Regulation

Registered nurses have a long tradition of concern about ethics, patient advocacy, safety, and quality of care. Beginning with the first clinical experience, the registered nurse must know the differences and necessary practice associated with privacy, confidentiality, and security. Just as for registered nurse colleagues, the Code of Ethics for Nurses With Interpretive Statements [ANA, 2001a] provides a framework for the informatics nurse. Although primarily focused on support activities for the healthcare environment, the informatics nurse has the obligation to be concerned about issues of confidentiality, security, and privacy surrounding the patient, clinician, and enterprise and the associated data, information, and knowledge.

The federal government's current focus on establishing the National Health Information Network (NHIN), electronic health record (EHR), personal health record, and regional health information

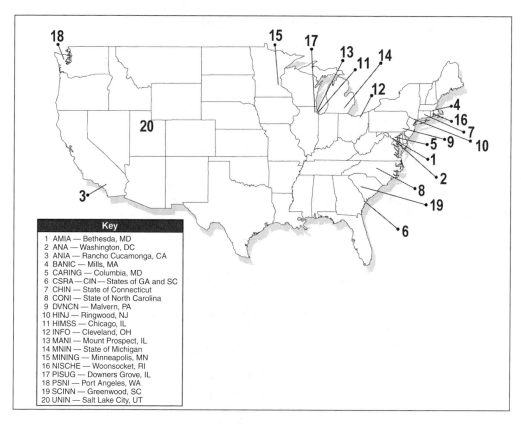

FIGURE 43.1 The figure shows a U.S. map with representative locations for some of these regional groups. The figure also lists the nursing informatics organizations that are affiliating with ANI.

organizations (RHIO) provides numerous ethical and regulatory issues [Thompson and Brailer, 2004]. For example, the current U.S. healthcare environment has yet to resolve the problem of clinical practice and licensure across state lines for individuals working with nurse call centers, telehealth applications, and electronic prescriptions. Another example is related to unequal distribution of resources, or the digital divide which is characterized by those without a working personal computer and high-speed access to the Internet at home.

Consider the ethical issues associated with the data and information management of genetic databases. Data integrity, appropriate database structuring, standardized terminologies and indexing processes, and correct representation of complex multidimensional structures and images pose new ethical issues. What assurances must be in place to prevent public dissemination of an individual's adverse genetic profile? Will that prevent these individuals from securing health insurance, cause termination from a job, or lead to discrimination in schools or the hiring process? Similarly, the move toward increased patient participation in clinical decision making continues to create tensions in the decision support and information systems development arenas. Informatics nurses join their colleagues in biomedical engineering and in clinical practice to identify and resolve such ethical questions.

43.6   Standards in Vocabularies and Data Sets

Nursing has been developing nomenclatures for over 24 years to address the nursing process components of diagnosis, interventions, and outcomes. Table 43.2 lists the ANA recognized terminologies supporting nursing practice in 2004. More recently the International Organization for Standardization (ISO) of

TABLE 43.2 ANA Recognized Terminologies Supporting Nursing
Practice, 2004

ABC codes

Clinical Care Classification (CCC) [Formerly Home Health Care Classification]
International Classification for Nursing Practice (ICNP®)
Logical Observation Identifiers Names and Codes (LOINC®)
NANDA-Nursing Diagnoses, Definitions, and Classification
Nursing Outcomes Classification (NOC)
Nursing Management Minimum Data Set (NMMDS)
Nursing Interventions Classification System (NIC)
Nursing Minimum Data Set (NMDS)
Omaha System
Patient Care Data Set (PCDS)
PeriOperative Nursing Data Set (PNDS)
SNOMED CT®

Geneva, Switzerland, recently published an international standard for nursing. The standard — Health Informatics: Integration of a Reference Terminology Model for Nursing — is the first step toward creating comparable nursing data across settings, organizations, and countries. Such data assists in identifying and implementing "best nursing practices" or determining how scarce nursing resources should be spent. The International Medical Informatics Association (IMIA) Nursing Informatics Working Group developed the standard in collaboration with the International Council of Nurses (ICN) [Saba et al., 2003]. This collaboration was accomplished as a result of the international network of nurses who in turn were developing standards for nomenclature and classifications within their respective countries. This group recognized the value of an international collaborative effort to compare quality, efficiencies, and outcomes of care resulting from nursing care that is delivered internationally.

In addition, numerous nurses have been working on other ISO TC-215 and Health Level Seven (HL7) standards, Logical Observation Identifiers Names and Codes (LOINC), and Systematized Nomenclature of Medicine (SNOMED) committees. Wherever health standards are being developed and applied, nurses are present on those committees and working groups to provide input that often includes consideration of professional nursing standards.

43.7 Clinical Information Systems

Healthcare information systems that adequately support nursing practice have not emerged over the past decades. Figure 43.2 identifies some of the system components, influencing factors, and relationships that have not been fully considered in describing the complexity of nursing, a profession that relies so heavily on evidence, knowledge, and critical thinking. Consequently the requisite detailed analysis and design processes have never begun or have failed to generate the appropriate and diverse information system components necessary for successful support for nurses and nursing practice.

Recent research has begun to identify the relationships of computer and information literacy of nurses and the use of information systems [McNeil, 2003]. Nurses' experience with different computer applications corresponds with higher confidence in using a new information system, according to a recent study [Dillon et al., 2003]. The study, which surveyed 139 nurses at a 450-bed regional hospital center, also found that this "self-efficacy" is higher, on average, for younger nurses and those with more advanced degrees.

Using a computer at home and having general computer skills, for example, were associated with higher levels of self-efficacy according to the researchers. Nurses' self-assessed ability to use word processing, conduct Internet searches, and use e-mail also corresponded with higher self-efficacy.

The study also found that "a younger age, a higher level of education, and a more positive attitude toward the new information system had a slight association with self-efficacy." "Improvement of nurses'

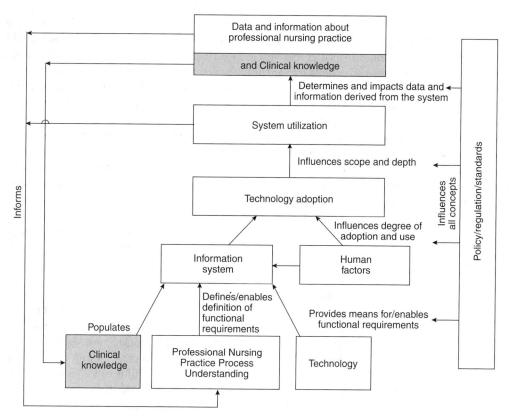

FIGURE 43.2   The organizing framework for clinical information systems: critical knowledge as the critical factor.

self-efficacy toward the system will not guarantee a successful implementation," the study concluded, "but it is expected that with a more organized and strategic approach to implementation, the adoption of a new information system will be enhanced."

43.8   Bridging Nursing and Engineering Specialties: The Bioinformatics Partnership of Nurses and Engineers

Bioinformatics by definition focuses on "how information is represented and transmitted in biological systems, starting at the molecular level" [Shortliffe et al., 2001]. Accepting the central goal of nursing informatics as improving the health of populations, communities, families, and individuals by optimizing information management and communication, it is clear that the intersection of these two fields — the biological systems of human beings and the applied/clinical practice of nursing — creates a synergy related to direct provision of care, and administrative, educational, and research priorities.

Bioinformatics focuses on the representation, communication, and management of information related to basic biological sciences and biological processes. It is readily dependent upon using integrative models to expand and disseminate the science as well as providing clinically relevant contributions. Although nursing predominantly focuses on aspects of clinical care, characteristics of nursing, especially in decision making, particularly position this discipline and its nursing informatics specialty as productive partners with bioinformatics. These nursing characteristics can contribute to the bridging of bench science with input on care needs, as well as the clinical significance of innovations put into real world practice.

Nursing contributes to the data, information, and knowledge supporting patients, families, and communities across all settings. Two key threads are significant to information related to the biological aspects of people (1) nursing is positioned to assess not only individual information, but also information related to families and communities and (2) this assessment (information access) occurs across all settings. The Human Genome Project is a key revolution illustrating the importance of information from the individual and family levels across all settings of care to the aggregate. Consider, for example, genetic diseases, pharmaceutical discoveries, and healthy aging.

Moreover, collaboration with nurse scientists offers additional information not commonly the focus of the medical record. Nursing by its very nature is context dependent and consequently has collected information related to the patient/family context, domain, as well as the environment and domain of healthcare delivery. The knowledge discovery in databases research strengthens informatics capacity to consider the interrelationships of cellular societal systems.

This collaborative capacity extends beyond the cellular focus of bioinformatics. Addressing the complexity of healthcare systems and process can benefit from the collaboration with nursing. As the central information broker across all settings, nursing can be a pivotal partner in examining and designing efficient safe care systems. Studying and extending the science of complex adaptive systems from cellular to societal levels is one example.

Nursing is well positioned to partner with bioinformatics and engineering to address the essential demands of the healthcare system. A substantial cadre of nursing informatics scientists has been prepared, some even with Ph.D.s in engineering. Specifically, there are a growing number of scientists in nursing informatics with knowledge discovery expertise, encompassing multiple Knowledge Discovery in Databases (KDD) methods, including complex adaptive systems in patient care and with the consumer. Nursing has maintained crucial expertise in knowledge representation and information messaging, both essential to bioinformatics, nursing, and the interface area between the two disciplines. And significantly, nursing informatics has established a national network to support bridging the disciplines.

43.8.1 Benefits of Using Information Systems in Patient Care

Two types of data are available related to the benefits of utilizing information systems in the delivery of patient care. Early in the last decade, researchers began assessing the value of computer terminals at the bedside or at the point of care. In one study of the impact of bedside terminals on the quality of nursing documentation, Marr et al. [1993] found that comprehensiveness of documentation measured by the presence or absence of components of the record was better with bedside terminals. They also found that timeliness of documentation was improved when performed closer to the actual time that care was delivered. Other benefits of nurses using computers to document practice were (1) the integration of care plans with nursing interventions, (2) calculation of specific acuity, and (3) automatic bills for nursing services.

The Nicholas E. Davies Award of Excellence for Electronic Health Records recognizes excellence in the implementation of EHRs in healthcare organizations and primary care practices. Established in 1995 this program has recognized 19 hospitals in the past 9 years. As part of the application process, organizations must document the financial impact of their implemented EHR. A 2001 winner, the University of Illinois at Chicago Medical Center, documented that during a two year period, $1.2 million of nurse time was reallocated from manual documentation tasks to direct hands-on patient care [CPRI-HOST, 2001]. Registered nurses in the charge nurse role gained 2.75 h per shift in the medication administration process.

Data are also available on the computerization of evidence-based practice recommendations [Saba and McCormick, 2005]. Although these data are sparse, existing publications cover a diverse range of topics from the integration of information technology with outcomes management, coding, and taxonomy issues relevant to outcomes, including standardized language and other issues tied to the nursing minimum data set, and the development of nursing-sensitive outcome measures from nursing care and interventions. Former studies focusing on outcomes suggest that nurses should serve on multidisciplinary teams and collaborate with others in building IT systems to improve organizational learning, use of evidence, and quality [McCormick, 2005].

Other reported studies of bedside terminals have documented the ease of use, elimination of redundant data, system support at the bedside, availability, currency of data, and access to expert systems. Use of clinical information systems have been shown to provide soft benefits related to improvements in patient safety, care provider communication, and workflow enhancements. Historically there have been few studies to show hard benefits of dollars saved, or a substantial decrease in care hours. However, as more nursing-focused software is implemented a positive return on investment (ROI) has been noted [Curtis, 2004]. Nursing and engineering must work together to articulate the shared benefits achieved with successful systems implementations.

43.9 Barriers to Creating an Effective Healthcare Information Infrastructure

The survey of nurse informaticists identified financial resources as the largest barrier to success in their role of implementing healthcare information infrastructures. This is consistent with the responses of chief information officers (CIOs) as reflected in the 15th Annual Leadership Survey [HIMSS, 2004]. Lack of user acceptance or administrative support, and software design that ignores current work-flow processes were also described as barriers. Healthcare CIOs in this survey have recognized the importance of a clinical champion by identifying the need to increase IT staff to address clinical issues.

A 1997 review of information technology use by nurses suggested that barriers include: lack of integration of nursing systems within hospital information systems, the need for a unified nursing language, and lack of point-of-care terminals [Bowles, 1997]. However, more recent reviews describe that these barriers are slowly being resolved [Androwich et al., 2003]. Additional barriers include lack of a standard design for clinical systems that would address the inconsistency of entering or extracting data from the end user's perspective [Hermann, 2004].

In another study recently undertaken by the Interagency Council on Information Resources for Nurses (ICIRN), the information literacy of nurses was surveyed Tanner et al. [2004]. Information literacy was identified as a nursing informatics competency for the nurse. Information literacy has been found to be an essential element in the application and use of evidence based practice (EBP). The study identified the gaps in knowledge and skills for identifying, accessing, retrieving, evaluating, and utilizing research evidence to provide best practice for patients. The study also reported that over 64% of nurses regularly need information, but 43% rated workplace information resources as totally inadequate or less than adequate. The three primary organizational constraints in the practice settings were identified as (1) the presence of other goals of higher priority, (2) difficulty recruiting and retaining staff, and (3) organizational budget for acquisition of information resources. Three personal barriers were identified (1) lack of understanding of organization or structure of electronic databases, (2) difficulty accessing information, and (3) lack of skills to use and synthesize evidence into practice.

Findings from another study indicated that nurses at every level and role exhibit large gaps in knowledge and competencies at each step in the information literacy process — from lack of awareness that they need information to lack of access or ability to successfully search and utilize information needed for practice, particularly in an electronic format [Pravikoff et al., 2003]. However, significantly more nurses who received their most recent nursing degree after 1990 acknowledged successful searches of evidence in the National Library of Medicine (NLM) Medline and Cumulative Index to Nursing and Allied Health Literature (CINAHL) when compared with those who graduated before 1990 [Tanner, 2000]. Thus, training in computer skills has been a barrier that may diminish with more nurses becoming computer literate in high school and college [Pierce, 2000]. The "tipping point" may be a generation gap.

Most nurses did not have training regarding computer use or typing skills in their nursing or college curriculum unless they returned to school for further education after 1990 [Gloe, 2004]. Therefore, the practicing nurse should be provided with opportunities for learning basic "keyboarding," that is, typing skills and computer basics such as how to use the mouse. This would lessen the anxiety for computer use. Nurses are caring for patients with greater acuity and requiring more documentation, thus creating higher stress than ever before. Adding the stress of computerization when one is totally unfamiliar with the computer can be a major challenge. Incorporating this challenge into their current workload may seem like an insurmountable task to nurses and could be a large barrier for EHR implementation. Thus, providing educational opportunities as well as designing user friendly applications for use by the nursing staff can lessen the stress and remove barriers.

Summarizing an Agency for Healthcare Research and Quality (AHRQ) conference examining quality research, the attendees asked if the primary barriers to achieving the NHIN are more political than technical. The participants identified the need for standards to govern the infrastructure, the lack of broad-based agreement among stakeholders of a system concept, and the legal concerns about privacy and confidentiality [Lang and Mitchell, 2004]. Vahey et al. [2004] summarized the need for additional research on the barriers to quality improvement that they defined as: lack of standardized measures, inadequate information systems to collect data, inadequate resources to pay for data collection and translation, and technological issues. As stated by others at the same conference [Lamb et al., 2004] the necessary demand and incentives are currently not in place to assure the development of information infrastructures that will support quality improvement.

Finally, in a monograph sponsored by AMIA in collaboration with the ANA, the major constraints to full implementation of the information infrastructure for nursing were identified as lack of: policy, regulation and standards, technology, information systems, human factors, technology adoption, and system utilization [Androwich et al., 2003]. Other barriers include lack of a positive ROI for the use of clinical documentation systems, and limited availability of applications that specifically support the work of nurses.

Many reports, such as those recently published by the Institute of Medicine (IOM), Committe on Quality in Health Care support the use of technology in reducing medical errors and encourage implementation of evidence-based healthcare practice. The results of these recent studies identify gaps and barriers that limit effecting these prescribed practices among nurses, the largest number of health care professionals who provide the greatest percentage of direct contact, time, and intensity with the consumer/patient.

43.9.1 Opportunities to Create an Effective Healthcare Information Infrastructure

Patient safety is a well-documented priority for healthcare organizations. This focus provides an opportunity for healthcare organizations to evaluate the use of information technology and the related infrastructure to deliver safe and effective patient care. Computerized provider order entry (CPOE), clinical information systems, and bar coded medication management are three top applications for healthcare organizations in the next several years as reported in the survey of CIOs [HIMSS, 2004b]. Nurses play a critical role, as almost three-quarters of respondents are involved with the implementation of their organization's clinical information system, 52% with the implementation of CPOE software, and 48% with implementation of an EMR. The extensive clinical background of nurse informaticists is valuable, as nurses have an intimate understanding of the workflow, environment, and procedures that are necessary to achieve success.

Another opportunity that could also be a potential barrier for creating an effective healthcare information infrastructure, relates to leadership and a clear strategic vision [Kennedy, 2004]. The complexity of creating a healthcare information infrastructure is immense and can only be developed once it has been fully defined. Several efforts have been initiated in this direction one at the conceptual level (i.e., IOM's definition of the Computer-based Patient Record) and the other at the detailed data level (i.e., HL7's Reference Data Model). Yet the missing link may be the discussion about how to distill this information into practical, usable models that can be applied to improve the work environment of the nurse and enhance patient safety. An innovative approach is needed to create a cohesive agenda across a very dynamic, complex healthcare delivery organization. Once an "effective" healthcare information infrastructure is defined, it could be recognized and promoted from both a nursing and collaborative health care model.

43.10 Research and Development Needs

The nursing profession has both a critical mass of nurses involved in information technology and experience with implementing technology and related systems. Yet there is a need to educate nurses involved with implementing and utilizing information infrastructures. The focus has shifted nationally from developing an information infrastructure, to using an information infrastructure to assure safe, effective, patient-centered, timely, efficient, and equitable care. Information technology is the critical tool to be used in the redesign of systems supporting the delivery of care to achieve the type of quality care recommended by the current federal leaders and the recent IOM reports.

The nursing profession is a participant in the delivery of care in the hospital and outpatient environment, and is centrally placed in community and home care. There is a need to create centers for evaluation of the barriers and benefits of information infrastructures. These centers should be located in academic centers or developed in cooperation with commercial developers of information systems. These centers should be multidisciplinary and nursing focused. Nurses must be involved in these types of research and evaluation efforts.

The National Institute on Nursing Research (NINR) developed priorities for research in nursing informatics in 1993. These included (a) formalization of nursing vocabularies, (b) design and management of databases for nursing information, (c) development of technologies to support nursing practice, (d) use of telecommunications technologies in nursing, (e) patient use of information, (f) identification of nurses' information needs, and (g) systems modeling and evaluation [NINR, 1993]. While NINR has funded a number of studies in these areas and achieved outcomes in advancing nursing informatics, the Institute has never received sufficient funds to disseminate the findings, translate them to practice, or expand the individual studies to the support of Centers of Excellence.

Other research has been recommended in the areas of (1) prototyping methodology to explore specific ways to realize innovations, (2) pilot tests of technology based innovations and new workflow processes, (3) analyses of successful and unsuccessful outcomes and change processes in the implementation of systems, and (4) demonstrations of the return on investment from nursing documentation on such areas as patient safety, errors, quality, effectiveness, and efficiencies [Androwich et al., 2003].

The Health Resources and Services Administration (HRSA) Division of Nursing has funded training in nursing informatics. Enhanced budgets would provide the necessary funds to expand those programs with a focus on the literacy gaps in nursing at both the academic levels and in practice areas.

According to a workgroup report to the American Academy of Nursing Technology and Work Force Conference, the ideal nursing care-delivery system enables staff nurses to increase their productivity, job satisfaction, and the quality of care by increasing the time spent on direct care activities [Sensmeier et al., 2002]. The report recommends that this system must include information technology that replaces the paper-based, administrative tasks with a paperless, point-of-care, computer-based patient record imbedded with intelligent, rules-based capabilities that automate the manual workflow processes, policies, and procedures, and that support the nurses' critical thinking. Research to explore these recommendations is needed.

Other target areas for practice-based research identified by the Boston Area Nursing Informatics Consortium (BANIC) [Kennedy, 2004] include, workflow and workplace design for point-of-care applications, creating a model for systems value at the point of care, clinical systems implementation, clinical documentation and utilization of standardized nursing language, clinical systems evaluation tools, consumer health systems, web-based education, and methods for evaluating applications, specifically CPOE and medication management.

The AHRQ has also funded research in nursing informatics and the impact on quality and evidence-based practice. One such study demonstrated that installing a computerized medical information management system in hospital intensive care units can significantly reduce the time spent by ICU nurses on documentation, giving them more time for direct patient care [AHRQ, 2003]. Follow-up studies are needed to validate these findings.

The AHRQ hosted a conference where nurses helped the Agency define research priorities. The conferees concurred that the sole reason to design and implement clinical information systems was to use the information to track, interpret, and improve quality of care. They identified information systems technology as the crucial bridge to translate research into practice [Lamb et al., 2004]. They suggested that a research emphasis should be placed on reducing the barriers to getting timely and credible information to the nurses. The group identified the gap between collecting data to measure quality, and using the data to improve the quality of care. They identified this as the greatest opportunity for achieving the ROI for developing systems. Information technology supported by evidence-based practice and patient safety initiatives is key to a quality agenda. However, the information technology is available, so the barriers to achieving its benefits must be evaluated and solutions developed so that direct providers and decision makers can implement systems [Lamb et al., 2004].

Conference participants recommended the following research goals relative to nursing informatics: (1) standardized quality indicators need development and measurement including nurse-sensitive measures from nursing care and interventions measures, and quality indicators to link care across settings, (2) improved risk adjustment methodologies, and (3) a national health information structure to inform quality improvement efforts [Vahey et al., 2004]. They further cited the need for integration and collaboration among stakeholders in conducting research on the information systems' needs to measure quality, improvements in patient safety, and risk and error reduction.

Since nursing practice is often absent in databases and systems of reimbursement from private and public sources, other recommended research has focused on the inclusion of nursing-sensitive quality indicators achieved from nursing care and interventions, in conjunction with the analysis of workforce and contributions of advanced practice nurses (nurse practitioners) [Brooten et al., 2004]. Lamb et al. [2004] stressed that the critical research question in the quality initiative involves the complex analysis of the interplay between information infrastructure systems, organization, financial and clinical practice features. Not only did this group recommend that AHRQ expand their research agenda for nursing sensitive areas, but they also recommended broader dissemination of the results of the impact of nursing staffing on achieving quality outcomes.

The Center for Disease Control and Prevention (CDC) has sponsored research in public health and biodefense information infrastructure. While nurses have been involved in implementing these programs, the impact of nursing research on these areas could benefit from additional funding.

The Center for Medicare and Medicaid Services (CMS) provides data from which health services research nurses have evaluated the impact of nursing care on quality, effectiveness, and efficiencies. Researchers have identified that quality indicators of care from the largest group of health care workers, namely nurses, are absent in the databases and subsequently the systems of reimbursement from CMS [Brooten et al., 2004]. The utilization of cooperative agreements and contracts for evaluation of the ROI for nursing information systems embedded in health care information systems has not been widespread. The pilots and demonstration studies recommended above could be facilitated by CMS contracts and grants. Models of incentives could be studied to determine how CMS could include nursing documentation data in health care records to evaluate quality, outcomes, and cost impacts. Constructing nursing-sensitive quality indicators from existing databases and establishing their validity needs further research. Medicare and Medicaid data are incomplete representations of nursing's contributions to quality outcomes. Lamb et al. further recommended that systems be created and maintained to assure that the quality data can be captured at the point of care and translated into useful clinical information to be applied by nurses and other health professionals [Lamb et al., 2004].

Finally, the National Library of Medicine has sponsored research that has helped advance the literacy and impact of nursing informatics. Further targeted funding for nursing informatics and consumer informatics would be required to accelerate the national health information infrastructure in the United States.

43.11 Summary

Development of an increased awareness of nursing activities in informatics has been the major objective in preparing this chapter. This awareness thereby promotes the establishment of better partnerships between engineers, biomedical engineers, and the nurses working in informatics as well as in practice, administration, research, and education. Wherever nurses are participating in health care, they can team with engineers to develop better solutions to improve health care processes and outcomes.

References

AHRQ (2003). Case Study Finds Computerized ICU Information System Can Significantly Reduce Time Spent by Nurses on Documentation. Press Release Date: October 10, 2003. http://www.ahrq.gov/news/press/pr2003/compicupr.htm

American Nurses Association (2001a). *Code of Ethics for Nurses with Interpretive Statements.* Washington, DC: American Nurses Publishing.

American Nurses Association (2001b). *Scope and Standards of Nursing Informatics Practice.* Washington, DC: American Nurses Publishing.

American Nurses Association (2003). *Nursing's Social Policy Statement,* 2nd ed. Washington, DC: American Nurses Publishing.

Androwich, I.M., Bickford, C.J., Button, P.S., Hunter, K.M., Murphy, J., and Sensmeier, J. (2003). *Clinical Information Systems: A Framework for Reaching the Vision.* Washington, DC: American Nurses Publishing.

Bowles, K.W. (1997). The benefits and barriers to nursing information systems. *Computers in Nursing* 15, 191–196.

Brooten, D., Youngblut, J.M., Kutcher, J., and Bobo, C. (2004). Quality and the nursing workforce: APNs, patient outcomes, and health care costs. *Nursing Outlook* 52, 45–52.

Committee on Quality of Health Care in America, Institute of Medicine. *Crossing the Quality Chasm: A New Health System for the 21st Century* (2001). Washington, DC: National Academy Press.

CPRI-HOST (2001). The Seventh Annual Nicholas E. Davies Award Proceedings, November.

Curtis, K. Personal correspondence, March 29, 2004.

Dillon, T.W., Lending, D., Crews, T.R., and Blankenship, R. (2003). Nursing self-efficacy of an integrated clinical and administrative information system. CIN: Computers, Informatics, Nursing, 21, 198–205.

Gloe, D. Personal correspondence, March 24, 2004.

Hermann, B. Personal correspondence, March 30, 2004.

HIMSS (2004a). HIMSS Nursing Informatics Survey, February 23, 2004. http://www.himss.org/content/files/nursing_info_survey2004.pdf

HIMSS (2004b). 15th Annual HIMSS Leadership Survey. http://www.himss.org/2004survey/ASP/index.asp

HIMSS (2004c). Nursing Informatics Groups form Alliance through HIMSS and AMIA to Provide Unified Structure. Press Release: Date October 19, 2004. AMIA and HIMSS. http://www.himss.org

Kennedy, M. Personal correspondence, March 30, 2004.

Lamb, G.S., Jennings, B.M., Mitchell, P.H., and Lang, N.M. (2004). Quality agenda: Priorities for action-recommendations of the American academy of nursing conference on health care quality. *Nursing Outlook* 52: 60–65.

Lang, N.M. and Mitchell, P.H. (2004). Guest editorial: Quality as an enduring an encompassing concept. *Nursing Outlook* 52: 1–2.

Marr, P., Duthie, E., and Glassman, K. (1993). Bedside terminals and quality of nursing documentation. *Computers in Nursing* 11, 176–182, 1993.

McNeil, B., Elfrink, V., Bickford, C., Pierce, S., Beyea, S., Averill, C., and Klappenback, C. (2003). Nursing information technology knowledge, skills, and preparation of student nurses, nursing faculty, and clinicians: a U.S. survey. *Journal of Nursing Education* 42: 341–359.

McCormick, K.A. (2005). Translating Evidence into Practice: Evidence, Clinical Practice Guidelines, and Automated Implementation Tools. In *Essential of Nursing Informatics*, 4th ed. Saba, V.K. and McCormick, K.A. New York: McGraw-Hill.

NINR. Report on Nursing Information, US PHS, 1993.

Pierce, S. (2000). Readiness for evidence-based practice: Information literacy needs of nursing faculty and students in a southern U.S. state. DAI, 62(12B), 5645. Accession no. AAI3035514.

Pravikoff, D., Pierce, S., and Tanner, A. (2003). Are nurses ready for evidence-based practice? *American Journal of Nursing* 103, 95–96.

Saba, V.K. and McCormick, K.A. (2005). *Essentials of Nursing Informatics*, 4th ed. New York: McGraw-Hill.

Saba, V., Coenen, A., McCormick, K., and Bakken, S. (2003). Nursing Language: Terminology Model for Nursing. *ISO Bulletin* September. http://www.iso.ch/iso/en/commcentre/isobulletin/articles/2003/pdf/terminology03-09.pdf

Sensmeier, J., Raiford, R., Taylor, S., and Weaver, C. (2002) Using Innovative Technology to Enhance Patient Care Delivery. American Academy of Nursing Technology and Work-force Conference, Washington, DC July 12–14 last accessed at: http://www.himss.org/content/files/AANNsgSummitHIMSSFINAL_18770.pdf

Shortliffe, E., Perreault, L., Wiederhold, G., and Fagan, L. (2001). *Medical Informatics: Computer Applications in Health Care and Biomedicine.* 2nd ed. New York: Springer-Verlag.

Tanner, A., Pierce, S., and Pravikoff, D. (2004) Readiness for Evidence-Based Practice: Information Literacy Needs of Nurses in the US. MedInfo 2004. 11 (Part 2) 936–940.

Tanner, A. (2000). Readiness for evidence-based practice: Information literacy needs of nursing faculty and students in a southern U.S. state. DAI 62(12B), 5647. Accession no. AAI303551.

Thompson, T.G. and Brailer, D.J. (2004). The Decade of Health Information Technology: Delivering Consumer-centric and Information-rich Health care. Framework for Strategic Action. U.S. Department of Health and Human Services.

Vahey, D.C., Swan, B.A., Lang, N.M., and Mitchell, P.H. (2004). Measuring and improving health care quality: Nursing's contribution to the state of the art. *Nursing Outlook* 52: 6–10.

44

Non-AI Decision Making

44.1 Analytical Models **44**-2
44.2 Decision Theoretic Models **44**-2
    Clinical Algorithms • Decision Trees • Influence Diagrams
44.3 Statistical Models **44**-4
    Database Search • Regression Analysis • Statistical Pattern
    Analysis • Bayesian Analysis • Dempster–Shafer Theory •
    Syntactic Pattern Analysis • Causal Modeling • Artificial
    Neural Networks
44.4 Summary **44**-8
References **44**-8

Ron Summers
Loughborough University

Derek G. Cramp
Ewart R. Carson
City University

Non-AI decision making can be defined as those methods and tools used to increase information content in the context of some specific clinical situation without having cause to refer to knowledge embodied in a computer program. Theoretical advances in the 1950s added rigor to this domain when Meehl argued that many clinical decisions could be made by statistical rather than intuitive means [1]. Evidence of this view was supported by Savage [2], whose theory of choice under uncertainty is still the classical and most elegant formulation of subjective Bayesian decision theory, and was very much responsible for reintroducing Bayesian decision analysis to clinical medicine. Ledley and Ludsted [3] provided further evidence that medical reasoning could be made explicit and represented in decision theoretic ways. Decision theory also provided the means for Nash to develop a "Logoscope," which might be considered as the first mechanical diagnostic aid [4].

An information system developed using non-AI decision-making techniques may comprise procedural or declarative knowledge. Procedural knowledge maps the decision-making process into the methods by which the clinical problems are solved or clinical decisions made. Examples of techniques that form a procedural knowledge base are those that are based on algorithmic analytical models, clinical algorithms, or decision trees. Information systems based on declarative knowledge comprise what can essentially be termed a database of facts about different aspects of a clinical problem; the causal relationships between these facts form a rich network from which explicit (say) cause–effect pathways can be determined. Semantic networks and causal probabilistic networks are perhaps the best examples of information systems based on declarative knowledge. There are other types of clinical decision aids, based purely on statistical methods applied to patient data, for example, classification analyses based on logistic regression, relative frequencies of occurrence, pattern-matching algorithms, or neural networks.

The structure of this chapter mirrors to some extent the different methods and techniques of non-AI decision making mentioned earlier. It is important to distinguish between analytical models based on quantitative or qualitative mathematical representations and decision theoretic methods typified by the use of clinical algorithms, decision trees, and set theory. Most of the latter techniques add to an information base by way of procedural knowledge. It is then that advantage can be taken of the many techniques that have statistical decision theoretic principles as their underpinning.

This section begins with a discussion of simple linear regression models and pattern recognition, but then more complex statistical techniques are introduced, for example, the use of Bayesian decision analysis, which leads to the introduction of causal probabilistic networks. The majority of these techniques add information by use of declarative knowledge. Particular applications are used throughout to illustrate the extent to which non-AI decision making is used in clinical practice.

44.1 Analytical Models

In the context of this chapter, the analytical models considered are qualitative and quantitative mathematical models that are used to predict future patient state based on present state and a historical representation of what has passed. Such models could be representations of system behavior that allow test signals to be used so that response of the system to various disturbances can be studied, thus making predictions of future patient state.

For example, Leaning et al. [5,6] produced a 19-segment quantitative mathematical model of the blood circulation to study the short-term effects of drugs on the cardiovascular system of normal, resting patients. The model represented entities such as the compliance, flow, and volume of model segments in what was considered a closed system. In total, the quantitative mathematical model comprised 61 differential equations and 159 algebraic equations. Evaluation of the model revealed that it was fit for its purpose in the sense of heuristic validity, that is, it could be used as a tool for developing explanations for cardiovascular control, particularly in relation to the central nervous system (CNS).

Qualitative models investigate time-dependent behavior by representing patient state trajectory in the form of a set of connected nodes, the links between the nodes reflecting transitional constraints placed on the system [7]. The types of decision making supported by this type of model are assessment and therapy planning. In diagnostic assessment, the precursor nodes and the pathway to the node (decision) of interest define the causal mechanisms of the disease process. Similarly, for therapy planning, the optimal plan can be set by investigation of the utility values associated with each link in the disease–therapy relationship. These utility values refer to a cost function, where cost can be defined as the monetary cost of providing the treatment and cost benefit to the patient in terms of efficiency, efficacy, and effectiveness of alternative treatment options. Both quantitative [8] and qualitative [9] analytical models can be realized in other ways to form the basis of rule-based systems; however that excludes their analysis in this chapter.

44.2 Decision Theoretic Models

44.2.1 Clinical Algorithms

The clinical algorithm is a procedural device that mimics clinical decision making by structuring the diagnostic or therapeutic decision processes in the form of a classification tree. The root of the tree represents some initial state, and the branches yield the different options available. For the operation of the clinical algorithm the choice points are assumed to follow branching logic with the decision function being a yes/no (or similar) binary choice. Thus, the clinical algorithm comprises a set of questions that must be collectively exhaustive for the chosen domain and the responses available to the clinician at each branch point must be mutually exclusive. These decision criteria pose rigid constraints on the type of medical problem that can be represented by this method, as the lack of flexibility is appropriate only for a certain set of well-defined clinical domains. Nevertheless, there is rich literature available; examples include the use of the clinical algorithm for acid–base disorders [10] and diagnosis of mental disorders [11]. A comprehensive guide to clinical algorithms can be found on the website of the American Academy of Family Physicians [12].

44.2.2 Decision Trees

A more rigorous use of classification tree representations than the clinical algorithm can be found in decision tree analysis. Although from a structural perspective, decision trees and clinical algorithms are similar in appearance, for decision tree analysis the likelihood and cost benefit for each choice are also calculated in order to provide a quantitative measure for each option available. This allows the use of optimization procedures to gauge the probability of success for the correct diagnosis being made or for a beneficial outcome from therapeutic action being taken. A further difference between the clinical algorithm and decision tree analysis is that the latter has more than one type of decision node (branch point): at decision nodes the clinician must decide on which choice (branch) is appropriate for the given clinical scenario; at chance nodes the responses available have no clinician control, for example, the response may be due to patient specific data; and outcome nodes define the chance nodes at the "leaves" of the decision tree. That is, they summarize a set of all possible clinical outcomes for the chosen domain.

The possible outcomes from each chance node must obey the rules of probability and sum to unity; the probability assigned to each branch reflects the frequency of that event occurring in a general patient population. It follows that these probabilities are dynamic, with accuracy increasing, as more evidence becomes available. A utility value can be added to each of the outcome scenarios. These utility measures reflect a trade-off between competing concerns, for example, survivability and quality of life, and may be assigned heuristically.

When the first edition of this chapter was written in 1995 it was noted that although a rich literature describing potential applications existed [13], the number of practical applications described was limited. The situation has changed and there has been an explosion of interest in applying decision analysis to clinical problems. Not only is decision analysis methodology well described [14–17] but there are also numerous articles appearing in mainstream medical journals, particularly *Medical Decision Making*. An important driver for this acceleration of interest has been the desire to contain costs of medical care, while maintaining clinical effectiveness and quality of care. Cost-effectiveness analysis is an extension of decision analysis and compares the outcome of decision options in terms of the monetary cost per unit of effectiveness. Thus, it can be used to set priorities for the allocation of resources and to decide between one or more treatment or intervention options. It is most useful when comparing treatments for the same clinical condition. Cost-effectiveness analysis and its implications are described very well elsewhere [18,19]. One reason for the lack of clinical applications using decision trees is that the underpinning software technologies remain relatively underdeveloped. Babič et al. [20] address this point by comparing decision tree software with other non-AI decision-making methods.

44.2.3 Influence Diagrams

In the 1960s researchers at Stanford Research Institute (SRI) proposed the use of influence diagrams as representational models when developing computer programs to solve decision problems. However, it was recognized somewhat later by decision analysts at SRI [21] that such diagrams could be used to facilitate communication with domain experts when eliciting information about complex decision problems. Influence diagrams are a powerful mode of graphic representation for decision modeling. They do not replace but complement decision trees and it should be noted that both are different graphical representations of the same mathematical model and operations. Recently, two exciting papers have been published that make the use of influence diagrams accessible to those interested in medical decision making [22,23].

44.3 Statistical Models

44.3.1 Database Search

Interrogation of large clinical databases yields statistical evidence of diagnostic value and in some representations form the basis of rule induction used to build expert systems [24]. These systems will not be discussed here. However, the most direct approach for clinical decision making is to determine the relative frequency of occurrence of an entity, or more likely group of entities, in the database of past cases. This enables a prior probability measure to be estimated [25]. A drawback of this simple, direct approach to problem solving is the apparent tautology of more evidence available leading to fewer matches in the database being found; this runs against common wisdom that more evidence leads to an increase in probability of a diagnosis being found. Further, the method does not provide a weight for each item of evidence to gauge those that are more significant for patient outcome.

With the completion of the Human Genome sequence there has been renewed interest in database search methods for finding data (e.g., single nucleotide polymorphisms — or more simply SNPs) in the many genetic database resources that are distributed throughout the world [26]. Vyas and Summers [27] provide both a summary of the issues surrounding the use of metadata to combine these dispersed data resources and suggest a solution via a semantic web-based knowledge architecture. It is clear that such methods of generating data will have an increasing impact on the advent of molecular medicine.

44.3.2 Regression Analysis

Logistic regression analysis is used to model the relationship between a response variable of interest and a set of explanatory variables. This is achieved by adjusting the regression coefficients, the parameters of the model, until a "best fit" to the data set is achieved. This type of model improves upon the use of relative frequencies, as logistic regression explicitly represents the extent to which elements of evidence are important in the value of the regression coefficients. An example of clinical use can be found in the domain of gastroenterology [28].

44.3.3 Statistical Pattern Analysis

The recognition of patterns in data can be formulated as a statistical problem of classifying the results of clinical findings into mutually exclusive but collectively exhaustive decision regions. In this way, not only can physiologic data be classified but also the pathology that they give rise to and the therapy options available to treat the disease. Titterington [29] describes an application in which patterns in a complex data set are recognized to enhance the care of patients with head injuries. Pattern recognition is also the cornerstone of computerized methods for cardiac rhythm analysis [30]. The methods used to distinguish patterns in data rely on discriminant analysis. In simple terms, this refers to a measure of separability between class populations.

In general, pattern recognition is a two-stage process as shown in Figure 44.1. The pattern vector, P, is an n-dimensional vector derived from the data set used. Let Ω_p be the pattern space, which is the set of all possible values P may assume, then the pattern recognition problem is formulated as finding a way of dividing Ω_p into mutually exclusive and collectively exhaustive regions. For example, in the analysis of the electrocardiogram the complete waveform may be used to perform classifications of diagnostic value. A complex decision function would probably be required in such cases. Alternatively (and if appropriate), the pattern vector can be simplified to investigation of sub features within a pattern. For cardiac arrhythmia analysis, only the R–R interval of the electrocardiogram is required, which allows a much simpler decision function to be used. This may be a linear or nonlinear transformation process:

$$X = \tau P$$

where X is termed the feature vector and τ is the transformation process.

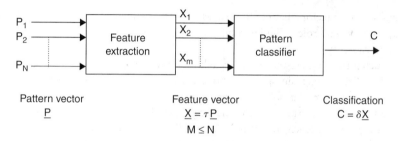

FIGURE 44.1   Pattern recognition.

Just as the pattern vector P belongs to a pattern space Ω_p, so the feature vector X belongs to a feature space Ω_X. As the function of feature extraction is to reduce the dimensionality of the input vector to the classifier, some information is lost. Classification of Ω_X can be achieved using numerous statistical methods including: discriminant functions (linear and polynomial), kernel estimation, k-nearest neighbor, cluster analysis, and Bayesian analysis.

44.3.4 Bayesian Analysis

Ever since their reinvestigation by Savage in 1954 [2], Bayesian methods of classification have provided one of the most popular approaches used to assist in clinical decision making. Bayesian classification is an example of a parametric method of estimating class-conditional probability density functions. Clinical knowledge is represented as a set of prior probabilities of diseases to be matched with conditional probabilities of clinical findings in a patient population with each disease. The classification problem becomes one of a choice of decision levels, which minimizes the average rate of misclassification or to minimize the maximum of the conditional average loss function (the so-called minmax criterion) when information about prior probabilities is not available. Formally, the optimal decision rule that minimizes the average rate of misclassification is called the Bayes rule; this serves as the inference mechanism that allows the probabilities of competing diagnoses to be calculated when patient specific clinical findings become available.

The great advantage of Bayesian classification is that a large clinical database of past cases is not required, thus allowing the time taken to reach a decision to be faster compared with other database search techniques; furthermore, classification errors due to the use of inappropriate clinical inferences are quantifiable. However, a drawback of this approach to clinical decision making is that the disease states are considered as complete and mutually exclusive, whereas in real life neither assumption may be true.

Nevertheless, Bayesian decision analysis functions as a basis for differential diagnosis and has been used successfully, for example, in the diagnosis of acute abdominal pain [31]. De Dombal first described this system in 1972, but it took another 20 years or so for it to be accepted via a multicenter multinational trial. The approach has been exploited in ILIAD; this is a commercially available [32] computerized diagnostic decision support system with some 850 to 990 frames in its knowledge base. As it is a Bayesian system, each frame has the prevalence of a disease for its prior probability. There is the possibility however, that the prevalence rates may not have general applicability. This highlights a very real problem, namely the validity of relating causal pathways in clinical thinking and connecting such pathways to a body of validated (true) evidence. Ideally, such evidence will come from randomized controlled clinical or epidemiological trials. However, such studies may be subject to bias.

To overcome this, Eddy et al. [33] devised the Confidence Profile Method. This is a set of quantitative techniques for interpreting and displaying the results of individual studies (trials), exploring the effects of any biases that might affect the internal validity of the study, adjusting for external validity, and, finally, combining evidence from several sources. This meta-analytical approach can formally incorporate experimental evidence and, in a Bayesian fashion, also the results of previous analytical studies or subjective judgments about specific factors that might arise when interpreting evidence. Influence diagram representations play an important role in linking results in published studies and estimates of probabilities and statements about causality.

Currently, much interest is being generated as to how, what is perceived as the Bayesian action-oriented approach can be used in determining health policy, where the problem is perceived to be a decision problem rather than a statistical problem, see for instance Lilford and Braunholz [34].

Bayesian analysis continues to be used in a wide range of clinical applications either as a single method or as part of a multimethod approach, for example, for insulin sensitivity [35], for understanding incomplete data sets [36], and has been used extensively for the analysis of clinical trials (e.g., see References 37 and 38).

Bayesian decision theory also provides a valuable framework for health care technology assessment. Bayesian methods have also become increasingly visible in places where they are being applied to the analysis of economic models [39], being applied particularly to two decision problems commonly encountered in pharmaco-economics and health technology assessment generally, namely: adoption and allocation.

Acceptability curves generated from Bayesian cost effectiveness analyses can be interpreted as the probability that the new intervention is cost effective at a given level of willingness-to-pay. For Bayesian methods applied to clinical trials with cost as well as efficacy data see O'Hagan and Stevens [40]. This probabilistic interpretation of study findings provides information that is more relevant and more transparent to decision makers. The Bayesian value of information analysis offers a decision-analytic framework to explore the conceptually separate decisions of whether a new technology should be adopted from the question of whether more research is required to inform this choice in the future [41,42]. Thus, it is a useful analytical framework for decision-makers who wish to achieve allocative efficacy.

The Bayesian approach has several advantages over the frequentist approach. First, it allows accumulation and updating of knowledge by using the prior distribution. Second, it yields more flexible inferences and emphasizes predictions rather than hypothesis testing. Third, probabilities involving multiple endpoints are relatively simply to estimate. Finally, it provides a solid theoretical framework for decision analyses.

44.3.5 Dempster–Shafer Theory

One way to overcome the problem of mutually exclusive disease states is to use an extension to Bayesian classification put forward by Dempster [43] and Shafer [44]. Here, instead of focusing on a single disorder, the method can deal with combinations of several diseases. The key concept used is that the set of all possible diseases is partitioned into n-tuples of possible disease state combinations.

A simple example will illustrate this concept. Suppose there is a clinical scenario in which four disease states describe the whole hypothesis space. Each new item of evidence will impact on all the possible subsets of the hypothesis space and is represented by a function, the basic probability assignment. This measure is a belief function that must obey the law of probability and sum to unity across the subsets impacted upon. In the example, all possible subsets comprise: one that has all four disease states in it; four, which have three of the four diseases as members; six, which have two diseases as members; and finally, four subsets that have a single disease as a member. Thus, when new evidence becomes available in the form of a clinical finding, only certain hypotheses, represented by individual subsets, may be favored.

44.3.6 Syntactic Pattern Analysis

As demonstrated earlier, a large class of clinical problem solving using statistical methods involves classification or diagnosis of disease states, selection of optimal therapy regimes, and prediction of patient outcome. However, in some cases the purpose of modeling is to reconstruct the input signal from the data available. This cannot be done by methods discussed thus far. The syntactic approach to pattern recognition uses a hierarchical decomposition of information and draws upon an analogy to the syntax of language. Each input pattern is described in terms of more simple sub-patterns, which themselves are

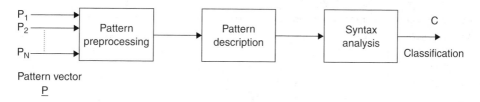

FIGURE 44.2   Syntactic pattern recognition system.

decomposed into simpler subunits, until the most elementary subpatterns, termed the pattern primitives, are reached. The pattern primitives should be selected so that they are easy to recognize with respect to the input signal. Rules that govern the transformation of pattern primitives back (ultimately) to the input signal are termed the grammar.

In this way a string grammar, G, which is easily representable in computer-based applications, can be defined:

$$G = \{V_T, V_N, S, P\}$$

where, V_T are the terminal variables (pattern primitives); V_N are the non-terminal variables; S is the start symbol; and P is the set of production rules, which specify the transformation between each level of the hierarchy. It is an important assumption that in set theoretic terms, the union of V_T and V_N is the total vocabulary of G, and the intersection of V_T and V_N is the null (empty) set.

A syntactic pattern recognition system therefore comprises three functional subunits (Figure 44.2): a preprocessor — this manipulates the input signal, P, into a form that can be presented to the pattern descriptor, the pattern descriptor that assigns a vocabulary to the signal, and the syntax analyzer that classifies the signal accordingly. This type of system has been used successfully to represent the electrocardiogram [45,46] and the electroencephalogram [47] and for representation of the carotid pulse wave [48].

44.3.7   Causal Modeling

A causal probabilistic network (CPN) is an acyclic multiply-connected graph, which at a qualitative level comprises nodes and arcs [49]. Nodes are the domain objects and may represent, for example, clinical findings, pathophysiologic states, diseases, or therapies. Arcs are the causal relationships between successive nodes and are directed links. In this way the node and arc structure represents a model of the domain. Quantification is expressed in the model by a conditional probability table being associated with each arc, allowing the state of each node to be represented as a binary value or more frequently as a continuous probability distribution.

In root nodes the conditional probability table reduces to a probability distribution of all its possible states.

A key concept of CPNs is that computation is reduced to a series of local calculations, using only one node and those that are linked to it in the network. Any node can be instantiated with an observed value; this evidence is then propagated through the CPN via a series of local computations. Thus, CPNs can be used in two ways: to instantiate the leaf nodes of the network with known patterns for given disorders to investigate expected causal pathways; or to instantiate the root nodes or nodes in the graphical hierarchy with, for example, test results to obtain a differential diagnosis. The former method has been used to investigate respiratory pathology [50], and the latter method has been read to obtain pathologic information from electromyography [51].

44.3.8   Artificial Neural Networks

Artificial neural networks (ANNs) mimic their biologic counterparts, although at the present time on a much smaller scale. The fundamental unit in the biological system is the neuron. This is a specialized cell that, when activated, transmits a signal to its connected neighbors. Both activation and transmission involve chemical transmitters, which cross the synaptic gap between neurons. Activation of the neuron takes place only when a certain threshold is reached. This biologic system is modeled in the representation of an artificial neural network. It is possible to identify three basic elements of the neuron model: a set of weighted connecting links that form the input to the neuron (analogous to neurotransmission across the synaptic gap), an adder for summing the input signals, and an activation function that limits the amplitude of the output of the neuron to the range (typically) -1 to $+1$. This activation function also has a threshold term that can be applied externally and forms one of the parameters of the neuron model. Many books are available which provide a comprehensive introduction to this class of model (e.g., see Reference 52).

ANNs can be applied to two categories of problems: prediction and classification. It is the latter that has caught the imagination of biomedical engineers for its similarity to diagnostic problem solving. For instance, the conventional management of patients with septicemia requires a diagnostic strategy that takes up to 18 to 24 h before initial identification of the causal microorganism. This can be compared to a method in which an ANN is applied to a large clinical database of past cases; the quest becomes one of seeking an optimal match between present clinical findings and patterns present in the recorded data. In this application, pattern matching is a nontrivial problem as each of the 5000 past cases has 51 data fields. It has been shown that for this problem the ANN method outperforms other statistical methods such as k-nearest neighbor [53].

The use of ANNs in clinical decision making is becoming widespread. A further example of their use in critical care medicine is given by Yamamura et al. [54]. ANNs are used in chronic and acute clinical episodes. An example of the former is their use in cancer survival predictions [55] and an example of the latter is their use in the emergency room to detect early onset of myocardial infarction [56].

44.4 Summary

This chapter has reviewed what are normally considered to be the major categories of approach available to support clinical decision making, which do not rely on what is classically termed artificial intelligence (AI). They have been considered under the headings of analytical, decision theoretic, and statistical models, together with their corresponding subdivisions. It should be noted, however, that the division into non-AI approaches and AI approaches that is adopted in this volume (see the Chapter entitled Expert Systems: Methods and Tools) is not totally clear-cut. In essence the range of approaches can in many ways be regarded as a continuum. There is no unanimity as to where the division should be placed and the separation adopted; here is but one of a number that is feasible. It is therefore desirable that the reader should consider these two chapters together and choose an approach that is relevant to the particular clinical context.

References

[1] Meehl, R. 1954. *Clinical versus Statistical Prediction*. Minnesota, University of Minnesota Press.

[2] Savage L.I. 1954. *The Foundations of Statistics*. New York, John Wiley & Sons.

[3] Ledley R.S. and Ludsted L.B. 1959. Reasoning foundations of medical diagnosis. *Science* 130: 9.

[4] Nash F.A. 1954. Differential diagnosis: an apparatus to assist the logical faculties. *Lancet* 4: 874.

[5] Leaning M.S., Pullen H.E., Carson E.R. et al. 1983. Modelling a complex biological system: the human cardiovascular system: 1. Methodology and model description. *Trans. Inst. Meas. Contr.* 5: 71.

[6] Leaning M.S., Pullen H.E., Carson E.R. et al. 1983. Modelling a complex biological system: the human cardiovascular system: 2. Model validation, reduction and development. *Trans. Inst. Meas. Contr.* 5: 87.

[7] Kuipers B.J. 1986. Qualitative simulation. *Artif. Intel.* 29: 289.

[8] Furukawa T., Tanaka H., and Hara S. 1987. FLUIDEX: A microcomputer-based expert system for fluid therapy consultations. In M.K. Chytil and R. Engelbrecht (Eds.), *Medical Expert Systems.* Wilmslow, Sigma Press, pp. 59–74.

[9] Bratko I., Mozetic J., and Lavrac N. 1988. In Michie D. and Bratko I. (Eds.), *Expert Systems: Automatic Knowledge Acquisition.* Reading, Mass. Addison-Wesley, pp. 61–83.

[10] Bleich H.L. 1972. Computer-based consultations: Electrolyte and acid–base disorders. *Am. J. Med.* 53: 285.

[11] McKenzie D.P., McGary P.D., Wallac et al. 1993. Constructing a minimal diagnostic decision tree. *Meth. Inform. Med.* 32: 161.

[12] http://www.aafp.org/x19449.xml (accessed February 2005).

[13] Pauker S.G. and Kassirer J.P. 1987. Decision analysis. *N. Engl. J. Med.* 316: 250.

[14] Weinstein M.C. and Fineberg H.V. 1980. *Clinical Decision Analysis.* London, W.B. Saunders.

[15] Watson S.R. and Buede D.M. 1994. *Decision Synthesis.* Cambridge, Cambridge University Press.

[16] Sox H.C., Blatt M.A., Higgins M.C., and Marton K.I. 1988. *Medical Decision Making.* Boston, Butterworth Heinemann.

[17] Llewelyn H. and Hopkins A. 1993. *Analysing How We Reach Clinical Decisions.* London, Royal College of Physicians.

[18] Gold M.R., Siegel J.E., Russell L.B., and Weinstein M.C. (Eds.) 1996. *Cost-Effectiveness in Health and Medicine.* New York, Oxford University Press.

[19] Sloan F.A. (Ed.) 1996. *Valuing Health Care.* Cambridge, Cambridge University Press.

[20] Babič S.H., Kokol P., Podgorelec V., Zorman M., Šprogar M., and Štiglic M.M. 2000. The art of building decision trees. *J. Med. Syst.* 24: 43–52.

[21] Owen D.L. 1984. The use of influence diagrams in structuring complex decision problems. In Howard R.A. and Matheson J.E. (Eds.), *Readings on the Principles and Applications of Decision Analysis,* Vol. 2. Menlo Park, CA, Strategic Decisions Group, pp. 763–772.

[22] Owens D.K., Shachter R.D., and Nease R.F. 1997. Representation and analysis of medical decision problems with influence diagrams. *Med. Decis. Mak.* 17: 241.

[23] Nease R.F. and Owens D.K. 1997. Use of influence diagrams to structure medical decisions. *Med. Decis. Mak.* 17: 263.

[24] Quinlan J.R. 1979. Rules by induction from large collections of examples. In D. Michie (Ed.), *Expert Systems in the Microelectronic Age.* Edinburgh, Edinburgh University Press.

[25] Gammerman A. and Thatcher A.R. 1990. Bayesian inference in an expert system without assuming independence. In M.C. Golumbic (Ed.), *Advances in Artificial Intelligence.* New York, Springer-Verlag, pp. 182–218.

[26] Goble C.A., Stevens R., and Ng S. 2001. Transparent access to multiple bioinformatics information sources. *IBM Syst. J.* 40: 532–551.

[27] Vyas H. and Summers R. 2004. Impact of semantic web on bioinformatics. In *Proceedings of the International Symposium of Santa Caterina on Challenges in the Internet and Interdisciplinary Research (SSCCII),* CD-ROM Proceedings.

[28] Spiegelhalter D.J. and Knill-Jones R.P. 1984. Statistical and knowledge-based approaches to clinical decision-support systems with an application in gastroenterology. *J. Roy. Stat. Soc.* A 147: 35.

[29] Titterington D.M., Murray G.D., Murray L.S. et al. 1981. Comparison of discriminant techniques applied to a complex set of head injured patients. *J. Roy. Stat. Soc.* A 144: 145.

[30] Morganroth J. 1984. Computer recognition of cardiac arrhythmias and statistical approaches to arrhythmia analysis. *Ann. NY Acad. Sci.* 432: 117.

[31] De Dombal F.T., Leaper D.J., Staniland J.R. et al. 1972. Computer-aided diagnosis of acute abdominal pain. *Br. Med. J.* 2: 9.

[32] *Applied Medical Informatics.* Salt Lake City, UT.

[33] Eddy D.M., Hasselblad V., and Shachter R. 1992. *Meta-Analysis by the Confidence Profile Methods.* London, Academic Press.

[34] Lilford R.J. and Braunholz D. 1996. The statistical basis of public policy: a paradigm shift is overdue. *Br. Med. J.* 313: 603.

[35] Agbaje O.F., Luzio S.D., Albarrak A.I.S., Lunn D.J., Owens D.R., and Hovorka R. 2003. Bayesian hierarchical approach to estimate insulin sensitivity by minimal model. *Clin. Sci.* 105: 551–560.

[36] Crawford S.L., Tennstedt S.L., and McKinlay J.B. 1995. Longitudinal care patterns for disabled elders: A Bayesian analysis of missing data. In Gatsonis C., Hodges J., and Kass R.E. (Eds.), *Case Studies in Bayesian Statistics*, Vol. 2. New York: Springer-Verlag, pp. 293–308.

[37] Lewis R.J. and Wears R.L. 1993. An introduction to the Bayesian analysis of clinical trials. *Ann. Emerg. Med.* 22: 1328–1336.

[38] Spiegelhalter D.J., Freedman L.S., and Parmar M.K.B. 1994. Bayesian approaches to randomised trials. *J. Roy. Stat. Soc.* A 157: 357–416.

[39] Parmigiani G. 2002. *Modeling in Medical Decision Making: A Bayesian Approach.* Chichester, Wiley.

[40] O'Hagan A. and Stevens J.W. 2003. Bayesian methods for design and analysis of cost-effectiveness trials in the evaluation of health care technologies. *Stat. Meth. Med. Res.* 11: 469–490.

[41] Claxton K. and Posnett J. 1996. An economic approach to clinical trial design and research priority setting. *Health Econ.* 5: 513–524.

[42] Claxton K. 1999. The irrelevance of inference: A decision making approach to the stochastic evaluation of health care technologies. *J. Health Econ.* 18: 341–364.

[43] Dempster A. 1967. Upper and lower probabilities induced by multi-valued mapping. *Ann. Math. Stat.* 38: 325.

[44] Shafer G. 1976. *A Mathematical Theory of Evidence.* Princeton, NJ, Princeton University Press.

[45] Belforte G., De Mori R., and Ferraris E. 1979. A contribution to the automatic processing of electrocardiograms using syntactic methods. *IEEE Trans. Biomed. Eng.* BME 26: 125.

[46] Birman K.P. 1982. Rule-based learning for more accurate ECG analysis. *IEEE Trans. Pat. Anal. Mach. Intell.* PAMI 4: 369.

[47] Ferber G. 1985. Syntactic pattern recognition of intermittant EEG activity. *Meth. Inf. Med.* 24: 79.

[48] Stockman G.C. and Kanal L.N. 1983. Problem reduction in representation for the linguistic analysis of waveforms. *IEEE Trans. Pat. Anal. Mach. Intel.* PAMI 5: 287.

[49] Andersen S.K., Jensen F.V., and Olesen K.G. 1987. *The HUGIN Core-Preliminary Considerations on Inductive Reasoning: Managing Empirical Information in AI Systems.* Riso, Denmark.

[50] Summers R., Andreassen S., Carson E.R. et al. 1993. A causal probabilistic model of the respiratory system. In *Proceedings of the IEEE 15th Annual Conference of the Engineering in Medicine and Biology Society.* New York, IEEE, pp. 534–535.

[51] Jensen F.V., Andersen S.K., Kjaerulff U. et al. 1987. MUNIN: On the case for probabilities in medical expert systems — a practical exercise. In Fox J., Fieschi M., and Engelbrecht R. (Eds.), *Proceedings of the Ist Conference European Society for AI in Medicine.* Heidelberg, Springer-Verlag, pp. 149–160.

[52] Haykin S. 1994. *Neural Networks: A Comprehensive Foundation.* New York, Macmillan.

[53] Worthy P.J., Dybowski R., Gransden W.R., et al. 1993. Comparison of learning vector quantisation and nearest neighbour for prediction of microorganisms associated with septicaemia. In: *Proceedings of the IEEE 15th Annual Conference of the Engineering in Medicine and Biology Society*, New York, IEEE, pp. 273–274.

[54] Yamamura S., Takehira R., Kawada K., Nishizawa K., Katayama S., Hirano M., and Momose Y. 2003. Application of artificial neural network modelling to identify severely ill patients whose aminoglycoside concentrations are likely to fall below therapeutic concentrations. *J. Clin. Pharm. Ther.* 28: 425–432.

[55] Burke H.B., Goodman P.H., and Rosen D.B. 1997. Artificial neural networks improve the accuracy of cancer survival prediction. *Cancer* 79: 857–862.

[56] Baxt W.G., Shofer F.S., Sites F.D., and Hollander J.E. 2002. A neural computational aid to the diagnosis of acute myocardial infarction. *Ann. Emerg. Med.* 39: 366–373.

45

Medical Informatics and Biomedical Emergencies: New Training and Simulation Technologies for First Responders

Joseph M. Rosen
Christopher Swift
Eliot B. Grigg
Matthew F. McKnight
Susan McGrath
Dennis McGrath
Peter Robbie
C. Everett Koop
Dartmouth-Hitchcock Medical Center

45.1 Asymmetric Warfare and Bioterrorism................. **45**-2
45.2 Disaster Management Paradigms...................... **45**-3
45.3 Disaster Response Paradigms **45**-5
45.4 Medical Informatics and Emergency Response........ **45**-6
45.5 Advanced Technologies................................. **45**-8
45.6 Conclusions **45**-9
References **45**-9

Delivering detection, diagnostic, and treatment information to first responders remains a central challenge in disaster management. This is particularly true in biomedical emergencies involving highly infectious agents. Adding inexpensive, established information technologies to existing response system will produce beneficial outcomes. In some instances, however, emerging technologies will be necessary to enable an immediate, continuous response. This article identifies and describes new training, education, and simulation technologies that will help first responders cope with bioterrorist events. The September 11 Commission report illuminated many of the errors leading to Al Qaeda's dramatic attacks in New York and Washington, DC Among them was a well-documented failure to coordinate intelligence within the federal bureaucracy. Yet the greatest failure noted by the Commissioners was a failure of policy — a failure of imagination [1]. Federal, state, and local officials must avoid similar myopia in working to secure the homeland. Responding to future attacks with Chemical, Biological, Radiological, Nuclear or Explosive (CBRNE) agents is one area where imagination and innovation will be necessary.

September 11 marked a watershed in Americans' understanding of the world and their place in it. Al Qaeda's attacks were audacious, innovative, and cruel. Yet they were also highly conventional. The use of civilian aircraft as guided missiles mimicked the fuel air bombs that the U.S. forces used to attack Osama bin Laden's training camps in 1998. September 11 was also a tactical strike. Notwithstanding the scale of suffering and destruction, it undermined neither the capacity of the United States to defend itself militarily, nor the public's will to wage defensive war [2].

From securing government buildings to screening airline passengers, much of the political debate stemming from the September 11 Commission report now focuses on preventing similar tactical strikes. This goal is laudable, but may not be practically attainable. U.S. intelligence and law enforcement agencies are neither omniscient nor omnipotent. Robust search and seizure capabilities will inevitably be restrained in a society that values civil rights and individual freedom. Even Russia, whose government retains extensive domestic intelligence gathering and surveillance powers, proved unable to interdict armed hostage takers at Moscow's Dubrovka theater and the Beslan primary school.

Against that backdrop, a reflexive focus on preventing *any* form of terrorism may detract attention and divert funding from preparations necessary to respond to a *strategic* terrorist attack. Policy makers and the American public should not lose sight of the big picture. It may not always be possible to preempt, much less prevent future terrorist attacks. It is possible, however, to ameliorate or mitigate the strategic effects of future attack through proper planning, resources, and training. With that object in mind, training local first responders for a full spectrum of CBRNE contingencies must remain foremost among the reforms considered in the wake of the September 11 Commission report. This examination of emerging training and simulation technologies endeavors to inform that debate.

This investigation proceeds in four stages. First, it addresses the political implications of CBRNE agents, with a particular focus on Biological Warfare (BW). Second, it compares and contrasts the incremental U.S. National Disaster Medical System (NDMS) with the flexible, net-centric disaster management model employed by German emergency personnel. Third, it examines the role of Information Technology (IT) and medical informatics in disaster response. Finally, it assesses the role of simulation technologies in developing and disseminating CBRNE disaster training tools across both legal and geographic jurisdictions.

45.1 Asymmetric Warfare and Bioterrorism

Epidemics played a major role in destabilizing great empires. Between 250 and 650 AD, the Roman empire "was assaulted by successive waves of pandemics that reduced the population by at least one-quarter . . ." [3]. Naturally occurring phenomena carried strategic implications. As the number of infections rose, the result was significantly reduced economic productivity, a declining agricultural and tax base, and severe shortages in military manpower. "Rome's greatest enemy cannot from within," observes medieval historian Norman F. Cantor, "but from biomedical plagues that the Romans could not possibly understand or combat" [3]. Germs, not the Goths, brought the Roman civilization to its knees.

A similar civilization collapse is improbable today. Contemporary scientific knowledge is infinitely more advanced that in the classical period. Economies are now digital and global, relying less and less on physical human labor. Had imperial Rome possessed an institution comparable to the Centers for Disease Control (CDC), its response to epidemiological crises may have proved more robust. Modern society's capacity to detect and contain epidemics does not render them harmless, however. Indeed, the very characteristics that make biological agents unwieldy and unpredictable as battlefield weapons — silence, incubation time, and uncontrollability — render them especially effective for terrorist attacks [4].

Four characteristics make BW preferable to nuclear, chemical, or even radiological weapons. First, they are easily concealed. Small containers and host carriers can carry enough pathogen to infect hundreds, if not thousands. Second, incubation periods enable silent dispersion and subsequent transmission within

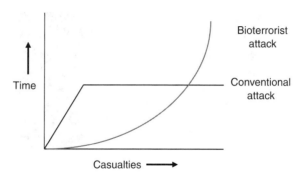

FIGURE 45.1 Conventional and bioterrorist attacks.

target populations. Initial cases would be almost indistinguishable from naturally occurring phenomena. Third, BW attacks threaten the very public health personnel necessary for effective detection, containment, and treatment — especially in high-density metropolitan areas. Those responsible for diagnosing and containing an agent are most likely to be infected by it. Finally, the longer a BW attack remains undetected, the more difficult it becomes to prevent continued proliferation. Unlike a static, conventional strike, the damage caused by a bioterrorist attack can grow geometrically [4] (see Figure 45.1).

Serious vulnerabilities exist. The 2000 TOPOFF exercises in Denver, Colorado, together with simulations run by Dartmouth College in 2001, indicated that BW attacks might threaten vital U.S. security interests [4]. Properly executed by a competent adversary, such an event could swiftly assume strategic dimensions. In 1993, for example, the Congressional Office of Technology Assessment (OTA) estimated that the aerosolized release of one hundred kilograms of anthrax in the Washington, DC area would produce between 130,000 and 3 million fatalities [5]. Although that analysis does not account for reforms undertaken during the last decade, it is still worth noting that scale of lethality reported by OTA is comparable to that from a thermonuclear bomb [5].

These simulations also revealed that existing local, state, and federal capabilities are ill suited for BW. Time lags in resources allocation and failure to distribute resources effectively within the disaster area proved highly problematic [6]. Such failings only exacerbate existing vulnerabilities. Swift detection, containment, and treatment are essential in mitigating both the tactical effects and strategic implications of a bioterrorist attack. Failure would concede control of the operational tempo to the contagion and those employing it as a weapon.

45.2 Disaster Management Paradigms

Although these threats are recognized within the U.S. Government, the current structure of the federal emergency response system remains insufficient. The situation is even more pronounced when one considers existing barriers to coordination between federal authorities and first responders at the state and local level. Recent studies by the Federation of American Scientists revealed that "physicians. Nurses, emergency medical workers, police and fire officials feel unprepared for a WMD emergency — particularly at the level of cities and counties" [7]. To address these apparent shortcomings, we must first rethink our approach to disaster response, as well as the manner in which we train first responders.

The U.S. Government established the National Disaster Management System (NDMS) in 1983. Drawing resources from the Federal Emergency Management Agency (FEMA), as well as the Departments of Defense (DOD), Health and Human Services (HHS), and Veterans Affairs (VA), the system concentrated sophisticated equipment and highly trained personnel in regional Disaster Management Assistance Teams (DMATs). HHS oversaw medical stockpiles. DOD provided transportation for medical evacuation. The VA would open regional medical centers, when needed, to mobilize DMAT teams [2] (see Figure 45.2).

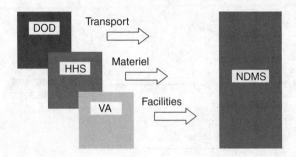

FIGURE 45.2   Cold war NDMS structure.

	Threat	Doctrine	Response	Structure
Cold war	Conventional	Evacuation	Escalating	Hierarchical
War on terror	Asymmetric	Isolation	Overwhelming	Net-centric

FIGURE 45.3   NDMS transformation.

NDMS was a product of the Cold War. Though designed for natural and transportation disasters, the infrastructure was also intended to support mass casualties evacuated from military operations outside the Continental United States (OCONUS). Were the Soviet Union to invade western Europe, the United States could accommodate the anticipated mass of NATO casualties. Unfortunately, NDMS was not designed with homeland security in mind, much less bioterrorism. In an age where intercontinental thermonuclear war represented the primary threat to U.S. security, there was little strategic value in responding to an attack in which most if not all the civilian casualties would be killed.

NDMS's Cold War roots are evident in three characteristics. First, the role of the federal government is to supplement state and local emergency response capabilities by providing triage, austere medical care, and casualty staging. Second, NDMS is an incremental, echelon-based system. The larger the casualty pool, the more DMATs deployed. Third, the chief mission of first responders is stabilization and evacuation. As currently configured, DMATs treat only 10% of all casualties on-scene, transporting the remaining 90% from the incident site to remote medical facilities operated by the VA and others.

This system is poorly configured for the challenges of catastrophic terrorism. The first problem is doctrinal. BW and other CBREN attacks will generally require swift isolation and decontamination. Though useful in earthquakes and airline disasters, a Cold War doctrine emphasizing swift patient evacuation could exacerbate crisis conditions. In the case of bioterrorism, delayed onset places greater emphasis on vaccination and restricted movement. New doctrines must bring the hospital to the patient, rather than the patient to the hospital (see Figure 45.3).

The second problem is architecture. In the current NDMS system, local first responders often encounter a disaster with minimal external support. State and federal resources become available only after the declaration of a state of emergency—a process that can take hours, if not days. The result is often a delayed operations tempo: by "the time a crisis is detected, the scale of it is appreciated, and federal resources are put into play, it may be too late" [2]. Staging disaster response may unintentionally cede the initiative to the adversary, allowing an event to escalate beyond the incident area, or to acquire public resonances several orders of magnitude greater than the scope of the actual event. Though "federal personnel [might] deal with the horrendous aftermath, [they] would not be involved in the direct response" [8].

The need for a continuous, integrated response is particularly evident in BW scenarios. At the tactical level, casualties must be isolated and the incident site contained. All should be treated on-site or screened before evacuation to remote medical facilities. In many instances, hospitals are likely to be the locus of pathogen detection, as well as a nexus for further infection. Absent adequate staging of personnel, equipment, and supplies, the confluence of treatment facility and incident cite could lead to broader contamination while compromising a node in the local public health network. Failure to maintain strict containment regimes will only exacerbate a pathogen's potential physical, psychological, and political effects.

Although some doctrinal reforms are underway, the NDMS's hierarchical architecture and incremental approach may prove unable to keep pace with anthropomorphic epidemics occurring simultaneously in multiple population centers. To ensure effective consequence management, U.S. emergency response paradigms must move beyond echelon-based care to a continuous care system in which "patients are followed by single or distinct groups or providers throughout the system" [2]. Ultimately, the goal must be "to have all resources, both system performance and human resources, available immediately wherever the bioattack is detected" [8].

45.3 Disaster Response Paradigms

A terrorist attack of national scope will inevitably initiate "a multi-agency operation requiring sophistic-ated (and sometimes chaotic) communications and coordination" [2]. Enhancing interoperability across function and geographic jurisdictions is now a primary objective for first responders and the federal agen-cies supporting them. Efforts to improve communications networks and enhance incident Command and Control (C^2) are now underway. Chief among them is the adoption of new NDMS doctrines for cite isolation and treatment. Also notable is the DOD's creation of a Northern Command (NORTHCOM), which plays a leading role in coordination capabilities among relevant federal, state, and local agencies.

Despite these efforts, however, first responder training often falls to a diverse collection of agencies possessing disparate sources of authority, funding, and information. The Department of Energy (DOE), for example, oversees training for nuclear and radiological attacks. HHS and the Centers for Disease Control (CDC) oversee bioterrorism programs. The Departments of Justice (DOJ) and Homeland Security (DHS) each provide a broad spectrum of grants and training programs for fire, law enforcement, and emergency medical personnel. The result is an unwieldy and extraordinarily complex bureaucratic web.

Congressional oversight displays similar stovepipes, with 79 committees and subcommittees, all 100 senators, "and at least 412 of the 435 House members" sharing "some degree of responsibility for homeland security operations" [9]. This broad balkanization presents two major challenges. First, it obstructs coordination and cooperation, both within the federal government and between Washington and the states. Second, it contributes to political confusion and policy failure. Absent a broad view of the entire homeland security apparatus, legislators are likely to respond to parochial interests rather than "develop a broad overview of homeland security priorities" [9].

Significant challenges also exist at the state and local level. Some 80% of U.S. first responders are unpaid volunteers [7]. Most training occurs under the auspices of local departments, sometimes either supported by state or regional academies. As such, the "level of preparedness often varies from jurisdiction to jurisdiction and from agency to agency" [10]. The result is a patchwork quilt that covers some areas, but leaves others woefully bare. "Absent better coordination and approaches to the dissemination of training materials," warns the Federation of American Scientists, "much of the investment [in Homeland Security] is likely to be wasted and decades could pass before the need is met" [7].

For a new disaster management paradigm to emerge, we must first identify the objectives sought and the characteristics necessary to achieve them. The 1998 crash of the high-speed InterCity Express (ICE) train 884 near Eschede, Germany provides a valuable model. Like the United States, Germany is a federal republic. Political authority is distributed among federal, state, and local officials. Disaster management is an interdepartmental endeavor involving numerous agencies with varied capabilities and legal jurisdictions. There is no centralized hierarchy responsible for emergency planning or response. Given these similar systems, one might also expect similar outcomes.

The German response to ICE 884 proved otherwise. Emergency personnel responded within 4 min of the train derailing. Within 8 min, first responders arrived on the scene, declared a disaster and issued

Massive casualties	
Fatalities	101 (96 died on impact; 5 in hospital)
Injuries	108
Overwhelming response	
Personnel	1800 (Rescue, police, and military)
Ground vehicles	100
Helicopters	39

FIGURE 45.4   InterCity Express 884.

mutual aid requests to neighboring emergency command centers. Within 15 min, 14 additional emergency physicians were en route to the incident site via rescue helicopters. Military units cleared landing zones. Commanders mobilized heavy-duty rescue equipment. The rescue operation took four short hours, during which time more than 1,800 personnel from various agencies evacuated all of the 108 injured victims. Only five died in hospital [11] (see Figure 45.4).

What then, are the primary differences between the U.S. and German disaster management paradigms? The first is organizational. Where the U.S. system is bifurcated and bureaucratized, the Germans employ an integrated, multifaceted approach drawing on prepositioned assets and previously agreed mutual-aid covenants. Where the U.S. approach stresses hierarchy, incremental response, and echelon-based care, the German system favors an immediate, overwhelming response in which all players know their assigned role and are trained to act in concert. Where the U.S. system stresses specialized skills, the German system trains first responders to operate in concert with colleagues from various professional and experiential backgrounds.

The second major difference is operational: namely, the extensive use of Health Information Systems (HIS). In Germany, each element in the disaster response system shares standardized disaster incident information. The result is a net-centric C^2 architecture in which emergency personnel, incident commanders, and remote medical facilities can accurately track both the dispatch of resources to the incident site, as well as anticipate care required following the evacuation of trauma victims. This ability to swiftly share and coordinate diagnostic, geographic, and logistical information across all of the responding agencies helps create a seamless and highly adaptable disaster response system while simultaneously reducing confusion and duplication. Incident commanders can command, rather than improvise.

45.4 Medical Informatics and Emergency Response

The use of medical informatics can be as simple as reporting as patient's condition to physicians en route to the hospital, or as complex as managing triage in a mass casualty, multiple-incident terrorist attack. In both instances, first responders collect, categorize, and communicate casualty information to other personnel in the disaster management system. In the latter scenario, however, the nature and scope of the events introduces a high degree of complexity and sensitivity, requiring careful management of patients and resources alike. Both instances use IT to significantly improve the richness and reach of available information (see Figure 45.5).

As evident in the case of ICE 884, the systematized collection, dissemination, and application of casualty information is necessary for triage and treatment in any conventional disaster. This is true even when information density is relatively low, as in a motor vehicle accident. In a major terrorist attack, however, medical informatics can assume strategic importance. Understanding the nature and location of the incident, the current condition of the victims, and the likely cause will each be critical prerequisites for

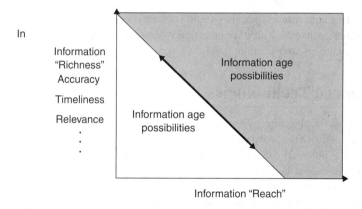

FIGURE 45.5   Information Richness and Reach. (Taken from D.S. Alberts, J.J. Gartska, R.E. Hayes, and D.A. Signori, *CCRO Publication Series*, 2001.)

successful consequence management. Providing that information in the face of significant information density may require a brute force scaling of current HIS systems, together with significant increases in telecommunications bandwidth [13]. It will also require significant investments in public health. Existing care systems must "be enhanced, rather than simply being augmented by DMATs that drop in after an attack is discovered" [2].

In large-scale, long-duration events, diagnostic information alone will not be sufficient. Also vital is geographic information regarding the location of casualties and incident sites, together with the position of both material and personnel. Ideally, a dynamic, integrated HIS system would be combining Global Positioning System (GPS) and Geographical Information System (GIS) technologies to provide first responders and incident commanders alike with a seamless data source. Likewise, logistical and environmental data would prove invaluable in tracking not only casualties, but also the potential spread of a biological, chemical, or radiological plume beyond the initial incident zone.

From GIS to HIS, effectively integrating and employing medical informatics will involve both hardware and software issues — issues that must be addressed in establishing interoperability and coordination across a broad spectrum of probable disaster situations. These new technologies will also require properly configured "wetware." To establish a net-centric disaster response domain, emergency personnel must first know how to use the systems in question, and be able to develop doctrines that codify best practices. Training, education, and simulation (TES) will each play a critical role in bringing new systems online.

It is axiomatic that highly trained personnel "are an essential element in delivering effective emergency medical care" [14]. Less obvious is the high degree of variation in training regimes, even within highly structured and closely regulated professions. In the case of clinical surgical education, for example, quality is often "quite unpredictable and depends mainly on the instructor and the particular cases to which the surgeon is exposed during his or her training" [15]. Similar patterns exist in other fields. Prior to September 11, the National Standard Curricula for Emergency Medical Technicians (EMTs) maintained by the U.S. Department of Transportation lacked detailed discussion of the resources, strategies, and techniques necessary in a CBRNE attack. Even in the wake of recent reforms, the complexity of the current training programs, together with the absence of a central clearinghouse for best practices, provides few reliable mechanisms for identifying, updating, and communicating response procedures [7]. Despite widespread recognition, federal initiatives to correct this oversight remain illusive.

The state of civilian emergency training stands in stark contrast with innovative programs in the military sphere. By 2007, Army medics training under the recently created "Healthcare occupational specialty will be certified at a civilian emergency medical technician level . . . and have the ability to treat chemical, biological and nuclear exposed casualties" [7]. Army Reserve and National Guard troops must meet the same requirements by 2009. While questions remain as to whether these reforms will promote the acquisition of true core competency, they could substantially increase the number of qualified EMTs available in both the civilian and military emergency response systems. This is a critical first step in mounting an instantaneous, overwhelming disaster response.

45.5 Advanced Technologies

Against this backdrop, the object in any first responder training program "must be to provide a core set of skills that should be useful to the broad set of people who may become involved in responding to a terrorist incident..." [7]. The potential cohort is as broad as it is diverse. First responders may be firefighters, police officers, EMTs and, at least in some instances, even military personnel. Each profession brings its own preconceptions and procedures to an incident site. Absent agreed frameworks for cooperation, commanders could find themselves managing those functional and jurisdictional differences in addition to the disaster itself.

There are three primary challenges in preparing first responders for Homeland Security missions. The first is establishing a uniform training regimen for personnel that may respond to terrorist strikes. The second is integrating medical informatics into training and response, so that each element in the disaster response system possesses the situational awareness necessary to contain events, treat victims, and minimize unnecessary casualties among emergency response personnel. The third challenge is training for interoperability, using the U.S. military's proven doctrine of "train as you fight, fight as you train."

TES technologies can play a central role in meeting each of these challenges. In recent years, both Fortune 500 Companies and the U.S. Department of Defense adopted Computer-Based Training (CBT), which now provides the most cost-effective method for standardizing the acquisition of basic cognitive knowledge. Trainees can develop more advanced skills through interactive videoconferencing and simulations, which reduce the time necessary for hands-on training and improve the knowledge they bring to drills in the field. By using standardized, computer-based curricula, small training cadres from the federal government could supplement local and regional programs whenever necessary (see Figure 45.6).

Simulation technologies could also play a central role. Just as war games are invaluable in military planning and training, simulated crisis scenarios will likely prove instrumental in teaching first responders to cope with a broad spectrum of disaster situations. In addition to providing cost-effective technologies for regular drills, Virtual Reality (VR) and Augmented Reality (AR) trainers would enable personnel from various professional and jurisdictional backgrounds to simulate different operational roles. Frontline firefighters or police officers might play incident commanders, while state and federal decision makers could be tasked with first responder duties. Likewise, fire, police, and medical personnel might swap duties, thus providing valuable opportunities for cross training while elevating each individual's understanding of the manner in which the various elements of the disaster management system operate.

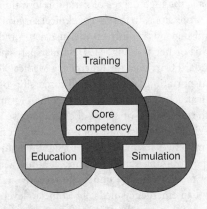

FIGURE 45.6   Training, Education and Simulation (TES).

Finally, these same technologies may also improve the use of medical informatics in crisis situations. The very hardware and software used for instruction purposes could carry real-time information regarding the condition, location, and status of victims in multiple casualty event. Combined with GPS and GIS technology, VR programs might link physicians in remote hospitals with first responders at the incident site — a particularly valuable interface in BW attacks and other CBRNE scenarios requiring swift treatment and effective containment [8].

Foremost among the beneficiaries of TES technologies would be large urban areas where daily operation tempos may limit the time available for continuing education. Rural and geographically isolated areas would also benefit, particularly from the dissemination of CBT software, which might be mailed to local fire and police stations on compact disks [16]. TES holds great promise at the state and federal level as well, particularly in intergovernmental planning and operations. Combined with remote communications platforms, databases, and sensor platforms, the same systems used to train and drill first responders could be employed within and among the various government agencies supporting personnel at the incident site. Broad dissemination of these C^2 nodes would dramatically enhance the flow and coordination of information in a multi-site, multi-event terrorist attack [8].

45.6 Conclusions

The objects of simulation-based training, drilling, and war-gaming are twofold. First, they will improve the "jointness" of disaster response and consequence management. Second, they will enhance the breadth and depth of existing capabilities, allowing local emergency personnel to respond in a much wider spectrum of potential crises.

As the threat of global terrorism grows, so does the need for a corps of fire, police, and EMTs trained to take the initiative in chaotic, dynamic events. The ideal first responder must be well rounded, an expert in his or her field, prepared for an eventuality and capable, when necessary, of working alone. These characteristics may be innate, but can also be learned. The human dimension is essential. Enabling local decision making is not only desirable, but a necessary first step in creating a net-centric crisis response paradigm in which other disaster information flows horizontally among all components of the Homeland Security architecture.

A centralized, federally controlled emergency management system is the ideal model. Instead, the optimal solution is to establish an operation milieu in which all elements of the Homeland Security architecture can most effectively employ their assets, information, and personnel. Establishing such a system demands more than just time and money. It will also require an institutional and technological transformation every bit as powerful and profound as the Revolution in Military Affairs (RMA) that transformed the U.S. military in the 1990s. That paradigm shift could take years — years that policy makers and the public may not have. While deeper reflection and greater imagination will be necessary to secure the homeland, implementing TES technologies and improving the use of medical informatics represent important near-term solutions.

References

[1] "The 9/11 Commission Report," National Commission on Terrorist Attacks Upon the United States, Washington, DC, July 22, 2004.

[2] J.M. Rosen, E. Grigg, S. McGrath, S. Lillibridge, and C.E. Koop, "Cybercare NDMS: An Improved Strategy for Biodefense Using Information Technologies," in *Integration of Health Telematics into Medical Practice*, M. Nerlich and U. Schaechinger, Eds. Amsterdam: IOS Press, 2003, pp. 95–114.

[3] N.F. Cantor, *In the Wake of the Plague: The Black Death and World It Made*. New York, NY: Free Press, 2001.

[4] J.M. Rosen, C.E. Koop, and E.B. Grigg, "Cybercare: A System for Confronting Bioterrorism," *The Bridge*, 32, 34–50, 2002.

[5] OTA, Proliferation of Weapons of Mass Destruction: Assessing the Risk, Government Printing Office, Washington, DC, 1999.

[6] J.M. Rosen, R. Gougelet, M. Mughal, and R. Hutchinson, "Conference Report of the Medical Disaster Conference," Dartmouth College, Hanover, NH, June 13–15, 2001.

[7] H. Kelly, V. Blackwood, M. Roper, G. Higgins, G. Klein, J. Tyler, D. Fletcher, H. Jenkins, A. Chisolm, and K. Squire, "Training Technology against Terror: Using Advanced Technology to Prepare America's Emergency Medical Personnel and First Responders for a Weapons of Mass Destruction Attack," Federation of American Scientists, Washington, DC, September 9, 2002.

[8] J.M. Rosen, E.B. Grigg, M.F. McKnight, C.E. Koop, S. Lillibridge, B.L. Kindberg, L. Hettinger, and R. Hutchinson, "Transforming Medicine for Biodefense and Healthcare Delivery: Developing a Dual-Use Doctrine that Utilizes Information Superiority and Network-Based Organization," *IEEE Eng. Med. Biol.*, 23, 89–101, 2004.

[9] "Homeland Security Oversight," in *The Washington Post*. Washington, DC, 2004, p. A18.

[10] M.F. Murphy, "Emergency Medical Services in Disaster," pp. 90–103.

[11] D. Langley, S. Michael Lockhardt, J. Michael Lockhardt, J.M. Rosen, and M.F. McKnight, "ICE 884: Response to Disaster," Durham, NH: Team Hill Studios, 2004.

[12] D.S. Alberts, J.J. Gartska, R.E. Hayes, and D.A. Signori, "Understanding Information Age Warfare," *CCRO Publication Series*, 2001.

[13] The authors wish to thank Jon Bowersox for this insight.

[14] S.L. Delp, P. Loan, C. Basdogan, and J.M. Rosen, "Surgical Simulation: An Emerging Technology for Training in Emergency Medicine," *Presence*, 6, 147–159, 1997.

[15] T. Lange, D.J. Indelicato, and J.M. Rosen, "Virtual Reality in Surgical Training," *Surg. Techn. Outcomes*, 9, 61–79, 2000.

[16] The prototype Virtual Terrorism Response Academy (VTRA) developed by Joseph Henderson and the Interactive Medical Laboratory at Dartmouth College operates on this principle.

V

Biomedical Sensors

Michael R. Neuman
Michigan Technological University

46 Physical Measurements
Michael R. Neuman **46**-1

47 Biopotential Electrodes
Michael R. Neuman **47**-1

48 Electrochemical Sensors
Chung-Chiun Liu **48**-1

49 Optical Sensors
Yitzhak Mendelson **49**-1

50 Bioanalytic Sensors
Richard P. Buck **50**-1

51 Biological Sensors for Diagnostics
Orhan Soykan **51**-1

S ENSORS CONVERT SIGNALS OF ONE type of quantity such as hydrostatic fluid pressure into an equivalent signal of another type of quantity, for example, an electrical signal. Biomedical sensors take signals representing biomedical variables and convert them into what is usually an electrical signal. As such, the biomedical sensor serves as the interface between a biologic and an electronic system and must function in such a way as to not adversely affect either of these systems. In considering biomedical sensors, it is necessary to consider both sides of the interface: the biologic and the electronic, since both biologic and electronic factors play an important role in sensor performance.

TABLE V.1   Classification of
Biomedical Sensors

Physical sensors
   Geometric
   Mechanical
   Thermal
   Hydraulic
   Electric
   Optical
Chemical sensors
   Gas
   Electrochemical
   Photometric
   Other physical and chemical methods
   Bioanalytic

Many different types of sensors can be used in biomedical applications. Table V.1 gives a general classification of these sensors. It is possible to categorize all sensors as being either physical or chemical. In the case of physical sensors, quantities such as geometric, mechanical, thermal, and hydraulic variables are measured. In biomedical applications these can include things such as muscle displacement, blood pressure, core body temperature, blood flow, cerebrospinal fluid pressure, and bone growth. Two types of physical sensors deserve special mention with regard to their biomedical application: sensors of electrical phenomena in the body, usually known as electrodes, play a special role as a result of their diagnostic and therapeutic applications. The most familiar of these are sensors used to obtain the electrocardiogram, an electrical signal produced by the heart. The other type of physical sensor that finds many applications in biology and medicine is the optical sensor. These sensors can use light to collect information, and, in the case of fiber optic sensors, light is the signal transmission medium as well.

The second major classification of sensing devices is chemical sensors. In this case the sensors are concerned with measuring chemical quantities such as identifying the presence of particular chemical compounds, detecting the concentrations of various chemical species, and monitoring chemical activities in the body for diagnostic and therapeutic applications. A wide variety of chemical sensors can be classified in many ways. One such classification scheme is illustrated in Table V.1 and is based upon the methods used to detect the chemical components being measured. Chemical composition can be measured in the gas phase using several techniques, and these methods are especially useful in biomedical measurements associated with the pulmonary system. Electrochemical sensors measure chemical concentrations or, more precisely, activities based on chemical reactions that interact with electrical systems. Photometric chemical sensors are optical devices that detect chemical concentrations based upon changes in light transmission, reflection, or color. The familiar litmus test is an example of an optical change that can be used to measure the acidity or alkalinity of a solution. Other types of physical chemical sensors such as the mass spectrometer use various physical methods to detect and quantify chemicals associated with biologic systems.

Although they are essentially chemical sensors, bioanalytic sensors are often classified as a separate major sensor category. These devices incorporate biologic recognition reactions such as enzyme–substrate, antigen–antibody, or ligand-receptor to identify complex biochemical molecules. The use of biologic reactions gives bioanalytic sensors high sensitivity and specificity in identifying and quantifying biochemical substances.

One can also look at biomedical sensors from the standpoint of their applications. These can be generally divided according to whether a sensor is used for diagnostic or therapeutic purposes in clinical medicine and for data collection in biomedical research. Sensors for clinical studies such as those carried out in the clinical chemistry laboratory must be standardized in such a way that errors that could result in an incorrect diagnosis or inappropriate therapy are kept to an absolute minimum. Thus these sensors must

TABLE V.2 Types of
Sensor-Subject Interfaces

Noncontacting (noninvasive)
Skin surface (contacting)
Indwelling (minimally invasive)
Implantable (invasive)

not only be reliable themselves, but appropriate methods must exist for testing the sensors that are a part of the routine use of the sensors for making biomedical measurements.

One can also look at biomedical sensors from the standpoint of how they are applied to the patient or research subject. Table V.2 shows the range of general approaches to attaching biomedical sensors. At the top of the list we have the method that involves the least interaction with the biologic object being studied; the bottom of the list includes sensors that interact to the greatest extent. Clearly if a measurement can be made equally well by a sensor that does not contact the subject being measured or by one that must be surgically implanted, the former is by far the most desirable. However, a sensor that is used to provide information to help control a device already surgically placed in the body to replace or assist a failing organ should be implanted, since this is the best way to communicate with the internal device.

You will notice in reading this section that the majority of biomedical sensors are essentially the same as sensors used in other applications. The unique part about biomedical sensors is their application. There are, however, special problems that are encountered by biomedical sensors that are unique to them. These problems relate to the interface between the sensor and the biologic system being measured. The presence of foreign materials, especially implanted materials, can affect the biologic environment in which they are located. Many biologic systems are designed to deal with foreign materials by making a major effort to eliminate them. The rejection reaction that is often discussed with regard to implanted materials or transplanted tissues is an example of this. Thus, in considering biomedical sensors, one must worry about this rejection phenomenon and how it will affect the performance of the sensor. If the rejection phenomenon changes the local biology or chemistry around the sensor, this can result in the sensor measuring phenomena associated with the reaction that it has produced as opposed to phenomena characteristic of the biologic system being studied.

Biologic systems can also affect sensor performance. This is especially true for indwelling and implanted sensors. Biologic tissue represents a hostile environment which can degrade sensor structure and performance. In addition to many corrosive ions, body fluids contain enzymes that break down complex molecules as a part of the body's effort to rid itself of foreign and toxic materials. These can attack the materials that make up the sensor and its package, causing the sensor to lose calibration or fail.

Sensor packaging is an especially important problem. The package must not only protect the sensor from the corrosive environment of the body, but it must allow that portion of the sensor that performs the actual measurement to communicate with the biologic system. Furthermore, because it is frequently desirable to have sensors be as small as possible, especially those that are implanted and indwelling, it is important that the packaging function be carried out without significantly increasing the size of the sensor structure. There are many measurements that can now be made on biological specimens ranging from molecules through cells and larger structures. These measurements involve specialized sensors and instrumentation systems that are necessary for these types of measurements and their ultimate application in diagnostic medicine. This section concludes with a chapter devoted to describing some of the more common of these measurements. Although there have been many improvements in sensor packaging, this remains a major problem in biomedical sensor research. High-quality packaging materials that do not elicit major foreign body responses from the biologic system are still being sought.

Another problem that is associated with implanted sensors is that once they are implanted, access to them is very limited. This requires that these sensors be highly reliable so that there is no need to repair or replace them. It is also important that these sensors be highly stable, since in most applications it is not possible to calibrate the sensor *in vivo*. Thus, sensors must maintain their calibration once they are implanted, and for applications such as organ replacement, this can represent a potentially long time, the remainder of the patient's life.

In the following sections we will look at some of the sensors described above in more detail. We will consider physical sensors with special sections on biopotential electrodes and optical sensors. We will also look at chemical sensors, including bioanalytic sensing systems.[1] Although it is not possible to cover the field in extensive detail in a handbook such as this, it is hoped that these sections can serve as an introduction to this important aspect of biomedical engineering and instrumentation.

---

[1] There are many measurements that can now be made on biological specimens ranging from molecules through cells and larger structures. These measurements involve specialized sensors and instrumentation systems that are necessary for these types of measurements and their ultimate application in diagnostic medicine. This section concludes with a chapter devoted to describing some of the more common of these measurements.

46

Physical
Measurements

46.1 Description of Sensors 46-2
    Linear and Angular Displacement Sensors • Inductance
    Sensors • Capacitive Sensors • Sonic and Ultrasonic
    Sensors • Velocity Measurement • Accelerometers • Force
    • Measurement of Fluid Dynamic Variables • Thermistors
    • Thermocouples
46.2 Biomedical Applications of Physical Sensors 46-16
References 46-17
Further Information 46-18

Michael R. Neuman
Michigan Technological University

Physical variables associated with biomedical systems are measured by a group of sensors known as physical sensors. Although many specific physical variables can be measured in biomedical systems, these can be categorized into a simple list as shown in Table 46.1. Sensors for these variables, whether they are measuring biomedical systems or other systems, are essentially the same. Thus, sensors of linear displacement can frequently be used equally well for measuring the displacement of the heart muscle during the cardiac cycle or the movement of a robot arm. There is, however, one notable exception regarding the similarity of these sensors: the packaging of the sensor and attachment to the system being measured. Although physical sensors used in nonbiomedical applications need to be packaged so as to be protected from their environment, few of these sensors have to deal with the harsh environment of biologic tissue, especially with the mechanisms inherent in this tissue for trying to eliminate the sensor as a foreign body. Another notable exception to this similarity of sensors for measuring physical quantities in biologic and nonbiologic systems are the sensors used for fluidic measurements such as pressure and flow. Special needs for these measurements in biologic systems have resulted in special sensors and instrumentation systems for these measurements that can be quite different from systems for measuring pressure and flow in nonbiologic environments.

In this chapter, we will attempt to review various examples of sensors used for physical measurement in biologic systems. Although it would be beyond the scope of this chapter to cover all these in detail, the principal sensors applied for biologic measurements will be described. Each section will include a brief description of the principle of operation of the sensor and the underlying physical principles, examples of some of the more common forms of these sensors for application in biologic systems, methods of signal processing for these sensors where appropriate, and important considerations for when the sensor is applied.

TABLE 46.1 Physical Variables and Sensors

Physical quantity	Sensor	Variable sensed
Geometric	Strain gauge	Strain
	LVDT	Displacement
	Ultrasonic transit time	Displacement
Kinematic	Velocimeter	Velocity
	Accelerometer	Acceleration
Force–Torque	Load cell	Applied force or torque
Fluidic	Pressure transducer	Pressure
	Flow meter	Flow
Thermal	Thermometer	Temperature
	Thermal flux sensor	Heat flux

TABLE 46.2 Comparison of Displacement Sensors

Sensor	Electrical variable	Measurement circuit	Sensitivity	Precision	Range
Variable resistor	Resistance	Voltage divider, ohmmeter, bridge, current source	High	Moderate	Large
Foil strain gauge	Resistance	Bridge	Low	Moderate	Small
Liquid metal strain gauge	Resistance	Ohmmeter, bridge	Moderate	Moderate	Large
Silicon strain gauge	Resistance	Bridge	High	Moderate	Small
Mutual inductance coils	Inductance	Impedance bridge, inductance meter	Moderate to high	Moderate to low	Moderate to large
Variable reluctance	Inductance	Impedance bridge, inductance meter	High	Moderate	Large
LVDT	Inductance	Voltmeter	High	High	High
Parallel plate capacitor	Capacitance	Impedance bridge, capacitance meter	Moderate to high	Moderate	Moderate to large
Sonic/ultrasonic	Time	Timer circuit	High	High	Large

46.1 Description of Sensors

46.1.1 Linear and Angular Displacement Sensors

A comparison of various characteristics of displacement sensors described in detail below is outlined in Table 46.2.

46.1.1.1 Variable Resistance Sensor

One of the simplest sensors for measuring displacement is a variable resistor similar to the volume control on an audio electronic device [1]. The resistance between two terminals on this device is related to the linear or angular displacement of a sliding tap along a resistance element. Precision devices are available that have a reproducible, linear relationship between resistance and displacement. These devices can be connected in circuits that measure resistance such as an ohmmeter or bridge, or they can be used as a part of a circuit that provides a voltage that is proportional to the displacement. Such circuits include the voltage divider (as illustrated in Figure 46.1a) or driving a known constant current through the resistance and measuring the resulting voltage across it. This sensor is simple and inexpensive and can be used for measuring relatively large displacements.

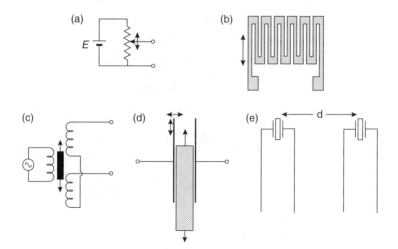

FIGURE 46.1 Examples of displacement sensors: (a) variable resistance sensor, (b) foil strain gauge, (c) linear variable differential transformer (LVDT), (d) parallel plate capacitive sensor, and (e) ultrasonic transit time displacement sensor.

There are some things to keep in mind when applying this type of displacement sensor. Since the circuit is a simple voltage divider, it is important that the electrical load on the output is very small such that there is very little current in the slider circuit. Significant current will introduce nonlinearities in the voltage vs. displacements characteristics. The sensor requires mechanical attachment to the structure being displaced and to some reference point, this can present difficulties in some biologic situations. Furthermore because the slider must move along the resistance element, this can introduce some friction that may alter the displacement.

46.1.1.2 Strain Gauge

Another displacement sensor based on an electrical resistance change is the strain gauge [2]. If a long narrow electrical conductor such as a piece of metal foil or a fine gauge wire is stretched within its elastic limit, it will increase in length and decrease in cross-sectional area. Because the electric resistance between both ends of this foil or wire can be given by

$$R = \rho \frac{l}{A}$$
(46.1)

where ρ is the electrical resistivity of the foil or wire material, l is its length, and A is its cross-sectional area, this stretching will result in an increase in resistance. The change in length can only be very small for the foil or wire to remain within its elastic limit, so the change in electric resistance will also be small. The relative sensitivity of this device is given by its gauge factor, γ, which is defined as

$$\gamma = \frac{\Delta R/R}{\Delta l/l}$$
(46.2)

where ΔR is the change in resistance when the structure is stretched by an amount Δl. Foil strain gauges are the most frequently applied and consist of a structure such as shown in Figure 46.1b. A piece of metal foil that is bonded to an insulating polymeric film such as polyimide that has a much greater compliance than the foil itself is chemically etched into the pattern shown in Figure 46.1b. When a strain is applied in the sensitive direction, the long direction of the individual elements of the strain gauge, the length of the gauge will be slightly increased, and this will result in an increase in the electrical resistance seen between the terminals. Since the displacement or strain that this structure can measure is quite small for it to remain within its elastic limit, it can only be used to measure small displacements such as occur as

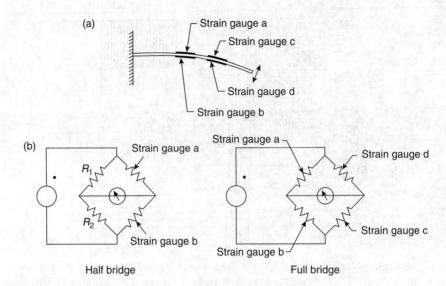

FIGURE 46.2   Strain gauges on a cantilever structure to provide temperature compensation: (a) cross-sectional view of the cantilever and (b) placement of the strain gauges in a half bridge or full bridge for temperature compensation and enhanced sensitivity.

loads are applied to structural beams. If one wants to increase the range of a foil strain gauge, one has to attach it to some sort of a mechanical impedance converter such as a cantilever beam. If the strain gauge is attached to one surface of the beam as shown in Figure 46.2a, a fairly large displacement at the unsupported end of the beam can be translated to a relatively small displacement on the beam's surface. It is possible for this structure to be used to measure larger displacements at the cantilever beam tip using a strain gauge bonded on the beam surface.

Because the electric resistance changes for a strain gauge are quite small, the measurement of this resistance change can be challenging. Generally, Wheatstone bridge circuits are used. It is important to note, however, that changes in temperature can also result in electric resistance changes that are of the same order of magnitude or even larger than the electric resistance changes due to the strain. Thus, it is important to temperature-compensate strain gauges in most applications. A simple method of temperature compensation is to use a double or quadruple strain gauge and a bridge circuit for measuring the resistance change. This is illustrated in Figure 46.2. If one can use the strain gauge in an application such as the cantilever beam application described above, one can place one or two of the strain gauge structures on the concave side of the beam and the other one or two on the convex side of the beam. Thus, as the beam deflects, the strain gauge on the convex side will experience tension, and that on the concave side will experience compression. By putting these gauges in adjacent arms of the Wheatstone bridge, their effects can double the sensitivity of the circuit in the case of the double strain gauge and quadruple it in the case where the entire bridge is made up of strain gauges on a cantilever. In addition to increased sensitivity, the bridge circuit minimizes temperatures effects on the strain measurements. Placing strain gauges that are on opposite sides of the beam in adjacent arms of the bridge results in a change in bridge output voltage when the beam is deflected. This occurs because the strain gauges on one side of the beam will increase in resistance while those on the other side will decrease in resistance when the beam is deflected. On the other hand, when the temperature of the beam changes, all of the strain gauges will have the same change in resistance, and this change will not affect the bridge output voltage.

In some applications it is not possible to place strain gauges so that one gauge is undergoing tension while the other is undergoing compression. In this case, the second strain gauge used for temperature compensation can be oriented such that its sensitive axis is in a direction where strain is minimal. Thus, it is still possible to have the temperature compensation by having two identical strain gauges at the same temperature in adjacent arms of the bridge circuit, but the sensitivity improvement described in the previous paragraph is not seen.

Another constraint imposed by temperature is that the material to which the strain gauge is attached and the strain gauge both have temperature coefficients of expansion. Thus, even if a gauge is attached to a structure under conditions of no strain, if the temperature is changed, the strain gauge could experience some strain due to the different expansion that it will have compared to the structure to which it is attached. To avoid this problem, strain gauges have been developed that have identical temperature coefficients of expansion to various common materials. In selecting a strain gauge, one should choose a device with thermal expansion characteristics as close as possible to those of the object upon which the strain is to be measured.

A more compliant structure that has found applications in biomedical instrumentation is the liquid metal strain gauge [3]. Instead of using a solid electric conductor such as the wire or metal foil, mercury confined to a compliant, thin wall, narrow bore elastomeric tube is used. The compliance of this strain gauge is determined by the elastic properties of the tube. Since only the elastic limit of the tube is of concern, this sensor can be used to detect much larger displacements than conventional strain gauges. Its sensitivity is roughly the same as a foil or wire strain gauge, but it is not as reliable. The mercury can easily become oxidized or small air gaps can occur in the mercury column. These effects make the sensor's characteristics noisy and sometimes results in complete failure.

Another variation on the strain gauge is the semiconductor strain gauge. These devices are frequently made out of pieces of silicon with strain gauge patterns formed using semiconductor microelectronic technology. The principal advantage of these devices is that their gauge factors can be more than 50 times greater than that of the solid and liquid metal devices. They are available commercially, but they are a bit more difficult to handle and attach to structures being measured due to their small size and brittleness.

46.1.2 Inductance Sensors

46.1.2.1 Mutual Inductance

The mutual inductance between two coils is related to many geometric factors, one of which is the separation of the coils. Thus, one can create a very simple displacement sensor by having two coils that are coaxial but with different separation. By driving one coil with an ac signal and measuring the voltage signal induced in the second coil, this voltage will be related to how far apart the coils are from one another. When the coils are close together, the mutual inductance will be relatively high, and so a higher voltage will be induced in the second coil; when the coils are more widely separated, the mutual inductance will be lower as will the induced voltage. The relationship between voltage and separation will be determined by the specific geometry of the coils and in general will not be a linear relationship with separation unless the change of displacement is relatively small. Nevertheless, this is a simple method of measuring separation that works reasonably well provided the coils remain coaxial. If there is movement of the coils transverse to their axes, it is difficult to separate the effects of transverse displacement from those of displacement along the axis.

46.1.2.2 Variable Reluctance

A variation on this sensor is the variable reluctance sensor wherein a single coil or two coils remain fixed on a form which allows a high reluctance material such as piece of iron to move into or out of the center of the coil or coils along their axis. Since the position of this core material determines the number of flux linkages through the coil or coils, this can affect the self-inductance or mutual inductance of the coils. In the case of the mutual inductance, this can be measured using the technique described in the previous paragraph, whereas self-inductance changes can be measured using various instrumentation circuits used for measuring inductance. This method is also a simple method for measuring displacements, but the characteristics are generally nonlinear, and the sensor often has only moderate precision.

46.1.2.3 Linear Variable Differential Transformer

By far the most frequently applied displacement transducer based upon inductance is the linear variable differential transformer (LVDT) [4]. This device is illustrated in Figure 46.1c and is essentially a three-coil variable reluctance transducer. The two secondary coils are situated symmetrically about and coaxial with the primary coil and connected such that the induced voltages in each secondary oppose each other. When a high-reluctance core is located in the center of the structure equidistant from each secondary coil, the voltage induced in each secondary will be the same. Since these voltages oppose one another, the output voltage from the device will be zero. As the core is moved closer to one or the other secondary coils, the voltages in each coil will no longer be equal, and there will be an output voltage proportional to the displacement of the core from the central, zero-voltage position. Because of the symmetry of the structure, this voltage is linearly related to the core displacement. When the core passes through the central, zero point, the phase of the output voltage from the sensor changes by 180°. Thus, by measuring the phase angle as well as the voltage, one can determine the position of the core. The circuit associated with the LVDT not only measures the voltage but often measures the phase angle as well.

Linear variable differential transformers are available commercially in many sizes and shapes. Depending on the configuration of the coils, they can measure displacements ranging from tens of micrometers through several centimeters.

46.1.3 Capacitive Sensors

Displacement sensors can be based upon measurements of capacitance as well as inductance. The fundamental principle of operation is the capacitance of a parallel plate capacitor as given by

$$C = e\frac{A}{d} \tag{46.3}$$

where e is the dielectric constant of the medium between the plates, d is the separation between the plates, and A is the cross-sectional area of the plates. Each of the quantities in Equation 46.3 can be varied to form a displacement transducer. By moving one of the plates with respect to the other, Equation 46.3 shows us that the capacitance will vary inversely with respect to the plate separation. This will give a hyperbolic capacitance–displacement characteristic. However, if the plate separation is maintained at a constant value and the plates are displaced laterally with respect to one another so that the area of overlap changes, this can produce a capacitance–displacement characteristic that can be linear, depending on the shape of the actual plates.

The third way that a variable capacitance transducer can measure displacement is by having a fixed parallel plate capacitor with a slab of dielectric material having a dielectric constant different from that of air that can slide between the plates (Figure 46.1d). The effective dielectric constant for the capacitor will depend on how much of the slab is between the plates and how much of the region between the plates is occupied only by air. This, also, can yield a transducer with linear characteristics.

The electronic circuitry used with variable capacitance transducers, is essentially the same as any other circuitry used to measure capacitance. As with the inductance transducers, this circuit can take the form of a bridge circuit or specific circuits that measure capacitive reactance.

46.1.4 Sonic and Ultrasonic Sensors

If the velocity of sound in a medium is constant, the time it takes a short burst of that sound energy to propagate from a source to a receiver will be proportional to the displacement between the two transducers. This is given by

$$d = cT \tag{46.4}$$

where c is the velocity of sound in the medium, T is the transit time, and d is the displacement. A simple system for making such a measurement is shown in Figure 46.1e [5]. A brief sonic or ultrasonic pulse is generated at the transmitting transducer and propagates through the medium. It is detected by the receiving transducer at time T after the burst was initiated. The displacement can then be determined by applying Equation 46.4.

In practice, this method is best used with ultrasound, since the wavelength is shorter, and the device will neither produce annoying sounds nor respond to extraneous sounds in the environment. Small piezoelectric transducers to generate and receive ultrasonic pulses are readily available. The electronic circuit used with this instrument carries out three functions (1) generation of the sonic or ultrasonic burst, (2) detection of the received burst, and (3) measurement of the time of propagation of the ultrasound. An advantage of this system is that the two transducers are coupled to one another only sonically. There is no physical connection as was the case for the other sensors described in this section.

46.1.5 Velocity Measurement

Velocity is the time derivative of displacement, and so all the displacement transducers mentioned above can be used to measure velocity if their signals are processed by passing them through a differentiator circuit. There are, however, two additional methods that can be applied to measure velocity directly.

46.1.5.1 Magnetic Induction

If a magnetic field that passes through a conducting coil varies with time, a voltage is induced in that coil that is proportional to the time-varying magnetic field. This relationship is given by

$$v = N \frac{d\phi}{dt} \tag{46.5}$$

where v is the voltage induced in the coil, N is the number of turns in the coil, and ϕ is the total magnetic flux passing through the coil (the product of the flux density and area within the coil). Thus a simple way to apply this principle is to attach a small permanent magnet to an object whose velocity is to be determined, and attach a coil to a nearby structure that will serve as the reference against which the velocity is to be measured. A voltage will be induced in the coil whenever the structure containing the permanent magnet moves, and this voltage will be related to the velocity of that movement. The exact relationship will be determined by the field distribution for the particular magnet and the orientation of the magnet with respect to the coil.

46.1.5.2 Doppler Ultrasound

When the receiver of a signal in the form of a wave such as electromagnetic radiation or sound is moving at a nonzero velocity with respect to the emitter of that wave, the frequency of the wave perceived by the receiver will be different than the frequency of the transmitter. This frequency difference, known as the Doppler shift, is determined by the relative velocity of the receiver with respect to the emitter and is given by

$$f_d = \frac{f_o u}{c} \tag{46.6}$$

where f_d is the Doppler frequency shift, f_o is the frequency of the transmitted wave, u is the relative velocity between the transmitter and receiver, and c is the velocity of sound in the medium. This principle can be applied in biomedical applications as a Doppler velocimeter. A piezoelectric transducer can be used as the ultrasound source with a similar transducer as the receiver. When there is no relative movement between the two transducers, the frequency of the signal at the receiver will be the same as that at the emitter, but when there is relative motion, the frequency at the receiver will be shifted according to Equation 46.6.

The ultrasonic velocimeter can be applied in the same way that the ultrasonic displacement sensor is used. In this case the electronic circuit produces a continuous ultrasonic wave and, instead of detecting

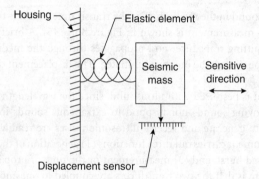

FIGURE 46.3   Fundamental structure of an accelerometer.

the transit time of the signal, now detects the frequency difference between the transmitted and received signals. This frequency difference can then be converted into a signal proportional to the relative velocity between the two transducers.

46.1.6 Accelerometers

Acceleration is the time derivative of velocity and the second derivative with respect to time of displacement. Thus, sensors of displacement and velocity can be used to determine acceleration when their signals are appropriately processed through differentiator circuits. In addition, there are direct sensors of acceleration based upon Newton's second law and Hooke's law. The fundamental structure of an accelerometer is shown in Figure 46.3. A known seismic mass is attached to the housing by an elastic element. As the structure is accelerated in the sensitive direction of the elastic element, a force is applied to that element according to Newton's second law. This force causes the elastic element to be distorted according to Hooke's law, which results in a displacement of the mass with respect to the accelerometer housing. This displacement is measured by a displacement sensor. The relationship between the displacement and the acceleration is found by combining Newton's second law and Hooke's law

$$a = \frac{k}{m}x \tag{46.7}$$

where x is the measured displacement, m is the known mass, k is the spring constant of the elastic element, and a is the acceleration. Any of the displacement sensors described above can be used in an accelerometer. The most frequently used displacement sensors are strain gauges or the LVDT. One type of accelerometer uses a piezoelectric sensor as both the displacement sensor and the elastic element. A piezoelectric sensor generates an electric signal that is related to the dynamic change in shape of the piezoelectric material as a force is applied. Thus, piezoelectric materials can only directly measure time varying forces. A piezoelectric accelerometer is, therefore, better for measuring changes in acceleration than for measuring constant accelerations. A principal advantage of piezoelectric accelerometers is that they can be made very small, which is useful in many biomedical applications. Very small and relatively inexpensive accelerometers are now made on a single silicon chip using microelectromechanical systems (MEMS) technology. An example is shown in Figure 46.4. A small piece of silicon is etched to give the paddle-like structure that is attached to the silicon frame at one end and is free to move with respect to the frame by flexing the "handle" of the paddle. This movement results in strains being induced on the surfaces of the "handle," and a strain gauge integrated into this handle structures detects the strain and converts it to an electrical signal. The paddle, itself serves as the seismic mass, and the "handle" is the elastic element.

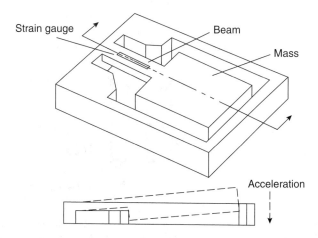

FIGURE 46.4 Example of a silicon chip accelerometer fabricated using MEMS technology. The lower figure shows the upward deflection of the seismic mass with a downward acceleration.

46.1.7 Force

Force is measured by converting the force to a displacement and measuring the displacement with a displacement sensor. The conversion takes place as a result of the elastic properties of a material. Applying a force to the material distorts the material's shape, and this distortion can be measured by a displacement sensor. For example, the cantilever structure shown in Figure 46.2a could be a force sensor. Applying a vertical force at the tip of the beam will cause the beam to deflect according to its elastic properties. This deflection can be detected using a displacement sensor such as a strain gauge as described previously.

A common form of force sensor is the load cell. This consists of a block of material with known elastic properties that has strain gauges attached to it. Applying a force to the load cell stresses the material, resulting in a strain that can be measured by the strain gauge. Applying Hooke's law, one finds that the strain is proportional to the applied force. The strain gauges on a load cell are usually in a half-bridge or full-bridge configuration to minimize the temperature sensitivity of the device. Load cells come in various sizes and configurations, and they can measure a wide range of forces.

46.1.8 Measurement of Fluid Dynamic Variables

The measurement of the fluid pressure and flow in both liquids and gases is important in many biomedical applications. These two variables, however, often are the most difficult variables to measure in biologic applications because of interactions with the biologic system and stability problems. Some of the most frequently applied sensors for these measurements are described in the following paragraphs.

46.1.8.1 Pressure Measurement

Sensors of pressure for biomedical measurements such as blood pressure [6] consist of a structure such as shown in Figure 46.5. In this case a fluid coupled to the fluid to be measured is housed in a chamber with a flexible diaphragm making up a portion of the wall, with the other side of the diaphragm at atmospheric pressure. When a pressure exists across the diaphragm, it will cause the diaphragm to deflect. This deflection is then measured by a displacement sensor. In the example in Figure 46.5, the displacement sensor consists of four fine-gauge wires drawn between a structure attached to the diaphragm and the housing of the pressure sensor so that these wires serve as strain gauges. When pressure causes the diaphragm to deflect, two of the fine-wire strain gauges will be extended by a small amount, and the other two will contract by the same amount. By connecting these wires into a bridge circuit, a voltage proportional to the deflection of the diaphragm and hence the pressure can be obtained.

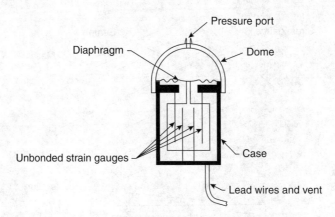

FIGURE 46.5 Structure of an unbonded strain gauge pressure sensor. (Reproduced from Neuman M.R. 1993. In R.C. Dorf (Ed.), *The Electrical Engineering Handbook,* Boca Raton, FL, CRC Press. With permission).

Semiconductor technology has been applied to the design of pressure transducers such that the entire structure can be fabricated from silicon. A portion of a silicon chip can be formed into a diaphragm and semiconductor strain gauges incorporated directly into that diaphragm to produce a small, inexpensive, and sensitive pressure sensor. Such sensors can be used as disposable, single-use devices for measuring blood pressure without the need for additional sterilization before being used on the next patient. This minimizes the risk of transmitting blood-borne infections in the cases where the transducer is coupled directly to the patient's blood for direct blood pressure measurement.

In using this type of sensor to measure blood pressure, it is necessary to couple the chamber containing the diaphragm to the blood or other fluids being measured. This is usually done using a small, flexible plastic tube known as a catheter, that can have one end placed in an artery of the subject while the other is connected to the pressure sensor. This catheter is filled with a physiologic saline solution so that the arterial blood pressure is coupled to the sensor diaphragm. This external blood-pressure-measurement method is used quite frequently in the clinic and research laboratory, but it has the limitation that the properties of the fluid in the catheter and the catheter itself can affect the measurement. For example, both ends of the catheter must be at the same vertical level to avoid a pressure offset due to hydrostatic effects. Also, the compliance of the tube will affect the frequency response of the pressure measurement. Air bubbles in the catheter or obstructions due to clotted blood or other materials can introduce distortion of the waveform due to resonance and damping. These problems can be minimized by utilizing a miniature semiconductor pressure transducer that is located at the tip of a catheter and can be placed in the blood vessel rather than being positioned external to the body. Such internal pressure sensors are available commercially and have the advantages of a much broader frequency response, no hydrostatic pressure error, and generally clearer signals than the external system.

Although it is possible to measure blood pressure using the techniques described above, this remains one of the major problems in biomedical sensor technology. Long-term stability of pressure transducers is not very good. This is especially true for pressure measurements of venous blood, cerebrospinal fluid, or fluids in the gastrointestinal tract, where pressures are usually relatively low. Long-term changes in baseline pressure for most pressure sensors require that they be frequently adjusted to be certain of zero pressure. Although this can be done relatively easily when the pressure transducer is located external to the body, this can be a major problem for indwelling or implanted pressure transducers. Thus, these transducers must be extremely stable and have low baseline drift to be useful in long-term applications. The packaging of the pressure transducer is also a problem that needs to be addressed, especially when the transducer is in contact with blood for long periods. Not only must the package be biocompatible, but it also must allow the appropriate pressure to be transmitted from the biologic fluid to the diaphragm. Thus, a material that is mechanically stable under corrosive and aqueous environments in the body is needed.

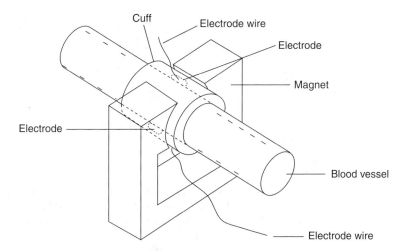

FIGURE 46.6 Fundamental structure of an electromagnetic flowmeter. (Reproduced from Neuman M.R. 1986. In J.D. Bronzino (Ed.), *Biomedical Engineering and Instrumentation: Basic Concepts and Applications,* Boston, PWS Publishers. With permission.)

46.1.8.2 Measurement of Flow

The measurement of true volummetric flow in the body represents one of the most difficult problems in biomedical sensing [7]. The sensors that have been developed measure velocity rather than volume flow, and they can only be used to measure flow if the velocity is measured for a tube of known cross-section. Thus, most flow sensors constrain the vessel to have a specific cross-sectional area.

The most frequently used flow sensor in biomedical systems is the electromagnetic flow meter illustrated in Figure 46.6. This device consists of a means of generating a magnetic field transverse to the flow vector in a vessel. A pair of very small biopotential electrodes are attached to the wall of the vessel such that the vessel diameter between them is at right angles to the direction of the magnetic field. As the blood flows in the structure, ions in the blood deflect in the direction of one or the other electrodes due to the magnetic field, and this results in a voltage across the electrodes that is given by

$$v = Blu \tag{46.8}$$

where B is the magnetic field, l is the distance between the electrodes, and u is the average instantaneous velocity of the fluid across the vessel. If the sensor constrains the blood vessel to have a specific diameter, then its cross-sectional area will be known, and multiplying this area by the velocity will give the volume flow.

Although d.c. flow sensors have been developed and are available commercially, the most desirable method is to use ac excitation of the magnetic field so that offset potential effects from the biopotential electrodes do not generate errors in this measurement.

Small ultrasonic transducers can also be attached to a blood vessel to measure flow as illustrated in Figure 46.7. In this case the transducers are oriented such that one transmits a continuous ultrasound signal that illuminates the blood. Cells within the blood diffusely reflect this signal in the direction of the second sensor so that the received signal undergoes a Doppler shift in frequency that is proportional to the velocity of the blood. By measuring the frequency shift and knowing the cross-sectional area of the vessel, it is possible to determine the flow.

Another method of measuring flow that has had biomedical application is the measurement of cooling of a heated object by convection. The object is usually a thermistor (see Section 46.1.8.3) placed either in a blood vessel or in tissue, and the thermistor serves as both the heating element and the temperature sensor. In one mode of operation, the amount of power required to maintain the thermistor at a temperature

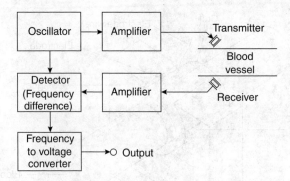

FIGURE 46.7 Structure of an ultrasonic Doppler flowmeter with the major blocks of the electronic signal processing system. The oscillator generates a signal that, after amplification, drives the transmitting transducer. The oscillator frequency is usually in the range of 1 to 10 MHz. The reflected ultrasound from the blood is sensed by the receiving transducer and amplified before being processed by a detector circuit. This block generates the frequency difference between the transmitted and received ultrasonic signals. This difference frequency can be converted into a voltage proportional to frequency, and hence flow velocity, by the frequency to voltage converter circuit.

TABLE 46.3 Properties of Temperature Sensors

Sensor	Form	Sensitivity	Stability	Range (°C)
Metal resistance thermometer	Coil of fine platinum wire	Low	High	−100 to 700
Thermistor	Bead, disk, chip, or rod	High	Moderate	−50 to 150
Thermocouple	Pair of wires	Low	High	−100 to >1500
Mercury in glass thermometer	Column of Hg in glass capillary	Moderate	High	−50 to 400
Silicon p–n diode	Electronic component	Moderate	High	−50 to 150

slightly above that of the blood upstream is measured. As the flow around the thermistor increases, more heat is removed from the thermistor by convection, and so more power is required to keep it at a constant temperature. Relative flow is then measured by determining the amount of power supplied to the thermistor.

In a second approach the thermistor is heated by applying a current pulse and then measuring the cooling curve of the thermistor as the blood flows across it. The thermistor will cool more quickly as the blood flow increases. Both these methods are relatively simple to achieve electronically, but both also have severe limitations. They are essentially qualitative measures and strongly depend on how the thermistor probe is positioned in the vessel being measured. If the probe is closer to the periphery or even in contact with the vessel wall, the measured flow will be different than if the sensor is in the center of the vessel.

46.1.8.3 Temperature

There are many different sensors of temperature [8], but three find particularly wide application to biomedical problems. Table 46.3 summarizes the properties of various temperature sensors, and these three, including metallic resistance thermometers, thermistors, and thermocouples, are described in the following paragraphs.

TABLE 46.4 Temperature Coefficient of Resistance for
Common Metals and Alloys

Metal or alloy	Resistivity at 20°C $\mu\Omega$-cm	Temperature coefficient of resistance (%/°C)
Platinum	9.83	0.3
Gold	2.22	0.368
Silver	1.629	0.38
Copper	1.724	0.393
Constantan (60% Cu, 40% Ni)	49.0	0.0002
Nichrome (80% Ni, 20% Cr)	108.0	0.013

Source: Pender H. and McIlwain K. 1957. *Electrical Engineers' Handbook,* 4th ed., New York, John Wiley & Sons.

46.1.8.4 Metallic Resistance Thermometers

The electric resistance of a piece of metal or wire generally increases as the temperature of that electric conductor increases. A linear approximation to this relationship is given by

$$R = R_0[1 + \alpha(T - T_0)] \tag{46.9}$$

where R_0 is the resistance at temperature T_0, α is the temperature coefficient of resistance, and T is the temperature at which the resistance is being measured. Most metals have temperature coefficients of resistance of the order of 0.1 to 0.4%/°C, as indicated in Table 46.4. The noble metals are preferred for resistance thermometers, since they do not corrode easily and, when drawn into fine wires, their cross-section will remain constant, thus avoiding drift in the resistance over time which could result in an unstable sensor. It is also seen from Table 46.4 that the noble metals, gold and platinum, have some of the highest temperature coefficients of resistance of the common metals.

Metal resistance thermometers are often fabricated from fine-gauge insulated wire that is wound into a small coil. It is important in doing so to make certain that there are not other sources of resistance change that could affect the sensor. For example, the structure should be utilized in such a way that no external strains are applied to the wire, since the wire could also behave as a strain gauge. Metallic films and foils can also be used as temperature sensors, and commercial products are available in the wire, foil, or film forms. The electric circuits used to measure resistance, and hence the temperature, are similar to those used with the wire or foil strain gauges. A bridge circuit is the most desirable, although ohmmeter circuits can also be used. It is important to make sure that the electronic circuit does not pass a large current through the resistance thermometer for that would cause self-heating due to the Joule conversion of electric energy to heat.

46.1.9 Thermistors

Unlike metals, semiconductor materials have an inverse relationship between resistance and temperature. This characteristic is very nonlinear and cannot be characterized by a linear equation such as for the metals. The thermistor is a semiconductor temperature sensor. Its resistance as a function of temperature is given by

$$R = R_0 e^{\beta\left[\frac{1}{T} - \frac{1}{T_0}\right]} \tag{46.10}$$

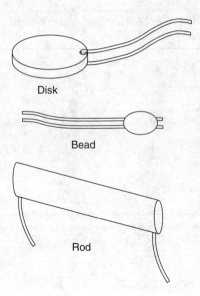

FIGURE 46.8   Common forms of thermistors.

where β is a constant determined by the materials that make up the thermistor. Thermistors can take a variety of forms and cover a large range of resistances. The most common forms used in biomedical applications are the bead, disk, or rod forms of the sensor as illustrated in Figure 46.8. These structures can be formed from a variety of different semiconductors ranging from elements such as silicon and germanium to mixtures of various semiconducting metallic oxides. Most commercially available thermistors are manufactured from the latter materials, and the specific materials as well as the process for fabricating them are closely held industrial secrets. These materials are chosen not only to have high sensitivity but also to have the greatest stability, since thermistors are generally not as stable as the metallic resistance thermometers. However, thermistors can be close to an order of magnitude more sensitive.

46.1.10 Thermocouples

When different regions of an electric conductor or semiconductor are at different temperatures, there is an electric potential between these regions that is directly related to the temperature differences. This phenomenon, known as the Seebeck effect, can be used to produce a temperature sensor known as a thermocouple by taking a wire of metal or alloy A and another wire of metal or alloy B and connecting them as shown in Figure 46.9. One of the junctions is known as the sensing junction, and the other is the reference junction. When these junctions are at different temperatures, a voltage proportional to the temperature difference will be seen at the voltmeter when metals A and B have different Seebeck coefficients. This voltage is roughly proportional to the temperature difference and can be represented over the relatively small temperature differences encountered in biomedical applications by the linear equation

$$V = S_{AB}(T_s - T_r) \tag{46.11}$$

where S_{AB} is the Seebeck coefficient for the thermocouple made up of metals A and B. Although this equation is a reasonable approximation, more accurate data are usually found in tables of actual voltages as a function of temperature difference. In some applications the voltmeter is located at the reference junction, and one uses some independent means such as a mercury in glass thermometer to measure the reference junction temperature. Where precision measurements are made, the reference junction is often placed in an environment of known temperature such as an ice bath. Electronic measurement of reference junction temperature can also be carried out and used to compensate for the reference junction

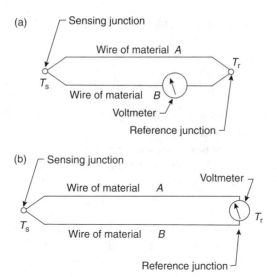

FIGURE 46.9 Circuit arrangement for a thermocouple showing the voltage-measuring device, the voltmeter, interrupting one of the thermocouple wires (a) and at the cold junction (b).

TABLE 46.5 Common Thermocouples

Type	Materials	Seebeck coefficient, $\mu V/^\circ C^a$	Temperature range (°C)
S	Platinum/platinum 10% rhodium	6	0 to 1700
T	Copper/constantan	50	−190 to 400
K	Chromel/alumel	41	−200 to 1370
J	Iron/constantan	53	−200 to 760
E	Chromel/constantan	78	−200 to 970

[a] Seebeck coefficient value is at a temperature of 25°C.

temperature so that the voltmeter reads a signal equivalent to what would be seen if the reference junction were at 0°C. This electronic reference junction compensation is usually carried out using a metal resistance temperature sensor to determine reference junction temperature.

The voltages generated by thermocouples used for temperature measurement are generally quite small being on the order of tens of microvolts per °C. Thus, for most biomedical measurements where there is only a small difference in temperature between the sensing and reference junction, very sensitive voltmeters or amplifiers must be used to measure these potentials. Thermocouples have been used in industry for temperature measurement for many years. Several standard alloys to provide optimal sensitivity and stability of these sensors have evolved. Table 46.5 lists these common alloys, the Seebeck coefficient for thermocouples of these materials at room temperature, and the full range of temperatures over which these thermocouples can be used.

Thermocouples can be fabricated in many different ways depending on their applications. They are especially suitable for measuring temperature differences between two structures, since the sensing junction can be placed on one while the other has the reference junction. Higher-output thermocouples or thermopiles can be produced by connecting several thermocouples in series. Thermocouples can be made from very fine wires that can be implanted in biologic tissues for temperature measurements, and it is also possible to place these fine-wire thermocouples within the lumen of a hypodermic needle to make short-term temperature measurements in tissue. Microfabrication technology has been made it possible to make thermocouples small enough to fit within a living cell.

46.2 Biomedical Applications of Physical Sensors

Just as it is not possible to cover the full range of physical sensors in this chapter, it is also impossible to consider the many biomedical applications that have been reported for these sensors. Instead, some representative examples will be given. These are summarized in Table 46.6 and will be briefly described in the following paragraphs.

Liquid metal strain gauges are especially useful in biomedical applications, because they are mechanically compliant and provide a better mechanical impedance match to most biomedical tissues than other types of strain gauges. By wrapping one of these strain gauges around a circumference of the abdomen, it will stretch and contract with the abdominal breathing movements. The signal from the strain gauge can then be used to monitor breathing in patients or experimental animals. The advantage of this sensor is its compliance so that it does not interfere with the breathing movements or substantially increase the required breathing effort.

One of the original applications of the liquid metal strain gauge was in limb plethysmography [3]. One or more of these sensors are wrapped around an arm or leg at various points and can be used to measure changes in circumference that are related to the cross-sectional area and hence the volume of the limb at those points. If the venous drainage from the limb is occluded, the limb volume will increase as it fills with blood. Releasing the occlusion allows the volume to return to normal. The rate of this decrease in volume can be monitored using the liquid metal strain gauges, and this can be used to identify venous blockage when the return to baseline volume is too slow.

Breathing movements, although not volume, can be seen using a simple magnetic velocity detector. By placing a small permanent magnet on the anterior side of the chest or abdomen and a flat, large-area coil on the posterior side opposite from the magnet, voltages are induced in the coil as the chest of abdomen moves during breathing. The voltage itself can be used to detect the presence of breathing movements, or it can be electronically integrated to give a signal related to displacement.

The LVDT is a displacement sensor that can be used for more precise applications. For example, it can be used in studies of muscle physiology where one wants to measure the displacement of a muscle or where one is measuring the isometric force generated by the muscle (using a load cell) and must ensure that there is no muscle movement. It can also be incorporated into other physical sensors such as a pressure sensor or a tocodynamometer, a sensor used to electronically "feel" uterine contractions of patients in labor or those at risk of premature labor and delivery.

TABLE 46.6 Examples of Biomedical Applications of Physical Sensors

Sensor	Application	Signal range	Reference
Liquid metal	Breathing movement	0–0.05 (strain)	
strain gauge	Limb plethysmography	0–0.02 (strain)	3
Magnetic displacement sensor	Breathing movement	0–10 mm	10
LVDT	Muscle contraction	0–20 mm	
	Uterine contraction sensor	0–5 mm	11
Load cell	Electronic scale	0–440 lbs (0–200 kg)	12
Accelerometer	Subject activity	0–20 m/sec^2	13
Miniature silicon pressure sensor	Intra-arterial blood pressure	0–50 Pa (0–350 mmHg)	
	Urinary bladder pressure	0–10 Pa (0–70 mmHg)	
	Intrauterine pressure	0–15 Pa (0–100 mmHg)	14
Electromagnetic flow sensor	Cardiac output (with integrator)	0–500 ml/min	
	Organ blood flow	0–100 ml/min	15

In addition to studying muscle forces, load cells can be used in various types of electronic scales for weighing patients or study animals. The simplest electronic scale consists of a platform placed on top of a load cell. The weight of any object placed on the platform will produce a force that can be sensed by the load cell. In some critical care situations in the hospital, it is important to carefully monitor the weight of a patient. For example, this is important in watching water balance in patients receiving fluid therapy. The electronic scale concept can be extended by placing a load cell under each leg of the patient's bed and summing the forces seen by each load cell to get the total weight of the patient and the bed. Since the bed weight remains fixed, weight changes seen will reflect changes in patient weight.

Accelerometers can be used to measure patient or research subject activity. By attaching a small accelerometer to the individual being studied, any movements can be detected. This can be useful in sleep studies where movement can help to determine the sleep state. Miniature accelerometers and recording devices can also be worn by patients to study activity patterns and determine effects of disease or treatments on patient activity [9].

Miniature silicon pressure sensors are used for the indwelling measurement of fluid pressure in most body cavities. The measurement of intra-arterial blood pressure is the most frequent application, but pressures in other cavities such as the urinary bladder and the uterus are also measured. The small size of these sensors and the resulting ease of introduction of the sensor into the cavity make these sensors important for these applications.

The electromagnetic flow sensor has been a standard method in use in the physiology laboratory for many years. Its primary application has been for measurement of cardiac output and blood flow to specific organs in research animals. New miniature inverted electromagnetic flow sensors make it possible to temporarily introduce a flow probe into an artery through its lumen to make clinical measurements.

The measurement of body temperature using instruments employing thermistors as the sensor has greatly increased in recent years. Rapid response times of these low-mass sensors make it possible to quickly assess patients' body temperatures so that more patients can be evaluated in a given period. This can then help to reduce health care costs. The rapid response time of low-mass thermistors makes them a simple sensor to be used for sensing breathing. By placing small thermistors near the nose and mouth, the elevated temperature of exhaled air can be sensed to document a breath [10].

The potential applications of physical sensors in medicine and biology are almost limitless. To be able to use these devices, however, scientists must first be familiar with the underlying sensing principles. It is then possible to apply these in a form that addresses the problems at hand.

References

[1] Doebelin E.O. 2003. *Measurement Systems: Applications and Design*, New York, McGraw-Hill.
[2] Dechow P.C. 1988. Strain gauges. In J. Webster (Ed.), *Encyclopedia of Medical Devices and Instrumentation*, pp. 2715–2721, New York, John Wiley & Sons.
[3] Whitney R.J. 1949. The measurement of changes in human limb-volume by means of a mercury-in-rubber strain gauge. *J. Physiol.* 109: 5.
[4] Schaevitz H. 1947. The linear variable differential transformer. *Proc. Soc. Stress Anal.* 4: 79.
[5] Stegall H.F., Kardon M.B., Stone H.L. et al. 1967. A portable simple sonomicrometer. *J. Appl. Physiol.* 23: 289.
[6] Geddes L.A. 1991. *Handbook of Blood Pressure Measurement*, Totowa, NJ, Humana.
[7] Roberts V.C. 1972. *Blood Flow Measurements*, Baltimore, Williams & Wilkins.
[8] Herzfeld C.M. (Ed). 1962. *Temperature: Its Measurement and Control in Science and Industry*, New York, Reinhold.
[9] Patterson S.M., Krantz D.S., Montgomery L.C. et al. 1993. Automated physical activity monitoring: validation and comparison with physiological and self-report measures. *Psychophysiology* 30: 296.
[10] Sekey, A. and Seagrave, C. 1981. Biomedical subminiature thermistor sensor for analog control by breath flow, *Biomater. Med. Dev. Artif. Org.* 9: 73–90.

[11] Angelsen B.A. and Brubakk A.O. 1976. Transcutaneous measurement of blood flow velocity in the human aorta. *Cardiovasc. Res.* 10: 368.

[12] Rolfe P. 1971. A magnetometer respiration monitor for use with premature babies. *Biomed. Eng.* 6: 402.

[13] Reddy N.P. and Kesavan S.K. 1988. Linear variable differential transformers. In J. Webster (Ed.), *Encyclopedia of Medical Devices and Instrumentation*, pp. 1800–1806, New York, John Wiley & Sons.

[14] Roe F.C. 1966. New equipment for metabolic studies. *Nurs. Clin. N. Am.* 1: 621.

[15] Fleming D.G., Ko W.H., and Neuman M.R. (Eds). 1977. *Indwelling and Implantable Pressure Transducers*, Cleveland, CRC Press.

[16] Wyatt D.G. 1971. Electromagnetic blood flow measurements. In B.W. Watson (Ed.), *IEE Medical Electronics Monographs*, London, Peregrinus.

[17] Bently, J.P. 2005. *Principles of Measurement Systems* 4th ed., Englewood Cliffs, N.J., Pearson Prentice-Hall.

[18] Webster J.G. 1999. *Mechanical Variables Measurement — Solid, Fluid, and Thermal*, Boca Raton, CRC Press.

[19] Michalski, L., Eckersdorf, K., Kucharski, J., and Mc Ghee, J. 2001. *Temperature Measurement*, 2nd ed., New York, John Wiley & Sons.

[20] Childs, P.R.N. 2001. *Practical Temperature Measurement*, Oxford, Butterworth-Heinemann.

Further Information

Good overviews of physical sensors are found in these books: Doebelin E.O. 1990. *Measurement Systems: Application and Design*, 4th ed., New York, McGraw-Hill; Harvey, G.F. (Ed.). 1969. *Transducer Compendium*, 2nd ed., New York, Plenum. One can also find good descriptions of physical sensors in chapters of two works edited by John Webster. Chapters 2, 7, and 8 of his textbook (1998) *Medical Instrumentation: Application and Design*, 3rd ed., New York, John Wiley & Sons, and several articles in his *Encyclopedia on Medical Devices and Instrumentation*, published by Wiley in 1988, cover topics on physical sensors.

Although a bit old, the text *Transducers for Biomedical Measurements* (New York, John Wiley & Sons, 1974) by Richard S.C. Cobbold, remains one of the best descriptions of biomedical sensors available. By supplementing the material in this book with recent manufacturers' literature, the reader can obtain a wealth of information on physical (and for that matter chemical) sensors for biomedical application.

The journals *IEEE Transactions on Biomedical Engineering* and *Medical and Biological Engineering and Computing* are good sources of recent research on biomedical applications of physical sensors. The journals *Physiological Measurement* and *Sensors and Actuators* are also good sources for this material as well as papers on the sensors themselves. The IEEE sensors Journal covers many different types of sensors, but biomedical devices are included in its scope.

47
Biopotential Electrodes

47.1 Sensing Bioelectric Signals 47-2
47.2 Electric Characteristics 47-4
47.3 Practical Electrodes for Biomedical Measurements ... 47-5
      Body-Surface Biopotential Electrodes • Intracavitary and
      Intratissue Electrodes • Microelectrodes • Electrodes
      Fabricated Using Microelectronic Technology
47.4 Biomedical Applications 47-11
      References 47-12
      Further Information 47-12

Michael R. Neuman
Michigan Technological University

Biologic systems frequently have electric activity associated with them. This activity can be a constant d.c. electric field, a constant flux of charge-carrying particles or current, or a time-varying electric field or current associated with some time-dependent biologic or biochemical phenomenon. Bioelectric phenomena are associated with the distribution of ions or charged molecules in a biologic structure and the changes in this distribution resulting from specific processes. These changes can occur as a result of biochemical reactions, or they can emanate from phenomena that alter local anatomy.

One can find bioelectric phenomena associated with just about every organ system in the body. Nevertheless, a large proportion of these signals are associated with phenomena that are at the present time not especially useful in clinical medicine and represent time-invariant, low-level signals that are not easily measured in practice. There are, however, several signals that are of diagnostic significance or that provide a means of electronic assessment to aid in understanding biologic systems. These signals, their usual abbreviations, and the systems they measure are listed in Table 47.1. Of these, the most familiar is the electrocardiogram, a signal derived from the electric activity of the heart. This signal is widely used in diagnosing disturbances in cardiac rhythm, signal conduction through the heart, and damage due to cardiac ischemia and infarction. The electromyogram is used for diagnosing neuromuscular diseases, and the electroencephalogram is important in identifying brain dysfunction and evaluating sleep. The other signals listed in Table 47.1 are currently of lesser diagnostic significance but are, nevertheless, used for studies of the associated organ systems.

Although Table 47.1 and the above discussion are concerned with bioelectric phenomena in animals and these techniques are used primarily in studying mammals, bioelectric signals also arise from plants [1]. These signals are generally steady-state or slowly changing, as opposed to the time-varying signals listed in Table 47.1. An extensive literature exists on the origins of bioelectric signals, and the interested reviewer is referred to the text by Plonsey and Barr for a general overview of this area [2].

TABLE 47.1 Bioelectric Signals Sensed by Biopotential Electrodes and Their Sources

Bioelectric signal	Abbreviation	Biologic source
Electrocardiogram	ECG	Heart — as seen from body surface
Cardiac electrogram	—	Heart — as seen from within
Electromyogram	EMG	Muscle
Electroencephalogram	EEG	Brain
Electrooptigram	EOG	Eye dipole field
Electroretinogram	ERG	Eye retina
Action potential	—	Nerve or muscle
Electrogastrogram	EGG	Stomach
Galvanic skin reflex	GSR	Skin

47.1 Sensing Bioelectric Signals

The mechanism of electric conductivity in the body involves ions as charge carriers. Thus, picking up bioelectric signals involves interacting with these ionic charge carriers and transducing ionic currents into electric currents required by wires and electronic instrumentation. This transducing function is carried out by electrodes that consist of electrical conductors in contact with the aqueous ionic solutions of the body. The interaction between electrons in the electrodes and ions in the body can greatly affect the performance of these sensors and requires that specific considerations be made in their application.

At the interface between an electrode and an ionic solution redox (oxidation–reduction), reactions need to occur for a charge to be transferred between the electrode and the solution. These reactions can be represented in general by the following equations:

$$C1C^{n+} + ne^- \tag{47.1}$$

$$A^{m-}1A + me^- \tag{47.2}$$

where n is the valence of cation material C, and m is the valence of anion material, A. For most electrode systems, the cations in solution and the metal of the electrodes are the same, so the atoms C are oxidized when they give up electrons and go into solution as positively charged ions. These ions are reduced when the process occurs in the reverse direction. In the case of the anion reaction, Equation 47.2, the directions for oxidation and reduction are reversed. For best operation of the electrodes, these two reactions should be reversible, that is, it should be just as easy for them to occur in one direction as the other.

The interaction between a metal in contact with a solution of its ions produces a local change in the concentration of the ions in solution near the metal surface. This causes charge neutrality not to be maintained in this region, which can result in causing the electrolyte surrounding the metal to be at a different electrical potential from the rest of the solution. Thus, a potential difference known as the half-cell potential is established between the metal and the bulk of the electrolyte. It is found that different characteristic potentials occur for different materials and different redox reactions of these materials. Some of these potentials are summarized in Table 47.2. These half-cell potentials can be important when using electrodes for low frequency or d.c. measurements.

The relationship between electric potential and ionic concentrations or, more precisely, ionic activities is frequently considered in electrochemistry. Most commonly two ionic solutions of different activity are separated by an ion-selective semipermeable membrane that allows one type of ion to pass freely through the membrane. It can be shown that an electric potential E will exist between the solutions on either side of the membrane, based upon the relative activity of the permeable ions in each of these solutions.

TABLE 47.2 Half-Cell Potentials for Materials and Reactions Encountered in Biopotential Measurement

Metal and reaction	Half-cell potential, V
$Al \rightarrow Al^{3+} + 3e^-$	−1.706
$Ni \rightarrow Ni^{2+} + 2e^-$	−0.230
$H_2 \rightarrow 2H^+ + 2e^-$	0.000 (by definition)
$Ag + Cl^- \rightarrow AgCl + e^-$	+0.223
$Ag \rightarrow Ag^+ + e^-$	+0.799
$Au \rightarrow Au^+ + e^-$	+1.680

This relationship is known as the Nernst equation

$$E = -\frac{RT}{nF} \ln\left(\frac{a_1}{a_2}\right) \tag{47.3}$$

where a_1 and a_2 are the activities of the ions on either side of the membrane, R is the universal gas constant, T is the absolute temperature, n is the valence of the ions, and F is the Faraday constant. More detail on this relationship can be found in Chapter 48.

When no electric current flows between an electrode and the solution of its ions or across an ion-permeable membrane, the potential observed should be the half-cell potential or the Nernst potential, respectively. If, however, there is a current, these potentials can be altered. The difference between the potential at zero current and the measured potentials while current is passing is known as the over voltage and is the result of an alteration in the charge distribution in the solution in contact with the electrodes or the ion-selective membrane. This effect is known as polarization and can result in diminished electrode performance, especially under conditions of motion. There are three basic components to the polarization over potential: the ohmic, the concentration, and the activation over potentials. More details on these over potentials can be found in electrochemistry or biomedical instrumentation texts [3].

Perfectly polarizable electrodes pass a current between the electrode and the electrolytic solution by changing the charge distribution within the solution near the electrode. Thus, no actual current crosses the electrode–electrolyte interface. Nonpolarized electrodes, however, allow the current to pass freely across the electrode–electrolyte interface without changing the charge distribution in the electrolytic solution adjacent to the electrode. Although these types of electrodes can be described theoretically, neither can be fabricated in practice. It is possible, however, to come up with electrode structures that closely approximate their characteristics.

Electrodes made from noble metals such as platinum are often highly polarizable. A charge distribution different from that of the bulk electrolytic solution is found in the solution close to the electrode surface. Such a distribution can create serious limitations when movement is present and the measurement involves low frequency or even d.c. signals. If the electrode moves with respect to the electrolytic solution, the charge distribution in the solution adjacent to the electrode surface will change, and this will induce a voltage change in the electrode that will appear as motion artifact in the measurement. Thus, for most biomedical measurements, nonpolarizable electrodes are preferred to those that are polarizable.

The silver–silver chloride electrode is one that has characteristics similar to a perfectly nonpolarizable electrode and is practical for use in many biomedical applications. The electrode (Figure 47.1a) consists of a silver base structure that is coated with a layer of the ionic compound silver chloride. Some of the silver chloride when exposed to light is reduced to metallic silver, so a typical silver–silver chloride electrode has finely divided metallic silver within a matrix of silver chloride on its surface. Since the silver chloride is relatively insoluble in aqueous solutions, this surface remains stable. Because there is minimal polarization associated with this electrode, motion artifact is reduced compared to polarizable electrodes such as the

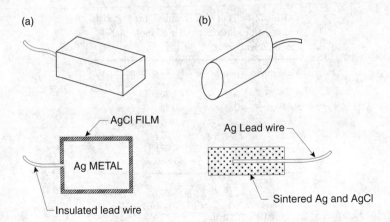

FIGURE 47.1   Silver–silver electrodes for biopotential measurements: (a) metallic silver with a silver chloride surface layer and (b) sintered electrode structure. The lower views show the electrodes in cross-section.

platinum electrode. Furthermore, due to the reduction in polarization, there is also a smaller effect of frequency on electrode impedance, especially at low frequencies.

Silver–silver chloride electrodes of this type can be fabricated by starting with a silver base and electrolytically growing the silver chloride layer on its surface [3]. Although an electrode produced in this way can be used for most biomedical measurements, it is not a robust structure, and pieces of the silver chloride film can be chipped away after repeated use of the electrode. A structure with greater mechanical stability is the sintered silver–silver chloride electrode in Figure 47.1b. This electrode consists of a silver lead wire surrounded by a sintered cylinder made up of finely divided silver and silver-chloride powder pressed together.

In addition to its nonpolarizable behavior, the silver–silver chloride electrode exhibits less electrical noise than the equivalent polarizable electrodes. This is especially true at low frequencies, and so silver–silver chloride electrodes are recommended for measurements involving very low voltages for signals that are made up primarily of low frequencies. A more detailed description of silver–silver chloride electrodes and methods to fabricate these devices can be found in Janz and Ives [5] and biomedical instrumentation textbooks [4].

47.2   Electric Characteristics

The electric characteristics of biopotential electrodes are generally nonlinear and a function of the current density at their surface. Thus, having the devices represented by linear models requires that they be operated at low potentials and currents.[1] Under these idealized conditions, electrodes can be represented by an equivalent circuit of the form shown in Figure 47.2. In this circuit R_d and C_d are components that represent the impedance associated with the electrode–electrolyte interface and polarization at this interface. R_s is the series resistance associated with interfacial effects and the resistance of the electrode materials themselves. The battery E_{hc} represents the half-cell potential described above. It is seen that the impedance of this electrode will be frequency dependent, as illustrated in Figure 47.3. At low frequencies the impedance is dominated by the series combination of R_s and R_d, whereas at higher frequencies C_d bypasses the effect of R_d so that the impedance is now close to R_s. Thus, by measuring the impedance of an electrode at high and low frequencies, it is possible to determine the component values for the equivalent circuit for that electrode.

---

[1]Or at least at an operating point where the voltage and current is relatively fixed.

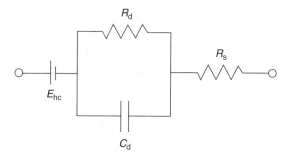

FIGURE 47.2 The equivalent circuit for a biopotential electrode.

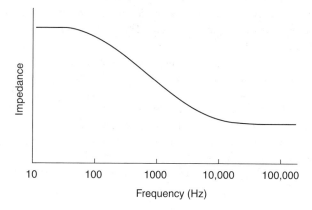

FIGURE 47.3 An example of biopotential electrode impedance as a function of frequency. Characteristic frequencies will be somewhat different for electrode different geometries and materials.

TABLE 47.3 The Effect of Electrode Properties on Electrode Impedance

Property	Change in property	Changes in electrode impedance
Surface area	↑	↓
Polarization	↑	↑ At low frequencies
Surface roughness	↑	↓
Radius of curvature	↑	↓
Surface contamination	↑	↑

↑ — increase in quantity; ↓ — decrease in property.

The electrical characteristics of electrodes are affected by many physical properties of these electrodes. Table 47.3 lists some of the more common physical properties of electrodes and qualitatively indicates how these can affect electrode impedance.

47.3 Practical Electrodes for Biomedical Measurements

Many different forms of electrodes have been developed for different types of biomedical measurements. To describe each of these would go beyond the constraints of this article, but some of the more commonly used electrodes are presented in this section. The reader is referred to the monograph by Geddes for more details and a wider selection of practical electrodes [6].

47.3.1 Body-Surface Biopotential Electrodes

This category includes electrodes that can be placed on the body surface for recording bioelectric signals. The integrity of the skin is not compromised when these electrodes are applied, and they can be used for short-term diagnostic recording such as taking a clinical electrocardiogram or long-term chronic recording such as occurs in cardiac monitoring.

47.3.1.1 Metal Plate Electrodes

The basic metal plate electrode consists of a metallic conductor in contact with the skin with a thin layer of an electrolyte gel between the metal and the skin to establish this contact. Examples of metal plate electrodes are seen in Figure 47.4a. Metals commonly used for this type of electrode include German silver (a nickel–silver alloy), silver, gold, and platinum. Sometimes these electrodes are made of a foil of the metal so as to be flexible, and sometimes they are produced in the form of a suction electrode (Figure 47.4b) to make it easier to attach the electrode to the skin to make a measurement and then move it to another point to repeat the measurement. These types of electrodes are used primarily for diagnostic recordings of biopotentials such as the electrocardiogram or the electroencephalogram. Metal disk electrodes with a gold surface in a conical shape such as shown in Figure 47.4c are frequently used for EEG recordings. The apex of the cone is open so that electrolyte gel or paste can be introduced to both make good contact between the electrode and the head and to allow this contact medium to be replaced should it dry out during its use. These types of electrodes were the primary types used for obtaining diagnostic electrocardiograms for many years. Today, disposable electrodes such as described in the next section are frequently used. These do not require as much preparation or strapping to the limbs as the older electrodes did, and since they are disposable, they do not need to be cleaned between applications to patients. Because they are usually silver–silver chloride electrodes, they have less noise and motion artifact than the metal electrodes.

47.3.1.2 Electrodes for Chronic Patient Monitoring

Long-term monitoring of biopotentials such as the electrocardiogram as performed by cardiac monitors places special constraints on the electrodes used to pick up the signals. These electrodes must have a stable interface between them and the body, and frequently nonpolarizable electrodes are, therefore, the best for this application. Mechanical stability of the interface between the electrode and the skin can help to reduce motion artifact, and so there are various approaches to reduce interfacial motion between the electrode and the coupling electrolyte or the skin. Figure 47.4d is an example of one approach to reduce motion artifact by recessing the electrode in a cup of electrolytic fluid or gel. The cup is then securely fastened to the skin surface using a double-sided adhesive ring. Movement of the skin with respect to the electrode may affect the electrolyte near the skin–electrolyte interface, but the electrode–electrolyte interface can be several millimeters away from this location, since it is recessed in the cup. The fluid movement is unlikely to affect the recessed electrode–electrolyte interface as compared to what would happen if the electrode was separated from the skin by just a thin layer of electrolyte.

The advantages of the recessed electrode can be realized in a simpler design that lends itself to mass production through automation. This results in low per-unit cost so that these electrodes can be considered disposable. Figure 47.4e illustrates such an electrode in cross section. The electrolyte layer now consists of an open-celled sponge saturated with a thickened (high-viscosity) electrolytic solution. The sponge serves the same function as the recess in the cup electrodes and is coupled directly to a silver–silver chloride electrode. Frequently, the electrode itself is attached to a clothing snap through an insulating-adhesive disk that holds the structure against the skin. This snap serves as the point of connection to a lead wire. Many commercial versions of these electrodes in various sizes are available, including electrodes with a silver–silver chloride interface or ones that use metallic silver as the electrode material.

A modification of this basic monitoring electrode structure is shown in Figure 47.4f. In this case the metal electrode is a silver foil with a surface coating of silver chloride. The foil gives the electrode increased flexibility to fit more closely over body contours. Instead of using the sponge, a hydrogel film (really a sponge on a microscopic level) saturated with an electrolytic solution and formed from materials that

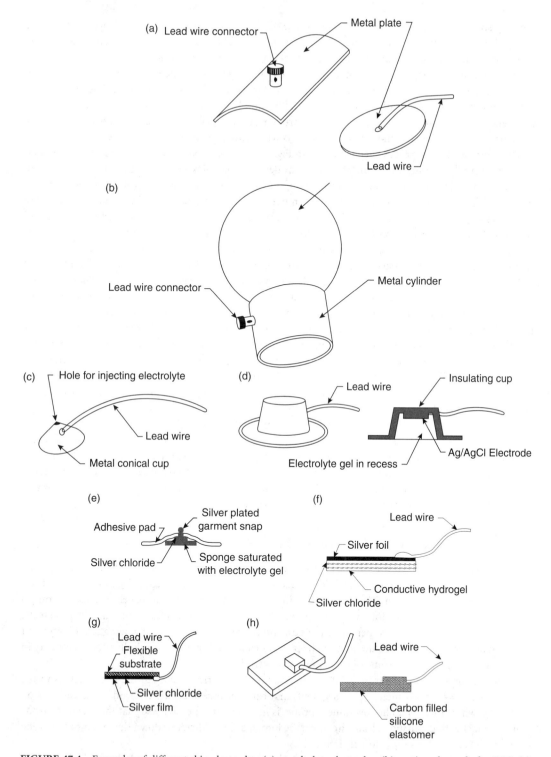

FIGURE 47.4 Examples of different skin electrodes: (a) metal plate electrodes, (b) suction electrode for ECG, (c) metal cup EEG electrode, (d) recessed electrode, (e) disposable electrode with electrolyte-impregnated sponge (shown in cross-section), (f) disposable hydrogel electrode (shown in cross-section), (g) thin-film electrode for use with neonates (shown in cross-section), (h) carbon-filled elastomer dry electrode.

are very sticky is placed over the electrode surface. The opposite surface of the hydrogel layer can be attached directly to the skin, and since it is very sticky, no additional adhesive is needed. The mobility and concentration of ions in the hydrogel layer is generally lower than for the electrolytic solution used in the sponge or the cup. This results in an electrode that has a higher source impedance as compared to these other structures. An important advantage of this structure is its ability to have the electrolyte stick directly on the skin. This greatly reduces interfacial motion between the skin surface and the electrolyte, and hence there is a smaller amount of motion artifact in the signal. This type of hydrogel electrode is, therefore, especially valuable in monitoring patients who move a great deal or during exercise.

Thin-film flexible electrodes such as shown in Figure 47.4g have been used for monitoring neonates. They are basically the same as the metal plate electrodes; only the thickness of the metal in this case is less than a micrometer. These metal films need to be supported on a flexible plastic substrate such as polyester or polyimide. The advantage of using only a thin metal layer for the electrode lies in the fact that these electrodes are x-ray transparent. This is especially important in infants where repeated placement and removal of electrodes, so that x-rays may be taken, can cause substantial skin irritation.

Electrodes that do not use artificially applied electrolyte solutions or gels and, therefore, are often referred to as dry electrodes have been used in some monitoring applications. These sensors as illustrated in Figure 47.4h can be placed on the skin and held in position by an elastic band or tape. They are made up of a graphite or metal-filled polymer such as silicone. The conducting particles are ground into a fine powder, and this is added to the silicone elastomer before it cures so to produce a conductive material with physical properties similar to that of the elastomer. When held against the skin surface, these electrodes establish contact with the skin without the need for an electrolytic fluid or gel. In actuality such a layer is formed by sweat under the electrode surface. For this reason these electrodes tend to perform better after they have been left in place for an hour or two so that this layer forms. Some investigators have found that placing a drop of physiologic saline solution on the skin before applying the electrode accelerates this process. This type of electrode has found wide application in home infant cardiorespiratory monitoring because of the ease with which it can be applied by untrained caregivers.

Dry electrodes are also used on some consumer products such as stationary exercise bicycles and treadmills to pick up an electrocardiographic signal to determine heart rate. When a subject grabs the metal contacts, there is generally enough sweat to establish good electrical contact so that a Lead I electrocardiogram can be obtained and used to determine the heart rate. The signals, however, are much noisier than those obtained from other electrodes described in this section.

47.3.2 Intracavitary and Intratissue Electrodes

Electrodes can be placed within the body for biopotential measurements. These electrodes are generally smaller than skin surface electrodes and do not require special electrolytic coupling fluid, since natural body fluids serve this function. There are many different designs for these internal electrodes, and only a few examples are given in the following paragraphs. Basically these electrodes can be classified as needle electrodes, which can be used to penetrate the skin and tissue to reach the point where the measurement is to be made, or they are electrodes that can be placed in a natural cavity or surgically produced cavity in tissue. Figure 47.5 illustrates some of these internal electrodes.

A catheter tip or probe electrode is placed in a naturally occurring cavity in the body such as in the gastrointestinal system. A metal tip or segment on a catheter makes up the electrode. The catheter or, in the case where there is no hollow lumen, probe, is inserted into the cavity so that the metal electrode makes contact with the tissue. A lead wire down the lumen of the catheter or down the center of the probe connects the electrode to the external circuitry.

The basic needle electrode shown in Figure 47.5b consists of a solid needle, usually made of stainless steel, with a sharp point. An insulating material coats the shank of the needle up to a millimeter or two of the tip so that the very tip of the needle remains exposed. When this structure is placed in tissue such as skeletal muscle, electrical signals can be picked up by the exposed tip. One can also make needle electrodes by running one or more insulated wires down the lumen of a standard hypodermic needle. The electrode

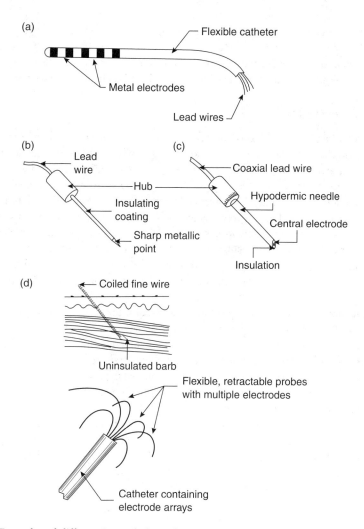

FIGURE 47.5 Examples of different internal electrodes: (a) catheter or probe electrode, (b) needle electrode, (c) coaxial needle electrode, (d) coiled wire electrode. (Reprinted with permission from Webster J.G. (Ed.). 1992. *Medical Instrumentation: Application and Design*, John Wiley & Sons, New York.)

as shown in Figure 47.5c is shielded by the metal of the needle and can be used to pick up very localized signals in tissue.

Fine wires can also be introduced into tissue using a hypodermic needle, which is then withdrawn. This wire can remain in tissue for acute or chronic measurements. Caldwell and Reswick [7] and Knutson et al. [12] have used fine coiled wire electrodes in skeletal muscle for several years without adverse effects.

The advantage of the coil is that it makes the electrode very flexible and compliant. This helps it and the lead wire to endure the frequent flexing and stretching that occurs in the body without breaking.

The relatively new clinical field of cardiac electrophysiology makes use of electrodes that can be advanced into the heart to identify aberrant regions of myocardium that cause life-threatening arrhythmias. These electrodes may be similar to the multiple electrode probe or catheter shown in Figure 47.5a or they might be much more elaborate such as the "umbrella" electrode array in Figure 47.5e. In this case the electrode array with multiple electrodes on each umbrella rib is advanced into the heart in collapsed form through a blood vessel in the same way as a catheter is passed into the heart. The umbrella is then opened in the heart such that the electrodes on the ribs contact the endocardium and are used to record and map intracardiac electrograms. Once the procedure is finished, the umbrella is collapsed and withdrawn through the blood vessel. A similar approach can be taken with an electrode array on the surface of a balloon. The collapsed balloon is advanced into one of the chambers of the heart and then distended. Simultaneous recordings are made from each electrode of the array, and then the balloon is collapsed and withdrawn [16,17].

47.3.3 Microelectrodes

The electrodes described in the previous paragraphs have been applied to studying bioelectric signals at the organism, organ, or tissue level but not at the cellular level. To study the electric behavior of cells, electrodes that are themselves smaller than the cells being studied need to be used. Three types of electrodes have been described for this purpose: etched metal electrodes, micropipette electrodes, and metal-film-coated micropipette electrodes. The metal microelectrode is essentially a subminiature version of the needle electrode described in the previous section (Figure 47.6a). In this case, a strong metal wire such as tungsten is used. One end of this wire is etched electrolytically to give tip diameters on the order of a few micrometers. The structure is insulated up to its tip, and it can be passed through the membrane of a cell to contact the cytosol. The advantage of this type of electrode is that it is both small and robust and can be used for neurophysiologic studies. Its principal disadvantage is the difficulty encountered in its fabrication and high source impedance.

The second and most frequently used type of microelectrode is the glass micropipette. This structure, as illustrated in Figure 47.6b consists of a fine glass capillary drawn to a very narrow point and filled with an electrolytic solution. The point can be as narrow as a fraction of a micrometer, and the dimensions of this electrode are strongly dependent on the skill of the individual drawing the tip. The electrolytic solution in the lumen serves as the contact between the interior of the cell through which the tip has been impaled and a larger conventional electrode located in the shank of the pipette. These electrodes also suffer from high source impedances and fabrication difficulty.

A combined form of these two types of electrodes can be achieved by depositing a metal film over the outside surface of a glass micropipette as shown in Figure 47.6c. In this case, the strength and smaller dimensions of the micropipette can be used to support films of various metals that are insulated by an additional film up to a point very close to the actual tip of the electrode structure. These electrodes have been manufactured in quantity and made available as commercial products. Since they combine

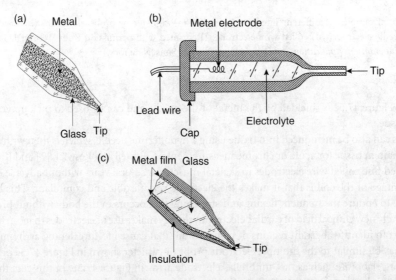

FIGURE 47.6 Microelectrodes: (a) metal, (b) micropipette, (c) thin metal film on micropipette. (Reprinted with permission from Webster J.C. (Ed.). 1992. *Medical Instrumentation: Application and Design*, Houghton Mifflin, Boston.)

the features of both the metal and the micropipette electrodes, they also suffer from many of the same limitations. They do, however, have the advantage of flexibility due to the capability of being able to make films of different metals on the micropipette surface without having to worry about the strength of the metal, as would be the case if the metal were used alone.

47.3.4 Electrodes Fabricated Using Microelectronic Technology

Modern microelectronic technology can be used to fabricate many different types of electrodes for specific biomedical applications. For example, dry electrodes with high source resistances or microelectrodes with similar characteristics can be improved by incorporating a microelectronic amplifier for impedance conversion right on the electrode itself. In the case of the conventional-sized electrodes, a metal disk 5 to 10 mm in diameter can have a high input impedance microelectronic amplifier configured as a follower integrated into the back of the electrode so that localized processing of the high source impedance signal can produce one of lower, more practical impedance for signal transmission [8]. Single- and multiple-element electrodes can be made from thin-film or silicon technology. Mastrototaro and colleagues have demonstrated probes for measuring intramyocardial potentials using thin, patterned gold films on polyimide or oxidised molybdenum substrates [9]. When electrodes are made from pieces of micromachined silicon, it is possible to integrate an amplifier directly into the electrode [10]. Multichannel amplifiers or multiplexers can be used with multiple electrodes on the same probe. Electrodes for contact with individual nerve fibers can be fabricated using micromachined holes in a silicon chip that are just big enough to pass a single growing axon. Electrical contacts on the sides of these holes can then be used to pick up electrical activity from these nerves [11]. These examples are just a few of the many possibilities that can be realized using microelectronics and three-dimensional micromachining technology to fabricate specialized electrodes.

47.4 Biomedical Applications

Electrodes can be used to perform a wide variety of measurements of bioelectric signals. An extensive review of this would be beyond the scope of this chapter, but some typical examples of applications are highlighted in Table 47.4. The most popular application for biopotential electrodes is in obtaining the electrocardiogram for diagnostic and patient-monitoring applications. A substantial commercial market exists for various types of electrocardiographic electrodes, and many of the forms described in the previous section are available commercially. Other electrodes for measuring bioelectric potentials for application in diagnostic medicine are indicated in Table 47.4. Research applications of biopotential electrodes are

TABLE 47.4 Examples of Applications of Biopotential Electrodes

Application	Biopotential	Type of electrode
Cardiac monitoring	ECG	Ag/AgCl with sponge
		Ag/AgCl with hydrogel
Infant cardiopulmonary monitoring	ECG impedance	Ag/AgCl with sponge
		Ag/AgCl with hydrogel
		Thin-film
		Filled elastomer dry
Sleep encephalography	EEG	Gold cups
		Ag/AgCl cups
		Active electrodes
Diagnostic muscle activity	EMG	Needle
Cardiac electrograms	Electrogram	Intracardiac probe
Implanted telemetry of biopotentials	ECG	Stainless steel wire loops
	EMG	Platinum disks
Eye movement	EOG	Ag/AgCl with hydrogel

highly varied and specific for individual studies. Although a few examples are given in Table 47.4, the field is far too broad to be completely covered here.

Biopotential electrodes are one of the most common biomedical sensors used in clinical medicine. Although their basic principle of operation is the same for most applications, they take on many forms and are used in the measurement of many types of bioelectric phenomena. They will continue to play an important role in biomedical instrumentation systems.

References

[1] Yoshida T., Hayashi K., and Toko K. (1988). The effect of anoxia on the spatial pattern of electric potential formed along the root. *Ann. Bot.* 62: 497.

[2] Plonsey R. and Barr R.C. (1988). *Bioelectricity*, New York, Plenum Press.

[3] Weast R.C. (Ed.) (1974). *Handbook of Chemistry and Physics*, 55th ed., Boca Raton, FL, CRC Press.

[4] Webster J.G. (Ed.) (1992). *Medical Instrumentation: Application and Design*, Boston, Houghton Mifflin.

[5] Janz G.I. and Ives D.J.G. (1968). Silver–silver chloride electrodes. *Ann. NY Acad. Sci.* 148: 210.

[6] Geddes L.A. (1972). *Electrodes and the Measurement of Bioelectric Events*, New York, John Wiley & Sons.

[7] Caldwell C.W. and Reswick J.B. (1975). A percutaneous wire electrode for chronic research use. *IEEE Trans. Biomed. Eng.* 22: 429.

[8] Ko W.H. and Hynecek J. (1974). Dry electrodes and electrode amplifiers. In H.A. Miller and D.C. Harrison (Eds.), *Biomedical Electrode Technology*, pp. 169–181, New York, Academic Press.

[9] Mastrototaro J.J., Massoud H.Z., Pilkington T.C. et al. (1992). Rigid and flexible thin-film microelectrode arrays for transmural cardiac recording. *IEEE Trans. Biomed. Eng.* 39: 271.

[10] Wise K.D., Najafi K., Ji J. et al. (1990). Micromachined silicon microprobes for CNS recording and stimulation. *Proc. Ann. Conf. IEEE Eng. Med. Biol. Soc.* 12: 2334.

[11] Edell D.J. (1986). A peripheral nerve information transducer for amputees: long-term multichannel recordings from rabbit peripheral nerves. *IEEE Trans. Biomed. Eng.* 33: 203.

[12] Knutson J.S., Naples G.G., Peckham P.H., and Keith M.W. (2002). Fracture rates and occurrences of infection and granuloma associated with percutaneous intramuscular electrodes in upper extremity functional electrical simulation applications. *J. Rehab. Res. Dev.* 39: 671–684.

[13] Ives J.R. (2005). New chronic EEG electrode for critical/intensive care unit monitoring. *J. Clin. Neurophysiol.* 22: 119–123

[14] Griss P., Tolvanen-Laakso H.K., Meriläinen P. et al. (2002). Characterization of micromachined spiked biopotential electrodes. *IEEE Trans. Biomed. Eng.* 49: 597–604.

[15] Konings K.T., Kirchhof C.I., Smeets J.R. et al. (1994). High-density mapping of electrically induced atrial fibrillation in humans. *Circulation* 89: 1665–1680.

[16] Rao L., He R., Ding C. et al. (2004). Novel noncontact catheter system for endocardial electrical and anatomical imaging. *Ann. Biomed. Eng.* 32: 573–584.

[17] Chen T.C., Parson I.D., and Downar E. (1991). The construction of endocardial balloon arrays for cardiac mapping. *Pacing. Clin. Electrophysiol.* 14: 470–479.

Further Information

Good overviews of biopotential electrodes are found in Geddes L.A. 1972. *Electrodes and the Measurement of Bioelectric Events*, New York, John Wiley & Sons; and Ferris C.D. 1974. *Introduction to Bioelectrodes*, New York, Plenum. Even though these references are more than 20 years old, they clearly cover the field, and little has changed since these books were written.

Overviews of biopotential electrodes are found in chapters of two works edited by John Webster. Chapter 5 of his textbook, Medical Instrumentation: Application and Design, covers the material of this chapter in more detail, and there is a section on "Bioelectrodes" in his *Encyclopedia on Medical Devices and Instrumentation*, published by Wiley in 1988.

The journals *IEEE Transactions on Biomedical Engineering and Medical and Biological Engineering and Computing* are good sources of recent research on biopotential electrodes.

48

Electrochemical Sensors

48.1 Conductivity/Capacitance
       Electrochemical Sensors **48**-1
48.2 Potentiometric Sensors **48**-3
48.3 Voltammetric Sensors **48**-4
48.4 Reference Electrodes **48**-5
48.5 Summary **48**-6
References **48**-6

Chung-Chiun Liu
Case Western Reserve University

Electrochemical sensors have been used extensively either as a whole or an integral part of a chemical and biomedical sensing element. For instance, blood gas (PO_2, PCO_2, and pH) sensing can be accomplished entirely by electrochemical means. Many important biomedical enzymatic sensors, including glucose sensors, incorporate an enzymatic catalyst and an electrochemical sensing element. The Clark type of oxygen sensor [Clark, 1956] is a well-known practical biomedical sensor based on electrochemical principles, an amperometric device. Electrochemical sensors generally can be categorized as conductivity/capacitance, potentiometric, amperometric, and voltammetric sensors. The amperometric and voltammetric sensors are characterized by their current–potential relationship with the electrochemical system and are less well-defined. Amperometric sensors can also be viewed as a subclass of voltammetric sensors.

Electrochemical sensors are essentially an electrochemical cell which employs a two- or three-electrode arrangement. Electrochemical sensor measurement can be made at steady-state or transient. The applied current or potential for electrochemical sensors may vary according to the mode of operation, and the selection of the mode is often intended to enhance the sensitivity and selectivity of a particular sensor. The general principles of electrochemical sensors have been extensively discussed in many electroanalytic references. However, many electroanalytic methods are not practical in biomedical sensing applications. For instance, dropping mercury electrode polarography is a well-established electroanalytic method, yet its usefulness in biomedical sensor development, particularly for potential *in vivo* sensing, is rather limited. In this chapter, we shall focus on the electrochemical methodologies which are useful in biomedical sensor development.

48.1 Conductivity/Capacitance Electrochemical Sensors

Measurement of the electric conductivity of an electrochemical cell can be the basis for an electrochemical sensor. This differs from an electrical (physical) measurement, for the electrochemical sensor measures the conductivity change of the system in the presence of a given solute concentration. This solute is often the sensing species of interest. Electrochemical sensors may also involve a measuring capacitative impedance resulting from the polarization of the electrodes and the faradaic or charge transfer processes.

It has been established that the conductance of a homogeneous solution is directly proportional to the cross-sectional area perpendicular to the electrical field and inversely proportional to the segment of solution along the electrical field. Thus, the conductance of this solution (electrolyte), G (Ω^{-1}), can be expressed as

$$G = \sigma A/L \qquad (48.1)$$

where A is the cross-sectional area (in cm^2), L is the segment of the solution along the electrical field (in cm), and σ (in $\Omega\,cm^{-1}$) is the specific conductivity of the electrolyte and is related quantitatively to the concentration and the magnitude of the charges of the ionic species. For a practical conductivity sensor, A is the surface of the electrode, and L is the distance between the two electrodes.

Equivalent and molar conductivities are commonly used to express the conductivity of the electrolyte. Equivalent conductance depends on the concentration of the solution. If the solution is a strong electrolyte, it will completely dissociate the components in the solution to ionic forms. Kohlrauch [MacInnes, 1939] found that the equivalent conductance of a strong electrolyte was proportional to the square root of its concentration. However, if the solution is a weak electrolyte which does not completely dissociate the components in the solution to respective ions, the above observation by Kohlrauch is not applicable.

The formation of ions leads to consideration of their contribution to the overall conductance of the electrolyte. The equivalent conductance of a strong electrolyte approaches a constant limiting value at infinite dilution, namely,

$$\Lambda_o = \Lambda_{\lim\to 0} = \lambda_0^+ + \lambda_0^- \qquad (48.2)$$

where Λ_0 is the equivalent conductance of the electrolyte at infinite dilution and λ_0^+ and λ_0^- are the ionic equivalent conductance of cations and anions at infinite dilution, respectively.

Kohlrauch also established the law of independent mobilities of ions at infinite dilution. This implies that Lo at infinite dilution is a constant at a given temperature and will not be affected by the presence of other ions in the electrolytes. This provides a practical estimation of the value of Λ_0 from the values of λ_0^+ and λ_0^-. As mentioned, the conductance of an electrolyte is influenced by its concentration. Kohlrausch stated that the equivalent conductance of the electrolyte at any concentration C in mol/l or any other convenient units can be expressed as

$$\Lambda = \Lambda_0 - \beta C^{0.5} \qquad (48.3)$$

where β is a constant depending on the electrolyte.

In general, electrolytes can be classified as weak electrolytes, strong electrolytes, and ion-pair electrolytes. Weak electrolytes only dissociate to their component ions to a limited extent, and the degree of the dissociation is temperature dependent. However, strong electrolytes dissociate completely, and Equation 48.3 is applicable to evaluate its equivalent conductance. Ion-pair electrolytes can by characterized by their tendency to form ion pairs. The dissociation of ion pairs is similar to that of a weak electrolyte and is affected by ionic activities. The conductivity of ion-pair electrolytes is often nonlinear related to its concentration.

The electrolyte conductance measurement technique, in principle, is relatively straightforward. However, the conductivity measurement of an electrolyte is often complicated by the polarization of the electrodes at the operating potential. Faradaic or charge transfer processes occur at the electrode surface, complicating the conductance measurement of the system. Thus, if possible, the conductivity electrochemical sensor should operate at a potential where no faradaic processes occur. Also, another important consideration is the formation of the double layer adjacent to each electrode surface when a potential is imposed on the electrochemical sensor. The effect of the double layer complicates the interpretation of the conductivity measurement and is usually described by the Warburg impedance. Thus, even in the absence of faradaic processes, the potential effect of the double layer on the conductance of the electrolyte must be carefully assessed. The influence of a faradaic process can be minimized by maintaining a high center constant, L/A, of the electrochemical conductivity sensor, so that the cell resistance lies in the region of 1 to 50 kΩ. This implies the desirable feature of a small electrode surface area and a relatively large distance between the two electrodes. Yet, a large electrode surface area enhances the accuracy of the measurement, since a large deviation from the null point facilitates the balance of the Wheatstone bridge, resulting in improvement of sensor sensitivity. These opposing features can be resolved by using a multiple-sensing electrode configuration in which the surface area of each electrode element is small compared to the distance between the electrodes. The multiple electrodes are connected in parallel, and the output of the sensor represents the total sum of the current through each pair of electrodes. In this mode of measurement, the effect of the double layer is included in the conductance measurement. The effects of both the double layers and the faradaic processes can be minimized by using a high-frequency, low-amplitude alternating current. The higher the frequency and the lower the amplitude of the imposed alternating current, the closer the measured value is to the true conductance of the electrolyte.

48.2   Potentiometric Sensors

When a redox reaction, Ox + Ze = Red, takes place at an electrode surface in an electrochemical cell, a potential may develop at the electrode–electrolyte interface. This potential may then be used to quantify the activity (on concentration) of the species involved in the reaction forming the fundamental of potentiometric sensors.

The above reduction reaction occurs at the surface of the cathode and is defined as a half-cell reaction. At thermodynamic equilibrium, the Nernst equation is applicable and can be expressed as:

$$E = E^\circ + \frac{RT}{ZF} \ln\left(\frac{a_{\text{ox}}}{a_{\text{red}}}\right), \tag{48.4}$$

where E and E° are the measured electrode potential and the electrode potential at standard state, respectively, a_{ox} and a_{red} are the activities of Ox (reactant in this case) and Red (product in this case), respectively; Z is the number of electrons transferred, F the Faraday constant, R the gas constant, and T the operating temperature in the absolute scale. In the electrochemical cell, two half-cell reactions will take place simultaneously. However, for sensing purposes, only one of the two half-cell reactions should involve the species of interest, and the other half-cell reaction is preferably reversible and noninterfering. As indicated in Equation 48.4, a linear relation exists between the measured potential E and the natural logarithm of the ratio of the activities of the reactant and product. If the number of electrons transferred, Z, is one, at ambient temperature (25°C or 298°K) the slope is approximately 60 mV/decade. This slope value governs the sensitivity of the potentiometric sensor.

Potentiometric sensors can be classified based on whether the electrode is inert or active. An inert electrode does not participate in the half-cell reaction and merely provides the surface for the electron transfer or provides a catalytic surface for the reaction. However, an active electrode is either an ion donor or acceptor in the reaction. In general, there are three types of active electrodes: the metal/metal ion, the metal/insoluble salt or oxide, and metal/metal chelate electrodes.

Noble metals such as platinum and gold, graphite, and glassy carbon are commonly used as inert electrodes on which the half-cell reaction of interest takes place. To complete the circuitry for the potentiometric sensor, the other electrode is usually a reference electrode on which a noninterference half-cell reaction occurs. Silver–silver chloride and calomel electrodes are the most commonly used reference electrodes. Calomel consists of $Hg/HgCl_2$ and is less desirable for biomedical systems in terms of toxicity.

An active electrode may incorporate chemical or biocatalysts and is involved as either an ion donor or acceptor in the half-cell reaction. The other half-cell reaction takes place on the reference electrode and should also be noninterfering.

If more than a single type of ion contributes to the measured potential in Equation 48.4, the potential can no longer be used to quantify the ions of interest. This is the interference in a potentiometric sensor. Thus, in many cases, the surface of the active electrode often incorporates a specific functional membrane which may be ion-selective, ion-permeable, or have ion-exchange properties. These membranes tend to selectivity permit the ions of interest to diffuse or migrate through. This minimizes the ionic interference.

Potentiometric sensors operate at thermodynamic equilibrium conditions. Thus, in practical potentiometric sensing, the potential measurement needs to be made under zero-current conditions. Consequently, a high-input impedance electrometer is often used for measurements. Also, the response time for a potentiometric sensor to reach equilibrium conditions in order to obtain a meaningful reading can be quite long. These considerations are essential in the design and selection of potentiometric sensors for biomedical applications.

48.3   Voltammetric Sensors

The current-potential relationship of an electrochemical cell provides the basis for voltammetric sensors. Amperometric sensors, that are also based on the current-potential relationship of the electrochemical cell, can be considered a subclass of voltammetric sensors. In amperometric sensors, a fixed potential is applied to the electrochemical cell, and a corresponding current, due to a reduction or oxidation reaction, is then obtained. This current can be used to quantify the species involved in the reaction. The key consideration of an amperometric sensor is that it operates at a fixed potential. However, a voltammetric sensor can operate in other modes such as linear cyclic voltammetric modes. Consequently, the respective current potential response for each mode will be different.

In general, voltammetric sensors examine the concentration effect of the detecting species on the current-potential characteristics of the reduction or oxidation reaction involved.

The mass transfer rate of the detecting species in the reaction onto the electrode surface and the kinetics of the faradaic or charge transfer reaction at the electrode surface directly affect the current-potential characteristics. This mass transfer can be accomplished through (a) an ionic migration as a result of an electric potential gradient, (b) a diffusion under a chemical potential difference or concentration gradient, and (c) a bulk transfer by natural or forced convection. The electrode reaction kinetics and the mass transfer processes contribute to the rate of the faradaic process in an electrochemical cell. This provides the basis for the operation of the voltammetric sensor. However, assessment of the simultaneous mass transfer and kinetic mechanism is rather complicated. Thus, the system is usually operated under definitive hydrodynamic conditions. Various techniques to control either the potential or current are used to simplify the analysis of the voltammetric measurement. A description of these techniques and their corresponding mathematical analyses are well documented in many texts on electrochemistry or electroanalysis [Adams, 1969; Bard and Faulkner, 1980; Lingane, 1958; Macdonald, 1977; Murray and Reilley, 1966].

A preferred mass transfer condition is total diffusion, which can be described by Fick's law of diffusion. Under this condition, the cell current, a measure of the rate of the faradaic process at an electrode, usually increases with increases in the electrode potential. This current approaches a limiting value when the rate of the faradaic process at the electrode surface reaches its maximum mass transfer rate. Under this condition, the concentration of the detecting species at the electrode surface is considered as zero and is diffusional mass transfer. Consequently, the limiting current and the bulk concentration of the detecting species can be related by

$$i = ZFkmC^*$$

(48.5)

where km is the mass transfer coefficient and C^* is the bulk concentration of the detecting species. At the other extreme, when the electrode kinetics are slow compared with the mass transfer rate, the electrochemical system is operated in the reaction kinetic control regime. This usually corresponds to a small overpotential. The limiting current and the bulk concentration of the detecting species can be related as

$$i = ZFkcC^* \tag{48.6}$$

where kc is the kinetic rate constant for the electrode process. Both Equation 48.5 and Equation 48.6 show the linear relationship between the limiting current and the bulk concentration of the detecting species. In many cases, the current does not tend to a limiting value with an increase in the electrode potential. This is because other faradaic or nonfaradaic processes become active, and the cell current represents the cumulative rates of all active electrode processes. The relative rates of these processes, expressing current efficiency, depend on the current density of the electrode. Assessment of such a system is rather complicated, and the limiting current technique may become ineffective.

When a voltammetric sensor operates with a small overpotential, the rate of faradaic reaction is also small; consequently, a high-precision instrument for the measurement is needed. An amperometric sensor is usually operated under limiting current or relatively small overpotential conditions. Amperometric sensors operate under an imposed fixed electrode potential. Under this condition, the cell current can be correlated with the bulk concentration of the detecting species (the solute). This operating mode is commonly classified as amperometric in most sensor work, but it is also referred to as the chronosuperometric method, since time is involved.

Voltammetric sensors can be operated in a linear or cyclic sweep mode. Linear sweep voltammetry involves an increase in the imposed potential linearly at a constant scanning rate from an initial potential to a defined upper potential limit. This is the so-called potential window. The current-potential curve usually shows a peak at a potential where the oxidation or reduction reaction occurs. The height of the peak current can be used for the quantification of the concentration of the oxidation or reduction species. Cyclic voltammetry is similar to the linear sweep voltammetry except that the electrode potential returns to its initial value at a fixed scanning rate. The cyclic sweep normally generates the current peaks corresponding to the oxidation and reduction reactions. Under these circumstances, the peak current value can relate to the corresponding oxidation or reduction reaction. However, the voltammogram can be very complicated for a system involving adsorption (nonfaradaic processes) and charge processes (faradaic processes). The potential scanning rate, diffusivity of the reactant, and operating temperature are essential parameters for sensor operation, similar to the effects of these parameters for linear sweep voltammograms. The peak current may be used to quantify the concentration of the reactant of interest, provided that the effect of concentration on the diffusivity is negligible. The potential at which the peak current occurs can be used in some cases to identify the reaction, or the reactant. This identification is based on the half-cell potential of the electrochemical reactions, either oxidation or reduction. The values of these half-cell reactions are listed extensively in handbooks and references.

The described voltammetric and amperometric sensors can be used very effectively to carry out qualitative and quantitative analyses of chemical and biochemical species. The fundamentals of this sensing technique are well established, and the critical issue is the applicability of the technique to a complex, practical environment, such as in whole blood or other biologic fluids. This is also the exciting challenge of designing a biosensor using voltammetric and amperometric principles.

48.4   Reference Electrodes

Potentiometric, voltammetric, and amperometric sensors employ a reference electrode. The reference electrode in the case of potentiometric and amperometric sensors serves as a counter electrode to complete the circuitry. In either case, the reaction of interest takes place at the surface of the working electrode, and this reaction is either an oxidation or reduction reaction. Consequently, the reaction at the counter electrode, that is, the reference electrode, is a separate reduction or oxidation reaction, respectively. It is necessary that the reaction occurring at the reference electrode does not interfere with the reaction at the working electrode. For practical applications, the reaction occurring at the reference electrode should be highly reversible and, as stated, does not contribute to the reaction at the working electrode. In electrochemistry, the hydrogen electrode is universally accepted as the primary standard with which other electrodes are compared. Consequently, the hydrogen electrode serves extensively as a standard reference. A hydrogen reference electrode is relatively simple to prepare. However, for practical applications hydrogen reference electrodes are too cumbersome to be useful in practice.

A class of electrode called the electrode of the second kind, which forms from a metal and its sparingly soluble metal salt, finds use as the reference electrode. The most common electrode of this type includes the calomel electrode, $Hg/HgCl_2$ and the silver–silver chloride electrode, $Ag/AgCl$. In biomedical applications, particularly in *in vivo* applications, $Ag/AgCl$ is more suitable as a reference electrode.

An $Ag/AgCl$ electrode can be small, compact, and relatively simple to fabricate. As a reference electrode, the stability and reproducibility of an $Ag/AgCl$ electrode is very important. Contributing factors to instability and poor reproducibility of $Ag/AgCl$ electrodes include the purity of the materials used, the aging effect of the electrode, the light effect, and so on. When in use, the electrode and the electrolyte interface contribute to the stability of the reference electrode. It is necessary that a sufficient quantity of Cl^- ions exists in the electrolyte when the $Ag/AgCl$ electrode serves as a reference. Therefore, other silver–silver halides such as $Ag/AgBr$ or Ag/AgI electrodes are used in cases where these other halide ions are present in the electrolyte.

In a voltammetric sensor, the reference electrode serves as a true reference for the working electrode, and no current flows between the working and reference electrodes. Nevertheless, the stability of the reference electrode remains essential for a voltammetric sensor.

48.5   Summary

Electrochemical sensors are used extensively in many biomedical applications including blood chemistry sensors, PO_2, PCO_2, and pH electrodes. Many practical enzymatic sensors, including glucose and lactate sensors, also employ electrochemical sensors as sensing elements. Electrochemically based biomedical sensors have found *in vivo* and *in vitro* applications. We believe that electrochemical sensors will continue to be an important aspect of biomedical sensor development.

References

Adams R.N. 1969. *Electrochemistry at Solid Electrodes*, New York, Marcel Dekker.

Bard A. and Faulkner L.R. 1980. *Electrochemical Methods*, New York, John Wiley & Sons.

Clark L.C. Jr. 1956. Monitor and control of blood and tissue oxygen tissues. *Trans. Am. Soc. Artif. Organs* 2: 41.

Lingane J.J. 1958. *Electroanalytical Chemistry*, New York, London, Interscience.

Macdonald D.D. 1977. *Transient Techniques in Electrochemistry*, New York, Plenum.

MacInnes D.A. 1939. *The Principles of Electrochemistry*, New York, Reinhold.

Murray R.W. and Reilley C.N. 1996. *Electroanalytical Principles*, New York-London, Interscience.

49

Optical Sensors

49.1 Instrumentation 49-2
      Light Source • Optical Elements • Photodetectors •
      Signal Processing
49.2 Optical Fibers 49-3
      Probe Configurations • Optical Fiber Sensors •
      Indicator-Mediated Transducers
49.3 General Principles of Optical Sensing 49-5
      Evanescent Wave Spectroscopy • Surface Plasmon Resonance
49.4 Applications 49-7
      Oximetry • Blood Gases • Glucose Sensors •
      Immunosensors
References 49-14

Yitzhak Mendelson
Worcester Polytechnic Institute

Optical methods are among the oldest and best-established techniques for sensing biochemical analytes. Instrumentation for optical measurements generally consists of a light source, a number of optical components to generate a light beam with specific characteristics and to direct this light to some modulating agent, and a photodetector for processing the optical signal. The central part of an optical sensor is the modulating component, and a major part of this chapter will focus on how to exploit the interaction of an analyte with optical radiation in order to obtain essential biochemical information.

The number of publications in the field of optical sensors for biomedical applications has grown significantly during the past two decades. Numerous scientific reviews and historical perspectives have been published, and the reader interested in this rapidly growing field is advised to consult these sources for additional details. This chapter will emphasize the basic concept of typical optical sensors intended for continuous *in vivo* monitoring of biochemical variables, concentrating on those sensors which have generally progressed beyond the initial feasibility stage and reached the promising stage of practical development or commercialization.

Optical sensors are usually based on optical fibers or on planar waveguides. Generally, there are three distinctive methods for quantitative optical sensing at surfaces:

1. The analyte directly affects the optical properties of a waveguide, such as evanescent waves (electromagnetic waves generated in the medium outside the optical waveguide when light is reflected from within) or surface plasmons (resonances induced by an evanescent wave in a thin film deposited on a waveguide surface).
2. An optical fiber is used as a plain transducer to guide light to a remote sample and return light from the sample to the detection system. Changes in the intrinsic optical properties of the medium itself are sensed by an external spectrophotometer.

3. An indicator or chemical reagent placed inside, or on, a polymeric support near the tip of the optical fiber is used as a mediator to produce an observable optical signal. Typically, conventional techniques, such as absorption spectroscopy and fluorimetry, are employed to measure changes in the optical signal.

49.1 Instrumentation

The actual implementation of instrumentation designed to interface with optical sensors will vary greatly depending on the type of optical sensor used and its intended application. A block diagram of a generic instrument is illustrated in Figure 49.1. The basic building blocks of such an instrument are the light source, various optical elements, and photodetectors.

49.1.1 Light Source

A wide selection of light sources are available for optical sensor applications. These include highly coherent gas and semiconductor diode lasers, broad spectral band incandescent lamps, and narrow-band, solid-state, light-emitting diodes (LEDs). The important requirement of a light source is obviously good stability. In certain applications, for example in portable instrumentation, LEDs have significant advantages over other light sources because they are small and inexpensive, consume lower power, produce selective wavelengths, and are easy to work with. In contrast, tungsten lamps provide a broader range of wavelengths, higher intensity, and better stability but require a sizable power supply and can cause heating problems inside the apparatus.

49.1.2 Optical Elements

Various optical elements are used routinely to manipulate light in optical instrumentation. These include lenses, mirrors, light choppers, beam splitters, and couplers for directing the light from the light source into the small aperture of a fiber optic sensor or a specific area on a waveguide surface and collecting the light from the sensor before it is processed by the photodetector. For wavelength selection, optical filters, prisms, and diffraction gratings are the most common components used to provide a narrow bandwidth of excitation when a broadwidth light source is utilized.

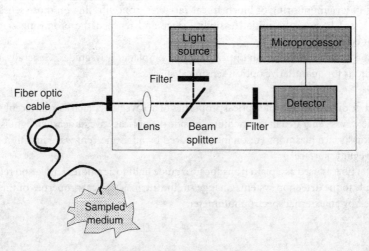

FIGURE 49.1 General diagram representing the basic building blocks of an optical instrument for optical sensor applications.

49.1.3 Photodetectors

In choosing photodetectors for optical sensors, a number of factors must be considered. These include sensitivity, detectivity, noise, spectral response, and response time. Photomultipliers and semiconductor quantum photodetectors, such as photoconductors and photodiodes, are both suitable. The choice, however, is somewhat dependent on the wavelength region of interest. Generally, both types give adequate performance. Photodiodes are usually more attractive because of the compactness and simplicity of the circuitry involved.

Typically, two photodetectors are used in optical instrumentation because it is often necessary to include a separate reference detector to track fluctuations in source intensity and temperature. By taking a ratio between the two detector readings, whereby a part of the light that is not affected by the measurement variable is used for correcting any optical variations in the measurement system, a more accurate and stable measurement can be obtained.

49.1.4 Signal Processing

Typically, the signal obtained from a photodetector provides a voltage or a current proportional to the measured light intensity. Therefore, either simple analog computing circuitry (e.g., a current-to-voltage converter) or direct connection to a programmable gain voltage stage is appropriate. Usually, the output from a photodetector is connected directly to a preamplifier before it is applied to sampling and analog-to-digital conversion circuitry residing inside a computer.

Quite often two different wavelengths of light are utilized to perform a specific measurement. One wavelength is usually sensitive to changes in the species being measured, and the other wavelength is unaffected by changes in the analyte concentration. In this manner, the unaffected wavelength is used as a reference to compensate for fluctuation in instrumentation over time. In other applications, additional discriminations, such as pulse excitation or electronic background subtraction utilizing synchronized lock-in amplifier detection, are useful, allowing improved selectivity and enhanced signal-to-noise ratio.

49.2 Optical Fibers

Several types of biomedical measurements can be made by using either plain optical fibers as a remote device for detecting changes in the spectral properties of tissue and blood or optical fibers tightly coupled to various indicator-mediated transducers. The measurement relies either on direct illumination of a sample through the endface of the fiber or by excitation of a coating on the side wall surface through evanescent wave coupling. In both cases, sensing takes place in a region outside the optical fiber itself. Light emanating from the fiber end is scattered or fluoresced back into the fiber, allowing measurement of the returning light as an indication of the optical absorption or fluorescence of the sample at the fiber optic tip.

Optical fibers are based on the principle of total internal reflection. Incident light is transmitted through the fiber if it strikes the cladding at an angle greater than the so-called critical angle, so that it is totally internally reflected at the core/cladding interface. A typical instrument for performing fiber optic sensing consists of a light source, an optical coupling arrangement, the fiber optic light guide with or without the necessary sensing medium incorporated at the distal tip, and a light detector.

A variety of high-quality optical fibers are available commercially for biomedical sensor applications, depending on the analytic wavelength desired. These include plastic, glass, and quartz fibers which cover the optical spectrum from the UV through the visible to the near IR region. On one hand, plastic optical fibers have a larger aperture and are strong, inexpensive, flexible, and easy to work with but have poor UV transmission below 400 nm. On the other hand, glass and quartz fibers have low attenuation and better transmission in the UV but have small apertures, are fragile, and present a potential risk in *in vivo* applications.

49.2.1 Probe Configurations

There are many different ways to implement fiber optic sensors. Most fiber optic chemical sensors employ either a single-fiber configuration, where light travels to and from the sensing tip in one fiber, or a double-fiber configuration, where separate optical fibers are used for illumination and detection. A single fiber optic configuration offers the most compact and potentially least expensive implementation. However, additional challenges in instrumentation are involved in separating the illuminating signal from the composite signal returning for processing.

The design of intravascular catheters requires special considerations related to the sterility and biocompatibility of the sensor. For example, intravascular fiberoptic sensors must be sterilizable and their material nonthrombogenic and resistant to platelet and protein deposition. Therefore, these catheters are typically made of materials covalently bound with heparin or antiplatelet agents. The catheter is normally introduced into the peripheral artery or vein via a cut-down and a slow heparin flush is maintained until the device is removed from the blood.

49.2.2 Optical Fiber Sensors

Advantages cited for fiber sensors include their small size and low cost. In contrast to electrical measurements, where the difference of two absolute potentials must be measured, fiber optics are self-contained and do not require an external reference signal. Because the signal is optical, there is no electrical risk to the patient, and there is no direct interference from surrounding electric or magnetic fields. Chemical analysis can be performed in real-time with almost an instantaneous response. Furthermore, versatile sensors can be developed that respond to multiple analytes by utilizing multiwavelength measurements.

Despite these advantages, optical fiber sensors exhibit several shortcomings. Sensors with immobilized dyes and other indicators have limited long-term stability, and their shelf life degrades over time. Moreover, ambient light can interfere with the optical measurement unless optical shielding or special time-synchronous gating is performed. As with other implanted or indrolling sensors, organic materials or cells can deposit on the sensor surface due to the biologic response to the presence of the foreign material. All of these problems can result in measurement errors.

49.2.3 Indicator-Mediated Transducers

Only a limited number of biochemical analytes have an intrinsic optical absorption that can be measured with sufficient selectivity directly by spectroscopic methods. Other species, particularly hydrogen, oxygen, carbon dioxide, and glucose, which are of primary interest in diagnostic applications, are not susceptible to direct photometry. Therefore, indicator-mediated sensors have been developed using specific reagents that are properly immobilized on the surface of an optical sensor.

The most difficult aspect of developing an optical biosensor is the coupling of light to the specific recognition element so that the sensor can respond selectively and reversibly to a change in the concentration of a particular analyte. In fiber-optic-based sensors, light travels efficiently to the end of the fiber where it exists and interacts with a specific chemical or biologic recognition element that is immobilized at the tip of the fiber optic. These transducers may include indicators and ionophores (i.e., ion-binding compounds) as well as a wide variety of selective polymeric materials. After the light interacts with the sample, the light returns through the same or a different optical fiber to a detector which correlates the degree of change with the analyte concentration.

Typical indicator-mediated fiber-optic-sensor configurations are shown schematically in Figure 49.2. In (a) the indicator is immobilized directly on a membrane positioned at the end of a fiber. An indicator in the form of a powder can be either glued directly onto a membrane, as shown in (b), or physically retained in position at the end of the fiber by a special permeable membrane (c), a tubular capillary/membrane (d), or a hollow capillary tube (e).

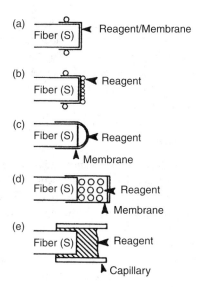

FIGURE 49.2 Typical configuration of different indicator-mediated fiber optic sensor tips. (Taken from Otto S. Wolfbeis, *Fiber Optic Chemical Sensors and Biosensors*, Vol. 1, CRC Press, Boca Raton, 1990.)

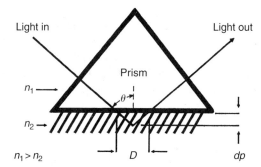

FIGURE 49.3 Schematic diagram of the path of a light ray at the interface of two different optical materials with index of refraction n_1 and n_2. The ray penetrates a fraction of a wave-length (dp) beyond the interface into the medium with the smaller refractive index.

49.3 General Principles of Optical Sensing

Two major optical techniques are commonly available to sense optical changes at sensor interfaces. These are usually based on evanescent wave and surface plasmon resonance principles.

49.3.1 Evanescent Wave Spectroscopy

When light propagates along an optical fiber, it is not confined to the core region but penetrates to some extent into the surrounding cladding region. In this case, an electromagnetic component of the light penetrates a characteristic distance (on the order of one wavelength) beyond the reflecting surface into the less optically dense medium where it is attenuated exponentially according to Beer–Lambert's law (Figure 49.3).

The evanescent wave depends on the angle of incidence and the incident wavelength. This phenomenon has been widely exploited to construct different types of optical sensors for biomedical applications. Because of the short penetration depth and the exponential decay of the intensity, the evanescent wave is absorbed mainly by absorbing compounds very close to the surface. In the case of particularly weak absorbing analytes, sensitivity can be enhanced by combining the evanescent wave principle with multiple internal reflections along the sides of an unclad portion of a fiber optic tip.

Instead of an absorbing species, a fluorophore can also be used. Light is absorbed by the fluorophore emitting detectable fluorescent light at a higher wavelength, thus providing improved sensitivity. Evanescent wave sensors have been applied successfully to measure the fluorescence of indicators in solution, for pH measurement, and in immunodiagnostics.

49.3.2 Surface Plasmon Resonance

Instead of the dielectric/dielectric interface used in evanescent wave sensors, it is possible to arrange a dielectric/metal/dielectric sandwich layer such that when monochromatic polarized light (e.g., from a laser source) impinges on a transparent medium having a metallized (e.g., Ag or Au) surface, light is absorbed within the plasma formed by the conduction electrons of the metal. This results in a phenomenon known as surface plasmon resonance (SPR). When SPR is induced, the effect is observed as a minimum in the intensity of the light reflected off the metal surface.

As is the case with the evanescent wave, an SPR is exponentially decaying into solution with a penetration depth of about 20 nm. The resonance between the incident light and the plasma wave depends on the angle, wavelength, and polarization state of the incident light and the refractive indices of the metal film and the materials on either side of the metal film. A change in the dielectric constant or the refractive index at the surface causes the resonance angle to shift, thus providing a highly sensitive means of monitoring surface reactions.

The method of SPR is generally used for sensitive measurement of variations in the refractive index of the medium immediately surrounding the metal film. For example, if an antibody is bound to or absorbed into the metal surface, a noticeable change in the resonance angle can be readily observed because of the change of the refraction index at the surface, assuming all other parameters are kept constant (Figure 49.4). The advantage of this concept is the improved ability to detect the direct interaction between antibody and antigen as an interfacial measurement.

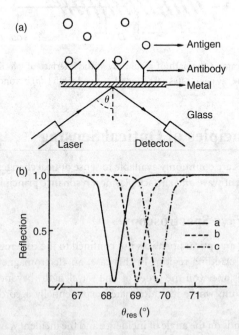

FIGURE 49.4 Surface plasmon resonance at the interface between a thin metallic surface and a liquid (a). A sharp decrease in the reflected light intensity can be observed in (b). The location of the resonance angle is dependent on the refractive index of the material present at the interface.

SPR has been used to analyze immunochemicals and to detect gases. The main limitation of SPR, however, is that the sensitivity depends on the optical thickness of the adsorbed layer, and, therefore, small molecules cannot be measured in very low concentrations.

49.4 Applications

49.4.1 Oximetry

Oximetry refers to the colorimetric measurement of the degree of oxygen saturation of blood, that is, the relative amount of oxygen carried by the hemoglobin in the erythrocytes, by recording the variation in the color of deoxyhemoglobin (Hb) and oxyhemoglobin (HbO_2). A quantitative method for measuring blood oxygenation is of great importance in assessing the circulatory and respiratory status of a patient.

Various optical methods for measuring the oxygen saturation of arterial (SaO_2) and mixed venous (SvO_2) blood have been developed, all based on light transmission through, or reflecting from, tissue and blood. The measurement is performed at two specific wavelengths: $l1$, where there is a large difference in light absorbance between Hb and HbO_2 (e.g., 660 nm red light), and $l2$, which can be an isobestic wavelength (e.g., 805 nm infrared light), where the absorbance of light is independent of blood oxygenation, or a different wavelength in the infrared region (>805 nm), where the absorbance of Hb is slightly smaller than that of HbO_2.

Assuming for simplicity that a hemolyzed blood sample consists of a two-component homogeneous mixture of Hb and HbO_2, and that light absorbance by the mixture of these two components is additive, a simple quantitative relationship can be derived for computing the oxygen saturation of blood:

$$\text{Oxygen saturation} = A - B\left[\frac{\text{OD}(\lambda_1)}{\text{OD}(\lambda_2)}\right] \tag{49.1}$$

where A and B are coefficients which are functions of the specific absorptivities of Hb and HbO_2, and OD is the corresponding absorbance (optical density) of the blood [4].

Since the original discovery of this phenomenon over 50 years ago, there has been progressive development in instrumentation to measure oxygen saturation along three different paths: bench-top oximeters for clinical laboratories, fiber optic catheters for invasive intravascular monitoring, and transcutaneous sensors, which are noninvasive devices placed against the skin.

49.4.1.1 Intravascular Fiber Optic SvO_2 Catheters

In vivo fiberoptic oximeters were first described in the early 1960s by Polanyi and Heir [1]. They demonstrated that in a highly scattering medium such as blood, where a very short path length is required for a transmittance measurement, a reflectance measurement was practical. Accordingly, they showed that a linear relationship exists between oxygen saturation and the ratio of the infrared-to-red (IR/R) light backscattered from the blood

$$\text{oxygen saturation} = a - b(\text{IR/R}) \tag{49.2}$$

where a and b are catheter-specific calibration coefficients.

Fiber optic SvO_2 catheters consist of two separate optical fibers. One fiber is used for transmitting the light to the flowing blood, and a second fiber directs the backscattered light to a photodetector. In some commercial instruments (e.g., Oximetrix), automatic compensation for hematocrit is employed utilizing three, rather than two, infrared reference wavelengths. Bornzin et al. [2] and Mendelson et al. [3] described a 5-lumen, 7.5F thermodilution catheter that is comprised of three unequally spaced optical fibers, each fiber 250 mm in diameter, and provides continuous SvO_2 reading with automatic corrections for hematocrit variations (Figure 49.5).

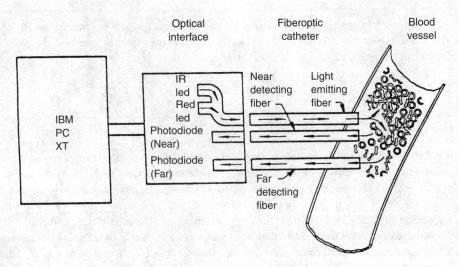

FIGURE 49.5 Principle of a three-fiber optical catheter for SvO$_2$/HCT measurement. (Taken from Bornzin G.A., Mendelson Y., Moran B.L., et al. 1987. *Proc. 9th Ann. Conf. Eng. Med. Bio. Soc.* pp. 807–809. With permission.)

Intravenous fiberoptic catheters are utilized in monitoring SvO$_2$ in the pulmonary artery and can be used to indicate the effectiveness of the cardiopulmonary system during cardiac surgery and in the ICU. Several problems limit the wide clinical application of intravascular fiberoptic oximeters. These include the dependence of the individual red and infrared backscattered light intensities and their ratio on hematocrit (especially for SvO$_2$ below 80%), blood flow, motion artifacts due to catheter tip "whipping" against the blood vessel wall, blood temperature, and pH.

49.4.1.2 Noninvasive Pulse Oximetry

Noninvasive monitoring of SaO$_2$ by pulse oximetry is a well-established practice in many fields of clinical medicine [4]. The most important advantage of this technique is the capability to provide continuous, safe, and effective monitoring of blood oxygenation at the patient's bedside without the need to calibrate the instrument before each use.

Pulse oximetry, which was first suggested by Aoyagi and colleagues [5] and Yoshiya and colleagues [6], relies on the detection of the time-variant photoplethysmographic signal, caused by changes in arterial blood volume associated with cardiac contraction. SaO$_2$ is derived by analyzing only the time-variant changes in absorbance caused by the pulsating arterial blood at the same red and infrared wavelengths used in conventional invasive type oximeters. A normalization process is commonly performed by which the pulsatile (a.c.) component at each wavelength, which results from the expansion and relaxation of the arterial bed, is divided by the corresponding nonpulsatile (d.c.) component of the photoplethysmogram, which is composed of the light absorbed by the blood-less tissue and the nonpulsatile portion of the blood compartment. This effective scaling process results in a normalized red/infrared ratio which is dependent on SaO$_2$ but is largely independent of the incident light intensity, skin pigmentation, skin thickness, and tissue vasculature.

Pulse oximeter sensors consist of a pair of small and inexpensive red and infrared LEDs and a single, highly sensitive, silicon photodetector. These components are mounted inside a reusable rigid spring-loaded clip, a flexible probe, or a disposable adhesive wrap (Figure 49.6). The majority of the commercially available sensors are of the transmittance type in which the pulsatile arterial bed, for example, ear lobe, fingertip, or toe, is positioned between the LEDs and the photodetector. Other probes are available for reflectance (backscatter) measurement where both the LEDs and photodetectors are mounted side-by-side facing the skin [7,8].

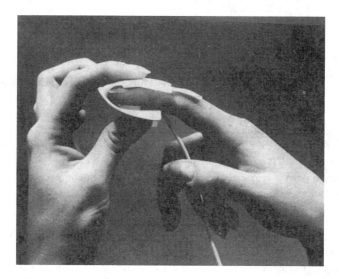

FIGURE 49.6 Disposable finger probe of a noninvasive pulse oximeter.

49.4.1.3 Noninvasive Cerebral Oximetry

Another substance whose optical absorption in the near infrared changes corresponding to its reduced and oxidized state is cytochrome aa3, the terminal member of the respiratory chain. Although the concentration of cytochrome aa3 is considerably lower than that of hemoglobin, advanced instrumentation including time-resolved spectroscopy and differential measurements is being used successfully to obtain noninvasive measurements of hemoglobin saturation and cytochrome aa3 by transilluminating areas of the neonatal brain [9–11].

49.4.2 Blood Gases

Frequent measurement of blood gases, that is, oxygen partial pressure (PO_2), carbon dioxide partial pressure (PCO_2), and pH, is essential to clinical diagnosis and management of respiratory and metabolic problems in the operating room and the ICU. Considerable effort has been devoted over the last two decades to developing disposable extracorporeal and in particular intravascular fiber optic sensors that can be used to provide continuous information on the acid-base status of a patient.

In the early 1970s, Lübbers and Opitz [12] originated what they called optodes (from the Greek, optical path) for measurements of important physiologic gases in fluids and in gases. The principle upon which these sensors was designed was a closed cell containing a fluorescent indicator in solution, with a membrane permeable to the analyte of interest (either ions or gases) constituting one of the cell walls. The cell was coupled by optical fibers to a system that measured the fluorescence in the cell. The cell solution would equilibrate with the PO_2 or PCO_2 of the medium placed against it, and the fluorescence of an indicator reagent in the solution would correspond to the partial pressure of the measured gas.

49.4.2.1 Extracorporeal Measurement

Following the initial feasibility studies of Lübbers and Opitz, Cardiovascular Devices (CDI, USA) developed a GasStat™ extracorporeal system suitable for continuous online monitoring of blood gases *ex vivo* during cardiopulmonary bypass operations. The system consists of a disposable plastic sensor connected inline with a blood loop through a fiber optic cable. Permeable membranes separate the flowing blood from the system chemistry. The CO_2-sensitive indicator consists of a fine emulsion of a bicarbonate buffer in a two-component silicone. The pH-sensitive indicator is a cellulose material to which hydroxypyrene trisulfonate (HPTS) is bonded covalently. The O_2-sensitive chemistry is composed of

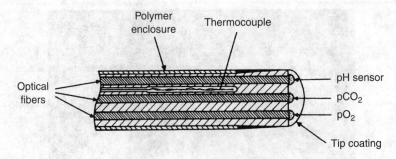

FIGURE 49.7 Structural diagram of an integrated fiber optic blood gas catheter. (Taken from Otto S. Wolfbeis, *Fiber Optic Chemical Sensors and Biosensors*, Vol. 2, CRC Press, Boca Raton, 1990.)

a solution of oxygen-quenching decacyclene in a one-component silicone covered with a thin layer of black PTFE for optical isolation and to render the measurement insensitive to the halothane anesthetic.

The extracorporeal device has two channels, one for arterial blood and the other for venous blood, and is capable of recording the temperature of the blood for correcting the measurements to 37°C. Several studies have been conducted comparing the specifications of the GasStat™ with that of intermittent blood samples analyzed on bench-top blood gas analyzers [13–15].

49.4.2.2 Intravascular Catheters

In recent years, numerous efforts have been made to develop integrated fiber optic sensors for intravascular monitoring of blood gases. Recent literature reports of sensor performance show considerable progress has been made mainly in improving the accuracy and reliability of these intravascular blood gas sensors [16–19], yet their performance has not yet reached a level suitable for widespread clinical application.

Most fiber optic intravascular blood gas sensors employ either a single- or double-fiber configuration. Typically, the matrix containing the indicator is attached to the end of the optical fiber as illustrated in Figure 49.7. Since the solubility of O_2 and CO_2 gases, as well as the optical properties of the sensing chemistry itself, are affected by temperature variations, fiber optic intravascular sensors include a thermo-couple or thermistor wire running alongside the fiber optic cable to monitor and correct for temperature fluctuations near the sensor tip. A nonlinear response is characteristic of most chemical indicator sensors, so they are designed to match the concentration region of the intended application. Also, the response time of the optode is somewhat slower compared to electrochemical sensors.

Intravascular fiber optic blood gas sensors are normally placed inside a standard 20-gauge catheter, which is sufficiently small to allow adequate spacing between the sensor and the catheter wall. The resulting lumen is large enough to permit the withdrawal of blood samples, introduction of a continuous heparin flush, and the recording of a blood pressure waveform. In addition, the optical fibers are encased in a protective tubing to contain any fiber fragments in case they break off.

49.4.2.3 pH Sensors

In 1976, Peterson et al. [20] originated the development of the first fiber optic chemical sensor for physiological pH measurement. The basic idea was to contain a reversible color-changing indicator at the end of a pair of optical fibers. The indicator, phenol red, was covalently bound to a hydrophilic polymer in the form of water-permeable microbeads. This technique stabilized the indicator concentration. The indicator beads were contained in a sealed hydrogen-ion-permeable envelope made out of a hollow cellulose tubing. In effect, this formed a miniature spectrophotometric cell at the end of the fibers and represented an early prototype of a fiber optic chemical sensor.

The phenol red dye indicator is a weak organic acid, and the acid form (un-ionized) and base form (ionized) are present in a concentration ratio determined by the ionization constant of the acid and the pH of the medium according to the familiar Henderson-Hasselbalch equation. The two forms of the dye have different optical absorption spectra, so the relative concentration of one of the forms, which varies as a function of pH, can be measured optically and related to variations in pH. In the pH sensor, green (560 nm) and red (longer than 600 nm) light emerging from the end of one fiber passes through the dye and is reflected back into the other fiber by light-scattering particles. The green light is absorbed by the base form of the indicator. The red light is not absorbed by the indicator and is used as an optical reference. The ratio of green to red light is measured and is related to pH by an S-shaped curve with an approximate high-sensitivity linear region where the equilibrium constant (pK) of the indicator matches the pH of the solution.

The same principle can also be used with a reversible fluorescent indicator, in which case the concentration of one of the indicator forms is measured by its fluorescence rather than absorbance intensity. Light in the blue or UV wavelength region excites the fluorescent dye to emit longer wavelength light, and the two forms of the dye may have different excitation or emission spectra to allow their distinction.

The original instrument design for a pH measurement was very simple and consisted of a tungsten lamp for fiber illumination, a rotating filter wheel to select the green and red light returning from the fiber optic sensor, and signal processing instrumentation to give a pH output based on the green-to-red ratio. This system was capable of measuring pH in the physiologic range between 7.0 and 7.4 with an accuracy and precision of 0.01 pH units. The sensor was susceptible to ionic strength variation in the order of 0.01 pH unit per 11% change in ionic strength.

Further development of the pH probe for practical use was continued by Markle and colleagues [21]. They designed the fiber optic probe in the form of a 25-gauge (0.5 mm OD) hypodermic needle, with an ion-permeable side window, using 75-μm-diameter plastic optical fibers. The sensor had a 90% response time of 30 s. With improved instrumentation and computerized signal processing and with a three-point calibration, the range was extended to ± 3 pH units, and a precision of 0.001 pH units was achieved.

Several reports have appeared suggesting other dye indicator systems that can be used for fiber optic pH sensing [22]. A classic problem with dye indicators is the sensitivity of their equilibrium constant to ionic strength. To circumvent this problem, Wolfbeis and Offenbacher [23] and Opitz and Lübbers [24] demonstrated a system in which a dual sensor arrangement can measure ionic strength and pH and simultaneously can correct the pH measurement for variations in ionic strength.

49.4.2.4 PCO$_2$ Sensors

The PCO$_2$ of a sample is typically determined by measuring changes in the pH of a bicarbonate solution that is isolated from the sample by a CO$_2$-permeable membrane but remains in equilibrium with the CO$_2$. The bicarbonate and CO$_2$, as carbonic acid, form a pH buffer system, and, by the Henderson–Hasselbalch equation, hydrogen ion concentration is proportional to the pCO$_2$ in the sample. This measurement is done with either a pH electrode or a dye indicator in solution.

Vurek [25] demonstrated that the same techniques can also be used with a fiber optic sensor. In his design, one plastic fiber carries light to the transducer, which is made of a silicone rubber tubing about 0.6 mm in diameter and 1.0 mm long, filled with a phenol red solution in a 35-mM bicarbonate. Ambient PCO$_2$ controls the pH of the solution which changes the optical absorption of the phenol red dye. The CO$_2$ permeates through the rubber to equilibrate with the indicator solution. A second optical fiber carries the transmitted signal to a photodetector for analysis. The design by Zhujun and Seitz [26] uses a PCO$_2$ sensor based on a pair of membranes separated from a bifurcated optical fiber by a cavity filled with bicarbonate buffer. The external membrane is made of silicone, and the internal membrane is HPTS immobilized on an ion-exchange membrane.

49.4.2.5 PO$_2$ Sensors

The development of an indicator system for fiber optic PO$_2$ sensing is challenging because there are very few known ways to measure PO$_2$ optically. Although a color-changing indicator would have been desirable, the development of a sufficiently stable indicator has been difficult. The only principle applicable to fiber optics appears to be the quenching effect of oxygen on fluorescence.

Fluorescence quenching is a general property of aromatic molecules, dyes containing them, and some other substances. In brief, when light is absorbed by a molecule, the absorbed energy is held as an excited electronic state of the molecule. It is then lost by coupling to the mechanical movement of the molecule (heat), reradiated from the molecule in a mean time of about 10 nsec (fluorescence), or converted into another excited state with much longer mean lifetime and then reradiated (phosphorescence). Quenching reduces the intensity of fluorescence and is related to the concentration of the quenching molecules, such as O_2.

A fiber optic sensor for measuring PO_2 using the principle of fluorescence quenching was developed by Peterson and colleagues [27]. The dye is excited at around 470 nm (blue) and fluoresces at about 515 nm (green) with an intensity that depends on the PO_2. The optical information is derived from the ratio of green fluorescence to the blue excitation light, which serves as an internal reference signal. The system was chosen for visible light excitation, because plastic optical fibers block light transmission at wavelengths shorter than 450 nm, and glass fibers were not considered acceptable for biomedical use.

The sensor was similar in design to the pH probe continuing the basic idea of an indicator packing in a permeable container at the end of a pair of optical fibers. A dye perylene dibutyrate, absorbed on a macroreticular polystyrene adsorbent, is contained in a oxygen-permeable porous polystyrene envelope. The ratio of green to blue intensity was processed according to the Stren–Volmer equation:

$$\frac{I_0}{I} = 1 + KPO_2 \tag{49.3}$$

where I and I_0 are the fluorescence emission intensities in the presence and absence of a quencher, respectively, and I is the Stern-Volmer quenching coefficient. This provides a nearly linear readout of PO_2 over the range of 0–150 mmHg (0–20 kPa), with a precision of 1 mmHg (0.13 kPa). The original sensor was 0.5 mm in diameter, but it can be made much smaller. Although its response time in a gas mixture is a fraction of a second, it is slower in an aqueous system, about 1.5 min for 90% response.

Wolfbeis et al. [28] designed a system for measuring the widely used halothane anesthetic which interferes with the measurement of oxygen. This dual-sensor combination had two semipermeable membranes (one of which blocked halothane) so that the probe could measure both oxygen and halothane simultaneously. The response time of their sensor, 15–20 sec for halothane and 10–15 sec for oxygen, is considered short enough to allow gas analysis in the breathing circuit. Potential applications of this device include the continuous monitoring of halothane in breathing circuits and in the blood.

49.4.3 Glucose Sensors

Another important principle that can be used in fiber optic sensors for measurements of high sensitivity and specificity is the concept of competitive binding. This was first described by Schultz et al. [29] to construct a glucose sensor. In their unique sensor, the analyte (glucose) competes for binding sites on a substrate (the lectin concanavalin A) with a fluorescent indicator-tagged polymer [fluorescein isothiocyanate (FITC)-dextran]. The sensor, which is illustrated in Figure 49.8, is arranged so that the substrate is fixed in a position out of the optical path of the fiber end. The substrate is bound to the inner wall of a glucose-permeable hollow fiber tubing (300 m O.D. × 200 m ID) and fastened to the end of an optical fiber. The hollow fiber acts as the container and is impermeable to the large molecules of the fluorescent indicator. The light beam that extends from the fiber "sees" only the unbound indictor in solution inside the hollow fiber but not the indicator bound on the container wall. Excitation light passes through the fiber and into the solution, fluorescing the unbound indicator, and the fluorescent light passes back along the same fiber to a measuring system. The fluorescent indicator and the glucose are in competitive binding equilibrium with the substrate. The interior glucose concentration equilibrates with its concentration exterior to the probe. If the glucose concentration increases, the indicator is driven off the substrate to increase the concentration of the indicator. Thus, fluorescence intensity as seen by the optical fiber follows the glucose concentration.

The response time of the sensor was found to be about 5 min. *In vivo* studies demonstrated fairly close correspondence between the sensor output and actual blood glucose levels. A time lag of about 5 min

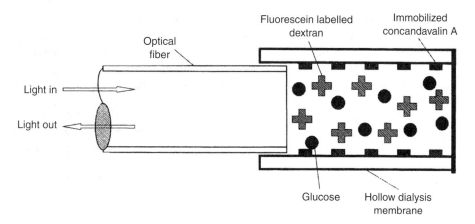

FIGURE 49.8   Schematic diagram of a competitive binding fluorescence affinity sensor for glucose measurement. (Taken from Schultz J.S., Mansouri S., and Goldstein I.J. 1982. *Diabetes Care* 5: 245. With permission.)

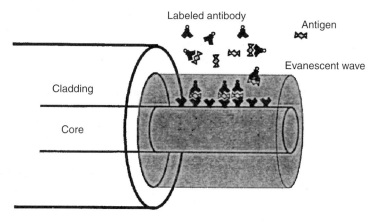

FIGURE 49.9   Basic principle of a fiber optic antigen-antibody sensor. (Taken from Anderson G.P., Golden J.P., and Ligler F.S. 1993. *IEEE Trans. Biomed. Eng.* 41: 578.)

was found and is believed to be due to the diffusion of glucose across the hollow fiber membrane and the diffusion of FTIC-dextran within the tubing.

In principle, the concept of competitive binding can be applied to any analysis for which a specific reaction can be devised. However, long-term stability of these sensors remains the major limiting factor that needs to be solved.

49.4.4 Immunosensors

Immunologic techniques offer outstanding selectivity and sensitivity through the process of antibody–antigen interaction. This is the primary recognition mechanism by which the immune system detects and fights foreign matter and has therefore allowed the measurement of many important compounds at trace levels in complex biologic samples.

In principle, it is possible to design competitive binding optical sensors utilizing immobilized antibodies as selective reagents and detecting the displacement of a labeled antigen by the analyte. Therefore, antibody-based immunologic optical systems have been the subject of considerable research [30–34]. In practice, however, the strong binding of antigens to antibodies and vice versa causes difficulties in constructing reversible sensors with fast dynamic responses.

Several immunologic sensors based on fiber optic waveguides have been demonstrated for monitoring antibody–antigen reactions. Typically, several centimeters of cladding are removed along the fiber's distal end, and the recognition antibodies are immobilized on the exposed core surface. These antibodies bind fluorophore-antigen complexes within the evanescent wave as illustrated in Figure 49.9. The fluorescent signal excited within the evanescent wave is then transmitted through the cladded fiber to a fluorimeter for processing.

Experimental studies have indicated that immunologic optical sensors can generally detect micromolar and even picomolar concentrations. However, the major obstacle that must be overcome to achieve high sensitivity in immunologic optical sensors is the nonspecific binding of immobilized antibodies.

References

[1] Polanyi M.L. and Heir R.M. 1962. *In vivo* oximeter with fast dynamic response. *Rev. Sci. Instrum.* 33: 1050.

[2] Bornzin G.A., Mendelson Y., Moran B.L. et al. 1987. Measuring oxygen saturation and hematocrit using a fiberoptic catheter. *Proc. 9th Ann. Conf. Eng. Med. Bio. Soc.* pp. 807–809.

[3] Mendelson Y., Galvin J.J., and Wang Y. 1990. *In vitro* evaluation of a dual oxygen saturation/hematocrit intravascular fiberoptic catheter. *Biomed. Instrum. Tech.* 24: 199.

[4] Mendelson Y. 1992. Pulse oximetry: Theory and application for noninvasive monitoring. *Clin. Chem.* 28: 1601.

[5] Aoyagi T., Kishi M., Yamaguchi K. et al. 1974. Improvement of the earpiece oximeter. *Jpn. Soc. Med. Electron. Biomed. Eng.* 90–91.

[6] Yoshiya I., Shimada Y., and Tanaka K. 1980. Spectrophotometric monitoring of arterial oxygen saturation in the fingertip. *Med. Biol. Eng. Comput.* 18: 27.

[7] Mendelson Y. and Solomita M.V. 1992. The feasibility of spectrophotometric measurements of arterial oxygen saturation from the scalp utilizing noninvasive skin reflectance pulse oximetry. *Biomed. Instrum. Technol.* 26: 215.

[8] Mendelson Y. and McGinn M.J. 1991. Skin reflectance pulse oximetry: *in vivo* measurements from the forearm and calf. *J. Clin. Monit.* 7: 7.

[9] Chance B., Leigh H., Miyake H. et al. 1988. Comparison of time resolved and un-resolved measurements of deoxyhemoglobin in brain. *Proc. Natl Acad. Sci. USA* 85: 4971.

[10] Jobsis F.F., Keizer J.H., LaManna J.C. et al. 1977. Reflection spectrophotometry of cytochrome aa3 *in vivo*. *Appl. Physiol: Respirat. Environ. Excerc. Physiol.* 43: 858.

[11] Kurth C.D., Steven I.M., Benaron D. et al. 1993. Near-infrared monitoring of the cerebral circulation. *J. Clin. Monit.* 9: 163.

[12] Lübbers D.W. and Opitz N. 1975. The pCO_2/pO_2-optode: a new probe for measurement of pCO_2 or pO_2 in fluids and gases. *Z. Naturforsch. C: Biosci.* 30C: 532.

[13] Clark C.L., O'Brien J., McCulloch J. et al. 1986. Early clinical experience with GasStat. *J. Extra Corporeal. Technol.* 18: 185.

[14] Hill A.G., Groom R.C., Vinansky R.P. et al. 1985. On-line or off-line blood gas analysis: Cost vs. time vs. accuracy. *Proc. Am. Acad. Cardiovasc. Perfusion* 6: 148.

[15] Siggaard-Andersen O., Gothgen I.H., Wimberley et al. 1988. Evaluation of the GasStat fluorescence sensors for continuous measurement of pH, pCO_2 and pO_3 during CPB and hypothermia. *Scand. J. Clin. Lab. Invest.* 48: 77.

[16] Zimmerman J.L. and Dellinger R.P. 1993. Initial evaluation of a new intra-arterial blood gas system in humans. *Crit. Care Med.* 21: 495.

[17] Gottlieb A. 1992. The optical measurement of blood gases — approaches, problems and trends: Fiber optic medical and fluorescent sensors and applications. *Proc. SPIE* 1648: 4.

[18] Barker S.L. and Hyatt J. 1991. Continuous measurement of intraarterial pHa, $PaCO_2$, and PaO_2 in the operation room. *Anesth. Analg.* 73: 43.

[19] Larson C.P., Divers G.A., and Riccitelli S.D. 1991. Continuous monitoring of PaO_2 and $PaCO_2$ in surgical patients. *Abstr. Crit. Care Med.* 19: 525.

[20] Peterson J.I., Goldstein S.R., and Fitzgerald R.V. 1980. Fiber optic pH probe for physiological use. *Anal. Chem.* 52: 864.

[21] Markle D.R., McGuire D.A., Goldstein S.R. et al. 1981. A pH measurement system for use in tissue and blood, employing miniature fiber optic probes. In D.C. Viano (Ed.), *Advances in Bioengineering*, p. 123, New York, American Society of Mechanical Engineers.

[22] Wolfbeis O.S., Furlinger E., Kroneis H. et al. 1983. Fluorimeter analysis: 1. A study on fluorescent indicators for measuring near neutral (physiological) pH values. *Fresenius' Z. Anal. Chem.* 314: 119.

[23] Wolfbeis O.S. and Offenbacher H. 1986. Fluorescence sensor for monitoring ionic strength and physiological pH values. *Sens. Actuat.* 9: 85.

[24] Opitz N. and Lübbers D.W. 1983. New fluorescence photomatrical techniques for simultaneous and continuous measurements of ionic strength and hydrogen ion activities. *Sens. Actuat.* 4: 473.

[25] Vurek G.G., Feustel P.J., and Severinghaus J.W. 1983. A fiber optic pCO_2 sensor. *Ann. Biomed. Eng.* 11: 499.

[26] Zhujun Z. and Seitz W.R. 1984. A carbon dioxide sensor based on fluorescence. *Anal. Chim. Acta* 160: 305.

[27] Peterson J.I., Fitzgerald R.V., and Buckhold D.K. 1984. Fiber-optic probe for *in vivo* measurements of oxygen partial pressure. *Anal. Chem.* 56: 62.

[28] Wolfbeis O.S., Posch H.E., and Kroneis H.W. 1985. Fiber optical fluorosensor for determination of halothane and/or oxygen. *Anal. Chem.* 57: 2556.

[29] Schultz J.S., Mansouri S., and Goldstein I.J. 1982. Affinity sensor: a new technique for developing implantable sensors for glucose and other metabolites. *Diabetes Care* 5: 245.

[30] Andrade J.D., Vanwagenen R.A., Gregonis D.E. et al. 1985. Remote fiber optic biosensors based on evanescent-excited fluoro-immunoassay: concept and progress. *IEEE Trans. Elect. Devices* ED-32: 1175.

[31] Sutherland R.M., Daehne C., Place J.F. et al. 1984. Optical detection of antibody–antigen reactions at a glass–liquid interface. *Clin. Chem.* 30: 1533.

[32] Hirschfeld T.E. and Block M.J. 1984. Fluorescent immunoassay employing optical fiber in a capillary tube. US Patent No. 4,447,546.

[33] Anderson G.P., Golden J.P., and Ligler F.S. 1993. An evanescent wave biosensor: Part I. Fluorescent signal acquisition from step-etched fiber optic probes. *IEEE Trans. Biomed. Eng.* 41: 578.

[34] Golden J.P., Anderson G.P., Rabbany S.Y. et al. 1994. An evanescent wave biosensor: Part II. Fluorescent signal acquisition from tapered fiber optic probes. *IEEE Trans. Biomed. Eng.* 41: 585.

50

Bioanalytic Sensors

50.1 Classification of Biochemical Reactions in the
Context of Sensor Design and Development 50-1
Introduction and Definitions • Classification of Recognition
Reactions and Receptor Processes
50.2 Classification of Transduction Processes — Detection
Methods 50-2
Calorimetric, Thermometric, and Pyroelectric Transducers •
Optical, Optoelectronic Transducers • Piezoelectric
Transducers • Electrochemical Transducers
50.3 Tables of Sensors from the Literature 50-8
50.4 Applications of Microelectronics in Sensor
Fabrication 50-8
References 50-10

Richard P. Buck
University of North Carolina

50.1 Classification of Biochemical Reactions in the Context of Sensor Design and Development

50.1.1 Introduction and Definitions

Since sensors generate a measurable material property, they belong in some grouping of transducer devices. Sensors specifically contain a recognition process that is characteristic of a material sample at the molecular-chemical level, and a sensor incorporates a transduction process (step) to create a useful signal. Biomedical sensors include a whole range of devices that may be chemical sensors, physical sensors, or some kind of mixed sensor.

Chemical sensors use chemical processes in the recognition and transduction steps. Biosensors are also chemical sensors, but they use particular classes of biological recognition/transduction processes. A pure physical sensor generates and transduces a parameter that does not depend on the chemistry per se, but is a result of the sensor responding as an aggregate of point masses or charges. All these when used in a biologic system (biomatrix) may be considered bioanalytic sensors without regard to the chemical, biochemical, or physical distinctions. They provide an "analytic signal of the biologic system" for some further use.

The chemical recognition process focuses on some molecular-level chemical entity, usually a kind of chemical structure. In classical analysis this structure may be a simple functional group: SiO — in a glass electrode surface, a chromophore in an indicator dye, or a metallic surface structure, such as silver metal that recognizes Ag+ in solution. In recent times, the biologic recognition processes have been better understood, and the general concept of recognition by receptor or chemoreceptor has come into fashion. Although these are often large molecules bound to cell membranes, they contain specific structures that

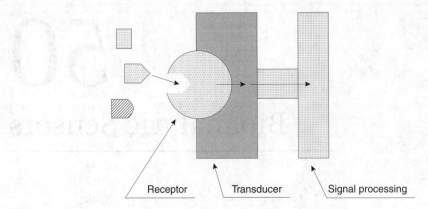

FIGURE 50.1   Generic bioanalytic sensor.

permit a wide variety of different molecular recognition steps including recognition of large and small species and of charged and uncharged species. Thus, chemoreceptor appears in the sensor literature as a generic term for the principal entity doing the recognition. For a history and examples, see References 1 to 6.

Biorecognition in biosensors has especially stressed "receptors" and their categories. Historically, application of receptors has not necessarily meant measurement directly of the receptor. Usually there are coupled chemical reactions, and the transduction has used measurement of the subsidiary products: change of pH, change of dissolved O_2, generation of H_2O_2, changes of conductivity, changes of optical adsorption, and changes of temperature. Principal receptors are enzymes because of their extraordinary selectivity. Other receptors can be the more subtle species of biochemistry: antibodies, organelles, microbes, and tissue slices, not to mention the trace level "receptors" that guide ants, such as pheromones, and other unusual species. A sketch of a generic bioanalytic sensor is shown in Figure 50.1.

50.1.2 Classification of Recognition Reactions and Receptor Processes

The concept of recognition in chemistry is universal. It almost goes without saying that all chemical reactions involved recognition and selection on the basis of size, shape, and charge. For the purpose of constructing sensors, general recognition based on these factors is not usually enough. Frequently in inorganic chemistry a given ion will react indiscriminantly with similar ions of the same size and charge. Changes in charge from unity to two, for example, do change the driving forces of some ionic reactions. By control of dielectric constant of phases, heterogeneous reactions can often be "tailored" to select divalent ions over monovalent ions and to select small versus large ions or vice versa.

Shape, however, has more special possibilities, and natural synthetic methods permit product control. Nature manages to use shape together with charge to build organic molecules, called enzymes, that have acquired remarkable selectivity. It is in the realm of biochemistry that these natural constructions are investigated and catalogued. Biochemistry books list large numbers of enzymes and other selective materials that direct chemical reactions. Many of these have been tried as the basis of selective sensors for bioanalytic and biomedical purposes. The list in Table 50.1 shows how some of the materials can be grouped into lists according to function and to analytic substrate, both organic and inorganic. The principles seem general, so there is no reason to discriminate against the inorganic substrates in favor or the organic substrates. All can be used in biomedical analysis.

50.2 Classification of Transduction Processes — Detection Methods

Some years ago, the engineering community addressed the topic of sensor classification — Richard M. White in *IEEE Trans. Ultra., Ferro., Freq. Control* (UFFC), UFFC-34 (1987) 124, and Wen H. Ko

TABLE 50.1 Recognition Reactions and Receptor Processes

1. Insoluble salt-based sensors
   a. $S^+ + R^-$ 1 (insoluble salt)
   Ion exchange with crystalline SR (homogeneous or heterogeneous crystals)

chemical signal S^{+n}	receptor R^{-n}
inorganic cations	inorganic anions
examples: Ag^+, Hg_2^{2+}, Pb^{2+}, Cd^{2+}, Cu^{2+}	$S^=$, $Se^{2=}$, SCN^-, I^-, Br^-, Cl^-

   b. $S^{-n} + R^{+n}$ 1SR (insoluble salt)
   Ion exchange with crystalline SR (homogeneous or heterogeneous crystals)

chemical signal S^{-n}	receptor R^{+n}
inorganic anions	inorganic cations
examples: F^-, $S^=$, $Se^{2=}$, SCN^-, I^-, Br^-, Cl^-	LaF_2^+, Ag^+, Hg_2^{2+}, Pb^{2+}, Cd^{2+}, Cu^{2+}

2. Solid ion exchanges
   a. $S^{+n} + R^{-n}$ (sites) lS^{+n} R^{-n} = SR (in ion exchanger phase)
   Ion exchange with synthetic ion exchangers containing negative fixed sites (homogeneous or heterogeneous, inorganic or organic materials)

chemical signal S^{+n}	receptor R^{-n}
inorganic and organic ions	inorganic and organic ion sites
examples: H^+, Na^+, K^+	silicate glass $Si\text{-}0^-$
H^+, Na^+, K^+, other M^{+n}	synthetic sulfonated, phosphorylated, EDTA-substituted polystyrenes

   b. $S^{-n} + R^{+n}$ (sites) $1S^{-n}$ R^{+n} = SR (in ion exchanger phase)
   Ion exchange with synthetic ion exchangers containing positive fixed sites (homogeneous or heterogeneous, inorganic or organic materials)

chemical signal S^{-n}	receptor R^{+n}
organic and inorganic ions	organic and inorganic ion sites
examples: hydrophobic anions	quaternized polystyrene

3. Liquid ion exchanger sensors with electrostatic selection
   a. $S^{-n} + R^{-n}$ (sites) lS^{+n} R^{-n} = SR (in ion exchanger phase)
   Plasticized, passive membranes containing mobile trapped negative fixed sites (homogeneous or heterogeneous, inorganic or organic materials)

chemical signal S^{+n}	receptor R^{-n}
inorganic and organic ions	inorganic and organic ion sites
examples: Ca^{2+}	diester of phosphoric acid or monoester of a phosphonic acid
M^{+n}	dinonylnaphthalene sulfonate and other organic, hydrophobic anions
R_1, R_2, R_3 R_4 N^+ and bis-Quaternary Cations cationic drugs tetrasubstituted arsonium$^-$	tetraphenylborate anion or substituted derivatives

   b. $S^{-n} + R^{+n}$ (sites) $1S^{-n}$ R^{+n} = SR (in ion exchanger phase)
   Plasticized, passive membranes containing mobile, trapped negative fixed sites (homogeneous or heterogeneous, inorganic or organic materials)

chemical signal S^{-n}	receptor R^{+n}
inorganic and organic ions	inorganic and organic sites
examples: anions, simple Cl^-, Br^-, ClO_4^-	quaternary ammonium cations: e.g., tridodecylmethyl-ammonium
anions, complex, drugs	quaternary ammonium cations: e.g., tridodecylmethyl-ammonium

(Continued)

TABLE 50.1 (Continued) Recognition Reactions and Receptor Processes

4. Liquid ion exchanger sensors with neutral (or charged) carrier selection
   a. $S^{+n} + X$ and R^{-n} (sites) $1S^{+n} X R^{-n} = SXR$ (in ion
   exchanger phase)
   Plasticized, passive membranes containing mobile, trapped negative fixed sites (homogeneous or heterogeneous,
   inorganic or organic materials)

chemical signal S^{+n}	receptor R^{-n}
inorganic and organic ions	inorganic and organic ion sites
examples: Ca^{2+}	$X =$ synthetic ionophore complexing agent selective to Ca^{2+}
	R^{-n} usually a substituted tetra phenylborate salt
Na^+, K^+, H^+	$X =$ selective ionophore complexing agent

   b. $S^{-n} + X$ and R^{+n} (sites) $1S^{-n} X R^{+n} = SXR$ (in ion
   exchanger phase)
   Plasticized, passive membranes containing mobile, trapped negative fixed sites (homogeneous or heterogeneous,
   inorganic or organic materials)

chemical signal S^{-n}	receptor R^{+n}
inorganic and organic ions	inorganic and organic ion sites
examples: $HPO_4^{2=}$	$R^{+n} =$ quaternary ammonium salt
	$X =$ synthetic ionophore complexing agent; aryl organotin compound or suggested cyclic polyamido-polyamines
HCO_3^-	$X =$ synthetic ionophore: trifluoro acetophenone
Cl^-	$X =$ aliphatic organotin compound

5. Bioaffinity sensors based on change of local electron densitites
   $S + R 1SR$

chemical signal S	receptor R
protein	dyes
saccharide	lectin
glycoprotein	
susbstrate	enzyme
inhibitor	Transferases
	Hydrolases (peptidases, esterases, etc.)
	Lyases
	Isomerases
	Ligases
prosthetic group	apoenzyme
antigen	antibody
hormone	"receptor"
substrate analogue	transport system

6. Metabolism sensors based on substrate consumption and product formation
   $S + R 1SR \rightarrow P + R$

chemical signal S	receptor R
substrate	enzyme
examples: lactate (SH_2)	hydrogenases catalyze hydrogen transfer from S to acceptor A (not molecular oxygen!) reversibly pyruvate + NADH +
$SH_2 + A 1S + AH_2$ lactate $+ NAD^+$	H^+ using lactate dehydrogenase
glucose (SH_2)	
$SH_2 + \frac{1}{2} O_2 1S + H_2O$ or	oxidases catalyze hydrogen transfer to molecular oxygen
$SH_2 + O_2 1S + H_2O_2$	using glucose oxidase
glucose $+ O_2$ 1gluconolactone $+ H_2O_2$	
reducing agents (S)	peroxidases catalyze oxidation of a substrate by H_2O_2 using horseradish peroxidase

(Continued)

TABLE 50.1 (Continued) Recognition Reactions and Receptor Processes

$2S + 2H^+ + H_2O_2\ 12S^+ + 2H_2O$	
$Fe^{2+} + H_2O_2 + 2H^+\ 1Fe^{3+} + 2H_2O$	
reducing agents	oxygenates catalyze substrate oxidations by molecular O_2
L-lactate + O_2 lactate + CO_2 + H_2O	
cofactor	organelle
inhibitor	microbe
activator	tissue slice
enzyme activity	

7. Coupled and hybrid systems using sequences, competition, anti-interference and amplification concepts and reactions.

8. Biomimetic sensors

chemical signal S	receptor R
sound	carrier-enzyme
stress	
light	

Source: Adapted from Scheller F., Schubert F. 1989. *Biosensors, #18 in Advances in Research Technologies (Beitrage zur Forschungstec technologies)*, Berlin, Akademie-Verlag, Amsterdam, Elsevier. Cosofret V.V., Buck R.P. 1992. *Pharmaceutical Applications of Membrane Sensors*, Boca Raton, FL, CRC Press.

in IEEE/EMBS Symposium Abstract T.1.1 84CH2068-5 (1984). It is interesting because the physical and chemical properties are given equal weight. There are many ideas given here that remain without embodiment. This list is reproduced as Table 50.2. Of particular interest in this section are "detection means used in sensors" and "sensor conversion phenomena." At present the principle transduction schemes use electrochemical, optical, and thermal detection effects and principles.

50.2.1 Calorimetric, Thermometric, and Pyroelectric Transducers

Especially useful for enzymatic reactions, the generation of heat (enthalpy change) can be used easily and generally. The enzyme provides the selectivity and the reaction enthalpy cannot be confused with other reactions from species in a typical biologic mixture. The ideal aim is to measure total evolved heat, that is, to perform a calorimetric measurement. In real systems there is always heat loss, that is, heat is conducted away by the sample and sample container so that the process cannot be adiabatic as required for a total heat evolution measurement. As a result, temperature difference before and after evolution is measured most often. It has to be assumed that the heat capacity of the specimen and container is constant over the small temperature range usually measured.

The simplest transducer is a thermometer coated with the enzyme that permits the selected reaction to proceed. Thermistors are used rather than thermometers or thermocouples. The change of resistance of certain oxides is much greater than the change of length of a mercury column or the microvolt changes of thermocouple junctions.

Pyroelectric heat flow transducers are relatively new. Heat flows from a heated region to a lower temperature region, controlled to occur in one dimension. The lower temperature side can be coated with an enzyme. When the substrate is converted, the lower temperature side is warmed. The pyroelectric material is from a category of materials that develops a spontaneous voltage difference in a thermal gradient. If the gradient is disturbed by evolution or adsorption of heat, the voltage temporarily changes.

In biomedical sensing, some of the solid-state devices based on thermal sensing cannot be used effectively. The reason is that the sensor itself has to be heated or is heated quite hot by catalytic surface reactions. Thus pellistors (oxides with catalytic surfaces and embedded platinum wire thermometer), chemiresistors, and "Figaro" sensor "smoke" detectors have not found many biologic applications.

TABLE 50.2 Detection Means and
Conversion Phenomena Used in Sensors

Detection means
  Biologic
  Chemical
  Electric, magnetic, or electromagnetic wave
  Heat, temperature
  Mechanical displacement of wave
  Radioactivity, radiation
  Other
Conversion phenomena
  Biologic
    Biochemical transformation
    Physical transformation
    Effect on test organism
    Spectroscopy
    Other
  Chemical
    Chemical transformation
    Physical transformation
    Electrochemical process
    Spectroscopy
    Other
  Physical
    Thermoelectric
    Photoelectric
    Photomagnetic
    Magnetoelectric
    Elastomagnetic
    Thermoelastic
    Elastoelectric
    Thermomagnetic
    Thermooptic
    Photoelastic
    Others

50.2.2   Optical, Optoelectronic Transducers

Most optical detection systems for sensors are small, that is, they occupy a small region of space because the sample size and volume are themselves small. This means that common absorption spectrophotometers and photofluorometers are not used with their conventional sample-containing cells, or with their conventional beam-handling systems. Instead light-conducting optical fibers are used to connect the sample with the more remote monochromator and optical readout system. The techniques still remain absorption spectrophotometry, fluorimetry including fluorescence quenching, and reflectometry.

The most widely published optical sensors use a miniature reagent contained or immobilized at the tip of an optical fiber. In most systems a permselective membrane coating allows the detected species to penetrate the dye region. The corresponding absorption change, usually at a sensitive externally preset wavelength, is changed and correlated with the sample concentration. Similarly, fluorescence can be stimulated by the higher-frequency external light source and the lower-frequency emission detected. Some configurations are illustrated in References 1 and 2. Fluorimetric detection of coenzyme A, NAD+/NADH, is involved in many so-called pyridine-linked enzyme systems. The fluorescence of NADH contained or immobilized can be a convenient way to follow these reactions. Optodes, miniature encapsulated dyes, can be placed *in vivo*. Their fluorescence can be enhanced or quenched and used to detect acidity, oxygen, and other species.

A subtle form of optical transduction uses the "peeled" optical fiber as a multiple reflectance cell. The normal fiber core glass has a refractive index greater than that of the exterior coating; there is a range of angles of entry to the fiber so that all the light beam remains inside the core. If the coating is removed and materials of lower index of refraction are coated on the exterior surface, there can be absorption by multiple reflections, since the evanescent wave can penetrate the coating. Chemical reagent can be added externally to create selective layers on the optical fiber.

Ellipsometry is a reflectance technique that depends on the optical constants and thickness of surface layer. For colorless layers, a polarized light beam will change its plane of polarization upon reflection by the surface film. The thickness can sometimes be determined when optical constants are known or approximated by constants of the bulk material. Antibody–antigen surface reaction can be detected this way.

50.2.3 Piezoelectric Transducers

Cut quartz crystals have characteristic modes of vibration that can be induced by painting electrodes on the opposite surfaces and applying a megaHertz ac voltage. The frequency is searched until the crystal goes into a resonance. The resonant frequency is very stable. It is a property of the material and maintains a value to a few parts per hundred million. When the surface is coated with a stiff mass, the frequency is altered. The shift in frequency is directly related to the surface mass for thin, stiff layers. The reaction of a substrate with this layer changes the constants of the film and further shifts the resonant frequency. These devices can be used in air, in vacuum, or in electrolyte solutions.

50.2.4 Electrochemical Transducers

Electrochemical transducers are commonly used in the sensor field. The main forms of electrochemistry used are potentiometry (zero-current cell voltage [potential difference measurements]), amperometry (current measurement at constant applied voltage at the working electrode), and ac conductivity of a cell.

50.2.4.1 Potentiometric Transduction

The classical generation of an activity-sensitive voltage is spontaneous in a solution containing both nonredox ions and redox ions. Classical electrodes of types 1, 2, and 3 respond by ion exchange directly or indirectly to ions of the same material as the electrode. Inert metal electrodes (sometimes called type 0) — Pt, Ir, Rh, and occasionally carbon C — respond by electrons exchange from redox pairs in solution. Potential differences are interfacial and reflect ratios of activities of oxidized to reduced forms.

50.2.4.2 Amperometric Transduction

For dissolved species that can exchange electrons with an inert electrode, it is possible to force the transfer in one direction by applying a voltage very oxidizing (anodic) or reducing (cathodic). When the voltage is fixed, the species will be, by definition, out of equilibrium with the electrode at its present applied voltage. Locally, the species (regardless of charge) will oxidize or reduce by moving from bulk solution to the electrode surface where they react. Ions do not move like electrons. Rather they diffuse from high to low concentration and do not usually move by drift or migration. The reason is that the electrolytes in solutions are at high concentrations, and the electric field is virtually eliminated from the bulk. The field drops through the first 1000 A at the electrode surface. The concentration of the moving species is from high concentration in bulk to zero at the electrode surface where it reacts. This process is called concentration polarization. The current flowing is limited by mass transport and so is proportional to the bulk concentration.

50.2.4.3 Conductometric Transducers

Ac conductivity (impedance) can be purely resistive when the frequency is picked to be about 1000 to 10,000 Hz. In this range the transport of ions is sufficiently slow that they never lose their uniform

TABLE 50.3   Chemical Sensors and Properties Documented in the
Literature

  I.   General topics including items II–V; selectivity, fabrication, data processing
 II.   Thermal sensors
III.   Mass sensors
      Gas sensors
      Liquid sensors
 IV.   Electrochemical sensors
      Potentiometric sensors
        Reference electrodes
        Biomedical electrodes
        Applications to cations, anions
        Coated wire/hybrids
        ISFETs and related
        Biosensors
        Gas sensors
      Amperometric sensors
        Modified electrodes
        Gas sensors
        Biosensors
          Direct electron transfer
          Mediated electron transfer
          Biomedical
      Conductimetric sensors
        Semiconducting oxide sensors
        Zinc oxide-based
        Chemiresistors
        Dielectrometers
  V.   Optical sensors
      Liquid sensors
      Biosensors
      Gas sensors

---

concentration. They simply quiver in space and carry current forward and backward each half cycle. In the lower and higher frequencies, the cell capacitance can become involved, but this effect is to be avoided.

50.3   Tables of Sensors from the Literature

The longest and most consistently complete references to the chemical sensor field is the review issue of Analytical Chemistry Journal. In the 1970s and 1980s these appeared in the April issue, but more recently they appear in the June issue. The editors are Jiri Janata and various colleagues [7–10]. Note all possible or imaginable sensors have been made according to the list in Table 50.2. A more realistic table can be constructed from the existing literature that describes actual devices. This list is Table 50.3. Book references are listed in Table 50.4 in reverse time order to about 1986. This list covers most of the major source books and many of the symposium proceedings volumes. The reviews [7–10] are a principal source of references to the published research literature.

50.4   Applications of Microelectronics in Sensor Fabrication

The reviews of sensors since 1988 cover fabrication papers and microfabrication methods and examples [7–10]. A recent review by two of the few chemical sensor scientists (chemical engineers) who also operate a microfabrication laboratory is C. C. Liu, Z.-R. Zhang. 1992. Research and development of chemical sensors using microfabrication techniques. *Selective Electrode* 14: 147.

TABLE 50.4 Books and Long Reviews Keyed to Items in Table 50.3 (Reviewed Since 1988 in Reverse Time Sequence)

I. **General Topics**

Yamauchi S. (ed). 1992. *Chemical Sensor Technology*, Vol 4, Tokyo, Kodansha Ltd.

Flores J.R., Lorenzo E. 1992. Amperometric biosensors, In M.R. Smyth, J.G. Vos (eds), *Comprehensive Analytical Chemistry*, Amsterdam, Elsevier

Vaihinger S., Goepel W. 1991. Multicomponent analysis in chemical sensing. In W. Goepel, J. Hesse, J. Zemel (eds), *Sensors*, Vol 2, Part 1, pp. 191–237, Weinheim, Germany, VCH Publishers

Wise D.L. (ed). 1991. *Bioinstrumentation and Biosensors*, New York, Marcel Dekker Scheller F., Schubert F. 1989. *Biosensors*, Basel, Switzerland, Birkhauser Verlag, see also [2].

Madou M., Morrison S.R. 1989. *Chemical Sensing with Solid State Devices*, New York, Academic Press.

Janata J. 1989. *Principles of Chemical Sensors*, New York, Plenum Press.

Edmonds T.E. (ed). 1988. *Chemical Sensors*, Glasgow, Blackie.

Yoda K. 1988. Immobilized enzyme cells. *Methods Enzymology*, 137: 61.

Turner A.P.F., Karube I., Wilson G.S. (eds). 1987. *Biosensors: Fundamentals and Applications*, Oxford, Oxford University Press.

Seiyama T. (ed). 1986. *Chemical Sensor Technology*, Tokyo, Kodansha Ltd.

II. **Thermal Sensors**

There are extensive research and application papers and these are mentioned in books listed under I. However, the up-to-date lists of papers are given in references 7 to 10.

III. **Mass Sensors**

There are extensive research and application papers and these are mentioned in books listed under I. However, the up-to-date lists of papers are given in references 7 to 10. Fundamentals of this rapidly expanding field are recently reviewed:

Buttry D.A., Ward M.D. 1992. Measurement of interfacial processes at electrode surfaces with the electrochemical quartz crystal microbalance, *Chemical Reviews* 92: 1355.

Grate J.W., Martin S.J., White R.M. 1993. Acoustic wave microsensors, Part 1, *Analyt Chem* 65: 940A; part 2, *Analyt. Chem.* 65: 987A.

Ricco A.T. 1994. SAW Chemical sensors, *The Electrochemical Society Interface Winter*: 38–44.

IVA. **Electrochemical Sensors — Liquid Samples**

Scheller F., Schmid R.D. (eds). 1992. *Biosensors: Fundamentals, Technologies and Applications*, GBF Monograph Series, New York, VCH Publishers.

Erbach R., Vogel A., Hoffmann B. 1992. Ion-sensitive field-effect structures with Langmuir-Blodgett membranes. In F. Scheller, R.D. Schmid (eds). *Biosensors: Fundamentals, Technologies, and Applications*, GBF Monograph 17, pp. 353–357, New York, VCH Publishers.

Ho May Y.K., Rechnitz G.A. 1992. An introduction to biosensors, In R.M. Nakamura, Y. Kasahara, G.A. Rechnitz (eds), *Immunochemical Assays and Biosensors Technology*, pp. 275–291, Washington, DC, American Society Microbiology.

Mattiasson B., Haakanson H. Immunochemically-based assays for process control, 1992. *Advances in Biochemical Engineering and Biotechnology* 46: 81.

Maas A.H., Sprokholt R. 1990. Proposed IFCC Recommendations for electrolyte measurements with ISEs in clinical chemistry, In A. Ivaska, A. Lewenstam, R. Sara (eds), *Contemporary Electroanalytical Chemistry, Proceedings of the ElectroFinnAnalysis International Conference on Electroanalytical Chemistry*, pp. 311–315, New York, Plenum.

Vanrolleghem P., Dries D., Verstreate W. RODTOX: Biosensor for rapid determination of the biochemical oxygen demand, 1990. In C. Christiansen, L. Munck, J. Villadsen (eds), *Proceedings of the 5th European Congress Biotechnology*, Vol 1, pp. 161–164, Copenhagen, Denmark, Munksgaard.

Cronenberg C., Van den Heuvel H., Van den Hauw M., Van Groen B. Development of glucose microelectrodes for measurements in biofilms, 1990. In C. Christiansen, L. Munck, J. Villadsen (eds), *Proceedings of the 5th European Congress Biotechnology*, Vol 1, pp. 548–551, Copenhagen, Denmark, Munksgaard.

Wise D.L. (ed). 1989. *Bioinstrumentation Research, Development and Applications*, Boston, MA, Butterworth-Heinemann.

Pungor E. (ed). 1989. *Ion-Selective Electrodes — Proceedings of the 5th Symposium* [Matrafured, Hungary 1988], Oxford, Pergamon.

Wang J. (ed). 1988. *Electrochemical Techniques in Clinical Chemistry and Laboratory Medicine*, New York, VCH Publishers.

Evans A. 1987. *Potentiometry and Ion-seiective Electrodes*, New York, Wiley.

Ngo T.T. (ed). 1987. *Electrochemical Sensors in Immunological Analysis*, New York, Plenum.

(Continued)

TABLE 50.4   (Continued) Books and Long Reviews Keyed to Items in Table 50.3

IVB.   **Electrochemical Sensors — Gas Samples**
　　　Sberveglieri G. (ed). 1992. *Gas Sensors*, Dordrecht The Netherlands, Kluwer.
　　　Moseley P.T., Norris J.O.W., Williams D.E. 1991. *Technology and Mechanisms of Gas Sensors*, Bristol, U.K., Hilger.
　　　Moseley P.T., Tofield B.D. (eds). 1989. *Solid State Gas Sensors*, Philadelphia, Taylor and Francis, Publishers.
V.　　**Optical Sensors**
　　　Coulet P.R., Blum L.J. Luminescence in biosensor design, 1991. In D.L. Wise, L.B. Wingard, Jr (eds). *Biosensors with Fiberoptics*, pp. 293–324, Clifton, N.J., Humana.
　　　Wolfbeis OS. 1991. Spectroscopic techniques, In O.S. Wolfbeis (ed). *Fiber Optic Chemical Sensors and Biosensors*, Vol 1, pp. 25–60. Boca Raton. FL, CRC Press.
　　　Wolfbeis O.S. 1987. Fibre-optic sensors for chemical parameters of interest in biotechnology, In R.D. Schmidt (ed). GBF (Gesellschaft fur Biotechnologische Forschung) *Monogr. Series*, Vol 10, pp. 197–206, New York, VCH Publishers.

References

[1] Janata J. 1989. *Principles of Chemical Sensors*, New York, Plenum.

[2] Scheller F. and Schubert F. 1989. *Biosensors, #18 in Advances in Research Technologies (Beitrage zur Forschungstechnologie)*, Berlin, Akademie-Verlag, Amsterdam, Elsevier (English translation).

[3] Turner A.P.F., Karube I., and Wilson G.S. 1987. *Biosensors: Fundamentals and Applications*, Oxford, Oxford University Press.

[4] Hall E.A.H. 1990. *Biosensors*, Milton Keynes, England, Open University Press.

[5] Eddoes M.J. 1990. Theoretical methods for analyzing biosensor performance. In A.E.G. Cass (ed), *Biosensor — A Practical Approach*, Oxford, IRL Press at Oxford University, Ch. 9, pp. 211–262.

[6] Cosofret V.V. and Buck R.P. 1992. *Pharmaceutical Applications of Membrane Sensors*, Boca Raton, FL, CRC Press.

[7] Janata J. and Bezegh A. 1988. Chemical sensors, *Analyt. Chem.* 60: 62R.

[8] Janata J. 1990. Chemical sensors, *Analyt. Chem.* 62: 33R.

[9] Janata J. 1992. Chemical sensors, *Analyt. Chem.* 66: 196R.

[10] Janata J. and Josowicz M., and DeVaney M. 1994. Chemical sensors, *Analyt. Chem.* 66: 207R.

51

Biological Sensors for Diagnostics

51.1	Diagnostics Industry......................................	**51**-1
51.2	Diagnostic Sensors for Measuring Proteins and Enzymes	**51**-1
	Spectrophotometry • Immunoassays • Mass Spectrometry • Electrophoresis • Chromatography	
51.3	Sensors for Measuring Nucleic Acids	**51**-7
	Enabling Technologies — DNA Extraction and Amplification • DNA/RNA probes • SNP Detection	
51.4	Sensors for Cellular Processes...........................	**51**-10
51.5	Personalized Medicine...................................	**51**-11
51.6	Final Comments	**51**-12
	References	**51**-12

Orhan Soykan
Medtronic, Inc.
Michigan Technological University

51.1 Diagnostics Industry

Many biologically relevant molecules can be measured from the samples taken from the body, which constitutes the foundation of the medical diagnostics industry. In 2003, the global clinical diagnostic market was more than U.S. $2 billion. Of that, sales of the laboratory instruments constituted slightly less than half, while the point of care systems and the diagnostic kits made up the rest. Even though this amount accounts for only a few percent of the total spending on health care, it continues to grow, and not surprisingly, a significant number of biomedical engineers are employed in the research, design, and manufacturing of these products.

Utilization of these devices for various functions is shown in Table 51.1.

In this chapter, we will discuss some examples to illustrate the principles and the technologies used for these measurements. They will be categorized in three groups (a) sensors for proteins and enzymes, (b) sensors for nucleic acids, and (c) sensors for cellular processes.

51.2 Diagnostic Sensors for Measuring Proteins and Enzymes

We are all born with the genes that we will carry throughout our lives, and our genetic makeup remains relatively constant except in parts of the immune and reproductive systems. Expression patterns of genes

TABLE 51.1   Diagnostics Industry by Discipline

Discipline	Percentage (%)
Clinical chemistry tests	42.0
Immunodiagnostics	30.6
Hematology/flow cytometry	7.7
Microbiology	6.9
Molecular diagnostics	5.8
Coagulation	3.4
Other	3.5

Source: Simonsen, M., *BBI Newsletter*, 27: pp. 221–228, 2004.

on the other hand are noting but constant. These changes can be due to aging, environmental and physiological conditions we experience, or due to diseases. Hence, many of the diseases can be detected by sensing the presence, or measuring the level of activity of proteins and enzymes in the tissue and blood for diagnostic purposes. In this section, we will review some of these techniques.

51.2.1 Spectrophotometry

Spectrophotometry utilizes the principle of atomic absorption to determine the concentration of a substance in a volume of solution. Transmission of light through a clear fluid containing an analyte has a reciprocal relationship to the concentration of the analyte, as shown in Figure 51.1b [2]. Percent transmission can be calculated as

$$\%T = \frac{I_T}{I_O} 100$$

where, I_T and I_O are intensities of transmitted and incident light respectively.

Absorption (A) can be defined as $A = -\log(\%T)$, which yields a linear relationship between absorption and the concentration (C) of the solute, as shown in Figure 51.1c.

A schematic diagram of a spectrophotometer is shown in Figure 51.1a. Light from an optical source is first passed through a monochromator, such as a prism or a diffraction grating. Then, a beam splitter produces two light beams where one passes through a cuvette containing the patient sample, and the other through a cuvette containing a reference solution. Intensities of the transmitted light beams are detected and compared to each other to determine the concentration of the analyte in the sample [3].

The exponential form of the Beer–Lambert law can be used to calculate the absorption of light passing through a solution.

$$\frac{I_T}{I_O} = e^{-A}$$

where I_T is the transmitted light intensity, I_O is the incident light intensity, and A is the absorption occurring in the light amplitude as it travels through the media.

Absorption in a cuvette can be calculated as follows:

$$A = abC$$

where a is the absorptivity coefficient, b is the optical path length in the solution, and C is the concentration of the colored analyte of interest.

If A_S and A_R are the absorption in the sample and the reference cuvettes, and the C_S and C_R are the analyte concentrations in the sample and reference cuvettes, then the concentration in the sample cuvette

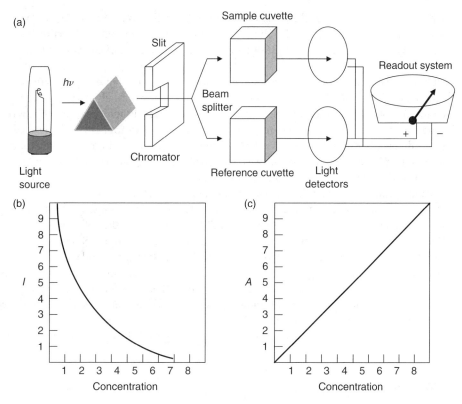

FIGURE 51.1 Principle of spectrophotometry: monochromated light is split into two beams and passed through a sample cuvette as well as a reference solution. Intensities of the transmitted light beams are compared to determine the concentration of the analyte in the sample. Lower two graphs show the percent transmission of light and absorption as a function of the concentration of the analyte of interest in a given solution.

can be calculated as follows:

$$\frac{A_S}{A_R} = \frac{C_S}{C_R} \Rightarrow C_S = \frac{A_S}{A_R} C_R = \frac{\log(I_R)}{\log(I_S)} C_R$$

where I_S and I_R are the intensity of the light transmitted through the cuvettes and detected by the photo-sensors.

A common use of spectrophotometry in clinical medicine is for the measurement of hemoglobin. Hemoglobin is made of heme, an iron compound, and globin, a protein. The iron gives blood its red color and the hemoglobin tests make use of this red color. A chemical is added to a sample of blood to make the red blood cells burst and to release the hemoglobin into the surrounding fluid, coloring it clear red. By measuring this color change using a spectrophotometer, and using the above equations, the concentration of hemoglobin in the blood can be determined [4,5].

For substances that are not colored, one can monitor the absorption at wavelengths that are outside of the visible spectrum, such as infrared and ultraviolet. Additionally, fluorescence spectroscopy can also be utilized.

51.2.2 Immunoassays

When the concentration of the analyte in the biological solution is too low for detection using spectrophotometry, more sensitive methods such as immunoassays are used for the measurement. Immunoassays utilize antibodies developed against the analyte of interest. Since the antigen and the antibody have a very specific interaction and has very high affinity toward each other, the resulting detection system also has a very high sensitivity. A specific example, the enzyme linked immunosorbent assay (ELISA), will be described here.

First, antibodies against the protein to be measured are developed in a host animal. For example, protein can be the human cardiac troponin-T (h-cT), which is a marker of myocardial infarction. Purified h-cT is injected into a rabbit to raise IgG molecules against h-cT, and these antibodies can either be recovered from the blood or produced recombinantly in a bioprocessor. A secondary antibody is also needed, which reacts with the first antibody and provides a colored solution. For example, this secondary antibody can be the goat antirabbit IgG antibody, which is tagged with a coloring compound or a fluorescent molecule. This second antibody can be used for any ELISA test that utilizes rabbit IgGs, regardless of the analyte, and such secondary antibodies are usually available commercially [6].

In the first step, a solution containing the protein of interest is placed on a substrate forming the sensor, such as a polystyrene dish. Then, the first antibody is added to the solution and allowed to react with the analyte. Unbound antibody is washed away and the second antibody is added. After a sufficient time is allowed for the second antibody to react with the first one, a second wash is performed to remove the unbound second antibody. Now the remaining solution contains the complexes formed by the protein of interest as well as the first and the second antibodies. Therefore, the color or the fluorescence produced is a function of the protein concentration. Figure 51.2 shows the steps used in an ELISA process. ELISAs are used for many clinical tests such as determining pregnancy or infectious disease tests such as detecting HIV. Its high sensitivity is due to the extremely high specificity of the antigen–antibody interaction [7,8].

51.2.3 Mass Spectrometry

Sometimes a test for more than one protein is needed and mass spectrometry is the method of choice for that purpose. A good example for this would be the use of tandem mass spectrometry to screen neonates for metabolic disorders such as amino acidemias (e.g., phenylketonuria — PKU), organic acidemias (e.g., propionic acidemia — PPA), and fatty acid oxidation disorders (e.g., Medium-chain acyl-CoA Dehydrogenase deficiency — MCAD) [9]. Although the price of this capital equipment could be high, costs of using it as a sensor is quite low (usually <U.S. $50.00 to screen for more than 20 metabolic disorders), and many states in the United States provide the service to newborns during the first week of life.

A mass spectrometer can be considered as a giant sensor, which measures the mass/charge (m/z) ratio as well as the relative abundance of multiple molecules in a given sample. Mass spectrometers consist of three main components: an ionization source, a physical separation environment, and a detector. Ionization of the molecules in the sample can be done by the deposition of energy from a laser source to remove an electron, a technique known as laser desorption ionization, which is depicted on the left side of Figure 51.3. Alternatively, it is possible to ionize molecules in a fluid flow by applying an electrical voltage to cause them to charge and subsequently spray, a technique known as electrospray ionization.

Following the ionization step, the molecules are sent into a physical separation chamber, where they are separated based on their m/z ratio. This can be achieved by first accelerating them in an electric field to give them a speed of

$$v = \sqrt{\frac{2Uz}{m}}$$

where U is the accelerating potential, z and m are the charge and the mass of the molecule respectively.

Since the velocity is a function of the mass, a determination of the mass of the molecules becomes possible in the physical separation environment. One option is to measure the time of flight in a flight tube, as shown in the middle section of Figure 51.3. This technique is known as the time-of-flight

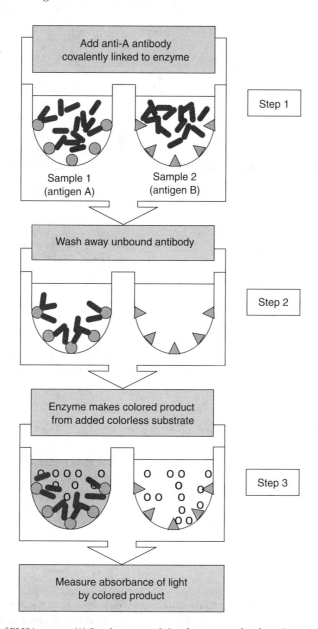

FIGURE 51.2   Steps of ELISA process (1) Specimen containing the target molecule antigen A, shown as round circles, is exposed to the primary antibody, shown as rectangular shapes. (2) Unbound antibody is washed, leaving the plate on the right hand side with no primary antibodies. (3) Secondary antibody depicted with oval shapes is added to the wells. (4) Unbound secondary antibody is also washed away, leaving the primary-secondary antibody complex along with the target molecule in the wells (step not shown). Test on the left plate would give a positive response to this test.

measurement, and makes use of the fact that larger molecules will fly slowly and require more time to cross the flight tube. Molecular mass can be calculated as

$$m = 2\frac{T^2}{L^2}Uz$$

where T is the flight time and L is the length of the flight tube.

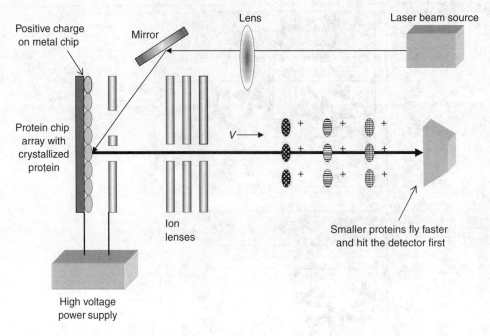

FIGURE 51.3 Mass spectrophotometry: proteins are released from the chip surface by the application of the laser pulse. A secondary pulse is used to charge the proteins, which are later accelerated in an electric field. A time-of-flight measurement can be used to determine the mass of the protein.

Alternatively, one can apply a fixed magnetic field, perpendicular to the flight path of the ions, and cause a deviation in the flight path of the moving ions to separate them.

Although the mass spectrometer can separate the molecules based on their molecular weight, additional analysis is needed to separate molecules with identical or similar masses. This can be achieved by tandem mass spectrometry, where the ions coming from the first spectrometer enter into an argon collision chamber, and the resulting molecular fragments are catalogued by a secondary mass spectrometer. By studying the fragments, composition of the original mixture and the relative amount of the ions in the solution can be calculated [10–12].

51.2.4 Electrophoresis

Electrophoresis can be used to obtain a rapid separation of the proteins. A typical apparatus used for this purpose is shown in Figure 51.4. Proteins are first exposed to negatively charged sodium dodecyl sulfate, or SDS, which binds to the hydrophobic regions of the proteins, and causes them to unfold. The mixtures are placed into the wells on top of vertically placed gel slabs, as shown in Figure 51.4. Application of the electric potential, usually on the order of hundreds of volts, across the gel creates a force to move the protein molecules downward. Mobility of the proteins in the gel is given by

$$\mu = \frac{Q}{6\pi r \eta}$$

where μ is the electrophoretic mobility (cm/sec), Q, the ionic charge (due to SDS), r, the radius of the protein, and η is the viscosity of the cellulose acetate or polyacrylamide gel.

Therefore, the movement of the ions within the gel is directly proportional to the applied voltage, and inversely proportional to the size of the protein. Gel electrophoresis is run for a fixed amount of time, allowing the small proteins to migrate further than the larger ones, resulting in their separation based on

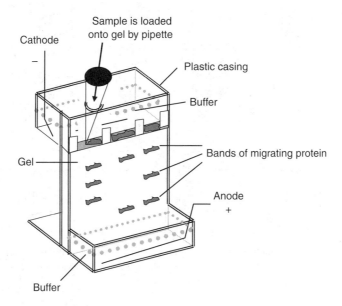

FIGURE 51.4 Gel electrophoresis: proteins loaded on the slab of gel are separated based on their size as they migrate under a constant electric field. Smaller proteins move faster and travel further than the larger ones.

their size. Coomassie blue or silver staining can be used to detect the bands across the gel to confirm the presence of proteins with known molecular masses.

Unlike mass spectroscopy, gel electrophoresis does not provide a quantitative value for the amount of given protein. However, it provides a low cost and relatively rapid method for the analysis of multiple proteins in a specimen, especially when implemented as a capillary electrophoresis system. Therefore, it has been used for the separation of enzymes (e.g., creatinine phosphokinase), mucopolysaccharides, plasma, serum, cerebrospinal fluid, urine, and other bodily fluids [13]. It is also used for quality control applications for the manufacturing of biological compounds to verify the purity or to examine the manufacturing yield [14].

51.2.5 Chromatography

Chromatography is also a simple technique that has applications in the toxicology and serum drug level measurements. In paper chromatography, a solution containing the analytes wicks up an absorbent paper for a period of time, and separation is achieved by the relative position of the analytes while the analyte and the solvent move up in the paper. A more precise technique known as column chromatography uses affinity columns, where the sample is applied to the top of the column and the fractionated molecules are eluted and collected at the bottom of the column (Figure 51.5). Since the smaller molecules with lower affinity to the column material will come out sooner than the larger molecules and ones with the higher affinity to the column, separation is achieved as a function of time. Further analysis can be done in the fractionated samples if desired.

51.3 Sensors for Measuring Nucleic Acids

Nucleic acids present in the body exist in the form of DNA and RNA. Determination of DNA sequences would allow the clinicians to determine the presence to congenital or genetically inherited diseases. On the other hand, measurement of RNA levels would indicate if gene is turned on or off. Discussions in this section focuses on the basics of few of the tools used in practice beginning with some enabling technologies.

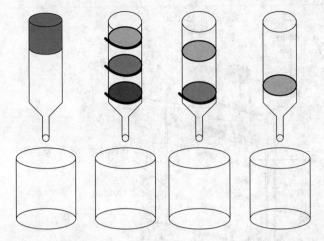

FIGURE 51.5 Affinity chromatography: a chemical column with relatively high affinity to proteins is loaded with a mixture of proteins, and allowed to run downward with the aid of gravity. Eluted fractions are collected in different tubes, each of which would contain different group of proteins.

TABLE 51.2 Genetic Code

1st base in codon	2nd base in codon: U	C	A	G	3rd base in codon
U	Phe	Ser	Tyr	Cys	U
	Phe	Ser	Tyr	Cys	C
	Leu	Ser	**STOP**	**STOP**	A
	Leu	Ser	**STOP**	Trp	G
C	Leu	Pro	His	Arg	U
	Leu	Pro	His	Arg	C
	Leu	Pro	Gln	Arg	A
	Leu	Pro	Gln	Arg	G
A	Ile	Thr	Asn	Ser	U
	Ile	Thr	Asn	Ser	C
	Ile	Thr	Lys	Arg	A
	Met	Thr	Lys	Arg	G
G	Val	Ala	Asp	Gly	U
	Val	Ala	Asp	Gly	C
	Val	Ala	Glu	Gly	A
	Val	Ala	Glu	Gly	G

Amino acids coded by three nucleic acid bases are shown as the entries of the table.

51.3.1 Enabling Technologies — DNA Extraction and Amplification

Cells in the human body contain the genetic material, DNA, which consists of a very long series of nucleic acids. Three nucleic acids in a row in the genome is called a codon, which determines the amino acid to be used when synthesizing a protein. This genetic code is shown in Table 51.2. Table 51.2 has $4^3 = 64$ entries, but since there are only 20 amino acids, many of the codons do code the same amino acid, a fact known as the redundancy of the genetic code. Therefore, a change in the genetic sequence may or may not cause a change in the protein synthesis. If the variation in the genetic sequence causes a change in the amino acid sequence altering the function of the protein, then an altered phenotype may emerge. Although the results of some of these changes are benign, such as different hair and eye colors, others are

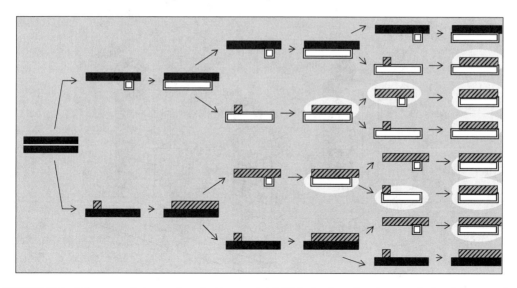

FIGURE 51.6 Polymerase chain reaction: double stranded DNA is first heated to denature the bonds between the two strands. In the second step, primers are allowed to attach to their complementary strands. In the third step, double stranded DNA is formed by the enzyme DNA Polymerase. Process is repeated many times, doubling the amount of DNA at each step.

not, such as increased susceptibility to various diseases. This genetic information can be read from the genes of interest. However, before that can be done, the DNA must be extracted and amplified.

Extraction of DNA from biological samples can be accomplished by precipitation or affinity methods [15]. Amplification of the amount of DNA is also needed before any sequence detection can be done. This can be done by a method known as polymerase chain reaction or PCR in short. This process is depicted in Figure 51.6. Briefly, original double stranded DNA molecules, shown as black rectangles, are heated to more than 90°C for separation. Afterward, DNA primers, shown as squares, as well as nucleic acids are added to the solution to initiate the DNA synthesis, forming two pairs of double stranded DNA at the end of the first cycle. The process is repeated for more than 30 times, doubling the amount of DNA at each step [16]. RNA can also be amplified using a similar process known as reverse transcription-polymerase chain reaction (RT-PCR) [17].

51.3.2 DNA/RNA probes

Gene chip arrays are being utilized as sensors to measure the level of gene expression to discover the genetic causes or to validate the presence of various disorders such as cancer. The most common form of these sensors is the RNA chips that consist of an array of probes. Each spot on the array contains multiple copies of a single genetic sequence immobilized to the sensor surface. These probe sequences are complementary to the RNA sequences being studied. Amplified RNA from the patient is labeled with a fluorescent dye, for example one that fluoresces red in this case. A second set of RNA, the reference RNA, with known concentration is labeled with another fluorescent dye, for example, green in this case. The RNA solutions are mixed and exposed to the sensor. Since sections of RNA from the patient and the reference are complementary to individual probe sequence, there would be a competitive binding during the exposure period (Figure 51.7). Following the incubation period, unbound RNA is removed, and the sensor array is exposed to a light source for the measurement of the fluorescence from each spot on the array. If a spot fluoresces red, the indication would be that the most of the RNA bound to this spot came from the patient, meaning that the patient is expressing this gene at high levels. On the other hand, a green fluorescence would indicate that the binding is from the reference RNA, and the patient is not expressing high levels of the gene. A yellow color would indicate a moderate gene expression, since some

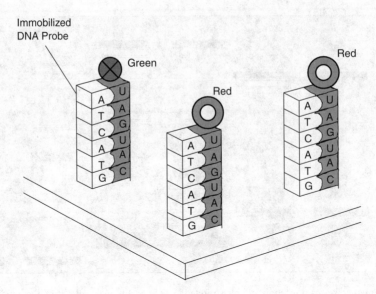

FIGURE 51.7 Gene array: reference RNA labeled with green fluorescence molecules compete with the RNA from the patient labeled with red fluorescent molecules to bind to the immobilized probes on the gene array.

of each type of RNA molecule must bind to the probe to produce the mixed response. The advantage of these sensors is the same as any other sensor array, which is the ability to probe a large number of genes simultaneously [18].

51.3.3 SNP Detection

Single nucleotide polymorphism, or SNP, occurs when only one nucleotide in the genetic sequence is altered. It could be a mutation, and it could be inherited from a parent. Reading a single nucleotide from the genome that had been substituted for another one might stop the reading process of that gene or cause a different protein to be synthesized. Thus detecting a SNP could be important in diagnosing genetically related diseases or a patient's tendency toward being more susceptible to this type of disease.

There are many methods developed for the detection of a SNP, and one of them will be described later, which is illustrated in Figure 51.8. In the first step, a primer consisting of 20 to 50 nucleic acids having a sequence complementary to the gene sequence adjacent to the SNP is synthesized and allowed to anneal to a single strand of the DNA from the patient. In the second step, terminal nucleic acids (A, T, C, and G) with different fluorescent tags are added allowing the double stand to grow by only one base pair. As the third step, the solution is exposed to a laser light for detecting the fluorescence to read the nucleic acid at the SNP location. Since the patient sample will contain two copies for each gene, one from each parent, the sensor might detect one or two nucleic acids for each SNP site [19].

Detection of SNPs can be used as a clinical test to diagnose various diseases. Some examples of these are SNPs for BRAC-1 gene to detect patients with high susceptibility to a type of breast cancer, and long-quantitative trait (QT) genes, which make patients prone to fatal cardiac arrhythmias [20,21].

51.4 Sensors for Cellular Processes

Flow cytometry is used to separate populations of cells in a mixture from one another by means of fluorescently labeled antibodies and DNA specific dyes. Antibodies used are usually against the molecules expressed on the cell surface, such as cell-surface receptors. The labeled cells are diluted in a solution and passed through a nozzle in a single-cell stream while being illuminated by a laser beam. Fluorescence

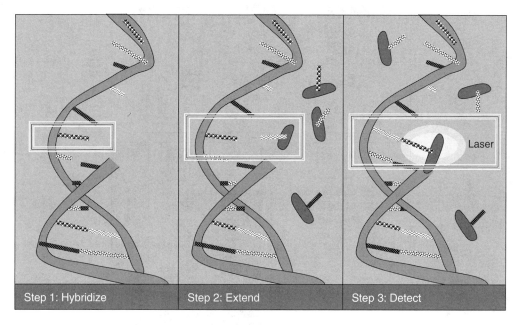

FIGURE 51.8 SNP detection by primer extension method: first the amplified DNA is hybridized to the primers that are specific to the genetic region of interest. Second, a labeled terminating base at the target SNP site extends the primer. Finally, the extended primer is read by fluorescence.

is detected by photomultiplier tubes (PMTs) with optical filters to determine the emission wavelength, which in turn helps to identify the surface receptors (Figure 51.9). Fluorescence data is used to measure the relative proportions of various cell types in the mixture, and to derive the diagnostic information [22].

Flow cytometry is commonly used in the clinical diagnostics, for immunophenotyping leukemia, counting stem cells for optimizing autologous transplants for the treatment of leukemia, counting CD4+/CD8+ lymphocytes in HIV-infected patients to determine the progression of the disease, and the analysis of stained DNA from solid tumors [23].

51.5 Personalized Medicine

Today the personalization of the treatment for the needs of individual patients is done by health care providers. In some cases, clinicians can neither predict reliably the best treatment pathway for a patient, nor anticipate the optimal drug regimen. However, it would be possible to improve the treatment and tailor the therapy to the specific needs of the patients if their genetic information is known. For example, some drugs are known to cause cardiac arrhythmias in patients with certain genotypes and should be avoided. It might be possible that in the future, patients coming to hospitals might be asked to bring their genome cards along with their insurance cards. Knowledge of the genome of individual patients would not only predict their medical vulnerabilities, but also help with the selection of their treatment [24].

Some of these studies have already begun. For example, in the United States, the Food and Drug Administration is already encouraging the pharmaceutical industry to submit the results of genomic tests when seeking approval for new drugs [25]. This new field of research is now being recognized as pharmacogenetics.

Another early application of personalized medicine is the use of microphysiometry, a device that measures the extracellular acidification rate of cells, to establish their sensitivity to chemotherapy [26].

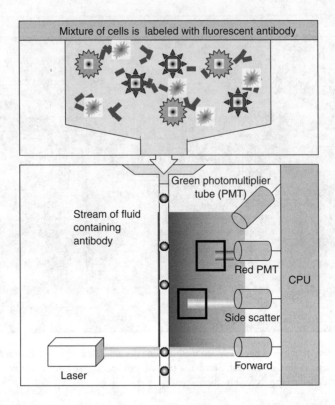

FIGURE 51.9   Flow cytometry: fluorescently labeled cells are passed in front of light detectors (labeled as PMTs in the figure) to detect their labeling color, which indicates the phenotype of the cell.

This sensor measures the chemosensitivity by comparing the acidification rate of cells treated with cyto-static agents, such as anticancer drugs, to that of nontreated cells, before a drug is prescribed to the patient.

51.6   Final Comments

As the aging of the population in the Western world, and the increase in the population of the World in general continues, the need for diagnostic procedures will also increase. Due to the need for cost containment, the emphasis will continue to shift from therapeutics to early diagnosis for prevention. Both of these factors will increase the need for diagnostic procedures and additional diagnostic technologies. While the basic methodology for the traditional diagnostics is becoming well established, the techniques needed for personalized medicine are still being developed, and the biomedical engineers will be able to participate in both the research and implementation aspects of these very important areas.

References

[1] Simonsen, M., Nucleic Acid Testing, Proteomics to drive future of diagnostics, *BBI Newsletter*, 27, 221–228, 2004.

[2] Skoog, D.A. and Leary, J.J., *Principles of Instrumental Analysis*, 4th ed., Saunders, Orlando, FL, 1992.

[3] Kellner, R., Mermet, J.-M., Otto, M., and Widmer, H.M., *Analytical Chemistry*, Wiley, Weinheim, GR, 1998.

[4] Kaplan, A., Jack, R., Opheim, K.E., Toivola, B., and Lyon, A.W., *Clinical Chemistry*, 4th ed., Williams & Wilkins, Malvern, PA, 1995.

[5] Burtis, C.A. and Ashwood, E.R., *Tietz Fundamentals of Clinical Chemistry*, 5th ed., W.N. Saunders, Philadelphia, PA, 2001.

[6] Alberts, B., Bray, D., Lewis, J., Raff, M., Roberts, K., and Watson, J.D., *Molecular Biology of the Cell*, 3rd ed., Garland, New York, NY, 1994,

[7] Liu, S., Boyer-Chatenet, L., Lu, H., and Jiang, S., Rapid and automated fluorescence-linked immunosorbent assay for high-throughput screening of HIV-1 fusion inhibitors targeting gp41. *J. Biomol. Screen.* 8, 685–693, 2003.

[8] Bandi, Z.L., Schoen, I., and DeLara, M., Enzyme-linked immunosorbent urine pregnancy tests, *Am. J. Clin. Pathol.*, 87, 236–242, 1987.

[9] Schulze, A., Lindner, M., Kohlmuller, D., Olgemoller, K., Mayatepek, E., and Hoffmann, G.F., Expanded newborn screening for inborn errors of metabolism by electrospray ionization-tandem mass spectrometry: results, outcome, and implications, *Pediatrics*, 111, 1399–1406, 2003.

[10] Liebler, D.C., *Introduction to Proteomics*, Humana Press, Totowa, NJ, 2002.

[11] Pennington, S.R. and Dunn, M.J., *Proteomics*, Springer-Verlag, New York, NY, 2001.

[12] Kambhampati, D., *Protein Microarray Technology*, Wiley, Heppenheim, GR, 2004.

[13] Chen, F.T., Liu, C.M., Hsieh, Y.Z., and Sternberg, J.C., Capillary electrophoresis — a new clinical tool, *Clin. Chem.*, 37, 14–19, 1991.

[14] Reilly, R.M., Scollard, D.A., Wang, J., Monda, H., Chen, P., Henderson, L.A., Bowen, B.M., and Vallis, K.A., A kit formulated under good manufacturing practices for labeling human epidermal growth factor with 111In for radiotherapeutic applications, *J. Nucl. Med.*, 45, 701–708, 2004.

[15] Bowtell, D. and Sambrook, J., *DNA Microarrays: A Molecular Cloning Manual*, Cold Spring Harbor Press, Cold Spring Harbor, NY, 2003.

[16] Malacinski, G.M., *Essentials of Molecular Biology*, 4th ed., Jones and Bartlett, Sudbury, MA, 2003.

[17] Stahlberg, A., Hakansson, J., Xian, X., Semb, H., and Kubista, M., Properties of the reverse transcription reaction in mRNA quantification, *Clin. Chem.*, 50, 509–515, 2004.

[18] Blalock, E., *A Beginner's Guide to Microarrays*, Kluwer, Dordrecht, NL, 2003.

[19] Kwok, P.-Y., *Single Nucleotide Polymorphisms: Methods and Protocols*, Humana, Totowa, NJ, 2003.

[20] Burke, W., Genomic medicine: genetic testing, *N. Engl. J. Med.*, 347, 1867–1875, 2002.

[21] Haack, B., Kupka, S., Ebauer, M., Siemiatkowska, A., Pfister, M., Kwiatkowska, J., Erecinski, J., Limon, J., Ochman, K., and Blin, N., Analysis of candidate genes for genotypic diagnosis in the long QT syndrome, *J. Appl. Genet.*, 45, 375–381, 2004.

[22] Lodish, H., Berk, A., Zipursky, S.L., Matsudaira, P., Baltimore, D., and Barnell, J., *Molecular Cell Biology*, 4th ed., W.H. Freeman, New York, NY, 2000.

[23] Rose, N.R., Friedman, H., and Fahey, J.L., *Manual of Clinical Laboratory Immunology*, 3rd ed., American Society for Microbiology, Washington, D.C., 1986.

[24] Brown, S.M., *Essentials of Medical Genomics*, Wiley, Hoboken, NJ, 2003.

[25] Guidance for Industry: Pharmacogenomic Data Submissions, U.S. Department of Health and Human Services, Food and Drug Administration, November 2003.

[26] Waldenmaier, D.S., Babarina, A., and Kischkel, F.C., Rapid *in vitro* chemosensitivity analysis of human colon tumor cell lines, *Toxicol. Appl. Pharmacol.*, 192, 237–245, 2003.

VI

Medical Instruments and Devices

Wolf W. von Maltzahn
Rensselaer Polytechnic Institute

52 Biopotential Amplifiers
Joachim H. Nagel 52-1

53 Bioelectric Impedance Measurements
Robert Patterson 53-1

54 Implantable Cardiac Pacemakers
Michael Forde, Pat Ridgely 54-1

55 Noninvasive Arterial Blood Pressure and Mechanics
Gary Drzewiecki 55-1

56 Cardiac Output Measurement
Leslie A. Geddes 56-1

57 External Defibrillators
Willis A. Tacker 57-1

58 Implantable Defibrillators
Edwin G. Duffin 58-1

59 Implantable Stimulators for Neuromuscular Control
Primoz Strojnik, P. Hunter Peckham 59-1

60 Respiration
Leslie A. Geddes **60**-1

61 Mechanical Ventilation
Khosrow Behbehani **61**-1

62 Essentials of Anesthesia Delivery
A. William Paulsen **62**-1

63 Electrosurgical Devices
Jeffrey L. Eggleston, Wolf W. von Maltzahn **63**-1

64 Biomedical Lasers
Millard M. Judy **64**-1

65 Instrumentation for Cell Mechanics
Nathan J. Sniadecki, Christopher S. Chen **65**-1

66 Blood Glucose Monitoring
David D. Cunningham **66**-1

67 Atomic Force Microscopy: Probing Biomolecular Interactions
Christopher M. Yip **67**-1

68 Parenteral Infusion Devices
Gregory I. Voss, Robert D. Butterfield **68**-1

69 Clinical Laboratory: Separation and Spectral Methods
Richard L. Roa **69**-1

70 Clinical Laboratory: Nonspectral Methods and Automation
Richard L. Roa **70**-1

71 Noninvasive Optical Monitoring
Ross Flewelling **71**-1

72 Medical Instruments and Devices Used in the Home
Bruce R. Bowman, Edward Schuck **72**-1

73 Virtual Instrumentation: Applications in Biomedical Engineering
Eric Rosow, Joseph Adam **73**-1

N OT TOO LONG AGO, the term *medical instrument* stood for simple hand-held instruments used by physicians for observing patients, examining organs, making simple measurements, or administering medication. These small instruments, such as stethoscopes, thermometers, tongue depressors, and a few surgical tools, typically fit into a physician's hand bag. Today's medical instruments are considerably more complicated and diverse, primarily because they incorporate electronic systems for sensing, transducing, manipulating, storing, and displaying data or information. Furthermore, medical specialists today request detailed and accurate measurements of a vast number of physiologic parameters for diagnosing illnesses and prescribe complicated procedures for treating these. As a result, the number

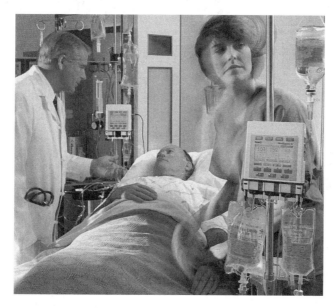

FIGURE VI.1 A typical IV infusion system.

of medical instruments and devices has grown from a few hundred a generation ago to more than 10,000 today, and the complexity of these instruments has grown at the same pace. The description of all these instruments and devices would fill an entire handbook by itself; however, due to the limited space assigned to this topic, only a selected number are described.

While medical instruments acquire and process information and data for monitoring patients and diagnosing illnesses, medical devices use electrical, mechanical, chemical, or radiation energy for achieving a desired therapeutic purpose, maintaining physiologic functions, or assisting a patient's healing process. To mention only a few functions, medical devices pump blood, remove metabolic waste products, destroy kidney stones, infuse fluids and drugs, stimulate muscles and nerves, cut tissue, administer anesthesia, alleviate pain, restore function, or warm tissue. Because of their complexity, medical devices are used mostly in hospitals and medical centers by trained personnel, but some also can be found in private homes operated by patients themselves or their caregivers.

This section on medical instruments and devices neither replaces a textbook on this subject nor presents the material in a typical textbook manner. The authors assume the reader to be interested in but not knowledgeable on the subject. Therefore, each chapter begins with a short introduction to the subject material, followed by a brief description of current practices and principles, and ends with recent trends and developments. Whenever appropriate, equations, diagrams, and pictures amplify and illustrate the topic, while tables summarize facts and data. The short reference section at the end of each chapter points toward further resource materials, including books, journal articles, patents, and company brochures.

The chapters in the first half of this section cover the more traditional topics of bioinstrumentation, such as biopotential amplifiers and noninvasive blood pressure, blood flow, and respiration monitors, while those of the second half focus more on recently developed instruments and devices such as pulse oximeters or home-care monitoring devices. Some of this latter material is new or hard to find elsewhere. A few traditional bioinstrumentation or electroencephalography have been omitted entirely because most textbooks on this subject give excellent introductions and reviews. Transducers, biosensors, and electrodes are covered in other sections of this *handbook*. Thus, this section provides an overview, albeit an incomplete one, of recent developments in the field of medical instruments and devices.

52

Biopotential Amplifiers

52.1 Basic Amplifier Requirements 52-1
    Interferences
52.2 Special Circuits.. 52-5
    Instrumentation Amplifier • Isolation Amplifier and Patient
    Safety • Surge Protection • Input Guarding • Dynamic
    Range and Recovery • Passive Isolation Amplifiers • Digital
    Electronics
52.3 Summary 52-13
Defining Terms 52-13
References 52-14
Further Information 52-14

Joachim H. Nagel
University of Stuttgart

Biosignals are recorded as potentials, voltages, and electrical field strengths generated by nerves and muscles. The measurements involve voltages at very low levels, typically ranging between 1 μV and 100 mV, with high source impedances and superimposed high level interference signals and noise. The signals need to be amplified to make them compatible with devices such as displays, recorders, or A/D converters for computerized equipment. Amplifiers adequate to measure these signals have to satisfy very specific requirements. They have to provide amplification selective to the physiological signal, reject superimposed noise and interference signals, and guarantee protection from damages through voltage and current surges for both patient and electronic equipment. Amplifiers featuring these specifications are known as *biopotential amplifiers*. Basic requirements and features, as well as some specialized systems, will be presented.

52.1 Basic Amplifier Requirements

The basic requirements that a biopotential amplifier has to satisfy are:

- The physiological process to be monitored should not be influenced in any way by the amplifier
- The measured signal should not be distorted
- The amplifier should provide the best possible separation of signal and interferences
- The amplifier has to offer protection of the patient from any hazard of electrical shock
- The amplifier itself has to be protected against damages that might result from high input voltages as they occur during the application of defibrillators or electrosurgical instrumentation

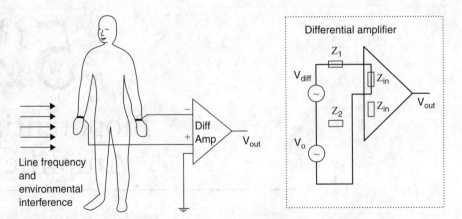

FIGURE 52.1 Typical configuration for the measurement of biopotentials. The biological signal appears between the two measuring electrodes at the right and left arm of the patient and is fed to the inverting and the noninverting inputs of the differential amplifier.

A typical configuration for the measurement of biopotentials is shown in Figure 52.1. Three electrodes, two of them picking up the biological signal and the third providing the reference potential, connect the subject to the amplifier. The input signal to the amplifier consists of five components (1) the desired biopotential, (2) undesired biopotentials, (3) a power line interference signal of 60 Hz (50 Hz in some countries) and its harmonics, (4) interference signals generated by the tissue/electrode interface, and (5) noise. Proper design of the amplifier provides rejection of a large portion of the signal interferences. The main task of the differential amplifier as shown in Figure 52.1 is to reject the line frequency interference that is electrostatically or magnetically coupled into the subject. The desired biopotential appears as a voltage between the two input terminals of the differential amplifier and is referred to as the *differential signal*. The line frequency interference signal shows only very small differences in amplitude and phase between the two measuring electrodes, causing approximately the same potential at both inputs, and thus appears only between the inputs and ground and is called the *common mode signal*. Strong rejection of the common mode signal is one of the most important characteristics of a good biopotential amplifier.

The **common mode rejection ratio (CMRR)** of an amplifier is defined as the ratio of the differential mode gain over the common mode gain. As seen in Figure 52.1, the rejection of the common mode signal in a biopotential amplifier is both a function of the amplifier CMRR and the source impedances Z_1 and Z_2. For the ideal biopotential amplifier with $Z_1 = Z_2$ and infinite CMRR of the differential amplifier, the output voltage is the pure biological signal amplified by G_D, the differential mode gain: $V_{out} = G_D \cdot V_{biol}$. With finite CMRR, the common mode signal is not completely rejected, adding the interference term $G_D \cdot V_c/\text{CMRR}$ to the output signal. Even in the case of an ideal differential amplifier with infinite CMRR, the common mode signal will not completely disappear unless the source impedances are equal. The common mode signal V_c causes currents to flow through Z_1 and Z_2. The related voltage drops show a difference if the source impedances are unequal, thus generating a differential signal at the amplifier input which, of course, is not rejected by the differential amplifier. With amplifier gain G_D and input impedance Z_{in}, the output voltage of the amplifier is:

$$V_{out} = G_D V_{biol} + \frac{G_D V_c}{\text{CMRR}} + G_D V_c \left(1 - \frac{Z_{in}}{Z_{in} + Z_1 - Z_2}\right) \tag{52.1}$$

The output of a real biopotential amplifier will always consist of the desired output component due to a differential biosignal, an undesired component due to incomplete rejection of common mode interference signals as a function of CMRR, and an undesired component due to source impedance unbalance allowing a small proportion of a common mode signal to appear as a differential signal to the amplifier. Since

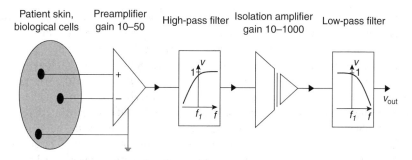

Patient skin, biological cells | Preamplifier gain 10–50 | High-pass filter | Isolation amplifier gain 10–1000 | Low-pass filter

FIGURE 52.2 Schematic design of the main stages of a biopotential amplifier. Three electrodes connect the patient to a preamplifier stage. After removing dc and low-frequency interferences, the signal is connected to an output low-pass filter through an isolation stage which provides electrical safety to the patient, prevents ground loops, and reduces the influence of interference signals.

source impedance unbalances of 5,000 to 10,000 Ω, mainly caused by electrodes, are not uncommon, and sufficient rejection of line frequency interferences requires a minimum CMRR of 100 dB, the input impedance of the amplifier should be at least 10^9 Ω at 60 Hz to prevent source impedance unbalances from deteriorating the overall CMRR of the amplifier. State-of-the-art biopotential amplifiers provide a CMRR of 120 to 140 dB.

In order to provide optimum signal quality and adequate voltage level for further signal processing, the amplifier has to provide a gain of 100 to 50,000 and needs to maintain the best possible signal-to-noise ratio. The presence of high level interference signals not only deteriorates the quality of the physiological signals, but also restricts the design of the biopotential amplifier. Electrode half-cell potentials, for example, limit the gain factor of the first amplifier stage since their amplitude can be several orders of magnitude larger than the amplitude of the physiological signal. To prevent the amplifier from going into saturation, this component has to be eliminated before the required gain can be provided for the physiological signal.

A typical design of the various stages of a biopotential amplifier is shown in Figure 52.2. The electrodes which provide the transition between the ionic flow of currents in biological tissue and the electronic flow of current in the amplifier, represent a complex electrochemical system that is described elsewhere in this handbook. The electrodes determine to a large extent the composition of the measured signal. The preamplifier represents the most critical part of the amplifier itself since it sets the stage for the quality of the biosignal. With proper design, the preamplifier can eliminate, or at least minimize, most of the signals interfering with the measurement of biopotentials.

In addition to electrode potentials and electromagnetic interferences, noise — generated by the amplifier and the connection between biological source and amplifier — has to be taken into account when designing the preamplifier. The total source resistance R_s, including the resistance of the biological source and all transition resistances between signal source and amplifier input, causes thermal voltage noise with a root mean square (rms) value of:

$$E_{rms} = \sqrt{4kTR_s B} \quad \text{(volt)} \tag{52.2}$$

where k = Boltzmann constant, T = absolute temperature, R_s = resistance in Ω, and B = bandwidth in Hz.

Additionally, there is the inherent amplifier noise. It consists of two frequency-dependent components, the internal voltage noise source e_n and the voltage drop across the source resistance R_s caused by an internal current noise generator i_n. The total input noise for the amplifier with a bandwidth of $B = f_2 - f_1$ is calculated as the sum of its three independent components:

$$E_{rms}^2 = \int_{f_1}^{f_2} e_n^2 df + R_s^2 \int_{f_1}^{f_2} i_n^2 df + 4kTR_s B \tag{52.3}$$

High signal-to-noise ratios thus require the use of very low noise amplifiers and the limitation of bandwidth. Current technology offers differential amplifiers with voltage noise of less than $10\,nV/\sqrt{Hz}$ and current noise less than $1\,pA/\sqrt{Hz}$. Both parameters are frequency dependent and decrease approximately with the square root of frequency. The exact relationship depends on the technology of the amplifier input stage. Field effect transistor (FET) preamplifiers exhibit about five times the voltage noise density compared to bipolar transistors but a current noise density that is about 100 times smaller.

The purpose of the high pass and low pass filters in Figure 52.2 is to eliminate interference signals like electrode half-cell potentials and preamplifier offset potentials and to reduce the noise amplitude by the limitation of the amplifier bandwidth. Since the biosignal should not be distorted or attenuated, higher order sharp-cutting linear phase filters have to be used. Active Bessel filters are preferred filter types due to their smooth transfer function. Separation of biosignal and interference is in most cases incomplete due to the overlap of their spectra.

The isolation stage serves the galvanic decoupling of the patient from the measuring equipment and provides safety from electrical hazards. This stage also prevents galvanic currents from deteriorating the signal-to-noise ratio especially by preventing ground loops. Various principles can be used to realize the isolation stage. Analog isolation amplifiers use either transformer, optical, or capacitive couplers to transmit the signal through the isolation barrier. Digital isolation amplifiers use a voltage/frequency converter to digitize the signal before it is transmitted easily by optical or inductive couplers to the output frequency/voltage converter. The most important characteristics of an isolation amplifier are low leakage current, isolation impedance, isolation voltage (or mode) rejection (IMR), and maximum safe isolation voltage.

52.1.1 Interferences

The most critical point in the measurement of biopotentials is the contact between electrodes and biological tissue. Both the electrode offset potential and the electrode/tissue impedance are subject to changes due to relative movements of electrode and tissue. Thus, two interference signals are generated as motion artifacts: the changes of the electrode potential and motion-induced changes of the voltage drop caused by the input current of the preamplifier. These motion artifacts can be minimized by providing high input impedances for the preamplifier, usage of non-polarized electrodes with low half-cell potentials such as Ag/AgCl electrodes, and by reducing the source impedance by use of electrode gel. Motion artifacts, interferences from external electromagnetic fields, and noise can also be generated in the wires connecting electrodes and amplifier. Reduction of these interferences is achieved by using twisted pair cables, shielded wires, and *input guarding*.

Recording of biopotentials is often done in an environment that is equipped with many electrical systems which produce strong electrical and magnetic fields. In addition to 60 Hz power line frequency and some strong harmonics, high frequency electromagnetic fields are encountered. At power line frequency, the electric and magnetic components of the interfering fields can be considered separately. Electrical fields are caused by all conductors that are connected to power, even with no flow of current. A current is capacitively coupled into the body where it flows to the ground electrode. If an isolation amplifier is used without patient ground, the current is capacitively coupled to ground. In this case, the body potential floats with a voltage of up to 100 V towards ground. Minimizing interferences requires increasing the distance between power lines and the body, use of isolation amplifiers, separate grounding of the body at a location as far away from the measuring electrodes as possible, and use of shielded electrode cables.

The magnetic field components produce eddy currents in the body. The amplifier, the electrode cable, and the body form an induction loop that is subject to the generation of an interference signal. Minimizing this interference signal requires increasing the distance between the interference source and patient, twisting the connecting cables, shielding of the magnetic fields, and relocating the patient to a place and orientation that offers minimum interference signals. In many cases, an additional narrow band-rejection filter (notch filter) is implemented as an additional stage in the biopotential amplifier to provide sufficient suppression of line frequency interferences.

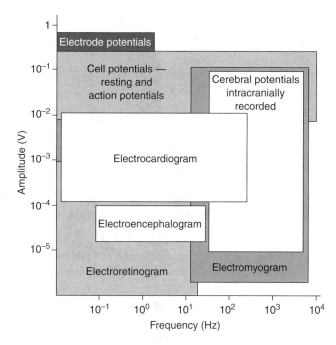

FIGURE 52.3 Amplitudes and spectral ranges of some important biosignals. The various biopotentials completely cover the area from 10^{-5} V to almost 1 V and from dc to 10 kHz.

In order to achieve optimum signal quality, the biopotential amplifier has to be adapted to the specific application. Based on the signal parameters, both appropriate bandwidth and gain factor are chosen. Figure 52.3 shows an overview of the most commonly measured biopotentials and specifies the normal ranges for amplitude and bandwidth.

A final requirement for biopotential amplifiers is the need for calibration. Since the amplitude of the biopotential often has to be determined very accurately, there must be provisions to easily determine the gain or the amplitude range referenced to the input of the amplifier. For this purpose, the gain of the amplifier must be well calibrated. In order to prevent difficulties with calibrations, some amplifiers that need to have adjustable gain use a number of fixed gain settings rather than providing a continuous gain control. Some amplifiers have a standard signal source of known amplitude built in that can be momentarily connected to the input by the push of a button to check the calibration at the output of the biopotential amplifier.

52.2 Special Circuits

52.2.1 Instrumentation Amplifier

An important stage of all biopotential amplifiers is the input preamplifier which substantially contributes to the overall quality of the system. The main tasks of the preamplifier are to sense the voltage between two measuring electrodes while rejecting the common mode signal, and minimizing the effect of electrode polarization overpotentials. Crucial to the performance of the preamplifier is the input impedance which should be as high as possible. Such a differential amplifier cannot be realized using a standard single **operational amplifier (op-amp)** design since this does not provide the necessary high input impedance. The general solution to the problem involves voltage followers, or noninverting amplifiers, to attain high input impedances. A possible realization is shown in Figure 52.4a. The main disadvantage of this circuit is that it requires high CMRR both in the followers and in the final op-amp. With the input buffers working at unity gain, all the common-mode rejection must be accomplished in the output amplifier,

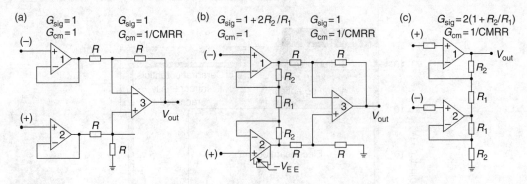

FIGURE 52.4 Circuit drawings for three different realizations of instrumentation amplifiers for biomedical applications. Voltage follower input stage (a), improved, amplifying input stage (b), and 2-op-amp version (c).

requiring very precise resistor matching. Additionally, the noise of the final op-amp is added at a low signal level, decreasing the signal-to-noise ratio unnecessarily. The circuit in Figure 52.4b eliminates this disadvantage. It represents the standard instrumentation amplifier configuration. The two input op-amps provide high differential gain and unity common-mode gain without the requirement of close resistor matching. The differential output from the first stage represents a signal with substantial relative reduction of the common-mode signal and is used to drive a standard differential amplifier which further reduces the common-mode signal. CMRR of the output op-amp as well as resistor matching in its circuit are less critical than in the follower type instrumentation amplifier. Offset trimming for the whole circuit can be done at one of the input op-amps. Complete instrumentation amplifier integrated circuits based on this standard instrumentation amplifier configuration are available from several manufacturers. All components except R_1, which determines the gain of the amplifier, and the potentiometer for offset trimming are contained on the integrated circuit chip. Figure 52.4c shows another configuration that offers high input impedance with only two op-amps. For good CMRR, however, it requires precise resistor matching.

In applications where dc and very low frequency biopotentials are not to be measured, it would be desirable to block those signal components at the preamplifier inputs by simply adding a capacitor working as a passive high-pass filter. This would eliminate the electrode offset potentials and permit a higher gain factor for the preamplifier *and thus a higher CMRR*. A capacitor between electrodes and amplifier input would, however, result in charging effects from the input bias current. Due to the difficulty of precisely matching capacitors for the two input leads, they would also contribute to an increased source impedance unbalance and thus reduce CMRR. Avoiding the problem of charging effects by adding a resistor between the preamplifier inputs and ground as shown in Figure 52.5a also results in a decrease of CMRR due to the diminished and mismatched input impedance. A 1% mismatch for two 1-MΩ resistors can already create a -60 dB loss in CMRR. The loss in CMRR is much greater if the capacitors are mismatched, which cannot be prevented in real systems. Nevertheless, such realizations are used where the specific situation allows. In some applications, a further reduction of the amplifier to a two-electrode amplifier configuration would be convenient, even at the expense of some loss in the CMRR. Figure 52.6 shows a preamplifier design working with two electrodes and providing ac coupling as proposed by Pallás-Areny and Webster [1990].

A third alternative of eliminating dc and low frequencies in the first amplifier stage is a directly coupled quasi-high-pass amplifier design, which maintains the high CMRR of dc coupled high input impedance instrumentation amplifiers [Song et al., 1998]. In this design, the gain determining resistor R_1 (Figure 52.5a) is replaced by a first order high-pass filter consisting of R_1 and a series capacitor C_f. The signal gain of the amplifier is

$$G = 1 + \frac{2R_2}{R_1 + \frac{1}{j\omega C}} \tag{52.4}$$

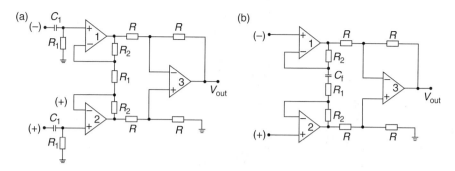

FIGURE 52.5 AC coupled instrumentation amplifier designs. The classical design using an RC high-pass filter at the inputs (a), and a high CMRR "quasi-high-pass" amplifier as proposed by Lu (b).

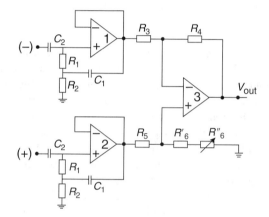

FIGURE 52.6 Composite instrumentation amplifier based on an ac-coupled first stage. The second stage is based on a one op-amp differential amplifier which can be replaced by an instrumentation amplifier.

Thus, dc gain is 1, while the high frequency gain remains at $G = 1 + 2R_2/R_1$. A realization using an off-the-shelf instrumentation amplifier (Burr-Brown INA 118) operates at low power (0.35 mA) with low offset voltage (11 μV typical) and low input bias current (1 nA typical), and offers a high CMRR of 118 dB at a gain of $G = 50$. The very high input impedance (10 GΩ) of the instrumentation amplifier renders it insensitive to fluctuations of the electrode impedance. Therefore, it is suitable for bioelectric measurements using pasteless electrodes applied to unprepared, that is, high impedance skin.

The preamplifier, often implemented as a separate device which is placed close to the electrodes or even directly attached to the electrodes, also acts as an impedance converter which allows the transmission of even weak signals to the remote monitoring unit. Due to the low output impedance of the preamplifier, the input impedance of the following amplifier stage can be low, and still the influence of interference signals coupled into the transmission lines is reduced.

52.2.2 Isolation Amplifier and Patient Safety

Isolation amplifiers can be used to break ground loops, eliminate source ground connections, and provide isolation protection to patient and electronic equipment. In a biopotential amplifier, the main purpose of the isolation amplifier is the protection of the patient by eliminating the hazard of electric shock resulting from the interaction among patient, amplifier, and other electric devices in the patient's environment, specifically defibrillators and electrosurgical equipment. It also adds to the prevention of line frequency interferences.

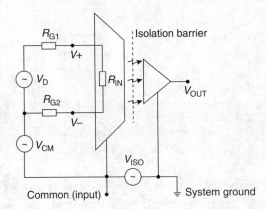

FIGURE 52.7   Equivalent circuit of an isolation amplifier. The differential amplifier on the left transmits the signal through the isolation barrier by a transformer, capacitor, or an opto-coupler.

Isolation amplifiers are realized in three different technologies: transformer isolation, capacitor isolation, and opto-isolation. An isolation barrier provides a complete galvanic separation of the input side, that is, patient and preamplifier, from all equipment on the output side. Ideally, there will be no flow of electric current across the barrier. The isolation-mode voltage is the voltage which appears across the isolation barrier, that is, between the input common and the output common (Figure 52.7). The amplifier has to withstand the largest expected isolation voltages without damage. Two isolation voltages are specified for commercial isolation amplifiers (1) the continuous rating and (2) the test voltage. To eliminate the need for longtime testing, the device is tested at about two times the rated continuous voltage. Thus, for a continuous rating of 2000 V, the device has to be tested at 4000 to 5000 V for a reasonable period of time.

Since there is always some leakage across the isolation barrier, the **isolation mode rejection ratio (IMRR)** is not infinite. For a circuit as shown in Figure 52.7, the output voltage is:

$$V_{\text{out}} = \frac{G}{R_{\text{G1}} + R_{\text{G2}} + R_{\text{IN}}} \left[V_{\text{D}} + \frac{V_{\text{CM}}}{\text{CMRR}} \right] + \frac{V_{\text{ISO}}}{\text{IMRR}} \tag{52.5}$$

where G is the amplifier gain, V_{D}, V_{CM}, and V_{ISO} are differential, common mode, and isolation voltages, respectively, and CMRR is the common mode rejection ratio for the amplifier [Burr-Brown, 1994].

Typical values of IMRR for a gain of 10 are 140 dB at dc, and 120 dB at 60 Hz with a source unbalance of 5000 Ω. The isolation impedance is approximately 1.8 pF $\parallel$ $10^{12}\Omega$.

Transformer coupled isolation amplifiers perform on the basis of inductive transmission of a carrier signal that is amplitude modulated by the biosignal. A synchronous demodulator on the output port reconstructs the signal before it is fed through a Bessel response low-pass filter to an output buffer. A power transformer, generally driven by a 400 to 900 kHz square wave, supplies isolated power to the amplifier.

Optically coupled isolation amplifiers can principally be realized using only a single LED and photodiode combination. While useful for a wide range of digital applications, this design has fundamental limitations as to its linearity and stability as a function of time and temperature. A matched photodiode design, as used in the Burr-Brown 3650/3652 isolation amplifier, overcomes these difficulties [Burr-Brown, 1994]. Operation of the amplifier requires an isolated power supply to drive the input stages. Transformer coupled low leakage current isolated dc/dc converters are commonly used for this purpose. In some particular applications, especially in cases where the signal is transmitted over a longer distance by fiber optics, for example, ECG amplifiers used for gated magnetic resonance imaging, batteries are used to power the amplifier. Fiber optic coupling in isolation amplifiers is another option that offers the advantage of higher flexibility in the placement of parts on the amplifier board.

Biopotential amplifiers have to provide sufficient protection from electrical shock to both user and patient. Electrical-safety codes and standards specify the minimum safety requirements for the equipment, especially the maximum leakage currents for chassis and patient leads, and the power distribution system [Webster, 1992; AAMI, 1993].

Special attention to patient safety is required in situations where biopotential amplifiers are connected to personal computers which are more and more often used to process and store physiological signals and data. Due to the design of the power supplies used in standard PCs permitting high leakage currents — an inadequate situation for a medical environment — there is a potential risk involved even when the patient is isolated from the PC through an isolation amplifier stage or optical signal transmission from the amplifier to the computer. This holds especially in those cases where, due to the proximity of the PC to the patient, an operator might touch patient and computer at the same time, or the patient might touch the computer. It is required that a special power supply with sufficient limitation of leakage currents is used in the computer, or that an additional, medical grade isolation transformer is used to provide the necessary isolation between power outlet and PC.

52.2.3 Surge Protection

The isolation amplifiers described in the preceding paragraph are primarily used for the protection of the patient from electric shock. Voltage surges between electrodes as they occur during the application of a defibrillator or electrosurgical instrumentation also present a risk to the biopotential amplifier. Biopotential amplifiers should be protected against serious damage to the electronic circuits. This is also part of the patient safety since defective input stages could otherwise apply dangerous current levels to the patient. To achieve this protection, voltage limiting devices are connected between each measuring electrode and electric ground. Ideally, these devices do not represent a shunt impedance and thus do not lower the input impedance of the preamplifier as long as the input voltage remains in a range considered safe for the equipment. They appear as an open circuit. As soon as the voltage drop across the device reaches a critical value V_b, the impedance of the device changes sharply and current passes through it to such an extent that the voltage cannot exceed V_b due to the voltage drop across the series resistor R as indicated in Figure 52.8.

Devices used for amplifier protection are diodes, Zener diodes, and gas-discharge tubes. Parallel silicon diodes limit the voltage to approximately 600 mV. The transition from nonconducting to conducting state is not very sharp, and signal distortion begins at about 300 mV which can be within the range of

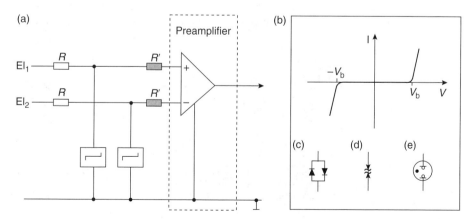

FIGURE 52.8 Protection of the amplifier input against high-voltage transients. The connection diagram for voltage-limiting elements is shown in panel (a) with two optional resistors R' at the input. A typical current–voltage characteristic is shown in panel (b). Voltage-limiting elements shown are the anti-parallel connection of diodes (c), anti-parallel connection of Zener diodes (d), and gas-discharge tubes (e).

input voltages depending on the electrodes used. The breakdown voltage can be increased by connecting several diodes in series. Higher breakdown voltages are achieved by Zener diodes connected back to back. One of the diodes will be biased in the forward direction and the other in the reverse direction. The breakdown voltage in the forward direction is approximately 600 mV, but the breakdown voltage in the reverse direction is higher, generally in the range of 3 to 20 V, with a sharper voltage–current characteristic than the diode circuit.

A preferred voltage-limiting device for biopotential amplifiers is the *gas-discharge tube*. Due to its extremely high impedance in the nonconducting state, this device appears as an open circuit until it reaches its breakdown voltage. At the breakdown voltage which is in the range of 50 to 90 V, the tube switches to the conducting state and maintains a voltage that is usually several volts less than the breakdown voltage. Though the voltage maintained by the gas-discharge tube is still too high for some amplifiers, it is low enough to allow the input current to be easily limited to a safe value by simple circuit elements such as resistors like the resistors R′ indicated in Figure 52.8a. Preferred gas discharge tubes for biomedical applications are miniature neon lamps which are very inexpensive and have a symmetric characteristic.

52.2.4 Input Guarding

The common mode input impedance and thus the CMRR of an amplifier can be greatly increased by guarding the input circuit. The common mode signal can be obtained by two averaging resistors connected between the outputs of the two input op-amps of an instrumentation amplifier as shown in Figure 52.9. The buffered common-mode signal at the output of op-amp 4 can be used as guard voltage to reduce the effects of cable capacitance and leakage.

In many modern biopotential amplifiers, the reference electrode is not grounded. Instead, it is connected to the output of an amplifier for the common mode voltage, op-amp 3 in Figure 52.10, which works as an inverting amplifier. The inverted common mode voltage is fed back to the reference electrode. This negative feedback reduces the common-mode voltage to a low value [Webster, 1992]. Electrocardiographs based on this principle are called driven-right-leg systems replacing the right leg ground electrode of ordinary electrocardiographs by an actively driven electrode.

52.2.5 Dynamic Range and Recovery

With an increase of either the common mode or differential input voltage there will be a point where the amplifier will overload and the output voltage will no longer be representative for the input voltage. Similarly, with a decrease of the input voltage, there will be a point where the noise components of the output voltage cover the output signal to a degree that a measurement of the desired biopotential is no

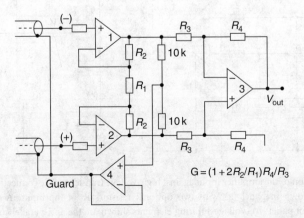

FIGURE 52.9   Instrumentation amplifier providing input guarding.

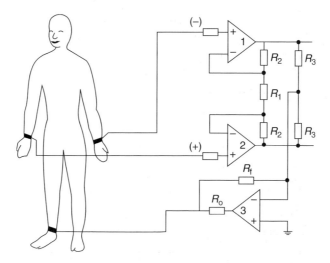

FIGURE 52.10 Driven-right-leg circuit reducing common-mode interference.

longer possible. The dynamic range of the amplifier, that is, the range between the smallest and largest possible input signal to be measured, has to cover the whole amplitude range of the physiological signal of interest. The required dynamic range of biopotential amplifiers can be quite large. In an application like fetal monitoring for example, two signals are recorded simultaneously from the electrodes which are quite different in their amplitudes: the fetal and the maternal ECG. While the maternal ECG shows an amplitude of up to 10 mV, the fetal ECG often does not reach more than 1 μV. Assuming that the fetal ECG is separated from the composite signal and fed to an analog/digital converter for digital signal processing with a resolution of 10 bit (signed integer), the smallest voltage to be safely measured with the biopotential amplifier is 1/512 μV or about 2 nV vs. 10 mV for the largest signal, or even up to 300 mV in the presence of an electrode offset potential. This translates to a dynamic range of 134 dB for the signals alone and 164 dB if the electrode potential is included in the consideration. Though most applications are less demanding, even such extreme requirements can be realized through careful design of the biopotential amplifer and the use of adequate components. The penalty for using less expensive amplifiers with diminished performance would be a potentially severe loss of information.

Transients appearing at the input of the biopotential amplifier, like voltage peaks from a cardiac pacemaker or a defibrillator, can drive the amplifier into saturation. An important characteristic for the amplifier is the time it takes to recover from such overloads. The recovery time depends on the characteristics of the transient, like amplitude and duration, the specific design of the amplifier, like bandwidth, and the components used. Typical biopotential amplifiers may take several seconds to recover from severe overload. The recovery time can be reduced by disconnecting the amplifier inputs at the discovery of a transient using an electronic switch.

52.2.6 Passive Isolation Amplifiers

Increasingly, biopotentials have to be measured within implanted devices and need to be transmitted to an external monitor or controller. Such applications include cardiac pacemakers transmitting the intracardiac ECG and functional electrical stimulation where, for example, action potentials measured at one eyelid serve to stimulate the other lid to restore the physiological function of a damaged lid at least to some degree. In these applications, the power consumption of the implanted biopotential amplifier limits the lifespan of the implanted device. The usual solution to this problem is an inductive transmission of power into the implanted device that serves to recharge an implanted battery. In applications where the size of the implant is of concern, it is desirable to eliminate the need for the battery and the related circuitry by using a quasi passive biopotential amplifier, that is, an amplifier that does not need a power supply.

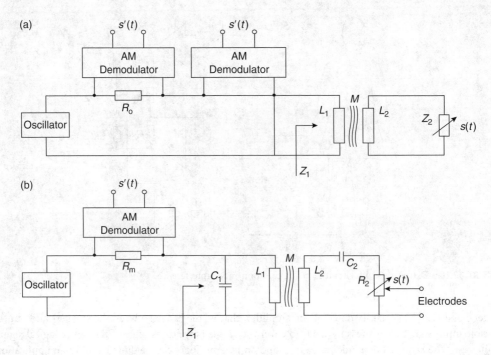

FIGURE 52.11 The *passive* isolation amplifier can be operated without the need for an isolated power supply. The biological source provides the power to modulate the load impedance of an inductive transformer. As an easy realization shown in panel (b), a FET can be directly connected to two electrodes. The source-drain resistance changes as a linear function of the biopotential which is then reflected by the input impedance of the transformer.

   The function of passive telemetric amplifiers for biopotentials is based on the ability of the biological source to drive a low power device such as a FET and the sensing of the biopotentials through inductive or acoustic coupling of the implanted and external devices [Nagel et al., 1982]. In an inductive system, a FET serves as a load to an implanted secondary LC-circuit which is stimulated inductively by an extracorporal oscillator (Figure 52.11). Depending on the special realization of the system, the biopotential is available in the external circuit from either an amplitude or frequency-modulated carrier-signal. The input impedance of the inductive transmitter as a function of the secondary load impedance Z_2 is given by:

$$Z_1 = j\omega L_1 + \frac{(\omega M)^2}{Z_2 + j\omega L_2} \tag{52.6}$$

In an amplitude-modulated system, the resistive part of the input-impedance Z_1 must change as a linear function of the biopotential. The signal is obtained as the envelope of the carrier signal, measured across a resistor R_m. A frequency-modulated system is realized when the frequency of the signal generator is determined at least in part by the impedance Z_1 of the inductive transmitter. In both cases, the signal-dependent changes of the secondary impedance Z_2 can be achieved by a junction-FET. Using the field effect transistor as a variable load resistance changing its resistance in proportion to the source-gate voltage which is determined by the electrodes of this two-electrode amplifier, the power supplied by the biological source is sufficient to drive the amplifier. The input impedance can be in the range of 10^{10} Ω.

   Optimal transmission characteristics are achieved with AM systems. Different combinations of external and implanted resonance circuits are possible to realize in an AM system, but primary parallel with secondary serial resonance yields the best characteristics. In this case, the input impedance is given by:

$$Z_1 = \frac{1}{j\omega C_1} + \left(\frac{L_1}{M}\right)^2 \cdot R_2 \tag{52.7}$$

The transmission factor $(L_1/M)^2$ is optimal since the secondary inductivity, that is, the implanted inductivity, can be small, only the external inductivity determines the transmission factor and the mutual inductivity should be small, a fact that favors the loose coupling that is inherent to two coils separated by skin and tissue. There are, of course, limits to M which cannot be seen from Equation 52.7. In a similar fashion, two piezoelectric crystals can be employed to provide the coupling between input and output.

This 2-lead isolation amplifier design is not limited to telemetric applications. It can also be used in all other applications where its main advantage lies in its simplicity and the resulting substantial cost savings as compared to other isolation amplifiers which require additional amplifier stages and an additional isolated power supply.

52.2.7 Digital Electronics

The ever increasing density of integrated digital circuits together with their extremely low power consumption permits digitizing and preprocessing of signals already on the isolated patient-side of the amplifiers, thus improving signal quality and eliminating the problems normally related to the isolation barrier, especially those concerning isolation voltage interferences and long-term stability of the isolation amplifiers. Digital signal transmission to a remote monitoring unit, a computer system, or computer network can be achieved without any risk of picking up transmission line interferences, especially when implemented with fiberoptical cables.

Digital techniques also offer an easy means of controlling the front-end of the amplifier. Gain factors can be easily adapted, and changes of the electrode potential resulting from electrode polarization or from interferences which might drive the differential amplifier into saturation can easily be detected and compensated.

52.3   Summary

Biopotential amplifiers are a crucial component in many medical and biological measurements, and largely determine the quality and information content of the measured signals. The extremely wide range of necessary specifications with regard to bandwidth, sensitivity, dynamic range, gain, CMRR, and patient safety leaves only little room for the application of general purpose biopotential amplifiers, and mostly requires the use of special purpose amplifiers.

Defining Terms

Common Mode Rejection Ratio (CMRR):   The ratio between the amplitude of a common mode signal and the amplitude of a differential signal that would produce the same output amplitude or as the ratio of the differential gain over the common-mode gain: CMRR $= G_D/G_{CM}$. Expressed in decibels, the common mode rejection is $20 \log_{10}$ CMRR. The common mode rejection is a function of frequency and source-impedance unbalance.

Isolation Mode Rejection Ratio (IMRR):   The ratio between the isolation voltage, V_{ISO}, and the amplitude of the isolation signal appearing at the output of the isolation amplifier, or as isolation voltage divided by output voltage V_{OUT} in the absence of differential and common mode signal: IMRR $= V_{ISO}/V_{OUT}$.

Operational Amplifier (op-amp):   A very high gain dc-coupled differential amplifier with single-ended output, high voltage gain, high input impedance, and low output impedance. Due to its high open-loop gain, the characteristics of an op-amp circuit only depend on its feedback network. Therefore, the integrated circuit op-amp is an extremely convenient tool for the realization of linear amplifier circuits [Horowitz and Hill, 1980].

References

AAMI, 1993. *AAMI Standards and Recommended Practices, Biomedical Equipment*, Vol. 2, 4th ed. AAMI, Arlington, VA.

Burr-Brown, 1994. *Burr-Brown Integrated Circuits Data Book, Linear Products*, Burr-Brown Corp., Tucson, AZ.

Horowitz, P. and Hill, W., 1980. *The Art of Electronics*, Cambridge University Press, Cambridge, UK.

Hutten, H. (Hrsg) 1992. *Biomedizinische Technik*, Springer-Verlag, Berlin.

Nagel, J., Ostgen, M., and Schaldach, M., 1982. *Telemetriesystem*, German Patent Application, P 3233240.8-15.

Pallás-Areny, R. and Webster, J.G., 1990. Composite Instrumentation Amplifier for Biopotentials. *Annals of Biomedical Engineering* 18, 251–262.

Strong, P., 1970. *Biophysical Measurements*, Tektronix, Inc., Beaverton, OR.

Webster, J.G., Ed., 1992. *Medical Instrumentation, Application and Design*, 2nd ed. Houghton Mifflin Company, Boston, MA.

Song, Y., Ozdamar, O., and Lu, C.C., 1998. Pasteless Electrode/Amplifier System for Auditory Brainstem Response (ABR) Recording. *Annals of Biomedical Engineering* 26, S-103.

Further Information

Detailed information on the realization of amplifiers for biomedical instrumentation and the availability of commercial products can be found in the references and in the Data Books and Application Notes of various manufacturers of integrated circuit amplifiers like Burr-Brown, Analog Devices, and Precision Monolithics Inc. as well as manufacturers of laboratory equipment like Gould and Grass.

53

Bioelectric Impedance Measurements

53.1 Measurement Methods **53**-1
53.2 Modeling and Formula Development **53**-3
53.3 Respiration Monitoring and Apnea Detection......... **53**-4
53.4 Peripheral Blood Flow **53**-5
53.5 Cardiac Measurements **53**-5
53.6 Body Composition (Single Frequency
       Measurement)... **53**-7
53.7 Impedance Spectroscopy **53**-7
53.8 Summary **53**-8
       Defining Terms **53**-8
       References **53**-8
       Further Information **53**-9

Robert Patterson
The University of Minnesota

Bioelectric tissue impedance measurements to determine or infer biological information have a long history dating back to before the turn of the century. The start of modern clinical applications of bioelectric impedance (BEI) measurements can be attributed in large part to the reports by Nyboer [1970]. BEI measurements are commonly used in **apnea** monitoring, especially for infants, and in the detection of venous **thrombus.** Many papers report the use of the BEI technique for peripheral blood flow, cardiac stroke volume, and body composition. Commercial equipment is available for these latter three applications, although the reliability, validity, and accuracy of these applications have been questioned and, therefore, have not received widespread acceptance in the medical community.

BEI measurements can be classified into two types. The first and most common application is in the study of the small pulsatile impedance changes associated with heart and respiratory action. The goal of this application is to give quantitative and qualitative information on the volume changes (**plethysmography**) in the lung, heart, peripheral arteries, and veins. The second application involves the determination of body characteristics such as total body fluid volume, inter and extra-cell volume, percent body fat, and cell and tissue viability. In this application, the total impedance is used and in some cases measured as a function of frequency, which is referred to as *impedance spectroscopy.*

53.1 Measurement Methods

Most single frequency BEI measurements are in the range of 50 to 100 kHz (at these frequencies no significant electrical shock hazard exists) using currents from 0.5 to 4 mA RMS. Currents at these levels

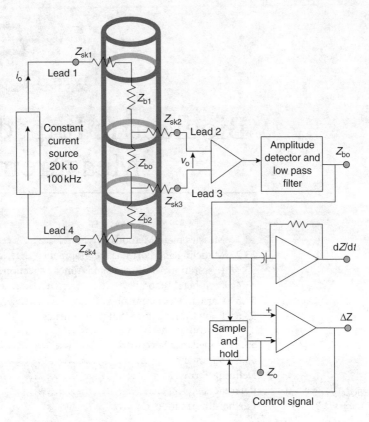

FIGURE 53.1 The four-electrode impedance measurement technique and the associated instrumentation.

are usually necessary to obtain a good signal-to-noise ratio when recording the small pulsatile changes that are in the range of 0.1 to 1% of the total impedance. The use of higher frequencies creates instrumentation design problems due to stray capacity.

BEI measurements in the 50–100 kHz range have typical skin impedance values 2–10 times the value of the underlying body tissue of interest depending on electrode area. In order to obtain BEI values that can be used to give quantitative biological information, the skin impedance contribution must be eliminated. This is accomplished by using the four electrode impedance measurement method shown in Figure 53.1, along with other signal processing blocks used in typical impedance plethysmographs.

Z_{bo} is the internal section of tissue we wish to measure. If we used two electrodes to make the measurement, we would include two skin impedances (i.e., Z_{sk1} and Z_{sk4}) and two internal tissue impedances (i.e., Z_{b1} and Z_{b2}) which would make it impossible to estimate an accurate value for Z_{bo}.

A constant current source supplies current, I_o, to the outside two electrodes 1 and 4. This current flows through the skin and body tissue independent of tissue and skin impedance values. The voltage V_o is measured across Z_{bo} with a voltage amplifier using electrodes 2 and 3. Assuming the output impedance of the current source is $\gg Z_{sk1} + Z_{b1} + Z_{bo} + Z_{b2} + Z_{sk4}$ and the input impedance of the voltage amplifier is $\gg Z_{sk2} + Z_{bo} + Z_{sk3}$, then

$$Z_{bo} = Z_o + \Delta Z, \qquad Z_o = V_o/I_o, \quad \text{and} \quad \Delta Z = \Delta V_o/I_o \tag{53.1}$$

where Z_o is the non-time-varying portion of the impedance and ΔZ is the impedance change typically-associated with the pulsation of blood in the region of measurement.

The output from the voltage pick-up amplifier (Figure 53.1) is connected to the amplitude detector and low pass filter which removes the high frequency carrier signal, which results in an output voltage proportional to $Z_{bo} \cdot Z_{bo}$ has a large steady part which is proportional to the magnitude of the tissue impedance (Z_0) and a small (0.1 to 1%) part, ΔZ, that represents the change due to respiratory or cardiac activity. In order to obtain a signal representing ΔZ, Z_0 must be removed from Z_{bo} and the signal amplified. This can be accomplished by capacity coupling or by subtracting a constant that represents Z_0. The latter is usually done because many applications require near dc response. The output of the ΔZ amplifier will be a waveform oscillating around zero volts. The output from the ΔZ amplifier controls the sample and hold circuit. When the ΔZ output exceeds a given value, usually plus or minus a few tenths of an ohm, the sample and hold circuit updates its value of Z_0. The output from the sample and hold circuit is subtracted from Z_{bo} by the ΔZ amplifier. The derivative of Z_{bo} is frequently obtained in instruments intended for cardiac use.

53.2 Modeling and Formula Development

To relate the ΔZ obtained on the thorax or peripheral limbs to the pulsatile blood volume change, the parallel column model, first described by Nyboer [1970], is frequently used (Figure 53.2). The model consists of a conducting volume with impedance Z_0 in parallel with a time-varying column with resistivity ρ, length L, and a time-varying cross-sectional area which oscillates from zero to a finite value. At the time in the cardiac cycle when the pulsatile volume is at a minimum, all of the conducting tissues and fluids are represented by the volume labeled Z_0. This volume can be a heterogeneous mixture of all of the non-time-varying tissues such as fat, bone, muscle, etc. in the region under measurement. The only information needed about this volume is its impedance Z_0 and that it is electrically in parallel with the small time varying column. During the cardiac cycle, the volume change in the right column starts with a zero cross-sectional area and increases in area until its volume equals the blood volume change. If the impedance of this volume is much greater than Z_0, then the following relation holds:

$$\Delta V = \rho(L^2/Z_0^2)\Delta Z \qquad (53.2)$$

where

ΔV = the pulsatile volume change with resistivity ρ
ρ = the resistivity of the pulsatile volume in Ω-cm (typically the resistivity of blood)
L = the length of the cylinder
Z_0 = the impedance measured when the pulsatile volume is at a minimum
ΔZ = the magnitude of the pulsatile impedance change.

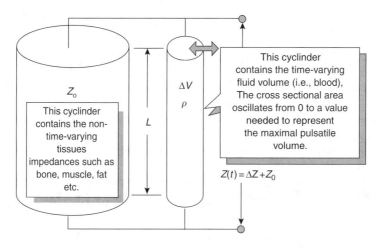

FIGURE 53.2 Parallel column model.

The resistivity of blood, ρ in Ω-cm, is a function of hematocrit (H) expressed as a percentage and can be calculated as $\rho = 67.919 \exp(0.0247H)$ [Mohapatra et al., 1977]. The typical value used for blood is 150 Ω-cm.

53.3   Respiration Monitoring and Apnea Detection

If the BEI is measured across the thorax, a variation of approximately 1 to 2 Ω/l of lung volume change is observed, which increases with inspiration. The most common position of the electrodes for respiratory measurements is on each side of the thorax along the midaxillary line. The largest signal is generally obtained at the level of the xiphsternal joint although a more linear signal is obtained higher up near the axilla [Geddes and Baker, 1989].

The problems encountered with the quantitative use of BEI for respiration volume are movement artifacts and the change in the response depending on whether diaphragmatic or intercostal muscles are used. For most applications, the most serious problem is body movement and positional changes artifacts which can cause impedance changes significantly larger than the change caused by respiration.

The determination of apnea or whether respiration has stopped [Neuman, 1988] in infants is one of the most widely used applications of BEI. For convenience and due to the lack of space on the thorax of infants, only two electrodes are used. These are placed at the mid-thoracic level along the midaxillary line and are also used to obtain the ECG. No effort is usually made to quantitate the volume change. Filtering is used to reduce movement artifacts and automatic gain controls and adaptive threshold detection is used in the breath detection circuits. Due to movement artifacts, the normal breath detection rate in infants is not highly reliable. When respiration stops, body movement ceases which eliminates the movement artifacts and then apnea can be detected. Ventation detection problems can occur if the airway is obstructed and the infant makes inspiratory movement efforts or cardiac-induced impedance changes are interpreted as a respiratory signal. Figure 53.3 shows a typical impedance measurement during an apneic period.

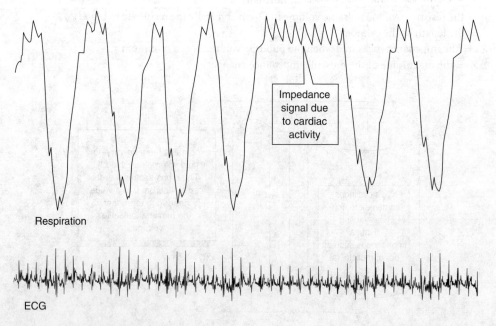

FIGURE 53.3   Example of BEI respiration signal and ECG.

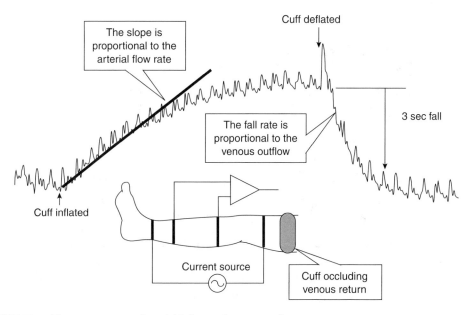

FIGURE 53.4   The measurement of arterial inflow and venous outflow.

53.4   Peripheral Blood Flow

BEI measurements are made on limbs to determine arterial blood flow into the limb or for the detection of venous **thrombosis**. In both applications, an occluding cuff is inflated above venous pressure to prevent outflow for a short period of time.

Figure 53.4 shows the typical electrode arrangement on the leg and the position of the occluding cuff. The cuff is rapidly inflated to 40 to 50 mmHg, which prevents venous outflow without significantly changing arterial inflow. The arterial inflow causes an increase in the volume of the limb. The slope of the initial impedance change as determined by the first three or four beats is used to measure the arterial flow rate. Equation 53.2 is used to calculate the volume change from the impedance change. The flow (the slope of the line in Figure 53.4) is determined by dividing the volume change by the time over which the impedance change was measured. The volume change that occurs after the impedance change reaches a plateau is a measure of the **compliance** of the venous system.

After the volume change of the leg has stabilized, the cuff is quickly deflated which results in an exponential decrease in volume. If a thrombosis exists in the veins, the time constant of the outflow lengthens. The initial slope, the time constant, and percentage change at 3 sec after cuff deflation have been used to quantitate the measurement. The percentage change at 3 sec has been reported to show the best agreement with **venograms**. The determination of deep venous thrombus is frequently made by combining the maximal volume change with the outflow rate. The agreement with a venogram is 94% for the detection of deep venous thrombus proximal to the knee [Anderson, 1988].

53.5   Cardiac Measurements

The measurements of chest impedance changes due to cardiac activity have been reported starting in 1930s. One of the most popular techniques, first reported by Patterson et al. [1964], for quantitative measurements uses band electrodes around the ends of the thorax as shown in Figure 53.5. Each heart beat causes a pulsatile decrease in impedance of 0.1 to 0.2 Ω (decreasing ΔZ and negative dZ/dt are shown in an upward direction). The empirical formula for stroke volume based on this method follows

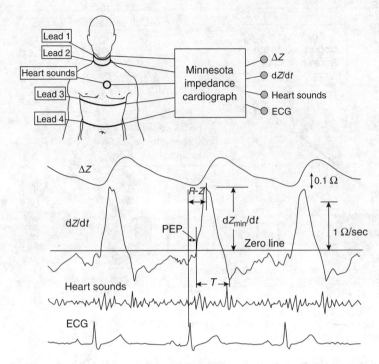

FIGURE 53.5   Impedance cardiographic waveforms.

from Equation 53.2:

$$\Delta V = \rho (L^2/Z_o^2)\, T\, dZ_{min}/dt \qquad\qquad (53.3)$$

where

ΔV = cardiac stroke volume (ml)
ρ = resistivity of blood (Ω-cm)
L = distance between the inner band electrodes (cm)
Z_o = base impedance (Ω)
dZ_{min}/dt = the magnitude of the largest negative derivative of the impedance change occurring during systole (Ω/sec)
T = systolic ejection time (sec)

Many studies have been conducted comparing the impedance technique with other standard methods of measuring stroke volume and cardiac output. In general, the correlation coefficient in subjects without valve problems or heart failure and with a stable circulatory system is 0.8 to 0.9. In patients with a failing circulatory system or valvular or other cardiovascular problems, the correlation coefficient may be less than 0.6 [Patterson, 1989].

Experimental physiological studies and computer modeling show that multiple sources contribute to the impedance signal. The anatomical regions that make significant contributions are the aorta, lungs, and atria. Recent studies have reported that the blood resistivity change with flow, pulsatile changes in the neck region, and the movement of the heart significantly contribute to the signal [Patterson et al., 1991; Wang and Patterson, 1995]. It appears that a number of different sources of the thoracic impedance change combine in a fortuitous manner to allow for a reasonable correlation between BEI measured stroke volume and other accepted techniques. However, in patients with cardiac problems where the contributions of the different sources may vary, the stroke volume calculated from BEI measurements may have significant error.

53.6 Body Composition (Single Frequency Measurement)

The percentage of body fat has been an important parameter in sports medicine, physical conditioning, weight loss programs, and predicting optimum body weight. To determine body composition, the body is configured as two parallel cylinders similar to the model described earlier. One cylinder is represented by fat and the other as fat-free body tissue. Since the resistivity of fat is much larger than muscle and other body fluids, the volume determined from the total body impedance measurement is assumed to represent the fat-free body volume. Studies have been conducted that calculate the fat-free body mass by determining the volume of the fat-free tissue cylinder using the impedance measured between the right hand and right foot, and using the subject's height as a measure of the cylinder's length with an empirical constant used to replace ρ [Lukaski et al., 1985]. Knowing the total weight and assuming body density factors, the percentage of body fat can be calculated as the difference between total weight and the weight of the fat-free tissue. Many studies have reported the correlation of the percentage of body fat calculated from BEI with other accepted standard techniques from approximately 0.88 to 0.98 [Schoeller and Kushner, 1989]. The physical model used for the equation development is a poor approximation to the actual body because it assumes a uniform cross-sectional area for the body between the hand the foot. Patterson [1989] pointed out the main problem with the technique: the measured impedance depends mostly on the characteristics of the arms and legs and not of the trunk. Therefore, determination of body fat with this method may often be inaccurate.

53.7 Impedance Spectroscopy

By measuring BEI over a range of frequencies (typically between 1 kHz and 1 MHz), the material properties of the tissues can be determined [Ackmann and Seitz, 1984]. Figure 53.6 shows the typical complex plane plot of the real and imaginary part of impedance and the model used to fit the data. R_E represents the extra-cellular space, R_I the intra-cellular space, and C_m the cell membrane. The parameter α is proportional to the angle of the suppression of the semicircle. It exists to account for the distribution of time constants in the tissue. At low frequencies, the current flows in the extra-cellular space and at high frequencies the current is capacitively passed across the cell membrane while the extra and intra cell spaces are in parallel.

Using these model parameters, studies have shown positive results in determining intra and extra-cellular fluid volumes [Kanai et al., 1987], body fat [De Lorenzo et al., 1997], tissue ischemica [Cinca et al., 1997] and cancerous tissues [Jossient, 1998].

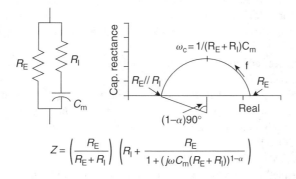

$$Z = \left(\frac{R_E}{R_E + R_I}\right)\left(R_I + \frac{R_E}{1 + (j\omega C_m(R_E + R_I))^{1-\alpha}}\right)$$

FIGURE 53.6   Typical impedance spectroscopy data, model, and the equation used to fit the data.

53.8 Summary

Electrical impedance instrumentation is not relatively costly, which has encouraged its possible application in many different areas. The impedance measurement is influenced by many different factors including geometry, tissue conductivity, and blood flow. Because of this complexity, it is difficult to reliably measure an isolated physiological parameter, which has been the principle factor limiting its use. The applications that are widely used in clinical medicine are apnea monitoring and the detection of venous thrombosis. The other applications described above will need more study before becoming a reliable and useful measurement.

Defining Terms

Apnea: A suspension of respiration.

Compliance: The volume change divided by the pressure change. The higher the compliance, the more easily the vessel will expand as pressure increases.

Plethysmography: The measurement of the volume change of an organ or body part.

Thrombosis: The formation of a thrombus.

Thrombus: A clot of blood formed within the heart or vessel.

Venogram: An x-ray image of the veins using an injected radiopaque contrast material.

References

Ackmann, J.J. and Seitz, M.A. (1984). Methods of complex impedance measurements in biologic tissue. *Crit. Rev. Biomed. Eng.* 11: 281–311.

Anderson, F.A. Jr. (1988). Impedance plethysmography, in J.G. Webster (Ed.) *Encyclopedia of Medical Devices and Instrumentation,* Wiley, New York, pp. 1632–1643.

Cinca, J., Warran, M., Carreno, A., Tresanchez, M., Armadans, L., Gomez, P., and Soler-Soler, J. (1997). Changes in myocardial electrical impedance induced by coronary artery occlusion in pigs with and without preconditioning. *Circulation* 96: 3079–3086.

De Lorenzo, A., Andreoi, A., Matthie, J., and Withers, P. (1997). Predicting body cell mass with bioimpedance by using theoretical methods: a technological review. *J. Appl. Physiol.* 82: 1542–1558.

Geddes, L.A. and Baker, L.E. (1989). *Principles of Applied Biomedical Instrumentation — Third Edition,* Wiley, New York, pp. 569–572.

Jossient, J. (1998). The impedivity of freshly excised human breast tissue. *Physiol. Meas.* 19: 61–75.

Kanai, H., Haeno, M., and Sakamoto, K. (1987). Electrical measurement of fluid distribution in human legs and arms. *Med. Prog. Technol.* 12: 159–170.

Lukaski, H.C., Johnson, P.E., Bolonchuk, W.W., and Lykken, G.I. (1985). Assessment of fat-free mass using bioelectric impedance measurements of the human body. *Am. J. Clin. Nutr.* 41: 810–817.

Mohapatra, S.N., Costeloe, K.L., and Hill, D.W. (1977). Blood resistivity and its implications for the calculations of cardiac output by the thoracic electrical impedance technique. *Intensive Care Med.* 3: 63.

Neuman, M.R. (1988). Neonatal monitoring, in J.G. Webster (Ed.) *Encyclopedia of Medical Devices and Instrumentation,* Wiley, New York, pp. 2020–2034.

Nyboer, J. (1970). *Electrical Impedance Plethysmography,* 2nd ed., Charles C. Thomas, Springfield, IL.

Patterson, R.P. (1989). Fundamentals of impedance cardiography, *IEEE Eng. Med. Biol. Mag.* 8: 35–38.

Patterson, R.P. (1989). Body fluid determinations using multiple impedance measurements, *IEEE Eng. Med. Biol. Mag.* 8: 16–18.

Patterson, R., Kubicek, W.G., Kinnen, E., Witsoe, D., and Noren, G. (1964). Development of an electrical impedance plethysmography system to monitor cardiac output. *Proc of the First Ann. Rocky Mountain Bioengineering Symposium,* pp. 56–71.

Patterson, R.P., Wang, L., and Raza, S.B. (1991). Impedance cardiography using band and regional electrodes in supine, sitting, and during exercise. *IEEE Trans. BME* 38: 393–400.

Schoeller, D.A. and Kushner, R.F. (1989). Determination of body fluids by the impedance technique. *IEEE Eng. Med. Biol. Mag.* 8: 19–21.

Wang, L. and Patterson, R.P. (1995). Multiple sources of the impedance cardiogram based on 3D finite difference human thorax models. *IEEE Trans. Biomed. Eng.* 42: 393–400.

Further Information

The book by Nyboer, *Electrical Impedance Plethysmography* contains useful background information. *The Encyclopedia of Medical Devices and Instrumentation* edited by J.G. Webster and *Principles of Applied Biomedical Instrumentation* by L.A. Geddes and L.E. Baker give a more in-depth description of many applications and describe some usual measurements.

54

Implantable Cardiac Pacemakers

54.1	Indications	**54**-2
54.2	Pulse Generators	**54**-3
	Sensing Circuit • Output Circuit • Timing Circuit • Telemetry Circuit • Power Source	
54.3	Leads	**54**-7
54.4	Programmers...	**54**-9
54.5	System Operation	**54**-9
54.6	Clinical Outcomes and Cost Implications	**54**-10
54.7	Conclusion	**54**-11
	Defining Terms...	**54**-11
	References	**54**-12
	Further Information	**54**-12

Michael Forde
Pat Ridgely
Medtronic, Inc.

The practical use of an implantable device for delivering a controlled, rhythmic electric stimulus to maintain the heartbeat is relatively recent: cardiac pacemakers have been in clinical use only slightly more than 30 years. Although devices have gotten steadily smaller over this period (from 250 g in 1960 to 25 g today), the technological evolution goes far beyond size alone. Early devices provided only single-chamber, asynchronous, nonprogrammable pacing coupled with questionable reliability and longevity. Today, advanced electronics afford dual-chamber multi*programmability*, diagnostic functions, rate response, data collection, and exceptional reliability, and lithium-iodine power sources extend longevity to upward of 10 years. Continual advances in a number of clinical, scientific, and engineering disciplines have so expanded the use of pacing that it now provides cost-effective benefits to an estimated 350,000 patients worldwide each year.

The modern pacing system is comprised of three distinct components: pulse generator, lead, and programmer (Figure 54.1). The pulse generator houses the battery and the circuitry which generates the stimulus and senses electrical activity. The lead is an insulated wire that carries the stimulus from the generator to the heart and relays intrinsic cardiac signals back to the generator. The programmer is a telemetry device used to provide two-way communications between the generator and the clinician. It can alter the therapy delivered by the pacemaker and retrieve diagnostic data that are essential for optimally titrating that therapy. Ultimately, the therapeutic success of the pacing prescription rests on the clinician's choice of an appropriate system, use of sound implant technique, and programming focused on patient outcomes.

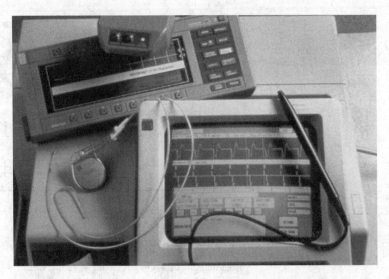

FIGURE 54.1   The pacing systems comprise a programmer, pulse generator, and lead. There are two programmers pictured above; one is portable, and the other is an office-based unit.

This chapter discusses in further detail the components of the modern pacing system and the significant evolution that has occurred since its inception. Our focus is on system design and operations, but we also briefly overview issues critical to successful clinical performance.

54.1   Indications

The decision to implant a permanent pacemaker for bradyarrhythmias usually is based on the major goals of symptom relief (at rest and with physical activity), restoration of functional capacity and quality of life, and reduced mortality. As with other healthcare technologies, appropriate use of pacing is the intent of indications guidelines established by Medicare and other third-party payors.

In 1984 and again in 1991, a joint commission of the American College of Cardiology and the American Heart Association established guidelines for pacemaker implantation (Committee on Pacemaker Implantation, 1991). In general, pacing is indicated when there is a dramatic slowing of the heart rate or a failure in the connection between the atria and ventricles resulting in decreased cardiac output manifested by such symptoms as syncope, light-headedness, fatigue, and exercise intolerance. Failure of impulse formation and/or conduction is the overriding theme of all pacemaker indications. There are four categories of pacing indications:

1. Heart block (e.g., complete heart block, symptomatic 2° AV block)
2. Sick sinus syndrome (e.g., symptomatic bradycardia, sinus arrest, sinus exit block)
3. Myocardial infarction (e.g., conduction disturbance related to the site of infarction)
4. Hypersensitive carotid sinus syndrome (e.g., recurrent syncope)

Within each of these four categories the ACC/AHA provided criteria for classifying a condition as group I (pacing is considered necessary), group II (pacing may be necessary), or group III (pacing is considered inappropriate).

New indications for cardiac pacing are being evaluated under the jurisdiction of the Food and Drug Administration. For example, **hypertrophic obstructive cardiomyopathy** (HOCM) is one of these new potential indications, with researchers looking at dual-chamber pacing as a means of reducing left ventricular outflow obstruction. Though efforts in these areas are ongoing and expanding, for now they remain unapproved as standard indications for pacing.

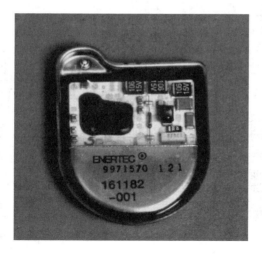

FIGURE 54.2   Internal view of pulse generator.

54.2   Pulse Generators

The pulse generator contains a power source, output circuit, sensing circuit, and a timing circuit (Figure 54.2). A telemetry coil is used to send and receive information between the generator and the programmer. **Rate-adaptive** pulse generators include the sensor components along with the circuit to process the information measured by the sensor.

Modern pacemakers use **CMOS circuit** technology. One to 2 kilobytes of read-only memory (ROM) are used to direct the output and sensing circuits; 16 to 512 bytes of random-access memory (RAM) are used to store diagnostic data. Some manufacturers offer fully RAM-based pulse generators, providing greater storage of diagnostic data and the flexibility for changing feature sets after implantation.

All components of the pulse generator are housed in a *hermetically* sealed titanium case with a connector block that accepts the lead(s). Because pacing leads are available with a variety of different connector sites and configurations, the pulse generator is available with an equal variety of connectors. The outer casing is laser-etched with the manufacturer, name, type (e.g., single- versus dual-chamber), model number, serial number, and the lead connection diagram for each identification. Once implanted, it may be necessary to use an x-ray to reveal the identity of the generator. Some manufacturers use radiopaque symbols and ID codes for this purpose, whereas others give their generators characteristic shapes.

54.2.1   Sensing Circuit

Pulse generators have two basic functions, pacing and sensing. Sensing refers to the recognition of an appropriate signal by the pulse generator. This signal is the intrinsic cardiac depolarization from the chamber or chambers in which the leads are placed. It is imperative for the sensing circuit to discriminate between these intracardiac signals and unwanted electrical interference such as far-field cardiac events, diastolic potentials, skeletal muscle contraction, and pacing stimuli. An intracardiac electrogram (Figure 54.3) shows the waveform as seen by the pacemaker; it is typically quite different from the corresponding event as shown on the surface ECG.

Sensing (and pacing) is accomplished with one of two configurations, bipolar and unipolar. In bipolar, the anode and cathode are close together, with the anode at the tip of the lead and the cathode a ring electrode about 2 cm proximal to the tip. In unipolar, the anode and cathode may be 5 to 10 cm apart. The anode is at the lead tip and the cathode is the pulse generator itself (usually located in the pectoral region).

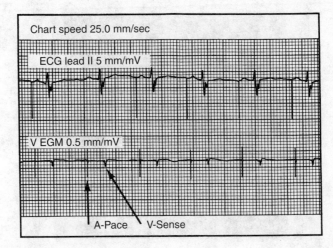

FIGURE 54.3 The surface ECG (ECG LEAD II) represents the sum total of the electrical potentials of all depolarizing tissue. The intracardiac electrogram (V EGM) shows only the potentials measured between the lead electrodes. This allows the evaluation of signals that may be hidden within the surface ECG.

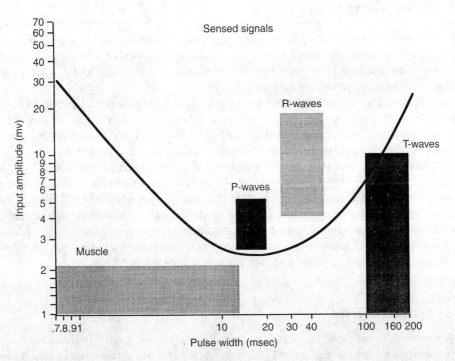

FIGURE 54.4 This is a conceptual depiction of the bandpass filter demonstrating the typical filtering of unwanted signals by discriminating between those with slew rates that are too low and/or too high.

In general, bipolar and unipolar sensing configurations have equal performance. A drawback of the unipolar approach is the increased possibility of sensing noncardiac signals: the large electrode separation may, for example, sense myopotentials from skeletal muscle movement, leading to inappropriate inhibition of pacing. Many newer pacemakers can be programmed to sense or pace in either configuration.

Once the electrogram enters the sensing circuit, it is scrutinized by a bandpass filter (Figure 54.4). The frequency of an R-wave is 10–30 Hz. The center frequency of most sensing amplifiers is 30 Hz. T-waves are slower, broad signals that are composed of lower frequencies (approximately 5 Hz or less). Far-field signals are also lower-frequency signals, whereas skeletal muscle falls in the range of 10–200 Hz.

At the implant, the voltage amplitude of the R-wave (and the P-wave, in the case of dual-chamber pacing) is measured to ensure the availability on an adequate signal. R-wave amplitudes are typically 5–25 mV, and P-wave amplitudes are 2–6 mV. The signals passing through the sense amplifier are compared to an adjustable reference voltage called the **sensitivity**. Any signal below the reference voltage is not sensed, and those above it are sensed. Higher-sensitivity settings (high-reference voltage) may lead to substandard sensing, and a lower reference voltage may result in oversensing. A minimum 2 : 1 safety margin should be maintained between the sensitivity setting and the amplitude of the intracardiac signal. The circuit is protected from extremely high voltages by a Zener diode.

The slope of the signal is also surveyed by the sensing circuit and is determined by the slew rate (the time rate of change in voltage). A slew rate that is too flat or too steep may be eliminated by the bandpass filter. On the average, the slew rate measured at implant should be between 0.75 and 2.50 V/sec.

The last line of defense in an effort to remove undesirable signals is to "blind" the circuit at specific times during the cardiac cycle. This is accomplished with blanking and refractory periods. Some of these periods are **programmable**. During the blanking period the sensing circuit is turned off, and during the refractory period the circuit can see the signal but does not initiate any of the basic timing intervals. Virtually all paced and sensed events begin concurrent blanking and refractory periods, typically ranging from 10 to 400 msec. These are especially helpful in dual-chamber pacemakers where there exists the potential for the pacing output of the atrial side to inhibit the ventricular pacing output, with dangerous consequences for patients in complete heart block.

Probably the most common question asked by the general public about pacing systems is the effect of electromagnetic interference (EMI) on their operation. EMI outside of the hospital is an infrequent problem, though patients are advised to avoid such sources of strong electromagnetic fields as arc welders, high-voltage generators, and radar antennae. Some clinicians suggest that patients avoid standing near antitheft devices used in retail stores. Airport screening devices are generally safe, though they may detect a pacemaker's metal case. Microwave ovens, ham radio equipment, video games, computers, and office equipment rarely interfere with the operation of modern pacemakers. A number of medical devices and procedures may on occasion do so, however; electrocautery, cardioversion and defibrillation, MRI, lithotripsy, diathermy, TENS units, and radiation therapy.

Pacemakers affected by interference typically respond with temporary loss of output or temporary reversion to asynchronous pacing (pacing at a fixed rate, with no inhibition from intrinsic cardiac events). The usual consequence for the patient is a return of the symptoms that originally led to the pacemaker implant.

54.2.2 Output Circuit

Pacing is the most significant drain on the pulse generator power source. Therefore, current drain must be minimized while maintaining an adequate safety margin between the **stimulation threshold** and the programmed output stimulus. Modern permanent pulse generators use constant voltage. The voltage remains at the programmed value while current fluctuates in relation to the source impedance.

Output energy is controlled by two programmable parameters, pulse amplitude and pulse duration. Pulse amplitudes range from 0.8 to 5 V and, in some generators, can be as high as 10 V (used for troubleshooting or for pediatric patients). Pulse duration can range from 0.05 to 1.5 msec. The prudent selection of these parameters will greatly influence the longevity of the pulse generator.

The output pulse is generated from the discharge of a capacitor charged by the battery. Most modern pulse generators contain a 2.8 V battery. The higher voltages are achieved using voltage multipliers (smaller capacitors used to charge the large capacitor). The voltage can be doubled by charging two smaller capacitors in parallel, with the discharge delivered to the output capacitor in series. Output pulses are emitted at a rate controlled by the timing circuit; output is commonly inhibited by sensed cardiac signals.

54.2.3 Timing Circuit

The timing circuit regulates such parameters as the pacing cycle length, refractory and blanking periods, pulse duration, and specific timing intervals between atrial and ventricular events. A crystal oscillator generating frequencies in the kHz range sends a signal to a digital timing and logic control circuit, which in turn operates internally generated clocks at divisions of the oscillatory frequency.

A rate-limiting circuit is incorporated into the timing circuit to prevent the pacing rate from exceeding an upper limit should a random component failure occur (an extremely rare event). This is also referred to as "runaway" protection and is typically 180 to 200 ppm.

54.2.4 Telemetry Circuit

Today's pulse generators are capable of both transmitting information from an RF antenna and receiving information with an RF decoder. This two-way communication occurs between the pulse generator and the programmer at approximately 300 Hz. Real-time telemetry is the term used to describe the ability of the pulse generator to provide information such as pulse amplitude, pulse duration, lead impedance, battery impedance, lead current, charge, and energy. The programmer, in turn, delivers coded messages to the pulse generator to alter any of the programmable features and to retrieve diagnostic data. Coding requirements reduce the likelihood of inappropriate programming alterations by environmental sources of radiofrequency and magnetic fields. It also prevents the improper use of programmers from other manufacturers.

54.2.5 Power Source

Over the years, a number of different battery technologies have been tried, including mercury-zinc, rechargeable silver-modified-mercuric-oxide-zinc, rechargeable nickel-cadmium, radioactive plutonium or promethium, and lithium with a variety of different cathodes. Lithium-cupric-sulfide and mercury-zinc batteries were associated with corrosion and early failure. Mercury-zinc produced hydrogen gas as a by-product of the battery reaction; the venting required made it impossible to hermetically seal the generator. This led to fluid infiltration followed by the risk of sudden failure.

The longevity of very early pulse generators was measured in hours. With the lithium-iodide technology now used, longevity has been reported as high as 15 years. The clinical desire to have a generator that is small and full-featured yet also long-lasting poses a formidable challenge to battery designers. One response by manufacturers has been to offer different models of generators, each offering a different balance between therapy, size, and longevity. Typical **battery capacity** is in the range of 0.8 to 3.0 amp-hours.

Many factors affect longevity, including pulse amplitude and duration, pacing rate, single- versus dual-chamber pacing, degree to which the patient uses the pacemaker, lead design, and static current drain from the sensing circuits. Improvements in lead design are often overlooked as a factor in improving longevity, but electrodes used in 1960 required a pulse generator output of 675 μJ for effective stimulation, whereas the electrodes of the 1990s need only 3 to 6 μJ.

Another important factor in battery design lies in the electrolyte that separates the anode and the cathode. The semisolid layer of lithium iodide that is used gradually thickens over the life of the cell, increasing the internal resistance of the battery. The voltage produced by lithium-iodine batteries is inversely related to this resistance and is linear from 2.8 V to approximately 2.4 V, representing about 90% of the usable battery life. It then declines exponentially to 1.8 V as the internal battery resistance increases from 10,000 to 40,000 Ω (Figure 54.5).

When the battery reaches between 2.0 and 2.4 V (depending on the manufacturer), certain functions of the pulse generator are altered so as to alert the clinician. These alterations are called the elective-replacement indicators (ERI). They vary from one pulse generator to another and include signature decreases in rate, a change to a specific pacing **mode**, pulse duration stretching, and the telemetered battery voltage. When the battery voltage reaches 1.8 V, the pulse generator may operate erratically or

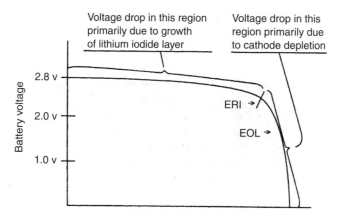

FIGURE 54.5   The initial decline in battery voltage is slow and then more rapid after the battery reaches the ERI voltage. An important aspect of battery design is the predictability of this decline so that timely generator replacement is anticipated.

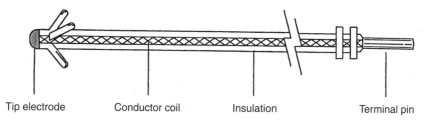

FIGURE 54.6   The four major lead components.

cease to function and is said to have reached "end of life." The time period between appearance of the ERI and end-of-life status averages about 3 to 4 months.

54.3   Leads

Implantable pacing leads must be designed not only for consistent performance within the hostile environment of the body but also for easy handling by the implanting physician. Every lead has four major components (Figure 54.6): the electrode, the conductor, the insulation, and the connector pin(s).

The electrode is located at the tip of the lead and is in direct contact with the myocardium. Bipolar leads have a tip electrode and a ring electrode (located about 2 cm proximal to the tip); unipolar leads have tip electrodes only. A small-radius electrode provides increased current density resulting in lower stimulation thresholds. The electrode also increases resistance at the electrode-myocardial interface, thus lowering the current drain further and improving battery longevity. The radius of most electrodes is 6 to 8 mm^2, though there are clinical trials underway using a "high-impedance" lead with a tip radius as low as 1.5 mm^2.

Small electrodes, however, historically have been associated with inferior sensing performance. Lead designers were able to achieve both good pacing and good sensing by creating porous-tip electrodes containing thousands of pores in the 20 to 100 μm range. The pores allow the ingrowth of tissue, resulting in the necessary increase in effective sensing area while maintaining a small pacing area. Some commonly used electrode materials include platinum-iridium. Elgiloy (an alloy of cobalt, iron, chromium, molybdenum, nickel, and manganese), platinum coated with platinized titanium, and vitreous or pyrolytic carbon coating a titanium or graphite core.

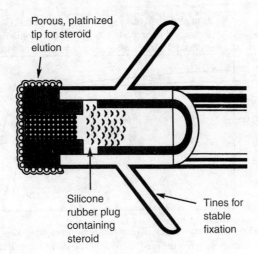

Porous, platinized
tip for steroid
elution

Silicone
rubber plug
containing
steroid

Tines for
stable
fixation

FIGURE 54.7   The steroid elution electrode.

Another major breakthrough in lead design is the steroid-eluting electrode. About 1 mg of a corticosteroid (dexamethasone sodium phosphate) is contained in a silicone core that is surrounded by the electrode material (Figure 54.7). The "leaking" of the steroid into the myocardium occurs slowly over several years and reduces the inflammation that results from the lead placement. It also retards the growth of the fibrous sack that forms around the electrode which separates it from viable myocardium. As a result, the dramatic rise in acute thresholds that is seen with nonsteroid leads over the 8 to 16 weeks postimplant is nearly eliminated. This makes it possible to program a lower pacing output, further extending longevity.

Once a lead has been implanted, it must remain stable (or fixated). The fixation device is either active or passive. The active fixation leads incorporate corkscrew mechanisms, barbs, or hooks to attach themselves to the myocardium. The passive fixation leads are held into place with tines that become entangled into the netlike lining (trabeculae) of the heart. Passive leads generally have better acute pacing and sensing performance but are difficult to remove chronically. Active leads are easier to remove chronically and have the advantage of unlimited placement sites. Some implanters prefer to use active-fixation leads in the atrium and passive-fixation leads in the ventricle.

The conductor carries electric signals to the pulse generator and delivers the pacing pulses to the heart. It must be strong and flexible to withstand the repeated flexing stress placed on it by the beating heart. The early conductors were a single, straight wire that was vulnerable to fracturing. They have evolved into coiled (for increased flexibility) multifilar (to prevent complete failure with partial fractures) conductors. The conductor material is a nickel alloy called MP35N. Because of the need for two conductors, bipolar leads are usually larger in diameter than unipolar leads. Current bipolar leads have a coaxial design that has significantly reduced the diameter of bipolar leads.

Insulation materials (typically silicone and polyurethane) are used to isolate the conductor. Silicone has a longer history and the exclusive advantage of being repairable. Because of low tear strength, however, silicone leads tend to be thicker than polyurethane leads. Another relative disadvantage of silicone is its high coefficient of friction in blood, which makes it difficult for two leads to pass through the same vein. A coating applied to silicone leads during manufacturing has diminished this problem.

A variety of generator-lead connector configurations and adapters are available. Because incompatibility can result in disturbed (or even lost) pacing and sensing, an international standards (IS-1) has been developed in an attempt to minimize incompatibility.

Leads can be implanted epicardially and endocardially. *Epicardial* leads are placed on the outer surface of the heart and require the surgical exposure of a small portion of the heart. They are used when venous occlusion makes it impossible to pass a lead transvenously, when abdominal placement of the pulse generator is needed (as in the case of radiation therapy to the pectoral area), or in children (to allow for growth). *Endocardial* leads are more common and perform better in the long term. These leads are passed through the venous system and into the right side of the heart. The subclavian or cephalic veins in the pectoral region are common entry sites. Positioning is facilitated by a thin, firm wire stylet that passes through the central lumen of the lead, stiffening it. Fluoroscopy is used to visualize lead positioning and to confirm the desired location.

Manufacturers are very sensitive to the performance reliability of the leads. Steady improvements in materials, design, manufacturing, and implant technique have led to reliability well in excess of 99% over 3-year periods.

54.4 Programmers

Noninvasive reversible alteration of the functional parameters of the pacemaker is critical to ongoing clinical management. For a pacing system to remain effective throughout its lifetime, it must be able to adjust to the patient's changing needs. The programmer is the primary clinical tool for changing settings, for retrieving diagnostic data, and for conducting noninvasive tests.

The pacing rate for programmable pacemakers of the early 1960s was adjusted via a Keith needle manipulated percutaneously into a knob on the side of the pacemaker; rotating the needle changed the pacing rate. Through the late 1960s and early 1970s, magnetically attuned reed switches in the pulse generator made it possible to noninvasively change certain parameters such as rate, output, sensitivity, and polarity. The application of a magnet could alter the parameters which were usually limited to only one of two choices. It was not until the late 1970s, when radiofrequency energy was incorporated as the transmitter of information, that programmability began to realize its full potential. Radiofrequency transmission is faster, provides bidirectional telemetry, and decreases the possibility of unintended programming from inappropriate sources.

Most manufacturers today are moving away from a dedicated proprietary instrument and toward a PC-based design. The newer designs are generally more flexible, more intuitive to use, and more easily updated when new devices are released. Manufacturers and clinicians alike are becoming more sensitive to the role that time-efficient programming can play in the productivity of pacing clinics, which may provide follow-up for as many as 500 to 1000 patients a year.

54.5 System Operation

Pacemakers have gotten steadily more powerful over the last three decades, but at the cost of steadily greater complexity. Manufacturers have come to realize the challenge that this poses for busy clinicians and have responded with a variety of interpretive aids (Figure 54.8).

Much of the apparent complexity of the timing rules that determine pacemaker operation is due to a design goal of mimicking normal cardiac function without interfering with it. One example is the dual-chamber feature that provides sequential stimulation of the atrium before the ventricle.

Another example is rate response, designed for patients who lack the normal ability to increase their heart rate in response to a variety of physical conditions (e.g., exercise). Introduced in the mid-1980s, rate-responsive systems use some sort of sensor to measure the change in a physical variable correlated to heart rate. The sensor output is signal-processed and then used by the output circuit to specify a target pacing rate. The clinician controls the aggressiveness of the rate increase through a variety of parameters (including a choice of transfer function); pacemaker-resident diagnostics provide data helpful in titrating the rate-response therapy.

The most common sensor is the activity sensor, which uses piezoelectric materials to detect vibrations caused by body movement. Systems using a transthoracic-impedance sensor to estimate pulmonary **minute ventilation** are also commercially available. Numerous other sensors (e.g., stroke volume, blood temperature or pH, oxygen saturation, preejection interval, right ventricular pressure) are in various

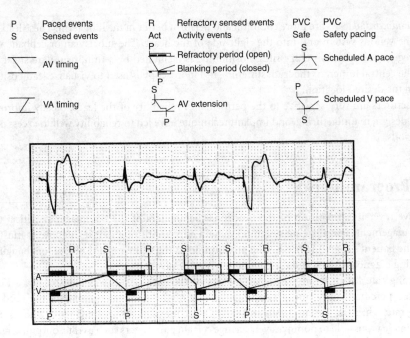

FIGURE 54.8 The Marker Channel Diagram is just one tool that makes interpretation of the ECG strip faster and more reliable for the clinician. It allows quick checking of the timing operations of the system.

stages of clinical research or have been market released outside the United States. Some of these systems are dual-sensor, combining the best features of each sensor in a single pacing system.

To make it easier to understand the gross-level system operation of modern pacemakers, a five-letter code has been developed by the North American Society of Pacing and Electrophysiology and the British Pacing and Electrophysiology Group [Bernstein et al., 1987]. The first letter indicates the chamber (or chambers) that are paced. The second letter reveals those chambers in which sensing takes place, and the third letter describes how the pacemaker will respond to a sensed event. The pacemaker will "inhibit" the pacing output when intrinsic activity is sensed or will "trigger" a pacing output based on a specific previously sensed event. For example, in DDD mode:

D: Pacing takes place in the atrium and the ventricle.

D: Sensing takes place in the atrium and the ventricle.

D: Both inhibition and triggering are the response to a sensed event. An atrial output is inhibited with an atrial-sensed event, whereas a ventricular output is inhibited with a ventricular-sensed event; a ventricular pacing output is triggered by an atrial-sensed event (assuming no ventricular event occurs during the A-V interval).

The fourth letter in the code is intended to reflect the degree of programmability of the pacemaker but is typically used to indicate that the device can provide rate response. For example, a DDDR device is one that is programmed to pace and sense in both chambers and is capable of sensor-driven rate variability. The fifth letter is reserved specifically for antitachycardia functions (Table 54.1).

Readers interested in the intriguing details of pacemaker timing operations are referred to the works listed at the end of this chapter.

54.6 Clinical Outcomes and Cost Implications

The demonstrable hemodynamic and symptomatic benefits provided by rate-responsive and dual-chamber pacing have led U.S. physicians to include at least one of these features in over three-fourths

TABLE 54.1   The NASPE/NPEG Code

Position	I	II	III	IV	V
Category	Chamber(s) paced	Chamber(s) sensed	Response to sensing	Programmability rate modulation	Antitachyarrhythmia function(s)
	O = None	O = None	O = None	O = None	O = None
	A = Atrium	A = Atrium	T = Triggered	P = Simple programmable	P = Packing
	V = Ventricle	V = Ventricle	I = Inhibited	M = Multiprogrammable	S = Shock
	D = Dual (A + V)	D = Dual (A + V)	D = Dual (T + I)	C = Communicating	D − Dual (P + S)
				R = Rate modulation	
Manufacturers' designation only	S = Single (A or V)	S = Single (A or V)			

Note: Positions I through III are used exclusively for antibradyarrhythmia function.
Source: From Bernstein A.D., et al., *PACE*, Vol. 10, July–Aug. 1987.

of implants in recent years. Also, new prospective data [Andersen et al., 1993] support a hypothesis investigated retrospectively since the mid-1980s: namely, that pacing the atrium in patients with sinus node dysfunction can dramatically reduce the incidence of such life-threatening complications as **congestive heart failure** and stroke associated with chronic **atrial fibrillation.** Preliminary analysis of the cost implications suggest that dual-chamber pacing is significantly cheaper to the U.S. healthcare system than is single-chamber pacing over the full course of therapy, despite the somewhat higher initial cost of implanting the dual-chamber system.

54.7   Conclusion

Permanent cardiac pacing is the beneficiary of three decades of advances in a variety of key technologies: biomaterials, electrical stimulation, sensing of bioelectrical events, power sources, microelectronics, transducers, signal analysis, and software development. These advances, informed and guided by a wealth of clinical experience acquired during that time, have made pacing a cost-effective cornerstone of cardiac arrhythmia management.

Defining Terms

Atrial fibrillation: An atrial arrhythmia resulting in chaotic current flow within the atria. The effective contraction of the atria is lost, allowing blood to pool and clot, leading to stroke if untreated.
Battery capacity: Given by the voltage and the current delivery. The voltage is a result of the battery chemistry, and current delivery (current × time) is measured in ampere hours and is related to battery size.
CMOS circuit: Abbreviation for complementary metallic oxide semiconductor, which is a form of semiconductor often used in pacemaker technology.
Congestive heart failure: The pathophysiologic state in which an abnormality of cardiac function is responsible for the failure of the heart to pump blood at a rate commensurate with the requirements of the body.
Endocardium: The inner lining of the heart.
Epicardium: The outer lining of the heart.
Hermeticity: The term, as used in the pacemaker industry, refers to a very low rate of helium gas leakage from the sealed pacemaker container. This reduces the chance of fluid intruding into the pacemaker generator and causing damage.

Hypertrophic obstructive cardiomyopathy: A disease of the myocardium characterized by thickening (hypertrophy) of the interventricular septum, resulting in the partial obstruction of blood from the left ventricle.

Minute ventilation: Respiratory rate × tidal volume (the amount of air taken in with each breath) = minute ventilation. This parameter is used as a biologic indicator for rate-adaptive pacing.

Mode: The type of pacemaker response to the patient's intrinsic heartbeat. The three commonly used modes are asynchronous, demand, and triggered.

Programmable: The ability to alter the pacemaker settings noninvasively. A variety of selections exist, each with its own designation.

Rate-adaptive: The ability to change the pacemaker stimulation interval caused by sensing a physiologic function other than the intrinsic atrial rhythm.

Sensitivity: A programmable setting that adjusts the reference voltage to which signals entering the sensing circuit are compared for filtering.

Stimulation threshold: The minimum output energy required to consistently "capture" (cause depolarization) of the heart.

References

Andersen H.R., Thuesen L., Bagger J.P. et al. (1993). Atrial versus ventricular pacing in sick sinus syndrome: a prospective randomized trial in 225 consecutive patients. *Eur. Heart. J.* 14: 252.

Bernstein A.D., Camm A.J., Fletcher R.D. et al. (1987). The NASPE/BPEG generic pacemaker code for antibradyarrhythmia and adaptive-rate pacing and antitachyarrhythmia devices. *PACE* 10: 794.

Committee on Pacemaker Implantation (1991). Guidelines for implantation of cardiac pacemakers and antiarrhythmic devices. *J. Am. Coll. Cardiol.* 18: 1.

Further Information

A good basic introduction to pacing from a clinical perspective is the third edition of *A Practical Guide to Cardiac Pacing* by H. Weston Moses, Joel Schneider, Brain Miller, and George Taylor (Little, Brown, 1991).

Cardiac Pacing (Blackwell Scientific, 1992), edited by Kenneth Ellenbogen, is an excellent intermediate treatment of pacing. The treatments of timing cycles and troubleshooting are especially good.

In-depth discussion of a wide range of pacing topics is provided by the third edition of *A Practice of Cardiac Pacing* by Seymour Furman, David Hayes, and David Holmes (Futura, 1993), and by *New Perspectives in Cardiac Pacing 3*, edited by Serge Barold and Jacques Mugica (Futura, 1993).

Detailed treatment of rate-responsive pacing is given in *Rate-Adaptive Cardiac Pacing: Single and Dual Chamber* by Chu-Pak Lau (Futura, 1993), and in *Rate-Adaptive Pacing*, edited by David Benditt (Blackwell Scientific, 1993).

The Foundations of Cardiac Pacing, Part I by Richard Sutton and Ivan Bourgeois (Futura, 1991) contains excellent illustrations of implantation techniques.

Readers seeking a historical perspective may wish to consult "Pacemakers, Pastmakers, and the Paced: An Informal History from A to Z," by Dwight Harken in the July/August 1991 issue of *Biomedical Instrumentation and Technology.*

PACE is the official journal of the North American Society of Pacing and Electrophysiology (NASPE) and of the International Cardiac Pacing and Electrophysiology Society. It is published monthly by Futura Publishing (135 Bedford Road, PO Box 418, Armonk, NY 10504 USA).

55

Noninvasive Arterial Blood Pressure and Mechanics

55.1	Introduction...	**55**-1
55.2	Long-Term Sampling Methods	**55**-2
	Vascular Unloading Principle • Occlusive Cuff Mechanics • Method of Korotkoff • Oscillometry • Derivative Oscillometry	
55.3	Pulse Dynamics Methods	**55**-8
	R-Wave Time Interval Technique • Continuous Vascular Unloading • Pulse Sensing • Arterial Tonometry • Flexible Diaphragm Tonometry	
55.4	Noninvasive Arterial Mechanics	**55**-12
55.5	Summary	**55**-14
	Acknowledgments..	**55**-14
	References	**55**-14

Gary Drzewiecki
Rutgers University

55.1 Introduction

The beginnings of noninvasive arterial pulse recording can be traced to the Renaissance. At that time, the Polish scientist, Strus (1555) had proposed that the arterial pulse possesses a waveform. Although instrumentation that he used was simple, he suggested that changes in the arterial pulse shape and strength may be related to disease conditions. Today, even though the technology is more advanced, noninvasive arterial blood pressure measurement still remains a challenge. Rigorous methods for extracting functional cardiovascular information from noninvasive pressure have been limited.

In this chapter, the most standard of noninvasive methods for arterial pressure measurements will be reviewed and future trends will be proposed. Two types of methods for noninvasive arterial pressure measurement may be defined; those that periodically sample and those that continuously record the pulse waveform. The sampling methods typically provide systolic and diastolic pressure and sometimes mean pressure. These values are collected over different heart beats during the course of 1 min. The continuous recording methods provide beat-to-beat measurements and often, the entire waveform. Some continuous methods only provide pulse pressure waveform and timing information.

The knowledge of systolic and diastolic pressure is fundamental for the evaluation of basic cardiovascular function and identifying disease. The choice of method depends on the type of study. For example, high blood pressure is a known precursor to many other forms of cardiovascular disease. A noninvasive method that samples blood pressure over the time course of months is usually adequate to study the progression of hypertension. The occlusive cuff-based methods fall into this category. These methods have been automated with recent instruments designed for ambulatory use [Graettinger et al., 1988]. Twenty-four to forty-eight hours ambulatory monitors have been applied to monitor the diurnal variation of a patient's blood pressure. This type of monitoring can alleviate the problem of "white coat hypertension," that is, the elevation of blood pressure associated with a visit to the physician's office [Pickering et al., 1988].

Short-term hemodynamic information obtained from the noninvasive arterial pulse waveform is a virtually untapped arena. While a great deal of knowledge has been gathered on the physics of the arterial pulse [Noordergraaf, 1978], it has been lacking in application because continuous pressure waveform monitors have not been available. A review of methods for continuous pulse monitoring that fill this gap will be provided.

Some applications for pulse monitoring can be found. In the recording time span of less than 1 min, the importance of the pressure waveform dominates, as well as beat-to-beat variations. This type of monitoring is critical in situations where blood pressure can alter quickly, such as due to trauma or anesthesia. Other applications for acute monitoring have been in aerospace, biofeedback, and lie detection. Moreover, pulse dynamics information becomes available such as wave reflection [Li, 1986]. Kelly et al. [1989] have shown that elevated systolic pressure can be attributed to pulse waveform changes due to a decrease in arterial compliance and increased wave reflection. Lastly, information on the cardiovascular control process can be obtained from pulse pressure variability [Omboni et al., 1993].

It has become increasingly popular to provide simultaneous recording of such variables as noninvasive blood pressure, oxygen saturation via pulse oximetry, body temperature, etc., in a single instrument. It is apparent that the advances in computer technology impinge on this practice, making it a clear trend. While this practice is likely to continue, the forefront of this approach will be those instruments that provide more than just a mere marriage of technology in a single design. It will be possible to extract functional information in addition to just pressure. As an example of this, a method for noninvasive measurement of the arterial pressure–lumen area curve will be provided.

55.2   Long-Term Sampling Methods

55.2.1   Vascular Unloading Principle

The vascular unloading principle is fundamental to all occlusive cuff-based methods of determining arterial blood pressure. It is performed by applying an external compression pressure or force to a limb such that it is transmitted to the underlying vessels. It is usually assumed that the external pressure and the tissue pressure (stress) are in equilibrium. The underlying vessels are then subjected to altered transmural pressure (internal minus external pressure) by varying the external pressure. It is further assumed [Marey, 1885] that the tension within the wall of the vessel is zero when transmural pressure is zero. Hence, the term vascular unloading originated.

Various techniques have been developed that attempt to detect vascular unloading. These generally rely on the fact that once a vessel is unloaded, further external pressure will cause it to collapse. In summary,

$$\text{If } P_a > P_c \Rightarrow \text{Lumen open}$$

or

$$\text{If } P_a > P_c \Rightarrow \text{Lumen closed}$$

where P_a is the arterial pressure and P_c is the cuff pressure. Most methods that employ the occlusive arm cuff rely on this principle and differ in the means of detecting whether the artery is open or closed. Briefly, some approaches are the skin flush, palpatory, Korotkoff (auscultatory), oscillometric, and ultrasound methods [Drzewiecki et al., 1987]. Of these, the methods of Korotkoff and oscillometry are in most common use and will be reviewed here.

The idea of using lumen opening and closure as an indication of blood pressure has survived since its introduction by Marey. This simple concept is complicated by the fact that lumen closure may not necessarily occur at zero transmural pressure. Instead, transmural pressure must be negative by 5 to 20 mmHg for complete closure. *In vitro* and *in vivo* human measurements have revealed that vessel buckling more closely approximates zero transmural pressure [Drzewiecki et al., 1997; Drzewiecki and Pilla, in press]. Buckling may be defined as the point at which the vessel switches from wall stretch to wall bending as a means of supporting its pressure load. The vessel is maximally compliant at this point and is approximately 25% open.

The validity of employing the buckling concept to blood pressure determination was tested. Sheth and Drzewiecki [1998] employed feedback control to regulate the pressure in a flexible diaphragm tonometer (see the section on *flexible diaphragm tonometer*). The buckling point was determined from the volume pulse. Thus, to detect vessel buckling, the derivative of the volume pulse with respect to mean pressure was computed. This was performed on a beat-to-beat basis. The feedback system was then used to adjust pressure such that this derivative was maximized, indicating the point of greatest instability. Thus, the underlying blood vessel was maintained in a constant state of buckling. According to the buckling theory, the transmural pressure should be nearly zero and tonometer pressure is equal to arterial pressure. A sample 2 min recording of noninvasive arterial pressure by this approach is shown (Figure 55.1). The method was capable of tracking the subject's blood pressure in response to a Valsalva maneuver in this same record. This test demonstrates the feasibility of employing buckling to measure blood pressure. This example also illustrates that beat-to-beat pressure can be obtained by this method without the necessity to occlude blood flow. This approach should be useful for pressure variability studies.

55.2.2 Occlusive Cuff Mechanics

The occlusive arm cuff has evolved more out of convenience than engineering design. As such, its mechanical properties are relatively unknown. The current version of the cuff is designed to encircle the upper arm. It consists of a flat rubber bladder connected to air supply tubing. The bladder is covered externally by cloth material with Velcro fasteners at either end for easy placement and removal. While the cuff encircles

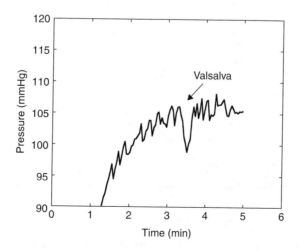

FIGURE 55.1   Application of arterial buckling to the continuous measurement of arterial pressure. The record shown tracks the subject's mean pressure in the brachial artery. The initial portion of the record illustrates the system as it locates the buckling point and the subject's blood pressure. The subject was directed to perform a brief Valsalva maneuver mid-way through the recording.

the entire arm, the bladder extends over approximately half the circumference. The bladder is pressurized with air derived from a hand pump, release valve, and manometer connected to the air supply tubing.

The cuff should accurately transmit pressure down to the tissue surrounding the brachial artery. A mechanical analysis revealed that the length of the cuff is required to be a specific fraction of the arm's circumference for pressure equilibrium [Alexander et al., 1977]. A narrow cuff resulted in the greatest error in pressure transmission and, thus, the greatest error in blood pressure determination. Geddes and Whistler [1978] experimentally examined the effect of cuff size on blood pressure accuracy for the Korotkoff method. Their measurements confirmed that a cuff-width-to-arm circumference ratio of 0.4 should be maintained. Cuff manufacturers, therefore, supply a range of cuff sizes appropriate for pediatric use up to large adults.

Another aspect of the cuff is its pressure response due to either internal air volume change or that of the limb. In this sense, the cuff can be thought of as a plethysmograph. It was examined by considering its pressure–volume characteristics. In an experiment, the cuff properties were isolated from that of the arm by applying it to a rigid cylinder of similar diameter [Drzewiecki et al., 1993]. Pressure–volume data were then obtained by injecting a known volume of air and noting the pressure. This was performed for a standard bladder cuff (13 cm width) over a typical range of blood pressure.

The cuff pressure–volume results for pressures less than 130 mmHg are nonlinear (Figure 55.2). For higher pressures, the data asymptotically approach a linear relationship. The cuff volume sensitivity, that

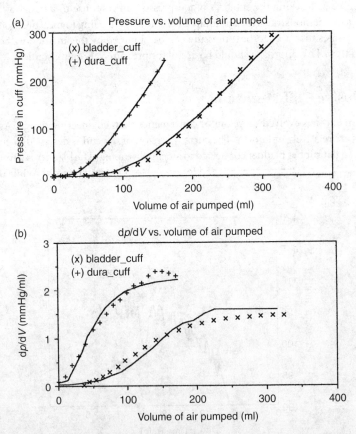

FIGURE 55.2 (a) Pressure–volume data obtained from two different occlusive arm cuffs. Inner surface of the cuff was fixed in this case to isolate cuff mechanics from that of the arm. (b) Derivative of the cuff pressure with respect to volume obtained from pressure–volume data of both cuffs. These curves indicate the pressure response of the cuff to volume change and are useful for plethysmography. Solid curves in both figures are the results of the occlusive cuff model.

is, its derivative with respect to volume, increased with cuff pressure (Figure 55.2). Above 130 mmHg, the cuff responded with nearly constant sensitivity.

A cuff mechanics theory was developed to explain the above cuff experiment [Drzewiecki et al., 1993]. Cuff mechanics was theorized to consist of two components. The first consists of the compressibility of air within the cuff. This was modeled using Boyle's gas law. The second component consists of elastic and geometric deformation of the cuff bladder. Cuff shape deformation proceeds at low pressures until the bladder reaches its final geometry, rendering a curved pressure–volume relationship. Then, elastic stretch of the rubber bladder takes over at high pressures, resulting in a nearly linear relationship. Solutions for this model are shown in comparison with the data in Figure 55.2 for two cuffs; a standard cuff and the Critikon Dura-cuf. This model was useful in linearizing the cuff for use as a plethysmograph and for application to oscillometry (below).

55.2.3 Method of Korotkoff

The auscultatory method or method of Korotkoff was introduced by the Russian army physician N. Korotkoff [1905]. In his experiments, Korotkoff discovered that sound emitted distally from a partially occluded limb. He realized that this sound was indicative of arterial flow and that together with the occlusive cuff could be used to determine blood pressure. The method, as employed today, utilizes a stethoscope placed distal to an arm cuff over the brachial artery at the antecubital fossa. The cuff is inflated to about 30 mmHg above systolic pressure and then allowed to deflate at a rate of 2 to 3 mm Hg/sec. With falling cuff pressure, sounds begin and slowly change their characteristics. The initial "tapping" sounds are referred to as Phase I Korotkoff sound and denote systolic pressure. The sounds increase in loudness during Phase II. The maximum intensity occurs in Phase III, where the tapping sound may be followed by a murmur due to turbulence. Finally, Phase IV Korotkoff sound is identified as muffled sound, and Phase V is the complete disappearance of sound. Phase IV is generally taken to indicate diastolic arterial pressure. But, Phase V has also been suggested to be a more accurate indication of diastolic pressure. This matter is a continued source of controversy. The long history of the Korotkoff sound provides much experimental information. For example, the frequency spectrum of sound, spatial variation along the arm, filtering effects, and timing are reviewed [Drzewiecki et al., 1989].

It is a long-held misconception that the origin of the Korotkoff sound is flow turbulence. Turbulence is thought to be induced by the narrowing of the brachial artery under an occlusive cuff as it is forced to collapse. There are arguments against this idea. First, the Korotkoff sounds do not sound like turbulence, that is, a murmur. Second, the Korotkoff sound can occur in low blood flow situations, while turbulence cannot. And, last, Doppler ultrasound indicates that peak flow occurs following the time occurrence of Korotkoff sound. An alternative theory suggests that the sound is due to nonlinear distortion of the brachial pulse, such that sound is introduced to the original pulse. This is shown to arise from flow limitation under the cuff in addition to curvilinear pressure–area relationship of the brachial artery [Drzewiecki et al., 1989]. Strong support for this theory comes from its ability to predict many of the Korotkoff sound's observable features.

The accuracy of the Korotkoff method is well known. London and London [1967] find that the Korotkoff method underestimates systolic pressure by 5 to 20 mmHg and overestimates diastolic pressure by 12 to 20 mmHg. However, certain subject groups, such as hypertensives or the elderly, can compound these errors [Spence et al., 1978]. In addition, it has been shown that the arm blood flow can alter the Korotkoff sound intensity and, thus, the accuracy of blood pressure measurement [Rabbany et al., 1993]. Disappearance of Korotkoff sound occurs early in Phase III for some subjects and is referred to as the auscultatory gap. This causes an erroneous indication of elevated diastolic pressure. The auscultatory gap error can be avoided by simply allowing cuff pressure to continue to fall, where the true Phase IV sounds return. This is particularly critical for automatic instruments to take into account. In spite of these errors, the method of Korotkoff is considered a documented noninvasive blood pressure standard by which other noninvasive methods may be evaluated [White et al., 1993].

The Korotkoff method is applicable to other vessels besides the brachial artery of the arm. For example, the temporal artery has been employed [Shenoy et al., 1993]. In this case, a pressure capsule is applied over the artery on the head in place of an occlusive cuff, to provide external pressure. This approach has been shown to be accurate and is applicable to aerospace. Pilots' cerebral vascular pressure often falls in high acceleration maneuvers, so that temporal artery pressure is a better indicator of this response.

55.2.4 Oscillometry

Oscillometric measurement of blood pressure predates the method of Korotkoff. The French physiologist Marey [1885] placed the arm within a compression chamber and observed that the chamber pressure fluctuated with the pulse. He also noted that the amplitude of pulsation varied with chamber pressure. Marey believed that the maximum pulsations or the onset of pulsations were associated with equality of blood pressure and chamber pressure. At that time, he was not certain what level of arterial pressure the maximum pulsations corresponded with. Recently, it has been demonstrated theoretically that the variation in cuff pressure pulsation is primarily due to the brachial artery buckling mechanics [Drzewiecki et al., 1994].

Today, oscillometry is performed using a standard arm cuff together with an in-line pressure sensor. Due to the requirement of a sensor, oscillometry is generally not performed manually, but, rather, with an automatic instrument. The recorded cuff pressure is high-pass-filtered above 1 Hz to observe the pulsatile oscillations as the cuff slowly deflates (Figure 55.3). It has been determined only recently that the maximum oscillations actually correspond with cuff pressure equal to mean arterial pressure (MAP) [Posey et al., 1969; Ramsey, 1979], confirming Marey's early idea. Systolic pressure is located at the point where the oscillations, O_s, are a fixed percentage of the maximum oscillations, O_m [Geddes et al., 1983]. In comparison with the intra-arterial pressure recordings, the systolic detection ratio is $O_s/O_m = 0.55$.

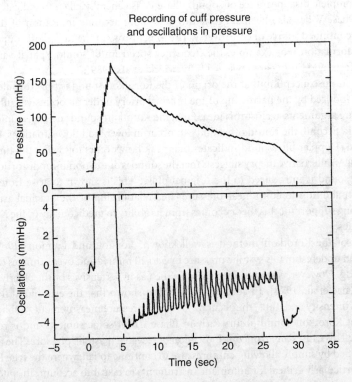

FIGURE 55.3 Sample recording of cuff pressure during oscillometric blood pressure measurement. Bottom panel shows oscillations in cuff pressure obtained by high pass filtering above 1/2 Hz.

Similarly, the diastolic pressure can be found as a fixed percentage of the maximum oscillations, as $O_d/O_m = 0.85$.

55.2.5 Derivative Oscillometry

The use of the oscillometric detection ratios to find systolic and diastolic pressure is an empirical approach. That is, the ratios are statistically valid over the population of subjects that form the total sample. This is a distinctly different approach than measuring blood pressure by detecting an event, such as the maximum in cuff pressure oscillations or the occurrence of Korotkoff sound. The event is constrained by the physics of arterial collapse under the cuff [Drzewiecki et al., 1994]. Therefore, it is more likely to be accurate under different conditions and, more importantly, for subjects outside of the sample population. In fact, the oscillometric determination of MAP is more accurate than systolic and diastolic pressures.

Drzewiecki et al. [1994] employed a model of oscillometry to evaluate the derivative of the oscillation amplitude curve (Figure 55.3) with respect to cuff pressure. When this derivative is plotted against cuff pressure, it was found that it reaches a maximum positive value. This occurred when cuff pressure equals diastolic pressure. Additionally, the minimum negative value was found to occur at systolic pressure. A measurement performed in our lab on a single subject illustrates the approach (Figure 55.4). The specific advantage offered is that the empirically based systolic and diastolic ratios are not necessary [Link, 1987]. This method may be referred to as derivative oscillometry.

Derivative oscillometry was evaluated experimentally in our lab. The values of systolic and diastolic pressures obtained by derivative oscillometry were compared with those obtained by the method of Korotkoff. Thirty recordings were obtained on normal subjects (Figure 55.5). The results indicated a high correlation of 0.93 between the two methods. Systolic mean error was determined to be 9% and diastolic mean error was −6%. Thus, derivative oscillometry was found to compare well with the method of Korotkoff in this preliminary evaluation. Before adopting derivative oscillometry, a more complete evaluation needs to be performed using a greater and more diverse subject population.

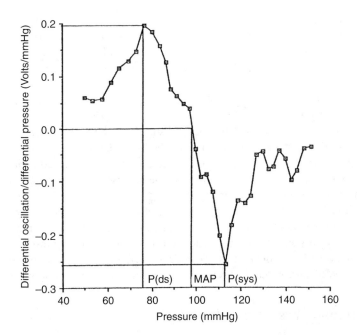

FIGURE 55.4 Method of derivative oscillometry. The derivative of cuff pressure oscillations data with respect to cuff pressure is shown from a single subject. The maximum and minimum values denote diastolic and systolic pressure, respectively. A zero derivative indicates MAP in this plot.

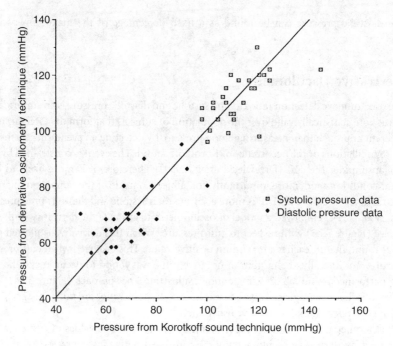

FIGURE 55.5 Experimental evaluation of derivative oscillometry using systolic and diastolic pressure from the method of Korotkoff as reference. The line indicates the result of linear regression to the data.

55.3   Pulse Dynamics Methods

55.3.1   R-Wave Time Interval Technique

One of the basic characteristics of pressure and flow under an occlusive cuff is that the pulse is apparently delayed with increasing cuff pressure. The R-wave of the ECG is often employed as a time reference. Arzbaecher et al. [1973] measured the time delay of the Korotkoff sound relative to the R-wave. They suggested that the curve obtained by plotting this data represents the rising portion of the arterial pulse waveform.

A Korotkoff sound model Drzewiecki et al., 1989 was employed to investigate the cuff delay effect. Time delay of the Korotkoff sound was computed relative to the proximal arterial pulse. Since the arterial pulse waveform was known in this calculation, the pressure-RK interval curve can be compared directly. The resemblance to a rising arterial pulse was apparent but some deviation was noted, particularly in the early portion of the RK interval curve. The model indicates that the pulse occurs earlier and with higher derivative than the true pulse waveform. In particular, the increased derivative that occurs at the foot of the pulse may mislead any study of wave propagation.

Recently, Sharir et al. [1993] performed comparisons of Doppler flow pulse delay and direct arterial pressure recordings. Their results confirm a consistent elevation in pulse compared with intra-arterial recording in the early portions of the wave. The average deviation was 10 mmHg in value. Hence, if accuracy is not important, this method can provide a reasonable estimate of blood pressure and its change. The commercial pulse watch has been a recent application of this approach.

55.3.2   Continuous Vascular Unloading

Penaz [1973] reasoned that if the cuff pressure could be continuously adjusted to equal the arterial pressure, the vessels would be in a constant state of vascular unloading. He employed mechanical feedback to continuously adjust the pressure in a finger chamber to apply this concept. The vascular volume was measured using photoplethysmography. When feedback was applied such that the vascular volume was held constant and at maximum pulsatile levels, the chamber pressure waveform was assumed to be equal to the arterial pressure.

Recent applications of the Penaz method have been developed by Wesseling et al. [1978] and Yamakoshi et al. [1980]. One instrument is commercially available as the FINAPRES [Ohmeda, Finapres, Englewood, CO]. These instruments have been evaluated in comparison with intra-arterial pressure recordings [Omboni et al., 1993]. Good waveform agreement has been obtained in comparison with intra-arterial measurements from the radial artery. But, it should be clear that the Penaz method employs finger pressure, which is a peripheral vascular location. This recording site is prone to pulse wave reflection effects and is therefore sensitive to the vascular flow resistance. It is anticipated that the technique would be affected by skin temperature, vasoactive drugs, and anesthetics. Moreover, mean pressure differences between the finger pulse and central aortic pressure should be expected.

55.3.3 Pulse Sensing

Pulse sensors attempt to measure the arterial pulse waveform from either the arterial wall deflection or force at the surface of the skin above a palpable vessel. Typically, these sensors are not directly calibrated in terms of pressure, but ideally respond proportionately to pressure. As such, they are primarily useful for dynamic information. While there are many designs available for this type of sensor, they generally fall into two categories. The first category is that of the volume sensor (Figure 55.6 [left]). This type of sensor relies on the adjacent tissues surrounding the vessel as a non-deflecting frame of reference as, for example, a photoplethysmograph. Skin deflections directly above the vessel are then measured relative to a reference frame to represent the arterial pressure. Several different transduction methods may be employed such as capacitive, resistive, inductive, optical, etc. Ideally, this type of sensor minimally restricts the motion of the skin so that contact force is zero. The drawback to pulse volume sensing is that the method responds to volume distention and *indirectly* to pressure. The nonlinear and viscoelastic nature of the vascular wall result in complex waveform alterations for this type of sensor that are difficult to correct in practice.

The second category is that of the pressure pulse sensor (Figure 55.6 [right]). This type of sensor measures stress due to arterial pressure transmitted though the skin above the pulse artery. The pressure pulse sensor requires that surface deflections are zero, as opposed to the volume sensor. Thus, the contact forces are proportionate to arterial pressure at the skin surface.

The differences in pulse waveforms that are provided by the above pulse recording techniques are clear in comparison with intra-arterial recordings [Van der Hoeven and Beneken, 1970]. In all cases, the pressure pulse method was found to provide superior waveform accuracy, free of the effects of vascular nonlinear viscoelasticity. Alternatively, the stiffness of the sensor can best characterize its pulse accuracy. High stiffness relative to the artery and surrounding tissue is required to best approximate the pressure pulse method.

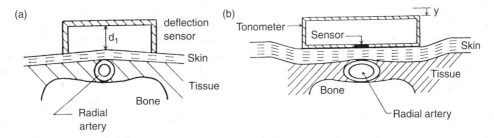

FIGURE 55.6   (a) Illustration of volume pulse method. (b) Illustration of pressure pulse method and arterial tonometry.

Arterial pulse recording is performed while the subject is stationary and refrains from moving the pulse location. But, it has become of interest to acquire ambulatory records. Without restraint, pulse recording is quite difficult due to motion artifact. For example, hand or finger motion can appear in recordings of the radial artery. A change in sensor positioning or acceleration can result in other types of artifact. The artifacts are often comparable in magnitude and frequency to the pulse, rendering simple filtering methods useless. Recently though, artifact cancellation techniques that employ sensor arrays have been applied with good success [Ciaccio et al., 1989].

55.3.4 Arterial Tonometry

Pulse sensing methods do not provide calibrated pressure. Arterial tonometry [Pressman and Newgard, 1963] is a pressure pulse method that can noninvasively record calibrated pressure in superficial arteries with sufficient bony support, such as the radial artery.

A tonometer is applied by first centering a contact stress sensor over the vessel. This is accomplished by repositioning the device until the largest pulse is detected. An array of sensors [Weaver et al., 1978] has been used to accomplish this electronically. Then, the tonometer is depressed towards the vessel. This leads to applanation of the vessel wall (Figure 55.6). If the vessel is not flattened sufficiently, the tonometer measures forces due to arterial wall tension and bending of the vessel. As depression is continued, the arterial wall is applanated further, but not so much as to occlude blood flow. At this intermediate position, wall tension becomes parallel to the tonometer sensing surface. Arterial pressure is then the remaining stress perpendicular to the surface and is measured by the sensor. This is termed the contact stress due to pressure. Ideally, the sensor should not measure skin shear (frictional) stresses. The contact stress is equal in magnitude to the arterial pressure when these conditions are achieved. The details of arterial tonometer calibration and design were analyzed by Drzewiecki et al. [1983, 1987]. In summary, tonometry requires that the contact stress sensor be flat, stiffer than the tissues, and small relative to the vessel diameter. Proper calibration can be attained either by monitoring the contact stress distribution (using a sensor array) or the maximum in measured pulse amplitude.

Recent research in tonometry has focused on miniaturization of semiconductor pressure sensor arrays [Weaver et al., 1978]. Alternatively, fiber optics have been employed by Drzewiecki [1985] and Moubarak et al. [1989], allowing extreme size reduction of the contact stress sensor. Commercial technology has been available (Jentow, Colin Electronics, Japan) and has been evaluated against intra-arterial records. Results indicate an average error of −5.6 mmHg for systolic pressure and −2.4 mmHg for diastole. Excellent pulse waveform quality is afforded by tonometry [Sato et al., 1993], making it a superior method for noninvasive pulse dynamics applications.

55.3.5 Flexible Diaphragm Tonometry

As an alternative to the high resolution tonometers under development, a new low resolution technology is introduced here. The basic advantage becomes one of cost, ease of positioning, and patient comfort, which is critical for long-term applications. In addition, while most tonometers have employed only the radial artery of the wrist for measurement, this technology is suitable for other superficial vessels and conforms to skin surface irregularities.

The flexible tonometer design applies the fact that tissue is incompressible in the short term [Bansal et al., 1994]. The concept is shown in Figure 55.7 using three tonometer volume compartments. These compartments are not physically separated and fluid can move between them. They are coupled to the skin and artery by means of the flexible diaphragm. When the arterial pressure exceeds that in the tonometer, the volume of the artery expands into V_b. Note also, that V_a and V_c must increase to take up this expansion since water is incompressible. To restore the tonometer to a flat surface, the total volume of the tonometer is increased (Figure 55.7). In response, the tonometer pressure increases and the artery flattens. At this point, the volume in each compartment is equal, the diaphragm is flat, and the tonometer pressure is equal to arterial pressure. Thus, by maintaining the equilibrium of the relative volume compartments,

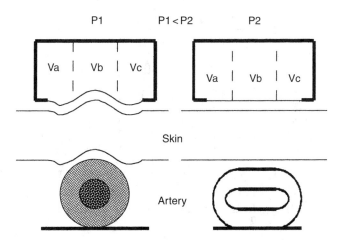

FIGURE 55.7 Concept of flexible diaphragm tonometry. P1 illustrates inappropriate level of pressure to provide arterial applanation tonometry. P2 indicates an increase in chamber volume so that the relative compartment volumes, V, are equal. In practice, relative compartment volumes are maintained constant via feedback control and applanation is continuous. Compartment pressure equals arterial pressure in P2.

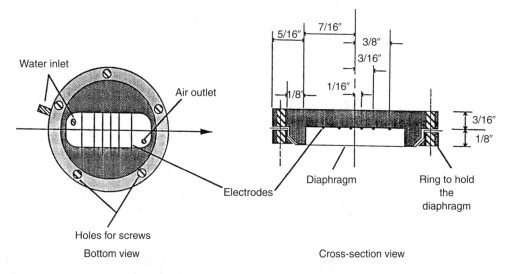

FIGURE 55.8 Design of a flexible diaphragm tonometer in accordance with the concept shown in Figure 55.7. Compartment volumes are obtained by means of impedance plethysmography. Electrode positions define the compartment boundaries.

applanation tonometry can be accomplished with a flexible diaphragm rather than a rigid one. In practice, instrumentation continuously adjusts the relative compartment volumes as arterial pressure changes.

A flexible diaphragm tonometer was machined from plexiglass (Figure 55.8). A rectangular channel was designed to contain saline. The front of the channel was sealed with a polyurethane sheet of 0.004 in. thickness. Two stainless steel electrodes were placed at each end of the channel. These were used to inject a current along the channel length. Near the center of the channel, four measuring electrodes were placed at equal spacing. Each pair of electrodes defined a volume compartment and the voltage across each pair was calibrated in terms of volume using impedance plethysmography. External to the tonometer, a saline-filled catheter was used to connect the channel to an electro-mechanical volume pump. The dynamics of the system were designed to possess appropriate frequency response.

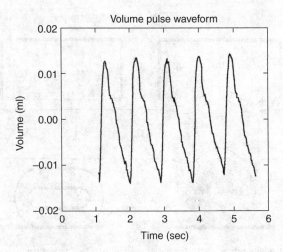

FIGURE 55.9 Sample of radial arterial volume recording from tonometer of Figure 55.8. Chamber pressure was fixed at 25 mmHg. Calibrated volume change is shown relative to the mean compartment volume.

Several beats of data were plotted from the volume pulse recordings of the flexible tonometer (Figure 55.9) for two adjacent compartments. The pulse volume is shown as a volume deviation from the mean compartment volume given a constant average tonometer pressure. The waveform shown illustrates the ability to provide calibrated noninvasive arterial volume information.

55.4 Noninvasive Arterial Mechanics

The flexible diaphragm tonometer and the occlusive cuff are capable of measuring volume in addition to pressure. Combining noninvasive measurements can extend the information provided by a single instrument, beyond that of blood pressure alone. Furthermore, functional information about the vasculature requires the simultaneous determination of pressure as well as geometry. In this section, the standard occlusive arm cuff will be employed as a plethysmograph to illustrate this concept.

The transmural pressure vs. lumen area (P–A) graph has been a convenient approach to analyze vessel function [Drzewiecki et al., 1997]. This curve can be applied to hemodynamics and portrays vessel function in a single graph. Unfortunately, its use has been limited to invasive studies or studies of isolated vessels where pressure can be experimentally controlled. The occlusive arm cuff offers a noninvasive solution to this problem by allowing the transmural pressure to be varied by altering the external pressure applied to a blood vessel. This approach has been used to noninvasively measure the transmural pressure vs. compliance relationship of the brachial artery [Mazhbich et al., 1983].

Drzewiecki and Pilla [1998] furthered the idea of noninvasively varying the transmural pressure by developing a cuff-based instrument that measures the P–A relationship. To perform the measurement, an occlusive arm cuff was pressurized by means of a diaphragm air pump. Cuff pressure was measured using a pressure sensor that provides pressure as an electronic signal. The pressure signal was input to a computer system via an analog-to-digital convertor for analysis. Two valves were used to control the flow of air. Initially, the valves were operated so that the pump inflated the cuff to well above the subject's systolic pressure. At that point, cuff air was recirculated through the pump. Under this condition, the mean cuff pressure remained constant, but the stroke volume of the pump resulted in cuff pressure oscillations at the frequency of the pump. Since the pump volume is a known quantity, it was used as a volume calibration source. The pump volume was divided by the cuff pressure oscillations due to the pump to yield the cuff compliance. With cuff compliance known, the cuff pressure arterial pulse was converted to a volume pulse by multiplying by cuff compliance. The pump was designed to operate at approximately 40 Hz, well

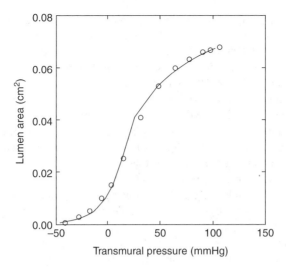

FIGURE 55.10 Arterial compliance obtained noninvasively by employing the occlusive arm cuff as a plethysmograph. Points are measured data. The solid curve is the model result obtained from Equation 55.1.

above the heart rate frequency components. This allowed the arterial pulse and pump pulse to be easily separated from the cuff pressure recording by using low pass and high pass digital filters with a cutoff frequency of 25 Hz.

The above procedure was repeated at every level of cuff pressure. The cuff pressure was released in steps of 5 to 10 mmHg until it was zero by briefly opening the release valve. The subject's pulse volume was divided by their pressure pulse (systolic minus diastolic pressures) to obtain the arterial compliance at every value of cuff pressure. The compliance per unit length was obtained by further dividing by the effective cuff length. The systolic, diastolic, and mean arterial pressures were evaluated by oscillometry and the Korotkoff method. Arterial compliance was then plotted for every value of transmural pressure (Figure 55.10). The compliance was then numerically integrated to obtain the corresponding brachial artery P–A curve. Since the vessel was collapsed for large negative transmural pressures, the initial constant of integration was chosen to be zero lumen area.

The arterial compliance curve possesses a maximum near zero transmural pressure. This point corresponds with the onset of vessel buckling. On either side of the buckling point, the vessel supports its pressure load differently. On the negative pressure side, the vessel partially collapses and undergoes wall bending. The compliance rapidly approaches zero during collapse. This occurs as the opposite walls of the vessel begin to contact each other and close the lumen. On the positive pressure side, the vessel supports its pressure load by wall stretch. The compliance slowly decreases with increasing pressure because of nonlinear wall elasticity. That is, the wall becomes stiffer with increasing stretch. The s-shaped lumen area curve is a consequence of these two different mechanisms. Preliminary studies of several subjects revealed that the shape of the noninvasive P–A curve is consistent for all subjects studied [Whitt and Drzewiecki, 1997; Drzewiecki and Pilla, 1998].

A mathematical model was developed that incorporates the fundamental physical and material properties that contribute to the collapsible P–A relationship [Drzewiecki et al., 1997; Drzewiecki and Pilla, 1998]. The basic form of the model is summarized by the following equation for transmural pressure:

$$P = -E((\lambda^{-1})^n - 1) + P_b + a(e^{b(\lambda - 1)} - 1) \tag{55.1}$$

where a and b are arterial elastance constants for distension, E is vessel elastance during collapse, and n is a constant that determines the rate of change of pressure with respect to change in area during collapse. The quantity λ, was defined as the extension ratio and is evaluated from the lumen area divided by the lumen area at the buckling point, A/A_b. The first hyperbolic term is the pressure due to collapse and wall bending. The second term is the buckling pressure and is found when $A = A_b$. The third exponential term represents the pressure due to wall stretch. Some overlap in the contribution of each term may occur near the buckling pressure. Depending on the vessel type and material, Equation 55.1 can be improved by limiting the extension ratio and its inverse to unity.

Equation 55.1 was employed to analyze the brachial artery $P–A$ data from each subject. The constants A_b and P_b were measured directly from the data as the point on the $P–A$ curve that corresponds with maximum compliance or buckling. Their values were inserted into Equation 55.1 for each subject, leaving the remaining constants to be found by nonlinear least squares regression (Marquardt–Levenberg algorithm). The model was evaluated for the subject shown in Figure 55.10 and corresponds with the solid line curve. Similar results were obtained for all subjects studied ($N = 10$), with the mean error of estimate less than 3 mmHg. The above study suggests that no other physical properties need to be added to model vascular collapse. Thus, it can be considered a valid model for further studies of vascular properties and blood pressure determination.

While the other terms of the model were found to vary from subject to subject, the buckling pressure was discovered to be relatively constant (10 mmHg ± 11). Hence, buckling may be the important vascular feature that permits noninvasive blood pressure measurement to be feasible and may be the common thread that links all noninvasive methods. This idea was first examined in our theoretical examination of oscillometry above [Drzewiecki et al., 1994]. The successful use of buckling itself as a method to find arterial pressure was also described here [Sheth and Drzewiecki, 1998]. The phenomenon of buckling is a general effect that occurs independent of the technique used to find arterial pressure. It will also be independent of the quantitative differences in the $P–A$ relationship of each specific subject.

55.5 Summary

Future research is open to noninvasive studies of how cardiovascular disease can alter blood vessel mechanics and the accuracy of blood pressure determination. The use of methods, such as occlusive cuff plethysmography together with blood pressure measurement and vascular mechanical modeling presented here, offers a means for noninvasive detection of the early stages of cardiovascular disease. Additionally, pulse dynamics and pressure variation offered by noninvasive pulse recording can provide new information about cardiovascular control.

Marey originally proposed that vessel closure is the important event that permits noninvasive blood pressure measurement. From the work presented here, this early concept is refocused to the instability of arterial buckling, or the *process* of closure, as the basic mechanism that enables noninvasive blood pressure determination.

Acknowledgments

The author wishes to express thanks to graduate students Vineet Bansal, Edward Ciaccio, Cindy Jacobs, James Pilla, Deepa Sheth, and Michael Whitt for their assistance with the experimental results presented here. The oscillometry studies were supported, in part, by Critikon, Inc., Tampa, FL and arterial tonometry was supported, in part, by IVAC Corp., San Diego, CA.

References

Alexander H., Cohen M., and Steinfeld L. (1977). Criteria in the choice of an occluding cuff for the indirect measurement of blood pressure. *Med. Biol. Eng. Comput.* 15: 2–10.

Arzbaecher R.C. and Novotney R.L. (1973). Noninvasive measurement of the arterial pressure contour in man. *Biblio. Cardiol.* 31: 63–69.

Bansal V., Drzewiecki G., and Butterfield R. (1994). Design of a flexible diaphragm tonometer. *Thirteenth S. Biomed. Eng. Conf.*, Washington, D.C., pp. 148–151.

Ciaccio E.J., Drzewiecki G.M., and Karam E. (1989). Algorithm for reduction of mechanical noise in arterial pulse recording with tonometry. *Proc. 15th Northeast Bioeng. Conf.*, Boston, pp. 161–162.

Drzewiecki G.M. (1985). The Origin of the Korotkoff Sound and Arterial Tonometry, Ph.D. dissertation. University of Pennsylvania, Philadelphia.

Drzewiecki G., Field S., Moubarak I., and Li J.K.-J. (1997). Vascular growth and collapsible pressure–area relationship. *Am. J. Physiol.* 273: H2030–H2043.

Drzewiecki G., Hood R., and Apple H. (1994). Theory of the oscillometric maximum and the systolic and diastolic detection ratios. *Ann. Biomed. Eng.* 22: 88–96.

Drzewiecki G.M., Karam E., Bansal V., Hood R., and Apple H. (1993). Mechanics of the occlusive arm cuff and its application as a volume sensor. *IEEE Trans. Biomed. Eng.* BME-40: 704–708.

Drzewiecki G.M., Melbin J., and Noordergraaf A. (1983). Arterial tonometry: review and analysis. *J. Biomech.* 16: 141–152.

Drzewiecki G.M., Melbin J., and Noordergraaf A. (1987). Noninvasive blood pressure recording and the genesis of Korotkoff sound. In *Handbook of Bioengineering*, S. Chien and R. Skalak. (eds.), pp. 8.1–8.36. New York, McGraw-Hill.

Drzewiecki G.M., Melbin J., and Noordergraaf A. (1989). The Korotkoff sound. *Ann. Biomed. Eng.* 17: 325–359.

Drzewiecki G. and Pilla J. (1998). Noninvasive measurement of the human brachial artery pressure–area relation in collapse and hypertension. *Ann. Biomed. Eng.* In press.

Graettinger W.F., Lipson J.L., Cheung D.G., and Weber M.A. (1988). Validation of portable noninvasive blood pressure monitoring devices: comparisons with intra-arterial and sphygmomanometer measurements. *Am. Heart J.* 116: 1155–1169.

Geddes L.A., Voelz M., Combs C., and Reiner D. (1983). Characterization of the oscillometric method for measuring indirect blood pressure. *Ann. Biomed. Eng.* 10: 271–280.

Geddes L.A. and Whistler S.J. (1978). The error in indirect blood pressure measurement with incorrect size of cuff. *Am. Heart J.* 96: 4–8.

Kelly R., Daley J., Avolio A., and O'Rourke M. (1989). Arterial dilation and reduced wave reflection — benefit of dilevalol in hypertension. *Hypertension* 14: 14–21.

Korotkoff N. (1905). On the subject of methods of determining blood pressure. *Bull. Imperial Mil. Med. Acad. (St. Petersburg)* 11: 365–367.

Li J.K.-J. (1986). Time domain resolution of forward and reflected waves in the aorta. *IEEE Trans. Biomed. Eng.* BME-33: 783–785.

Link W.T. (1987). Techniques for obtaining information associated with an individual's blood pressure including specifically a stat mode technique. US Patent #4,664,126.

London S.B. and London R.E. (1967). Comparison of indirect blood pressure measurements (Korotkoff) with simultaneous direct brachial artery pressure distal to cuff. *Adv. Intern. Med.* 13: 127–142.

Marey E.J. (1885). La Methode Graphique dans les Sciences Experimentales et Principalement en Physiologie et en Medicine. Masson, Paris.

Maurer A. and Noordergraaf A. (1976). Korotkoff sound filtering for automated three-phase measurement of blood pressure. *Am. Heart J.* 91: 584–591.

Mazhbich B.J. (1983). Noninvasive determination of elastic properties and diameter of human limb arteries. *Pflugers Arch.* 396: 254–259.

Moubarak I.F., Drzewiecki G.M., and Kedem J. (1989). Semi-invasive fiber — optic tonometer. *Proc. 15th Boston Northeast Bioeng. Conf.*, Boston, pp. 167–168.

Noordergraaf A. (1978). *Circulatory System Dynamics*. New York, Academic Press.

Omboni S., Parati G., Frattol A., Mutti E., Di Rienzo M., Castiglioni P., and Mancia G. (1993). Spectral and sequence analysis of finger blood pressure variability: comparison with analysis of intra-arterial recordings. *Hypertension* 22: 26–33.

Penaz J. (1973). Photoelectric measurement of blood pressure, volume, and flow in the finger. *Dig. 10th Intl. Conf. Med. Eng.*, Dresden, Germany, p. 104.

Pickering T., James G., Boddie C., Harshfield G., Blank S., and Laragh J. (1988). How common is white coat hypertension? *JAMA* 259: 225–228.

Posey J.A., Geddes L.A., Williams H., and Moore A.G. (1969). The meaning of the point of maximum oscillations in cuff pressure in the indirect measurement of blood pressure. Part 1. *Cardiovasc. Res. Cent. Bull.* 8: 15–25.

Pressman G.L. and Newgard P.M. (1963). A transducer for the continuous external measurement of arterial blood pressure. *IEEE Trans. Biomed. Eng.* BME-10: 73–81.

Rabbany S.Y., Drzewiecki G.M., and Noordergraaf A. (1993). Peripheral vascular effects on auscultatory blood pressure measurement. *J. Clin. Monitoring* 9: 9–17.

Ramsey III M. (1979). Noninvasive blood pressure determination of mean arterial pressure. *Med. Biol. Eng. Comput.* 17: 11–18.

Sato T., Nishinaga M., Kawamoto A., Ozawa T., and Takatsuji H. (1993). Accuracy of a continuous blood pressure monitor based on arterial tonometry. *Hypertension* 21: 866–874.

Sharir T., Marmor A., Ting C.-T., Chen J.-W., Liu C.-P., Chang M.-S., Yin F.C.P., and Kass D.A. (1993). Validation of a method for noninvasive measurement of central arterial pressure. *Hypertension* 21: 74–82.

Shenoy D., von Maltzahn W.W., and Buckley J.C. (1993). Noninvasive blood pressure measurement on the temporal artery using the auscultatory method. *Ann. Biomed. Eng.* 21: 351–360.

Sheth D. and Drzewiecki G. (1998). Using vessel buckling for continuous determination of arterial blood pressure. *Ann. Biomed. Eng.* 26: S–70.

Spence J.D., Sibbald W.J., and Cape R.D. (1978). Pseudohypertension in the elderly. *Clin. Sci. Mol. Med.* 55: 399s–402s.

Strus J. (1555). Sphygmicae artis jam mille ducentos annos peritae et desideratae, Libri V a Josephi Struthio Posnanience, medico recens conscripti, Basel. (As transcribed by A. Noordergraaf, Univ. of Pennsylvania, Philadelphia, PA).

Van der Hoeven G.M.A. and Beneken J.E.W. (1970). A reliable transducer for the recording of the arterial pulse wave. *Prog. Rep. 2. Inst. Med. Phys.* TNO, Utrecht.

Wesseling K.H., de Wit B., Snoeck B., Weber J.A.P., Hindman B.W., Nijland R., and Van der Hoeven G.M.A. (1978). An implementation of the Penaz method for measuring arterial blood pressure in the finger and the first results of an evaluation. *Prog. Rep. 6. Inst. Med. Phys.* TNO, Utrecht.

Weaver C.S., Eckerle J.S., Newgard P.M., Warnke C.T., Angell J.B., Terry S.C., and Robinson J. (1978). A study of noninvasive blood pressure measurement technique. In *Noninvasive Cardiovascular Measurements. Soc. Photo-Opt. Instr. Eng.* 167: 89.

Westerhof N., Bosman F., DeVries C.J., and Noordergraaf A. (1969). Analog studies of the human systemic arterial tree. *J. Biomech.* 2: 121–143.

White W.W., Berson A.S., Robbins C., Jamieson M.J., Prisant M., Roccella E., and Sheps S.G. (1993). National standard for measurement of resting and ambulatory blood pressures with automated sphygmomanometers. *Hypertension* 21: 504–509.

Whitt M. and Drzewiecki G. (1997). Repeatability of brachial artery area measurement. *Ann. Biomed. Eng.* 25: S-12.

Yamakoshi K., Shimazu H., and Togawa T. (1980). Indirect measurement of instantaneous arterial blood pressure in the human finger by the vascular unloading technique. *IEEE Trans. Biomed. Eng.* BME-27: 150.

56

Cardiac Output Measurement

-Dilution Method **56**-1
  • Thermal Dilution Method • Indicator
on
hod **56**-5
Fraction **56**-7
Dilution Method for Ejection Fraction
.... **56**-10

' the right or left ventricular per unit of time. It
alized by division by body surface area in square
iac index. Cardiac output is sometimes normalized
gram. A typical resting value for a wide variety of

ained athletes, cardiac output can increase fivefold
ncreases, venous return increases, and the ejection
ts have a low resting heart rate, and the time for the
less than that for subjects who are not physically fit.
 methods of measuring cardiac output. Of equal
tput is the left-ventricular ejection fraction (stroke
the ability of the left ventricle to pump blood.

d is based on the upstream injection of a detectable
ration-time curve, which is called a *dilution curve.*
ith all the blood flowing through the central mixing
hes may be slightly different in shape, they all have

Figure 56.1a illustrates the injection of m g of indicator into an idealized flowing stream having the same velocity across the diameter of the tube. Figure 56.1b shows the dilution curve recorded downstream. Because of the flow-velocity profile, the cylinder of indicator and fluid becomes teardrop in shape, as shown in Figure 56.1c. The resulting dilution curve has a rapid rise and an exponential fall, as shown in

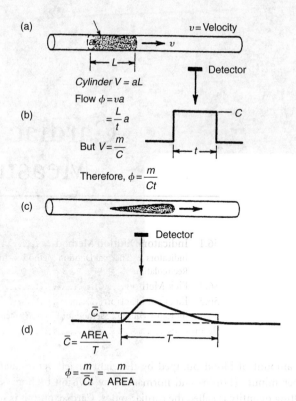

FIGURE 56.1 Genesis of the indicator-dilution curve.

Figure 56.1d. However, the area of the dilution curve is the same as that shown in Figure 56.1a. Derivation of the flow equation is shown in Figure 56.1, and the flow is simply the amount of indicator (m g) divided by the area of the dilution curve (g/mL × sec), which provides the flow in mL/sec.

56.1.1 Indicators

Before describing the various indicator-dilution methods, it is useful to recognize that there are two types of indicator, diffusible and nondiffusible. A diffusible indicator will leak out of the capillaries. A nondiffusible indicator is retained in the vascular system for a time that depends on the type of indicator. Whether cardiac output is overestimated with a diffusible indicator depends on the location of the injection and measuring sites. Table 56.1 lists many of the indictors that have been used for measuring cardiac output and the types of detectors used to obtain the dilution curve. It is obvious that the indicator selected must be detectable and not alter the flow being measured. Importantly, the indicator must be nontoxic and sterile.

When a diffusible indicator is injected into the right heart, the dilution curve can be detected in the pulmonary artery, and there is no loss of indicator because there is no capillary bed between these sites; therefore the cardiac output value will be accurate.

56.1.2 Thermal Dilution Method

Chilled 5% dextrose in water (D5W) or 0.9% NaCl can be used as indicators. The dilution curve represents a transient reduction in pulmonary artery blood temperature following injection of the indicator into the right atrium. Figure 56.2 illustrates the method and a typical thermodilution curve. Note that the indicator is really negative calories. The thermodilution method is based on heat exchange measured in calories, and the flow equation contains terms for the specific heat (C) and the specific gravity (S) of the indicator (i) and blood (b). The expression employed when a #7F thermistor-tipped catheter is used

TABLE 56.1 Indicators

Material	Detector	Retention data
Evans blue (T1824)	Photoelectric 640 μ	50% loss in 5 days
Indocyanine green	Photoelectric 800 μ	50% loss in 10 min
Coomassie blue	Photoelectric 585–600 μ	50% loss in 15–20 min
Saline (5%)	Conductivity cell	Diffusible[a]
Albumin 1^{131}	Radioactive	50% loss in 8 days
Na^{24}, K^{42}, D_2O, DHO	Radioactive	Diffusible[a]
Hot-cold solutions	Thermodetector	Diffusible[a]

[a] It is estimated that there is about 15% loss of diffusible indicators during the first pass through the lungs.

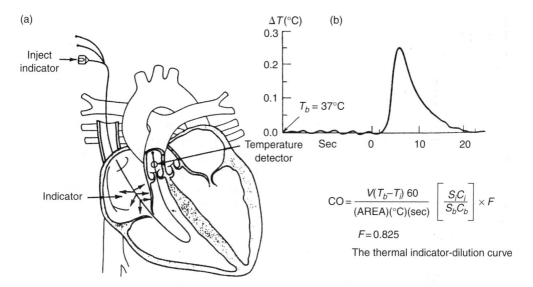

FIGURE 56.2   The thermodilution method (a) and a typical dilution curve (b).

and chilled D5W is injected into the right atrium is as follows:

$$CO = \left[\frac{V(T_b - T_i)60}{A} \right] \left[\frac{S_i C_i}{S_b C_b} \right] F \qquad (56.1)$$

where

V = Volume of indicator injected in mL
T_b = Temperature (average of pulmonary artery blood in (°C)
T_i = Temperature of the indicator (°C)
60 = Multiplier required to convert mL/sec into mL/min
A = Area under the dilution curve in (sec × °C)
S = Specific gravity of indicator (i) and blood (b)
C = Specific heat of indicator (i) and blood (b)
($S_i C_i / S_b C_b$ = 1.08 for 5% dextrose and blood of 40% packed-cell volume)
F = Empiric factor employed to correct for heat transfer through the injection catheter (for a #7F catheter, F = 0.825 [2]).

Entering these factors into the expression gives

$$CO = \frac{V(T_b - T_i)53.46}{A} \qquad (56.2)$$

where CO = cardiac output in mL/min

$$53.46 = 60 \times 1.08 \times 0.825$$

To illustrate how a thermodilution curve is processed, cardiac output is calculated below using the dilution curve shown in Figure 56.2.

$V = 5$ ml of 5% dextrose in water
$T_b = 37°C$
$T_i = 0°C$
$A = 1.59°C$ s
$CO = \dfrac{5(37 - 0)53.46}{1.59} = 6220$ mL/min

Although the thermodilution method is *the standard in clinical medicine*, it has a few disadvantages. Because of the heat loss through the catheter wall, several series 5-mL injections of indicator are needed to obtain a consistent value for cardiac output. If cardiac output is low, that is, the dilution curve is very broad, it is difficult to obtain an accurate value for cardiac output. There are respiratory-induced variations in PA blood temperature that confound the dilution curve when it is of low amplitude. Although room-temperature D5W can be used, chilled D5W provides a better dilution curve and a more reliable cardiac output value. Furthermore, it should be obvious that if the temperature of the indicator is the same as that of blood, there will be no dilution curve.

56.1.3 Indicator Recirculation

An ideal dilution curve shown in Figure 56.2 consists of a steep rise and an exponential decrease in indicator concentration. Algorithms that measure the dilution-curve area have no difficulty with such a curve. However, when cardiac output is low, the dilution curve is typically low in amplitude and very broad. Often the descending limb of the curve is obscured by recirculation of the indicator or by low-amplitude artifacts. Figure 56.3a is a dilution curve in which the descending limb is obscured by recirculation of the indicator. Obviously it is difficult to determine the practical end of the curve, which is often specified as the time when the indicator concentration has fallen to a chosen percentage (e.g., 1%) of the maximum amplitude (C_{max}). Because the descending limb represents a good approximation of a decaying exponential curve (e^{-kt}), fitting the descending limb to an exponential allows reconstruction of the curve without a recirculation error, thereby providing a means for identifying the end for what is called the *first pass of the indicator*.

In Figure 56.3b, the amplitude of the descending limb of the curve in Figure 56.3a has been plotted on semilogarithmic paper, and the exponential part represents a straight line. When recirculation appears, the data points deviate from the straight line and therefore can be ignored, and the linear part (representing the exponential) can be extrapolated to the desired percentage of the maximum concentration, say 1% of C_{max}. The data points representing the extrapolated part were replotted on Figure 56.3a to reveal the dilution curve undistorted by recirculation.

Commercially available indicator-dilution instruments employ digitization of the dilution curve. Often the data beyond about 30% of C_{max} are ignored, and the exponential is computed on digitally extrapolated data.

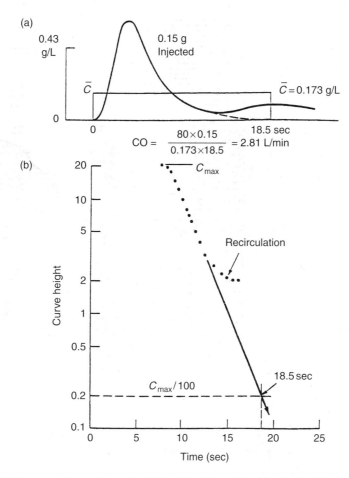

FIGURE 56.3   Dilution curve obscured by recirculation (a) and a semilogarithmic plot of the descending limb (b).

56.2   Fick Method

The Fick method *employs oxygen as the indicator* and the increase in oxygen content of venous blood as it passes through the lungs, along with the respiratory oxygen uptake, as the quantities that are needed to determine cardiac output (CO = O_2 uptake/$A - VO_2$ difference). Oxygen uptake (mL/min) is measured at the airway, usually with an oxygen-filled spirometer containing a CO_2 absorber. The $A - VO_2$ difference is determined from the oxygen content (mL/100 mL blood) from any arterial sample and the oxygen content (mL/100 mL) of pulmonary arterial blood. The oxygen content of blood used to be difficult to measure. However, the new blood–gas analyzers that measure, pH, pO_2, pCO_2, hematocrit, and hemoglobin provide a value for O_2 content by computation using the oxygen-dissociation curve.

There is a slight technicality involved in determining the oxygen uptake because oxygen is consumed at body temperature but measured at room temperature in the spirometer. Consequently, the volume of O_2 consumed per minute displayed by the spirometer must be multiplied by a factor, F. Therefore the Fick equation is

$$CO = \frac{O_2 \text{ uptake/min}(F)}{A - VO_2 \text{ difference}} \qquad (56.3)$$

Figure 56.4 is a spirogram showing a tidal volume riding on a sloping baseline that represents the resting expirating level (REL). The slope identifies the oxygen uptake at room temperature. In this subject,

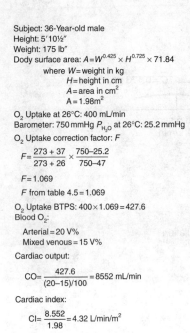
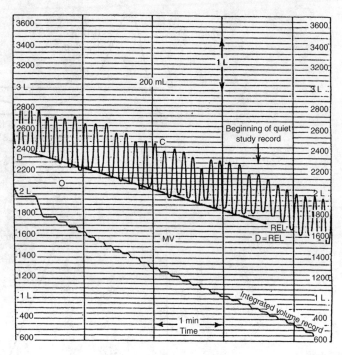

FIGURE 56.4 Measurement of oxygen uptake with a spirometer (*right*) and the method used to correct the measured volume (*left*).

the uncorrected oxygen consumption was 400 mL/min at 26°C in the spirometer. With a barometric pressure of 750 mmHg, the conversion factor F to correct this volume to body temperature (37°C) and saturated with water vapor is

$$F = \frac{273 + 37}{273 + T_s} \times \frac{P_b - PH_2O}{P_b - 47} \tag{56.4}$$

where T_s is the spirometer temperature, P_b is the barometric pressure, and PH_2O at T_s is obtained from the water-vapor table (Table 56.2).

A sample calculation for the correction factor F is given in Figure 56.4, which reveals a value for F of 1.069. However, it is easier to use Table 56.3 to obtain the correction factor. For example, for a spirometer temperature of 26°C and a barometric pressure of 750 mmHg, $F = 1.0691$.

Note that the correction factor F in this case is only 6.9%. The error encountered by not including it may be less than the experimental error in making all other measurements.

The example selected shows that the $A - VO_2$ difference is 20–15 mL/100 mL blood and that the corrected O_2 uptake is 400×1.069; therefore the cardiac output is:

$$CO = \frac{400 \times 1.069}{(20 - 15)/100} = 8552 \text{ mL/min} \tag{56.5}$$

The Fick method does not require the addition of a fluid to the circulation and may have value in such a circumstance. However, its use requires stable conditions because an average oxygen uptake takes many minutes to obtain.

TABLE 56.2   Vapor Pressure of Water

Temp. °C	0.0	0.2	0.4	0.6	0.8
15	12.788	12.953	13.121	13.290	13.461
16	13.634	13.809	13.987	14.166	14.347
17	14.530	14.715	14.903	15.092	15.284
18	15.477	15.673	15.871	16.071	16.272
19	16.477	16.685	16.894	17.105	17.319
20	17.535	17.753	17.974	18.197	18.422
21	18.650	18.880	19.113	19.349	19.587
22	19.827	20.070	20.316	20.565	20.815
23	21.068	21.324	21.583	21.845	22.110
24	22.377	22.648	22.922	23.198	23.476
25	23.756	24.039	24.326	24.617	24.912
26	25.209	25.509	25.812	26.117	26.426
27	26.739	27.055	27.374	27.696	28.021
28	28.349	28.680	29.015	29.354	29.697
29	30.043	30.392	30.745	31.102	31.461
30	31.825	32.191	32.561	32.934	33.312
31	33.695	34.082	34.471	34.864	35.261
32	35.663	36.068	36.477	36.891	37.308
33	37.729	38.155	38.584	39.018	39.457
34	39.898	40.344	40.796	41.251	41.710
35	42.175	42.644	43.117	43.595	44.078
36	44.563	45.054	45.549	46.050	46.556
37	47.067	47.582	48.102	48.627	49.157
38	49.692	50.231	50.774	51.323	51.879
39	42.442	53.009	53.580	54.156	54.737
40	55.324	55.910	56.510	57.110	57.720
41	58.340	58.960	59.580	60.220	60.860

56.3   Ejection Fraction

The ejection fraction (EF) is one of the most convenient indicators of the ability of the left (or right) ventricle to pump the blood that is presented to it. Let v be the stroke volume (SV) and V be the end-diastolic volume (EDV); the ejection fraction is v/V or SV/EDV.

Measurement of ventricular diastolic and systolic volumes can be achieved radiographically, ultrasonically, and by the use of an indicator that is injected into the left ventricle where the indicator concentration is measured in the aorta on a beat-by-beat basis.

56.3.1   Indicator-Dilution Method for Ejection Fraction

Holt [1] described the method of injecting an indicator into the left ventricular during diastole and measuring the stepwise decrease in aortic concentration with successive beats (Figure 56.5). From this concentration-time record, end-diastolic volume, stroke volume, and ejection fraction can be calculated. No assumption need be made about the geometric shape of the ventricle. The following describes the theory of this fundamental method.

Let V be the end-diastolic ventricular volume. Inject m gm of indicator into this volume during diastole. The concentration (C_1) of indicator in the aorta for the first beat is m/V. By knowing the amount of indicator (m) injected and the calibration for the aortic detector, C_1 is established, and ventricular end-diastolic volume $V = m/C_1$.

After the first beat, the ventricle fills, and the amount of indicator left in the left ventricle is $m - mv/V$. The aortic concentration (C_2) for the second beat is therefore $m - mV/V = m(1 - v/V)$. Therefore

TABLE 56.3 Correction Factor F for Standardization of Collected Volume

°C/P_B	640	650	660	670	680	690	700	710	720	730	740	750	760	770	780
15	1.1388	1.1377	1.1367	1.1358	1.1348	1.1339	1.1330	1.1322	1.1314	1.1306	1.1298	1.1290	1.1283	1.1276	1.1269
16	1.1333	1.1323	1.1313	1.1304	1.1295	1.1286	1.1277	1.1269	1.1260	1.1253	1.1245	1.1238	1.1231	1.1224	1.1217
17	1.1277	1.1268	1.1258	1.1249	1.1240	1.1232	1.1224	1.1216	1.1208	1.1200	1.1193	1.1186	1.1179	1.1172	1.1165
18	1.1222	1.1212	1.1203	1.1194	1.1186	1.1178	1.1170	1.1162	1.1154	1.1147	1.1140	1.1133	1.1126	1.1120	1.1113
19	1.1165	1.1156	1.1147	1.1139	1.1131	1.1123	1.1115	1.1107	1.1100	1.1093	1.1086	1.1080	1.1073	1.1067	1.1061
20	1.1108	1.1099	1.1091	1.1083	1.1075	1.1067	1.1060	1.1052	1.1045	1.1039	1.1032	1.1026	1.1019	1.1013	1.1008
21	1.1056	1.1042	1.1034	1.1027	1.1019	1.1011	1.1004	1.0997	1.0990	1.0984	1.0978	1.0971	1.0965	1.0960	1.0954
22	1.0992	1.0984	1.0976	1.0969	1.0962	1.0955	1.0948	1.0941	1.0935	1.0929	1.0923	1.0917	1.0911	1.0905	1.0900
23	1.0932	1.0925	1.0918	1.0911	1.0904	1.0897	1.0891	1.0884	1.0878	1.0872	1.0867	1.0861	1.0856	1.0850	1.0845
24	1.0873	1.0866	1.0859	1.0852	1.0846	1.0839	1.0833	1.0827	1.0822	1.0816	1.0810	1.0805	1.0800	1.0795	1.0790
25	1.0812	1.0806	1.0799	1.0793	1.0787	1.0781	1.0775	1.0769	1.0764	1.0758	1.0753	1.0748	1.0744	1.0739	1.0734
26	1.0751	1.0745	1.0738	1.0732	1.0727	1.0721	1.0716	1.0710	1.0705	1.0700	1.0696	1.0691	1.0686	1.0682	1.0678
27	1.0688	1.0682	1.0677	1.0671	1.0666	1.0661	1.0656	1.0651	1.0646	1.0641	1.0637	1.0633	1.0629	1.0624	1.0621
28	1.0625	1.0619	1.0614	1.0609	1.0604	1.0599	1.0595	1.0591	1.0586	1.0582	1.0578	1.0574	1.0570	1.0566	1.0563
29	1.0560	1.0555	1.0550	1.0546	1.0541	1.0537	1.0533	1.0529	1.0525	1.0521	1.0518	1.0514	1.0511	1.0507	1.0504
30	1.0494	1.0490	1.0486	1.0482	1.0478	1.0474	1.0470	1.0467	1.0463	1.0460	1.0456	1.0453	1.0450	1.0447	1.0444

Source: From Kovach J.C., Paulos P., and Arabadjis C. 1955. *J. Thorac. Surg.* **29**: 552.

$V_s = FV_c$, where V_s is the standardized condition and V_c is the collected condition:

$$V = \frac{1 + 37/273}{1 + t°C/273} \times \frac{P_B - PH_2O}{P_B - 47} \quad V_c = FV_c$$

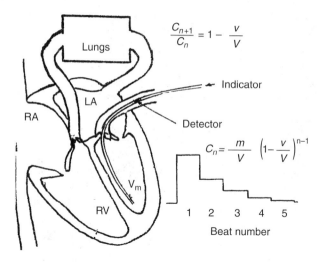

FIGURE 56.5 The saline method of measuring ejection fraction, involving injection of m g of NaCl into the left ventricle and detecting the aortic concentration (C) on a beat-by-beat basis.

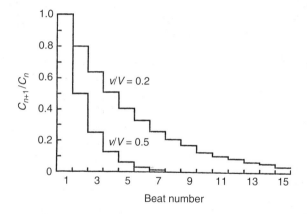

FIGURE 56.6 Stepwise decrease in indicator concentration (C) vs. beat number for ejection fraction (v/V) of 0.5 and 0.2.

the aortic concentration (C_2) for the second beat is

$$C_2 = \frac{m}{V}\left[1 - \frac{v}{V}\right] \tag{56.6}$$

By continuing the process, it is easily shown that the aortic concentration (C_n) for the nth beat is

$$C_n = \frac{m}{V}\left[1 - \frac{v}{V}\right]^{n-1} \tag{56.7}$$

Figure 56.6 illustrates the stepwise decrease in aortic concentration for ejection fractions (v/V) of 0.2 and 0.5, that is, 20% and 50%.

It is possible to determine the ejection fraction from the concentration ratio for two successive beats. For example,

$$C_n = \frac{m}{V}\left[1 - \frac{v}{V}\right]^{n-1} \tag{56.8}$$

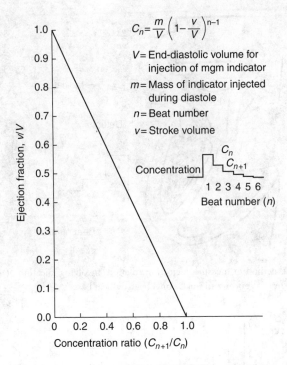

FIGURE 56.7   Ejection fraction (v/V) vs. the ratio of concentrations for successive beats (C_{n+1}/C_n).

$$C_n + 1 = \frac{m}{V}\left[1 - \frac{v}{V}\right]^n \tag{56.9}$$

$$\frac{C_{n+1}}{C_n} = 1 - \frac{v}{V} \tag{56.10}$$

from which

$$\frac{v}{V} = 1 - \frac{C_{n+1}}{C_n} \tag{56.11}$$

where v/V is the ejection fraction and C_{n+1}/C_n is the concentration ratio for two successive beats, for example, C_2/C_1 or C_3/C_2. Figure 56.7 illustrates the relationship between the ejection fraction v/V and the ratio of C_{n+1}/C_n. Observe that the detector need not be calibrated as long as there is a linear relationship between detector output and indicator concentration in the operating range.

References

[1] Holt, J.P. (1956). Estimation of the residual volume of the ventricle of the dog heart by two indicator-dilution techniques. *Circ. Res.* 4: 181.
[2] Weissel, R.D., Berger, R.L., and Hechtman, H.B. (1975). Measurement of cardiac output by thermodilution. *N. Engl. J. Med.* 292: 682.

57

External Defibrillators

57.1 Mechanism of Fibrillation **57**-1
57.2 Mechanism of Defibrillation **57**-2
57.3 Clinical Defibrillators **57**-3
57.4 Electrodes **57**-5
57.5 Synchronization **57**-6
57.6 Automatic External Defibrillators **57**-6
57.7 Defibrillator Safety **57**-8
References **57**-9
Further Information **57**-9

Willis A. Tacker
Purdue University

Defibrillators are devices used to supply a strong electric shock (often referred to as a *countershock*) to a patient in an effort to convert excessively fast and ineffective heart rhythm disorders to slower rhythms that allow the heart to pump more blood. External defibrillators have been in common use for many decades for emergency treatment of life-threatening cardiac rhythms as well as for elective treatment of less threatening rapid rhythms. Figure 57.1 shows an external defibrillator.

Cardiac arrest occurs in more than 500,000 people annually in the United States, and more than 70% of the out-of-hospitals are due to cardiac arrhythmia treatable with defibrillators. The most serious arrhythmia treated by a defibrillator is ventricular fibrillation. Without rapid treatment using a defibrillator, ventricular fibrillation causes complete loss of cardiac function and death within minutes. Atrial fibrillation and the more organized rhythms of atrial flutter and ventricular tachycardia can be treated on a less emergent basis. Although they do not cause immediate death, their shortening of the interval between contractions can impair filling of the heart chambers and thus decrease cardiac output. Conventionally, treatment of ventricular fibrillation is called *defibrillation*, whereas treatment of the other tachycardias is called *cardioversion*.

57.1 Mechanism of Fibrillation

Fibrillation is chaotic electric excitation of the myocardium and results in loss of coordinated mechanical contraction characteristic of normal heart beats. Description of mechanisms leading to, and maintaining, fibrillation and other rhythm disorders are reviewed elsewhere [1] and are beyond the scope of this chapter. In summary, however, these rhythm disorders are commonly held to be a result of reentrant excitation pathways within the heart. The underlying abnormality that leads to the mechanism is the combination of conduction block of cardiac excitation plus rapidly recurring depolarization of the membranes of the cardiac cells. This leads to rapid repetitive propagation of a single excitation wave or of multiple

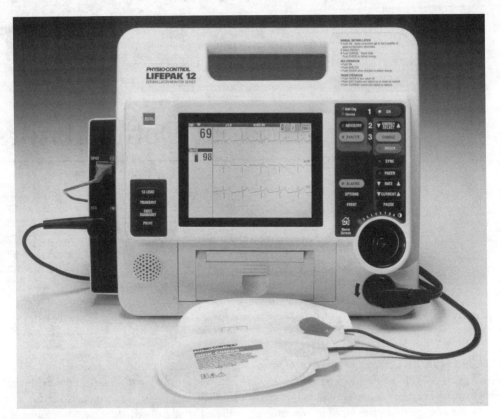

FIGURE 57.1 Photograph of a trans-chest defibrillator. (Provided by Physio-Control Corporation. With permission.)

excitatory waves throughout the heart. If the waves are multiple, the rhythm may degrade into total loss of synchronization of cardiac fiber contraction. Without synchronized contraction, the chamber affected will not contract, and this is fatal in the case of ventricular fibrillation. The most common cause of these conditions, and therefore of these rhythm disorders, is cardiac ischemia or infarction as a complication of atherosclerosis. Additional relatively common causes include other cardiac disorders, drug toxicity, electrolyte imbalances in the blood, hypothermia, and electric shocks (especially from alternating current).

57.2   Mechanism of Defibrillation

The corrective measure is to extinguish the rapidly occurring waves of excitation by simultaneously depolarizing most of the cardiac cells with a strong electric shock. The cells then can simultaneously repolarize themselves, and thus they will be back in phase with each other.

Despite years of intensive research, there is still no single theory for the mechanism of defibrillation that explains all the phenomena observed. However, it is generally held that the defibrillating shock must be adequately strong and have adequate duration to affect most of the heart cells. In general, longer duration shocks require less current than shorter duration shocks. This relationship is called the strength–duration relationship and is demonstrated by the curve shown in Figure 57.2. Shocks of strength and duration above and to the right of the current curve (or above the energy curve) have adequate strength to defibrillate, whereas shocks below and to the left do not. From the exponentially decaying current curve an energy curve can also be determined (also shown in Figure 57.2), which is high at very short durations due to

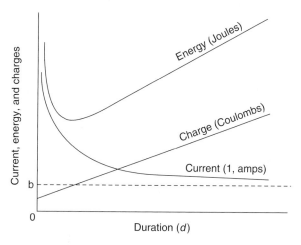

FIGURE 57.2   Strength–duration curves for current, energy, and charge. Adequate current shocks are above and to the right of the current curve. (Modified from Tacker W.A. and Geddes L.A. 1980. *Electrical Defibrillation*, Boca Raton, FL, CRC Press. With permission.)

high current requirements at short durations, but which is also high at longer durations due to additional energy being delivered as the pulse duration is lengthened at nearly constant current. Thus, for most electrical waveforms there is a minimum energy for defibrillation at approximate pulse durations of 3 to 8 msec. A strength–duration charge curve can also be determined as shown in Figure 57.2, which demonstrates that the minimum charge for defibrillation occurs at the shortest pulse duration tested. Very-short-duration pulses are not used, however, since the high current and voltage required is damaging to the myocardium. It is also important to note that excessively strong or long shocks may cause immediate refibrillation, thus failing to restore the heart function.

In practice, for a shock applied to electrodes on the skin surface of the patient's chest, durations are on the order of 3 to 10 msec and have an intensity of a few thousand volts and tens of amperes. The energy delivered to the subject by these shocks is selectable by the operator and is on the order of 50 to 360 J for most defibrillators. The exact shock intensity required at a given duration of electric pulse depends on several variables, including the intrinsic characteristics of the patient (such as the underlying disease problem or presence of certain drugs and the length of time the arrhythmia has been present), the techniques for electrode application, and the particular rhythm disorder being treated (more organized rhythms require less energy than disorganized rhythms).

57.3   Clinical Defibrillators

Defibrillator design has resulted from medical and physiologic research and advances in hardware technology. It is estimated that for each minute that elapses between onset of ventricular fibrillation and the first shock application, survival to leave hospital decreases by about 10%. The importance of rapid response led to development of portable, battery-operated defibrillators and more recently to automatic external defibrillators (AEDs) that enable emergency responders to defibrillate with minimal training.

All clinical defibrillators used today store energy in capacitors. Desirable capacitor specifications include small size, light weight, and capability to sustain several thousands of volts and many charge-discharge cycles. Energy storage capacitors account for at least one pound and usually several pounds of defibrillator weight. Energy stored by the capacitor is calculated from

$$W_s = \frac{1}{2}CE^2 \qquad\qquad (57.1)$$

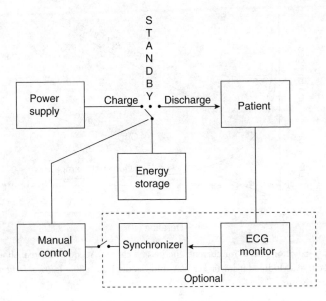

FIGURE 57.3   Block diagram of a typical defibrillator. (From Feinberg B. 1980. *Handbook Series in Clinical Laboratory Science,* Vol. 2, Boca Raton, FL, CRC Press. With permission.)

where W_s = stored energy in joules, C = capacitance in farads, and E = voltage applied to the capacitor. Delivered energy is expressed as

$$W_d = W_s \times \left(\frac{R}{R_i + R} \right) \tag{57.2}$$

where W_d = delivered energy, W_s = stored energy, R = subject resistance, and R_i = device resistance.

Figure 57.3 shows a block diagram for defibrillators. Most have a built-in monitor and synchronizer (dashed lines in Figure 57.3). Built-in monitoring speeds up diagnosis of potentially fatal arrhythmias, especially when the ECG is monitored through the same electrodes that are used to apply the defibrillating shock. The great preponderance of defibrillators for trans-chest defibrillation deliver shocks with either a damped sinusoidal waveform produced by discharge of an RCL circuit or a truncated exponential decay waveform (sometimes called trapezoidal). Basic components of exemplary circuits for damped sine waveform and trapezoidal waveform defibrillators are shown in Figure 57.4 and Figure 57.5. The shape of the waveforms generated by RCL defibrillators depend on the resistance of the patient as well as the energy storage capacitance and resistance and inductance of the inductor. When discharged into a 50-Ω load (to stimulate the patient's resistance), these defibrillators produce either a critically damped sine waveform or a slightly underdamped sine waveform (i.e., having a slight reversal of waveform polarity following the main waveform) into the 50-Ω load.

The exact waveform can be determined by application of Kirkchoff's voltage law to the circuit

$$L \frac{di}{dt} + (R_i + R)i + \frac{1}{C} \int i dt = 0 \tag{57.3}$$

where L = inductance in H, i = instantaneous current in amperes, t = time in seconds, R_i = device resistance, R = subject resistance, and C = capacitance. From this, the second-order differential equation describes the RCL defibrillator.

$$L \frac{d^2 i}{dt^2} + (R_i + R) \frac{di}{dt} + \frac{1}{C} i = 0 \tag{57.4}$$

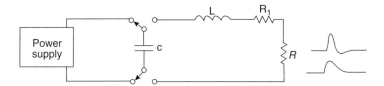

FIGURE 57.4   Resister–capacitor–inductor defibrillator. The patient is represented by R. (Modified from Feinberg B. 1980. *Handbook Series in Clinical Laboratory Science,* Vol. 2, Boca Raton, FL, CRC Press. With permission.)

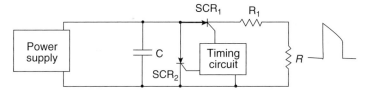

FIGURE 57.5   Trapezoidal wave defibrillator. The patient is represented by R. (Modified from Feinberg B. 1980. *Handbook Series in Clinical Laboratory Science,* Vol. 2, Boca Raton, FL, CRC Press. With permission.)

Trapezoidal waveform (actually, these are truncated exponential decay waveform) defibrillators are also used clinically. The circuit diagram in Figure 57.4 is exemplary of one design for producing such a waveform. Delivered energy calculation for this waveform is expressed as

$$W_\mathrm{d} = 0.5I_\mathrm{i}^2 R \left[\frac{d}{\log_e \left(\frac{I_\mathrm{i}}{I_\mathrm{f}} \right)} \right] \left[1 - \left(\frac{I_\mathrm{f}}{I_\mathrm{i}} \right)^2 \right] \qquad (57.5)$$

where W_d = delivered energy, I_i = initial current in amperes, I_f = final current, R = resistance of the patient, and d = pulse duration in seconds. Both RCL and trapezoidal waveforms defibrillate effectively. Implantable defibrillators now use alternative waveforms such as a biphasic exponential decay waveform, in which the polarity of the electrodes is reversed part way through the shock. Use of the biphasic waveform has reduced the shock intensity required for implantable defibrillators but has not yet been extended to trans-chest use except on an experimental basis.

RCL defibrillators are the most widely available. They store up to about 440 J and deliver up to about 360 J into a patient with 50-Ω impedance. Several selectable energy intensities are available, typically from 5 to 360 J, so that pediatric patients, very small patients, or patients with easily converted arrhythmias can be treated with low-intensity shocks. The pulse duration ranges from 3 to 6 msec. Because the resistance (R) varies between patients (25 to 150 Ω) and is part of the RCL discharge circuit, the duration and damping of the pulse also varies; increasing patient impedance lengthens and dampens the pulse. Figure 57.6 shows waveforms from RCL defibrillators with critically damped and with underdamped pulses.

57.4   Electrodes

Electrodes for external defibrillation are metal and from 70 to 100 cm^2 in surface area. They must be coupled to the skin with an electrically conductive material to achieve low impedance across the electrode-patient interface. There are two types of electrodes: hand-held (to which a conductive liquid or solid gel is applied) and adhesive, for which an adhesive conducting material holds the electrode in place. Hand-held electrodes are reusable and are pressed against the patient's chest by the operator during shock delivery. Adhesive electrodes are disposable and are applied to the chest before the shock delivery and left in place for reuse if subsequent shocks are needed. Electrodes are usually applied with both electrodes on the

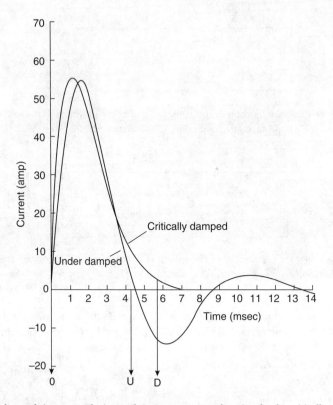

FIGURE 57.6   The damped sine wave. The interval *O–D* represents a duration for the critically and overdamped sine waves. By time *D*, more than 99% of the energy has been delivered. *O–U* is taken as the duration for an underdamped sine wave. (Modified from Tacker W.A. and Geddes L.A. 1980. *Electrical Defibrillation*, Boca Raton, FL, CRC Press. With permission.)

anterior chest as shown in Figure 57.7 or in anterior-to-posterior (front-to-back) position, as shown in Figure 57.8.

57.5   Synchronization

Most defibrillators for trans-chest use have the feature of synchronization, which is an electronic sensing and triggering mechanism for application of the shock during the QRS complex of the ECG. This is required when treating arrhythmias other than ventricular fibrillation, because inadvertent application of a shock during the *T* wave of the ECG often produces ventricular fibrillation. Selection by the operator of the synchronized mode of defibrillator operation will cause the defibrillator to automatically sense the QRS complex and apply the shock during the QRS complex. Furthermore, on the ECG display, the timing of the shock on the QRS is graphically displayed so the operator can be certain that the shock will not fall during the *T* wave (see Figure 57.9).

57.6   Automatic External Defibrillators

Automatic external defibrillators (AEDs) are defibrillators that automatically or semiautomatically recognize and treat rapid arrhythmias, usually under emergency conditions. Their operation requires less training than operation of manual defibrillators because the operator need not know which ECG waveforms indicate rhythms requiring a shock. The operator applies adhesive electrodes from the AED to the

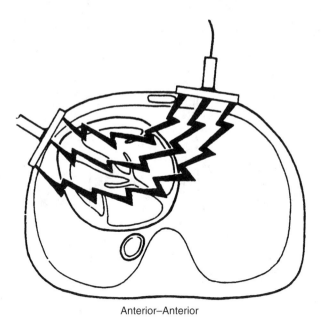

Anterior–Anterior

FIGURE 57.7   Cross-sectional view of the chest showing position for standard anterior wall (precordial) electrode placement. Lines of presumed current flow are shown between the electrodes on the skin surface. (Modified from Tacker W.A. [ed]. 1994. *Defibrillation of the Heart: ICDs, AEDs and Manual,* St. Louis, Mosby-Year Book. With permission.)

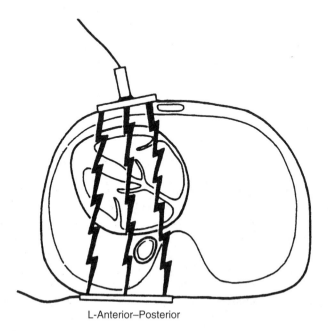

L-Anterior–Posterior

FIGURE 57.8   Cross-sectional view of the chest showing position for front-to-back electrode placement. Lines of presumed current flow are shown between the electrodes on the skin surface. (Modified from Tacker W.A. [ed]. 1994. *Defibrillation of the Heart: ICDs, AEDs and Manual,* St. Louis, Mosby-Year Book. With permission.)

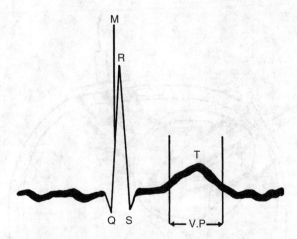

FIGURE 57.9   Timing mark (*M*) as shown on a synchronized defibrillator monitor. The *M* designates when a shock will be applied in the cardiac cycle. The *T* wave must be avoided, since a shock during the vulnerable period (V.P.) may fibrillate the ventricles. This tracing shows atrial fibrillation as identified by the irregular wavy baseline of the ECG. (Modified from Feinberg B. 1980. *Handbook Series in Clinical Laboratory Science*, Vol. 2, Boca Raton, FL, CRC Press. With permission.)

patient and turns on the AED, which monitors the ECG and determines by built-in signal processing whether or not and when to shock the patient. In a completely automatic mode, the AED does not have a manual control as shown in Figure 57.3 but instead has an automatic control. In semiautomatic mode, the operator must confirm the shock advisory from the AED to deliver the shock. AEDs have substantial potential for improving the chances of survival from cardiac arrest because they enable emergency personnel, who typically reach the patient before paramedics do, to deliver defibrillating shocks. Furthermore, the reduced training requirements make feasible the operation of AEDs in the home by a family member of a patient at high risk of ventricular fibrillation.

57.7   Defibrillator Safety

Defibrillators are potentially dangerous devices because of their high electrical output characteristics. The danger to the patient of unsynchronized shocks has already been presented, as has the synchronization design to prevent inadvertent precipitation of fibrillation by a cardioversion shock applied during the *T* wave.

There are other safety issues. Improper technique may result in accidental shocking of the operator or other personnel in the vicinity, if someone is in contact with the electric discharge pathway. This may occur if the operator is careless in holding the discharge electrodes or if someone is in contact with the patient or with a metal bed occupied by the subject when the shock is applied. Proper training and technique is necessary to avoid this risk.

Another safety issue is that of producing damage to the patient by application of excessively strong or excessively numerous shocks. Although cardiac damage has been reported after high-intensity and repetitive shocks to experimental animals and human patients, it is generally held that significant cardiac damage is unlikely if proper clinical procedures and guidelines are followed.

Failure of a defibrillator to operate correctly may also be considered a safety issue, since inability of a defibrillator to deliver a shock in the absence of a replacement unit means loss of the opportunity to resuscitate the patient. A recent review of defibrillator failures found that operator errors, inadequate defibrillator care and maintenance, and, to a lesser extent, component failure accounted for the majority of defibrillator failures [7].

References

[1] Tacker, W.A. Jr. (ed.). (1994). *Defibrillation of the Heart: ICDs, AEDs, and Manual.* St. Louis, Mosby-Year Book.

[2] Tacker, W.A. Jr. and Geddes, L.A. (1980). *Electrical Defibrillation.* Boca Raton, FL, CRC Press.

[3] Emergency Cardiac Care Committees, American Heart Association (1992). Guidelines for cardiopulmonary resuscitation and emergency cardiac care. *JAMA* 268: 2199.

[4] American National Standard ANSI/AAMI DF2 (1989). (second edition, revision of ANSI/AAMI DF2-1981) Safety and performance standard: cardiac defibrillator devices.

[5] Canadian National Standard CAN/CSA C22.2 No. 601.2.4-M90 (1990). Medical electrical equipment, part 2: particular requirements for the safety of cardiac defibrillators and cardiac defibrillator/monitors.

[6] International Standard IEC 601-2-4 (1983). Medical electrical equipment, part 2: particular requirements for the safety of cardiac defibrillators and cardiac defibrillator/monitors.

[7] Cummins, R.O., Chesemore, K., White, R.D., and the Defibrillator Working Group (1990). Defibrillator failures: causes of problems and recommendations for improvement. *JAMA* 264: 1019.

Further Information

Detailed presentation of material on defibrillator waveforms, algorithms for ECG analysis, and automatic defibrillation using AEDs, electrodes, design, clinical use, effects of drugs on shock strength required to defibrillate, damage due to defibrillator shocks, and use of defibrillators during open-thorax surgical procedures or trans-esophageal defibrillation are beyond the scope of this chapter. Also, the historical aspects of defibrillation are not presented here. For more information, the reader is referred to the publications at the end of this chapter [1–3]. For detailed description of specific defibrillators with comparisons of features, the reader is referred to articles from *Health Devices*, a monthly publication of ECRI, 5200 Butler Pike, Plymouth Meeting, Pa USA. For American, Canadian, and European defibrillator standards, the reader is referred to published standards [3–6] and Charbonnier's discussion of standards [1].

58

Implantable Defibrillators

58.1	Pulse Generators	**58**-1
58.2	Electrode Systems ("Leads")	**58**-2
58.3	Arrhythmia Detection	**58**-4
58.4	Arrhythmia Therapy	**58**-5
58.5	Implantable Monitoring	**58**-6
58.6	Follow-Up	**58**-7
58.7	Economics	**58**-7
58.8	Conclusion	**58**-8
	Acknowledgments	**58**-8
	References	**58**-8

Edwin G. Duffin
Medtronic, Inc.

The implantable cardioverter defibrillator (ICD) is a therapeutic device that can detect ventricular tachycardia or fibrillation and automatically deliver high-voltage (750 V) shocks that will restore normal sinus rhythm. Advanced versions also provide low-voltage (5 to 10 V) pacing stimuli for painless termination of ventricular tachycardia and for management of bradyarrhythmias. The proven efficacy of the automatic implantable defibrillator has placed it in the mainstream of therapies for the prevention of sudden arrhythmic cardiac death.

The implantable defibrillator has evolved significantly since first appearing in 1980. The newest devices can be implanted in the patient's pectoral region and use electrodes that can be inserted transvenously, eliminating the traumatic thoracotomy required for placement of the earlier epicardial electrode systems. Transvenous systems provide rapid, minimally invasive implants with high assurance of success and greater patient comfort. Advanced arrhythmia detection algorithms offer a high degree of sensitivity with reasonable specificity, and extensive monitoring is provided to document performance and to facilitate appropriate programming of arrhythmia detection and therapy parameters. Generator longevity can now exceed 4 years, and the cost of providing this therapy is declining.

58.1 Pulse Generators

The implantable defibrillator consists of a primary battery, high-voltage capacitor bank, and sensing and control circuitry housed in a hermetically sealed titanium case. Commercially available devices weigh between 197 and 237 g and range in volume from 113 to 145 cm^3. Clinical trials are in progress on devices with volumes ranging from 178 to 60 cm^3 and weights between 275 and 104 g. Further size reductions will be achieved with the introduction of improved capacitor and integrated circuit technologies and lead systems offering lower pacing and defibrillation thresholds. Progress should parallel that made with antibradycardia pacemakers that have evolved from 250-g, nonprogrammable, VOO units with 600-μJ pacing outputs to 26-g, multiprogrammable, DDDR units with dual 25-μJ outputs.

Implantable defibrillator circuitry must include an amplifier, to allow detection of the millivolt-range cardiac electrogram signals; noninvasively programmable processing and control functions, to evaluate the sensed cardiac activity and to direct generation and delivery of the therapeutic energy; high-voltage switching capability; dc–dc conversion functions to step up the low battery voltages; random access memories, to store appropriate patient and device data; and radiofrequency telemetry systems, to allow communication to and from the implanted device. Monolithic integrated circuits on hybridized substrates have made it possible to accomplish these diverse functions in a commercially acceptable and highly reliable form.

Defibrillators must convert battery voltages of approximately 6.5 to the 600–750 V needed to defibrillate the heart. Since the conversion process cannot directly supply this high voltage at current strengths needed for defibrillation, charge is accumulated in relatively large (Ý85–120 μF effective capacitance) aluminum electrolytic capacitors that account for 20 to 30% of the volume of a typical defibrillator. These capacitors must be charged periodically to prevent their dielectric from deteriorating. If this is not done, the capacitors become electrically leaky, yielding excessively long charge times and delay of therapy. Early defibrillators required that the patient return to the clinic periodically to have the capacitors reformed, whereas newer devices do this automatically at preset or programmable times. Improved capacitor technology, perhaps ceramic or thin-film, will eventually offer higher storage densities, greater shape variability for denser component packaging, and freedom from the need to waste battery capacity performing periodic reforming charges. Packaging density has already improved from 0.03 J/cm^3 for devices such as the early cardioverter to 0.43 J/cm^3 with some investigational ICDs. Capacitors that allow conformal shaping could readily increase this density to more than 0.6 J/cm^3.

Power sources used in defibrillators must have sufficient capacity to provide 50–400 full energy charges (Ý34 J) and 3 to 5 years of bradycardia pacing and background circuit operation. They must have a very low internal resistance in order to supply the relatively high currents needed to charge the defibrillation capacitors in 5–15 S. This generally requires that the batteries have large surface area electrodes and use chemistries that exhibit higher rates of internal discharge than those seen with the lithium iodide batteries used in pacemakers. The most commonly used defibrillator battery chemistry is lithium silver vanadium oxide.

58.2   Electrode Systems ("Leads")

Early implantable defibrillators utilized patch electrodes (typically a titanium mesh electrode) placed on the surface of the heart, requiring entry through the chest (Figure 58.1). This procedure is associated with approximately 3 to 4% perioperative mortality, significant hospitalization time and complications, patient discomfort, and high costs. Although subcostal, subxiphoid, and thoracoscopic techniques can minimize the surgical procedure, the ultimate solution has been development of fully transvenous lead systems with acceptable defibrillation thresholds.

Currently available transvenous leads are constructed much like pacemaker leads, using polyurethane or silicone insulation and platinum–iridium electrode materials. Acceptable thresholds are obtained in 67 to 95% of patients, with mean defibrillation thresholds ranging from 10.9 to 18.1 J. These lead systems use a combination of two or more electrodes located in the right ventricular apex, the superior vena cava, the coronary sinus, and sometimes, a subcutaneous patch electrode is placed in the chest region. These leads offer advantages beyond the avoidance of major surgery. They are easier to remove should there be infections or a need for lead system revision. The pacing thresholds of current transvenous defibrillation electrodes are typically 0.96±0.39 V, and the electrogram amplitudes are on the order of 16.4±6.4 mV. The eventual application of steroid-eluting materials in the leads should provide increased pacing efficiency

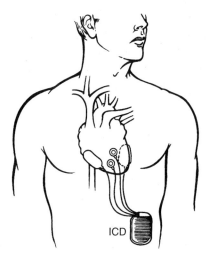

FIGURE 58.1   Epicardial ICD systems typically use two or three large defibrillating patch electrodes placed on the epicardium of the left and right ventricles and a pair of myocardial electrodes for detection and pacing. The generator is usually placed in the abdomen. (Copyright Medtronic, Inc. With permission.)

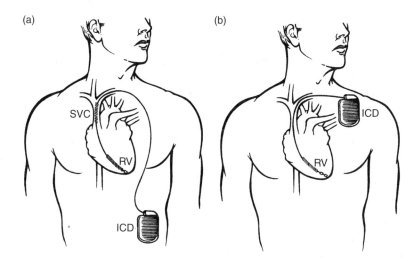

FIGURE 58.2   The latest transvenous fibrillation systems employ a single catheter placed in the right ventricular apex. In panel (a) a single transvenous catheter provides defibrillation electrodes in the superior vena cava and in the right ventricle. This catheter provides a single pace/sense electrode which is used in conjunction with the right ventricular high-voltage defibrillation electrode for arrhythmia detection and antibradycardia/antitachycardia pacing (a configuration that is sometimes referred to as *integrated bipolar*). With pulse generators small enough to be placed in the pectoral region, defibrillation can be achieved by delivering energy between the generator housing and one high-voltage electrode in the right ventricle (analogous to unipolar pacing) as is shown in panel (b). This catheter provided bipolar pace/sense electrodes for arrhythmia detection and antibradycardia/antitachycardia pacing. (Copyright Medtronic, Inc. With permission.)

with transvenous lead systems, thereby reducing the current drain associated with pacing and extending pulse generator longevity.

Lead systems are being refined to simplify the implant procedures. One approach is the use of a single catheter having a single right ventricular low-voltage electrode for pacing and detection, and a pair of high-voltage defibrillation electrodes spaced for replacement in the right ventricle and in the superior vena cava (Figure 58.2a). A more recent approach parallels that used for unipolar pacemakers.

A single right-ventricular catheter having bipolar pace/sense electrodes and one right ventricular high-voltage electrode is used in conjunction with a defibrillator housing that serves as the second high-voltage electrode (Figure 58.2b). Mean biphasic pulse defibrillation thresholds with the generator-electrode placed in the patient's left pectoral region are reported to be 9.8 ± 6.6 J ($n = 102$). This approach appears to be practicable only with generators suitable for pectoral placement, but such devices will become increasingly available.

58.3 Arrhythmia Detection

Most defibrillator detection algorithms rely primarily on heart rate to indicate the presence of a treatable rhythm. Additional refinements sometimes include simple morphology assessments, as with the probability density function, and analysis of rhythm stability and rate of change in rate.

The *probability density function* evaluates the percentage of time that the filtered ventricular electrogram spends in a window centered on the baseline. The rate-of-change-in-rate or *onset* evaluation discriminates sinus tachycardia from ventricular tachycardia on the basis of the typically gradual acceleration of sinus rhythms vs. the relatively abrupt acceleration of many pathologic tachycardias. The *rate stability* function is designed to bar detection of tachyarrhythmias as long as the variation in ventricular rate exceeds a physician-programmed tolerance, thereby reducing the likelihood of inappropriate therapy delivery in response to atrial fibrillation. This concept appears to be one of the more successful detection algorithm enhancements.

Because these additions to the detection algorithm reduce sensitivity, some defibrillator designs offer a supplementary detection mode that will trigger therapy in response to any elevated ventricular rate of prolonged duration. These *extended-high-rate* algorithms bypass all or portions of the normal detection screening, resulting in low specificity for rhythms with prolonged elevated rates such as exercise-induced sinus tachycardia. Consequently, use of such algorithms generally increases the incidence of inappropriate therapies.

Improvements in arrhythmia detection specificity are desirable, but they must not decrease the excellent sensitivity offered by current algorithms. The anticipated introduction of defibrillators incorporating dual-chamber pacemaker capability will certainly help in this quest, since it will then be possible to use atrial electrograms in the rhythm classification process. It would also be desirable to have a means of evaluating the patient's hemodynamic tolerance of the rhythm, so that the more comfortable pacing sequences could be used as long as the patient was not syncopal yet branch quickly to a definitive shock should the patient begin to lose consciousness.

Although various enhanced detection processes have been proposed, many have not been tested clinically, in some cases because sufficient processing power was not available in implantable systems, and in some cases because sensor technology was not yet ready for chronic implantation. Advances in technology may eventually make some of these very elegant proposals practicable. Examples of proposed detection enhancements include extended analyses of cardiac event timing (PR and RR stability, AV interval variation, temporal distribution of atrial electrogram intervals and of ventricular electrogram intervals, timing differences and/or coherency of multiple ventricular electrograms, ventricular response to a provocative atrial extrastimuli), electrogram waveform analyses (paced depolarization integral, morphology analyses of right ventricular or atrial electrograms), analyses of hemodynamic parameters (right-ventricular pulsatile pressure, mean right atrial and mean right ventricular pressures, wedge coronary sinus pressure, static right ventricular pressure, right atrial pressure, right ventricular stroke volume, mixed venous oxygen saturation and mixed venous blood temperature, left ventricular impedance, intramyocardial pressure gradient, aortic and pulmonary artery flow), and detection of physical motion.

Because defibrillator designs are intentionally biased to overtreat in preference to the life-threatening consequences associated with failure to treat, there is some incidence of inappropriate therapy delivery. Unwarranted therapies are usually triggered by supraventricular tachyarrhythmias, especially atrial fibrillation, or sinus tachycardia associated with rates faster than the ventricular tachycardia detection rate threshold. Additional causes include nonsustained ventricular tachycardia, oversensing of T waves, double counting of R waves and pacing stimuli from brady pacemakers, and technical faults such as loose leadgenerator connections or lead fractures.

Despite the bias for high detection sensitivity, undersensing does occur. It has been shown to result from inappropriate detection algorithm programming, such as an excessively high tachycardia detection rate; inappropriate amplifier gain characteristics; and electrode designs that place the sensing terminals too close to the high-voltage electrodes with a consequent reduction in electrogram amplitude following shocks. Undersensing can also result in the induction of tachycardia should the amplifier gain control algorithm result in undersensing of sinus rhythms.

58.4 Arrhythmia Therapy

Pioneering implantable defibrillators were capable only of defibrillation shocks. Subsequently, synchronized cardioversion capability was added. Antibradycardia pacing had to be provided by implantation of a standard pacemaker in addition to the defibrillator, and, if antitachycardia pacing was prescribed, it was necessary to use an antitachycardia pacemaker. Several currently marketed implantable defibrillators offer integrated ventricular demand pacemaker function and tiered antiarrhythmia therapy (pacing/cardioversion/defibrillation). Various burst and ramp antitachycardia pacing algorithms are offered, and they all seem to offer comparably high success rates. These expanded therapeutic capabilities improve patient comfort by reducing the incidence of shocks in conscious patients, eliminate the problems and discomfort associated with implantation of multiple devices, and contribute to a greater degree of success, since the prescribed regimens can be carefully tailored to specific patient needs. Availability of devices with antitachy pacing capability significantly increases the acceptability of the implantable defibrillator for patients with ventricular tachycardia.

Human clinical trials have shown that biphasic defibrillation waveforms are more effective than monophasic waveforms, and newer devices now incorporate this characteristic. Speculative explanations for biphasic superiority include the large voltage change at the transition from the first to the second phase or hyperpolarization of tissue and reactivation of sodium channels during the initial phase, with resultant tissue conditioning that allows the second phase to more readily excite the myocardium.

Antitachycardia pacing and cardioversion are not uniformly successful. There is some incidence of ventricular arrhythmia acceleration with antitachycardia pacing and cardioversion, and it is also not unusual for cardioversion to induce atrial fibrillation that in turn triggers unwarranted therapies. An ideal therapeutic solution would be one capable of preventing the occurrence of tachycardia altogether. Prevention techniques have been investigated, among them the use of precisely timed subthreshold stimuli, simultaneous stimulation at multiple sites, and pacing with elevated energies at the site of the tachycardia, but none has yet proven practical.

The rudimentary VVI antibradycardia pacing provided by current defibrillators lacks rate responsiveness and atrial pacing capability. Consequently, some defibrillator patients require implantation of a separate dual-chamber pacemaker for hemodynamic support. It is inevitable that future generations of defibrillators will offer dual-chamber pacing capabilities.

Atrial fibrillation, occurring either as a consequence of defibrillator operation or as a natural progression in many defibrillator patients, is a major therapeutic challenge. It is certainly possible to adapt implantable defibrillator technology to treat atrial fibrillation, but the challenge is to do so without causing the patient undue discomfort. Biphasic waveform defibrillation of acutely induced atrial fibrillation has been demonstrated in humans with an 80% success rate at 0.4 J using *epicardial* electrodes. Stand-alone atrial defibrillators are in development, and, if they are successful, it is likely that this capability would be integrated into the mainstream ventricular defibrillators as well. However, most conscious patients find shocks above 0.5 J to be very unpleasant, and it remains to be demonstrated that a clinically acceptable energy level will be efficacious when applied with transvenous electrode systems to spontaneously occurring atrial fibrillation. Moreover, a stand-alone atrial defibrillator either must deliver an atrial shock with complete assurance of appropriate synchronization to ventricular activity or must restrict the therapeutic energy delivery to atrial structures in order to prevent inadvertent induction of a malignant ventricular arrhythmia.

58.5 Implantable Monitoring

Until recently, defibrillator data recording capabilities were quite limited, making it difficult to verify the adequacy of arrhythmia detection and therapy settings. The latest devices record electrograms and diagnostic channel data showing device behavior during multiple tachyarrhythmia episodes. These devices also include counters (number of events detected, success and failure of each programmed therapy, and so on) that present a broad, though less specific, overview of device behavior (Figure 58.3). Monitoring capability in some of the newest devices appears to be the equivalent of 32 Kbytes of random access memory, allowing electrogram waveform records of approximately 2-min duration, with some opportunity for later expansion by judicious selection of sampling rates and data compression techniques. Electrogram storage has proven useful for documenting false therapy delivery due to atrial fibrillation, lead fractures, and sinus

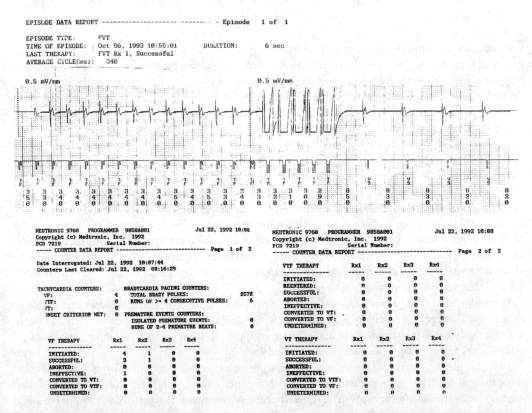

FIGURE 58.3 Typical data recorded by an implantable defibrillator include stored intracardiac electrograms with annotated markers indicating cardiac intervals, paced and sensed events, and device classification of events (TF = fast tachycardia; TP = antitachy pacing stimulus; VS = sensed nontachy ventricular event). In the example, five rapid pacing pulses convert a ventricular tachycardia with a cycle length of 340 msec into sinus rhythm with a cycle length of 830 msec. In the lower portion of the figure is an example of the summary data collected by the ICD, showing detailed counts of the performance of the various therapies (Rx) for ventricular tachycardia (VT), fast ventricular (VTF), and ventricular (VF). (Copyright Medtronic, Inc. With permission.)

tachycardia, determining the triggers of arrhythmias; documenting rhythm accelerations in response to therapies; and demonstrating appropriate device behavior when treating asymptomatic rhythms.

Electrograms provide useful information by themselves, yet they cannot indicate how the device interpreted cardiac activity. Increasingly, electrogram records are being supplemented with event markers that indicate how the device is responding on a beat-by-beat basis. These records can include measurements of the sensed and paced intervals, indication as to the specific detection zone an event falls in, indication of charge initiation, and other device performance data.

58.6 Follow-Up

Defibrillator patients and their devices require careful follow-up. In one study of 241 ICD patients with epicardial lead systems, 53% of the patients experienced one or more complications during an average exposure of 24 months. These complications included infection requiring device removal in 5%, postoperative respiratory complications in 11%, postoperative bleeding and/or thrombosis in 4%, lead system migration or disruption in 8%, and documented inappropriate therapy delivery, most commonly due to atrial fibrillation, in 22%. A shorter study of 80 patients with transvenous defibrillator systems reported no postoperative pulmonary complications, transient nerve injury (1%), asymptomatic subclavian vein occlusion (2.5%), pericardial effusion (1%), subcutaneous patch pocket hematoma (5%), pulse generator pocket infection (1%), lead fracture (1%), and lead system dislodgement (10%). During a mean follow-up period of 11 months, 7.5% of the patients in this series experienced inappropriate therapy delivery, half for atrial fibrillation and the rest for sinus tachycardia.

Although routine follow-up can be accomplished in the clinic, detection and analysis of transient events depends on the recording capabilities available in the devices or on the use of various external monitoring equipment.

58.7 Economics

The annual cost of ICD therapy is dropping as a consequence of better longevity and simpler implantation techniques. Early generators that lacked programmability, antibradycardia pacing capability, and event recording had 62% survival at 18 months and 2% at 30 months. Some recent programmable designs that include VVI pacing capability and considerable event storage exhibit 96.8% survival at 48 months. It has been estimated that an increase in generator longevity from 2 to 5 years would lower the cost per life-year saved by 55% in a hypothetical patient population with a 3-year sudden mortality of 28%. More efficient energy conversion circuits and finer line-width integrated circuit technology with smaller, more highly integrated circuits and reduced current drains will yield longer-lasting defibrillators while continuing the evolution to smaller volumes.

Cost of the implantation procedure is clearly declining as transvenous lead systems become commonplace. Total hospitalization duration, complication rates, and use of costly hospital operating rooms and intensive care facilities all are reduced, providing significant financial benefits. One study reported requiring half the intensive care unit time and a reduction in total hospitalization from 26 to 15 days when comparing transvenous to epicardial approaches. Another center reported a mean hospitalization stay of 6 days for patients receiving transvenous defibrillation systems.

Increasing sophistication of the implantable defibrillators paradoxically contributes to cost efficacy. Incorporation of single-chamber brady pacing capability eliminates the cost of a separate pacemaker and lead for those patients who need one. Eventually even dual-chamber pacing capability will be available. Programmable detection and therapy features obviate the need for device replacement that was required when fixed parameter devices proved to be inappropriately specified or too inflexible to adapt to a patient's physiologic changes.

Significant cost savings may be obtained by better patient selection criteria and processes, obviating the need for extensive hospitalization and costly electrophysiologic studies prior to device implantation in some patient groups. One frequently discussed issue is the prophylactic role that implantable defibrillators will or should play. Unless a means is found to build far less expensive devices that can be placed with minimal time and facilities, the life-saving yield for prophylactic defibrillators will have to be high if they are to be cost-effective. This remains an open issue.

58.8 Conclusion

The implantable defibrillator is now an established and powerful therapeutic tool. The transition to pectoral implants with biphasic waveforms and efficient yet simple transvenous lead systems is simplifying the implant procedure and drastically reducing the number of unpleasant VF inductions required to demonstrate adequate system performance These advances are making the implantable defibrillator easier to use, less costly, and more acceptable to patients and their physicians.

Acknowledgments

Portions of this text are derived from Duffin E.G. and Barold S.S. 1994. Implantable cardioverter-defibrillators: an overview and future directions, Chapter 28 of I. Singer (ed), Implantable Cardioverter-Defibrillator, and are used with permission of Futura Publishing Company, Inc.

References

Josephson, M. and Wellens H. (eds). (1992). *Tachycardias: Mechanisms and Management.* Mount Kisco, NY, Futura Publishing.

Kappenberger, L. and Lindemans, F. (eds). (1992). *Practical Aspects of Staged Therapy Defibrillators.* Mount Kisco, NY, Futura Publishing.

Singer, I. (ed.). (1994). *Implantable Cardioverter-Defibrillator.* Mount Kisco, NY, Futura Publishing.

Tacker, W. (ed.). (1994). *Defibrillation of the Heart: ICD's, AED's, and Manual.* St. Louis, Mosby.

Memorial issue on implantable defibrillators honoring Michel Mirowski. *PACE,* 14: 865.

59

Implantable Stimulators for Neuromuscular Control

59.1 Functional Electrical Stimulation...................... **59**-1
59.2 Technology for Delivering Stimulation Pulses to
      Excitable Tissue **59**-2
59.3 Stimulation Parameters **59**-2
59.4 Implantable Neuromuscular Stimulators **59**-3
      Receiving Circuit • Power Supply • Data Retrieval • Data
      Processing • Output Stage
59.5 Packaging of Implantable Electronics **59**-6
59.6 Leads and Electrodes **59**-7
59.7 Safety Issues of Implantable Stimulators.............. **59**-7
59.8 Implantable Stimulators in Clinical Use **59**-9
      Peripheral Nerve Stimulators • Stimulators of Central
      Nervous System
59.9 Future of Implantable Electrical Stimulators **59**-10
      Distributed Stimulators • Sensing of Implantable
      Transducer-Generated and Physiological Signals
59.10 Summary **59**-11
Defining Terms **59**-12
References **59**-12
Further Information **59**-14

Primoz Strojnik
P. Hunter Peckham
Case Western Reserve University

59.1 Functional Electrical Stimulation

Implantable stimulators for neuromuscular control are the technologically most advanced versions of functional electrical stimulators. Their function is to generate contraction of muscles, which cannot be controlled volitionally because of the damage or dysfunction in the neural paths of the central nervous system (CNS). Their operation is based on the electrical nature of conducting information within nerve fibers, from the neuron cell body (soma), along the axon, where a travelling action potential is the carrier of excitation. While the action potential is naturally generated chemically in the head of the axon, it may also be generated artificially by depolarizing the neuron membrane with an electrical pulse. A train of electrical impulses with certain amplitude, width, and repetition rate, applied to a muscle innervating nerve (a motor neuron) will cause the muscle to contract, very much like in natural excitation. Similarly, a train of electrical pulses applied to the muscular tissue close to the motor point will cause muscle contraction by stimulating the muscle through the neural structures at the motor point.

59.2   Technology for Delivering Stimulation Pulses to Excitable Tissue

A practical system used to stimulate a nerve consists of three components (1) a *pulse generator* to generate a train of pulses capable of depolarizing the nerve, (2) a **lead wire**, the function of which is to deliver the pulses to the stimulation site, and (3) an *electrode*, which delivers the stimulation pulses to the excitable tissue in a safe and efficient manner.

In terms of location of the above three components of an electrical stimulator, stimulation technology can be described in the following terms:

Surface or transcutaneous stimulation, where all three components are outside the body and the electrodes are placed on the skin above or near the motor point of the muscle to be stimulated. This method has been used extensively in medical rehabilitation of nerve and muscle. Therapeutically, it has been used to prevent atrophy of paralyzed muscles, to condition paralyzed muscles before the application of functional stimulation, and to generally increase the muscle bulk. As a functional tool, it has been used in rehabilitation of plegic and paretic patients. Surface systems for functional stimulation have been developed to correct drop-foot condition in hemiplegic individuals [Liberson, 1961], for hand control [Rebersek, 1973], and for standing and stepping in individuals with **paralysis** of the lower extremities [Kralj and Bajd, 1989]. This fundamental technology was commercialized by Sigmedics, Inc. [Graupe, 1998]. The inability of surface stimulation to reliably excite the underlying tissue in a repeatable manner and to selectively stimulate deep muscles has limited the clinical applicability of surface stimulation.

Percutaneous stimulation employs electrodes which are positioned inside the body close to the structures to be stimulated. Their lead wires permanently penetrate the skin to be connected to the external pulse generator. State of the art embodiments of percutaneous electrodes utilize a small-diameter insulated stainless steel lead that is passed through the skin. The electrode structure is formed by removal of the insulation from the lead and subsequent modification to ensure stability within the tissue. This modification includes forming barbs or similar anchoring mechanisms. The percutaneous electrode is implanted using a hypodermic needle as a trochar for introduction. As the needle is withdrawn, the anchor at the electrode tip is engaged into the surrounding tissue and remains in the tissue. A connector at the skin surface, next to the skin penetration point, joins the percutaneous electrode lead to the hardwired external stimulator. The penetration site has to be maintained and care must be taken to avoid physical damage of the lead wires. In the past, this technology has helped develop the existing implantable systems, and it may be used for short and long term, albeit not permanent, stimulation applications [Marsolais, 1986; Memberg, 1993].

The term *implantable stimulation* refers to stimulation systems in which all three components, pulse generator, lead wires, and electrodes, are permanently surgically implanted into the body and the skin is solidly closed after the implantation procedure. Any interaction between the implantable part and the outside world is performed using telemetry principles in a contact-less fashion. This chapter is focused on implantable neuromuscular stimulators, which will be discussed in more detail.

59.3   Stimulation Parameters

In functional **electrical stimulation**, the typical stimulation waveform is a train of rectangular pulses. This shape is used because of its effectiveness as well as relative ease of generation. All three parameters of a stimulation train, that is, frequency, amplitude, and pulse-width, have effect on muscle contraction. Generally, the stimulation frequency is kept as low as possible, to prevent muscle fatigue and to conserve stimulation energy. The determining factor is the muscle fusion frequency at which a smooth muscle response is obtained. This frequency varies; however, it can be as low as 12 to 14 Hz and as high as 50 Hz. In most cases, the stimulation frequency is kept constant for a certain application. This is true both for surface as well as implanted electrodes.

With surface electrodes, the common way of modulating muscle force is by varying the stimulation pulse amplitude at a constant frequency and pulse width. The stimulation amplitudes may be as low as 25 V at 200 μsec for the stimulation of the peroneal nerve and as high as 120 V or more at 300 μsec for activation of large muscles such as the gluteus maximus.

In implantable stimulators and electrodes, the stimulation parameters greatly depend on the implantation site. When the electrodes are positioned on or around the target nerve, the stimulation amplitudes are on the order of a few milliamperes or less. Electrodes positioned on the muscle surface (epimysial electrodes) or in the muscle itself (intramuscular electrodes), employ up to ten times higher amplitudes. For muscle force control, implantable stimulators rely either on pulse-width modulation or amplitude modulation. For example, in upper extremity applications, the current amplitude is usually a fixed paramter set to 16 or 20 mA, while the muscle force is modulated with pulse-widths within 0 to 200 μsec.

59.4   Implantable Neuromuscular Stimulators

Implantable stimulation systems use an encapsulated pulse generator that is surgically implanted and has subcutaneous leads that terminate at electrodes on or near the desired nerves. In low power consumption applications such as the cardiac pacemaker, a primary battery power source is included in the pulse generator case. When the battery is close to depletion, the pulse generator has to be surgically replaced.

Most implantable systems for neuromuscular application consist of an external and an implanted component. Between the two, an inductive radio-frequency link is established, consisting of two tightly coupled resonant coils. The link allows transmission of power and information, through the skin, from the external device to the implanted pulse generator. In more advanced systems, a back-telemetry link is also established, allowing transmission of data outwards, from the implanted to the external component.

Ideally, implantable stimulators for neuromuscular control would be stand alone, totally implanted devices with an internal power source and integrated sensors detecting desired movements from the motor cortex and delivering stimulation sequences to appropriate muscles, thus bypassing the neural damage. At the present developmental stage, they still need a control source and an external controller to provide power and stimulation information. The control source may be either operator driven, controlled by the user, or triggered by an event such as the heel-strike phase of the gait cycle. Figure 59.1 depicts a neuromuscular prosthesis developed at the Case Western Reserve University (CWRU) and Cleveland Veterans Affairs Medical Center for the restoration of hand functions using an implantable neuromuscular stimulator. In this application, the patient uses the shoulder motion to control opening and closing of the hand.

The internal electronic structure of an implantable neuromuscular stimulator is shown in Figure 59.2. It consists of receiving and data retrieval circuits, power supply, data processing circuits, and output stages.

59.4.1   Receiving Circuit

The stimulator's receiving circuit is an LC circuit tuned to the resonating frequency of the external transmitter, followed by a rectifier. Its task is to provide the raw DC power from the received **rf** signal and at the same time allow extraction of stimulation information embedded in the rf carrier. There are various encoding schemes allowing simultaneous transmission of power and information into an implantable electronic device. They include amplitude and frequency modulation with different modulation indexes as well as different versions of digital encoding such as Manchester encoding where the information is

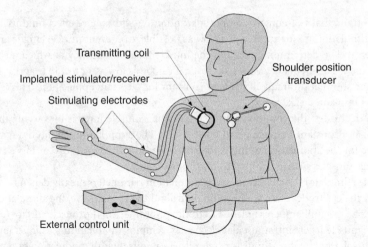

FIGURE 59.1   Implanted FES hand grasp system.

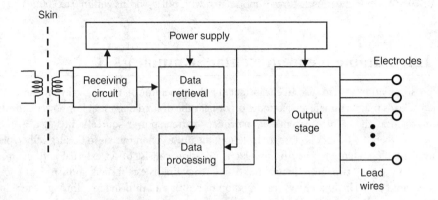

FIGURE 59.2   Block diagram of an implantable neuromuscular stimulator.

hidden in a logic value transition position rather than the logic value itself. Synchronous and asynchronous clock signals may be extracted from the modulated carrier to drive the implant's logic circuits.

The use of radiofrequency transmission for medical devices is regulated and in most countries limited to certain frequencies and radiation powers. (In the United States, the use of the rf space is regulated by the Federal Communication Commission [FCC].) Limited rf transmission powers as well as conservation of power in battery operated external controllers dictate high coupling efficiencies between the transmitting and receiving antennas. Optimal coupling parameters cannot be uniformly defined; they depend on application particularities and design strategies.

59.4.2 Power Supply

The amount of power delivered into an implanted electronic package depends on the coupling between the transmitting and the receiving coil. The coupling is dependent on the distance as well as the alignment between the coils. The power supply circuits must compensate for the variations in distance for different users as well as for the alignment variations due to skin movements and consequent changes in relative coil-to-coil position during daily usage. The power dissipated on power supply circuits must not raise the overall implant case temperature.

In implantable stimulators that require stimulation voltages in excess of the electronics power supply voltages (20 to 30 V), the stimulation voltage can be provided directly through the receiving coil. In that case, voltage regulators must be used to provide the electronics supply voltage (usually 5 V), which heavily taxes the external power transmitter and increases the implant internal power dissipation.

59.4.3 Data Retrieval

Data retrieval technique depends on the data-encoding scheme and is closely related to power supply circuits and implant power consumption. Most commonly, amplitude modulation is used to encode the in-going data stream. As the high quality factor of resonant LC circuits increases the efficiency of power transmission, it also effectively reduces the transmission bandwidth and therefore the transmission data rate. Also, high quality circuits are difficult to amplitude modulate since they tend to continue oscillating even with power removed. This has to be taken into account when designing the communication link in particular for the start-up situation when the implanted device does not use the power for stimulation and therefore loads the transmitter side less heavily, resulting in narrower and higher resonant curves. The load on the receiving coil may also affect the low pass filtering of the received rf signal.

Modulation index (m) or depth of modulation affects the overall energy transfer into the implant. At a given rf signal amplitude, less energy is transferred into the implanted device when 100% modulation is used ($m = 1$) as compared to 10% modulation ($m = 0.053$). However, retrieval of 100% modulated signal is much easier than retrieval of a 10% modulated signal.

59.4.4 Data Processing

Once the information signal has been satisfactorily retrieved and reconstructed into logic voltage levels, it is ready for logic processing. For synchronous data processing a clock signal is required. It can be generated locally within the implant device, reconstructed from the incoming data stream, or can be derived from the rf carrier. A crystal has to be used with a local oscillator to assure stable clock frequency. Local oscillator allows for asynchronous data transmission. Synchronous transmission is best achieved using Manchester data encoding. Decoding of Manchester encoded data recovers the original clock signal, which was used during data encoding. Another method is using the downscaled rf carrier signal as the clock source. In this case, the information signal has to be synchronized with the rf carrier. Of course, 100% modulation scheme cannot be used with carrier-based clock signal. Complex command structure used in multichannel stimulators requires intensive data decoding and processing and consequently extensive electronic circuitry. Custom-made, application specific circuits (ASIC) are commonly used to minimize the space requirements and optimize the circuit performance.

59.4.5 Output Stage

The output stage forms stimulation pulses and defines their electrical characteristics. Even though a mere rectangular pulse can depolarize a nervous membrane, such pulses are not used in clinical practice due to their noxious effect on the tissue and **stimulating electrodes**. These effects can be significantly reduced by charge balanced stimulating pulses where the cathodic stimulation pulse is followed by an anodic pulse containing the same electrical charge, which reverses the electrochemical effects of the cathodic pulse. Charge balanced waveforms can be assured by capacitive coupling between the pulse generator and stimulation electrodes. Charge balanced stimulation pulses include symmetrical and asymmetrical waveforms with anodic phase immediately following the cathodic pulse or being delayed by a short, 20 to 60 μsec interval.

The output stages of most implantable neuromuscular stimulators have constant current characteristics, meaning that the output current is independent on the electrode or tissue impedance. Practically, the constant current characteristics ensure that the same current flows through the excitable tissues regardless of the changes that may occur on the electrode-tissue interface, such as the growth of fibrous tissue around the electrodes. Constant current output stage can deliver constant current only within the supply voltage — compliance voltage. In neuromuscular stimulation, with the electrode impedance being on the order of 1 kΩ, and the stimulating currents in the order of 20 mA, the compliance voltage must be above

20 V. Considering the voltage drops and losses across electronic components, the compliance voltage of the output stage may have to be as high as 33 V.

The stimulus may be applied through either monopolar or bipolar electrodes. The monopolar electrode is one in which a single active electrode is placed near the excitable nerve and the return electrode is placed remotely, generally at the implantable unit itself. Bipolar electrodes are placed at the stimulation site, thus limiting the current paths to the area between the electrodes. Generally, in monopolar stimulation the active electrode is much smaller than the return electrode, while bipolar electrodes are the same size.

59.5   Packaging of Implantable Electronics

Electronic circuits must be protected from the harsh environment of the human body. The packaging of implantable electronics uses various materials, including polymers, metals, and ceramics. The encapsulation method depends somewhat on the electronic circuit technology. Older devices may still use discrete components in a classical form, such as leaded transistors and resistors. The newer designs, depending on the sophistication of the implanted device, may employ application-specific integrated circuits (ASICs) and thick film hybrid circuitry for their implementation. Such circuits place considerable requirements for hermeticity and protection on the implanted circuit packaging.

Epoxy encapsulation was the original choice of designers of implantable neuromuscular stimulators. It has been successfully used with relatively simple circuits using discrete, low impedance components. With epoxy encapsulation, the receiving coil is placed around the circuitry to be "potted" in a mold, which gives the implant the final shape. Additionally, the epoxy body is coated with silicone rubber that improves the **biocompatibility** of the package. Polymers do not provide an impermeable barrier and therefore cannot be used for encapsulation of high density, high impedance electronic circuits. The moisture ingress ultimately will reach the electronic components, and surface ions can allow electric shorting and degradation of leakage-sensitive circuitry and subsequent failure.

Hermetic packaging provides the implant electronic circuitry with a long-term protection from the ingress of body fluids. Materials that provide hermetic barriers are metals, ceramics, and glasses. Metallic packaging generally uses a titanium capsule machined from a solid piece of metal or deep-drawn from a piece of sheet metal. Electrical signals, such as power and stimulation, enter and exit the package through hermetic feedthroughs, which are hermetically welded onto the package walls. The **feedthrough** assembly utilizes a ceramic or glass insulator to allow one or more wires to exit the package without contact with the package itself. During the assembly procedures, the electronic circuitry is placed in the package and connected internally to the feedthroughs, and the package is then welded closed. Tungsten Inert Gas (TIG), electron beam, or laser welding equipment is used for the final closure. Assuming integrity of all components, hermeticity with this package is ensured. This integrity can be checked by detecting gas leakage from the capsule. Metallic packaging requires that the receiving coil be placed outside the package to avoid significant loss of rf signal or power, thus requiring additional space within the body to accommodate the volume of the entire implant. Generally, the hermetic package and the receiving antenna are jointly imbedded in an epoxy encapsulant, which provides electric isolation for the metallic antenna and stabilizes the entire implant assembly. Figure 59.3 shows such an implantable stimulator designed and made by the CWRU/Veterans Administration Program. The hermetic package is open, displaying the electronic **hybrid circuit**. More recently, alumina-based ceramic packages have been developed that allow hermetic sealing of the electronic circuitry together with enclosure of the receiving coil [Strojnik, 1994]. This is possible due to the rf transparency of ceramics. The impact of this type of enclosure is still not fully investigated. The advantage of this approach is that the volume of the implant can be reduced, thus minimizing the biologic response, which is a function of volume. Yet, an unexplored issue of this packaging method is the effect of powerful electromagnetic fields on the implant circuits, lacking the protection of the metal enclosure. This is a particular concern with high gain (EMG, ENG, or EKG sensing) amplifiers, which in the future may be included in the implant package as part of back-telemetry circuits. Physical strength of ceramic packages and their resistance to impact will also require future investigation.

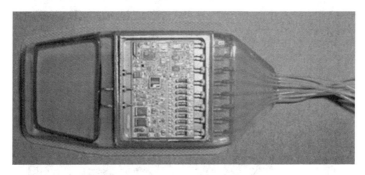

FIGURE 59.3 Photograph of a multichannel implantable stimulator telemeter. Hybrid circuit in titanium package is shown exposed. Receiving coil (left) is imbedded in epoxy resin together with titanium case. Double feedthroughs are seen penetrating titanium capsule wall on the right.

59.6 Leads and Electrodes

Leads connect the pulse generator to the electrodes. They must be sufficiently flexible to move across the joints while at the same time sufficiently sturdy to last for the decades of the intended life of the device. They must also be stretchable to allow change of distance between the pulse generator and the electrodes, associated with body movements. Ability to flex and to stretch is achieved by coiling the lead conductor into a helix and inserting the helix into a small-diameter silicone tubing. This way, both flexing movements and stretching forces exerted on the lead are attenuated, while translated into torsion movements and forces exerted on the coiled conductor. Using multi-strand rather than solid conductors further enhances the longevity. Several individually insulated multi-strand conductors can be coiled together, thus forming a multiple conductor lead wire. Most lead configurations include a connector at some point between the implant and the terminal electrode, allowing for replacement of the implanted receiver or leads in the event of failure. The connectors used have been either single pin in-line connectors located somewhere along the lead length or a multiport/multilead connector at the implant itself. Materials used for lead wires are stainless steels, MP35N (Co, Cr, Ni alloy), and noble metals and their alloys.

Electrodes deliver electrical charge to the stimulated tissues. Those placed on the muscle surface are called epimysial, while those inserted into the muscles are called intramuscular. Nerve stimulating electrodes are called epineural when placed against the nerve, or cuff electrodes when they encircle the nerve. Nerve electrodes may embrace the nerve in a spiral manner individually, or in an array configuration. Some implantable stimulation systems merely use exposed lead-wire conductor sutured to the epineurium as the electrode. Generally, nerve electrodes require approximately one-tenth of the energy for muscle activation as compared to muscle electrodes. However, they require more extensive surgery and may be less selective, but the potential for neural damage is greater than, for example, nerve encircling electrodes.

Electrodes are made of corrosion resistant materials, such as noble metals (platinum or iridium) and their alloys. For example, a platinum–iridium alloy consisting of 10% iridium and 90% platinum is commonly used as an electrode material. Epimysial electrodes developed at CWRU use Ø4 mm Pt90Ir10 discs placed on Dacron reinforced silicone backing. CWRU intramuscular electrodes employ a stainless steel lead-wire with the distal end de-insulated and configured into an electrode tip. A small, umbrella-like anchoring barb is attached to it. With this arrangement, the diameter of the electrode tip does not differ much from the lead wire diameter and this electrode can be introduced into a deep muscle with a trochar-like insertion tool. Figure 59.4 shows enlarged views of these electrodes.

59.7 Safety Issues of Implantable Stimulators

The targeted lifetime of implantable stimulators for neuromuscular control is the lifetime of their users, which is measured in tens of years. Resistance to premature failure must be assured by manufacturing

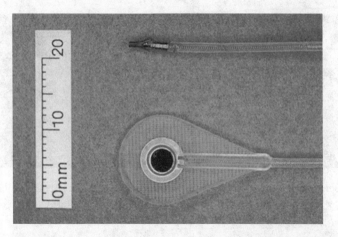

FIGURE 59.4 Implantable electrodes with attached lead wires. Intramuscular electrode (top) has stainless steel tip and anchoring barbs. Epimysial electrode has PtIr disk in the center and is backed by silicone-impregnated Dacron mesh.

processes and testing procedures. Appropriate materials must be selected that will withstand the working environment. Protection against mechanical and electrical hazards that may be encountered during the device lifetime must be incorporated in the design. Various procedures are followed and rigorous tests must be performed during and after its manufacturing to assure the quality and reliability of the device.

- *Manufacturing and testing* — Production of implantable electronic circuits and their encapsulation in many instances falls under the standards governing production and encapsulation of integrated circuits. To minimize the possibility of failure, the implantable electronic devices are manufactured in controlled clean-room environments, using high quality components and strictly defined manufacturing procedures. Finished devices are submitted to rigorous testing before being released for implantation. Also, many tests are carried out during the manufacturing process itself. To assure maximum reliability and product confidence, methods, tests, and procedures defined by military standards, such as MILSTD-883, are followed.
- *Bio-compatibility* — Since the implantable stimulators operate surgically implanted in living tissue, an important part of their design has to be dedicated to biocompatibility, that is, their ability to dwell in living tissue without disrupting the tissue in its functions, creating adverse tissue response, or changing its own properties due to the tissue environment. Elements of biocompatibility include tissue reaction to materials, shape, and size, as well as electrochemical reactions on stimulation electrodes. There are known biomaterials used in the making of implantable stimulators. They include stainless steels, titanium and tantalum, noble metals such as platinum and iridium, as well as implantable grades of selected epoxy and silicone-based materials.
- *Susceptibility to electromagnetic interference (EMI) and electrostatic discharge (ESD)* — Electromagnetic fields can disrupt the operation of electronic devices, which may be lethal in situations with life support systems, but they may also impose risk and danger to users of neuromuscular stimulators. Emissions of EMI may come from outside sources; however, the external control unit is also a source of electromagnetic radiation. Electrostatic discharge shocks are not uncommon during the dry winter season. These shocks may reach voltages as high as 15 kV and more. Sensitive electronic components can easily be damaged by these shocks unless protective design measures are taken. The electronic circuitry in implantable stimulators is generally protected by the metal case. However, the circuitry can be damaged through the feedthroughs either by handling or during the implantation procedure by the electrocautery equipment. ESD damage may happen even after implantation when long lead-wires are utilized. There are no standards directed specifically towards implantable electronic devices. The general standards put in place for

electromedical equipment by the International Electrotechnical Commission provide guidance. The specifications require survival after 3 kV and 8 kV ESD discharges on all conductive and nonconductive accessible parts, respectively.

59.8 Implantable Stimulators in Clinical Use

59.8.1 Peripheral Nerve Stimulators

- *Manipulation* — Control of complex functions for movement, such as hand control, requires the use of many channels of stimulation. At the Case Western Reserve University and Cleveland VAMC, an eight-channel stimulator has been developed for grasp and release [Smith, 1987]. This system uses eight channels of stimulation and a titanium-packaged, thick-film hybrid circuit as the pulse generator. The implant is distributed by the Neurocontrol Corporation (Cleveland, OH) under the name of Freehand®. It has been implanted in approximately 150 patients in the United States, Europe, Asia, and Australia. The implant is controlled by a dual-microprocessor external unit carried by the patient with an input control signal provided by the user's remaining volitional movement. Activation of the muscles provides two primary grasp patterns and allows the person to achieve functional performance that exceeds his or her capabilities without the use of the implanted system. This system received pre-market approval from the FDA in 1998.

- *Locomotion* — The first implantable stimulators were designed and implanted for the correction of the foot drop condition in hemiplegic patients. Medtronic's Neuromuscular Assist (NMA) device consisted of an rf receiver implanted in the inner thigh and connected to a cuff electrode embracing the peroneal nerve just beneath the head of fibula at the knee [McNeal, 1977; Waters 1984]. The Ljubljana peroneal implant had two versions [Vavken, 1976; Strojnik, 1987] with the common feature that the implant–rf receiver was small enough to be implanted next to the peroneal nerve in the fossa poplitea region. Epineural stimulating electrodes were an integral part of the implant. This feature and the comparatively small size make the Ljubljana implant a precursor of the micro-stimulators described in Section 59.9. Both NMA and the Ljubljana implants were triggered and synchronized with gait by a heel switch.

  The same implant used for hand control and developed by the CWRU has also been implanted in the lower extremity musculature to assist incomplete quadriplegics in standing and transfer operations [Triolo, 1996]. Since the design of the implant is completely transparent, it can generate any stimulation sequence requested by the external controller. For locomotion and transfer-related tasks, stimulation sequences are preprogrammed for individual users and activated by the user by means of pushbuttons. The implant (two in some applications) is surgically positioned in the lower abdominal region. Locomotion application uses the same electrodes as the manipulation system; however, the lead wires have to be somewhat longer.

- *Respiration* — Respiratory control systems involve a two-channel implantable stimulator with electrodes applied bilaterally to the phrenic nerve. Most of the devices in clinical use were developed by Avery Laboratories (Dobelle Institute) and employed discrete circuitry with epoxy encapsulation of the implant and a nerve cuff electrode. Approximately 1000 of these devices have been implanted in patients with respiratory disorders such as high-level tetraplegia [Glenn, 1986]. Activation of the phrenic nerve results in contraction of each hemidiaphragm in response to electrical stimulation. In order to minimize damage to the diaphragms during chronic use, alternation of the diaphragms has been employed, in which one hemidiaphragm will be activated for several hours followed by the second. A review of existing systems was given by Creasy et al. [1996]. Astrotech of Finland also recently introduced a phrenic stimulator. More recently, DiMarco [1997] has investigated use of CNS activation of a respiratory center to provide augmented breathing.

- *Urinary control* — Urinary control systems have been developed for persons with spinal cord injury. The most successful of these devices has been developed by Brindley [1982] and is manufactured by Finetech, Ltd. (England). The implanted receiver consists of three separate stimulator devices, each with its own coil and circuitry, encapsulated within a single package. The sacral roots (S2, S3, and S4) are placed within a type of encircling electrode, and stimulation of the proper roots will generate contraction of both the bladder and the external sphincter. Cessation of stimulation results in faster relaxation of the external sphincter than of the bladder wall, which then results in voiding. Repeated trains of pulses applied in this manner will eliminate most urine, with only small residual amounts remaining. Approximately 1500 of these devices have been implanted around the world. This technology also has received FDA pre-market approval and is currently distributed by NeuroControl Corporation.

- *Scoliosis treatment* — Progressive lateral curvature of the adolescent vertebral column with simultaneous rotation is known as idiopathic scoliosis. Electrical stimulation applied to the convex side of the curvature has been used to stop or reduce its progression. Initially rf powered stimulators have been replaced by battery powered totally implanted devices [Bobechko, 1979; Herbert, 1989]. Stimulation is applied intermittently, stimulation amplitudes are under 10.5 V (510 Ω), and frequency and pulsewidth are within usual FES parameter values.

59.8.2 Stimulators of Central Nervous System

Some stimulation systems have electrodes implanted on the surface of the central nervous system or in its deep areas. They do not produce functional movements; however, they "modulate" a pathological motor brain behavior and by that stop unwanted motor activity or abnormality. Therefore, they can be regarded as stimulators for neuromuscular control.

- *Cerebellar stimulation* — Among the earliest stimulators from this category are cerebellar stimulators for control of reduction of effects of cerebral palsy in children. Electrodes are placed on the cerebellar surface with the leads penetrating cranium and dura. The pulse generator is located subcutaneously in the chest area and produces intermittent stimulation bursts. There are about 600 patients using these devices [Davis, 1997].
- *Vagal stimulation* — Intermittent stimulation of the vagus nerve with 30 sec on and five min off has been shown to reduce frequency of epileptic seizures. A pacemaker-like device, developed by Cyberonics, is implanted in the chest area with a bipolar helical electrode wrapped around the left vagus nerve in the neck. The stimulation sequence is programmed (most often parameter settings are 30 Hz, 500 μsec, 1.75 mA); however, patients have some control over the device using a hand-held magnet [Terry, 1991]. More than 3000 patients have been implanted with this device, which received the pre-marketing approval (PMA) from the FDA in 1997.
- *Deep brain stimulation* — Recently, in 1998, an implantable stimulation device (Activa by Medtronic) was approved by the FDA that can dramatically reduce uncontrollable tremor in patients with Parkinson's disease or essential tremor [Koller, 1997]. With this device, an electrode array is placed stereotactically into the ventral intermediate nucleus of thalamic region of the brain. Lead wires again connect the electrodes to a programmable pulse generator implanted in the chest area. Application of high frequency stimulation (130 Hz, 60 to 210 μsec, 0.25 to 2.75 V) can immediately suppress the patient's tremor.

59.9 Future of Implantable Electrical Stimulators

59.9.1 Distributed Stimulators

One of the major concerns with multichannel implantable neuromuscular stimulators is the multitude of leads that exit the pulse generator and their management during surgical implantation. Routing of multiple leads virtually increases the implant size and by that the burden that an implant imposes on the tissue. A solution to that may be distributed stimulation systems with a single outside controller and multiple single-channel implantable devices implanted throughout the structures to be stimulated.

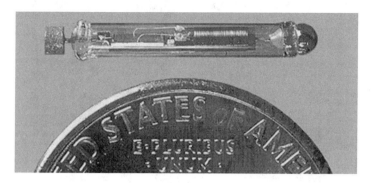

FIGURE 59.5   Microstimulator developed at A.E. Mann Foundation. Dimensions are roughly 2 × 16 mm. Electrodes at the ends are made of tantalum and iridium, respectively.

This concept has been pursued both by the Alfred E. Mann Foundation [Strojnik, 1992; Cameron, 1997] and the University of Michigan [Ziaie, 1997]. Micro-injectable stimulator modules have been developed that can be injected into the tissue, into a muscle, or close to a nerve through a lumen of a hypodermic needle. A single external coil can address and activate a number of these devices located within its field, on a pulse-to-pulse basis. A glass-encapsulated microstimulator developed at the AEMF is shown in Figure 59.5.

59.9.2 Sensing of Implantable Transducer-Generated and Physiological Signals

External command sources such as the shoulder-controlled joystick utilized by the Freehand® system impose additional constraints on the implantable stimulator users, since they have to be donned by an attendant. Permanently implanted control sources make neuro-prosthetic devices much more attractive and easier to use. An implantable joint angle transducer (IJAT) has been developed at the CWRU that consists of a magnet and an array of magnetic sensors implanted in the distal and the proximal end of a joint, respectively [Smith, 1998]. The sensor is connected to the implantable stimulator package, which provides the power and also transmits the sensor data to the external controller, using a back-telemetry link. Figure 59.6 shows a radiograph of the IJAT implanted in a patient's wrist. Myoelectric signals (MES) from muscles not affected by paralysis are another attractive control source for implantable neuromuscular stimulators. Amplified and bin-integrated EMG signal from uninvolved muscles, such as the sterno-cleido-mastoid muscle, has been shown to contain enough information to control an upper extremity neuroprosthesis [Scott, 1996]. EMG signal is being utilized by a multichannel stimulator-telemeter developed at the CWRU, containing 12 stimulator channels and 2 MES channels integrated into the same platform [Strojnik, 1998].

59.10   Summary

Implantable stimulators for neuromuscular control are an important tool in rehabilitation of paralyzed individuals with preserved neuro-muscular apparatus, as well as in the treatment of some neurological disorders that result in involuntary motor activity. Their impact on rehabilitation is still in its infancy; however, it is expected to increase with further progress in microelectronics technology, development of smaller and better sensors, and with improvements of advanced materials. Advancements in neuro-physiological science are also expected to bring forward wider utilization of possibilities offered by implantable neuromuscular stimulators.

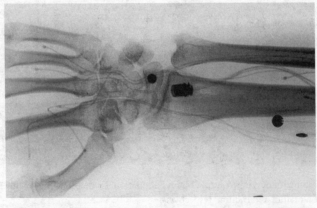

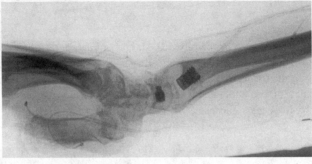

FIGURE 59.6 Radiograph of the joint angle transducer (IJAT) implanted in the wrist. The magnet is implanted in the lunate bone (top) while the magnetic sensor array is implanted in the radius. Leads going to the implant case can be seen as well as intramuscular and epimysial electrodes with their individual lead wires.

Defining Terms

Biocompatibility: Ability of a foreign object to coexist in a living tissue.

Electrical stimulation: Diagnostic, therapeutic, and rehabilitational method used to excite motor nerves with the aim of contracting the appropriate muscles and obtain limb movement.

EMG activity: Muscular electrical activity associated with muscle contraction and production of force.

Feedthrough: Device that allows passage of a conductor through a hermetic barrier.

Hybrid circuit: Electronic circuit combining miniature active and passive components on a single ceramic substrate.

Implantable stimulator: Biocompatible electronic stimulator designed for surgical implantation and operation in a living tissue.

Lead wire: Flexible and strong insulated conductor connecting pulse generator to stimulating electrodes.

Paralysis: Loss of power of voluntary movement in a muscle through injury to or disease to its nerve supply.

Stimulating electrode: Conductive device that transfers stimulating current to a living tissue. On its surface, the electric charge carriers change from electrons to ions or vice versa.

rf-radiofrequency: Pertaining to electromagnetic propagation of power and signal in frequencies above those used in electrical power distribution.

References

Bobechko, W.P., Herbert, M.A., and Friedman, H.G. 1979. Electrospinal instrumentation for scoliosis: current status. *Orthop. Clin. North. Am.* 10: 927.

Brindley, G.S., Polkey, C.E., and Rushton, D.N. 1982. Sacral anterior root stimulators for bladder control in paraplegia. *Paraplegia* 20: 365.

Cameron, T., Loeb, G.E., Peck, R.A., Schulman, J.H., Strojnik, P., and Troyk, P.R. 1997. Micromodular implants to provide electrical stimulation of paralyzed muscles and limbs. *IEEE Trans. Biomed. Eng.* 44: 781.

Creasey, G., Elefteriades, J., DiMarco, A., Talonen, P., Bijak, M., Girsch, W., and Kantor, C. 1996. Electrical stimulation to restore respiration. *J. Rehab. Res. Dev.* 33: 123.

Davis, R.: 1997. Cerebellar stimulation for movement disorders. In P.L. Gildenberg and R.R. Tasker (eds), *Textbook of Stereotactic and Functional Neurosurgery*, McGraw-Hill, New York.

DiMarco, A.F., Romaniuk, J.R., Kowalski, K.E., and Supinski, G.S. 1997. Efficacy of combined inspiratory intercostal and expiratory muscle pacing to maintain artificial ventilation. *Am. J. Respir. Crit. Care Med.* 156: 122.

Glenn, W.W., Phelps, M.L., Elefteriades, J.A., Dentz, B., and Hogan, J.F. 1986. Twenty years of experience in phrenic nerve stimulation to pace the diaphragm pacing. *Clin. Electrophysiol.* 9: 780.

Graupe, D. and Kohn, K.H. 1998. Functional neuromuscular stimulator for short-distance ambulation by certain thoracic-level spinal-cord-injured paraplegics. *Surg. Neurol.* 50: 202.

Herbert, M.A. and Bobechko, W.P. 1989. Scoliosis treatment in children using a programmable, totally implantable muscle stimulator (ESI). *IEEE Trans. Biomed. Eng.* 36: 801.

Koller, W., Pahwa, R., Busenbark, K., Hubble, J., Wilkinson, S., Lang, A., Tuite, P., Sime, E., Lazano, A., Hauser, R., Malapira, T., Smith, D., Tarsy, D., Miyawaki, E., Norregaard, T., Kormos, T., and Olanow, C.W. 1997. High-frequency unilateral thalamic stimulation in the treatment of essential and parkinsonian tremor. *Ann. Neurol.* 42: 292.

Kralj, A. and Bajd, T. 1989. *Functional Electrical Stimulation: Standing and Walking After Spinal Cord Injury*, CRC Press, Inc., Boca Raton, FL.

Liberson, W.T., Holmquest, H.J., Scot, D., and Dow, M. 1961. Functional electrotherapy: stimulation of the peroneal nerve synchronized with the swing phase of the gait of hemiplegic patients. *Arch. Phys. Med. Rehab.* 42: 101.

Marsolais, E.B. and Kobetic, R. 1986. Implantation techniques and experience with percutaneous intramuscular electrodes in lower extremities. *J. Rehab. Res. Dev.* 23: 1.

McNeal, D.R., Waters, R., and Reswick, J. 1977. Experience with implanted electrodes. *Neurosurgery* 1: 228.

Memberg, W., Peckham, P.H., Thorpe, G.B., Keith, M.W., and Kicher, T.P. 1993. An analysis of the reliability of percutaneous intramuscular electrodes in upper extremity FNS applications. *IEEE Trans. Biomed. Eng.* 1: 126.

Rebersek, S. and Vodovnik, L. 1973. Proportionally controlled functional electrical stimulation of hand. *Arch. Phys. Med. Rehab.* 54: 378.

Scott, T.R.D., Peckham, P.H., and Kilgore, K.L. 1996. Tri-state myoelectric control of bilateral upper extremity neuroprosthesies for tetraplegic individuals. *IEEE Trans. Rehab. Eng.* 2: 251.

Smith, B., Peckham, P.H., Keith, M.W., and Roscoe, D.D. 1987. An externally powered, multichannel, implantable stimulator for versatile control of paralyzed muscle. *IEEE Trans. Biomed. Eng.* 34: 499.

Smith, B., Tang, Johnson, M.W., Pourmehdi, S., Gazdik, M.M., Buckett, J.R., and Peckham, P.H. 1998. An externally powered, multichannel, implantable stimulator-telemeter for control of paralyzed muscle. *IEEE Trans. Biomed. Eng.* 45: 463.

Strojnik, P., Pourmehdi, S., and Peckham, P. 1998. Incorporating FES control sources into implanatable stimulators. *Proc. 6th Vienna International Workshop on Functional Electrostimulation*, Vienna, Austria.

Strojnik, P., Meadows, P., Schulman, J.H., and Whitmoyer, D. 1994. Modification of a cochlear stimulation system for FES applications. *Basic Appl. Myology.* BAM 4: 129.

Strojnik, P., Acimovic, R., Vavken, E., Simic, V., and Stanic, U. 1987. Treatment of drop foot using an implantable peroneal underknee stimulator. *Scand. J. Rehab. Med.* 19: 37.

Strojnik, P., Schulman, J., Loeb, G., and Troyk, P. 1992. Multichannel FES system with distributed microstimulators. *Proc. 14th Ann. Int. Conf. IEEE*, MBS, Paris, p. 1352.

Terry, R.S., Tarver, W.B., and Zabara, J. 1991. The implantable neurocybernetic prosthesis system. *Pacing Clin. Electrophysiol.* 14: 86.

Triolo, R.J., Bieri, C., Uhlir, J., Kobetic, R., Scheiner, A., and Marsolais, E.B. 1996. Implanted functional neuromuscular stimulation systems for individuals with cervical spinal cord injuries: clinical case reports. *Arch. Phys. Med. Rehabil.* 77: 1119.

Vavken, E. and Jeglic, A. 1976. Application of an implantable stimulator in the rehabilitation of paraplegic patients. *Int. Surg.* 61: 335–339.

Waters, R.L., McNeal, D.R., and Clifford, B. 1984. Correction of footdrop in stroke patients via surgically implanted peroneal nerve stimulator. *Acta Orthop. Belg.* 50: 285.

Ziaie, B., Nardin, M.D., Coghlan, A.R., and Najafi, K. 1997. A single-channel implantable microstimulator for functional neuromuscular stimulation. *IEEE Trans. Biomed. Eng.* 44: 909.

Further Information

Additional references on early work in FES which augment peer review publications can be found in Proceedings from Conferences in Dubrovnik and Vienna. These are the External Control of Human Extremities and the Vienna International Workshop on Electrostimulation, respectively.

60

Respiration

60.1 Lung Volumes **60**-1

60.2 Pulmonary Function Tests **60**-1
Dynamic Tests • The Pneumotachograph •
The Nitrogen-Washout Method for Measuring FRC

60.3 Physiologic Dead Space **60**-9

References **60**-10

Leslie A. Geddes
Purdue University

60.1 Lung Volumes

The amount of air flowing into and out of the lungs with each breath is called the tidal volume (TV). In a typical adult this amounts to about 500 ml during quiet breathing. The respiratory system is capable of moving much more air than the tidal volume. Starting at the *resting expiratory level* (REL in Figure 60.1), it is possible to inhale a volume amounting to about seven times the tidal volume; this volume is called the *inspiratory capacity* (IC). A measure of the ability to inspire more than the tidal volume is the *inspiratory reserve volume* (IRV), which is also shown in Figure 60.1. Starting from REL, it is possible to forcibly exhale a volume amounting to about twice the tidal volume; this volume is called the *expiratory reserve volume* (ERV). However, even with the most forcible expiration, it is not possible to exhale all the air from the lungs; a *residual volume* (RV) about equal to the expiratory reserve volume remains. The sum of the expiratory reserve volume and the residual volume is designated the *functional residual capacity* (FRC). The volume of air exhaled from a maximum inspiration to a maximum expiration is called the *vital capacity* (VC). The *total lung capacity* (TLC) is the total air within the lungs, that is, that which can be moved in a vital-capacity maneuver plus the residual volume. All except the residual volume can be determined with a volume-measuring instrument such as a spirometer connected to the airway.

60.2 Pulmonary Function Tests

In addition to the static lung volumes just identified, there are several time-dependent volumes associated with the respiratory act. The *minute volume* (MV) is the volume of air per breath (tidal volume) multiplied by the respiratory rate (R), that is, MV = (TV) R. It is obvious that the same minute volume can be produced by rapid shallow or slow deep breathing. However, the effectiveness is not the same, because not all the respiratory air participates in gas exchange, there being a dead space volume. Therefore the alveolar ventilation is the important quantity which is defined as the tidal volume (TV) minus the dead space (DS) multiplied by the respiratory rate R, that is, alveolar ventilation = (TV − DS) R. In a normal adult subject, the dead space amounts to about 150 ml, or 2 ml/kg.

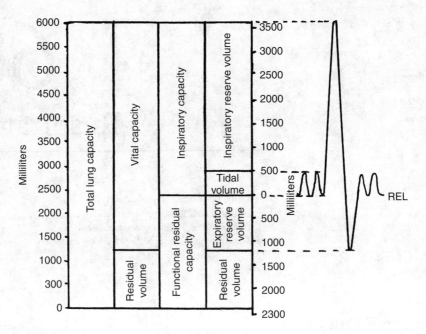

FIGURE 60.1   Lung volumes.

60.2.1 Dynamic Tests

Several timed respiratory volumes describe the ability of the respiratory system to move air. Among these are *forced vital capacity* (FVC), *forced expiratory volume* in t sec (FEV_t), the *maximum ventilatory volume* (MVV), which was previously designated the *maximum breathing capacity* (MBC), and the *peak flow* (PF). These quantities are measured with a spirometer without valves and CO_2 absorber or with a pneumotachograph coupled to an integrator.

60.2.1.1 Forced Vital Capacity

Forced vital capacity (FVC) is shown in Figure 60.2 and is measured by taking the maximum inspiration and forcing all of the inspired air out as rapidly as possible. Table 60.1 presents normal values for males and females.

60.2.1.2 Forced Expiratory Volume

Forced expiratory volume in t seconds (FEV_t) is shown in Figure 60.2, which identifies $FEV_{0.5}$ and $FEV_{1.0}$, and Table 60.1 presents normal values for $FEV_{1.0}$.

60.2.1.3 Maximum Voluntary Ventilation

Maximum voluntary ventilation (MVV) is the volume of air moved in 1 min when breathing as deeply and rapidly as possible. The test is performed for 20 sec and the volume scaled to a 1-min value; Table 60.1 presents normal values.

60.2.1.4 Peak Flow

Peak flow (PF) in l/min is the maximum flow velocity attainable during an FEV maneuver and represents the maximum slope of the expired volume–time curve (Figure 60.2); typical normal values are shown in Table 60.1.

60.2.1.5 The Water-Sealed Spirometer

The water-sealed spirometer was the traditional device used to measure the volume of air moved in respiration. The Latin word *spirare* means to breathe. The most popular type of spirometer consists of

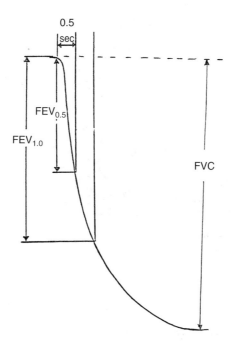

FIGURE 60.2 The measurement of timed forced expiratory volume (FEV_t) and forced vital capacity (FVC).

TABLE 60.1 Dynamic Volumes

Males
   FVC (l) = 0.133H − 0.022A − 3.60(SEE = 0.58)[a]
   FEV1 (l) = 0.094H − 0.028A − 1.59(SEE = 0.52)[a]
   MVV (l/min) = 3.39H − 1.26A − 21.4(SEE = 29)[a]
   PF (l/min) = (10.03 − 0.038A)H[b]
Females
   FVC (l) = 0.111H − 0.015A − 3.16(SD = 0.42)[c]
   FEV1 (l) = 0.068H − 0.023A − 0.92(SD = 0.37)[c]
   MVV (l/min) = 2.05H − 0.57A − 5.5(SD = 10.7)[c]
   PF (l/min) = (7.44 − 0.0183A)H[c]

H = height in inches, A = age in years, l = liters,
l/min = liters per minute, SEE = standard error of
estimate, SD = standard deviation
[a] Kory, Callahan, Boren, Syner (1961). *Am. J. Med.*
   30: 243.
[b] Leiner, Abramowitz, Small, Stenby, Lewis (1963).
   Am. Rev. Resp. Dis. 88: 644.
[c] Lindall, Medina, Grismer (1967). *Am. Rev. Resp. Dis.*
   95: 1061.

a hollow cylinder closed at one end, inverted and suspended in an annular space filled with water to provide an air-tight seal. Figure 60.3 illustrates the method of suspending the counterbalanced cylinder (bell), which is free to move up and down to accommodate the volume of air under it. Movement of the bell, which is proportional to volume, is usually recorded by an inking pen applied to a graphic record which is caused to move with a constant speed. Below the cylinder, in the space that accommodates the volume of air, are inlet and outlet breathing tubes. At the end of one or both of these tubes is a check valve designed to maintain a unidirectional flow of air through the spirometer. Outside the spirometer the two breathing tubes are brought to a Y tube which is connected to a mouthpiece. With a pinch clamp placed

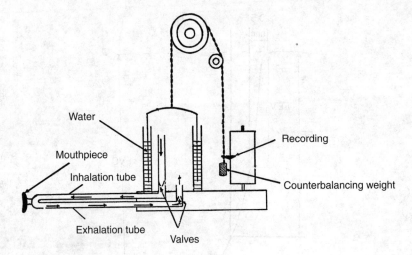

FIGURE 60.3   The simple spirometer.

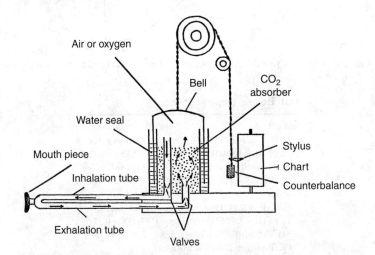

FIGURE 60.4   The spirometer with CO_2 absorber and a record of oxygen uptake (Figure 60.5).

on the nose, inspiration diminishes the volume of air under the bell, which descends, causing the stylus to rise on the graphic record. Expiration produces the reverse effect. Thus, starting with the spirometer half-filled, quiet respiration causes the bell to rise and fall. By knowing the "bell factor," the volume of air moved per centimeter excursion of the bell, the volume change can be quantitated. Although a variety of flowmeters are now used to measure respiratory volumes, the spirometer with a CO_2 absorber is ideally suited to measure oxygen uptake.

60.2.1.6   Oxygen Uptake

A second and very important use for the water-filled spirometer is measurement of oxygen used per unit of time, designated the O_2 *uptake.* This measurement is accomplished by incorporating a soda-lime, carbon-dioxide absorber into the spirometer as shown in Figure 60.4a. Soda-lime is a mixture of calcium hydroxide, sodium hydroxide, and silicates of sodium and calcium. The exhaled carbon dioxide combines with the soda-lime and becomes solid carbonates. A small amount of heat is liberated by this reaction.

Starting with a spirometer filled with oxygen and connected to a subject, respiration causes the bell to move up and down (indicating tidal volume) as shown in Figure 60.5. With continued respiration

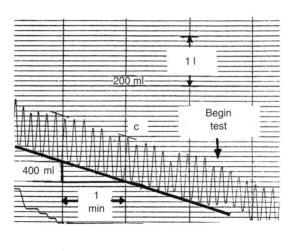

$$V_{BTPS} = V_{MEAS} \times F$$

$$F = \frac{273 + 37}{273 + T} \times \frac{P_B - P_{H2O}}{P_B - 47}$$

$$V_{MEAS} = 400\,ml \ @ \ 26°C = T$$
$$(P_B = 750\ mmHg)$$

$$F = \frac{273 + 37}{273 + 26} \times \frac{750 - 25.2*}{750 - 47}$$

$$= 1.069$$

$$V_{BTPS} = 400 \times 1.069$$

$$= 427.6\,ml$$

FIGURE 60.5   Oxygen consumption.

the baseline of the recording rises, reflecting disappearance of oxygen from under the bell. By measuring the slope of the baseline on the spirogram, the volume of oxygen consumed per minute can be determined. Figure 60.5 presents a typical example along with calculation.

60.2.1.7   The Dry Spirometer

The water-sealed spirometer was the most popular device for measuring the volumes of respiratory gases; however, it is not without its inconveniences. The presence of water causes corrosion of the metal parts. Maintenance is required to keep the device in good working order over prolonged periods. To eliminate these problems, manufacturers have developed dry spirometers. The most common type employs a collapsible rubber or plastic bellows, the expansion of which is recorded during breathing. The earlier rubber models had a decidedly undesirable characteristic which caused their abandonment. When the bellows was in its mid-position, the resistance to breathing was a minimum; when fully collapsed, it imposed a slight negative resistance; and when fully extended it imposed a slight positive resistance to breathing. Newer units with compliant plastic bellows minimize this defect.

60.2.2   The Pneumotachograph

The pneumotachograph is a device which is placed directly in the airway to measure the velocity of air flow. The volume per breath is therefore the integral of the velocity–time record during inspiration or expiration. Planimetric integration of the record, or electronic integration of the velocity–time signal, yields the tidal volume. Although tidal volume is perhaps more easily recorded with the spirometer, the dynamics of respiration are better displayed by the pneumotachograph, which offers less resistance to the air stream and exhibits a much shorter response time — so short in most instruments that cardiac impulses are often clearly identifiable in the velocity–time record.

If a specially designed resistor is placed in a tube in which the respiratory gases flow, a pressure drop will appear across it. Below the point of turbulent flow, the pressure drop is linearly related to air-flow velocity. The resistance may consist of a wire screen or a series of capillary tubes; Figure 60.6 illustrates both types. Detection and recording of this pressure differential constitutes a pneumotachogram; Figure 60.7

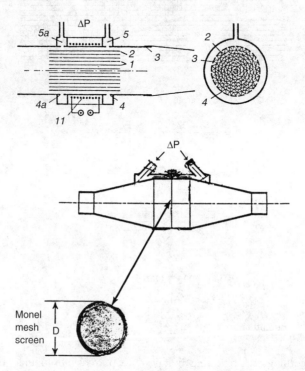

FIGURE 60.6   Pneumotachographs.

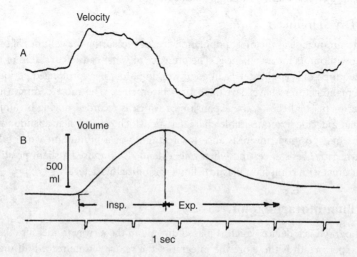

FIGURE 60.7   Velocity (A) and volume changes (B) during normal, quiet breathing; B is the integral of A.

presents a typical air–velocity record, along with the spirogram, which is the integral of the flow signal. The small-amplitude artifacts in the pneumotachogram are cardiac impulses.

For human application, linear flow rates up to 200 l/min should be recordable with fidelity. The resistance to breathing depends upon the flow rate, and it is difficult to establish an upper limit of tolerable resistance. Silverman and Whittenberger [1950] stated that a resistance of 6 mm H_2O is perceptible to human subjects. Many of the high-fidelity pneumotachographs offer 5 to 10 mm H_2O resistance at 100 and 200 l/min. It would appear that such resistances are acceptable in practice.

Response times of 15 to 40 msec seem to be currently in use. Fry and coworkers [1957] analyzed the dynamic characteristics of three types of commercially available, differential-pressure pneumotachographs which employed concentric cylinders, screen mesh, and parallel plates for the air resistors. Using a high-quality, differential-pressure transducer with each, they measured total flow resistance ranging from 5 to 15 cm H_2O. Frequency response curves taken on one model showed fairly uniform response to 40 Hz; the second model showed a slight increase in response at 50 Hz, and the third exhibited a slight drop in response at this frequency.

60.2.3   The Nitrogen-Washout Method for Measuring FRC

The *functional residual capacity* (FRC) and the *residual volume* (RV) are the only lung compartments that cannot be measured with a volume-measuring device. Measuring these requires use of the nitrogen analyzer and application of the dilution method.

Because nitrogen does not participate in respiration, it can be called a *diluent*. Inspired and expired air contain about 80% nitrogen. Between breaths, the FRC of the lungs contains the same concentration of nitrogen as in environmental air, that is, 80%. By causing a subject to inspire from a spirometer filled with 100% oxygen and to exhale into a second collecting spirometer, all the nitrogen in the FRC is replaced by oxygen, that is, the nitrogen is "washed out" into the second spirometer. Measurement of the concentration of nitrogen in the collecting spirometer, along with a knowledge of its volume, permits calculation of the amount of nitrogen originally in the functional residual capacity and hence allows calculation of the FRC, as now will be shown.

Figure 60.8 illustrates the arrangement of equipment for the nitrogen-washout test. Note that two check valves, (I, EX) are on both sides of the subject's breathing tube, and the nitrogen meter is connected to the mouthpiece. Valve V is used to switched the subject from breathing environmental air to the measuring system. The left-hand spirometer contains 100% oxygen, which is inhaled by the subject via valve I. Of course, a nose clip must be applied so that all the respired gases flow through the breathing tube connected

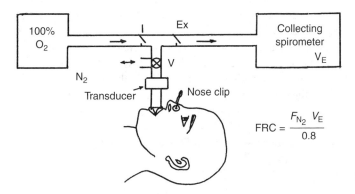

FIGURE 60.8   Arrangement of equipment for the nitrogen-washout technique. Valve V allows the subject to breathe room air until the test is started. The test is started by operating valve V at the end of a normal breath, that is, the subject starts breathing 100% O_2 through the inspiratory valve (I) and exhales the N_2 and O_2 mixture into a collecting spirometer via the expiratory valve EX.

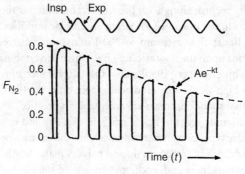

FIGURE 60.9 The nitrogen washout curve.

to the mouthpiece. It is in this tube that the sampling inlet for the nitrogen analyzer is located. Starting at the resting expiratory level, inhalation of pure oxygen causes the nitrogen analyzer to indicate zero. Expiration closes valve I and opens valve EX. The first expired breath contains nitrogen derived from the FRC (diluted by the oxygen which was inspired); the nitrogen analyzer indicates this percentage. The exhaled gases are collected in the right-hand spirometer. The collecting spirometer and all the interconnecting tubing was first flushed with oxygen to eliminate all nitrogen. This simple procedure eliminates the need for applying corrections and facilitates calculation of the FRC. With continued breathing, the nitrogen analyzer indicates less and less nitrogen because it is being washed out of the FRC and is replaced by oxygen. Figure 60.9 presents a typical record of the diminishing concentration of expired nitrogen throughout the test. In most laboratories, the test is continued until the concentration of nitrogen falls to about 1%. The nitrogen analyzer output permits identification of this concentration. In normal subjects, virtually all the nitrogen can be washed out of the FRC in about 5 min.

If the peaks on the nitrogen washout record are joined, a smooth exponential decay curve is obtained in normal subjects. A semilog of N_2 vs. time provides a straight line. In subjects with trapped air, or poorly ventilated alveoli, the nitrogen-washout curve consists of several exponentials as the multiple poorly ventilated regions give up their nitrogen. In such subjects, the time taken to wash out all the nitrogen usually exceeds 10 min. Thus, the nitrogen concentration–time curve provides useful diagnostic information on ventilation of the alveoli.

If it is assumed that all the collected (washed-out) nitrogen was uniformly distributed within the lungs, it is easy to calculate the FRC. If the environmental air contains 80% nitrogen, then the volume of nitrogen in the functional residual capacity is 0.8 (FRC). Because the volume of expired gas in the collecting spirometer is known, it is merely necessary to determine the concentration of nitrogen in this volume. To do so requires admitting some of this gas to the inlet valve of the nitrogen analyzer. Note that this concentration of nitrogen (F_{N_2}) exists in a volume which includes the volume of air expired (V_E) plus the original volume of oxygen in the collecting spirometer (V_0) at the start of the test and the volume of the tubing (V_t) leading from the expiratory collecting valve. It is therefore advisable to start with an empty collecting spirometer ($V_0 = 0$). Usually the tubing volume (V_t) is negligible with respect to the volume of expired gas collected in a typical washout test. In this situation the volume of nitrogen collected is $V_E F_{N_2}$, where F_{N_2} is the fraction of nitrogen within the collected gas. Thus, 0.80 (FRC) $= F_{N_2} (V_E)$. Therefore

$$\text{FRC} = \frac{F_{N_2} V_E}{0.80} \tag{60.1}$$

It is important to note that the value for FRC so obtained is at ambient temperature and pressure and is saturated with water vapor (ATPS). In respiratory studies, this value is converted to body temperature and saturated with water vapor (BTPS).

In the example shown in Figure 60.9, the washout to 1% took about 44 breaths. With a breathing rate of 12/min, the washout time was 220 sec. The volume collected (V_E) was 22 l and the concentration of nitrogen in this volume was 0.085 (F_{N_2}); therefore

$$\text{FRC} = \frac{0.085 \times 22,000}{0.80} = 2,337 \text{ ml} \tag{60.2}$$

60.3 Physiologic Dead Space

The volume of ventilated lung that does not participate in gas exchange is the physiologic dead space (V_d). It is obvious that the physiologic dead space includes anatomic dead space, as well as the volume of any alveoli that are not perfused. In the lung, there are theoretically four types of alveoli, as shown in Figure 60.10. The normal alveolus (A) is both ventilated and perfused with blood. There are alveoli that are ventilated but not perfused (B); such alveoli contribute significantly to the physiologic dead space. There are alveoli that are not ventilated but perfused (C); such alveoli do not provide the exchange of respiratory gases. Finally, there are alveoli that are both poorly ventilated and poorly perfused (D); such alveoli contain high CO_2 and N_2 and low O_2. These alveoli are the last to expel their CO_2 and N_2 in washout tests.

Measurement of physiologic dead space is based on the assumption that there is almost complete equilibrium between alveolar pCO_2 and pulmonary capillary blood. Therefore, the arterial pCO_2 represents mean alveolar pCO_2 over many breaths when an arterial blood sample is drawn for analysis of pCO_2. The Bohr equation for physiologic dead space is

$$V_d = \left[\frac{paCO_2 - pECO_2}{paCO_2} \right] V_E \tag{60.3}$$

In this expression, $paCO_2$ is the partial pressure in the arterial blood sample which is withdrawn slowly during the test; $pECO_2$ is the partial pressure of CO_2 in the volume of expired air; V_E is the volume of expired air per breath (tidal volume).

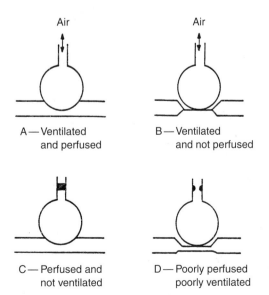

FIGURE 60.10 The four types of alveoli.

In a typical test, the subject would breathe in room air and exhale into a collapsed (Douglas) bag. The test is continued for 3 min or more, and the number of breaths is counted in that period. An arterial blood sample is withdrawn during the collection period. The pCO_2 in the expired gas is measured, and then the volume of expired gas is measured by causing it to flow into a spirometer or flowmeter by collapsing the collecting bag.

In a typical 3-min test, the collected volume is 33 l, and the pCO_2 in the expired gas is 14.5 mmHg. During the test, the pCO_2 in the arterial blood sample was 40 mmHg. The number of breaths was 60; therefore, the average tidal volume was 33,000/60 = 550 ml. The physiologic dead space (V_d) is:

$$V_d = \left[\frac{40 - 14.5}{40} \right] 550 = 350 \text{ ml} \tag{60.4}$$

It is obvious that an elevated physiological dead space indicates lung tissue that is not perfused with blood.

References

Fry D.I., Hyatt R.E., and McCall C.B. 1957. Evaluation of three types of respiratory flowmeters. *Appl. Physiol.* 10: 210.

Silverman L. and Whittenberger J. 1950. Clinical pneumotachograph. *Meth. Med. Res.* 2: 104.

61

Mechanical Ventilation

61.1 Introduction... **61**-1
61.2 Negative-Pressure Ventilators **61**-2
61.3 Positive-Pressure Ventilators **61**-3
61.4 Ventilation Modes **61**-3
   Mandatory Ventilation • Spontaneous Ventilation
61.5 Breath Delivery Control **61**-6
   Mandatory Volume Controlled Inspiratory Flow Delivery •
   Pressure Controlled Inspiratory Flow Delivery • Expiratory
   Pressure Control in Mandatory Mode • Spontaneous Breath
   Delivery Control
61.6 Summary **61**-10
Defining Terms **61**-10
References **61**-11

Khosrow Behbehani
The University of Texas at Arlington
The University of Texas
Southwestern Medical Center

61.1 Introduction

This chapter presents an overview of the structure and function of mechanical ventilators. Mechanical ventilators, which are often also called respirators, are used to artificially ventilate the lungs of patients who are unable to naturally breathe from the atmosphere. In almost 100 years of development, many mechanical ventilators with different designs have been developed [Mushin et al., 1980; Philbeam, 1998]. The very early devices used bellows that were manually operated to inflate the lungs. Today's respirators employ an array of sophisticated components such as microprocessors, fast response servo valves, and precision transducers to perform the task of ventilating the lungs. The changes in the design of ventilators have come about as the result of improvements in engineering the ventilator components and the advent of new therapy modes by clinicians. A large variety of ventilators are now available for short-term treatment of acute respiratory problems as well as long-term therapy for chronic respiratory conditions.

It is reasonable to broadly classify today's ventilators into two groups. The first and indeed the largest group encompasses the intensive care respirators used primarily in hospitals to support patients following certain surgical procedures or assist patients with acute respiratory disorders. The second group includes less complicated machines that are primarily used at home to treat patients with chronic respiratory disorders.

The level of engineering design and sophistication for the intensive care ventilators is higher than the ventilators used for chronic treatment. However, many of the engineering concepts employed in designing

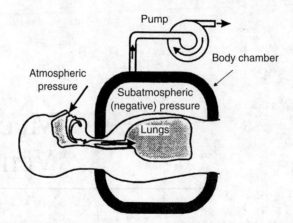

FIGURE 61.1   A simplified illustration of a negative-pressure ventilator.

intensive care ventilators can also be applied in the simpler chronic care units. Therefore, this presentation focuses on the design of intensive care ventilators; the terms respirator, mechanical ventilator, or ventilator that will be used from this point on refer to the intensive care unit respirators.

At the beginning, the designers of mechanical ventilators realized that the main task of a respirator was to ventilate the lungs in a manner as close to natural respiration as possible. Since natural inspiration is a result of negative pressure in the pleural cavity generated by distention of the diaphragm, designers initially developed ventilators that created the same effect. These ventilators are called *negative-pressure ventilators*. However, more modern ventilators use pressures greater than atmospheric pressures to ventilate the lungs; they are known as *positive-pressure ventilators*.

61.2   Negative-Pressure Ventilators

The principle of operation of a negative-pressure respirator is shown in Figure 61.1. In this design, the flow of air to the lungs is created by generating a negative pressure around the patient's thoracic cage. The negative pressure moves the thoracic walls outward expanding the intra-thoracic volume and dropping the pressure inside the lungs. The pressure gradient between the atmosphere and the lungs causes the flow of atmospheric air into the lungs. The inspiratory and expiratory phases of the respiration are controlled by cycling the pressure inside the body chamber between a sub-atmospheric level (inspiration) and the atmospheric level (exhalation). Flow of the breath out of the lungs during exhalation is caused by the recoil of thoracic muscles.

Although it may appear that the negative-pressure respirator incorporates the same principles as natural respiration, the engineering implementation of this concept has not been very successful. A major difficulty has been in the design of a chamber for creating negative pressure around the thoracic walls. One approach has been to make the chamber large enough to house the entire body with the exception of the head and neck. Using foam rubber around the patient's neck, one can seal the chamber and generate a negative pressure inside the chamber. This design configuration, commonly known as the iron lung, was tried back in the 1920s and proved to be deficient in several aspects. The main drawback was that the negative pressure generated inside the chamber was applied to the chest as well as the abdominal wall, thus creating a venous blood pool in the abdomen and reducing cardiac output.

More recent designs have tried to restrict the application of the negative pressure to the chest walls by designing a chamber that goes only around the chest. However, this has not been successful because obtaining a seal around the chest wall (Figure 61.1) is difficult.

Negative-pressure ventilators also made the patient less accessible for patient care and monitoring. Further, synchronization of the machine cycle with the patient's effort has been difficult and they are also

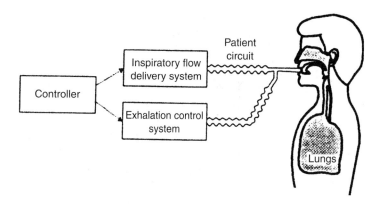

FIGURE 61.2   A simplified diagram of the functional blocks of a positive-pressure ventilator.

typically noisy and bulky [McPherson and Spearman, 1990]. These deficiencies of the negative-pressure ventilators have led to the development of the positive-pressure ventilators.

61.3 Positive-Pressure Ventilators

Positive-pressure ventilators generate the inspiratory flow by applying a positive pressure (greater than the atmospheric pressure) to the airways. Figure 61.2 shows a simplified block diagram of a positive-pressure ventilator. During inspiration, the inspiratory flow delivery system creates a positive pressure in the tubes connected to the patient airway, called **patient circuit**, and the exhalation control system closes a valve at the outlet of the tubing to the atmosphere. When the ventilator switches to exhalation, the inspiratory flow delivery system stops the positive pressure and the exhalation system opens the valve to allow the patient's exhaled breath to flow to the atmosphere. The use of a positive pressure gradient in creating the flow allows treatment of patients with high lung resistance and low compliance. As a result, positive-pressure ventilators have been very successful in treating a variety of breathing disorders and have become more popular than negative-pressure ventilators.

Positive-pressure ventilators have been employed to treat patients ranging from neonates to adults. Due to anatomical differences between various patient populations, the ventilators and their modes of treating infants are different than those for adults. Nonetheless, their fundamental design principles are similar and adult ventilators comprise a larger percentage of ventilators manufactured and used in clinics. Therefore, the emphasis here is on the description of adult positive-pressure ventilators. Also, the concepts presented will be illustrated using a microprocessor-based design example, as almost all modern ventilators use microprocessor instrumentation.

61.4 Ventilation Modes

Since the advent of respirators, clinicians have devised a variety of strategies to ventilate the lungs based on patient conditions. For instance, some patients need the respirator to completely take over the task of ventilating their lungs. In this case, the ventilator operates in **mandatory mode** and delivers mandatory breaths. On the other hand, some patients are able to initiate a breath and breathe on their own, but may need oxygen-enriched air flow or slightly elevated airway pressure. When a ventilator assists a patient who is capable of demanding a breath, the ventilator delivers spontaneous breaths and operates in **spontaneous mode**. In many cases, it is first necessary to treat the patient with mandatory ventilation and as the patient's condition improves spontaneous ventilation is introduced; it is used primarily to wean the patient from mandatory breathing.

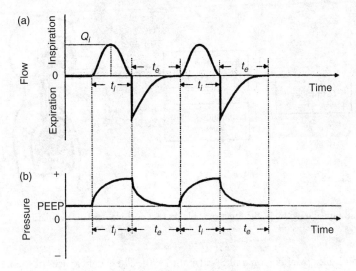

FIGURE 61.3 (a) Inspiratory flow for a controlled mandatory volume controlled ventilation breath, (b) airway pressure resulting from the breath delivery with a non-zero PEEP.

61.4.1 Mandatory Ventilation

Designers of adult ventilators have employed two rather distinct approaches for delivering mandatory breaths: **volume controlled ventilation** and **pressure controlled ventilation**. Volume controlled ventilation, which presently is more popular, refers to delivering a specified tidal volume to the patient during the inspiratory phase. Pressure controlled ventilation, however, refers to raising the airway pressure to a level, set by the therapist, during the inspiratory phase of each breath. Regardless of the type, a ventilator operating in mandatory mode must control all aspects of breathing such as tidal volume, respiration rate, inspiratory flow pattern, and oxygen concentration of the breath. This is often labeled as **controlled mandatory ventilation (CMV)**.

Figure 61.3 shows the flow and pressure waveforms for a volume controlled ventilation (CMV). In this illustration, the inspiratory flow waveform is chosen to be a half sinewave. In Figure 61.3a, t_i is the inspiration duration, t_e is the exhalation period, and Q_i is the amplitude of inspiratory flow. The ventilator delivers a tidal volume equal to the area under the flow waveform in Figure 61.3a at regular intervals $(t_i + t_e)$ set by the therapist. The resulting pressure waveform is shown in Figure 61.3b. It is noted that during volume controlled ventilation, the ventilator delivers the same volume irrespective of the patient's respiratory mechanics. However, the resulting pressure waveform such as the one shown in Figure 61.3b, will be different among patients. Of course, for safety purposes, the ventilator limits the maximum applied airway pressure according to the therapist's setting.

As can be seen in Figure 61.3b, the airway pressure at the end of exhalation may not end at atmospheric pressure (zero gauge). The **positive end expiratory pressure (PEEP)** is sometimes used to keep the alveoli from collapsing during expiration [Norwood, 1990]. In other cases, the expiration pressure is allowed to return to the atmospheric level.

Figure 61.4a shows a plot of the pressure and flow during a mandatory pressure controlled ventilation. In this case, the respirator raises and maintains the airway pressure at the desired level independent of patient airway compliance and resistance. The level of pressure during inspiration, P_i, is set by the therapist. While the ventilator maintains the same pressure trajectory for patients with different respiratory resistance and compliance, the resulting flow trajectory, shown in Figure 61.4b, will depend on the respiratory mechanics of each patient.

In the following, the presentation will focus on volume ventilators, as they are more common. Further, in a microprocessor-based ventilator, the mechanism for delivering mandatory volume and pressure

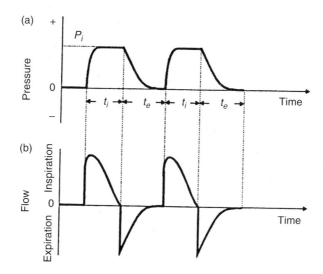

FIGURE 61.4 (a) Inspiratory pressure pattern for a controlled mandatory pressure controlled ventilation breath, (b) airway flow pattern resulting from the breath delivery. Note that PEEP is zero.

controlled ventilation have many similar main components. The primary difference lies in the control algorithms governing the delivery of breaths to the patient.

61.4.2 Spontaneous Ventilation

An important phase in providing respiratory therapy to a recovering pulmonary patient is weaning the patient from the respirator. As the patient recovers and gains the ability to breathe independently, the ventilator must allow the patient to initiate a breath and control the breath rate, flow rate, and the tidal volume. Ideally, when a respirator is functioning in the spontaneous mode, it should let the patient take breaths with the same ease as breathing from the atmosphere. This, however, is difficult to achieve because the respirator does not have an infinite gas supply or an instantaneous response. In practice, the patient generally has to exert more effort to breathe spontaneously on a respirator than from the atmosphere. However, patient effort is reduced as the ventilator response speed increases [McPherson, 1990]. Spontaneous ventilation is often used in conjunction with mandatory ventilation since the patient may still need breaths that are delivered entirely by the ventilator. Alternatively, when a patient can breathe completely on his own but needs oxygen-enriched breath or elevated airway pressure, spontaneous ventilation alone may be used.

As in the case of mandatory ventilation, several modes of spontaneous ventilation have been devised by therapists. Two of the most important and popular spontaneous breath delivery modes are described below.

61.4.2.1 Continuous Positive Airway Pressure (CPAP) in Spontaneous Mode

In this mode, the ventilator maintains a positive pressure at the airway as the patient attempts to inspire. Figure 61.5 illustrates a typical airway pressure waveform during CPAP breath delivery. The therapist sets the sensitivity level lower than PEEP. When the patient attempts to breathe, the pressure drops below the sensitivity level and the ventilator responds by supplying breathable gases to raise the pressure back to the PEEP level. Typically, the PEEP and sensitivity levels are selected such that the patient will be impelled to exert effort to breathe independently. As in the case of the mandatory mode, when the patient exhales the ventilator shuts off the flow of gas and opens the exhalation valve to allow the exhaled gases to flow into the atmosphere.

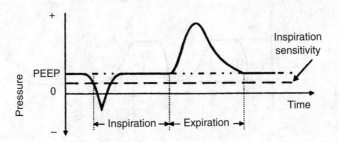

FIGURE 61.5   Airway pressure during a CPAP spontaneous breath delivery.

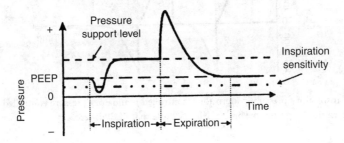

FIGURE 61.6   Airway pressure during a pressure support spontaneous breath delivery.

61.4.2.2   Pressure Support in Spontaneous Mode

This mode is similar to the CPAP mode with the exception that during the inspiration the ventilator attempts to maintain the patient airway pressure at a level above PEEP. In fact, CPAP may be considered a special case of **pressure support** ventilation in which the support level is fixed at the atmospheric level.

Figure 61.6 shows a typical airway pressure waveform during the delivery of a pressure support breath. In this mode, when the patient's airway pressure drops below the therapist-set sensitivity line, the ventilator inspiratory breath delivery system raises the airway pressure to the **pressure support level** (>PEEP), selected by the therapist. The ventilator stops the flow of breathable gases when the patient starts to exhale and controls the exhalation valve to achieve the set PEEP level.

61.5   Breath Delivery Control

Figure 61.7 shows a simplified block diagram for delivering mandatory or spontaneous ventilation. Compressed air and oxygen are normally stored in high pressure tanks ($\cong$1400 kPa) that are attached to the inlets of the ventilator. In some ventilators, an air compressor is used in place of a compressed air tank. Manufacturers of mechanical respirators have designed a variety of blending and metering devices [McPherson, 1990]. The primary mission of the device is to enrich the inspiratory air flow with the proper level of oxygen and to deliver a tidal volume according to the therapist's specifications. With the introduction of microprocessors for control of metering devices, electromechanical valves have gained popularity [Puritan-Bennett, 1987]. In Figure 61.7, the air and oxygen valves are placed in closed feedback loops with the air and oxygen flow sensors. The microprocessor controls each the valves to deliver the desired inspiratory air and oxygen flows for mandatory and spontaneous ventilation. During inhalation, the exhalation valve is closed to direct all the delivered flows to the lungs. When exhalation starts, the microprocessor actuates the exhalation valve to achieve the desired PEEP level. The airway pressure sensor, shown on the right side of Figure 61.7, generates the feedback signal necessary for maintaining the desired PEEP (in both mandatory and spontaneous modes) and airway pressure support level during spontaneous breath delivery.

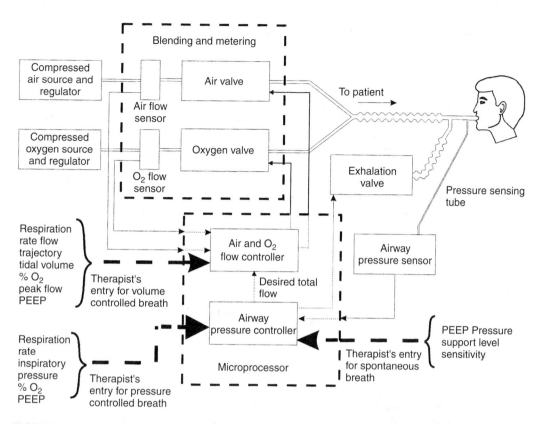

FIGURE 61.7   A simplified block diagram of a control structure for mandatory and spontaneous breath delivery.

61.5.1   Mandatory Volume Controlled Inspiratory Flow Delivery

In a microprocessor-controlled ventilator (Figure 61.7), the electronically actuated valves open from a closed position to allow the flow of blended gases to the patient. The control of flow through each valve depends on the therapist's specification for the mandatory breath. That is, the clinician must specify the following parameters for delivery of CMV breaths (1) respiration rate; (2) flow waveform; (3) tidal volume; (4) oxygen concentration (of the delivered breath); (5) peak flow; and (6) PEEP, as shown in the lower left side of Figure 61.7. It is noted that the PEEP selected by the therapist in the mandatory mode is only used for control of exhalation flow; that will be described in the following section. The microprocessor utilizes the first five of the above parameters to compute the total desired inspiratory flow trajectory. To illustrate this point, consider the delivery of a tidal volume using a half sinewave as shown in Figure 61.3. If the therapist selects a tidal volume of V_t (L), a respiration rate of n breaths per minute (bpm), the amplitude of the respirator flow, Q_i(L/s), then the total desired inspiratory flow, $Q_d(t)$, for a single breath, can be computed from the following equation:

$$Q_d(t) = \begin{cases} Q_i \sin \frac{\pi t}{t_i}, & 0 \le t < t_i \\ 0, & t_i < t \le t_e \end{cases} \tag{61.1}$$

where t_i signifies the duration of inspiration and is computed from the following relationship:

$$t_i = \frac{V_t}{2Q_i} \tag{61.2}$$

The duration of expiration in seconds is obtained from

$$t_e = \frac{60}{n} - t_i \tag{61.3}$$

The ratio of inspiratory to expiratory periods of a mandatory breath is often used for adjusting the respiration rate. This ratio is represented by $I:E$ **(ratio)** and is computed as follows. First, the inspiratory and expiratory periods are normalized with respect to t_i. Hence, the normalized inspiratory period becomes unity and the normalized expiratory period is given by $R = t_e/t_i$. Then, the $I:E$ **ratio** is simply expressed as $1:R$.

To obtain the desired oxygen concentration in the delivered breath, the microprocessor computes the discrete form of $Q_d(t)$ as $Q_d(k)$ where k signifies the kth sample interval. Then, the total desired flow, $Q_d(k)$, is partitioned using the following relationships:

$$Q_{da}(k) = \frac{(1 - m)Q_d(k)}{(1 - c)} \tag{61.4}$$

and

$$Q_{dx}(k) = \frac{(m - c)Q_d(k)}{(1 - c)} \tag{61.5}$$

where k signifies the sample interval, $Q_{da}(k)$ is the desired air flow (the subscript da stands for desired air), $Q_{dx}(k)$ is the desired oxygen flow (the subscript dx stands for desired oxygen), m is the desired oxygen concentration, and c is the oxygen concentration of the ventilator air supply.

A number of control design strategies may be appropriate for the control of the air and oxygen flow delivery valves. A simple controller is the proportional plus integral controller that can be readily implemented in a microprocessor. For example, the controller for the air valve has the following form:

$$I(k) = K_p E(k) + K_i A(k) \tag{61.6}$$

where $E(k)$ and $A(k)$ are given by

$$E(k) = Q_{da}(k) - Q_{sa}(k) \tag{61.7}$$

$$A(k) = A(k - 1) + E(k) \tag{61.8}$$

where $I(k)$ is the input (voltage or current) to the air valve at the kth sampling interval, $E(k)$ is the error in the delivered flow, $Q_{da}(k)$ is the desired air flow, $Q_{sa}(k)$ is the sensed or actual air flow (the subscript sa stands for sensed air flow), $A(k)$ is the integral (rectangular integration) part of the controller, and K_p and K_i are the controller proportionality constants. It is noted that the above equations are applicable to the control of either the air or oxygen valve. For control of the oxygen flow valve, $Q_{dx}(k)$ replaces $Q_{da}(k)$ and $Q_{sx}(k)$ replaces $Q_{sa}(k)$ where $Q_{sx}(k)$ represents the sensed oxygen flow (the subscript sx stands for sensed oxygen flow).

The control structure shown in Figure 61.7 provides the flexibility of quickly adjusting the percentage of oxygen in the enriched breath gases. That is, the controller can regulate both the total flow and the percent oxygen delivered to the patient. Since the internal volume of the flow control valve is usually small (<50 ml), the desired change in the oxygen concentration of the delivered flow can be achieved within one inspiratory period. In actual clinical applications, rapid change of percent oxygen from one breath to another is often desirable, as it reduces the waiting time for the delivery of the desired oxygen concentration. A design similar to the one shown in Figure 61.7 has been successfully implemented in a microprocessor-based ventilator [Behbehani, 1984] and is deployed in hospitals around the world.

61.5.2 Pressure Controlled Inspiratory Flow Delivery

The therapist entry for pressure-controlled ventilation is shown in Figure 61.7 (lower left-hand side). In contrast to the volume-controlled ventilation where $Q_d(t)$ was computed directly from the operator's entry, the total desired flow is generated by a closed loop controller labeled as Airway Pressure Controller in Figure 61.7. This controller uses the therapist-selected inspiratory pressure, respiration rate, and the I:E ratio to compute the desired inspiratory pressure trajectory. The trajectory serves as the controller reference input. The controller then computes the flow necessary to make the actual airway pressure track the reference input. Assuming a proportional-plus-integral controller, the governing equations are

$$Q_d(k) = C_p E_p(k) + C_i A_p(k) \tag{61.9}$$

where Q_d is the computed desired flow, C_p and C_i are the proportionality constants, k represents the sample interval, and $E_p(k)$ and $A_p(k)$ are computed using the following equations:

$$E_p(k) = P_d(k) - P_s(k) \tag{61.10}$$

$$A_p(k) = A_p(k-1) + E_p(k) \tag{61.11}$$

where $E_p(k)$ is the difference between the desired pressure trajectory, $P_d(k)$, and the sensed airway pressure, $P_s(k)$, the parameter $A_p(k)$ represents the integral portion of the controller. Using Q_d from Equation 61.9, the control of air and O_2 valves is accomplished in the same manner as in the case of volume-controlled ventilation described earlier (Equation 61.4 through Equation 61.8).

61.5.3 Expiratory Pressure Control in Mandatory Mode

It is often desirable to keep the patient's lungs inflated at the end of expiration at a pressure greater than atmospheric level [Norwood, 1990]. That is, rather than allowing the lungs to deflate during the exhalation, the controller closes the exhalation valve when the airway pressure reaches the PEEP level. When expiration starts, the ventilator terminates flow to the lungs; hence, the regulation of the airway pressure is achieved by controlling the flow of patient exhaled gases through the exhalation valve.

In a microprocessor-based ventilator, an electronically actuated valve can be employed that has adequate dynamic response ($\cong 20$ msec rise time) to regulate PEEP. For this purpose, the pressure in the patient breath delivery circuit is measured using a pressure transducer (Figure 61.7). The microprocessor will initially open the exhalation valve completely to minimize resistance to expiratory flow. At the same time, it will sample the pressure transducer's output and start to close the exhalation valve as the pressure begins to approach the desired PEEP level. Since the patient's exhaled flow is the only source of pressure, if the airway pressure drops below PEEP, it cannot be brought back up until the next inspiratory period. Hence, an overrun (i.e., a drop to below PEEP) in the closed-loop control of PEEP cannot be tolerated.

61.5.4 Spontaneous Breath Delivery Control

The small diameter ($\cong 5$ mm) pressure sensing tube, shown on the right side of Figure 61.7, pneumatically transmits the pneumatic pressure signal from the patient airway to a pressure transducer placed in the ventilator. The output of the pressure transducer is amplified, filtered, and then sampled by the microprocessor. The controller receives the therapist's inputs regarding the spontaneous breath characteristics such as the PEEP, sensitivity, and oxygen concentration, as shown on the lower right-hand side of Figure 61.7. The desired airway pressure is computed from the therapist entries of PEEP, pressure support level, and sensitivity. The multiple-loop control structure shown in Figure 61.7 is used to deliver a CPAP or a pressure support breath. The sensed proximal airway pressure is compared with the desired airway pressure. The airway pressure controller computes the total inspiratory flow level required to raise the airway pressure to the desired level. This flow level serves as the reference input or total desired flow for the flow control loop. Hence, in general, the desired total flow trajectory for the spontaneous breath delivery may be different for each inspiratory cycle. If the operator has specified oxygen concentration greater than 21.6% (the atmospheric air oxygen concentration of the ventilator air supply), the controller will partition the total required flow into the air and oxygen flow rates using Equation 61.4 and Equation 61.5. The flow controller then uses the feedback signals from air and oxygen flow sensors and actuates the air and oxygen valves to deliver the desired flows.

For a microprocessor-based ventilator, the control algorithm for regulating the airway pressure can also be a proportional plus integral controller [Behbehani, 1984; Behbehani and Watanabe, 1986]). In this case, the governing equations are identical to Equation 61.9 through Equation 61.11.

If a non-zero PEEP level is specified, the same control strategy as the one described for mandatory breath delivery can be used to achieve the desired PEEP.

61.6 Summary

Today's mechanical ventilators can be broadly classified into negative-pressure and positive-pressure ventilators. Negative-pressure ventilators do not offer the flexibility and convenience that positive-pressure ventilators provide; hence, they have not been very popular in clinical use. Positive-pressure ventilators have been quite successful in treating patients with pulmonary disorders. These ventilators operate in either mandatory or spontaneous mode. When delivering mandatory breaths, the ventilator controls all parameters of the breath such as tidal volume, inspiratory flow waveform, respiration rate, and oxygen content of the breath. Mandatory breaths are normally delivered to the patients that are incapable of breathing on their own. In contrast, spontaneous breath delivery refers to the case where the ventilator responds to the patient's effort to breathe independently. Therefore, the patient can control the volume and the rate of the respiration. The therapist selects the oxygen content and the pressure at which the breath is delivered. Spontaneous breath delivery is typically used for patients who are on their way to full recovery, but are not completely ready to breathe from the atmosphere without mechanical assistance.

Defining Terms

Continuous positive airway pressure (CPAP): A spontaneous ventilation mode in which the ventilator maintains a constant positive pressure, near or below PEEP level, in the patient's airway while the patient breathes at will.

I : E ratio: The ratio of normalized inspiratory interval to normalized expiratory interval of a mandatory breath. Both intervals are normalized with respect to the inspiratory period. Hence, the normalized inspiratory period is always unity.

Mandatory mode: A mode of mechanically ventilating the lungs where the ventilator controls all breath delivery parameters such as tidal volume, respiration rate, flow waveform, etc.

Patient circuit: A set of tubes connecting the patient airway to the outlet of a respirator.

Positive end expiratory pressure (PEEP): A therapist-selected pressure level for the patient airway at the end of expiration in either mandatory or spontaneous breathing.

Pressure controlled ventilation: A mandatory mode of ventilation where during the inspiration phase of each breath, a constant pressure is applied to the patient's airway independent of the patient's airway resistance and/or compliance respiratory mechanics.

Pressure support: A spontaneous breath delivery mode during which the ventilator applies a positive pressure greater than PEEP to the patient's airway during inspiration.

Pressure support level: Refers to the pressure level, above PEEP, that the ventilator maintains during the spontaneous inspiration.

Spontaneous mode: A ventilation mode in which the patient initiates and breathes from the ventilator-supplied gas at will.

Volume controlled ventilation: A mandatory mode of ventilation where the volume of each breath is set by the therapist and the ventilator delivers that volume to the patient independent of the patient's airway resistance and/or compliance respiratory mechanics.

References

Behbehani, K. (1984). PLM-Implementation of a Multiple Closed-Loop Control Strategy for a Microprocessor-Controlled Respirator. *Proc. ACC Conf.*, pp. 574–576.

Behbehani, K. and Watanabe, N.T. (1986). A New Application of Digital Computer Simulation in the Design of a Microprocessor-Based Respirator. *Summer Simulation Conf.*, pp. 415–420.

McPherson, S.P. and Spearman, C.B. (1990). *Respiratory Therapy Equipment*, 4th ed., C.V. Mosby Co., St. Louis, MO.

Norwood, S. (1990). Physiological Principles of Conventional Mechanical Ventilation. In *Clinical Application of Ventilatory Support*, Kirby, R.R., Banner, M.J., and Downs, J.B., Eds., Churchill Livingstone, New York, pp. 145–172.

Pilbeam, S.P. (1998). *Mechanical Ventilation: Physiological and Clinical Applications*, 3rd ed., Mosby, St. Louis, MO.

Puritan-Bennett 7200 Ventilator System Series, "Ventilator, Options and Accessories," Part No. 22300A, Carlsbad, CA, September 1990.

62

Essentials of Anesthesia Delivery

62.1 Gases Used During Anesthesia and Their Sources **62**-3
　　　Oxygen • Air (78% N_2, 21% O_2, 0.9% Ar, 0.1% Other Gases)
　　　• Nitrous Oxide • Carbon Dioxide • Helium
62.2 Gas Blending and Vaporization System **62**-5
62.3 Breathing Circuits.. **62**-7
62.4 Gas Scavenging Systems **62**-8
62.5 Monitoring the Function of the Anesthesia Delivery
　　　System **62**-8
62.6 Monitoring the Patient **62**-10
　　　Control of Patient Temperature • Monitoring the Depth of
　　　Anesthesia • Anesthesia Computer-Aided Record Keeping •
　　　Alarms • Ergonomics • Simulation in Anesthesia •
　　　Reliability
Further Information **62**-12

A. William Paulsen
Emory University

The intent of this chapter is to provide an introduction to the practice of anesthesiology and to the technology currently employed. Limitations on the length of this work and the enormous size of the topic require that this chapter rely on other elements within this Handbook and other texts cited as general references for many of the details that inquisitive minds desire and deserve.

The practice of anesthesia includes more than just providing relief from pain. In fact, pain relief can be considered a secondary facet of the specialty. In actuality, the modern concept of the safe and efficacious delivery of anesthesia requires consideration of three fundamental tenets, which are ordered here by relative importance:

1. Maintenance of vital organ function
2. Relief of pain
3. Maintenance of the "internal milieu"

The first, maintenance of vital organ function, is concerned with preventing damage to cells and organ systems that could result from inadequate supply of oxygen and other nutrients. The delivery of blood and cellular substrates is often referred to as perfusion of the cells or tissues. During the delivery of an anesthetic, the patient's "vital signs" are monitored in an attempt to prevent inadequate tissue perfusion. However, the surgery itself, the patient's existing pathophysiology, drugs given for the relief of pain, or even the management of blood pressure may compromise tissue perfusion. Why is adequate perfusion of tissues a higher priority than providing relief of pain for which anesthesia is named? A rather obvious extreme example is that without cerebral perfusion, or perfusion of the spinal cord, delivery of an anesthetic is not necessary. Damage to other organ systems may result in a range of complications from delaying the patient's recovery to diminishing their quality of life to premature death.

In other words, the primary purpose of anesthesia care is to maintain adequate delivery of required substrates to each organ and cell, which will hopefully preserve cellular function. The second principle of anesthesia is to relieve the pain caused by surgery. Chronic pain and suffering caused by many disease states is now managed by a relatively new sub-specialty within anesthesia, called Pain Management.

The third principle of anesthesia is the maintenance of the internal environment of the body, for example, the regulation of electrolytes (sodium, potassium, chloride, magnesium, calcium, etc.), acid-base balance, and a host of supporting functions on which cellular function and organ system communications rest.

The person delivering anesthesia may be an Anesthesiologist (physician specializing in anesthesiology), an Anesthesiology Physician Assistant (a person trained in a medical school at the masters level to administer anesthesia as a member of the care team lead by an Anesthesiologist), or a nurse anesthetist (a nurse with Intensive Care Unit experience that has additional training in anesthesia provided by advanced practice nursing programs). There are three major categories of anesthesia provided to patients (1) general anesthesia; (2) conduction anesthesia; and (3) monitored anesthesia care. General anesthesia typically includes the intravenous injection of anesthetic drugs that render the patient unconscious and paralyze their skeletal muscles. Immediately following drug administration a plastic tube is inserted into the trachea and the patient is connected to an electropneumatic system to maintain ventilation of the lungs. A liquid anesthetic agent is vaporized and administered by inhalation, sometimes along with nitrous oxide, to maintain anesthesia for the surgical procedure. Often, other intravenous agents are used in conjunction with the inhalation agents to provide what is called a balanced anesthetic.

Conduction anesthesia refers to blocking the conduction of pain and possibly motor nerve impulses travelling along specific nerves or the spinal cord. Common forms of conduction anesthesia include spinal and epidural anesthesia, as well as specific nerve blocks, for example, axillary nerve blocks. In order to achieve a successful conduction anesthetic, local anesthetic agents such as lidocaine, are injected into the proximity of specific nerves to block the conduction of electrical impulses. In addition, sedation may be provided intravenously to keep the patient comfortable while he/she is lying still for the surgery.

Monitored anesthesia care refers to monitoring the patient's vital signs while administering sedatives and analgesics to keep the patient comfortable, and treating complications related to the surgical procedure. Typically, the surgeon administers topical or local anesthetics to alleviate the pain.

In order to provide the range of support required, from the paralyzed mechanically ventilated patient to the patient receiving monitored anesthesia care, a versatile anesthesia delivery system must be available to the anesthesia care team. Today's anesthesia delivery system is composed of six major elements:

1. The primary and secondary sources of gases (O_2, air, N_2O, vacuum, gas scavenging, and possibly CO_2 and helium)
2. The gas blending and vaporization system
3. The breathing circuit (including methods for manual and mechanical ventilation)
4. The excess gas scavenging system that minimizes potential pollution of the operating room by anesthetic gases
5. Instruments and equipment to monitor the function of the anesthesia delivery system
6. Patient monitoring instrumentation and equipment

The traditional anesthesia machine incorporated elements 1, 2, 3, and more recently 4. The evolution to the anesthesia delivery system adds elements 5 and 6. In the text that follows, references to the "anesthesia machine" refer to the basic gas delivery system and breathing circuit as contrasted with the "anesthesia delivery system" which includes the basic "anesthesia machine" and all monitoring instrumentation.

62.1 Gases Used During Anesthesia and Their Sources

Most inhaled anesthetic agents are liquids that are vaporized in a device within the anesthesia delivery system. The vaporized agents are then blended with other breathing gases before flowing into the breathing circuit and being administered to the patient. The most commonly administered form of anesthesia is called a balanced general anesthetic, and is a combination of inhalation agent plus intravenous analgesic drugs. Intravenous drugs often require electromechanical devices to administer an appropriately controlled flow of drug to the patient.

Gases needed for the delivery of anesthesia are generally limited to oxygen (O_2), air, nitrous oxide (N_2O), and possibly helium (He) and carbon dioxide (CO_2). Vacuum and gas scavenging lines are also required. There needs to be secondary sources of these gases in the event of primary failure or questionable contamination. Typically, primary sources are those supplied from a hospital distribution system at 345 kPa (50 psig) through gas columns or wall outlets. The secondary sources of gas are cylinders hung on yokes on the anesthesia delivery system.

62.1.1 Oxygen

Oxygen provides an essential metabolic substrate for all human cells, but it is not without dangerous side effects. Prolonged exposure to high concentrations of oxygen may result in toxic effects within the lungs that decrease diffusion of gas into and out of the blood, and the return to breathing air following prolonged exposure to elevated O_2 may result in a debilitating explosive blood vessel growth in infants. Oxygen is usually supplied to the hospital in liquid form (boiling point of $-183°C$), stored in cryogenic tanks, and supplied to the hospital piping system as a gas. The efficiency of liquid storage is obvious since 1 l of liquid becomes 860 l of gas at standard temperature and pressure. The secondary source of oxygen within an anesthesia delivery system is usually one or more E cylinders filled with gaseous oxygen at a pressure of 15.2 MPa (2200 psig).

62.1.2 Air (78% N_2, 21% O_2, 0.9% Ar, 0.1% Other Gases)

The primary use of air during anesthesia is as a diluent to decrease the inspired oxygen concentration. The typical primary source of medical air (there is an important distinction between "air" and "medical air" related to the quality and the requirements for periodic testing) is a special compressor that avoids hydrocarbon based lubricants for purposes of medical air purity. Dryers are employed to rid the compressed air of water prior to distribution throughout the hospital. Medical facilities with limited need for medical air may use banks of H cylinders of dry medical air. A secondary source of air may be available on the anesthesia machine as an E cylinder containing dry gas at 15.2 MPa.

62.1.3 Nitrous Oxide

Nitrous oxide is a colorless, odorless, and non-irritating gas that does not support human life. Breathing more than 85% N_2O may be fatal. N_2O is not an anesthetic (except under hyperbaric conditions), rather it is an analgesic and an amnestic. There are many reasons for administering N_2O during the course of an anesthetic including: enhancing the speed of induction and emergence from anesthesia; decreasing the concentration requirements of potent inhalation anesthetics (i.e., halothane, isoflurane, etc.); and as an essential adjunct to narcotic analgesics. N_2O is supplied to anesthetizing locations from banks of H cylinders that are filled with 90% liquid at a pressure of 5.1 MPa (745 psig). Secondary supplies are available on the anesthesia machine in the form of E cylinders, again containing 90% liquid. Continual exposure to low levels of N_2O in the workplace has been implicated in a number of medical problems including spontaneous abortion, infertility, birth defects, cancer, liver and kidney disease, and others. Although there is no conclusive evidence to support most of these implications, there is a recognized need to scavenge all waste anesthetic gases and periodically sample N_2O levels in the workplace to maintain the lowest possible levels consistent with reasonable risk to the operating room personnel and cost to the institution [Dorsch and Dorsch, 1998]. Another gas with analgesic properties similar to N_2O is xenon, but its use is experimental, and its cost is prohibitive at this time.

62.1.4 Carbon Dioxide

Carbon dioxide is colorless and odorless, but very irritating to breathe in higher concentrations. CO_2 is a byproduct of human cellular metabolism and is not a life-sustaining gas. CO_2 influences many physiologic processes either directly or through the action of hydrogen ions by the reaction $CO_2 + H_2O \leftrightarrow H_2CO_3 \leftrightarrow H^+ + HCO_3^-$. Although not very common in the U.S. today, in the past CO_2 was administered during anesthesia to stimulate respiration that was depressed by anesthetic agents and to cause increased blood flow in otherwise compromised vasculature during some surgical procedures. Like N_2O, CO_2 is supplied as a liquid in H cylinders for distribution in pipeline systems or as a liquid in E cylinders that are located on the anesthesia machine.

62.1.5 Helium

Helium is a colorless, odorless, and non-irritating gas that will not support life. The primary use of helium in anesthesia is to enhance gas flow through small orifices as in asthma, airway trauma, or tracheal stenosis. The viscosity of helium is not different from other anesthetic gases (refer to Table 62.1) and is therefore of no benefit when airway flow is laminar. However, in the event that ventilation must be performed through abnormally narrow orifices or tubes which create turbulent flow conditions, helium is the preferred carrier gas. Resistance to turbulent flow is proportional to the density rather than viscosity of the gas and helium is an order of magnitude less dense than other gases. A secondary advantage of helium is that it has a large specific heat relative to other anesthetic gases and therefore can carry the heat from laser surgery out of the airway more effectively than air, oxygen, or nitrous oxide.

TABLE 62.1 Physical Properties of Gases Used During Anesthesia

Gas	Molecular wt.	Density (g/l)	Viscosity (cp)	Specific heat (KJ/Kg°C)
Oxygen	31.999	1.326	0.0203	0.917
Nitrogen	28.013	1.161	0.0175	1.040
Air	28.975	1.200	0.0181	1.010
Nitrous oxide	44.013	1.836	0.0144	0.839
Carbon dioxide	44.01	1.835	0.0148	0.850
Helium	4.003	0.1657	0.0194	5.190

TABLE 62.2 Physical Properties of Currently Available Volatile Anesthetic Agents

Agent generic name	Boiling point (°C at 760 mmHg)	Vapor pressure (mmHg at 20°C)	Liquid density (g/ml)	MAC[a] (%)
Halothane	50.2	243	1.86	0.75
Enflurane	56.5	175	1.517	1.68
Isoflurane	48.5	238	1.496	1.15
Desflurane	23.5	664	1.45	6.0
Sevoflurane	58.5	160	1.51	2.0

[a]Minimum alveolar concentration is the percentage of the agent required to provide surgical anesthesia to 50% of the population in terms of a cummulative dose response curve. The lower the MAC, the more potent the agent.

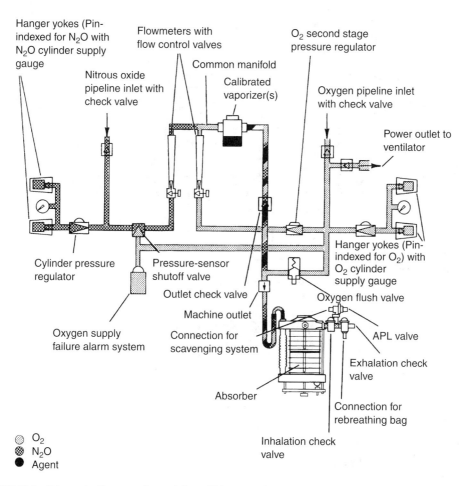

Hanger yokes (Pin-
indexed for N₂O with
N₂O cylinder supply
gauge

Flowmeters with
flow control valves

O₂ second stage
pressure regulator

Nitrous oxide
pipeline inlet with
check valve

Common manifold

Calibrated
vaporizer(s)

Oxygen pipeline inlet
with check valve

Power outlet to
ventilator

Cylinder pressure
regulator

Pressure-sensor
shutoff valve

Outlet check valve

Machine outlet

Hanger yokes (Pin-
indexed for O₂) with
O₂ cylinder
supply gauge

Oxygen flush valve

Oxygen supply
failure alarm system

Connection for
scavenging system

APL valve

Exhalation check
valve

Absorber

Connection for
rebreathing bag

○ O₂
⊛ N₂O
● Agent

Inhalation check
valve

FIGURE 62.1   Schematic diagram of gas piping within a simple two-gas (oxygen and nitrous oxide) anesthesia machine.

62.2   Gas Blending and Vaporization System

The basic anesthesia machine utilizes primary low pressure gas sources of 345 kPa (50 psig) available from wall or ceiling column outlets, and secondary high pressure gas sources located on the machine as pictured schematically in Figure 62.1. Tracing the path of oxygen in the machine demonstrates that oxygen comes from either the low pressure source, or from the 15.2 MPa (2200 psig) high pressure yokes via cylinder pressure regulators and then branches to service several other functions. First and foremost, the second stage pressure regulator drops the O_2 pressure to approximately 110 kPa (16 psig) before it enters the needle valve and the rotameter type flowmeter. From the flowmeter O_2 mixes with gases from other flowmeters and passes through a calibrated agent vaporizer where specific inhalation anesthetic agents are vaporized and added to the breathing gas mixture. Oxygen is also used to supply a reservoir canister that sounds a reed alarm in the event that the oxygen pressure drops below 172 kPa (25 psig). When the oxygen pressure drops to 172 kPa or lower, then the nitrous oxide pressure sensor shutoff valve closes and N_2O is prevented from entering its needle valve and flowmeter and is therefore eliminated from the breathing gas mixture. In fact, all machines built in the U.S. have pressure sensor shutoff valves installed in the lines to every flowmeter, except oxygen, to prevent the delivery of a hypoxic gas mixture in the event of an oxygen pressure failure. Oxygen may also be delivered to the common gas outlet or machine outlet via a momentary normally closed flush valve that typically provides a flow of 65 to 80 l of O_2 per min directly

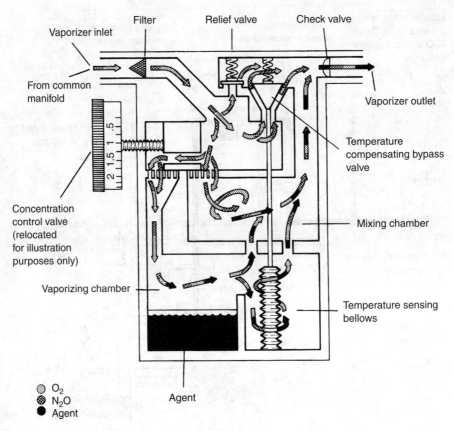

FIGURE 62.2 Schematic diagram of a calibrated in-line vaporizer that uses the flow-over technique for adding anesthetic vapor to the breathing gas mixture.

into the breathing circuit. Newer machines are required to have a safety system for limiting the minimum concentration of oxygen that can be delivered to the patient to 25%. The flow paths for nitrous oxide and other gases are much simpler in the sense that after coming from the high pressure regulator or the low pressure hospital source, gas is immediately presented to the pressure sensor shutoff valve from where it travels to its specific needle valve and flowmeter to join the common gas line and enter the breathing circuit.

Currently all anesthesia machines manufactured in the United States use only calibrated flow-through vaporizers, meaning that all of the gases from the various flowmeters are mixed in the manifold prior to entering the vaporizer. Any given vaporizer has a calibrated control knob that, once set to the desired concentration for a specific agent, will deliver that concentration to the patient. Some form of interlock system must be provided such that only one vaporizer may be activated at any given time. Figure 62.2 schematically illustrates the operation of a purely mechanical vaporizer with temperature compensation. This simple flow-over design permits a fraction of the total gas flow to pass into the vaporizing chamber where it becomes saturated with vapor before being added back to the total gas flow. Mathematically this is approximated by:

$$F_A = \frac{Q_{VC} * P_A}{P_B * (Q_{VC} + Q_G) - P_A * Q_G}$$

where F_A is the fractional concentration of agent at the outlet of the vaporizer, Q_G is the total flow of gas entering the vaporizer, Q_{VC} is the amount of Q_G that is diverted into the vaporization chamber, P_A is the vapor pressure of the agent, and P_B is the barometric pressure.

From Figure 62.2, the temperature compensator would decrease Q_{VC} as temperature increased because vapor pressure is proportional to temperature. The concentration accuracy over a range of clinically expected gas flows and temperatures is approximately ± 15%. Since vaporization is an endothermic process, anesthetic vaporizers must have sufficient thermal mass and conductivity to permit the vaporization process to proceed independent of the rate at which the agent is being used.

62.3   Breathing Circuits

The concept behind an effective breathing circuit is to provide an adequate volume of a controlled concentration of gas to the patient during inspiration, and to carry the exhaled gases away from the patient during exhalation. There are several forms of breathing circuits which can be classified into two basic types (1) open circuit, meaning no rebreathing of any gases and no CO_2 absorber present; and (2) closed circuit, indicating presence of CO_2 absorber and some rebreathing of other gases. Figure 62.3 illustrates the Lack modification of a Mapleson open circuit breathing system. There are no valves and no CO_2 absorber. There is a great potential for the patient to rebreath their own exhaled gases unless the fresh gas inflow is two to three times the patient's minute volume. Figure 62.4 illustrates the most popular form of breathing circuit, the circle system, with oxygen monitor, circle pressure gage, volume monitor

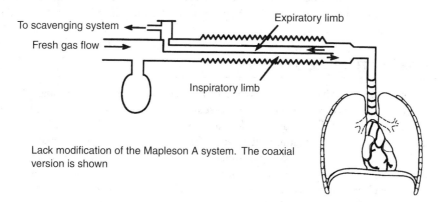

Lack modification of the Mapleson A system. The coaxial version is shown

FIGURE 62.3   An example of an open circuit breathing system that does not use unidirectional flow valves or contain a carbon dioxide absorbent.

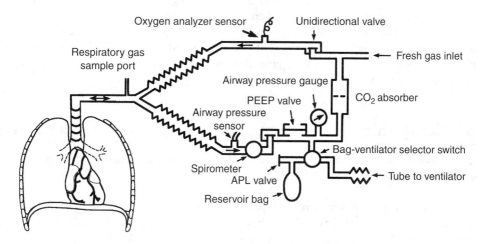

FIGURE 62.4   A diagram of a closed circuit circle breathing system with unidirectional valves, inspired oxygen sensor, pressure sensor, and CO_2 absorber.

(spirometer), and airway pressure sensor. The circle is a closed system, or semi-closed when the fresh gas inflow exceeds the patient's requirements. Excess gas evolves into the scavenging device, and some of the exhaled gas is rebreathed after having the CO_2 removed. The inspiratory and expiratory valves in the circle system guarantee that gas flows to the patient from the inspiratory limb and away from the patient through the exhalation limb. In the event of a failure of either or both of these valves, the patient will rebreath exhaled gas that contains CO_2, which is a potentially dangerous situation.

There are two forms of mechanical ventilation used during anesthesia (1) volume ventilation, where the volume of gas delivered to the patient remains constant regardless of the pressure that is required; and (2) pressure ventilation, where the ventilator provides whatever volume to the patient that is required to produce some desired pressure in the breathing circuit. Volume ventilation is the most popular since the volume delivered remains theoretically constant despite changes in lung compliance. Pressure ventilation is useful when compliance losses in the breathing circuit are high relative to the volume delivered to the lungs.

Humidification is an important adjunct to the breathing circuit because it maintains the integrity of the cilia that line the airways and promote the removal of mucus and particulate matter from the lungs. Humidification of dry breathing gases can be accomplished by simple passive heat and moisture exchangers inserted into the breathing circuit at the level of the endotracheal tube connectors, or by elegant dual servo electronic humidifiers that heat a reservoir filled with water and also heat a wire in the gas delivery tube to prevent rain-out of the water before it reaches the patient. Electronic safety measures must be included in these active devices due to the potential for burning the patient and the fire hazard.

62.4 Gas Scavenging Systems

The purpose of scavenging exhaled and excess anesthetic agents is to reduce or eliminate the potential hazard to employees who work in the environment where anesthetics are administered, including operating rooms, obstetrical areas, special procedures areas, physician's offices, dentist's offices, and veterinarian's surgical suites. Typically more gas is administered to the breathing circuit than is required by the patient, resulting in the necessity to remove excess gas from the circuit. The scavenging system must be capable of collecting gas from all components of the breathing circuit, including adjustable pressure level valves, ventilators, and sample withdrawal type gas monitors, without altering characteristics of the circuit such as pressure or gas flow to the patient. There are two broad types of scavenging systems as illustrated in Figure 62.5: the open interface is a simple design that requires a large physical space for the reservoir volume, and the closed interface with an expandable reservoir bag and which must include relief valves for handling the cases of no scavenged flow and great excess of scavenged flow.

Trace gas analysis must be performed to guarantee the efficacy of the scavenging system. The National Institutes of Occupational Safety and Health (NIOSH) recommends that trace levels of nitrous oxide be maintained at or below 25 parts per million (ppm) time weighted average and that halogenated anesthetic agents remain below 2 ppm.

62.5 Monitoring the Function of the Anesthesia Delivery System

The anesthesia machine can produce a single or combination of catastrophic events, any one of which could be fatal to the patient:

1. Delivery of a hypoxic gas mixture to the patient
2. The inability to adequately ventilate the lungs by not producing positive pressure in the patient's lungs, by not delivering an adequate volume of gas to the lungs, or by improper breathing circuit connections that permit the patient's lungs to receive only rebreathed gases
3. The delivery of an overdose of an inhalational anesthetic agent

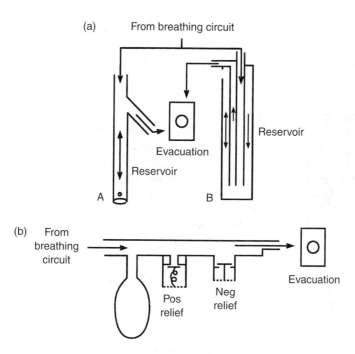

FIGURE 62.5 Examples of (a) open and (b) closed gas scavenger interfaces. The closed interface requires relief valves in the event of scavenging flow failure.

The necessary monitoring equipment to guarantee proper function of the anesthesia delivery system includes at least:

- Inspired Oxygen Concentration monitor with absolute low level alarm of 19%
- Airway Pressure Monitor with alarms for:
    1. Low pressure indicative of inadequate breathing volume and possible leaks
    2. Sustained elevated pressures that could compromise cardiovascular function
    3. High pressures that could cause pulmonary barotrauma
    4. Subatmospheric pressure that could cause collapse of the lungs
- Exhaled Gas Volume Monitor
- Carbon Dioxide Monitor (capnography)
- Inspired and Exhaled Concentration of anesthetic agents by any of the following:
    1. Mass spectrometer
    2. Raman spectrometer
    3. Infrared or other optical spectrometer

A mass spectrometer is a very useful cost-effective device since it alone can provide capnography, inspired and exhaled concentrations of all anesthetic agents, plus all breathing gases simultaneously (O_2, N_2, CO_2, N_2O, Ar, He, halothane, enflurane, isoflurane, desflurane, and suprane). The mass spectrometer is unique in that it may be tuned to monitor an assortment of exhaled gases while the patient is asleep, including (1) ketones for detection of diabetic ketoacidosis; (2) ethanol or other marker in the irrigation solution during transurethral resection of the prostate for early detection of the TURP syndrome, which results in a severe dilution of blood electrolytes; and (3) pentanes during the evolution of a heart attack, to mention a few.

Sound monitoring principles require (1) earliest possible detection of untoward events (before they result in physiologic derangements); and (2) specificity that results in rapid identification and resolution of the problem. An extremely useful rule to always consider is "*never monitor the anesthesia delivery system performance through the patient's physiologic responses.*" That is, never intentionally use a device like a pulse oximeter to detect a breathing circuit disconnection since the warning is very late and there is no specific information provided that leads to rapid resolution of the problem.

62.6 Monitoring the Patient

The anesthetist's responsibilities to the patient include: providing relief from pain and preserving all existing normal cellular function of all organ systems. Currently the latter obligation is fulfilled by monitoring essential physiologic parameters and correcting any substantial derangements that occur before they are translated into permanent cellular damage. The inadequacy of current monitoring methods can be appreciated by realizing that most monitoring modalities only indicate damage after an insult has occurred, at which point the hope is that it is reversible or that further damage can be prevented.

Standards for basic intraoperative monitoring of patients undergoing anesthesia, that were developed and adopted by the American Society of Anesthesiologists, became effective in 1990. Standard I concerns the responsibilities of anesthesia personnel, while Standard II requires that the patient's oxygenation, ventilation, circulation, and temperature be evaluated continually during all anesthetics. The following list indicates the instrumentation typically available during the administration of anesthetics.

Electrocardiogram	Non-invasive or invasive blood pressure
Pulse oximetry	Temperature
Urine output	Nerve stimulators
Cardiac output	Mixed venous oxygen saturation
Electroencephalogram (EEG)	Transesophageal echo cardiography (TEE)
Evoked potentials	Coagulation status

Blood gases and electrolytes (pO_2, pCO_2, pH, BE, Na^+, K^+, Cl^-, Ca^{++}, and glucose)

Mass spectrometry, Raman spectrometry, or infrared breathing gas analysis

62.6.1 Control of Patient Temperature

Anesthesia alters the thresholds for temperature regulation and the patient becomes unable to maintain normal body temperature. As the patient's temperature falls even a few degrees toward room temperature, several physiologic derangements occur (1) drug action is prolonged; (2) blood coagulation is impaired; and (3) post-operative infection rate increases. On the positive side, cerebral protection from inadequate perfusion is enhanced by just a few degrees of cooling. Proper monitoring of core body temperature and forced hot air warming of the patient is essential.

62.6.2 Monitoring the Depth of Anesthesia

There are two very unpleasant experiences that patients may have while undergoing an inadequate anesthetic (1) the patient is paralyzed and unable to communicate their state of discomfort, and they are feeling the pain of surgery and are aware of their surroundings; (2) the patient may be paralyzed, unable to communicate, and is aware of their surroundings, but is not feeling any pain. The ability to monitor the depth of anesthesia would provide a safeguard against these unpleasant experiences. However, despite numerous instruments and approaches to the problem it remains elusive. Brain stem auditory evoked responses have come the closest to depth of anesthesia monitoring, but it is difficult to perform, is expensive, and is not possible to perform during many types of surgery. A promising new technology, called bi-spectral index (BIS monitoring) is purported to measure the level of patient awareness through multivariate analysis of a single channel of the EEG.

62.6.3 Anesthesia Computer-Aided Record Keeping

Conceptually, every anesthetist desires an automated anesthesia record keeping system. Anesthesia care can be improved through the feedback provided by correct record keeping, but today's systems have an enormous overhead associated with their use when compared to standard paper record keeping. No doubt that automated anesthesia record keeping reduces the drudgery of routine recording of vital signs, but to enter drugs and drips and their dosages, fluids administered, urine output, blood loss, and other data requires much more time and machine interaction than the current paper system. Despite attempts to use every input/output device ever produced by the computer industry from keyboards to bar codes to voice and handwriting recognition, no solution has been found that meets wide acceptance. Tenants of a successful system must include:

1. The concept of a user transparent system, which is ideally defined as requiring no communication between the computer and the clinician (far beyond the concept of user friendly), and therefore that is intuitively obvious to use even to the most casual users
2. Recognition of the fact that educational institutions have very different requirements from private practice institutions
3. Real time hard copy of the record produced at the site of anesthetic administration that permits real time editing and notation
4. Ability to interface with a great variety of patient and anesthesia delivery system monitors from various suppliers
5. Ability to interface with a large number of hospital information systems
6. Inexpensive to purchase and maintain

62.6.4 Alarms

Vigilance is the key to effective risk management, but maintaining a vigilant state is not easy. The practice of anesthesia has been described as moments of shear terror connected by times of intense boredom. Alarms can play a significant role in redirecting one's attention during the boredom to the most important event regarding patient safety, but only if false alarms can be eliminated, alarms can be prioritized, and all alarms concerning anesthetic management can be displayed in a single clearly visible location.

62.6.5 Ergonomics

The study of ergonomics attempts to improve performance by optimizing the relationship between people and their work environment. Ergonomics has been defined as a discipline which investigates and applies information about human requirements, characteristics, abilities, and limitations to the design, development, and testing of equipment, systems, and jobs [Loeb, 1993]. This field of study is only in its infancy and examples of poor ergonomic design abound in the anesthesia workplace.

62.6.6 Simulation in Anesthesia

Complete patient simulators are hands-on realistic simulators that interface with physiologic monitoring equipment to simulate patient responses to equipment malfunctions, operator errors, and drug therapies. There are also crisis management simulators. Complex patient simulators, which are analogous to flight simulators, are currently being marketed for training anesthesia personnel. The intended use for these complex simulators is currently being debated in the sense that training people to respond in a preprogrammed way to a given event may not be adequate training.

62.6.7 Reliability

The design of an anesthesia delivery system is unlike the design of most other medical devices because it is a life support system. As such, its core elements deserve all of the considerations of the latest fail-safe technologies. Too often in today's quest to apply microprocessor technology to everything, trade-offs are made among reliability, cost, and engineering elegance. The most widely accepted anesthesia machine designs continue to be based upon simple ultra-reliable mechanical systems with an absolute minimum of catastrophic failure modes. The replacement of needle valves and rotameters, for example, with microprocessor controlled electromechanical valves can only introduce new catastrophic failure modes. However, the inclusion of microprocessors can enhance the safety of anesthesia delivery if they are implemented without adding catastrophic failure modes.

Further Information

Blitt, C.D. and Hines, R.L., Eds. (1995). *Monitoring in Anesthesia and Critical Care Medicine*, 3rd ed. Churchill Livingstone, New York.

Dorsch, J.A. and Dorsch, S.E. (1998). *Understanding Anesthesia Equipment*, 4th ed. Williams and Wilkins, Baltimore, MD.

Ehrenwerth, J. and Eisenkraft, J.B. (1993). *Anesthesia Equipment: Principles and Applications.* Mosby, St. Louis, MO.

Gravenstein N. and Kirby, R.R., Eds. (1996). *Complications in Anesthesiology*, 2nd ed. Lippincott-Raven, Philadelphia, PA.

Loeb, R. (1993). Ergonomics of the anesthesia workplace. *STA Interface* 4: 18.

Miller, R.D. Ed. (1999). *Anesthesia*, 5th ed. Churchill Livingstone, New York.

Miller, R.D. Ed. (1998). *Atlas of Anesthesia.* Churchill Livingstone, New York.

Saidman, L.J. and Smith, N.T., Eds. (1993). *Monitoring in Anesthesia*, 3rd ed. Butterworth-Heinemann, Stoneham, MA.

63

Electrosurgical Devices

63.1	Theory of Operation	**63**-2
63.2	Monopolar Mode	**63**-2
63.3	Bipolar Mode	**63**-4
63.4	ESU Design	**63**-4
63.5	Active Electrodes	**63**-6
63.6	Dispersive Electrodes	**63**-6
63.7	ESU Hazards	**63**-6
63.8	Recent Developments	**63**-8
	Defining Terms	**63**-8
	References	**63**-8
	Further Information	**63**-9

Jeffrey L. Eggleston
Valleylab, Inc.

Wolf W. von Maltzahn
Whitaker Foundation

An electrosurgical unit (ESU) passes high-frequency electric currents through biologic tissues to achieve specific surgical effects such as cutting, **coagulation**, or **desiccation**. Although it is not completely understood how electrosurgery works, it has been used since the 1920s to cut tissue effectively while at the same time controlling the amount of bleeding. Cutting is achieved primarily with a continuous sinusoidal waveform, whereas coagulation is achieved primarily with a series of sinusoidal wave packets. The surgeon selects either one of these waveforms or a blend of them to suit the surgical needs. An electrosurgical unit can be operated in two modes, the monopolar mode and the bipolar mode. The most noticeable difference between these two modes is the method in which the electric current enters and leaves the tissue. In the monopolar mode, the current flows from a small **active electrode** into the surgical site, spreads through the body, and returns to a large **dispersive electrode** on the skin. The high current density in the vicinity of the active electrode achieves tissue cutting or coagulation, whereas the low current density under the dispersive electrode causes no tissue damage. In the bipolar mode, the current flows only through the tissue held between two forceps electrodes. The monopolar mode is used for both cutting and coagulation. The bipolar mode is used primarily for coagulation.

This chapter begins with the theory of operation for electrosurgical units, outlines various modes of operation, and gives basic design details for electronic circuits and electrodes. It then describes how improper application of electrosurgical units can lead to hazardous situations for both the operator and the patient and how such hazardous situations can be avoided or reduced through proper monitoring methods. Finally, the chapter gives an update on current and future developments and applications.

63.1   Theory of Operation

In principle, electrosurgery is based on the rapid heating of tissue. To better understand the thermo-dynamic events during electrosurgery, it helps to know the general effects of heat on biologic tissue. Consider a tissue volume that experiences a temperature increase from normal body temperature to 45°C within a few seconds. Although the cells in this tissue volume show neither microscopic nor macroscopic changes, some cytochemical changes do in fact occur. However, these changes are reversible, and the cells return to their normal function when the temperature returns to normal values. Above 45°C, irreversible changes take place that inhibit normal cell functions and lead to cell death. First, between 45°C and 60°C, the proteins in the cell lose their quaternary configuration and solidify into a glutinous substance that resembles the white of a hard-boiled egg. This process, termed *coagulation*, is accompanied by tissue blanching. Further increasing the temperature up to 100°C leads to tissue drying; that is, the aqueous cell contents evaporate. This process is called *desiccation*. If the temperature is increased beyond 100°C, the solid contents of the tissue reduce to carbon, a process referred to as *carbonization*. Tissue damage depends not only on temperature, however, but also on the length of exposure to heat. Thus, the overall temperature-induced tissue damage is an integrative effect between temperature and time that is expressed mathematically by the Arrhenius relationship, where an exponential function of temperature is integrated over time [1].

In the monopolar mode, the active electrode either touches the tissue directly or is held a few millimeters above the tissue. When the electrode is held above the tissue, the electric current bridges the air gap by creating an electric discharge arc. A visible arc forms when the electric field strength exceeds 1 kV/mm in the gap and disappears when the field strength drops below a certain threshold level.

When the active electrode touches the tissue and the current flows directly from the electrode into the tissue without forming an arc, the rise in tissue temperature follows the bioheat equation

$$T - T_0 = \frac{1}{\sigma \rho c} J^2 t \qquad (63.1)$$

where T and T_0 are the final and initial temperatures (K), σ is the electrical conductivity (S/m), ρ is the tissue density (kg/m^3), c is the specific heat of the tissue (Jkg^{-1}K^{-1}), J is the current density (A/m^2), and t is the duration of heat applications [1]. The bioheat equation is valid for short application times where secondary effects such as heat transfer to surrounding tissues, blood perfusion, and metabolic heat can be neglected. According to Equation 63.1, the surgeon has primarily three means of controlling the cutting or coagulation effect during electrosurgery: the contact area between active electrode and tissue, the electrical current density, and the activation time. In most commercially available electrosurgical generators, the output variable that can be adjusted is power. This power setting, in conjunction with the output power vs. tissue impedance characteristics of the generator, allow the surgeon some control over current. Table 63.1 lists typical output power and mode settings for various surgical procedures. Table 63.2 lists some typical impedance ranges seen during use of an ESU in surgery. The values are shown as ranges because the impedance increases as the tissue dries out, and at the same time, the output power of the ESU decreases. The surgeon may control current density by selection of the active electrode type and size.

63.2   Monopolar Mode

A continuous sinusoidal waveform cuts tissue with very little hemostasis. This waveform is simply called *cut* or *pure cut*. During each positive and negative swing of the sinusoidal waveform, a new discharge arc forms and disappears at essentially the same tissue location. The electric current concentrates at this tissue location, causing a sudden increase in temperature due to resistive heating. The rapid rise in temperature then vaporizes intracellular fluids, increases cell pressure, and ruptures the cell membrane, thereby parting the tissue. This chain of events is confined to the vicinity of the arc, because from there the electric current

TABLE 63.1   Typical ESU Power Settings for Various
Surgical Procedures

Power-level range	Procedures
Low power	
<30 W cut	Neurosurgery
<30 W coag	Dermatology
	Plastic surgery
	Oral surgery
	Laparoscopic sterilization
	Vasectomy
Medium power	
30–150 W cut	General surgery
30–70 W coag	Laparotomies
	Head and neck surgery (ENT)
	Major orthopedic surgery
	Major vascular surgery
	Routine thoracic surgery
	Polypectomy
High power	
>150 W cut	Transurethral resection procedures (TURPs)
>70 W coag	Thoracotomies
	Ablative cancer surgery
	Mastectomies

Note: Ranges assume the use of a standard blade electrode.
Use of a needle electrode, or other small current-
concentrating electrode, allows lower settings to be used;
users are urged to use the lowest setting that provides the
desired clinical results.

TABLE 63.2   Typical Impedance Ranges Seen During
Use of an ESU in Surgery

Cut mode application	Impedance range (Ω)
Prostate tissue	400–1700
Oral cavity	1000–2000
Liver tissue	
Muscle tissue	
Gall bladder	1500–2400
Skin tissue	1700–2500
Bowel tissue	2500–3000
Periosteum	
Mesentery	3000–4200
Omentum	
Adipose tissue	3500–4500
Scar tissue	
Adhesions	
Coag Mode Application	
Contact coagulation to stop bleeding	100–1000

spreads to a much larger tissue volume, and the current density is no longer high enough to cause resistive heating damage. Typical output values for ESUs, in cut and other modes, are shown in Table 63.3.

Experimental observations have shown that more hemostasis is achieved when cutting with an interrupted sinusoidal waveform or amplitude modulated continuous waveform. These waveforms are typically

TABLE 63.3 Typical Output Characteristics of ESUs

	Output voltage range open circuit, $V_{peak-peak}$, V	Output power range, W	Frequency, kHz	Crest factor (V_{Peak}/V_{rms})	Duty cycle %
Monopolar modes					
Cut	200–5000	1–400	300–1750	1.4–2.1	100
Blend	1500–5800	1–300	300–1750	2.1–6.0	25–80
Desiccate	400–6500	1–200	240–800	3.5–6.0	50–100
Fulgurate/spray	6000–12000	1–200	300–800	6.0–20.0	10–70
Bipolar mode					
Coagulate/desiccate	200–1000	1–70	300–1050	1.6–12.0	25–100

called *blend* or *blended cut.* Some ESUs offer a choice of blend waveforms to allow the surgeon to select the degree of hemostasis desired.

When a continuous or interrupted waveform is used in contact with the tissue and the output voltage current density is too low to sustain arcing, desiccation of the tissue will occur. Some ESUs have a distinct mode for this purpose called *desiccation* or *contact coagulation.*

In noncontact coagulation, the duty cycle of an interrupted waveform and the crest factor (ratio of peak voltage to rms voltage) influence the degree of hemostasis. While a continuous waveform reestablishes the arc at essentially the same tissue location concentrating the heat there, an interrupted waveform causes the arc to reestablish itself at different tissue locations. The arc seems to dance from one location to the other raising the temperature of the top tissue layer to coagulation levels. These waveforms are called *fulguration* or *spray.* Since the current inside the tissue spreads very quickly from the point where the arc strikes, the heat concentrates in the top layer, primarily desiccating tissue and causing some carbonization. During surgery, a surgeon can easily choose between cutting, coagulation, or a combination of the two by activating a switch on the grip of the active electrode or by use of a footswitch.

63.3 Bipolar Mode

The bipolar mode concentrates the current flow between the two electrodes, requiring considerably less power for achieving the same coagulation effect than the monopolar mode. For example, consider coagulating a small blood vessel with 3-mm external diameter and 2-mm internal diameter, a tissue resistivity of 360 Ωcm, a contract area of 2×4 mm^2, and a distance between the forceps tips of 1 mm. The tissue resistance between the forceps is 450 Ω as calculated from $R = \rho L/A$, where ρ is the resistivity, L is the distance between the forceps, and A is the contact area. Assuming a typical current density of 200 mA/cm^2, then a small current of 16 mA, a voltage of 7.2 V, and a power level of 0.12 W suffice to coagulate this small blood vessel. In contrast, during monopolar coagulation, current levels of 200 mA and power levels of 100 W or more are not uncommon to achieve the same surgical effect. The temperature increase in the vessel tissue follows the bioheat equation, Equation 63.1. If the specific heat of the vessel tissue is 4.2 Jkg^{-1}K^{-1} and the tissue density is 1 g/cm^3, then the temperature of the tissue between the forceps increases from 37 to 57°C in 5.83 sec. When the active electrode touches the tissue, less tissue damage occurs during coagulation, because the charring and carbonization that accompanies **fulguration** is avoided.

63.4 ESU Design

Modern ESUs contain building blocks that are also found in other medical devices, such as microprocessors, power supplies, enclosures, cables, indicators, displays, and alarms. The main building blocks unique to ESUs are control input switches, the high-frequency power amplifier, and the safety monitor. The first two will be discussed briefly here, and the latter will be discussed later.

Control input switches include front panel controls, footswitch controls, and handswitch controls. In order to make operating an ESU more uniform between models and manufacturers, and to reduce the possibility of operator error, the ANSI/AAMI HF-18 standard [2] makes specific recommendations concerning the physical construction and location of these switches and prescribes mechanical and electrical performance standards. For instance, front panel controls need to have their function identified by a permanent label and their output indicated on alphanumeric displays or on graduated scales; the pedals of foot switches need to be labeled and respond to a specified activation force; and if the active electrode handle incorporates two finger switches, their position has to correspond to a specific function. Additional recommendations can be found in Reference 2.

Four basic high-frequency power amplifiers are in use currently; the somewhat dated vacuum tube/spark gap configuration, the parallel connection of a bank if bipolar power transistors, the hybrid connection of parallel bipolar power transistors cascaded with metal oxide silicon field effect transistors (MOSFETs), and the bridge connection of MOSFETs. Each has unique properties and represents a stage in the evolution of ESUs.

In a vacuum tube/spark gap device, a tuned-plate, tuned-grid vacuum tube oscillator is used to generate a continuous waveform for use in cutting. This signal is introduced to the patient by an adjustable isolation transformer. To generate a waveform for fulguration, the power supply voltage is elevated by a step-up transformer to about 1600 V rms which then connects to a series of spark gaps. The voltage across the spark gaps is capacitively coupled to the primary of an isolation transformer. The RLC circuit created by this arrangement generates a high crest factor, damped sinusoidal, interrupted waveform. One can adjust the output power and characteristics by changing the turns ratio or tap on the primary and/or secondary side of the isolation transformer, or by changing the spark gap distance.

In those devices that use a parallel bank of bipolar power transistors, the transistors are arranged in a Class A configuration. The bases, collectors, and emitters are all connected in parallel, and the collective base node is driven through a current-limiting resistor. A feedback RC network between the base node and the collector node stabilizes the circuit. The collectors are usually fused individually before the common node connects them to one side of the primary of the step-up transformer. The other side of the primary is connected to the high-voltage power supply. A capacitor and resistor in parallel to the primary create a resonance tank circuit that generates the output waveform at a specific frequency. Additional elements may be switched in and out of the primary parallel RLC to alter the output power and waveform for various electrosurgical modes. Small-value resistors between the emitters and ground improve the current sharing between transistors. This configuration sometimes requires the use of matched sets of high-voltage power transistors.

A similar arrangement exists in amplifiers using parallel bipolar transistors cascaded with a power MOSFET. This arrangement is called a *hybrid cascode amplifier*. In this type of amplifier, the collectors of a group if bipolar transistors are connected, via protection diodes, to one side of the primary of the step-up output transformer. The other side of the primary is connected to the high-voltage power supply. The emitters of two or three bipolar transistors are connected, via current limiting resistors, to the drain of an enhancement mode MOSFET. The source of the MOSFET is connected to ground, and the gate of the MOSFET is connected to a voltage-snubbing network driven by a fixed amplitude pulse created by a high-speed MOS driver circuit. The bases of the bipolar transistors are connected, via current control RC networks, to a common variable base voltage source. Each collector and base is separately fused. In cut modes, the gate drive pulse is a fixed frequency, and the base voltage is varied according to the power setting. In the coagulation modes, the base voltage is fixed and the width of the pulses driving the MOSFET is varied. This changes the conduction time of the amplifier and controls the amount of energy imparted to the output transformer and its load. In the coagulation modes and in high-power cut modes, the bipolar power transistors are saturated, and the voltage across the bipolar/MOSFET combination is low. This translates to high efficiency and low power dissipation.

The most common high-frequency power amplifier in use is a bridge connection of MOSFETs. In this configuration, the drains of a series of power MOSFETs are connected, via protection diodes, to one side of the primary of the step-up output transformer. The drain protection diodes protect the MOSFETs against the negative voltage swings of the transformer primary. The other side of the transformer primary is connected to the high-voltage power supply. The sources of the MOSFETs are connected to ground. The gate of each MOSFET has a resistor connected to ground and one to its driver circuitry. The resistor to ground speeds up the discharge of the gate capacitance when the MOSFET is turned on while the gate series resistor eliminates turn-off oscillations. Various combinations of capacitors and/or LC networks can be switched across the primary of the step-up output transformer to obtain different waveforms. In the cut mode, the output power is controlled by varying the high-voltage power supply voltage. In the coagulation mode, the output power is controlled by varying the on time of the gate drive pulse.

63.5   Active Electrodes

The monopolar active electrode is typically a small flat blade with symmetric leading and trailing edges that is embedded at the tip of an insulated handle. The edges of the blade are shaped to easily initiate discharge arcs and to help the surgeon manipulate the incision; the edges cannot mechanically cut tissue. Since the surgeon holds the handle like a pencil, it is often referred to as the "pencil." Many pencils contain in their handle one or more switches to control the electrosurgical waveform, primarily to switch between cutting and coagulation. Other active electrodes include needle electrodes, loop electrodes, and ball electrodes. Needle electrodes are used for coagulating small tissue volumes like in neurosurgery or plastic surgery. Loop electrodes are used to resect nodular structures such as polyps or to excise tissue samples for pathologic analysis. An example would be the LLETZ procedure where the transition zone of the cervix is excised. Electrosurgery at the tip of an endoscope or laparoscope requires yet another set of active electrodes and specialized training of the surgeon.

63.6   Dispersive Electrodes

The main purpose of the dispersive electrode is to return the high-frequency current to the electrosurgical unit without causing harm to the patient. This is usually achieved by attaching a large electrode to the patient's skin away from the surgical site. The large electrode area and a small contact impedance reduce the current density to levels where tissue heating is minimal. Since the ability of a dispersive electrode to avoid tissue heating and burns is of primary importance, dispersive electrodes are often characterized by their *heating factor*. The heating factor describes the energy dissipated under the dispersive electrode per Ω of impedance and is equal to I^2t, where I is the rms current and t is the time of exposure. During surgery a typical value for the heating factor is $3\,A^2s$, but factors of up to $9\,A^2s$ may occur during some procedures [3].

Two types of dispersive electrodes are in common use today, the resistive type and the capacitive type. In disposable form, both electrodes have a similar structure and appearance. A thin, rectangular metallic foil has an insulating layer on the outside, connects to a gel-like material on the inside, and may be surrounded by an adhesive foam. In the resistive type, the gel-like material is made of an adhesive conductive gel, whereas in the capacitive type, the gel is an adhesive dielectric nonconductive gel. The adhesive foam and adhesive gel layer ensure that both electrodes maintain good skin contact to the patient, even if the electrode gets stressed mechanically from pulls on the electrode cable. Both types have specific advantages and disadvantages. Electrode failures and subsequent patient injury can be attributed mostly to improper application, electrode dislodgment, and electrode defects rather than to electrode design.

63.7   ESU Hazards

Improper use of electrosurgery may expose both the patient and the surgical staff to a number of hazards. By far the most frequent hazards are electric shock and undesired burns. Less frequent are undesired neuromuscular stimulation, interference with pacemakers or other devices, electrochemical effects from direct currents, implant heating, and gas explosions [1,4].

Current returns to the ESU through the dispersive electrode. If the contact area of the dispersive electrode is large and the current exposure time short, then the skin temperature under the electrode does not rise above 45°C, which has been shown to be the maximum safe temperature [5]. However, to include a safety margin, the skin temperature should not rise more than 6°C above the normal surface temperature of 29 to 33°C. The current density at any point under the dispersive electrode has to be significantly below the recognized burn threshold of 100 mA/cm^2 for 10 sec.

To avoid electric shock and burns, the American National Standard for Electrosurgical Devices [2] requires that "any electrosurgical generator that provides for a dispersive electrode and that has a rated output power of greater than 50 W shall have at least one patient circuit safety monitor." The most common safety monitors are the contact quality monitor for the dispersive electrode and the patient circuit monitor. A contact quality monitor consists of a circuit to measure the impedance between the two sides of a split dispersive electrode and the skin. A small high-frequency current flows from one section of the dispersive electrode through the skin to the second section of the dispersive electrode. If the impedance between these two sections exceeds a certain threshold, or changes by a certain percentage, an audible alarm sounds, and the ESU output is disabled.

Patient circuit monitors range from simple to complex. The simple ones monitor electrode cable integrity while the complex ones detect any abnormal condition that could result in electrosurgical current flowing in other than normal pathways. Although the output isolation transformer present in most modern ESUs usually provides adequate patient protection, some potentially hazardous conditions may still arise. If a conductor to the dispersive electrode is broken, undesired arcing between the broken conductor ends may occur, causing fire in the operating room and serious patient injury. Abnormal current pathways may also arise from capacitive coupling between cables, the patient, operators, enclosures, beds, or any other conductive surface or from direct connections to other electrodes connected to the patient. The patient circuit monitoring device should be operated from an isolated power source having a maximum voltage of 12 V rms. The most common device is a cable continuity monitor. Unlike the contact quality monitor, this monitor only checks the continuity of the cable between the ESU and the dispersive electrode and sounds an alarm if the resistance in that conductor is greater than 1 kΩ. Another implementation of a patient circuit monitor measures the voltage between the dispersive electrode connection and ground. A third implementation functions similarly to a ground fault circuit interrupter (GFCI) in that the current in the wire to the active electrode and the current in the wire to the dispersive electrode are measured and compared with each other. If the difference between these currents is greater than a preset threshold, the alarm sounds and the ESU is disconnected.

There are other sources of undesired burns. Active electrodes get hot when they are used. After use, the active electrode should be placed in a protective holster, if available, or on a suitable surface to isolate it from the patient and surgical staff. The correct placement of an active electrode will also prevent the patient and/or surgeon from being burned if an inadvertent activation of the ESU occurs (e.g., someone accidentally stepping on a foot pedal). Some surgeons use a practice called *buzzing the hemostat* in which a small bleeding vessel is grasped with a clamp or hemostat and the active electrode touched to the clamp while activating. Because of the high voltages involved and the stray capacitance to ground, the surgeon's glove may be compromised. If the surgical staff cannot be convinced to eliminate the practice of buzzing hemostats, the probability of burns can be reduced by use of a cut waveform instead of a coagulation waveform (lower voltage), by maximizing contact between the surgeon's hand and the clamp, and by not activating until the active electrode is firmly touching the clamp.

Although it is commonly assumed that neuromuscular stimulation ceases or is insignificant at frequencies above 10 kHz, such stimulation has been observed in anesthetized patients undergoing certain electrosurgical procedures. This undesirable side effect of electrosurgery is generally attributed to nonlinear events during the electric arcing between the active electrode and tissue. These events rectify the high-frequency current leading to both dc and low-frequency current components. These current components can reach magnitudes that stimulate nerve and muscle cells. To minimize the probability of unwanted neuromuscular stimulation, most ESUs incorporate in their output circuit a high-pass filter that suppresses dc and low-frequency current components.

The use of electrosurgery means the presence of electric discharge arcs. This presents a potential fire hazard in an operating room where oxygen and flammable gases may be present. These flammable gases may be introduced by the surgical staff (anesthetics or flammable cleaning solutions), or may be generated within the patients themselves (bowel gases). The use of disposable paper drapes and dry surgical gauze also provides a flammable material that may be ignited by sparking or by contact with a hot active electrode. Therefore, prevention of fires and explosions depends primarily on the prudence and judgment of the ESU operator.

63.8   Recent Developments

Electrosurgery is being enhanced by the addition of a controlled column of argon gas in the path between the active electrode and the tissue. The flow of argon gas assists in clearing the surgical site of fluid and improves visibility. When used in the coagulation mode, the argon gas is turned into a plasma allowing tissue damage and smoke to be reduced, and producing a thinner, more flexible eschar. When used with the cut mode, lower power levels may be used.

Many manufacturers have begun to include sophisticated computer-based systems in their ESUs that not only simplify the use of the device but also increase the safety of patient and operator [6]. For instance, in a so-called soft coagulation mode, a special circuit continuously monitors the current between the active electrode and the tissue and turns the ESU output on only after the active electrode has contacted the tissue. Furthermore, the ESU output is turned off automatically, once the current has reached a certain threshold level that is typical for coagulated and desiccated tissue. This feature is also used in a bipolar mode termed *autobipolar*. Not only does this feature prevent arcing at the beginning of the procedure, but it also keeps the tissue from being heated beyond 70°C. Some devices offer a so-called power-peak-system that delivers a very short power peak at the beginning of electrosurgical cutting to start the cutting arc. Other modern devices use continuous monitoring of current and voltage levels to make automatic power adjustments in order to provide for a smooth cutting action from the beginning of the incision to its end. Some manufacturers are developing waveforms and instruments designed to achieve specific clinical results such as bipolar cutting tissue lesioning, and vessel sealing. With the growth and popularity of laparoscopic procedures, additional electrosurgical instruments and waveforms tailored to this surgical specialty should also be expected.

Increased computing power, more sophisticated evaluation of voltage and current waveforms, and the addition of miniaturized sensors will continue to make ESUs more user-friendly and safer.

Defining Terms

Active electrode: Electrode used for achieving desired surgical effect.
Coagulation: Solidification of proteins accompanied by tissue whitening.
Desiccation: Drying of tissue due to the evaporation of intracellular fluids.
Dispersive electrode: Return electrode at which no electrosurgical effect is intended.
Fulguration: Random discharge of sparks between active electrode and tissue surface in order to achieve coagulation and/or desiccation.
Spray: Another term for *fulguration*. Sometimes this waveform has a higher crest factor than that used for fulguration.

References

[1] Pearce John A. 1986. *Electrosurgery*, New York, John Wiley.
[2] American National Standard for Electrosurgical Devices. 1994. HF18, American National Standards Institute.

[3] Gerhard Glen C. 1988. Electrosurgical unit. In J.G. Webster (Ed.), *Encyclopedia of Medical Devices and Instrumentation*, Vol. 2, pp. 1180–1203, New York, John Wiley.

[4] Gendron Francis G. 1988. *Unexplained Patient Burns: Investigating Latrogenic Injuries*, Brea, CA, Quest Publishing.

[5] Pearce J.A., Geddes L.A., and Van Vleet J.F. et al. 1983. Skin burns from electrosurgical current. *Med. Instrum.* 17: 225.

[6] Haag R. and Cuschieri A. 1993. Recent advances in high-frequency electrosurgery: development of automated systems. *J. R. Coll. Surg. Ednb.* 38: 354.

[7] LaCourse J.R., Miller W.T. III, and Vogt M. et al. 1985. Effect of high frequency current on nerve and muscle tissue. *IEEE Trans. Biomed. Eng.* 32: 83.

Further Information

American National Standards Institute, 1988. International Standard, Medical Electrical Equipment, Part 1: General Requirements for Safety, IEC 601-1, 2nd ed., New York.

American National Standards Institute, 1991. International Standard, Medical Electrical Equipment, Part 2: Particular Requirements for the Safety of High Frequency Surgical Equipment, IEC 601-2-2, 2nd ed., New York.

National Fire Protection Association, 1993. Standard for Health Care Facilities, NFPA 99.

64

Biomedical Lasers

64.1 Interaction and Effects of UV–IR Laser Radiation on
Biologic Tissues **64**-2
Scattering in Biologic Tissue • Absorption in Biologic Tissue
64.2 Penetration and Effects of UV–IR Laser Radiation
into Biologic Tissue **64**-3
64.3 Effects of Mid-IR Laser Radiation **64**-4
64.4 Effects of Near-IR Laser Radiation **64**-4
64.5 Effects of Visible-Range Laser Radiation **64**-5
64.6 Effects of UV Laser Radiation.......................... **64**-5
64.7 Effects of Continuous and Pulsed IR–Visible Laser
Radiation and Associated Temperature Rise **64**-5
64.8 General Description and Operation of Lasers **64**-6
64.9 Biomedical Laser Beam Delivery Systems **64**-7
Optical Fiber Transmission Characteristics • Mirrored
Articulated Arm Characteristics • Optics for Beam Shaping
on Tissues • Features of Routinely Used Biomedical Lasers •
Other Biomedical Lasers
Defining Terms **64**-11
References **64**-11
Further Information **64**-13

Millard M. Judy
Baylor Research Institute

Approximately 20 years ago the CO_2 laser was introduced into surgical practice as a tool to photothermally ablate, and thus to incise and to debulk, soft tissues. Subsequently, three important factors have led to the expanding biomedical use of laser technology, particularly in surgery. These factors are (1) the increasing understanding of the wave-length selective interaction and associated effects of **ultraviolet-infrared (UV– IR) radiation** with biologic tissues, including those of acute damage and long-term healing, (2) the rapidly increasing availability of lasers emitting (essentially monochromatically) at those wavelengths that are strongly absorbed by molecular species within tissues, and (3) the availability of both optical fiber and lens technologies as well as of endoscopic technologies for delivery of the laser radiation to the often remote internal treatment site. Fusion of these factors has led to the development of currently available biomedical laser systems.

This chapter briefly reviews the current status of each of these three factors. In doing so, each of the following topics will be briefly discussed:

1. The physics of the interaction and the associated effects (including clinical efforts) of UV–IR radiation on biologic tissues
2. The fundamental principles that underlie the operations and construction of all lasers

3. The physical properties of the optical delivery systems used with the different biomedical lasers for delivery of the laser beam to the treatment site
4. The essential physical features of those biomedical lasers currently in routine use ranging over a number of clinical specialties, and brief descriptions of their use
5. The biomedical uses of other lasers used surgically in limited scale or which are currently being researched for applications in surgical and diagnostic procedures and the photosensitized inactivation of cancer tumors

In this review, effort is made in the text and in the last section to provide a number of key references and sources of information for each topic that will enable the reader's more in-depth pursuit.

64.1 Interaction and Effects of UV–IR Laser Radiation on Biologic Tissues

Electromagnetic radiation in the UV–IR spectral range propagates within biologic tissues until it is either scattered or absorbed.

64.1.1 Scattering in Biologic Tissue

Scattering in matter occurs only at the boundaries between regions having different optical refractive indices and is a process in which the energy of the radiation is conserved [Van de Hulst, 1957]. Since biologic tissue is structurally inhomogeneous at the microscopic scale, for example, both subcellular and cellular dimensions, and at the macroscopic scale, for example, cellular assembly (tissue) dimensions, and predominantly contains water, proteins, and lipids, all different chemical species, it is generally regarded as a scatterer of UV–IR radiation. The general result of scattering is deviation of the direction of propagation of radiation. The deviation is strongest when wavelength and scatterer are comparable in dimension (Mie scattering) and when wavelength greatly exceeds particle size (Rayleigh scattering) [Van de Hulst, 1957]. This dimensional relationship results in the deeper penetration into biologic tissues of those longer wavelengths which are not absorbed appreciably by pigments in the tissues. This results in the relative transparency of nonpigmented tissues over the visible and near-IR wavelength ranges.

64.1.2 Absorption in Biologic Tissue

Absorption of UV–IR radiation in matter arises from the wavelength-dependent resonant absorption of radiation by molecular electrons of optically absorbing molecular species [Grossweiner, 1989]. Because of the chemical inhomogeneity of biologic tissues, the degree of absorption of incident radiation strongly depends upon its wavelength. The most prevalent or concentrated UV–IR absorbing molecular species in biologic tissues are listed in Table 64.1 along with associated high-absorbance wavelengths. These species include the peptide bonds; the phenylalanine, tyrosine, and tryptophan residues of proteins, all of which absorb in the UV range; oxy- and deoxyhemoglobin of blood which absorb in the visible to near-IR range; melanin, which absorbs throughout the UV to near-IR range, which decreasing absorption occurring with increasing wavelength; and water, which absorbs maximally in the mid-IR range [Hale and Querry, 1973; Miller and Veitch, 1993; White et al., 1968]. Biomedical lasers and their emitted radiation wavelength values also are tabulated also in Table 64.1. The correlation between the wavelengths of clinically useful lasers and wavelength regions of absorption by constituents of biological tissues is evident. Additionally, exogenous light-absorbing chemical species may be intentionally present in tissues. These include:

1. Photosensitizers, such as porphyrins, which upon excitation with UV-visible light initiate photo-chemical reactions which are cytotoxic to the cells of the tissue, for example, a cancer which concentrates the photosensitizer relative to surrounding tissues [Spikes, 1989]

TABLE 64.1 UV–IR-Radiation-Absorbing Constituent of Biological Tissues and Biomedical Laser Wavelengths

		Optical absorption			
Constituent	Tissue type	Wavelength[a] (nm)	Relative[b] strength	Laser type	Wavelength (nm)
Proteins	All				
Peptide bond		<220 (r)	+++++++	ArF	193
Amino acid					
Residues					
Tryptophan		220–290 (r)	+		
Tyrosine		220–290 (r)	+		
Phenylalanine		220–2650 (r)	+		
Pigments					
Oxyhemoglobin	Blood	414 (p).	+++	Ar ion	488–514.5
	vascular tissues	537 (p).	++	frequency	532
		575 (p).	++	doubled	
		970 (p).	+	Nd:YAG	
		(690–1100) (r)		Diode	810
				Nd:YAG	1064
Deoxyhemoglobin	Blood	431 (p)	+++	Dye	400–700
	vascular tissues	554 (p)	++	Nd:YAG	1064
Melanin	Skin	220–1000 (r)	++++	Ruby	693
Water	All	2.1 (p)	+++	Ho:YAG	2100
		3.02 (p)	+++++++	Er:YAG	2940
		>2.94 (r)	++++	CO_2	10,640

[a] (p): Peak absorption wavelength; (r): wavelength range.
[b] The number of + signs qualitatively ranks the magnitude of the optical absorbtion.

2. Dyes such as indocyanine green which, when dispersed in a concentrate fibrin protein gel can be used to localize 810 nm *GaAlAs* diode laser radiation and the associated heating to achieve localized thermal denaturation and bonding of collagen to effect joining or welding of tissue [Bass et al., 1992; Oz et al., 1989]
3. Tattoo pigments including graphite (black) and black, blue, green, and red organic dyes [Fitzpatrick, 1994; McGillis et al., 1994]

64.2 Penetration and Effects of UV–IR Laser Radiation into Biologic Tissue

Both scattering and absorption processes affect the variations of the intensity of radiation with propagation into tissues. In the absence of scattering, absorption results in an exponential decrease of radiation intensity described simply by Beers law [Grossweiner, 1989]. With appreciable scattering present, the decrease in incident intensity from the surface is no longer monotonic. A maximum in local internal intensity is found to be present due to efficient back-scattering, which adds to the intensity of the incoming beam as shown, for example, by Miller and Veitch [1993] for visible light penetrating into the skin and by Rastegar et al. [1992] for 1.064 μm *Nd:YAG* laser radiation penetrating into the prostate gland. Thus, the relative contributions of absorption and scattering of incident laser radiation will stipulate the depth in a tissue at which the resulting tissue effects will be present. Since the absorbed energy can be released in a number of different ways including thermal vibrations, fluorescence, and resonant electronic energy transfer according to the identity of the absorber, the effects on tissue are in general different. Energy release from both hemoglobin and melanin pigments and from water is by molecular vibrations resulting in a local temperature rise. Sufficient continued energy absorption and release can result in local temperature increases which, as energy input increases, result in protein denaturation (41 to 65°C), water evaporation and boiling (up to $\simeq$300°C under confining pressure of tissue), thermolysis of proteins, generation of gaseous decomposition products and of carbonaceous residue or char ($\geq$300°C). The generation of residual char is minimized by sufficiently rapid energy input to support rapid gasification reactions. The clinical effect of this chain of thermal events is tissue ablation. Much smaller values of energy input result in coagulation of tissues due to protein denaturation.

Energy release from excited exogenous photosensitizing dyes is via formation of free-radical species or energy exchange with itinerant dissolved molecular oxygen [Spikes, 1989]. Subsequent chemical reactions following free-radical formation or formation of an activated or more reactive form of molecular oxygen following energy exchange can be toxic to cells with takeup of the photosensitizer.

Energy release following absorption of **visible (VIS) radiation** by fluorescent molecular species, either endogenous to tissue or exogenous, is predominantly by emission of longer wavelength radiation [Lakowicz, 1983]. Endogenous fluorescent species include tryptophan, tyrosine, phenylalanine, flavins, and metal-free porphyrins. Comparison of measured values of the intensity of fluorescence emission from hyperplastic (transformed precancerous) cervical cells to cancerous cervical cells with normal cervical epithelial cells shows a strong potential for diagnostic use in the automated diagnosis and staging of cervical cancer [Mahadevan et al., 1993].

64.3 Effects of Mid-IR Laser Radiation

Because of the very large absorption by water of radiation with wavelength in the IR range $\geq$2.0 μm, the radiation of *Ho:YAG, Er: YAG , and CO_2* lasers is absorbed within a very short distance of the tissue surface, and scattering is essentially unimportant. Using published values of the water absorption coefficient [Hale and Querry, 1973] and assuming an 80% water content and that the decrease in intensity is exponential with distance, the depth in the "average" soft tissue at which the intensity has decreased to 10% of the incident value (the optical penetration depth) is estimated to be 619, 13, and 170 μm, respectively, for Ho:YAG, Er:YAG, and CO_2 laser radiation. Thus, the absorption of radiation from these laser sources and thermalization of this energy results essentially in the formation of a surface heat source. With sufficient energy input, tissue ablation through water boiling and tissue thermolysis occur at the surface. Penetration of heat to underlying tissues is by diffusion alone; thus, the depth of coagulation of tissue below the surface region of ablation is limited by competition between thermal diffusion and the rate of descent of the heated surface impacted by laser radiation during ablation of tissue. Because of this competition, coagulation depths obtained in soft biologic tissues with use of mid-IR laser radiation are typically $\leq$205 to 500 μm, and the ability to achieve sealing of blood vessels leading to hemostatic ("bloodless") surgery is limited [Judy et al., 1992; Schroder et al., 1987].

64.4 Effects of Near-IR Laser Radiation

The 810-nm and 1064-μm radiation, respectively, of the GaAlAs diode laser and Nd:YAG laser penetrate more deeply into biologic tissues than the radiation of longer-wavelength IR lasers. Thus, the resulting thermal effects arise from absorption at greater depth within tissues, and the depths of coagulation and degree of hemostasis achieved with these lasers tend to be greater than with the longer-wavelength IR lasers. For example, the optical penetration depths (10% incident intensity) for 810-nm and 1.024-μm radiation are estimated to be 4.6 and $\simeq$8.6 mm respectively in canine prostate tissue [Rastegar et al., 1992]. Energy deposition of 3600 J from each laser onto the urethral surface of the canine prostate results in maximum coagulation depths of 8 and 12 mm respectively using diode and Nd:YAG lasers [Motamedi et al., 1993]. Depths of optical penetration and coagulation in porcine liver, a more vascular tissue than prostate gland, of 2.8 and $\simeq$9.6 mm, respectively, were obtained with a Nd:YAG laser beam, and of 7 and 12 mm respectively with an 810-nm diode laser beam [Rastegar et al., 1992]. The smaller penetration depth obtained with 810-nm diode radiation in liver than in prostate gland reflects the effect of greater vascularity (blood content) on near-IR propagation.

64.5 Effects of Visible-Range Laser Radiation

Blood and vascular tissues very efficiently absorb radiation in the visible wavelength range due to the strong absorption of hemoglobin. This absorption underlies, for example, the use of:

1. The argon ion laser (488 to 514.5 nm) in the localized heating and thermal coagulation of the vascular choroid layer and adjacent retina, resulting in the anchoring of the retina in treatment of retinal detachment [Katoh and Peyman, 1988].
2. The argon ion laser (488 to 514.5 nm), frequency-doubled Nd:YAG laser (532 nm), and dye laser radiation (585 nm) in the coagulative treatment of cutaneous vascular lesions such as port wine stains [Mordon et al., 1993].
3. The argon ion (488 to 514.5 nm) and frequency-doubled Nd:YAG lasers (532 nm) in the ablation of pelvic endometrial lesions which contain brown iron-containing pigments Keye et al., 1983].

Because of the large absorption by hemoglobin and iron-containing pigments, the incident laser radiation is essentially absorbed at the surface of the blood vessel or lesion, and the resulting thermal effects are essentially local [Miller and Veitch, 1993].

64.6 Effects of UV Laser Radiation

Whereas exposure of tissue to IR and visible-light-range laser energy result in removal of tissue by thermal ablation, exposure to *argon fluoride (ArF)* laser radiation of 193-nm wavelength results predominantly in ablation of tissue initiated by a photochemical process [Garrison and Srinivasan, 1985]. This ablation arises from repulsive forces between like-charged regions of ionized protein molecules that result from ejection of molecular electrons following UV photon absorption [Garrison and Srinivasan, 1985]. Because the ionization and repulsive processes are extremely efficient, little of the incident laser energy escapes as thermal vibrational energy, and the extent of thermal coagulation damage adjacent to the site of incidence is very limited [Garrison and Srinivasan, 1985]. This feature and the ability to tune very finely the fluence emitted by the ArF laser so that micrometer depths of tissue can be removed have led to ongoing clinical trials to investigate the efficiency of the use of the ArF laser to selectively remove tissue from the surface of the human cornea for correction of short-sighted vision to eliminate the need for corrective eyewear [Van Saarloos and Constable, 1993].

64.7 Effects of Continuous and Pulsed IR–Visible Laser Radiation and Associated Temperature Rise

Heating following absorption of IR-visible laser radiation arises from molecular vibration during loss of the excitation energy and initially is manifested locally within the exposed region of tissue. If incidence of the laser energy is maintained for a sufficiently long time, the temperature within adjacent regions of biologic tissue increases due to heat diffusion. The mean squared distance $\langle X^2 \rangle$ over which appreciable heat diffusion and temperature rise occur during exposure time t can be described in terms of the thermal diffusion time τ by the equation:

$$\langle X^2 \rangle = \tau t \tag{64.1}$$

where τ is defined as the ratio of the thermal conductivity to the product of the heat capacity and density. For soft biologic tissues τ is approximately 1×10^3 cm^2 sec^{-1} [Meijering et al., 1993]. Thus, with continued energy input, the distance over which thermal diffusion and temperature rise occurs increases. Conversely, with use of pulsed radiation, the distance of heat diffusion can be made very small; for example, with exposure to a 1-μsec pulse, the mean thermal diffusion distance is found to be approximately 0.3 μm, or about 3 to 10% of a biologic cell diameter. If the laser radiation is strongly absorbed and the ablation of tissues is efficient, then little energy diffuses away from the site of incidence, and lateral thermally induced coagulation of tissue can be minimized with pulses of short duration. The effect of limiting lateral thermal damage is desirable in the cutting of cornea [Hibst et al., 1992] and sclera of the eye [Hill et al., 1993], and joint cartilage [Maes and Sherk, 1994], all of which are avascular (or nearly so, with cartilage), and the hemostasis arising from lateral tissue coagulation is not required.

64.8   General Description and Operation of Lasers

Lasers emit a beam of intense electromagnetic radiation that is essentially monochromatic or contains at most a few nearly monochromatic wavelengths and is typically only weakly divergent and easily focused into external optical systems. These attributes of laser radiation depend on the key phenomenon which underlies laser operation, that of light amplification by stimulated emission of radiation, which in turn gives rise to the acronym *LASER*.

In practice, a laser is generally a generator of radiation. The generator is constructed by housing a light-emitting medium within a cavity defined by mirrors which provide feedback of emitted radiation through the medium. With sustained excitation of the ionic or molecular species of the medium to give a large density of excited energy states, the spontaneous and attendant stimulated emission of radiation from these states by photons of identical wavelength (a lossless process), which is amplified by feedback due to photon reflection by the cavity mirrors, leads to the generation of a very large photon density within the cavity. With one cavity mirror being partially transmissive, say 0.1 to 1%, a fraction of the cavity energy is emitted as an intense beam. With suitable selection of a laser medium, cavity geometry, and peak wavelengths of mirror reflection, the beam is also essentially monochromatic and very nearly collimated.

Identity of the lasing molecular species or laser medium fixes the output wavelength of the laser. Laser media range from gases within a tubular cavity, organic dye molecules dissolved in a flowing inert liquid carrier and heat sink, to impurity-doped transparent crystalline rods (solid state lasers) and semiconducting diode junctions [Lengyel, 1971]. The different physical properties of these media in part determine the methods used to excite them into lasing states.

Gas-filled, or gas lasers are typically excited by dc or rf electric current. The current either ionizes and excites the lasing gas, for example, argon, to give the electronically excited and lasing Ar+ ion, or ionizes a gaseous species in a mixture also containing the lasing species, for example, N_2, which by efficient energy transfer excites the lasing molecular vibrational states of the CO_2 molecule.

Dye lasers and so-called solid-state lasers are typically excited by intense light from either another laser or from a flash lamp. The excitation light wavelength range is selected to ensure efficient excitation at the absorption wavelength of the lasing species. Both excitation and output can be continuous, or the use of a pulsed flashlamp or pulsed exciting laser to pump a solid-state or dye laser gives pulsed output with high peak power and short pulse duration of 1 μsec to 1 msec. Repeated excitation gives a train of pulses. Additionally, pulses of higher peak power and shorter duration of approximately 10 nsec can be obtained from solid lasers by intracavity Q-switching [Lengyel, 1971]. In this method, the density of excited states is transiently greatly increased by impeding the path between the totally reflecting and partially transmitting mirror of the cavity interrupting the stimulated emission process. Upon rapid removal of the impeding device (a beam-interrupting or -deflecting device), stimulated emission of the very large population of excited lasing states leads to emission of an intense laser pulse. The process can give single pulses or can be repeated to give a pulse train with repetition frequencies typically ranging from 1 Hz to 1 kHz.

Gallium aluminum (GaAlAs) lasers are, as are all semiconducting diode lasers, excited by electrical current which creates excited hole-electron pairs in the vicinity of the diode junction. Those carrier pairs are the lasing species which emit spontaneously and with photon stimulation. The beam emerges parallel to the function with the plane of the function forming the cavity and thin-layer surface mirrors providing reflection. Use of continuous or pulsed excitation current results in continuous or pulsed output.

64.9   Biomedical Laser Beam Delivery Systems

Beam delivery systems for biomedical lasers guide the laser beam from the output mirror to the site of action on tissue. Beam powers of up to 100 W are transmitted routinely. All biomedical lasers incorporate a coaxial aiming beam, typically from a HeNe laser (632.8 nm) to illuminate the site of incidence on tissue.

Usually, the systems incorporate two different beam-guiding methods, either (1) a flexible fused silica (SiO_2) optical fiber or light guide, generally available currently for laser beam wavelengths between $\simeq$400 nm and $\simeq$2.1 μm, where SiO_2 is essentially transparent and (2) an articulated arm having beam-guiding mirrors for wavelengths greater than circa 2.1 μm (e.g., CO_2 lasers), for the Er:YAG and for pulsed lasers having peak power outputs capable of causing damage to optical fiber surfaces due to ionization by the intense electric field (e.g., pulsed ruby). The arm comprises straight tubular sections articulated together with high-quality power-handling dielectric mirrors at each articulation junction to guide the beam through each of the sections. Fused silica optical fibers usually are limited to a length of 1 to 3 m and to wavelengths in the visible-to-low midrange IR (<2.1 μm), because longer wavelengths of IR radiation are absorbed by water impurities (<2.9 μm) and by the SiO_2 lattice itself (wavelengths >5 μm), as described by Levi [1980].

Since the flexibility, small diameter, and small mechanical inertia of optical fibers allow their use in either flexible or rigid endoscopes and offer significantly less inertia to hand movement, fibers for use at longer IR wavelengths are desired by clinicians. Currently, researchers are evaluating optical fiber materials transparent to longer IR wavelengths. Material systems showing promise are fused Al_2O_3 fibers in short lengths for use with near-3-μm radiation of the Er:YAG laser and Ag $halide$ fibers in short lengths for use with the CO_2 laser emitting at 10.6 μm [Merberg, 1993]. A flexible hollow Teflon waveguide 1.6 mm in diameter having a thin metal film overlain by a dielectric layer has been reported recently to transmit 10.6 μm CO_2 radiation with attenuation of 1.3 and 1.65 dB/m for straight and bent (5-mm radius, 90-degree bend) sections, respectively [Gannot et al., 1994].

64.9.1   Optical Fiber Transmission Characteristics

Guiding of the emitted laser beam along the optical fiber, typically of uniform circular cross-section, is due to total internal reflection of the radiation at the interface between the wall of the optical fiber core and the cladding material having refractive index n_1 less than that of the core n_2 [Levi, 1980]. Total internal reflection occurs for any angle of incidence θ of the propagating beam with the wall of the fiber core such that $\theta > \theta_c$ where

$$\sin \theta_c = \left(\frac{n_1}{n_2} \right) \tag{64.2}$$

or in terms of the complementary angle α_c

$$\cos \alpha_c = \left(\frac{n_1}{n_2} \right) \tag{64.3}$$

For a focused input beam with apical angle α_m incident upon the flat face of the fiber as shown in Figure 64.1, total internal reflection and beam guidance within the fiber core will occur [Levi, 1980] for

$$\mathrm{NA} = \sin(\alpha_m/2) \leq \left[n_2^2 - n_1^2 \right]^{0.5} \tag{64.4}$$

where NA is the numerical aperture of the fiber.

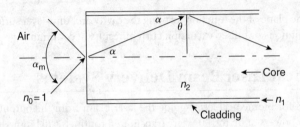

FIGURE 64.1 Critical reflection and propagation within an optical fiber.

This relationship ensures that the critical angle of incidence of the interface is not exceeded and that total internal reflection occurs [Levi, 1980]. Typical values of NA for fused SiO_2 fibers with polymer cladding are in the range of 0.36 to 0.40. The typical values of $\alpha_m = 14$ degrees used to insert the beam of the biomedical laser into the fiber is much smaller than those values ($\simeq 21$ to 23 degrees) corresponding to typical NA values. The maximum value of the propagation angle α typically used in biomedical laser systems is $\simeq 4.8$ degrees.

Leakage of radiation at the core–cladding interface of the fused SiO_2 fiber is negligible, typically being 0.3 dB/m at 400 nm and 0.01 dB/m at 1.064 μm. Bends along the fiber length always decrease the angle of the incidence at the core–cladding interface. Bends do not give appreciable losses for values of the bending radius sufficiently large that the angle of incidence θ of the propagating beam in the bent core does not becomes less than θ_c at the core–cladding interface [Levi, 1980]. The relationship given by Levi [1980] between the bending radius r_b, the fiber core radius r_0, the ratio (n_2/n_1) of fiber core to cladding refractive indices, and the propagation angle α in Figure 64.1 which ensures that the beam does not escape is

$$\frac{n_1}{n_2} > \frac{1-\rho}{1+\rho} \cos\alpha \tag{64.5}$$

where $\rho = (r_0/r_b)$. The inequality will hold for all $\alpha \le \alpha_c$ provided that

$$\frac{n_1}{n_2} \le \frac{1-\rho}{1+\rho} \tag{64.6}$$

Thus, the critical bending radius r_{bc} is the value of r_b such that Equation 64.6 is an equality. Use of Equation 64.6 predicts that bends with radii ≥ 12, 18, and 30 mm, respectively, will not result in appreciable beam leakage from fibers having 400-, 600-, and 1000-μm diameter cores, which are typical in biomedical use. Thus, use of fibers in flexible endoscopes usually does not compromise beam guidance.

Because the integrity of the core–cladding interface is critical to beam guiding, the clad fiber is encased typically in a tough but flexible protective fluoropolymer buffer coat.

64.9.2 Mirrored Articulated Arm Characteristics

Typically two or three relatively long tubular sections or arms of 50 to 80 cm length make up the portion of the articulated arm that extends from the laser output fixturing to the handpiece, endoscope, or operating microscope stage used to position the laser beam onto the tissue proper. Mirrors placed at the articulation of the arms and within the articulated handpiece, laparoscope, or operating microscope stage maintain the centration of the trajectory of the laser beam along the length of the delivery system. Dielectric multilayer mirrors [Levi, 1980] are routinely used in articulated devices. Their low high reflectivity $\le 99.9 +\%$ and power-handling capabilities ensure efficient power transmission down the arm. Mirrors in articulated devices typically are held in kinetically adjustable mounts for rapid stable alignment to maintain beam concentration.

64.9.3   Optics for Beam Shaping on Tissues

Since the rate of heating on tissue, and hence rates of ablation and coagulation, depends directly on energy input per unit volume of tissue, selection of ablation and coagulation rates of various tissues is achieved through control of the energy density (J/cm^2 or W sec/cm^2) of the laser beam. This parameter is readily achieved through use of optical elements such as discrete focusing lenses placed in the handpiece or rigid endoscope which control the spot size upon the tissue surface or by affixing a so-called contact tip to the end of an optical fiber. These are conical or spherical in shape with diameters ranging from 300 to 1200 μm and with very short focal lengths. The tip is placed in contact with the tissue and generates a submillimeter-sized focal spot in tissue very near the interface between the tip and tissue. One advantage of using the contact tip over a focused beam is that ablation proceeds with small lateral depth of attendant coagulation [Judy et al., 1993a]. This is because the energy of the tightly focused beam causes tissue thermolysis essentially at the tip surface and because the resulting tissue products strongly absorb the beam resulting in energy deposition and ablation essentially at the tip surface. This contrasts with the radiation penetrating deeply into tissue before thermolysis which occurs with a less tightly focused beam from a free lens or fiber. An additional advantage with the use of contact tips in the perception of the surgeon is that the kinesthetics of moving a contact tip along a resisting tissue surface more closely mimics the "touch" encountered in moving a scalpel across the tissue surface.

Recently a class of optical fiber tips has been developed which laterally directs the beam energy from a silica fiber [Judy et al., 1993b]. These tips, either a gold reflective micromirror or an angled refractive prism, offer a lateral angle of deviation ranging from 35 to 105 degrees from the optical fiber axis (undeviated beam direction). The beam reflected from a plane micromirror is unfocused and circular in cross-section, whereas the beam from a concave mirror and refractive devices is typically elliptical in shape, fused with distal diverging rays. Fibers with these terminations are currently finding rapidly expanding, large-scale application in coagulation (with 1.064-μm Nd:YAG laser radiation) of excess tissue lining the urethra in treatment of benign prostatic hypertrophy [Costello et al., 1992]. The capability for lateral beam direction may offer additional utility of these terminated fibers in other clinical specialties.

64.9.4   Features of Routinely Used Biomedical Lasers

Currently four lasers are in routine large-scale clinical biomedical use to ablate, dissect, and to coagulate soft tissue. Two, the carbon dioxide (CO_2) and argon ion (Ar-ion) lasers, are gas-filled lasers. The other two employ solid-state lasing media. One is the Neodymium–yttrium–aluminum–garnet (Nd:YAG) laser, commonly referred to as a solid-state laser, and the other is the gallium–aluminum arsenide (GaAlAs) semiconductor diode laser. Salient features of the operating characteristics and biomedical applications of those lasers are listed in Table 64.2 to Table 64.5. The operational descriptions are typical of the lasers currently available commercially and do not represent the product of any single manufacturer.

64.9.5   Other Biomedical Lasers

Some important biomedical lasers have smaller-scale use or currently are being researched for biomedical application. The following four lasers have more limited scales of surgical use:

The Ho:YAG (Holmium:YAG) laser, emitting pulses of 2.1 μm wavelength and up to 4 J in energy, used in soft tissue ablation in arthroscopic (joint) surgery (FDA approved).

The Q-switched Ruby ($Cr:Al_2O_3$) laser, emitting pulses of 694-nm wavelength and up to 2 J in energy is used in dermatology to disperse black, blue, and green tattoo pigments and melanin in pigmented lesions (not melanoma) for subsequent removal by phagocytosis by macrophages (FDA approved).

The flashlamp pumped pulsed dye laser emitting 1- to 2-J pulses at either 577- or 585-nm wavelength (near the 537–577 absorption region of blood) is used for treatment of cutaneous vascular lesions and melanin pigmented lesions except melanoma. Use of pulsed radiation helps to localize the thermal damage to within the lesions to obtain low damage of adjacent tissue.

The following lasers are being investigated for clinical uses.

1. The Er:YAG laser, emitting at 2.94 μm near the major water absorption peak (OH stretch), is currently being investigated for ablation of tooth enamel and dentin (Li et al., 1992)
2. Dye lasers emitting at 630 to 690 nm are being investigated for application as light sources for exciting dihematoporphyrin ether or benzoporphyrin derivatives in investigation of the efficacy of these photosensitives in the treatment of esophageal, bronchial, and bladder carcinomas for the FDA approved process

TABLE 64.2 Operating Characteristics of Principal Biomedical Lasers

Characteristics	Ar ion laser	CO_2 laser
Cavity medium	Argon gas, 133 Pa	10% CO_2 10% Ne, 80% He; 1330 Pa
Lasing species	Ar+ ion	CO_2 molecule
Excitation	Electric discharge, continuous	Electric discharge, continuous, pulsed
Electric input	208 V_{AC}, 60 A	110 V_{AC}, 15 A
Wall plug efficiency	$\simeq$0.06%	$\simeq$10%
characteristics	Nd:YAG laser	GaAlAs diode laser
Cavity medium	Nd-dopted YAG	n-p junction, GaAlAs diode
Lasing species	Nd3t in YAG lattice	Hole-electron pairs at diode junction
Excitation	Flashlamp, continuous, pulsed	Electric current, continuous pulsed
Electric input	208/240 V_{AC}, 30 A continuous 110 V_{AC}, 10 A pulsed	110 V_{AC}, 15A
Wall plug efficiency	$\simeq$1%	$\simeq$ 23%

TABLE 64.3 Output Beam Characteristics of Ar-Ion and CO_2 Biomedical Lasers

Output characteristics	Argon laser	CO_2 laser
Output power	2–8 W, continuous	1–100 W, continuous
Wavelength (sec)	Multiple lines (454.6–528.7 nm), 488, 514.5 dominant	10.6 μm
Electromagnetic wave propagation mode	TEM_{∞}	TEM_{∞}
Beam guidance, shaping	Fused silica optical fiber with contact tip or flat-ended for beam emission, lensed handpiece. Slit lamp with ocular lens	Flexible articulated arm with mirrors; lensed handpiece or mirrored microscope platen

TABLE 64.4 Output Beam Characteristics of Nd:YAG and GaAlAs Diode Biomedical Lasers

Output characteristics	Nd:YAG lasers	GaAlAs diode laser
Output power	1–100 W continuous at 1.064 millimicron 1–36 W continuous at 532 nm (frequency doubled with KTP)	1–25 W continuous
Wavelength(sec)	1.064 μm/532 nm	810 nm
Electromagnetic wave propagation modes	Mixed modes	Mixed modes
Beam guidance and shaping	Fused SiO_2 optical fiber with contact tip directing mirrored or refracture tip	Fused SiO_2 optical fiber with contact tip or laterally directing mirrored or refracture tip

TABLE 64.5 Clinical Uses of Principal Biomedical Lasers

Ar-ion laser	*CO$_2$ laser*
Pigmented (vascular) soft-tissue ablation in gynecology; general and oral sugery; otolaryngology; vascular lesion coagulation in dermatology; retinal coagulation in ophthalmology	Soft-tissue ablation — dissection and bulk tissue removal in dermatology; gynecology; general, oral, plastic, and neurosurgery; otolaryngology; podiatry; urology
Nd:YAG laser	*GaAlAs diode laser*
Soft-tissue, particularly pigmented vascular tissue, ablation — dissection and bulk tissue removal — in dermatology; gastroenterology; gynecology; general, arthroscopic, neuro-plastic, and thoracic surgery; urology; posterior capsulotomy (ophthalmology) with pulsed 1.064 millimicron and ocular lens	Pigmented (vascular) soft-tissue ablation — dissection and bulk removal in gynecology; gastroenterology, general, surgery, and urology; FDA approval for otolaryngology and thoracic surgery pending

Defining Terms

Biomedical Laser Radiation Ranges

Infrared (IR) radiation: The portion of the electromagnetic spectrum within the wavelength range 760 nm–1 mm, with the regions 760 nm–1.400 μm and 1.400–10.00 μm, respectively, called the near- and mid-IR regions.

Ultraviolet (UV) radiation: The portion of the electromagnetic spectrum within the wavelength range 100–400 nm.

Visible (VIS) radiation: The portion of the electromagnetic spectrum within the wavelength range 400–760 nm.

Laser Medium Nomenclature

Argon fluoride (ArF): Argon fluoride eximer laser (an eximer is a diatomic molecule which can exist only in an excited state).

Ar ion: Argon ion.

CO$_2$: Carbon dioxide.

Cr:Al$_2$0$_3$: Ruby laser.

Er:YAG: Erbium yttrium aluminum garnet.

GaAlAs: Gallium aluminum laser.

HeNe: Helium neon laser.

Ho:YAG: Holmium yttrium aluminum garnet.

Nd:YAG: Neodymium yttrium aluminum garnet.

Optical Fiber Nomenclature

Ag halide: Silver halide, halide ion, typically bromine (Br) and chlorine (Cl).

Fused silica: Fused SiO$_2$.

References

Bass L.S., Moazami N., Pocsidio J. et al. (1992). Change in type I collagen following laser welding. *Lasers Surg. Med.* 12: 500.

Costello A.J., Johnson D.E., and Bolton D.M. (1992). Nd:YAG laser ablation of the prostate as a treatment for benign prostate hypertrophy. *Lasers Surg. Med.* 12: 121.

Fitzpatrick R.E. (1993). Comparison of the Q-switched ruby, Nd:YAG, and alexandrite lasers in tattoo removal. *Lasers Surg. Med.* (Suppl.) 6: 52.

Gannot I., Dror J., Calderon S. et al. (1994). Flexible waveguides for IR laser radiation and surgery applications. *Lasers Surg. Med.* 14: 184.

Garrison B.J. and Srinivasan R. (1985). Laser ablation of organic polymers: microscopic models for photochemical and thermal processes. *J. Appl. Physiol.* 58: 2909.

Grossweiner L.I. (1989). Photophysics. In K.C. Smith (Ed.), *The Science of Photobiology*, pp. 1–47. New York, Plenum.

Hale G.M. and Querry M.R. (1973). Optical constants of water in the 200 nm to 200 μm wavelength region. *Appl. Opt.* 12: 555.

Hibst R., Bende T., and Schröder D. (1992). Wet corneal ablation by Er:YAG laser radiation. *Lasers Surg. Med.* (Suppl.) 4: 56.

Hill R.A., Le M.T., Yashiro H. et al. (1993). Ab-interno erbium (Er:YAG) laser sclerostomy with iridotomy in dutch cross rabbits. *Lasers Surg. Med.* 13: 559.

Judy M.M., Matthews J.L., Aronoff B.L. et al. (1993a). Soft tissue studies with 805 nm diode laser radiation: thermal effects with contact tips and comparison with effects of 1064 nm. Nd:YAG laser radiation. *Lasers Surg. Med.* 13: 528.

Judy M.M., Matthews J.L., Gardetto W.W. et al. (1993b). Side firing laser-fiber technology for minimally invasive transurethral treatment of benign prostate hyperplasia. *Proc. Soc. Photo-Opt. Instr. Eng. (SPIE)* 1982: 86.

Judy M.M., Matthews J.L., Goodson J.R. et al. (1992). Thermal effects in tissues from simultaneous coaxial CO_2 and Nd:YAG laser beams. *Lasers Surg. Med.* 12: 222.

Katoh N. and Peyman G.A. (1988). Effects of laser wavelengths on experimental retinal detachments and retinal vessels. *Jpn. J. Ophthalmol.* 32: 196.

Keye W.R., Matson G.A., and Dixon J. (1983). The use of the argon laser in treatment of experimental endometriosis. *Fertil. Steril.* 39: 26.

Lakowicz J.R. (1983). *Principles of Fluorescence Spectroscopy.* New York, Plenum.

Lengyel B.A. (1971). *Lasers.* New York, John Wiley.

Levi L. (1980). *Applied Optics,* Vol. 2. New York, John Wiley.

Li Z.Z., Code J.E., and Van de Merve W.P. (1992). Er:YAG laser ablation of enamel and dentin of human teeth: determination of ablation rates at various fluences and pulse repetition rates. *Lasers Surg. Med.* 12: 625.

Maes K.E. and Sherk H.H. (1994). Bone and meniscal ablation using the erbium YAG laser. *Lasers Surg. Med.* (Suppl.) 6: 31.

Mahadevan A., Mitchel M.F., Silva E. et al. (1993). Study of the fluorescence properties of normal and neoplastic human cervical tissue. *Lasers Surg. Med.* 13: 647.

McGillis S.T., Bailin P.L., Fitzpatrick R.E. et al. (1994). Successful treatments of blue, green, brown and reddish-brown tattoos with the Q-switched alexandrite laser. *Laser Surg. Med.* (Suppl.) 6: 52.

Meijering L.J.T., VanGermert M.J.C., Gijsbers G.H.M. et al. (1993). Limits of radial time constants to approximate thermal response of tissue. *Lasers Surg. Med.* 13: 685.

Merberg G.N. (1993). Current status of infrared fiberoptics for medical laser power delivery. *Lasers Surg. Med.* 13: 572.

Miller I.D. and Veitch A.R. (1993). Optical modeling of light distributions in skin tissue following laser irradiation. *Lasers Surg. Med.* 13: 565.

Mordon S., Beacco C., Rotteleur G. et al. (1993). Relation between skin surface temperature and minimal blanching during argon, Nd:YAG 532, and cw dye 585 laser therapy of port-wine stains. *Lasers Surg. Med.* 13: 124.

Motamedi M., Torres J.H., Cammack T. et al. (1993). Thermodynamics of cw laser interaction with prostatic tissue: effects of simultaneous cooling on lesion size. *Lasers Surg. Med.* (Suppl.) 5: 64.

Oz M.C., Chuck R.S., Johnson J.P. et al. (1989). Indocyanine green dye-enhanced welding with a diode laser. *Surg. Forum* 40: 316.

Rastegar S., Jacques S.C., Motamedi M. et al. (1992). Theoretical analysis of high-power diode laser (810 nm) and Nd:YAG laser (1064 nm) for coagulation of tissue: predictions for prostate coagulation. *Proc. Soc. Photo-Opt. Instr. Eng. (SPIE)* 1646: 150.

Schroder T., Brackett K., and Joffe S. (1987). An experimental study of effects of electrocautery and various lasers on gastrointestinal tissue. *Surgery* 101: 691.

Spikes J.D. (1989). Photosensitization. In K.C. Smith (Ed.), *The Science of Photobiology*, 2nd ed., pp. 79–110. New York, Plenum.

Van de Hulst H.C. (1957). *Light Scattering by Small Particles.* New York, John Wiley.

Van Saarloos P.P. and Constable I.J. (1993). Improved eximer laser photorefractive keratectomy system. *Lasers Surg. Med.* 13: 189.

White A., Handler P., and Smith E.L. (1968). *Principles of Biochemistry*, 4th ed. New York, McGraw-Hill.

Further Information

Current research on the optical, thermal, and photochemical interactions of radiation and their effect on biologic tissues, are published routinely in the journals: *Laser in Medicine and Surgery, Lasers in the Life Sciences,* and *Photochemistry Photobiology* and to a lesser extent in *Applied Optics and Optical Engineering.*

Clinical evaluations of biomedical laser applications appear in *Lasers and Medicine and Surgery* and in journals devoted to clinical specialties such as *Journal of General Surgery, Journal of Urology, Journal of Gastroenterological Surgery.*

The annual symposium proceedings of the biomedical section of the Society of Photo-Optical Instrumentation Engineers (SPIE) contain descriptions of new and current research on application of lasers and optics in biomedicine.

The book *Lasers* (a second edition by Bela A. Lengyel), although published in 1971, remains a valuable resource on the fundamental physics of lasers—gas, dye solid-state, and semiconducting diode. A more recent book, *The Laser Guidebook* by Jeffrey Hecht, published in 1992, emphasizes the technical characteristics of the gas, diode, solid-state, and semiconducting diode lasers.

The *Journal of Applied Physics, Physical Review Letters,* and *Applied Physics Letters* carry descriptions of the newest advances and experimental phenomena in lasers and optics.

The book *Safety with Lasers and Other Optical Sources* by David Sliney and Myron Wolbarsht, published in 1980, remains a very valuable resource on matters of safety in laser use.

Laser safety standards for the United States are given for all laser uses and types in the American National Standard (ANSI) Z136.1-1993, Safe Use of Lasers.

65

Instrumentation for Cell Mechanics

65.1 Background **65**-1
65.2 Cellular Mechanics...................................... **65**-2
65.3 Scaling Laws **65**-4
65.4 Measurement of Cellular Force **65**-5
        Membrane Wrinkling • Traction Force Microscopy •
        Micro-Cantilever Force Sensors
65.5 Conclusion **65**-9
Acknowledgments... **65**-10
References **65**-10

Nathan J. Sniadecki
Christopher S. Chen
University of Pennsylvania

65.1 Background

Mechanical forces are essential to life at the microscale — from tethering at the junctions between cells that compose a tissue to externally applied loads arising in the cellular environment. Consider the perturbations from acoustic sounds that affect the mechanosensors on auditory hair cells in the inner ear, the contractile forces that a dividing cell imparts on itself in order to split into two daughter cells during cytokinesis, or the bone and muscle loss that occurs from the reduced loads in microgravity [1,2]. Mechanical forces are particularly important in the cardiovascular and musculoskeletal systems [3]. Increased shear stress in the blood flow leads to the dilation and restructuring of blood vessels [4]. The immune response of leukocytes requires that they adhere to and transmigrate through the endothelial barrier of blood vessels [5]. The forces required between leukocytes and endothelium, and between neighboring endothelial cells, in order to execute such complex events have become an important avenue of research [6,7]. Arterial hypertension causes the underlying vessel walls to constrict, preventing local aneurysms and vessel failure [3]. Long-term exposure to such hypertension leads to increased thickening and stiffing of the vessel walls causing vessel stenosis. In the skeletal system, exercise-induced compressive forces increase bone and cartilage mass and strength while subnormal stresses, from bedrest, immobilization, or space travel, results in decreased bone mass [2]. Despite the clear demonstration that mechanical forces are an essential factor in the daily life of many cells and tissues, the underlying question remains to understand how these forces exert their effects.

A key insight to these areas of study has been that nearly all of the adaptive processes are regulated at the cellular level. That is, many of the tissue responses to forces are actually cellular responses. The contraction and hyperproliferation of smooth muscle cells embedded within the arteries in response to hypertension causes the vessel wall constriction and thickening. Changes in bone mass result from both changes in the production of new bone cells and the metabolic capacity of the existing bone cells. For example, mesenchymal stems cells have been found to differentiate into bone-producing osteoblasts if they are allowed to experience mechanical stresses generated between the individual cells and their local surroundings, but become fat-storing adipocytes when such stresses are eliminated [8]. Thus, an understanding of the importance of forces to medicine and biology must first derive from a better characterization of the forces acting at the single cell level. To begin to explore and characterize the forces experienced and generated by cells (cellular forces), engineers are taking a two-pronged approach. First, they are developing a better understanding of the cell as a mechanical object; and second, they are employing new tools for analyzing cellular forces in the micro and nanoscale.

The measurement of cellular forces is a difficult task because cells are active. That is, they continually change and adapt their mechanical structure in response to their surroundings. The primary mechanical elements in cells are polymers of proteins — in particular, actin, tubulin, and intermediate filament proteins — that are collectively called the cytoskeleton. These cytoskeletal scaffolding structures are continually disassembling and reassembling, realigning, renetworking, contracting, and lengthening. Perhaps one of the most fascinating and simultaneously challenging aspects of characterizing these mechanical rearrangements is that they often occur in direct response to mechanical perturbations. If one pulls on a corner of a cell to measure its material response, it will adjust to the perturbation with reinforcement at the point of applied force. If one places a cell on a soft substrate, it will adjust its shape to achieve a balance between its contractile forces generated by its cytoskeleton and the adhesion forces at its extracellular foundation. The dynamic response of cells to such forces makes the characterization of the natural state of cells difficult. Nonetheless, one of the major goals of mechanobiology is not only to characterize cellular mechanics, but also to identify the mechanism by which cells sense, transduce, and respond to mechanical forces. Whether the mechanosensor itself is an individual protein, a network of structures, or some novel control process remains to be determined. Due to the intimate interaction between the properties of the cell and the techniques used to measure them, we will first provide a brief introduction to the mechanics of the cells themselves, followed by the techniques used to measure the forces that they generate. In addition, since cells are quite small, we will provide a brief discussion of scaling laws and emphasize the technical challenges associated with measuring forces at this length scale.

65.2 Cellular Mechanics

The behavior and function of a cell is dependent to a large degree on the cytoskeleton which consists of three polymer filament systems — microfilaments, intermediate filaments, and microtubules. Acting together as a system, these cytoskeleton filament proteins serve as the scaffolding in the cytoplasm of the cell that (1) supports the delicate cell membrane, (2) tethers and secures organelles in position or guide their transport through the cytoplasm, and (3) in conjunction with various motor proteins, the machinery that provides force necessary for locomotion or protrusion formation [1]. Microfilaments are helical polymers formed from actin that organize into parallel bundles for filopodia extensions and contractile stress fibers or into extensively cross-linked networks at the leading edge of a migrating cell and throughout the cell cortex that supports the cell membrane (Figure 65.1b). Microtubules have tubulin subunits and form long, hollow cylinders that emanate from a single centrosome, which is located near the nucleus (Figure 65.1c). Of the three types of cytoskeletal filaments, microtubules have the higher bending resistance and act to resist compression [9]. Intermediate filaments form extensive networks within the cytoplasm that extend circumferentially from the meshwork structure that surrounds the nucleus (Figure 65.1d). These rope-like filaments are easy to bend but difficult to break. They are particularly predominant in the cytoplasm of cells that are subject to mechanical stress, which highlights their role in tissue-strengthening [10]. Since these three subcellular structures have distinct mechanical properties and varying concentrations between cells, the measured cellular forces and mechanical properties of a particular cell may not be the same as the next cell.

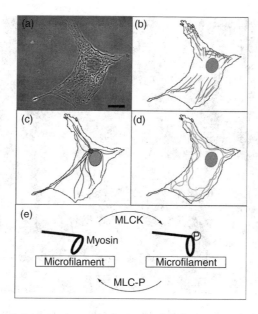

FIGURE 65.1 Cells have cytoskeletal structures that determine their force generation machinery. (a) Phase contract image of 3T3 fibroblast (bar: 10 μm). The diagram shows the general shape and location of (b) microfilaments, (c) microtubules, and (d) intermediate filaments. (e) Schematic of conventional actomyosin motor for cellular forces.

Microfilaments, when coupled with the motor protein myosin, generate the cellular forces that influence the function of the cell and surrounding tissue. Often, skeletal muscle cells come to mind when one thinks of cellular force generation. Cardiac muscle, striated muscle, smooth muscle, and myoepithelial cells, all of which originate from a common precursor myoblast cell, employ a contractile system involving actin as the filament and myosin as the motor protein. Myosin binds to the microfilaments and moves along it in a step-wise linear ratchet mechanism as a means to generate contractile force. Although well studied in muscle, the same actomyosin contractile apparatus found in skeletal muscle cells is present in nearly all cell types. Myosin changes its structure during cycles of phosphorylation, regulated by myosin light chain kinase (MLCK) and myosin light chain phosphatase (MLC-P), to create power strokes that advance the head of the protein along the filament (Figure 65.1e). Each cycle advances the myosin head about 5 nm along the actin filament and produces an average force of 3 to 4 pN [11]. The interaction of myosin and actin is not a constant machine but instead is cycled as dictated by the upstream signaling pathways that regulate MLCK and MLC-P.

A highly researched aspect of cellular forces that highlight their dynamic nature is cell locomotion. These forces, aptly named traction forces, are medically relevant for the metastasis of cancer and occurs when a sessile cell develops the ability to migrate from the tumor and into the bloodstream. Additionally, embryonic development, tissue formation, and wound healing exemplify the physiological relevance of cell migration. The mechanism that generates cell locomotion depends on the coordination of changes in cell shape, via restructuring of the cytoskeletal filaments, and shifting of adhesion sites to the extracellular matrix. When a cell moves forward, it extends a protrusion at the leading edge via microtubule formation and actin polymerization to create new adhesion sites, which are called focal adhesions or focal contacts (Figure 65.2). These nonuniformly distributed, punctate structures link the cytoskeletal filaments and the motor proteins to the substrate and are present at both ends of a migrating cell. After forming new attachments, the cell contracts to move the cell body forward by disassembling contacts at the back end. The locomotion is continued in a treadmill fashion of front protrusion and rear contraction. On account of its dynamic response, a cell does not have uniform mechanical properties and certainly cannot be regarded as a Hookean material with time-independent and linear material properties. As a result, a classical continuum model for the cell has not provided significant insight into the basis for the mechanical properties of a cell.

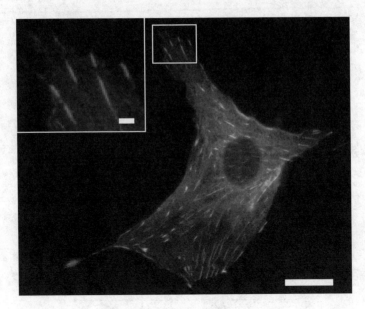

FIGURE 65.2   Immunofluorescence staining of focal adhesions (bar: 10 μm, inset bar: 2 μm).

To understand both the signaling pathways that control these cytoskeletal processes and the resultant mechanics of cell force-generation, researchers have begun to develop methods to measure these forces. To coordinate a global response with other cells of the tissue to a particular stimulus, there exists a complex mechanism of communication between the cells within a tissue. Often cellular signaling, or communication, is mediated by the release of soluble chemicals or growth factors. When these chemicals diffuse across populations of cells, each cell detects the signal via specific receptors and responds accordingly. One of the most challenging aspects of studying cellular mechanics, however, is that cells are also able to detect physical changes even under a constant chemical environment, and respond with changes in cellular function or mechanical state. The sensing and translation of mechanical signals into a functional biochemical signal is known as mechanotransduction. One of the sites in which mechanotransduction occurs is at focal adhesions. A critical engineering challenge in understanding how cells sense and control cellular forces is to characterize the nanonewton forces at these adhesion sites, and correlate these forces with the intercellular signaling response of mechanotransduction.

Based on these insights about the cells and their intracellular structure, it is clear that how one chooses to measure cellular forces can affect the measurements themselves. Since the mechanical properties of a cell are non-Hookean, one can consider the cell to have a history or a memory. Similar to hysteresis of materials, the loadings of forces on a cell have a time-dependent response and so a cell is often modeled as a viscoelastic material — a soft glassy material. As a result, the procedural conditions of a particular experiment must be examined for a time-dependent response. Thus, the observer needs to consider whether to measure the range of forces exerted by one cell to obtain the direct time-response but with a limited data population, or to interrogate a large number of cells with many cellular forces and only report the average value, thereby disregarding the effect that transitions between loading conditions have on a cell. These considerations should act as a simple warning that one must treat each new system, device, and resulting data on cellular mechanics with a healthy degree of guarded skepticism. Despite such concerns, investigators have begun to develop numerous tools that ultimately will address these issues.

65.3   Scaling Laws

In addition to the difficulty in measuring the nanonewton-scale forces that cells exert on the extracellular matrix or at cellular interconnects, the spots where these forces are applied are subcellular (micrometer and nanometer-scale) in dimension. Microscale detection is required in order to measure the different traction forces that are applied at the front vs. the back of a migrating cells. Moreover, since mechanical stresses appear to be sensed and applied at individual focal adhesions (ranging in size from 0.1 to 2 μm^2), it is pertinent to have spatial resolution in the submicron range (Figure 65.2). To obtain the microscale measurement power for studying cellular mechanics, researchers have turned to new techniques and tools. However, in their development, one must consider the impact of scaling laws on the design of the tool. At the micrometer or nanometer scale, the ratio of surface area to volume dramatically differs from the length scale to which we are accustomed. Thus, surface forces dominate over body forces since the former scales with the inverse of the square of the length (L^{-2}) while the later scales with the inverse of the length to the third power (L^{-3}). For example, adhesion forces and fluid shear forces are often more critical to the function of a cell than those of gravity [2,4]. The microscale forces that compose the environment of a cell are difficult to measure with the types of tools that are typically used at the macroscale.

Not only must the designer of these new tools consider the types of forces they want to measure, but also how they will transfer the data to some readable form. Using a microscope to read the measurements from the tool is a noninvasive technique that does not require direct connections to the substrate. However, the technique does require that the substrate be optically transparent, which limits materials available for fabrication, and has optical limitations in resolving below hundreds of nanometers. Despite the limitations, coupling microscopy with a force sensor does provide improved measurement read-out capabilities over other techniques such as electronics, which have sensitivity limitations due to the low signal to noise ratio from thermal and charge fluctuations in the aqueous environment and integration complexity in constructing the electrical components on the same substrate as the force sensors.

In scaling down to the cellular level, the development of the measuring instruments becomes dependent on experimental materials and microfabrication. Typical hard materials used in strain gauges and springs do not bend under nanonewton loadings with the same displacement that is required for measurement sensitivity. On account of this, soft materials are employed in the construction of the microsensors, even though these thin-film materials are not as fully characterized as their bulk material counterparts. Additionally, as the surface to volume ratio increases at the microscale, the effect of the different chemical composition at the surface of the material, such as the native oxide layers of iron, copper, or silicon, may have more dramatic effects on the overall material properties. In building devices with these materials, the microfabrication techniques used must have good reliability for repeatable and uniform measurements on the device. Even though the equipment used in microfabrication is engineered to deposit material with uniform properties and thickness across the device, tolerance issues are still pertinent because of the topological effect that a micrometer defect can have on the environment that the cell senses. Most of the microsensors are made one at a time or in limited batches and consistency in the fabrication methods is critical for repeatable measurements. In conclusion, the devices detailed in the following sections are powerful measurement tools for detecting the nanoscale cellular forces but are still prototypes, in which consistency in their construction is important to corroborating the scientific discoveries that they provide.

65.4 Measurement of Cellular Force

Studying the forces that cells exert on their microenvironment and their corresponding biological mechanisms generally involve culturing cells on flexible substrates that the cells physically deform when applying their contraction or traction forces. When the stiffness of the substrate has been characterized, then optical measurement of the substrate distortion reports the cellular force. A relationship between force and displacement holds whether the substrate is a film of polyacrylamide gel that distorts under the force of a contracting cell adhered to it or silicone microcantilevers that are deflected under the forces of a migrating cell. In the early 1980s, Albert Harris first pioneered the method of measuring cellular forces on thin films of silicone that wrinkled upon the force of the adherent cells and has since evolved into devices that use microfabrication techniques to obtain improved precision of their force sensors.

65.4.1 Membrane Wrinkling

The thin membranes of liquid silicon rubber were cross-linked when exposed briefly to flame so that a thin skin of rubber was cured to ~1 μm thickness on top of the remaining liquid rubber that served as the lubricant layer between the glass coverslip [12,13]. Cells could be cultured on the silicone rubber, which is optically transparent and nontoxic, and as they spread on the skin surface, the adhesion forces they applied to the skin were strong enough to produce wrinkles and fold in the skin (Figure 65.3a). Directly underneath the cell, the wrinkles were circumferential with the cell boundary indicating that compressive forces created the folds in the membrane. At areas surrounding the adherent cell, the wrinkles projected out along radial lines from the cell boundary along the axes of tension forces. No observation of the cell pushing against the silicone membrane has been observed. This technique was a breakthrough in that cellular forces had not been experimentally observed and that qualitative measurement of the different regions of compression and tension could be observed simultaneously.

The membrane wrinkling technique has recently been improved upon with an additional fabrication step to reduce the stiffness of the substrate for increased wrinkles and folds and semi-quantitative

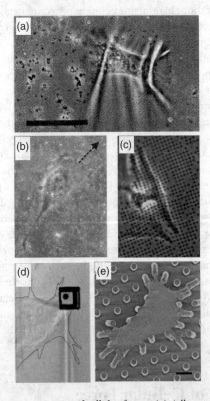

FIGURE 65.3 Techniques for the measurement of cellular forces. (a) Adherent fibroblast cell exerts forces strong enough to wrinkle the underlying silicone rubber membrane (black bar: 50 μm). (Reproduced from Harris, A.K., P. Wild, and D. Stopak, *Science*, 1980, **208**: 177–179.) (b) Traction forces from migrating fibroblast (arrow indicates direction) are measured from the displacement of fluorescent microparticles embedded in a polyacrylamide substrate. (Reproduced from Munevar, S., Y.-L. Wang, and M. Dembo, *Biophys. J.*, 2001, **80**: 1744–1757.) (c) Contracting fibroblast distorts the regular array of micropatterned fluorescent dots. (Reproduced from Balaban, N.Q. et al., *Nat. Cell Biol.*, 2001, **3**: 466–472.) (d) Bending of horizontal microcantilever locally reports the traction force of a subcellular region during fibroblast migration. (Reproduced from Galbraith, C.G. and M.P. Sheetz, *Proc. Natl Acad. Sci.*, USA, 1997, **94**: 9114–9118.) (e) Local contraction forces of smooth muscle cell are measured with an array of vertical elastomeric microcantilevers that deflect under cellular forces (black bar: 10 μm). (From Tan, J.L. et al., *Proc. Natl Acad. Sci.*, USA, 2003, **100**: 1484–1489. With permission.)

measurement of cellular forces in the hundreds of nanonewtons range. After the flame curing, the membranes were exposed to UV irradiation to weaken the cross-linking of the silicon sheets [14,15]. Applying a known tip-force from a glass pipette on the surface of the membrane and measuring the resultant wrinkles correlated the distortion and force relationship. Specifically, the researchers determined that the length of the wrinkles formed from the pipette was linear with the applied force and called it the "wrinkle stiffness." Using this new technique, they observed that cytokinesis occurs through increased contractility at the equator of the cell, near the cleavage furrow. The traction force drops as the two daughter cells pinch apart. The newly formed cells migrate away from each other resulting in an increase in traction wrinkles until a strong enough force is generated to rupture the intercellular junction. The observed elastic recoil when the daughter cells break their junction causes them to rapidly separate and there is a relaxation in the surrounding wrinkles. Furthermore, the increased number of wrinkles in this technique allows for the measure of the different subcellular forces that occur during live cell migration. At the lamellipodium of a migrating cell, the wrinkles were radial and remain anchored to spots, possibly focal adhesion, as the cell advanced forward. Once these spots were located at the boundary between the lamellipodium and cell body, the wrinkles transitioned to compressive wrinkles. At the rear of the cell, the wrinkle forces diminished slower than the decreasing cell contact area so that the shear stress of the cell increased to pull it forward. The forces that occur at different regions of a cells attachment to the substrate reveal the coordination between pulling forces at the front of the cell and detachment forces that act against the migrating cell.

The membrane wrinkling technique is sensitive to cellular forces and can monitor the force changes at regions of interest within the adhesion area of a cell over time, but it is only a qualitative technique. It does not have adequate subcellular force resolution to measure the applied forces at the focal adhesions. Quantification of the force by means of the "wrinkle stiffness" is not an accurate measurement of forces due to the nonlinear lengthening of the wrinkles when forces are applied at multiple locations on the membrane. Moreover, the chaotic buckling of the membrane has a low repeatability, which makes matching the wrinkle patterns or lengths between experiments inaccurate.

65.4.2 Traction Force Microscopy

To address these issues, traction force microscopy, a technique employing a nonwrinkling elastic substrate, was developed for cell mechanics [16]. The device layout is similar to Harris et al. in that a thin, highly compliant polymer membrane is cured on a glass coverslip on which cells are cultured, except that the membrane is not allowed to wrinkle. In addition to silicone rubber, polyacrylamide membranes have been used as the flexible membrane for cell attachment [17,18]. Instead of wrinkles, fluorescent beads with nanometer diameter were embedded into the material during the fabrication to act as displacement markers (Figure 65.3b). Fixing the sides of the membrane to the edges of the coverslip enables a prestress to be added to the membrane, which suppresses the wrinkling but enables adequate flexibility to allow in-plane traction forces to create visible displacements of the beads. Subtracting the position of the beads under the forces that the cell exerts and the position once the cell was removed from the surface determined the small movements of the beads between the two states, that is, relative displacement field. The corresponding force mapping of the cell is translated from the displacement field, which involves complex mathematical methods requiring the use of a supercomputer. The results provide spatial resolution of $\sim 5 \mu$m to measure the forces at smaller areas underneath the cell.

In obtaining the corresponding force map, the beads do not move as an ideal spring, in which the displacement is directly proportional to the applied force. Instead, many beads move in response to a single traction force because of the continuous membrane and their movement diminishes as a function of distance from the point of traction. As a result, many force mappings may be possible solutions for the measured displacement field. Appropriate constraints must be applied to the calculation for the solution to converge to a proper solution. Additionally, the displacement beads are discrete markers that are randomly seeded with a nonuniform density, resulting in the lack of displacement information in regions of the cell. To postulate on the magnitude and direction of the forces in the area between beads, a grid meshing approximation is superimposed on the cell area during the force calculation in order to solve for the force and displacement relationship at all regions. In fact, the placement of mesh nodes in these sparse areas leads to an ill-posed problem in solving for the force map because often more force points are introduced than there are displacement data due to the random seeding of beads underneath the cell area. Despite these limitations, the solution for the membrane displacement is well addressed in linear elastic theory [19]. The membrane can be regarded as a semi-infinite space of an incompressible, elastic material with tangential forces applied only at the boundary plane. Under these assumptions, the displacement field, $d(\mathbf{m})$, and the stress field, $T(r)$ are related by an integral relation:

$$d_i(\mathbf{m}) = \iint G_{ij}(\mathbf{m} - \mathbf{r}) T_j(\mathbf{r}) \, d\mathbf{r} \qquad (65.1)$$

where $i, j \leq 2$ for the two-dimensional half-space and $G_{ij}(\mathbf{m} - \mathbf{r})$ is Green's function that relates the displacement at position $\mathbf{m}$ resulting from the point force at position $\mathbf{r}$. Obtaining the stress field requires inverting Equation 65.1, which is not always a unique solution because often there are not enough beads to determine all the force points. To address this problem, regularization schemes are used to apply additional criteria in selecting the solution of the inversion operation. These criteria include incorporating the constraint that the sum of all of the traction forces must balance, that the forces are only applied at the limited points of focal adhesions, and that the least complex solution be used.

In contrast to the random seeding of beads, microfabricated regular arrays of fluorescent beads have been imprinted onto the elastomeric substrate for improved force tracking [23]. The deformation of the marker pattern on the substrate is readily observed under the microscopy during the recording of a cell's forces (Figure 65.3c). The patterns are formed with Si and GaAs molds to create sub-micron spot diameters with 2 to 30 μm spacing. The calculation for the force mapping is similar to the random seeding but with significant reduction in the number of possible solutions due to the uniform density of displacement markers throughout the cell area. The simplification of the problem makes the calculation readily attainable on a standard PC. Moreover, the regular pattern improved measurement power of the technique to a force resolution of 2 nN.

65.4.3 Micro-Cantilever Force Sensors

In the previous methods, the use of a continuous membrane for measuring cell forces has the inherent disadvantage that the discrete forces applied at the focal adhesions are convoluted with distribution of displacements. Since the force calculation is not direct, constraints and selection criteria are required in order to solve for the appropriate force mapping. The lack of a direct, linear technique to transduce the physical substrate deformation into unique traction force readings has necessitated the use of microfabricated devices to measure cellular forces. An innovative approach is the use of microcantilevers that act as force transducers. The first demonstration of these sensors is a horizontal cantilever fabricated on a silicon wafer where the cell bends the cantilever in the plane of the traction force as it migrates across it (Figure 65.3d) [20,21]. Since the sensor is mechanically decoupled from the substrate, the deflection of the cantilever directly reports only the local force. The simple spring equation relates the visually measured deflection of the cantilever beam, δ to the cellular traction force:

$$F = K\delta \qquad (65.2)$$

where K is the measured spring constant for the cantilever. The devices are constructed out of a polysilicon thin-film that is deposited on top of a phosphosilicate glass sacrificial layer. Once the sacrificial layer is etched away, the beam is freestanding and fully deflected under the force of a cell. These fabrication steps are labor-intensive and expensive, hence these devices are often reused between experiments. Even though this technique has quick force calculation, the horizontal design of the cantilever restricts the measurements to forces along one axis and only a single location on the cell.

Modifying the design to a high-density array of vertical cantilevers improved both the spatial resolution of the force sensor and the scope of possible experiments [22]. With each cantilever placed perpendicular to the plane of traction forces, the spacing between each sensor is significantly reduced (Figure 65.3e). These devices are made from silicone rubber that has cylindrical cantilevers formed from a microfabricated mold. The cost per device is inexpensive once the reusable mold has been built and so the devices are disposable. The tips of the cantilevers are coated with extracellular matrix proteins so that cells attach and spread across several cantilevers. The bending of the posts is easily measured under a microscope as the cells probe the tips and apply traction forces. As with the horizontal design, the deflection of the posts is related by a simple relationship between force and displacement:

$$F = \left(\frac{3EI}{L^3} \right) \delta \tag{65.3}$$

where E is the modulus of elasticity of the silicone rubber, I is the moment of inertia, and L is the length of the cantilevers. However, the deflection of the post is not limited to one axis, the force reported is a true vector quantity in which force mappings are possible with an equivalent resolution to those from traction force microscopy. With the close proximity between sensors and measuring independence between them, the array of vertical cantilevers can examine cells at a higher population density than previous methods. Moreover, the technique allows for more relevant studies than previously possible because the forces of large monolayers of cells can be measured. This technique does expose the cell to a topology that is not akin to *in vitro* conditions, which may have an affect on its biological response.

65.5 Conclusion

The mechanical force that cells experience in the environment directly regulate their function in healthy tissue. Through the sensing of these forces, cells interact with these mechanical signals through biological responses and mechanical force generation of their cytoskeletal structures and motor proteins. The engineering of deformable substrates to measure the cellular forces has provided powerful insight into the protein interactions associated with mechanotransduction. However, despite these advances, these devices have several issues that need to be addressed in order to overcome their limitations. First, one needs to consider how the cell reacts to the new environment that the tooling presents it. The nonplanar topology and high compliance of the vertical microcantilever substrate may cause the cell to react to an environment that is physiologically irrelevant. Additionally, chemical composition of substrate or deposited extracellular matrix may have a direct effect on what signaling pathways are activated during its mechanical response. Second, since the devices used in cellular mechanics studies are prototypes, they may be lacking in adequate calibration between samples or quality control in device fabrication. These variations are significant if the cell population studied is not sufficiently large, as in the case of expensive or labor-intensive techniques. Lastly, the construction of these devices needs to be simple enough so that widespread use is possible. A large collective effort can be used to screen the numerous protein interactions that occur during the mechanotransduction signaling pathways. In this manner, the understanding of the interaction between mechanical forces and biological response can provide valuable insight into the treatment of diseased states of tissue or cancer.

To achieve this goal, there are many future directions that the techniques described can be advanced to. Foremost is the integration of cellular mechanics instrumentation with other fluorescent microscopy techniques, such as fluorescent recovery after photobleaching (FRAP), GFP protein-labeling, and fluorescent resonant emission transfer (FRET). These optical techniques allow one to detect proteins at the single molecular level, and in combination with force mapping, provide a correlation between molecular activity and observable mechanics. The incorporation of nanotechnology materials or devices may provide powerful new sensors that improve both spatial resolution and force measurement. Since the size of a focal adhesion is ten to hundreds of nanometers and the force of a single actomyosin motor is few piconewtons, the ability to resolve these structures would provide greater insight into the mechanical behavior of cells. Additionally, the constructions of three-dimensional measurement techniques, be it in gels or more complex sensing devices, would extend the current two-dimensional understanding of force mechanics into an environment more pertinent to cellular interactions in living tissue. One early attempt has been made where two traction force substrates have been used to sandwich a cell while providing some understanding of three-dimensional forces, the substrates are still planar and constrain how the cell organizes its cytoskeleton and adhesions along those planes. Lastly, strong exploration into the development of devices or techniques that are usable for *in vivo* studies of mechanotransduction would open new areas of treatment for diseases in the cardiovascular and skeletal systems.

Acknowledgments

This work was in part funded by NIH grants, EB00262 and HL73305. NJS was supported by the NRSA — Ruth Kirschtein Postdoctoral Fellowship.

References

[1] Alberts, B. et al., *Molecular Biology of the Cell.* 4th ed., 2002, New York, NY: Garland Science.

[2] Cowin, S.C., On mechanosensation in bone under microgravity. *Bone*, 1998, **22**: 119S–125S.

[3] Chen, C.S., J. Tan, and J. Tien, Mechanotrandsuction at cell–matrix and cell–cell contacts *Ann. Rev. Biomed. Eng.*, 2004, **6**: 275–302.

[4] Davies, P.F., Flow-mediate endothelial mechanotransduction. *Phys. Rev.*, 1995, **75**: 519–560.

[5] Johnson-Leger, C., M. Aurrand-Lions, and B.A. Imhof, The parting of the endothelium: miracle, or simply a junctional affair? *J. Cell Sci.*, 2000, **113**: 921–933.

[6] Worthylake, R.A. and K. Burridge, Leukocyte transendothelial migration: orchestrating the underlying molecular machinery. *Curr. Opin. Cell Biol.*, 2001, **13**: 569–577.

[7] Dudek, S.M. and J.G.N. Garcia, Cytoskeletal regulation of pulmonary vascular permeability. *J. Appl. Physiol.*, 2001, **91**: 1487–1500.

[8] McBeath, R. et al., Cell shape, cytoskeletal tension, and RhoA regulate stem cell lineage commitment. *Develop. Cell*, 2004, **6**: 483–495.

[9] Ingber, D.E., Tensegrity I. Cell structure and hierarchical systems biology. *J. Cell Sci.*, 2003, **116**: 1157–1173.

[10] Couloumbe, P.A. and P. Wong, Cytoplasmic intermediate filaments revealed as dynamic and multipurpose scaffolds. *Nat. Cell Biol.*, 2004, **6**: 699–706.

[11] Finer, J.T., R.M. Simmons, and J.A. Spudich, Single myosin molecule mechanics: piconewton forces and nanometre steps. *Nature*, 1994, **368**: 113–119.

[12] Harris, A.K., P. Wild, and D. Stopak, Silicone rubber substrata: a new wrinkle in the study of cell locomotion. *Science*, 1980, **208**: 177–179.

[13] Harris, A.K., Tissue culture cells on deformable substrata: biomechanical implications. *J. Biomech. Eng.*, 1984, **106**: 19–24.

[14] Burton, K. and D.L. Taylor, Traction forces of cytokinesis measured with optically modified elastic substrate. *Nat. Cell Biol.*, 1997, **385**: 450–454.

[15] Burton, K., J.H. Park, and D.L. Taylor, Keratocytes generate traction froces in two phase. *Mol. Biol. Cell*, 1999, **10**: 3745–3769.

[16] Lee, J. et al., Traction forces generated by locomoting keratocytes. *J. Cell Biol.*, 1994, **127**: 1957–1964.

[17] Dembo, M. and Y.-L. Wang, Stresses at the cell-to-substrate interface during locomotion of fibroblasts. *Biophys. J.*, 1999, **76**: 2307–2316.

[18] Munevar, S., Y.-L. Wang, and M. Dembo, Traction force microscopy of migrating normal and H-ras transformed 3T3 fibroblasts. *Biophys. J.*, 2001, **80**: 1744–1757.

[19] Dembo, M. et al., Imaging the traction stresses exerted by locomoting cells with the elastic substratum method. *Biophys. J.*, 1996, **70**: 2008–2022.

[20] Balaban, N.Q. et al., Force and focal adhesion assembly: a close relationship studied using elastic micropatterned substrates. *Nat. Cell Biol.*, 2001, **3**: 466–472.

[21] Galbraith, C.G. and M.P. Sheetz, A micromachined device provides a new bend on fibroblast traction forces. *Proc. Natl Acad. Sci. USA*, 1997, **94**: 9114–9118.

[22] Galbraith, C.G. and M.P. Sheetz, Keratocytes pull with similar forces on their dorsal and ventral surfaces. *J. Cell Biol.*, 1999, **147**: 1313–1323.

[23] Tan, J.L. et al., Cells lying on a bed of microneedles: an approach to isolate mechanical force. *Proc. Natl Acad. Sci. USA*, 2003. **100**: 1484–1489.

66

Blood Glucose Monitoring

66.1 Medicine and Historical Methods **66**-2
66.2 Development of Colorimetric Test Strips and Optical Reflectance Meters **66**-2
66.3 Emergence of Electrochemical Strips.................. **66**-5
66.4 Improvements in User Interactions with the System and Alternate Site Testing **66**-6
66.5 Future Directions **66**-9
Defining Terms.. **66**-9
References **66**-9
Further Reading **66**-10

David D. Cunningham
Abbott Diagnostics

The availability of blood glucose monitoring devices for home use has significantly impacted the treatment of diabetes with the American Diabetes Association currently recommending that Type 1 insulin-dependent diabetic individuals perform blood glucose testing four times per day. Less than optimal outcomes are associated with high and low blood glucose levels. Injection of too much insulin without enough food lowers blood sugar into the hypoglycemic range, glucose below 60 mg/dL, resulting in mild confusion or in more severe cases loss of consciousness, seizure, and coma. On the other hand, long-term high blood sugar levels lead to diabetic complications such as eye, kidney, heart, nerve, or blood vessel disease [The Diabetes Control and Complications Trial Research Group, 1993]. Complications were tracked in a large clinical study showing that an additional 5 years of life, 8 years of sight, 6 years free from kidney disease, and 6 years free of amputations can be expected for a diabetic following tight glucose control vs. the standard regimen [The Diabetes Control and Complications Trial Research Group, 1996]. This compelling need for simple, accurate glucose measurements has lead to continuous improvements in sample test strips, electronic meters, and sample acquisition techniques. Some of the landmarks in glucose testing are shown in Table 66.1. Glucose monitoring systems are now available from a number of companies through pharmacy and mail-order outlets without a prescription. The remainder of the chapter comprises a history of technical developments with an explanation of the principles behind optical and electrochemical meters including examples of the chemical reactions used in commercial products.

TABLE 66.1 Landmarks in Glucose Monitoring

1941 — Effervescent tablet test for glucose in urine
1956 — Dip and read test strip for glucose in urine
1964 — Dry reagent blood glucose test strip requiring timing, wash step, and
      visual comparison to a color chart
1970 — Meter to read reflected light from a test strip, designed for use in the doctor's office
1978 — Major medical literature publications on home blood glucose monitoring
      with portable meters
1981 — Finger lancing device automatically lances and retracts tip
1986 — Electrochemical test strip and small meter in the form of a pen
1997 — Multiple test strip package for easy loading into meter
2001 — Integrated alternate-site glucose monitoring for painless, one-step testing

66.1 Medicine and Historical Methods

Diabetes is an ancient disease that was once identified by the attraction of ants to the urine of an affected individual. Later, physicians would often rely on the sweet taste of the urine in diagnosing the disease. Once the chemical reducing properties of glucose were discovered, solutions of a copper salt and dye, typically o-toluidine, were used for laboratory tests, and by the 1940s the reagents had been formulated into tablets for use in test tubes of urine. More specific tests were developed using glucose oxidase which could be impregnated on a dry paper strip. The reaction of glucose with glucose oxidase produces hydrogen peroxide which can subsequently react with a colorless dye precursor in the presence of hydrogen peroxide to form a visible color (see Equation 66.3). The first enzyme-based test strips required the addition of the sample to the strip for 1 min and subsequent washing of the strip. Visual comparison of the color on the test strip to the color on a chart was required to estimate the glucose concentration. However, measurement of glucose in urine is not adequate since only after the blood glucose level is very high for several hours does glucose "spill-over" into the urine. Other physiological fluids such as sweat and tears are not suitable because the glucose level is much lower than in blood.

Whole blood contains hemoglobin inside the red blood cells that can interfere with the measurement of color on a test strip. In order to prevent staining of the test strip with red blood cells, an ethyl cellulose layer was applied over the enzyme and dye impregnated paper on a plastic support [Mast, 1967]. Previously, in a commercially available test strip, the enzymes and dye were incorporated into a homogeneous water-resistant film that prevented penetration of red blood cells into the test strips and enabled their easy removal upon washing [Rey et al., 1971]. Through various generations of products, the formulations of the strips were improved to eliminate the washing/wiping steps and electronic meters were developed to measure the color.

66.2 Development of Colorimetric Test Strips and Optical Reflectance Meters

Optically based strips are generally constructed with various layers which provide a support function, a reflective function, an analytical function, and a sample-spreading function as illustrated in Figure 66.1. The support function serves as a foundation for the dry reagent and may also contain the reflective function. Otherwise, insoluble, reflective, or scattering materials such as TiO_2, $BaSO_4$, MgO, or ZnO are added to the dry reagent formulation. The analytical function contains the active enzyme. The reaction schemes used in several commercial products are described in greater detail in the following paragraphs. The spreading function must rapidly disperse the sample laterally after application and quickly form

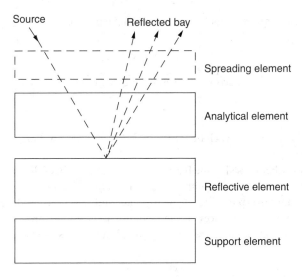

FIGURE 66.1 Basic functions of a reflectance-based test strip. (From Henning T.P. and Cunningham, D.D. 1998, *Commercial Biosensors*, John Wiley & Sons, pp. 3–46. With permission.)

a uniform sample concentration on the analytically active portion of the strip. Swellable films and semi-permeable membranes, particularly glass fiber fleece has been used to spread and separate plasma from whole blood. Upon formation of the colored reaction product, the amount of diffuse light reflected from the analytical portion of the strip decreases according to the following equation:

$$\%R = (I_u/I_s)R_s \tag{66.1}$$

where I_u is the reflected light from the sample, I_s is the reflected light from a standard, and R_s is the percent reflectivity of the standard. The Kubelka–Munk equation gives the relationship in a more useful form.

$$C \, \alpha K/S = (1 - R)^2/2R \tag{66.2}$$

where C is concentration, K is the absorption coefficient, S is the scattering coefficient, and R is the percent reflectance divided by 100.

The analytical function of the strip is based on an enzyme reaction with glucose and subsequent color forming reactions. Although the most stable enzyme is chosen for product development, some loss in activity occurs during manufacturing due to factors such as pH, temperature, physical sheer stress, organic solvents, and various other denaturing actions or agents. Additional inactivation occurs during the storage of the product. In general, sufficient enzyme and other reagents are incorporated into the strip so that the assay reactions near completion in a conveniently short time. Reagent formulations often include thickening agents, builders, emulsifiers, dispersion agents, pigments, plasticisers, pore formers, wetting agents and the like. These materials provide a uniform reaction layer required for good precision and accuracy. The cost of the materials in the strip must be low since it is only used once.

The glucose oxidase/peroxidase reaction scheme used in the Lifescan ONE TOUCH® [Phillips et al., 1990] and SureStep™ test strips follows. Glucose oxidase catalyzes the oxidation of glucose forming gluconic acid and hydrogen peroxide. The oxygen concentration in blood (ca. 0.3 mM) is much lower than the glucose concentration (3 to 35 mM), hence oxygen from the atmosphere must diffuse into the test strip to bring the reaction to completion. Peroxidase catalyzes the reaction of the hydrogen peroxide with 3-methyl-2-benzothiazolinone hydrazone (MBTH) and 3-dimethylaminobenzoic acid (DMAB).

A naphthalene sulfonic acid salt replaces DMAB in the SureStep strip.

$$\text{glucose + oxygen} \xrightarrow{\text{GOx}} \text{gluconic acid} + H_2O_2$$ (66.3)

$$H_2O_2 + MBTH + DMAB \xrightarrow{\text{peroxidase}} MBTH\text{–}DMAB \text{ (blue)}$$

The hexokinase reaction scheme used in the Bayer GLUCOMETER ENCORE™ test strip is shown below. Hexokinase, ATP, and magnesium react with glucose to produce glucose-6-phosphate. The glucose-6-phosphate reacts with glucose-6-phosphate dehydrogenase and NAD^+ to produce NADH. The NADH then reacts with diaphorase and reduces the tetrazolium indicator to produce a brown compound (formazan). The reaction sequence requires three enzymes but is insensitive to oxygen.

$$\text{glucose + ATP} \underset{Mg^{+2}}{\xrightarrow{\text{HK}}} \text{G-6-P + ADP}$$ (66.4)

$$\text{G-6-P} + NAD^+ \xrightarrow{\text{G-6-PDH}} \text{6-PG} + NADH + H^+$$

$$NADH + \text{tetrazolium} \xrightarrow{\text{diaphorase}} \text{formazan (brown)} + NAD^+$$

The reaction scheme used in the Roche Accu-Chek® Instant™ strip is shown below [Hoenes et al., 1995]. *Bis*-(2-hydroxy-ethyl)-(4-hydroximinocyclohex-2,5-dienylidene) ammonium chloride (BHEHD) is reduced by glucose to the corresponding hydroxylamine derivative and further to the corresponding diamine under the catalytic action of glucose oxidase. Note that while oxygen is not required in the reaction, oxygen in the sample may compete with the intended reaction creating an oxygen dependency. The diamine reacts with a 2,18-phosphomolybdic acid salt to form molybdenum blue.

$$\text{glucose + BHEHD} \xrightarrow{\text{GOx}} \text{diamine}$$ (66.5)

$$P_2Mo_{18}O_{62}^{-6} + \text{diamine} \longrightarrow MoO_{2.0}(OH) \text{ to } MoO_{2.5}(OH)_{0.5} \text{(molybdenum blue)}$$

The reaction scheme used in the Roche Accu-Chek® Easy™ Test strip is shown below [Freitag, 1990]. Glucose oxidase reacts with ferricyanide and forms potassium ferric ferrocyanide (Prussian Blue). Again, oxygen is not required but may compete with the intended reaction.

$$\text{glucose + GOD(ox)} \rightarrow \text{GOD (red)}$$

$$\text{GOD (red)} + [Fe(CN)_6]^{-3} \rightarrow \text{GOD (ox)} + [Fe(CN)_6]^{-4}$$ (66.6)

$$3[Fe(CN)_6]^{-4} + 4FeCl_3 \rightarrow Fe_4[Fe(CN)_6]_3 \text{ Prussian Blue}$$

Optical test strips and reflectance meters typically require 3–15 μL of blood and read out an answer in 10–30 sec. A significant technical consideration in the development of a product is the measurement

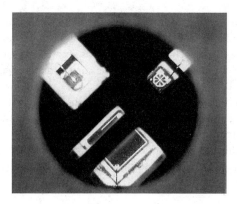

FIGURE 66.2   Photograph of light emitting diodes and photodetector on the OneTouch meter. Photodetector at bottom (blue), 635 nm light emitting diode at top left, 700 nm light emitting diode at top right. Optics viewed through the 4.5 mm hole in the strip after removal of the reagent membrane. Courtesy of John Grace.

of samples spanning the range of red blood cell concentrations (percent hematocrit) typically found in whole blood. Common hematocrit and glucose ranges are 30–55% and 40–500 mg/dL (2.2–28 mM), respectively. The Lifescan ONE TOUCH® meter contains two light emitting diodes (635 and 700 nm) which allows measurement of the color due to red blood cells and the color due to the dye. Reflectance measurements from both LEDs are measured with a single photodetector as shown in Figure 66.2. All glucose meters measure the detector signal at various timepoints and if the curve shape is not within reasonable limits an error message is generated. Some meters measure and correct for ambient temperature. Of course, optical systems are subject to interference from ambient light conditions and may not work in direct sunlight. Optical systems have gradually lost market share to electrochemical systems which were introduced commercially in 1987. Optical test strips generally require a larger blood sample and take longer to produce the result. Presently, optical reflectance meters are more costly to manufacture, require larger batteries, and are more difficult to calibrate than electrochemical meters.

66.3   Emergence of Electrochemical Strips

Electrochemical systems are based on the reaction of an electrochemically active mediator with an enzyme. The mediator is oxidized at a solid electrode with an applied positive potential. Electrons will flow between the mediator and electrode surface when a minimum energy is attained. The energy of the electrons in the mediator is fixed based on the chemical structure but the energy of the electrons in the solid electrode can changed by applying a voltage between the working electrode and a second electrode. The rate of the electron transfer reaction between the mediator and a working electrode surface is given by the Butler–Volmer equation [Bard and Faulkner, 1980]. When the potential is large enough the mediator reaching the electrode reacts rapidly and the reaction becomes diffusion controlled. The current from a diffusion limited reaction follows the Cottrell equation,

$$i = (nFAD^{1/2}C)/(\pi^{1/2}t^{1/2}) \tag{66.7}$$

where i is current, n is number of electrons, F is Faradays constant, A is electrode area, C is the concentration, D is the diffusion coefficient, and t is time. The current from a diffusion-controlled electrochemical reaction will decay away as the reciprocal square root of time. This means that the maximum electrochemical signal occurs at short times as opposed to color forming reactions where the color becomes more intense with time. The electrochemical method relies on measuring the current from the electron transfer between the electrode and the mediator. However, when a potential is first applied to the electrode the dipole moments of solvent molecules will align with the electric field on the surface of the electrode causing a current to flow. Thus, at very short times this charging current interferes with the analytical measurement. Electrochemical sensors generally apply a potential to the electrode surface and measure the current after the charging current has decayed sufficiently. With small volumes of sample, coulometric analysis can be used to measure the current required for complete consumption of glucose.

The reaction scheme used in the first commercial electrochemical test strip from MediSense is shown below. Electron transfer rates between the reduced form of glucose oxidase and ferricinium ion derivatives are very rapid compared with the unwanted side-reaction with oxygen [Cass et al., 1984]. Electrochemical oxidation of ferrocene is performed at 0.6 V. Oxidation of interferences, such as ascorbic acid and acetaminophen present in blood, are corrected for by measuring the current at a second electrode on the strip that does not contain glucose oxidase.

$$\text{glucose} + \text{GOx (oxidized)} \rightarrow \text{gluconolactone} + \text{Gox (reduced)}$$

$$\text{GOx (reduced)} + \text{ferricinium}^+ \rightarrow \text{GOx (oxidized)} + \text{ferrocene} \tag{66.8}$$

$$\text{ferrocene} \rightarrow \text{ferricinium}^+ + \text{electron (reaction at solid electrode surface)}$$

The reaction scheme used in the Abbott Laboratories MediSense Products Precision-Xtra and Sof-Tact test strips follows. The glucose dehydrogenase (GDH) enzyme does not react with oxygen and the phenanthroline quinine mediator can be oxidized at 0.2 V, which is below the oxidation potential of most interfering substances.

$$\text{glucose} + \text{GDH/NAD}^+ \rightarrow \text{GDH/NADH} + \text{gluconolactone}$$

$$\text{GDH/NADH} + \text{PQ} \rightarrow \text{GDH/NAD}^+ + \text{PQH}_2 \tag{66.9}$$

$$\text{PQH}_2 \rightarrow \text{PQ} + \text{electrons (reaction at solid electrode surface)}$$

The working electrode on most commercially available electrochemical strips is made by screen printing a conductive carbon ink on a plastic substrate, however, a more expensive noble metal foil is also used. Many of the chemistries described above are used on more than one brand of strip from the company. The package insert provided with the test strips describes the test principle and composition. Generally, test strips are manufactured, tested, and assigned a calibration code. The calibration code provided with each package of strips must be manually entered into the meter by the user. However, some high-end meters now automatically read the calibration code from the strips. Meters designed for use in the hospital have bar code readers to download calibration, quality control, and patient information. Test strips are supplied in bottles or individual foil wrappers to protect them from moisture over their shelf-life, typically about 1 year. The task of opening and inserting individual test strips into the meter has been minimized by packaging multiple test strips in the form of a disk shaped cartridge or a drum that is placed into the meter.

66.4 Improvements in User Interactions with the System and Alternate Site Testing

Both Type 1 and Type 2 diabetic individuals do not currently test as often as recommended by physicians so systems developed in the last few years have aimed to improve compliance with physician recommendations while maintaining accuracy. Historically, the biggest source of errors in glucose testing involved interaction of the user with the system. Blood is typically collected by lancing the edge of the end of the finger to a depth of about 1.5 mm. Squeezing or milking is required to produce a hanging drop of blood. The target area on test strips is clearly identified by design. A common problem is smearing a drop of blood on top of a strip resulting in a thinner than normal layer of blood over part of the strip and a low

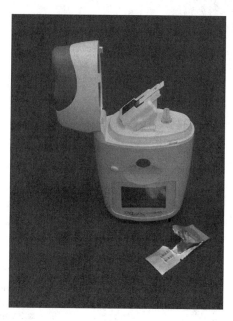

FIGURE 66.3 Sof-Tact meter with cover opened to load test strip and lancet. Test strip is inserted into an electrical connector. The hole in the opposite end of the test strip allows the lancet to pass through. The white cylindrical lancet is loaded into the lancet tip holder in the housing. To perform a test, the cover is closed, the gray area of the cover placed against the skin and blue button depressed.

reading. Many strips now require that the blood drop be applied to the end or side of the strip where capillary action is used to fill the strip. Partial filling can be detected electrochemically or by observation of the fill window on the strip. The small capillary space in the TheraSense electrochemical strip requires only 300 nl of blood.

Progressively thinner diameter lancets have come to the market with current sizes typically in the 28 to 31 gauge range. Most lancets are manufactured with three grinding steps to give a tri-level point. After loading the lancet into the lancing device, a spring system automatically lances and retracts the point. The depth of lancing is commonly adjustable through the use of several settings on the device or use of a different end-piece cap. Unfortunately, the high density of nerve endings on the finger make the process painful and some diabetic individuals do not test as often as they should due to the pain and residual soreness caused by fingersticks. Recently, lancing devices have been designed to lance and apply pressure on the skin of body sites other than the finger, a process termed "**alternate site testing**." Use of alternate site sampling lead to the realization that capillary blood from alternate sites can have slightly different glucose and hematocrit values than blood from a fingerstick due to the more arterial nature of blood in the fingertips. The pain associated with lancing alternate body sites is typically rated as painless most of the time and less painful than a fingerstick over 90% of the time. A low volume test strip, typically one microliter or less, is required to measure the small blood samples obtained from alternate sites. Some care and technique is required to obtain an adequate amount of blood and transfer it into the strips when using small blood samples.

One alternate site device, the Abbott/MediSense Sof-Tact meter, automatically extracts and transfers blood to the test strip (see Figure 66.3). The device contains a vacuum pump, a lancing device, and a test strip that is automatically indexed over the lancet wound after lancing. The vacuum turns off after sufficient blood enters the strip to make an electrical connection. The key factors and practical limits of blood extraction using a vacuum combined with skin stretching were investigated to assure that sufficient blood could be obtained for testing [Cunningham et al., 2002]. The amount of blood extracted increases with the application of heat or vacuum prior to lancing, the level of vacuum, the depth of lancing, the time

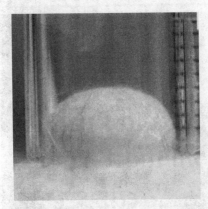

FIGURE 66.4 Photograph of skin on the forearm stretching up into a glass tube upon application of vacuum. Markings on tube at right in 1 mm increments. Courtesy of Douglas Young.

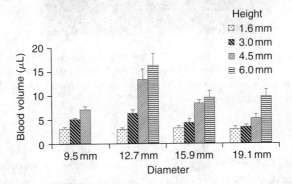

FIGURE 66.5 Effect of skin stretching by vacuum on blood volume extracted from lancet wounds on the forearm. Mean blood volume ± SE in 30 sec with −7.5 psig vacuum for nosepieces of different inner diameter and inside step height. (From Cunningham D.D. et al., 2002. *J. Appl. Physiol.* 92: 1089–1096. With permission.)

of collection, and the amount of skin stretching (see Figure 66.4). Particularly important is the diameter and height that skin is allowed to stretch into a nosepiece after the application of a vacuum as shown in Figure 66.5. A vacuum combined with skin stretching increases blood extraction by increasing the lancet wound opening, increasing the blood available for extraction by vasodilatation, and reducing the venous return of blood through the capillaries. The electrochemical test strip used with the meter can be inserted into a secondary support and used with a fingerstick sample when the battery is low.

The size of a meter is often determined by the size of the display although electrochemical meters can be made smaller than reflectance meters. The size and shape of one electrochemical meter, with a relatively small display, is indistinguishable from a standard ink pen. All meters store recent test results in memory and many allow downloading of the results to a computer. Advanced software functions are supplied with some meters to allow entry of exercise, food, and insulin doses, and a PDA-meter combination is on the market. Two combined insulin dosing-glucose meters are available. One combines an insulin injection pen with an electrochemical glucose meter, and the other combines a continuous insulin infusion pump with an electrochemical glucose meter using telemetry for downloading the glucose measurements into the insulin pump memory. The variety of meters available in the market is mainly driven by the need to satisfy the desires of various customer segments which are driven by different factors, such as cost, ease of use, or incorporation of a specific design or functional feature.

66.5   Future Directions

Several approaches to continuous glucose sensing are being actively pursued based on the desire to obtain better glucose control through a combination of sensing and insulin administration. The most advanced is an electrochemical needle sensor that is inserted through the skin into the subcutaneous fat layer [Feldman et al., 2003]. A second approach is to porate the skin and extract interstitial fluid for measurements with a miniature sensor [Gebhart et al., 2003]. With either of these approaches, infection becomes a concern after a few days. Longer term sensing may involve surgical implantation of a battery-operated unit although many issues remain with the long-term sensor stability and the biocompatibility of various materials of construction. One 24-h device, the GlucoWatch based on transdermal reverese iontophoresis [Kurnick et al., 1998] gained FDA approval but acceptance of the device in the market has been poor due to the need to calibrate the device with multiple fingersticks and poor precision and accuracy. A number of noninvasive spectroscopic approaches have been described, however, the amount of clinical data reported to date is very limited [Khalil, 1999]. Continuous sensing devices coupled with insulin delivery will almost certainly have a significant impact on the treatment of diabetes in the future [Siegel and Ziaie, 2004]. Less certain is the timing for the market launch of specific devices, the form and function of winning technologies, and the realization of commercial success.

Defining Terms

Alternate site testing: Lancing sites other than the finger to obtain blood in a less painful manner. The small volume of blood obtained from alternate sites requires use of a test strip requiring one microliter or less of blood.

Type 1 Diabetes: The immune system destroys insulin-producing islet cells in the pancreas, usually in children and young adults, hence regular injections of insulin are required (also referred to as juvenile diabetes).

Type 2 Diabetes: A complex disease based on gradual resistance to insulin and diminished production of insulin. Treatment often progresses from oral medications to insulin injections as disease progresses. Also referred to as adult onset diabetes and noninsulin dependent diabetes mellitus (NIDDM).

References

Bard A.J. and Faulkner L.R. 1980. *Electrochemical Methods*, John Wiley & Sons, New York, pp. 103, 143.

Cass A., Davis G., Francis G., Hill H., Aston W., Higgins I., Plotkin E., Scott L., and Turner A. 1984. Ferrocene-mediated enzyme electrode for amperometric determination of glucose. *Anal. Chem.*, 56: 667.

The Diabetes Control and Complications Trial Research Group, 1993. The effect of intensive treatment of diabetes on the development and progression of long-term complications in insulin-dependent diabetes mellitus. *N. Engl. J. Med.* 329: 977.

The Diabetes Control and Complications Trial Research Group, 1996. Lifetime benefits and costs of intensive therapy as practiced in the diabetes control and complications Trial. *J. Amer. Med. Assoc.* 276: 1409.

Feldman B., Brazg R., Schwartz S., and Weinstein R. 2003. A continuous glucose sensor based on wired enzyme technology — results from a 3-day trial in patients with type 1 diabetes. *Diabetes Technol. Ther.* 5: 769.

Freitag H. 1990. Method and reagent for determination of an analyte via enzymatic means using a ferricyanide/ferric compound system. U.S. Patent 4,929,545.

Gebhart S., Faupel M., Fowler R., Kapsner C., Lincoln D., McGee V., Pasqua J., Steed L., Wangsness M., Xu F., and Vanstory M. 2003. Glucose sensing in transdermal body fluid collected under continuous vacuum pressure via micropores in the stratum corneum. *Diabetes Technol. Ther.* 5: 159.

Hoenes J., Wielinger H., and Unkrig V. 1995. Use of a soluble salt of a heteropoly acid for the determination of an analyte, a corresponding method of determination as well as a suitable agent thereof. U.S. Patent 5,382,523

Khalil O.S. 1999. Spectroscopic and clinical aspects of noninvasive glucose measurements. *Clin. Chem.* 45: 165.

Kurnik R.T., Berner B., Tamada J., and Potts R.O. 1998. Design and simulation of a reverse iontophoretic glucose monitoring device. *J. Electrochem. Soc.* 145: 4199.

Mast R.L. 1967. Test article for the detection of glucose. U.S. Patent 3,298,789.

Phillips R., McGarraugh G., Jurik F., and Underwood R. 1990. Minimum procedure system for the determination of analytes. U.S. Patent 4,935,346.

Rey H., Rieckman P., Wiellager H., and Rittersdorf W. 1971 Diagnostic agent. U.S. Patent 3,630,957.

Siegel R.A. and Ziaie B. 2004. Biosensing and drug delivery at the microscale. *Adv. Drug Deliv. Rev.* 56: 121.

Further Reading

Ervin K.R. and Kiser E.J. 1999. Issues and implications in the selection of blood glucose monitoring technologies. *Diabetes Technol. Ther.* 1: 3.

Henning T.P. and Cunningham D.D. 1998. Biosensors for personal diabetes management, in *Commercial Biosensors*, Ramsey G., Ed., John Wiley & Sons, pp. 3–46.

Test results of glucose meters are often compared with results from a reference method and presented in the form of a Clark Error Grid that defines zones with different clinical implications. Clarke W.L., Cox D.C., Gonder-Frederick L.A., Carter W. and Pohl S.L. 1987. Evaluating clinical accuracy of systems for self-Monitoring of blood glucose. *Diabetes Care* 10: 622–628.

Error Grid Analysis has recently been extended for evaluation of continuous glucose monitoring sensors. Kovatchev B.P., Gonder-Frederick L.A., Cox D.J., and Clarke W.L. 2004. Evaluating the accuracy of continuous glucose-monitoring sensors. *Diabetes Care* 27: 1922.

Reviews and descriptions of many marketed products are available on-line at: www.childrenwithdiabetes.com.

Interviews of several people involved with the initial development of the blood glucose meters are available on-line at: www.mendosa.com/history.htm.

67

Atomic Force Microscopy: Probing Biomolecular Interactions

67.1 Introduction... **67**-1
67.2 Background **67**-2
67.3 SPM Basics **67**-2
67.4 Imaging Mechanisms **67**-3
Contact • Noncontact • Intermittent Contact •
Applications
67.5 Imaging.. **67**-6
67.6 Crystallography **67**-6
Protein Aggregation and Fibril Formation • Membrane
Protein Structure and Assemblies
67.7 Force Spectroscopy **67**-9
Fundamentals • Single Molecule Force Spectroscopy •
Force Volume • Pulsed Force Mode
67.8 Binding Forces **67**-11
Mechanical Properties • Coupled Imaging • Near-Field —
SNOM/NSOM • Evanescent-Wave — TIRF (Total Internal
Reflection
Fluorescence Microscopy)
67.9 Summary **67**-15
References **67**-15

Christopher M. Yip
University of Toronto

67.1 Introduction

Discerning and understanding structure–function relationships is often predicated on our ability to measure these properties on a variety of length scales. Fundamentally, nanotechnology and nanoscience might be arguably based on the precept that we need to understand how interactions occur at the atomic and molecular length scales if we are to truly understand how to manipulate processes and structures and ultimately control physical/chemical/electronic properties on more bulk macroscopic length scales. There is a clear need to understanding the pathways and functional hierarchy involved in the development of complex architectures from their simple building blocks. In order to study such phenomena at such a basic level, we need tools capable of performing measurements on these same length scales. If we can couple these capabilities with the ability to map these attributes against a real-space image of such structures, in real-time and hopefully, under real-world conditions, this would provide the researcher with a particularly powerful and compelling set of approaches to characterizing interactions and structures.

Powerful functional imaging tools such as single molecule fluorescence and nonlinear optical micro-scopies such as CARS and SHG through to the various electron microscopies (SEM/TEM/STEM) provide a powerful suite of tools for characterizing phenomena under a vast range of conditions and situations. What many of these techniques lack, however, is the ability to acquire true real-space, real-time informa-tion about surface structures on near-molecular length scales, and, in the case of many of these techniques, in the absence of specific labeling strategies. Atomic force microscopy (AFM), or more correctly, scanning probe microscopy (SPM) has come into the forefront as one of the most powerful tools for characterizing molecular scale phenomena and interactions and in particular, their contribution to the development of macroscopic mechanical properties, structures, and ultimately function.

This review will explore some of the recent advances in scanning probe microscopy, including the funda-mentals of SPM, where it has been applied in the context of biomolecular structures and functions — from single molecules to large aggregates and complexes — and introduce some new innovations in the field of correlated imaging tools designed to address many of the key limitations of this family of techniques.

67.2 Background

Scanning probe microscopy is founded on a fundamentally simple principle — by raster-scanning a sharp tip over a surface, and monitoring tip–sample interactions, which can range in scope from repulsive to attractive forces to local variations in temperature and viscoelasticity, it is possible to generate real-space images of surfaces with near-molecular scale (and in some cases, atomic scale) resolution. One can reasonably describe these images as isosurfaces of a parameter as a function of (x, y, z) space.

Since its inception in the mid-1980s, SPM has become a very well-accepted technique for characterizing surfaces and interfacial processes with nanometer-scale resolution and precision [Hansma et al., 1988; Lillehei and Bottomley, 2000; Poggi et al., 2002, 2004]. Emerging from efforts in the semi-conductor and physics fields, SPM has perhaps made its greatest impact in the biological sciences and the fields of soft materials [Engel and Muller, 2000]. What has really driven its use in these fields has been its perhaps unique ability to acquire such high resolution data, both spatial and most recently force, in real-time and often *in situ*. This growth has been fostered by a wealth of SPM-based imaging modes, including intermittent contact or tapping mode [Moller et al., 1999], and recently force spectroscopy and force volume imaging techniques [Florin et al., 1994b] [Rief et al., 1997b; Heinz and Hoh, 1999b; Oesterfelt et al., 1999], [Brown and Hoh, 1997; A-Hassan et al., 1998; Walch et al., 2000]. These attributes are particularly compelling for the study of protein assembly at surfaces, ranging from polymers through metals to model-supported planar lipid bilayers and live cell membranes [Pelling et al., 2004].

67.3 SPM Basics

Similar to a technique known as stylus profilometry, including very early work by Young on the "Topo-graphiner" [Young et al., 1971], scanning probe microscopy is a rather simple concept. As you raster-scan a sharp tip and a surface past each other, you monitor any number of tip–surface interactions. One can then generate a surface contour map that reflects relative differences in interaction intensity as a function of surface position. Precise control over the tip–sample separation distance through the use of piezoelec-tric scanners and sophisticated feedback control schemes is what provides the SPM technique with its high spatial and force resolution.

Based on the scanning tunneling microscope (STM), which operates on the principle of measuring the tunneling current between two conducting surfaces separated by a very small distance. [Binnig et al., 1982],

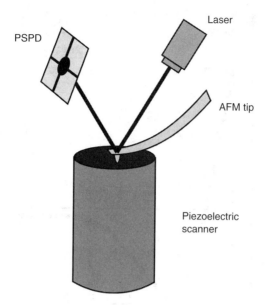

FIGURE 67.1 In AFM, a typically pyramidal silicon nitride tip is positioned over a sample. The relative motion between the tip and sample is controlled by a piezoelectric scanner. In this image, the sample is mounted to the scanner so the sample moves relative to a fixed tip. The reflection of a laser focused onto the back of the AFM tip is monitored on a four-quadrant position sensitive photodiode (PSPD). As the AFM tip is raster-scanned over the sample surface, variations in tip-sample interactions result in (vertical and lateral) deflection of the tip. This deflection is reflected in movement of the laser spot on the PSPD and is used to produce a three-dimensional topographical image of the surface.

atomic force microscopy is predicated on mapping local variations in the intermolecular and interatomic forces between the tip and the sample being scanned [Binnig et al., 1986]. In a conventional AFM, the surface is scanned with a nominally atomically sharp tip, typically pyramidal in shape, which is mounted on the underside of an extremely sensitive cantilever. The theoretical force sensitivity of these tips is on the order of 10^{-14} newtons (N), although practical limitations reduce this value to $\sim10^{-10}$ N. The resolution of an SPM is highly dependent on the nature of the sample, with near-atomic scale resolution often achievable on atomically flat surfaces (crystals) while soft, and often mobile interfaces, such as cells or membranes, are often challenging to image with a typical resolution in these cases of ~5 to 10 nm, depending on what you are imaging.

The relative motion of the tip and sample is controlled through the use of piezoelectric crystal scanners. The user sets the desired applied force (or amplitude dampening in the case of the intermittent contact imaging techniques). Deviations from these set point values are picked up as *error* signals on a four-quadrant position sensitive photodetector (PSPD), and then fed into the main computer (Figure 67.1). The error signal provided to the instrument is then used to generate a feedback signal that is used as the input to the feedback control software. The tip–sample separation distance is then dynamically changed in real-time and adjusted according to the error signal. While detection of the deflection signal is the simplest feedback signal, there are a host of other feedback signals that could be used to control the tip–sample mapping, including tip oscillation (amplitude/phase).

67.4 Imaging Mechanisms

67.4.1 Contact

During imaging, the AFM tracks gradients in interaction forces, either attractive or repulsive, between the tip and the surface (Figure 67.2). Similar to how the scanning tunneling microscope mapped out

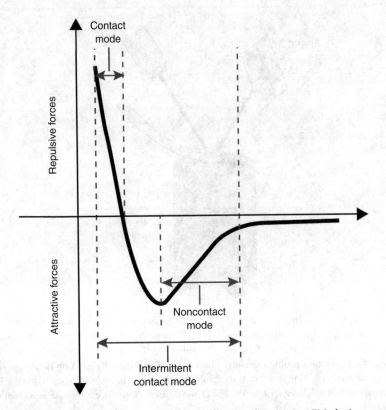

FIGURE 67.2 Tip-sample interaction forces vs tip-sample separation distance. In AFM, the instrument can operate in a number of different modes, based on the nature of the forces felt by the tip as it approaches the surface. When the instrument is operated in *non-contact* mode, the tip-sample separation is maintained so that the tip only feel an attractive interaction with the surface. In *contact* mode, the tip-sample interaction is repulsive. In *intermittent contact* mode, the tip alternates between sensing attractive and repulsive interactions with the surface. This is often achieved by vertically oscillating the tip during scanning.

local variations in tip–sample tunneling current, the AFM uses this force gradient to generate an iso-force surface image. In contact mode imaging, the tip–sample interaction is maintained at a specific, user defined load. It is this operating mode that arguably provides the best resolution for imaging of surfaces and structures. It also provides direct access to so-called friction force imaging where transient twisting of the cantilever during scanning can be used to develop maps of relative surface friction [Magonov and Reneker, 1997; Paige, 2003]. The ability to quantitate such data is limited due to difficulties in determining the torsional stiffness of the cantilevers, a determination that is further exacerbated by the shape of the cantilever. In contact mode imaging, this image represents either a constant attractive, or repulsive, tip–sample force, that is chosen by the user. Incorrect selection of this load can result in damage to the surface when the applied force is higher than what the surface can withstand, or poor tracking when the chosen set point load is too low. Subtle manipulation of these imaging forces affords the user the unique ability to both probe local structure and determine the response of the structure to the applied force.

67.4.2 Noncontact

In noncontact mode imaging, the AFM tip is actively oscillated near its resonance frequency at a distance of tens to hundreds of Angstroms away from sample surface. The resulting image represents an isosurface corresponding to regions of constant amplitude dampening. As the forces between the tip and the surface are very small, noncontact mode AFM is ideally suited for imaging softer samples such as proteins, surfactants, or membranes. In this mode, one often uses cantilevers with a higher spring constant that those employed during normal contact mode imaging. The net result is a very small feedback signal, which can make instrument control difficult and imaging challenging [Dinte et al., 1996; Lvov et al., 1998].

67.4.3 Intermittent Contact

This method, in which the tip alternates from the repulsive to the attractive regions of the tip–sample interaction curve, has become the method of choice currently for most AFM-basing imaging. In early contact mode work, it was quickly realized that poorly adhering molecules could be rapidly displaced by the sweeping motion of the AFM cantilever. This "snow-plow" effect has been largely ameliorated by vertically oscillating the tip during imaging, which removes (to a large extent) the lateral forces present during contact mode imaging. As the vertical oscillations occur at a drive frequency that is several orders of magnitude higher than the actual raster-scanning frequency, it is possible to obtain comparable lateral and vertical resolution as the continuous contact techniques. Since one detects the relative damping of the tip's free vertical oscillation during imaging, an intermittent contact mode AFM image can be viewed as an iso-energy dissipation landscape. Intermittent contact imaging provides access to other imaging modes, including phase imaging, which measures the phase shift between the applied and detected tip oscillations. This derivative signal is particularly useful for tracking spatial distributions of the relative modulus, viscoelasticity, and adhesive characteristics of surfaces, and has proven to be very powerful for studying polymeric materials [Fritzsche and Henderson, 1997; Hansma et al., 1997; Magonov et al., 1997; Magonov and Reneker, 1997; Magonov and Heaton, 1998; Noy et al., 1998b; Magonov and Godovsky, 1999; Nagao and Dvorak, 1999; Holland and Marchant, 2000; Paige, 2003] [Winkler et al., 1996; Brandsch et al., 1997; Czajkowsky et al., 1998; Noy et al., 1998a; Walch et al., 2000; Opdahl et al., 2001; Scott and Bhushan, 2003]. Recent work has shown that phase imaging is particularly useful for studying biological systems, including adsorbed proteins and supported lipid bilayers, even in the absence of topographic contrast [Argaman et al., 1997; Holland and Marchant, 2000; Krol et al., 2000; Deleu et al., 2001].

In intermittent contact imaging, the cantilever can be oscillated either acoustically or magnetically. In the first case, the cantilever is vertically oscillated by a piezoelectric crystal typically mounted under the cantilever. In air, this is typically a single resonance frequency. In fluid imaging, coupling of the cantilever motion with the fluid, and the fluid cell, can result in a complex power spectrum with multiple apparent resonant peaks. In this case, choosing the appropriate peak to operate with can be difficult and experience is often the best guide. Selection of the appropriate cantilever for intermittent contact imaging will depend on the physical imaging environment (air/fluid). In air, one typically uses the so-called diving board tips, which have a relatively high resonance peak of ∼250 kHz (depending on the manufacturer). In fluid, viscous coupling between the tip and the surrounding fluid results in an increase in the apparent resonant frequency of the tip. This allow for the use of the conventional V-shaped contact-mode cantilevers. In magnetic mode, the AFM tip/cantilever assembly can be placed in an oscillating magnetic field [Lindsay et al., 1993; Florin et al., 1994a; Han et al., 1996]. In this case, the silicon nitride AFM tip is coated with a thin magnetic film and it is the interaction of this film with the field that induces the tip oscillations. This is a fundamentally cleaner approach; however, there can be issues, including the tip coating affecting the spatial resolution of the AFM, the quality of the coating, and the nature of the sample.

67.4.4 Applications

The breadth of possible applications for scanning probe microscopy seems almost endless. As has been described earlier, the concepts underlying the instrument itself are, arguably, quite simple and to date, the software that drives the instrumentation and the technology itself is effectively turnkey. This does not mean that SPM itself is a very simple tool — it is critical that the user has a good grasp of the physical principles that underpin how an SPM image itself is generated. Similarly, the user must have a good understanding of the nature of their samples, and how they might behave during imaging — an aspect that is of particular interest to those investigating cellular phenomena. In the following sections, we will explore how SPM/AFM-based investigations have provided novel insights into the structure and function of biomolecular assemblies. We focus on a few specific areas, rather than attempting to cover the whole scope of the field. A careful look at the recent reviews by Bottomley et al., will give the reader a sense of the range of topics that are being studied by this and related techniques [Lillehei and Bottomley, 2000, 2001; Poggi et al., 2002, 2004].

SPM has made inroads in a number of different arenas, which can be separated into several key areas (1) imaging; (2) force spectroscopy; and (3) nanomechanical property measurement. We note that it would be difficult to cover all possible applications of this technique and we will restrict our focus to *in situ* studies of biomolecular systems.

67.5 Imaging

The real-space imaging capabilities, coupled with the ability to simultaneously display derivative images, such as phase (viscoelasticity), friction, and temperature is perhaps the most attractive attribute of the scanning probe microscope. In the case of biomolecules, it is the ability to perform such imaging but in buffer media, under a variety of solution conditions and temperatures, in real-time that has really powered the acceptance of this technique by the biomedical community [Conway et al., 2000; Moradian-Oldak et al., 2000; Oesterhelt et al., 2000a; Rochet et al., 2000; Trottier et al., 2000]. Such capabilities are allowing researchers to gain a glimpse of the mechanics and dynamics of protein assembly and function, and the role of extrinsic factors, such as pH, temperature, or other ligands on these processes [Thompson et al., 2000]. For example, *in situ* SPM has been used successfully to visualize and characterize voltage and pH-dependent conformational changes in two-dimensional arrays of OmpF [Moller et al., 1999] while a number of groups have used *in situ* SPM to characterize transcription and DNA-complex formation [Hun Seong et al., 2002; Mukherjee et al., 2002; Seong et al., 2002; Tahirov et al., 2002; Rivetti et al., 2003].

The raster-scanning action of the tip does, however, complicate *in situ* imaging. At the very least, if a process occurs faster than the time required to capture a single image, the SPM may in fact miss the event, or worse, in fact create an artifact associated with the motion of the object. The magnitude of this effect obviously depends on the kinetics of the processes under study. Accordingly, there can be a significant time lag between the first and last scan lines in an SPM image. This is particularly important when one is viewing live cell data where scan times are necessarily slow ($\sim$1 Hz) [Cho et al., 2002; Jena, 2002]. New advances in tip and controller technology are now helping to improve the stability of the instrument under high scan-rate conditions. For instance, special cantilevers are often required when one begins to approach TV scan rates in the SPM. These may include tips with active piezoelectric elements. A particularly useful, and low-cost option for improving time resolution is to simply disable one of the scanning directions so that the AFM image is a compilation of line scans taken at the same location as a function of time [Petsev et al., 2000]. This would therefore generate an isosurface wherein one of the image axes reflects time and not position.

67.6 Crystallography

In situ SPM has been used with great success to study the mechanisms associated with crystal growth [Ward, 2001], from amino acids [Manne et al., 1993], to zeolite crystallization [Agger et al., 2003], and biomineralization [Costa and Maquis, 1998; Teng et al., 1998; Wen et al., 2000]. For protein crystals, studies have ranged from early investigations of lysozyme [Durbin and Feher, 1996], to insulin [Yip et al., 2000], antibodies [Kuznetsov et al., 2000; Plomp et al., 2003], and recently the mechanisms of protein crystal repair [Plomp et al., 2003]. The advantages of SPM for characterizing protein crystallization mechanisms have been very well elucidated in a review by McPherson et al. [2000]. It is worth mentioning that the high spatial and temporal resolution capabilities of the SPM are ideal for examining and measuring the thermodynamic parameters for these processes. These range from local variations in free energy and their correlation with conventional models of crystal growth to a recent study of apoferritin in which step advancement rates were correlated with the product of the density of surface kink sites and the frequency of attachment [Yau and Vekilov, 2000].

A particular challenge for SPM studies of crystal growth is that interpreting the data paradoxically often requires that one already have a known crystal structure or a related isoform for comparison of packing motifs and molecular orientation. Recently the focus has shifted toward understanding the growth process. The ability to perform extended duration *in situ* imaging presents the crystallographer with the unique opportunity of directly determining the mechanisms and kinetics of crystal nucleation and growth. [McPherson et al., 2000; Yau et al., 2000; Yau and Vekilov, 2000; Day et al., 2001; Ko et al., 2001; Kuznetsov et al., 2001a–c; Lucas et al., 2001; McPherson et al., 2001; Yau et al., 2001; Yau and Vekilov, 2001; Chen and Vekilov, 2002; Malkin et al., 2002; Plomp et al., 2002, 2003]. This is arguably a consequence of the inability of the SPM to acquire true real-space three-dimensional images of the interior regions of the proteins. Often, the proteins will appear as amorphous blob to the AFM, even when packed into a lattice and it is therefore difficult to assign a specific secondary structure to the protein. In related work, dissolution studies of small molecule crystals have been very enlightening. Recent work by Danesh et al., resolved the difference between various crystal polymorphs including face-specific dissolution rates for drug candidates [Danesh et al., 2000a, b, 2001] while Guo et al. [2002] examined the effect of specific proteins on the crystallization of calcium oxalate monohydrate. In a particularly interesting study, Frincu et al. [2004] investigated cholesterol crystallization from bile solutions using calcite as a model substrate. In this chapter, the authors were able to use *in situ* SPM to characterize the role of specific substrate interactions in driving the initial nucleation events associated with cholesterol crystallization. Extended-duration imaging allowed the researchers to characterize the growth rates and the onset of Ostwald ripening under physiological conditions. They were able to confirm their observations and models by calculating the interfacial energies associated with the attachment of the cholesterol crystal to the calcite substrate. It is this rather powerful combination of *in situ* real-time characterization with theoretical modeling that has made *in situ* SPM a particularly compelling technique for studying self-assembly at interfaces.

67.6.1 Protein Aggregation and Fibril Formation

In a related context, the self-assembly of proteins into fibrillar motifs has been an area of active research for many years, owing in large part to the putative links to diseases such as Alzheimer's, Huntingtin's, and even diabetes in the context of *in vitro* insulin fibril formation [Waugh et al., 1950; Foster et al., 1951]. *In situ* studies of aggregation and fibrillogenesis by SPM have included collagen [Baselt et al., 1993; Cotterill et al., 1993; Gale et al., 1995; Watanabe et al., 1997; Taatjes et al., 1999], and spider silk [Li et al., 1994; Gould et al., 1999; Miller et al., 1999; Oroudjev et al., 2002]. The clinical implications of fibril and plaque formation and the fact that *in situ* SPM is perhaps the only means of acquiring real-space information on these processes and structures that clinically cannot be easily assayed has driven recent investigations of insulin amyloid polypeptide (IAPP), amylin, beta-amyloid, and synuclein [Harper et al., 1997a, b; Yang et al., 1999; Huang et al., 2000; Roher et al., 2000; McLaurin et al., 2002; Parbhu et al., 2002; Yip et al., 2002; Gorman et al., 2003].

Perhaps driven more by an applied technology perspective, *in situ* SPM has provided unique insights into the role of the nucleating substrate on directing the kinetics, orientation, and structure of the emerging fibril. As noted by Kowalewski in their investigation of beta-amyloid formation on different surfaces, chemically and structurally dissimilar substrate may in fact facilitate growth biasing the apparent kinetics and orientation of the aggregate [Kowalewski and Holtzman, 1999]. Since SPM imaging requires a supporting substrate, there is often a tacit assumption that this surface is passive and would not adversely influence the aggregation or growth process. However, what has become immediately obvious from a number of studies is that these surfaces can, and do, alter the nucleation and growth patterns [Yang et al., 2002; Wang et al., 2003]. Characterization, either theoretical or experimental using the *in situ* capabilities of the SPM, will, in principle, identify how the local physical/electronic/chemical nature of the surface will drive fibril formation [Sherrat et al., 2004]. However, it is clearly important that one be aware of this substrate-directing effect. One must ensure that appropriate controls were in place, or performed, so that the aggregate as seen by the SPM is clearly the responsible agent for nucleation. All of this certainly brings up the questions of (1) is the aggregate observed by these *in situ* tools truly the causative agent; (2) what role is the substrate playing in the aggregation or assembly pathway. The first point is a particularly compelling one when it concerns studies of protein adsorption and assembly. While the SPM can certainly resolve nanometer-sized objects, there always remains a question as to whether the object resolved by SPM is the smallest stable structure or whether there may be a solution species that is in fact smaller. Correlating solution with surface self-assembly mechanisms and structures, especially in the context of biomolecular complexes and phenomena, can be challenging and often one must resort to complementary, corroborative tools such as light scattering.

67.6.2 Membrane Protein Structure and Assemblies

One area in which scanning probe microscopy has made a significant impact has been in the structural characterization of membrane dynamics and protein–membrane interactions and assembly. Supported planar lipid bilayers are particularly attractive as model cell membranes [Sackmann, 1996] and recent work has provided very detailed insights of their local dynamics and structure [Dufrene and Lee, 2000; Jass et al., 2000; Leonenko et al., 2000; Richter et al., 2003], as well as the dynamics of domain formation [Rinia et al., 1999; McKiernan et al., 2000; Yuan et al., 2000; Giocondi et al., 2001b]. Exploiting the *in situ* high resolution imaging capabilities of the SPM, workers have been able to follow thermal phase transitions (gel–fluid) in supported bilayers [Giocondi et al., 2001b; Muresan et al., 2001; Tokumasu et al., 2002], and Langmuir–Blodgett films [Nielsen et al., 2000]. Recently, thermal transitions in mixed composition supported bilayers have been studied by *in situ* SPM [Giocondi et al., 2001a; Giocondi and Le Grimellec, 2004] where the so-called ripple phase domains were seen to form as the system entered the gel–fluid coexistence regime [Leidy et al., 2002].

In situ SPM has also been particularly useful for investigating the dynamics of the so-called lipid raft structures. For example, Rinia et al., investigated the role of cholesterol in the formation of rafts using a complex mixture of dioleoylphosphatidylcholine (DOPC), sphingomyelin (SpM), and cholesterol as the model membrane [Rinia and de Kruijff, 2001]. They were able to demonstrate that the room temperature phase separation seen in the SpM/DOPC bilayers, in the absence of cholesterol, at room temperature was simply a consequence of the gel-state SpM and fluid-state DOPC domains. As the cholesterol content increased, the authors reported the formation of SpM/cholesterol-rich domains or "lipid rafts" within the (DOPC) fluid domains. In related work, Van Duyl et al. [2003] observed similar domain formation for (1 : 1) SpM/DOPC SPBs containing 30 mol% cholesterol [van Duyl et al., 2003].

The effect of dynamically changing the cholesterol levels on raft formation and structure was reported by Lawrence et al. [2003]. By adding either water-soluble cholesterol or methyl-β-cyclodextrin (Mβ-CD), a cholesterol-sequestering agent, the authors were able to directly resolve the effect of adding or removing cholesterol on domain structure and dynamics, including a biphasic response to cholesterol level that was seen as a transient formation of raft domains as the cholesterol level was reduced.

The relative ease with which SPBs can be formed has prompted studies of reconstituted membrane proteins, including ion channels and transmembrane receptors [Lal et al., 1993; Puu et al., 1995, 2000; Takeyasu et al., 1996; Neff et al., 1997; Bayburt et al., 1998; Rinia et al., 2000; Fotiadis et al., 2001; Yuan and Johnston, 2001; Slade et al., 2002]. The premise here is that the SPB provides a membrane-mimicking environment for the protein allowing it to adopt a nominally native orientation at the bilayer surface. It is difficult to know a priori which way the receptor molecules will be oriented in the final supported bilayer since reconstitution occurs via freeze–thaw or sonication into the vesicle/liposome suspension [Radler et al., 1995; Puu and Gustafson, 1997; Jass et al., 2000; Reviakine and Brisson, 2000]. Often one relies on a statistical analysis of local surface topographies, which presumes that there is a distinct difference in the size and shape of the extra- and intracellular domains.

The SPBs have also been used as effective substrates in a vast number of AFM studies of the interactions between protein molecules and membrane surfaces. These studies have included membrane-active and membrane-associated proteins. Peptide-induced changes in membrane morphology and membrane disruption has been directly observed in SPBs in the presence of the amphipathic peptides; filipin, amphotericin B, and mellitin [Santos et al., 1998; Steinem et al., 2000; Milhaud et al., 2002]. In related work, the N-terminal domain of the capsid protein cleavage product of the flock house virus (FHV), has found to cause the formation of interdigitated domains upon exposure of the supported lipid bilayers to the soluble peptide [Janshoff et al., 1999].

Peptide–membrane interactions are also thought to be critical to the mechanism of neurodegenerative diseases such as Alzheimer's (AD) and Parkinson's (PD). For example, studies of α-synuclein with supported lipid bilayers revealed the gradual formation and growth of defects within the SPB [Jo et al., 2000]. Interestingly, the use of a mutant form of the -synuclein protein revealed a qualitatively slower rate of bilayer disruption. We conducted an analogous experiment to investigate the interaction between the amyloid-β (Aβ) peptide with SPBs prepared from a total brain lipid mixture [Yip and McLaurin, 2001]. Interestingly, *in situ* SPM revealed that the association of monomeric Aβ1-40 peptide with the SPB's resulted in rapid formation of fibrils followed by membrane disruption. Control experiments performed with pure component DMPC bilayers revealed similar membrane disruption however the mechanism was qualitatively different with the formation of amorphous aggregates rather than well-formed fibrils.

67.7 Force Spectroscopy

67.7.1 Fundamentals

Although most often used for imaging, by disabling the x- and y-scan directions and monitoring the tip deflection in the z-direction, the AFM is capable of measuring protein–protein and ligand–receptor binding forces, often with sub-piconewton resolution. The ability to detect such low forces is due to the low spring constant of the AFM cantilever (0.60 to 0.06 N/m). In these AFM force curve measurements, the tip is modeled as a Hookian spring whereby the amount of tip deflection (Δz) is directly related to the attractive/repulsive forces (F) acting on the tip through the tip spring constant (k). At the start of the force curve, the AFM tip is held at a null position of zero deflection out of contact with the sample surface. The tip–sample separation distance is gradually reduced and then enlarged using a triangular voltage cycle applied to the piezoelectric scanner. This will bring the tip into and out of contact with the sample surface. As the piezo extends, the sample surface contacts the AFM tip causing the tip to deflect upward until a maximum applied force is reached and the scanner then begins to retract. We should note that when the gradient of the attractive force between the tip and sample exceeds the spring constant of the tip, the tip will "jump" into contact with the sample surface. As the scanner retracts, the upward tip deflection is reduced until it reaches the null position. As the sample continues to move away from the tip, attractive forces between the tip and the surface hold the tip in contact with the surface and the tip begins to deflect in the opposite direction. The tip continues to deflect downward until the restoring force of the tip cantilever overcomes the attractive forces and the tip jumps out of contact with the sample surface (E), thereby providing us with an estimate of the tip–sample unbinding force, given as:

$$F = -k\Delta z$$

This force spectroscopy approach has found application ranging from mapping effect of varying ionic strength on the interactions between charged surfaces [Butt, 1991; Ducker et al., 1991; Senden and Drummond, 1995; Bowen et al., 1998; Liu et al., 2001; Tulpar et al., 2001; Lokar and Ducker, 2002; Mosley et al., 2003; Lokar and Ducker, 2004] [Ducker and Cook, 1990; Ducker et al., 1991, 1994; Butt et al., 1995; Manne and Gaub, 1997; Toikka and Hayes, 1997; Zhang et al., 1997; Hodges, 2002], to studying electrostatic forces at crystal surfaces [Danesh et al., 2000c; Muster and Prestidge, 2002].

67.7.2 Single Molecule Force Spectroscopy

The idea of mapping forces at surfaces rapidly lead to the concept of chemically modifying the SPM tips with ligands so that specific intermolecular interactions can be measured — *single molecule force spectroscopy* [Noy et al., 1995]. In principle, if we can measure the forces associated with the binding of a ligand to its complementary receptor, we may be able to correlate these forces with association energies [Leckband, 2000]. By tethering a ligand of interest, in the correct orientation, to the force microscope tip and bringing the now-modified tip into contact with an appropriately functionalized surface, one can now conceivably directly measure the attractive and repulsive intermolecular forces between single molecules as a function of the tip–sample separation distance. The vertical tip jump during pull-off can be used to estimate the interaction force, which can be related to the number of binding sites, adhesive contact area, and the molecular packing density of the bound molecules. In the case of biomolecular systems, multiple intermolecular interactions exist and both dissociation and (re)association events may occur on the time scale of the experiment resulting in broad retraction curve with discrete, possibly quantized, pull-off events. This approach has been used to investigate a host of interaction forces between biomolecules [Florin et al., 1994b; Hinterdorfer et al., 1996b; Rief et al., 1997a; Smith and Radford, 2000], and DNA–nucleotide interactions [Lee et al., 1994].

Although estimates of the adhesive interaction forces may be obtained from the vertical tip excursions during the retraction phase of the force curve, during pull-off, the width and shape of the retraction curve reflects entropically unfavorable molecular unfolding and elongation processes.

Although simple in principle, it was soon recognized that the force spectroscopy experiment was highly sensitive to sampling conditions. For example, it is now well recognized that the dynamics of the measurement will significantly influence the shape of the unbinding curve. It is well known that the rate of ligand–receptor dissociation increases with force resulting in a logarithmic dependence of the unbinding force with rate [Bell, 1978] and studies have shown that single molecule techniques, such as AFM, clearly sample an interaction energy landscape [Strunz et al., 2000]. It is therefore clear that forces measured by the AFM cannot be trivially related to binding affinities [Merkel et al., 1999]. Beyond these simple sampling rate dependence relationships, we must also be aware of the dynamics of the tip motion during the acquisition phase of the measurement. In particular, when these interactions are mapped in fluid media, one must consider the hydrodynamic drag associated with the (rapid) motion of the tip through the fluid [Janovjak et al., 2004]. This drag effect can be considerable when factored into the interaction force determination.

Another key consideration is that in single molecule force spectroscopy, the ligands of interest are necessarily immobilized at force microscope tips and sample surfaces. In principle, this approach will allow one to directly measure or evaluate the spatial relationship between the ligand and its corresponding receptor site. For correct binding to occur, the ligands of interest must be correctly oriented, have the appropriate secondary and tertiary structure, and be sufficiently flexible (or have sufficiently high unrestricted mobility) that they can bind correctly. An appropriate immobilization strategy would therefore require a priori information about the ligand's sequence, conformation, and the location of the binding sites [Wagner, 1998; Wadu-Mesthrige et al., 2000]. Strategies that have worked in the past include N-nitrilo-triacetic acid linkages [Schmitt et al., 2000] and His-tags to preferentially orient ligands at surface [Ill et al., 1993; Thomson et al., 1999]. More recent efforts have focused on the use of polyethylene glycol tethers to help extend the ligands away from the tip [Kada et al., 2001; Nevo et al., 2003; Stroh et al., 2004], a strategy that has proven to be quite reliable and robust [Hinterdorfer et al., 1996a; Raab et al., 1999; Schmidt et al., 1999; Baumgartner et al., 2000a,b].

67.7.3 Force Volume

Acquiring force curves at each point on an image plane provides a means of acquiring so-called force volume maps, a data-intensive imaging approach capable of providing a map of relative adhesion forces and charge densities across surfaces [Gad et al., 1997; Radmacher, 1997; Heinz and Hoh, 1999b]

[Heinz and Hoh, 1999a; Shellenberger and Logan, 2002]. This approach has been used successfully to examine polymer surfaces and surfaces under fluid [Mizes et al., 1991; van der Werf et al., 1994], as well as live cells [Gad et al., 1997; Nagao and Dvorak, 1998; Walch et al., 2000].

67.7.4 Pulsed Force Mode

As indicated earlier, force volume measurements are very time-consuming and this has led to the development of pulsed force mode imaging [Rosa-Zeiser et al., 1997]. Capable of rapidly acquiring topographic, elasticity, and adhesion data, pulsed force mode operates by sampling selected regions of the force–distance curve during contact-mode imaging. During image scanning, an additional sinusoidal oscillation imparted to the tip brings the tip in- and out-of contact with the surface at each point of the image. Careful analysis of the pulsed force spectrum can yield details about surface elasticity and adhesion [Okabe et al., 2000; Zhang et al., 2000a,b; Fujihira et al., 2001; Schneider et al., 2002; Kresz et al., 2004; Stenert et al., 2004]. Compared with the ~Hz sample rates present in conventional force volume imaging, in pulsed force mode, spectra are acquired on kHz sampling rates. Although this helps to resolve the issue related to the speed of data acquisition, one must clearly consider the possibilities associated (possible) rate-dependence of the adhesion forces, and as indicated in the previous section, the hydrodynamic forces would play a larger role.

67.8 Binding Forces

As discussed earlier, force spectroscopy samples regions of an energy landscape wherein the strength of a bond (and its lifetime) is highly dependent on the rate with which the spectra are collected [Evans and Ritchie, 1999] [Strunz et al., 2000]. At low loading rates, intermolecular bonds have long lifetimes but exhibit small unbinding forces, while at high loading rates, the same bonds will have shorter lifetimes and larger unbinding forces. In the case of biomolecular complexes, since multiple interactions are involved in stabilizing the binding interface, the dissociation pathway of a ligand–receptor complex will exhibit a number of unbinding energy barriers. This would suggest that one could in fact, sample any number of dissociation pathways, each with its own set of transitional bonding interactions.

For the majority of single molecule force microscopy studies, individual ligands have been either randomly adsorbed onto or directly attached to the AFM tip through covalent bond formation. Covalent binding of a molecule to the tip offers a more stable "anchor" during force measurements as a covalent bond is ~10 times stronger than a typical ligand–receptor bond [Grandbois et al., 1999]. Covalent binding also facilitates oriented attachment of the ligand as compared to random adsorption where the orientation of the ligand on the tip surface must be statistically inferred. These advantages are tempered with the challenges present in immobilizing molecules to surfaces such as the AFM tip. As mentioned earlier, oriented ligands have been tethered covalently to AFM tips through use of flexible poly(ethylene-glycol) (PEG)-linkers [Hinterdorfer et al., 1996b]. In this way, the peptide or ligand is extended away from the tip surface, which provides it with sufficient flexibility and conformational freedom for it to reorient and sample conformational space. Heterobifunctional PEG derivatives have provided the necessary synthetic flexibility for coupling a host of different ligands to the AFM tips. [Haselgrubler et al., 1995; Hinterdorfer et al., 1996b] [Willemsen et al., 1998] [Raab et al., 1999; Baumgartner et al., 2000a; Kada et al., 2001; Wielert-Badt et al., 2002; Nevo et al., 2003].

The field of single molecule force spectroscopy comprises two theme areas — the first pertains to mapping or measuring forces between discrete molecules. For example, a number of groups have investigated antibody–antigen interactions [Ros et al., 1998; Allen et al., 1999] and have shown that these unbinding forces may correlate with thermal dissociation rates [Schwesinger et al., 2000]. Force spectroscopy has been used to study the energetics of protein adsorption [Gergely et al., 2000]. Although the high force sensitivity of this approach is exceptionally attractive, it is equally important to recognize key experimental considerations, including the use of appropriate controls. Recently, a number of computational approaches, including steered molecular dynamics [Lu and Schulten, 1999; Marszalek et al., 1999; Baerga-Ortiz et al., 2000; Lu and Schulten, 2000; Isralewitz et al., 2001; Altmann et al., 2002; Gao et al., 2002a,b, 2003; Carrion-Vazquez et al., 2003], Monte Carlo simulations [Clementi et al., 1999], and graphical energy function analyses [Qian and Shapiro, 1999] have been used to simulate these dissociation experiments.

Force spectroscopy is also being applied to study protein-unfolding pathways. It was recognized in the early work that was done during the retraction phase of the AFM force curve, the molecule is subjected to a high tensile stress, and can undergo reversible elongation and unfolding. Careful control over the applied load (and the degree of extension) will allow one to probe molecular elasticity and the energetics involved in the unfolding/folding process [Vesenka et al., 1993; Engel et al., 1999; Fisher et al., 1999; Fotiadis et al., 2002] [Müller et al., 1998; Oesterhelt et al., 2000b; Rief et al., 2000; Best and Clarke, 2002; Muller et al., 2002; Oberhauser et al., 2002; Oroudjev et al., 2002; Rief and Grubmuller, 2002; Zhang et al., 2002; Carrion-Vazquez et al., 2003; Hertadi et al., 2003; Kellermayer et al., 2003; Williams et al., 2003; Janovjak et al., 2004; Schwaiger et al., 2004]. Past studies have included investigations of titin [Oberhauser et al., 2001], IgG phenotypes [Carrion-Vazquez et al., 1999], various polysaccharides [Marszalek et al., 1999], and spider silk proteins [Becker et al., 2003].

By bringing the AFM tip into contact with the surface-adsorbed molecules, and carefully controlling the rate and extent of withdrawal from the surface, it is now possible to resolve transitions that may be ascribed to unfolding of individual protein domains. Others have employed this "forced unfolding" approach to look at spectrin [Rief et al., 1999; Lenne et al., 2000], lysozyme [Yang et al., 2000], and DNA [Clausen-Schaumann et al., 2000]. Caution needs to be exercised during such experiments. Often the protein of interest is allowed to simply absorb to the substrate to form a film. Force curves performed on these films are then conducted in random locations and the retraction phase of the curve analyzed for elongation and unbinding events. This is a highly statistical approach and somewhat problematic. In such a configuration, the general premise is that the tip will bind to the protein somewhere and that if enough samples are acquired, there will be a statistically relevant number of curves that will exhibit the anticipated number of unbinding and unfolding events. What is fundamentally challenging here is that there is no a priori means of knowing where the tip will bind to the protein, which would obviously affect its ability to under extension, and it is difficult to assess the interactions between the protein and the supporting substrate or possibly other entangled proteins.

Where single molecule imaging comes to the forefront is in the combination of imaging and single molecule force spectroscopy. In the past, force spectroscopy has relied heavily on random sampling of the immobilized proteins, often without direct imaging of the selected protein. Recently, Raab et al. combined dynamic force microscopy, wherein a magnetically coated AFM tip is oscillated in close proximity to a surface by analternating magnetic field. This enabled the researchers to apply what they termed "recognition imaging" to facilitate mapping of individual molecular recognition sites on a surface [Raab et al., 1999]. In recognition imaging, specific binding events are detected through dampening of the amplitude of oscillation of the ligand-modified tip due to specific binding of the antibody on the tip to an antigen on the surface. The resulting AFM antibody–antigen recognition image will display regions of enhanced contrast that can be identified as possible binding sites or domains. In an excellent demonstration of the coupled imaging and force spectroscopy, Oesterhelt et al., studied the unfolding of bacteriorhodopsin by directly adsorbing native purple membrane to a surface, imaging the trimeric structure of the BR, and then carefully pulling on a selected molecule [Oesterhelt et al., 2000a]. This allowed them to resolve the force required to destabilize the BR helices from the membrane and by reimaging the same area, show that extraction occurred two helices at a time.

Computationally, these phenomena are most often modeled as worm-like chains [Zhang and Evans, 2001]. To assess what exactly "forced unfolding" involves, Paci and Karplus examined the role of topology and energetics on protein unfolding via externally applied forces and compared it against the more traditional thermal unfolding pathways [Paci and Karplus, 2000].

67.8.1 Mechanical Properties

The use of the AFM/SPM as a nanomechanical tester has certainly blossomed. For example, over the past 10 years, AFM-based nanoindentation has been used to determine the elastic modulus of polymers [Weisenhorn et al., 1993], biomolecules [Vinckier et al., 1996; Laney et al., 1997; Lekka et al., 1999; Parbhu et al., 1999; Suda et al., 1999] [Cuenot et al., 2000], cellular and tissue surfaces [Shroff et al., 1995; Mathur et al., 2000; Velegol and Logan, 2002; Touhami et al., 2003; Alhadlaq et al., 2004; Ebenstein and Pruitt, 2004], pharmaceutical solids [Liao and Wiedmann, 2004] and even teeth [Balooch et al., 2004]. What is particularly challenging in these applications is the need for careful consideration when extrapolating bulk moduli against the nanoindentation data. Often the classical models need to be adjusted in order to compensate for the small (nanometer) contact areas involved in the indentation [Landman et al., 1990]. A particularly important consideration with AFM-based nanoindentation is the sampling geometry. While traditional indentation instrumentation applies a purely vertical load on the sample, by virtue of the cantilever arrangement of the AFM system, there is also a lateral component to the indentation load. This leads to an asymmetry in the indentation profile. This asymmetry can make it difficult to compare AFM-based nanoindentation with traditional approaches using a center-loaded system. Often this effect is nullified by the use of a spherical tip with a well-defined geometry; however, this entails a further compromise in the ability to perform imaging prior to the indentation process. This effect has been extensively covered in the literature, especially in the context of polymer blends and composite materials [Van Landringham et al., 1997a–c, 1999; Bogetti et al., 1999; Bischel et al., 2000]. Other considerations include the relative stiffness of the AFM cantilever, the magnitude of the applied load, tip shape that plays a significant role in the indentation process, and possibly the dwell-time. In many cases, the relatively soft cantilever will allow one to perform more precise modulus measurements including the ability to image prior to, and immediately after, an indentation measurement. At an even more pragmatic level, determining the stiffness both in-plane and torsional, of the cantilever can be challenging, with approaches ranging from the traditional end-mass to new techniques based on thermal noise and resonant frequency shifts [Cleveland et al., 1993; Hutter and Bechhoefer, 1993; Bogdanovic et al., 2000]. Accurate determination of these values is essential in order for the correct assessment of the local stiffness to be made.

67.8.2 Coupled Imaging

While AFM/SPM is certainly a powerful tool for following structure and dynamics at surfaces under a wide variety of conditions, it can only provide relative information within a given imaging frame. It similarly cannot confirm (easily) that the structure being imaged is in fact the protein of interest. It could in fact be said that SPM images are artefactual until proven otherwise. This confirmation step can involve some *in situ* control, which might be a change in pH or T, or introduction of another ligand or reagent that would cause a change in the same that could be resolved by the SPM. Absent an *in situ* control, or in fact as an adjunct, careful shape/volume analysis is often conducted to characterize specific features in a sample. Image analysis and correlation tools and techniques are often exploited for postacquisition analysis. There has always been an obvious need to techniques or tools that can provide this complementary information, ideally in a form that could be readily integrated into the SPM.

Optical imaging represents perhaps the best tool for integration with scanning probe microscopy. This is motivated by the realization that there are a host of very powerful single molecule optical imaging techniques capable of addressing many of the key limitations of SPM, such as the ability to resolve dynamic events on millisecond time scales. Recent advances in confocal laser scanning (CLSM) and total internal reflectance fluorescence (TIRFM) techniques have enabled single molecule detection with subdiffraction limited images [Ambrose et al., 1999; Sako et al., 2000a,b; Osborne et al., 2001; Ludes and Wirth, 2002; Sako and Uyemura, 2002; Borisenko et al., 2003; Cannone et al., 2003; Michalet et al., 2003; Wakelin and Bagshaw, 2003].

67.8.3 Near-Field — SNOM/NSOM

In the family of scanning probe microscopes, perhaps the best example of an integrated optical-SPM system are the scanning near-field (or near-field scanning) optical microscopes (SNOM or NSOM), which use near-field excitation of the sample to obtained subdiffraction limited images with spatial resolution comparable to conventional scanning probe microscopes [Muramatsu et al., 1995; Sekatskii et al., 2000; de Lange et al., 2001; Edidin 2001; Harris 2003]. NSOM has been used successfully in single molecule studies of dyes [Betzig and Chichester, 1993], proteins [Moers et al., 1995; Garcia-Parajo et al., 1999; van Hulst et al., 2000], and the structure of lignin and ion channels [Ianoul et al., 2004; Micic et al., 2004]. NSOM imaging has also provided insights into ligand-induced clustering of the ErbB2 receptor, a member of the epidermal growth factor (EGF) receptor tyrosine kinase family, in the membrane of live cells [Nagy et al., 1999]. Fluorescence lifetime imaging by NSOM has been used to examine the energy and electron-transfer processes of the light harvesting complex (LHC II) [Hosaka and Saiki, 2001; Sommer and Franke, 2002] in intact photosynthetic membranes [Dunn et al., 1994]. NSOM has also been used to monitor the fluorescence resonance energy transfer (FRET) between single pairs of donor and acceptor fluorophores on dsDNA molecules [Ha et al., 1996]. Challenges that face the NSOM community arguably lie in the robust design of the imaging tips [Burgos et al., 2003; Prikulis et al., 2003].

67.8.4 Evanescent-Wave — TIRF (Total Internal Reflection Fluorescence Microscopy)

Time resolved single molecule imaging can be difficult and in the case of the AFM, one may question whether the local phenomena imaged by AFM is specific to that particular imaging location. This is especially true for studies of dynamic phenomena since the scanning action of the AFM tip effectively acts to increase mass transfer into the imaging volume. Recently, combined AFM/TIRF techniques have been used to study force transmission [Mathur et al., 2000] and single-particle manipulation [Nishida et al., 2002] in cells. These studies helped to address a particularly challenging aspect of scanning probe microscopy, which was that SPM/AFM can only (realistically) infer data about the upper surface of structures and that data on the underside of a structure, for instance the focal adhesions of a cell, are largely invisible to the SPM tip. In the case of cell adhesion, one might be interested in how a cell responds to a local stress applied to its apical surface by monitoring changes in focal adhesion density and size. Using a combined AFM-TIRF system, it then becomes possible to directly interrogate the basal surface of the cell (by TIRF) while applying a load or examining the surface topography of the cell by *in situ* AFM. We recently reported on the design and use of a AFM — objective-based TIRF-based instrument for the study of supported bilayer systems [Shaw et al., 2003]. By coupling these two instruments together we were able to identify unequivocally the gel and fluid domains in a mixed dPOPC/dPPC system. What was particularly compelling was the observation of $\sim$10 to 20% difference in the lateral dimension of the features as resolved by TIRF and AFM. While this likely reflects the inherent diffraction limited nature of TIRFM, we can in fact use the AFM data to confirm the real-space size of the structures that are responsible for the fluorescence image contrast. This combined system also provided another interesting insight. The nonuniform fluorescence intensity across the domains resolved by TIRF may reflect a nonuniform distribution of NBD-PC within dPOPC. It may also be linked to the time required to capture a TIRF image relative to the AFM imaging. At a typical scan rate of 2 Hz, it would require $\sim$4 min to capture a conventional 512×512 pixel AFM image, compared with the $\sim$30 frame/sec video imaging rate of the TIRF camera system. As such the TIRFM system represents an excellent means of visualizing and capturing data that occur on time scales faster than what can be readily resolved by the AFM. This further suggests that the differences in fluorescence intensity may reflect real-time fluctuations in the structure of the lipid bilayer that are not detected (or detectable) by AFM imaging. In a particularly intriguing experiment that used TIRF as an excitation source rather than in an imaging mode, Hugel and others were able to measure the effect of a conformational change on the relative stiffness of a photosensitive polymer

[Hugel et al., 2002]. By irradiating the sample *in situ*, they were able to initiate a *cis–trans* conformational change that resulted in a change in the backbone conformation of the polymer.

67.9 Summary

As can be readily seen in the brief survey of the SPM field, it is clearly expanding both in terms of technique and range of applications. The systems are becoming more ubiquitous and certainly more approachable by the general user; however, what is clearly important is that care must be taken in data interpretation, instrument control, and sample preparation. For example, early studies of intermolecular forces often did not exercise the same level of control over their sampling conditions as is commonplace today and this clearly impacts critical analysis of the resulting force spectra. Recognizing the limitations of the tools and hopefully developing strategies that help to overcome these limitations represent a key goal for many SPM users.

New innovations in integrated single molecule correlated functional imaging tools will certainly continue to drive advances in this technology. As we have seen, fluorescence imaging, either as NSOM/TIRF/CSLM, when coupled with SPM provides an excellent *in situ* tool for characterizing biomolecular interactions and phenomena. Unfortunately, such a scheme requires specific labeling strategies and it would be preferable to effect such measurements in the absence of a label. Recent work has focused on near-field vibrational microscopy to acquire both IR and Raman spectra on nanometer length scales [Knoll et al., 2001; Hillenbrand et al., 2002; Anderson and Gaimari, 2003], while a combined Raman-SPM system was used to characterize the surface of an insect compound eye [Anderson and Gaimari, 2003]. These exciting new developments are clear evidence that the field of SPM is not a mature one but one that in fact continues to accelerate.

References

A-Hassan, E., Heinz, W.F., Antonik, M., D'Costa, N.P., Nageswaran, S., Schoenenberger, C.-A., and Hoh, J.H. (1998). Relative microelastic mapping of living cells by atomic force microscopy. *Biophys. J.* 74: 1564–1578.

Agger, J.R., Hanif, N., Cundy, C.S., Wade, A.P., Dennison, S., Rawlinson, P.A., and Anderson, M.W. (2003). Silicalite crystal growth investigated by atomic force microscopy. *J. Am. Chem. Soc.* 125: 830–839.

Alhadlaq, A., Elisseeff, J.H., Hong, L., Williams, C.G., Caplan, A.I., Sharma, B., Kopher, R.A., Tomkoria, S., Lennon, D.P., Lopez, A. et al. (2004). Adult stem cell driven genesis of human-shaped articular condyle. *Ann. Biomed. Eng.* 32: 911–923.

Allen, S., Davies, J., Davies, M.C., Dawkes, A.C., Roberts, C.J., Tendler, S.J., and Williams, P.M. (1999). The influence of epitope availability on atomic-force microscope studies of antigen-antibody interactions. *Biochem. J.* 341: 173–178.

Altmann, S.M., Grunberg, R.G., Lenne, P.F., Ylanne, J., Raae, A., Herbert, K., Saraste, M., Nilges, M., and Horber, J.K. (2002). Pathways and intermediates in forced unfolding of spectrin repeats. *Structure (Camb.)* 10: 1085–1096.

Ambrose, W.P., Goodwin, P.M., and Nolan, J.P. (1999). Single-molecule detection with total internal reflectance excitation: comparing signal-to-background and total signals in different geometries. *Cytometry* 36: 224–231.

Anderson, M.S. and Gaimari, S.D. (2003). Raman-atomic force microscopy of the ommatidial surfaces of dipteran compound eyes. *J. Struct. Biol.* 142: 364–368.

Argaman, M., Golan, R., Thomson, N.H., and Hansma, H.G. (1997). Phase imaging of moving DNA molecules and DNA molecules replicated in the atomic force microscope. *Nucleic Acids Res.* 25: 4379–4384.

Baerga-Ortiz, A., Rezaie, A.R., and Komives, E.A. (2000). Electrostatic dependence of the thrombin-thrombomodulin interaction. *J. Mol. Biol.* 296: 651–658.

Balooch, G., Marshall, G.W., Marshall, S.J., Warren, O.L., Asif, S.A., and Balooch, M. (2004). Evaluation of a new modulus mapping technique to investigate microstructural features of human teeth. *J. Biomech.* 37: 1223–1232.

Baselt, D.R., Revel, J.P., and Baldeschwieler, J.D. (1993). Subfibrillar structure of type I collagen observed by atomic force microscopy. *Biophys. J.* 65: 2644–2655.

Baumgartner, W., Hinterdorfer, P., Ness, W., Raab, A., Vestweber, D., Schindler, H., and Drenckhahn, D. (2000a). Cadherin interaction probed by atomic force microscopy. *Proc. Natl Acad. Sci. USA* 97: 4005–4010.

Baumgartner, W., Hinterdorfer, P., and Schindler, H. (2000b). Data analysis of interaction forces measured with the atomic force microscope. *Ultramicroscopy* 82: 85–95.

Bayburt, T.H., Carlson, J.W., and Sligar, S.G. (1998). Reconstitution and imaging of a membrane protein in a nanometer-size phospholipid bilayer. *J. Struct. Biol.* 123: 37–44.

Becker, N., Oroudjev, E., Mutz, S., Cleveland, J.P., Hansma, P.K., Hayashi, C.Y., Makarov, D.E., and Hansma, H.G. (2003). Molecular nanosprings in spider capture-silk threads. *Nat. Mater.* 2: 278–283.

Bell, G.I. (1978). Models for the specific adhesion of cells to cells. *Science* 200: 618–627.

Best, R.B. and Clarke, J. (2002). What can atomic force microscopy tell us about protein folding? *Chem. Commun. (Camb.)*: 183–192.

Betzig, E. and Chichester, R.J. (1993). Single molecules observed by near-field scanning optical microscopy. *Science* 262: 1422–1425.

Binnig, G., Quate, C.F., and Gerber, C. (1986). Atomic force microscope. *Phys. Rev. Lett.* 56: 930–933.

Binnig, G., Rohrer, H., Gerber, C., and Weibel, E. (1982). Tunneling through a controllable vacuum gap. *Rev. Modern Phys.* 59: 178–180.

Bischel, M.S., Van Landringham, M.R., Eduljee, R.F., Gillespie, J.W.J., and Schultz, J.M. (2000). On the use of nanoscale indentation with the AFM in the identification of phases in blends on linear low density polyethylene and high density polyethylene. *J. Mat. Sci.* 35: 221–228.

Bogdanovic, G., Meurk, A., and Rutland, M.W. (2000). Tip friction–torsional spring constant determination. *Colloids Surf. B Biointerfaces* 19: 397–405.

Bogetti, T.A., Wang, T., Van Landringham, M.R., Eduljee, R.F., and Gillespie, J.W.J. (1999). Characterization of nanoscale property variations in polymer composite systems: Part 2 — Finite element modeling. *Composites Part A* 30: 85–94.

Borisenko, V., Lougheed, T., Hesse, J., Fureder-Kitzmuller, E., Fertig, N., Behrends, J.C., Woolley, G.A., and Schutz, G.J. (2003). Simultaneous optical and electrical recording of single gramicidin channels. *Biophys. J.* 84: 612–622.

Bowen, W.R., Hilal, N., Lovitt, R.W., and Wright, C.J. (1998). Direct measurement of interactions between adsorbed protein layers using an atomic force microscope. *J. Colloid. Interface Sci.* 197: 348–352.

Brandsch, R., Bar, G., and Whangbo, M.-H. (1997). On the factors affecting the contrast of height and phase images in tapping mode atomic force microscopy. *Langmuir* 13: 6349–6353.

Brown, H.G. and Hoh, J.H. (1997). Entropic exclusion by neurofilament sidearms: a mechanism for maintaining interfilament spacing. *Biochemistry* 36: 15035–15040.

Burgos, P., Lu, Z., Ianoul, A., Hnatovsky, C., Viriot, M.L., Johnston, L.J., and Taylor, R.S. (2003). Near-field scanning optical microscopy probes: a comparison of pulled and double-etched bent NSOM probes for fluorescence imaging of biological samples. *J. Microsc.* 211: 37–47.

Butt, H. (1991). Measuring electrostatic, van der Waals, and hydration forces in electrolyte solutions with an atomic force microscope. *Biophys. J.* 60: 1438–1444.

Butt, H.-J., Jaschke, M., and Ducker, W. (1995. Measuring surface forces in aqueous electrolyte solution with the atomic force microscopy. *Bioelectrochem. Bioenerg.* 38: 191–201.

Cannone, F., Chirico, G., and Diaspro, A. (2003). Two-photon interactions at single fluorescent molecule level. *J. Biomed. Opt.* 8: 391–395.

Carrion-Vazquez, M., Li, H., Lu, H., Marszalek, P.E., Oberhauser, A.F., and Fernandez, J.M. (2003). The mechanical stability of ubiquitin is linkage dependent. *Nat. Struct. Biol.*

Carrion-Vazquez, M., Marszalek, P.E., Oberhauser, A.F., and Fernandez, J.M. (1999). Atomic force microscopy captures length phenotypes in single proteins. *Proc. Natl Acad. Sci. USA* 96: 11288–11292.

Chen, K. and Vekilov, P.G. (2002). Evidence for the surface-diffusion mechanism of solution crystallization from molecular-level observations with ferritin. *Phys. Rev. E Stat. Nonlin. Soft Matter Phys.* 66: 021606.

Cho, S.J., Quinn, A.S., Stromer, M.H., Dash, S., Cho, J., Taatjes, D.J., and Jena, B.P. (2002). Structure and dynamics of the fusion pore in live cells. *Cell Biol. Int.* 26: 35–42.

Clausen-Schaumann, H., Rief, M., Tolksdorf, C., and Gaub, H.E. (2000). Mechanical stability of single DNA molecules. *Biophys. J.* 78: 1997–2007.

Clementi, C., Carloni, P., and Maritan, A. (1999). Protein design is a key factor for subunit–subunit association. *Proc. Natl Acad. Sci. USA* 96: 9616–9621.

Cleveland, J.P., Manne, S., Bocek, D., and Hansma, P.K. (1993). A nondestructive method for determining the spring constant of cantilevers for scanning force microscopy. *Rev. Sci. Instrum.* 64: 403–405.

Conway, K.A., Harper, J.D., and Lansbury, P.T., Jr. (2000). Fibrils formed *in vitro* from alpha-synuclein and two mutant forms linked to Parkinson's disease are typical amyloid. *Biochemistry* 39: 2552–2563.

Costa, N. and Maquis, P.M. (1998). Biomimetic processing of calcium phosphate coating. *Med. Eng. Phys.* 20: 602–606.

Cotterill, G.F., Fergusson, J.A., Gani, J.S., and Burns, G.F. (1993). Scanning tunnelling microscopy of collagen I reveals filament bundles to be arranged in a left-handed helix. *Biochem. Biophys. Res. Commun.* 194: 973–977.

Cuenot, S., Demoustier-Champagne, S., and Nysten, B. (2000). Elastic modulus of polypyrrole nanotubes. *Phys. Rev. Lett.* 85: 1690–1693.

Czajkowsky, D.M., Allen, M.J., Elings, V., and Shao, Z. (1998). Direct visualization of surface charge in aqueous solution. *Ultramicroscopy* 74: 1–5.

Danesh, A., Chen, X., Davies, M.C., Roberts, C.J., Sanders, G.H., Tendler, S.J., Williams, P.M., and Wilkins, M.J. (2000a). The discrimination of drug polymorphic forms from single crystals using atomic force microscopy. *Pharm. Res.* 17: 887–890.

Danesh, A., Chen, X., Davies, M.C., Roberts, C.J., Sanders, G.H.W., Tendler, S.J.B., and Williams, P.M. (2000b). Polymorphic discrimination using atomic force microscopy: distinguishing between two polymorphs of the drug cimetidine. *Langmuir* 16: 866–870.

Danesh, A., Connell, S.D., Davies, M.C., Roberts, C.J., Tendler, S.J., Williams, P.M., and Wilkins, M.J. (2001). An *in situ* dissolution study of aspirin crystal planes (100) and (001) by atomic force microscopy. *Pharm. Res.* 18: 299–303.

Danesh, A., Davies, M.C., Hinder, S.J., Roberts, C.J., Tendler, S.J., Williams, P.M., and Wilkins, M.J. (2000c). Surface characterization of aspirin crystal planes by dynamic chemical force microscopy. *Anal. Chem.* 72: 3419–3422.

Day, J., Kuznetsov, Y.G., Larson, S.B., Greenwood, A., and McPherson, A. (2001). Biophysical studies on the RNA cores of satellite tobacco mosaic virus. *Biophys. J.* 80: 2364–2371.

de Lange, F., Cambi, A., Huijbens, R., de Bakker, B., Rensen, W., Garcia-Parajo, M., van Hulst, N., and Figdor, C.G. (2001). Cell biology beyond the diffraction limit: near-field scanning optical microscopy. *J. Cell Sci.* 114: 4153–4160.

Deleu, M., Nott, K., Brasseur, R., Jacques, P., Thonart, P., and Dufrene, Y.F. (2001). Imaging mixed lipid monolayers by dynamic atomic force microscopy. *Biochim. Biophys. Acta* 1513: 55–62.

Dinte, B.P., Watson, G.S., Dobson, J.F., and Myhra, S. (1996). Artefacts in non-contact mode force microscopy: the role of adsorbed moisture. *Ultramicroscopy* 63: 115–124.

Ducker, W.A. and Cook, R.F. (1990). Rapid measurement of static and dynamic surface forces. *Appl. Phys. Lett.* 56: 2408–2410.

Ducker, W.A., Senden, T.J., and Pashley, R.M. (1991). Direct measurement of colloidal forces using an atomic force microscope. *Nature* 353: 239–241.

Ducker, W.A., Xu, Z., and Israelachvili, J.N. (1994). Measurements of hydrophobic and DLVO forces in bubble-surface interactions in aqueous solutions. *Langmuir* 10: 3279–3289.

Dufrene, Y.F. and Lee, G.U. (2000). Advances in the characterization of supported lipid films with the atomic force microscope. *Biochim. Biophys. Acta* 1509: 14–41.

Dunn, R.C., Holtom, G.R., Mets, L., and Xie, X.S. (1994). Near-field imaging and fluorescence lifetime measurement of light harvesting complexes in intact photosynthetic membranes. *J. Phys. Chem.* 98: 3094–3098.

Durbin, S.D. and Feher, G. (1996). Protein crystallization. *Annu. Rev. Phys. Chem.* 47: 171–204.

Ebenstein, D.M. and Pruitt, L.A. (2004). Nanoindentation of soft hydrated materials for application to vascular tissues. *J. Biomed. Mater. Res.* 69A: 222–232.

Edidin, M. (2001). Near-field scanning optical microscopy, a siren call to biology. *Traffic* 2: 797–803.

Engel, A., Gaub, H.E., and Muller, D.J. (1999). Atomic force microscopy: a forceful way with single molecules. *Curr. Biol.* 9: R133–136.

Engel, A. and Muller, D.J. (2000). Observing single biomolecules at work with the atomic force microscope. *Nat. Struct. Biol.* 7: 715–718.

Evans, E. and Ritchie, K. (1999). Strength of a weak bond connecting flexible polymer chains. *Biophys. J.* 76: 2439–2447.

Fisher, T.E., Marszalek, P.E., Oberhauser, A.F., Carrion-Vazquez, M., and Fernandez, J.M. (1999). The micro-mechanics of single molecules studied with atomic force microscopy. *J. Physiol.* 520: 5–14.

Florin, E.-L., Radmacher, M., Fleck, B., and Gaub, H.E. (1994a). Atomic force microscope with magnetic force modulation. *Rev. Sci. Instrum.* 65: 639–643.

Florin, E.L., Moy, V.T., and Gaub, H.E. (1994b). Adhesion forces between individual ligand–receptor pairs. *Science* 264: 415–417.

Foster, G.E., Macdonald, J., and Smart, J.V. (1951). The assay of insulin *in vitro* by fibril formation and precipitation. *J. Pharm. Pharmacol.* 3: 897–904.

Fotiadis, D., Jeno, P., Mini, T., Wirtz, S., Muller, S.A., Fraysse, L., Kjellbom, P., and Engel, A. (2001). Structural characterization of two aquaporins isolated from native spinach leaf plasma membranes. *J. Biol. Chem.* 276: 1707–1714.

Fotiadis, D., Scheuring, S., Muller, S.A., Engel, A., and Muller, D.J. (2002). Imaging and manipulation of biological structures with the AFM. *Micron* 33: 385–397.

Frincu, M.C., Fleming, S.D., Rohl, A.L., and Swift, J.A. (2004). The epitaxial growth of cholesterol crystals from bile solutions on calcite substrates. *J. Am. Chem. Soc.* 126: 7915–7924.

Fritzsche, W. and Henderson, E. (1997). Mapping elasticity of rehydrated metaphase chromosomes by scanning force microscopy. *Ultramicroscopy* 69: 191–200.

Fujihira, M., Furugori, M., Akiba, U., and Tani, Y. (2001). Study of microcontact printed patterns by chemical force microscopy. *Ultramicroscopy* 86: 75–83.

Gad, M., Itoh, A., and Ikai, A. (1997). Mapping cell wall polysaccharides of living microbial cells using atomic force microscopy. *Cell. Biol. Int.* 21: 697–706.

Gale, M., Pollanen, M.S., Markiewicz, P., and Goh, M.C. (1995). Sequential assembly of collagen revealed by atomic force microscopy. *Biophys. J.* 68: 2124–2128.

Gao, M., Craig, D., Lequin, O., Campbell, I.D., Vogel, V., and Schulten, K. (2003). Structure and functional significance of mechanically unfolded fibronectin type III1 intermediates. *Proc. Natl Acad. Sci. USA* 100: 14784–14789.

Gao, M., Craig, D., Vogel, V., and Schulten, K. (2002a). Identifying unfolding intermediates of FN-III(10) by steered molecular dynamics. *J. Mol. Biol.* 323: 939–950.

Gao, M., Wilmanns, M., and Schulten, K. (2002b). Steered molecular dynamics studies of titin i1 domain unfolding. *Biophys. J.* 83: 3435–3445.

Garcia-Parajo, M.F., Veerman, J.A., Segers-Nolten, G.M., de Grooth, B.G., Greve, J., and van Hulst, N.F. (1999). Visualising individual green fluorescent proteins with a near field optical microscope. *Cytometry* 36: 239–246.

Gergely, C., Voegel, J., Schaaf, P., Senger, B., Maaloum, M., Horber, J.K., and Hemmerle, J. (2000). Unbinding process of adsorbed proteins under external stress studied by atomic force microscopy spectroscopy. *Proc. Natl Acad. Sci. USA* 97: 10802–10807.

Giocondi, M.-C., Vie, V., Lesniewska, E., Milhiet, P.-E., Zinke-Allmang, M., and Le Grimellec, C. (2001a). Phase topology and growth of single domains in lipid bilayers. *Langmuir* 17: 1653–1659.

Giocondi, M.C. and Le Grimellec, C. (2004). Temperature dependence of the surface topography in dimyristoylphosphatidylcholine/distearoylphosphatidylcholine multibilayers. *Biophys. J.* 86: 2218–2230.

Giocondi, M.C., Pacheco, L., Milhiet, P.E., and Le Grimellec, C. (2001b). Temperature dependence of the topology of supported dimirystoyl-distearoyl phosphatidylcholine bilayers. *Ultramicroscopy* 86: 151–157.

Gorman, P.M., Yip, C.M., Fraser, P.E., and Chakrabartty, A. (2003). Alternate aggregation pathways of the Alzheimer beta-amyloid peptide: abeta association kinetics at endosomal pH. *J. Mol. Biol.* 325: 743–757.

Gould, S.A., Tran, K.T., Spagna, J.C., Moore, A.M., and Shulman, J.B. (1999). Short and long range order of the morphology of silk from Latrodectus hesperus (Black Widow) as characterized by atomic force microscopy. *Int. J. Biol. Macromol.* 24: 151–157.

Grandbois, M., Beyer, M., Rief, M., Clausen-Schaumann, H., and Gaub, H.E. (1999). How strong is a covalent bond? *Science* 283: 1727–1730.

Guo, S., Ward, M.D., and Wesson, J.A. (2002). Direct visualization of calcium oxalate monohydrate crystallization and dissolution with atomic force microscopy and the role of polymeric additives. *Langmuir* 18: 4282–4291.

Ha, T., Enderle, T., Ogletree, D.F., Chemla, D.S., Selvin, P.R., and Weiss, S. (1996). Probing the interaction between two single molecules: fluorescence resonance energy transfer between a single donor and a single acceptor. *Proc. Natl Acad. Sci. USA* 93: 6264–6268.

Han, W., Lindsay, S.M., and Jing, T. (1996). A magnetically driven oscillating probe microscope for operation in liquids. *Appl. Phys. Lett.* 69: 4111–4113.

Hansma, H.G., Kim, K.J., Laney, D.E., Garcia, R.A., Argaman, M., Allen, M.J., and Parsons, S.M. (1997). Properties of biomolecules measured from atomic force microscope images: a review. *J. Struct. Biol.* 119: 99–108.

Hansma, P.K., Elings, V., Marti, O., and Bracker, C.E. (1988). Scanning tunneling microscopy and atomic force microscopy: application to biology and technology. *Science* 242: 209–216.

Harper, J.D., Lieber, C.M., and Lansbury, P.T., Jr. (1997a). Atomic force microscopic imaging of seeded fibril formation and fibril branching by the Alzheimer's disease amyloid-beta protein. *Chem. Biol.* 4: 951–959.

Harper, J.D., Wong, S.S., Lieber, C.M., and Lansbury, P.T. (1997b). Observation of metastable Abeta amyloid protofibrils by atomic force microscopy. *Chem. Biol.* 4: 119–125.

Harris, C.M. (2003). Shedding light on NSOM. *Anal. Chem.* 75: 223A–228A.

Haselgrubler, T., Amerstorfer, A., Schindler, H., and Gruber, H.J. (1995). Synthesis and applications of a new poly(ethylene glycol) derivative for the crosslinking of amines with thiols. *Bioconjug. Chem.* 6: 242–248.

Heinz, W.F. and Hoh, J.H. (1999a). Relative surface charge density mapping with the atomic force microscope. *Biophys. J.* 76: 528–538.

Heinz, W.F. and Hoh, J.H. (1999b). Spatially resolved force spectroscopy of biological surfaces using the atomic force microscope. *Trends Biotechnol.* 17: 143–150.

Hertadi, R., Gruswitz, F., Silver, L., Koide, A., Koide, S., Arakawa, H., and Ikai, A. (2003). Unfolding mechanics of multiple OspA substructures investigated with single molecule force spectroscopy. *J. Mol. Biol.* 333: 993–1002.

Hillenbrand, R., Taubner, T., and Keilmann, F. (2002). Phonon-enhanced light matter interaction at the nanometre scale. *Nature* 418: 159–162.

Hinterdorfer, P., Baumgartner, W., Gruber, H.J., and Schilcher, K. (1996a). Detection and localization of individual antibody-antigen recognition events by atomic force microscopy. *Proc. Natl Acad. Sci. USA* 93: 3477–3481.

Hinterdorfer, P., Baumgartner, W., Gruber, H.J., Schilcher, K., and Schindler, H. (1996b). Detection and localization of individual antibody-antigen recognition events by atomic force microscopy. *Proc. Natl Acad. Sci. USA* 93: 3477–3481.

Hodges, C.S. (2002). Measuring forces with the AFM: polymeric surfaces in liquids. *Adv. Colloid Interface Sci.* 99: 13–75.

Holland, N.B. and Marchant, R.E. (2000). Individual plasma proteins detected on rough biomaterials by phase imaging AFM. *J. Biomed. Mater. Res.* 51: 307–315.

Hosaka, N. and Saiki, T. (2001). Near-field fluorescence imaging of single molecules with a resolution in the range of 10 nm. *J. Microsc.* 202: 362–364.

Huang, T.H., Yang, D.S., Plaskos, N.P., Go, S., Yip, C.M., Fraser, P.E., and Chakrabartty, A. (2000). Structural studies of soluble oligomers of the Alzheimer beta-amyloid peptide. *J. Mol. Biol.* 297: 73–87.

Hugel, T., Holland, N.B., Cattani, A., Moroder, L., Seitz, M., and Gaub, H.E. (2002). Single-molecule optomechanical cycle. *Science* 296: 1103–1106.

Hun Seong, G., Kobatake, E., Miura, K., Nakazawa, A., and Aizawa, M. (2002). Direct atomic force microscopy visualization of integration host factor-induced DNA bending structure of the promoter regulatory region on the Pseudomonas TOL plasmid. *Biochem. Biophys. Res. Commun.* 291: 361–366.

Hutter, J.L. and Bechhoefer, J. (1993). Calibration of atomic-force microscope tips. *Rev. Sci. Instrum.* 64: 1868–1873.

Ianoul, A., Street, M., Grant, D., Pezacki, J., Taylor, R.S., and Johnston, L.J. (2004). Near-field scanning fluorescence microscopy study of ion channel clusters in cardiac myocyte membranes. *Biophys. J.*

Ill, C.R., Keivens, V.M., Hale, J.E., Nakamura, K.K., Jue, R.A., Cheng, S., Melcher, E.D., Drake, B., and Smith, M.C. (1993). A COOH-terminal peptide confers regiospecific orientation and facilitates atomic force microscopy of an IgG1. *Biophys. J.* 64: 919–924.

Isralewitz, B., Gao, M., and Schulten, K. (2001). Steered molecular dynamics and mechanical functions of proteins. *Curr. Opin. Struct. Biol.* 11: 224–230.

Janovjak, H., Struckmeier, J., and Muller, D.J. (2004). Hydrodynamic effects in fast AFM single-molecule force measurements. *Eur. Biophys. J.*

Janshoff, A., Bong, D.T., Steinem, C., Johnson, J.E., and Ghadiri, M.R. (1999). An animal virus-derived peptide switches membrane morphology: possible relevance to nodaviral tranfection processes. *Biochemistry* 38: 5328–5336.

Jass, J., Tjarnhage, T., and Puu, G. (2000). From liposomes to supported, planar bilayer structures on hydrophilic and hydrophobic surfaces: an atomic force microscopy study. *Biophys. J.* 79: 3153–3163.

Jena, B.P. (2002). Fusion pore in live cells. *News Physiol. Sci.* 17: 219–222.

Jo, E., McLaurin, J., Yip, C.M., St George-Hyslop, P., and Fraser, P.E. (2000). α-synuclein membrane interactions and lipid specificity. *J. Biol. Chem.* 275: 34328–34334.

Kada, G., Blayney, L., Jeyakumar, L.H., Kienberger, F., Pastushenko, V.P., Fleischer, S., Schindler, H., Lai, F.A., and Hinterdorfer, P. (2001). Recognition force microscopy/spectroscopy of ion channels: applications to the skeletal muscle Ca2+ release channel (RYR1). *Ultramicroscopy* 86: 129–137.

Kellermayer, M.S., Bustamante, C., and Granzier, H.L. (2003). Mechanics and structure of titin oligomers explored with atomic force microscopy. *Biochim. Biophys. Acta* 1604: 105–114.

Knoll, A., Magerle, R., and Krausch, G. (2001). Tapping mode atomic force microscopy on polymers: where is the true sample surface? *Macromolecules* 34: 4159–4165.

Ko, T.P., Kuznetsov, Y.G., Malkin, A.J., Day, J., and McPherson, A. (2001). X-ray diffraction and atomic force microscopy analysis of twinned crystals: rhombohedral canavalin. *Acta Crystallogr. D Biol. Crystallogr.* 57: 829–839.

Kowalewski, T. and Holtzman, D.M. (1999). *In situ* atomic force microscopy study of Alzheimer's beta-amyloid peptide on different substrates: new insights into mechanism of beta-sheet formation. *Proc. Natl Acad. Sci. USA* 96: 3688–3693.

Kresz, N., Kokavecz, J., Smausz, T., Hopp, B., Csete, A., Hild, S., and Marti, O. (2004). Investigation of pulsed laser deposited crystalline PTFE thin layer with pulsed force mode AFM. *Thin Solid Films* 453–454: 239–244.

Krol, S., Ross, M., Sieber, M., Kunneke, S., Galla, H.J., and Janshoff, A. (2000). Formation of three-dimensional protein-lipid aggregates in monolayer films induced by surfactant protein B. *Biophys. J.* 79: 904–918.

Kuznetsov, Y.G., Larson, S.B., Day, J., Greenwood, A., and McPherson, A. (2001a). Structural transitions of satellite tobacco mosaic virus particles. *Virology* 284: 223–234.

Kuznetsov, Y.G., Malkin, A.J., Lucas, R.W., and McPherson, A. (2000). Atomic force microscopy studies of icosahedral virus crystal growth. *Colloids Surf. B Biointerfaces* 19: 333–346.

Kuznetsov, Y.G., Malkin, A.J., Lucas, R.W., Plomp, M., and McPherson, A. (2001b). Imaging of viruses by atomic force microscopy. *J. Gen. Virol.* 82: 2025–2034.

Kuznetsov, Y.G., Malkin, A.J., and McPherson, A. (2001c). Self-repair of biological fibers catalyzed by the surface of a virus crystal. *Proteins* 44: 392–396.

Lal, R., Kim, H., Garavito, R.M., and Arnsdorf, M.F. (1993). Imaging of reconstituted biological channels at molecular resolution by atomic force microscopy. *Am. J. Physiol.* 265: C851–C856.

Landman, U., Luedtke, W.D., Burnham, N.A., and Colton, R.J. (1990). Atomistic mechanisms and dynamics of adhesion, nanoindentation, and fracture. *Science* 248: 454–461.

Laney, D.E., Garcia, R.A., Parsons, S.M., and Hansma, H.G. (1997). Changes in the elastic properties of cholinergic synaptic vesicles as measured by atomic force microscopy. *Biophys. J.* 72: 806–813.

Lawrence, J.C., Saslowsky, D.E., Edwardson, J.M., and Henderson, R.M. (2003). Real-time analysis of the effects of cholesterol on lipid raft behavior using atomic force microscopy. *Biophys. J.* 84: 1827–1832.

Leckband, D. (2000). Measuring the forces that control protein interactions. *Annu. Rev. Biophys. Biomol. Struct.* 29: 1–26.

Lee, G.U., Chrisey, L.A., and Colton, R.J. (1994). Direct measurement of the forces between complementary strands of DNA. *Science* 266: 771–773.

Leidy, C., Kaasgaard, T., Crowe, J.H., Mouritsen, O.G., and Jorgensen, K. (2002). Ripples and the formation of anisotropic lipid domains: imaging two-component supported double bilayers by atomic force microscopy. *Biophys. J.* 83: 2625–2633.

Lekka, M., Laidler, P., Gil, D., Lekki, J., Stachura, Z., and Hrynkiewicz, A.Z. (1999). Elasticity of normal and cancerous human bladder cells studied by scanning force microscopy. *Eur. Biophys. J.* 28: 312–316.

Lenne, P.F., Raae, A.J., Altmann, S.M., Saraste, M., and Horber, J.K. (2000). States and transitions during forced unfolding of a single spectrin repeat. *FEBS Lett.* 476: 124–128.

Leonenko, Z.V., Carnini, A., and Cramb, D.T. (2000). Supported planar bilayer formation by vesicle fusion: the interaction of phospholipid vesicles with surfaces and the effect of gramicidin on bilayer properties using atomic force microscopy. *Biochim. Biophys. Acta* 1509: 131–147.

Li, S.F., McGhie, A.J., and Tang, S.L. (1994). New internal structure of spider dragline silk revealed by atomic force microscopy. *Biophys. J.* 66: 1209–1212.

Liao, X. and Wiedmann, T.S. (2004). Characterization of pharmaceutical solids by scanning probe microscopy. *J. Pharm. Sci.* 93: 2250–2258.

Lillehei, P.T. and Bottomley, L.A. (2000). Scanning probe microscopy. *Anal. Chem.* 72: 189R–196R.

Lillehei, P.T. and Bottomley, L.A. (2001). Scanning force microscopy of nucleic acid complexes. *Meth. Enzymol.* 340: 234–251.

Lindsay, S.M., Lyubchenko Yu, L., Tao, N.J., Li, Y.Q., Oden, P.I., Derose, J.A., and Pan, J. (1993). Scanning tunneling microscopy and atomic force microscopy studies of biomaterials at a liquid–solid interface. *J. Vac. Sci. Technol. A* 11: 808–815.

Liu, J.-F., Min, G., and Ducker, W.A. (2001). AFM study of cationic surfactants and cationic polyelectrolyutes at the silica-water interface. *Langmuir* 17: 4895–4903.

Lokar, W.J. and Ducker, W.A. (2002). Proximal adsorption of dodecyltrimethylammonium bromide to the silica-electrolyte solution interface. *Langmuir* 18: 3167–3175.

Lokar, W.J. and Ducker, W.A. (2004). Proximal adsorption at glass surfaces: ionic strength, pH, chain length effects. *Langmuir* 20: 378–388.

Lu, H. and Schulten, K. (1999). Steered molecular dynamics simulations of force-induced protein domain unfolding. *Proteins* 35: 453–463.

Lu, H. and Schulten, K. (2000). The key event in force-induced unfolding of Titin's immunoglobulin domains. *Biophys. J.* 79: 51–65.

Lucas, R.W., Kuznetsov, Y.G., Larson, S.B., and McPherson, A. (2001). Crystallization of Brome mosaic virus and T = 1 Brome mosaic virus particles following a structural transition. *Virology* 286: 290–303.

Ludes, M.D. and Wirth, M.J. (2002). Single-molecule resolution and fluorescence imaging of mixed-mode sorption of a dye at the interface of C18 and acetonitrile/water. *Anal. Chem.* 74: 386–393.

Lvov, Y., Onda, M., Ariga, K., and Kunitake, T. (1998). Ultrathin films of charged polysaccharides assembled alternately with linear polyions. *J. Biomater. Sci. Polym. Ed.* 9: 345–355.

Magonov, S. and Godovsky, Y. (1999). Atomic force microscopy, part 8: visualization of granular nanostructure in crystalline polymers. *Am. Lab.* 1999: 52–58.

Magonov, S. and Heaton, M.G. (1998). Atomic force microscopy, part 6: recent developments in AFM of polymers. *Am. Lab.* 30.

Magonov, S.N., Elings, V., and Whangbo, M.-H. (1997). Phase imaging and stiffness in tapping mode AFM. *Surface Sci.* 375: L385–L391.

Magonov, S.N. and Reneker, D.H. (1997). Characterization of polymer surfaces with atomic force microscopy. *Annu. Rev. Mater. Sci.* 27: 175–222.

Malkin, A.J., Plomp, M., and McPherson, A. (2002). Application of atomic force microscopy to studies of surface processes in virus crystallization and structural biology. *Acta Crystallogr. D Biol. Crystallogr.* 58: 1617–1621.

Manne, S., Cleveland, J.P., Stucky, G.D., and Hansma, P.K. (1993). Lattice resolution and solution kinetics on surfaces of amino acid crystals: an atomic force microscope study. *J. Cryst. Growth (Netherlands)* 130: 333–340.

Manne, S. and Gaub, H.E. (1997). Force microscopy: measurement of local interfacial forces and surface stresses. *Curr. Opin. Colloid Interface Sci.* 2: 145–152.

Marszalek, P.E., Lu, H., Li, H., Carrion-Vazquez, M., Oberhauser, A.F., Schulten, K., and Fernandez, J.M. (1999). Mechanical unfolding intermediates in titin modules. *Nature* 402: 100–103.

Mathur, A.B., Truskey, G.A., and Reichert, W.M. (2000). Atomic force and total internal reflection fluorescence microscopy for the study of force transmission in endothelial cells. *Biophys. J.* 78: 1725–1735.

McKiernan, A.E., Ratto, T.V., and Longo, M.L. (2000). Domain growth, shapes, and topology in cationic lipid bilayers on mica by fluorescence and atomic force microscopy. *Biophys. J.* 79: 2605–2615.

McLaurin, J., Darabie, A.A., and Morrison, M.R. (2002). Cholesterol, a modulator of membrane-associated Abeta-fibrillogenesis. *Ann. NY Acad. Sci.* 977: 376–383.

McPherson, A., Malkin, A.J., Kuznetsov, Y.G., and Plomp, M. (2001). Atomic force microscopy applications in macromolecular crystallography. *Acta Crystallogr. D Biol. Crystallogr.* 57: 1053–1060.

McPherson, A., Malkin, A.J., and Kuznetsov Yu, G. (2000). Atomic force microscopy in the study of macromolecular crystal growth. *Annu. Rev. Biophys. Biomol. Struct.* 29: 361–410.

Merkel, R., Nassoy, P., Leung, A., Ritchie, K., and Evans, E. (1999). Energy landscapes of receptor–ligand bonds explored with dynamic force spectroscopy. *Nature* 397: 50–53.

Michalet, X., Kapanidis, A.N., Laurence, T., Pinaud, F., Doose, S., Pflughoefft, M., and Weiss, S. (2003). The power and prospects of fluorescence microscopies and spectroscopies. *Annu. Rev. Biophys. Biomol. Struct.* 32: 161–182.

Micic, M., Radotic, K., Jeremic, M., Djikanovic, D., and Kammer, S.B. (2004). Study of the lignin model compound supramolecular structure by combination of near-field scanning optical microscopy and atomic force microscopy. *Colloids Surf. B Biointerfaces* 34: 33–40.

Milhaud, J., Ponsinet, V., Takashi, M., and Michels, B. (2002). Interactions of the drug amphotericin B with phospholipid membranes containing or not ergosterol: new insight into the role of ergosterol. *Biochim. Biophys. Acta* 1558: 95–108.

Miller, L.D., Putthanarat, S., Eby, R.K., and Adams, W.W. (1999). Investigation of the nanofibrillar morphology in silk fibers by small angle X-ray scattering and atomic force microscopy. *Int. J. Biol. Macromol.* 24: 159–165.

Mizes, H.A., Loh, K.-G., Miller, R.J.D., Ahujy, S.K., and Grabowski, G.A. (1991). Submicron probe of polymer adhesion with atomic force microscopy. Dependence on topography and material inhomogenities. *Appl. Phys. Lett.* 59: 2901–2903.

Moers, M.H., Ruiter, A.G., Jalocha, A., and van Hulst, N.F. (1995). Detection of fluorescence in situ hybridization on human metaphase chromosomes by near-field scanning optical microscopy. *Ultramicroscopy* 61: 279–283.

Moller, C., Allen, M., Elings, V., Engel, A., and Muller, D.J. (1999). Tapping-mode atomic force microscopy produces faithful high-resolution images of protein surfaces. *Biophys. J.* 77: 1150–1158.

Moradian-Oldak, J., Paine, M.L., Lei, Y.P., Fincham, A.G., and Snead, M.L. (2000). Self-assembly properties of recombinant engineered amelogenin proteins analyzed by dynamic light scattering and atomic force microscopy. *J. Struct. Biol.* 131: 27–37.

Mosley, L.M., Hunter, K.A., and Ducker, W.A. (2003). Forces between colloid particles in natural waters. *Environ. Sci. Technol.* 37: 3303–3308.

Mukherjee, S., Brieba, L.G., and Sousa, R. (2002). Structural transitions mediating transcription initiation by T7 RNA polymerase. *Cell* 110: 81–91.

Müller, D.J., Fotiadis, D., and Engel, A. (1998). Mapping flexible protein domains at subnanometer resolution with the atomic force microscope. *FEBS Lett.* 430: 105–111.

Muller, D.J., Kessler, M., Oesterhelt, F., Moller, C., Oesterhelt, D., and Gaub, H. (2002). Stability of bacteriorhodopsin alpha-helices and loops analyzed by single-molecule force spectroscopy. *Biophys. J.* 83: 3578–3588.

Muramatsu, H., Chiba, N., Umemoto, T., Homma, K., Nakajima, K., Ataka, T., Ohta, S., Kusumi, A., and Fujihira, M. (1995). Development of near-field optic/atomic force microscope for biological materials in aqueous solutions. *Ultramicroscopy* 61: 265–269.

Muresan, A.S., Diamant, H., and Lee, K.Y. (2001). Effect of temperature and composition on the formation of nanoscale compartments in phospholipid membranes. *J. Am. Chem. Soc.* 123: 6951–6952.

Muster, T.H. and Prestidge, C.A. (2002). Face specific surface properties of pharmaceutical crystals. *J. Pharm. Sci.* 91: 1432–1444.

Nagao, E. and Dvorak, J.A. (1998). An integrated approach to the study of living cells by atomic force microscopy. *J. Microsc.* 191: 8–19.

Nagao, E. and Dvorak, J.A. (1999). Phase imaging by atomic force microscopy: analysis of living homoiothermic vertebrate cells. *Biophys. J.* 76: 3289–3297.

Nagy, P., Jenei, A., Kirsch, A.K., Szollosi, J., Damjanovich, S., and Jovin, T.M. (1999). Activation-dependent clustering of the erbB2 receptor tyrosine kinase detected by scanning near-field optical microscopy. *J. Cell. Sci.* 112: 1733–1741.

Neff, D., Tripathi, S., Middendorf, K., Stahlberg, H., Butt, H.J., Bamberg, E., and Dencher, N.A. (1997). Chloroplast F0F1 ATP synthase imaged by atomic force microscopy. *J. Struct. Biol.* 119: 139–148.

Nevo, R., Stroh, C., Kienberger, F., Kaftan, D., Brumfeld, V., Elbaum, M., Reich, Z., and Hinterdorfer, P. (2003). A molecular switch between alternative conformational states in the complex of Ran and importin beta1. *Nat. Struct. Biol.* 10: 553–557.

Nielsen, L.K., Bjornholm, T., and Mouritsen, O.G. (2000). Fluctuations caught in the act. *Nature* 404: 352.

Nishida, S., Funabashi, Y., and Ikai, A. (2002). Combination of AFM with an objective-type total internal reflection fluorescence microscope (TIRFM) for nanomanipulation of single cells. *Ultramicroscopy* 91: 269–274.

Noy, A., Frisbie, C.D., Rozsnyai, L.F., Wrighton, M.S., and Leiber, C.M. (1995). Chemical force microscopy: exploiting chemically-modified tips to quantify adhesion, friction, and functional group distributions in molecular assemblies. *J. Am. Chem. Soc.* 117: 7943–7951.

Noy, A., Sanders, C.H., Vezenov, D.V., Wong, S.S., and Lieber, C.M. (1998a). Chemically-sensitive imaging in tapping mode by chemical force microscopy: relationship between phase lag and adhesion. *Langmuir* 14: 1508–1511.

Noy, A., Sanders, C.H., Vezenov, D.V., Wong, S.S., and Lieber, C.M. (1998b). Chemically-sensitive imaging in tapping mode by chemical force microscopy: relationship between phase lag and adhesion. *Langmuir* 14: 1508–1511.

Oberhauser, A.F., Badilla-Fernandez, C., Carrion-Vazquez, M., and Fernandez, J.M. (2002). The mechanical hierarchies of fibronectin observed with single-molecule AFM. *J. Mol. Biol.* 319: 433–447.

Oberhauser, A.F., Hansma, P.K., Carrion-Vazquez, M., and Fernandez, J.M. (2001). Stepwise unfolding of titin under force-clamp atomic force microscopy. *Proc. Natl Acad. Sci. USA* 98: 468–472.

Oesterfelt, F., Rief, M., and Gaub, H.E. (1999). Single molecule force spectroscopy by AFM indicates helical structure of poly(ethylene-glycol) in water. *New J. Phys.* 1: 6.1–6.11.

Oesterhelt, F., Oesterhelt, D., Pfeiffer, M., Engel, A., Gaub, H.E., and Muller, D.J. (2000a). Unfolding pathways of individual bacteriorhodopsins. *Science* 288: 143–146.

Oesterhelt, F., Oesterhelt, D., Pfeiffer, M., Engel, A., Gaub, H.E., and Müller, D.J. (2000b). Unfolding pathways of individual bacteriorhodopsins. *Science* 288: 143–146.

Okabe, Y., Furugori, M., Tani, Y., Akiba, U., and Fujihira, M. (2000). Chemical force microscopy of microcontact-printed self-assembled monolayers by pulsed-force-mode atomic force microscopy. *Ultramicroscopy* 82: 203–212.

Opdahl, A., Hoffer, S., Mailhot, B., and Somorjai, G.A. (2001). Polymer surface science. *Chem. Rec.* 1: 101–122.

Oroudjev, E., Soares, J., Arcdiacono, S., Thompson, J.B., Fossey, S.A., and Hansma, H.G. (2002). Segmented nanofibers of spider dragline silk: atomic force microscopy and single-molecule force spectroscopy. *Proc. Natl Acad. Sci. USA* 99: 6460–6465.

Osborne, M.A., Barnes, C.L., Balasubramanian, S., and Klenerman, D. (2001). Probing DNA surface attachment and local environment using single molecule spectroscopy. *J. Phys. Chem. B.* 105: 3120–3126.

Paci, E. and Karplus, M. (2000). Unfolding proteins by external forces and temperature: the importance of topology and energetics. *Proc. Natl Acad. Sci. USA* 97: 6521–6526.

Paige, M.F. (2003). A comparison of atomic force microscope friction and phase imaging for the characterization of an immiscible polystyrene/poly(methyl methacrylate) blend film. *Polymer* 44: 6345–6352.

Parbhu, A., Lin, H., Thimm, J., and Lal, R. (2002). Imaging real-time aggregation of amyloid beta protein (1-42) by atomic force microscopy. *Peptides* 23: 1265–1270.

Parbhu, A.N., Bryson, W.G., and Lal, R. (1999). Disulfide bonds in the outer layer of keratin fibers confer higher mechanical rigidity: correlative nano-indentation and elasticity measurement with an AFM. *Biochemistry* 38: 11755–11761.

Pelling, A.E., Sehati, S., Gralla, E.B., Valentine, J.S., and Gimzewski, J.K. (2004). Local nanomechanical motion of the cell wall of Saccharomyces cerevisiae. *Science* 305: 1147–1150.

Petsev, D.N., Thomas, B.R., Yau, S., and Vekilov, P.G. (2000). Interactions and aggregation of apoferritin molecules in solution: effects of added electrolytes. *Biophys. J.* 78: 2060–2069.

Plomp, M., McPherson, A., and Malkin, A.J. (2003). Repair of impurity-poisoned protein crystal surfaces. *Proteins* 50: 486–495.

Plomp, M., Rice, M.K., Wagner, E.K., McPherson, A., and Malkin, A.J. (2002). Rapid visualization at high resolution of pathogens by atomic force microscopy: structural studies of herpes simplex virus-1. *Am. J. Pathol.* 160: 1959–1966.

Poggi, M.A., Bottomley, L.A., and Lillehei, P.T. (2002). Scanning probe microscopy. *Anal. Chem.* 74: 2851–2862.

Poggi, M.A., Gadsby, E.D., Bottomley, L.A., King, W.P., Oroudjev, E., and Hansma, H. (2004). Scanning probe microscopy. *Anal. Chem.* 76: 3429–3444.

Prikulis, J., Murty, K.V., Olin, H., and Kall, M. (2003). Large-area topography analysis and near-field Raman spectroscopy using bent fibre probes. *J. Microsc.* 210: 269–273.

Puu, G., Artursson, E., Gustafson, I., Lundstrom, M., and Jass, J. (2000). Distribution and stability of membrane proteins in lipid membranes on solid supports. *Biosens. Bioelectron.* 15: 31–41.

Puu, G. and Gustafson, I. (1997). Planar lipid bilayers on solid supports from liposomes — factors of importance for kinetics and stability. *Biochim. Biophys. Acta* 1327: 149–161.

Puu, G., Gustafson, I., Artursson, E., and Ohlsson, P.A. (1995). Retained activities of some membrane proteins in stable lipid bilayers on a solid support. *Biosens. Bioelectron.* 10: 463–476.

Qian, H. and Shapiro, B.E. (1999). Graphical method for force analysis: macromolecular mechanics with atomic force microscopy. *Proteins* 37: 576–581.

Raab, A., Han, W., Badt, D., Smith-Gill, S.J., Lindsay, S.M., Schindler, H., and Hinterdorfer, P. (1999). Antibody recognition imaging by force microscopy. *Nat. Biotechnol.* 17: 901–905.

Radler, J., Strey, H., and Sackmann, E. (1995). Phenomenology and kinetics of lipid bilayer spreading on hydrophilic surfaces. *Langmuir* 11: 4539–4548.

Radmacher, M. (1997). Measuring the elastic properties of biological samples with the AFM. *IEEE Eng. Med. Biol. Mag.* 16: 47–57.

Reviakine, I. and Brisson, A. (2000). Formation of supported phospholipid bilayers from unilamellar vesicles investigated by atomic force microscopy. *Langmuir* 16: 1806–1815.

Richter, R., Mukhopadhyay, A., and Brisson, A. (2003). Pathways of lipid vesicle deposition on solid surfaces: a combined QCM-D and AFM study. *Biophys. J.* 85: 3035–3047.

Rief, M., Gautel, M., and Gaub, H.E. (2000). Unfolding forces of titin and fibronectin domains directly measured by AFM. *Adv. Exp. Med. Biol.* 481: 129–136; discussion 137–141.

Rief, M., Gautel, M., Oesterhelt, F., Fernandez, J.M., and Gaub, H.E. (1997a). Reversible unfolding of individual titin immunoglobulin domains by AFM. *Science* 276: 1109–1112.

Rief, M. and Grubmuller, H. (2002). Force spectroscopy of single biomolecules. *Chemphyschem* 3: 255–261.

Rief, M., Oesterhelt, F., Heymann, B., and Gaub, H.E. (1997b). Single molecule force spectroscopy on polysaccharides by atomic force microscopy. *Science* 275: 1295–1297.

Rief, M., Pascual, J., Saraste, M., and Gaub, H.E. (1999). Single molecule force spectroscopy of spectrin repeats: low unfolding forces in helix bundles. *J. Mol. Biol.* 286: 553–561.

Rinia, H.A. and de Kruijff, B. (2001). Imaging domains in model membranes with atomic force microscopy. *FEBS Lett.* 504: 194–199.

Rinia, H.A., Demel, R.A., van der Eerden, J.P., and de Kruijff, B. (1999). Blistering of langmuir-blodgett bilayers containing anionic phospholipids as observed by atomic force microscopy. *Biophys. J.* 77: 1683–1693.

Rinia, H.A., Kik, R.A., Demel, R.A., Snel, M.M.E., Killian, J.A., van Der Eerden, J.P.J.M., and de Kruijff, B. (2000). Visualization of highly ordered striated domains induced by transmembrane peptides in supported phosphatidylcholine bilayers. *Biochemistry* 39: 5852–5858.

Rivetti, C., Vannini, N., and Cellai, S. (2003). Imaging transcription complexes with the Atomic Force Microscope. *Ital. J. Biochem.* 52: 98–103.

Rochet, J.C., Conway, K.A., and Lansbury, P.T., Jr. (2000). Inhibition of fibrillization and accumulation of prefibrillar oligomers in mixtures of human and mouse alpha-synuclein. *Biochemistry* 39: 10619–10626.

Roher, A.E., Baudry, J., Chaney, M.O., Kuo, Y.M., Stine, W.B., and Emmerling, M.R. (2000). Oligomeriza-tion and fibril assembly of the mayloid-beta protein. *Biochim. Biophys. Acta* 1502: 31–43.

Ros, R., Schwesinger, F., Anselmetti, D., Kubon, M., Schafer, R., Pluckthun, A., and Tiefenauer, L. (1998). Antigen binding forces of individually addressed single-chain Fv antibody molecules. *Proc. Natl Acad. Sci. USA* 95: 7402–7405.

Rosa-Zeiser, A., Weilandt, E., Hild, S., and Marti, O. (1997). The simultaneous measurement of elastic, electrostatic and adhesive properties by scanning force microscopy: pulsed force mode operation. *Meas. Sci. Technol.* 8: 1333–1338.

Sackmann, E. (1996). Supported membranes: scientific and practical applications. *Science* 271: 43–48.

Sako, Y., Hibino, K., Miyauchi, T., Miyamoto, Y., Ueda, M., and Yanagida, T. (2000a). Single-molecule imaging of signaling molecules in living cells. *Single Mol.* 2: 159–163.

Sako, Y., Minoghchi, S., and Yanagida, T. (2000b). Single-molecule imaging of EGFR signalling on the surface of living cells. *Nat. Cell. Biol.* 2: 168–172.

Sako, Y. and Uyemura, T. (2002). Total internal reflection fluorescence microscopy for single-molecule imaging in living cells. *Cell Struct. Funct.* 27: 357–365.

Santos, N.C., Ter-Ovanesyan, E., Zasadzinski, J.A., Prieto, M., and Castanho, M.A. (1998). Filipin-induced lesions in planar phospholipid bilayers imaged by atomic force microscopy. *Biophys. J.* 75: 1869–1873.

Schmidt, T., Hinterdorfer, P., and Schindler, H. (1999). Microscopy for recognition of individual biomolecules. *Microsc. Res. Tech.* 44: 339–346.

Schmitt, L., Ludwig, M., Gaub, H.E., and Tampe, R. (2000). A metal-chelating microscopy tip as a new toolbox for single-molecule experiments by atomic force microscopy. *Biophys. J.* 78: 3275–3285.

Schneider, M., Zhu, M., Papastavrou, G., Akari, S., and Mohwald, H. (2002). Chemical pulsed-force microscopy of single polyethyleneimine molecules in aqueous solution. *Langmuir* 18: 602–606.

Schwaiger, I., Kardinal, A., Schleicher, M., Noegel, A.A., and Rief, M. (2004). A mechanical unfolding intermediate in an actin-crosslinking protein. *Nat. Struct. Mol. Biol.* 11: 81–85.

Schwesinger, F., Ros, R., Strunz, T., Anselmetti, D., Guntherodt, H.J., Honegger, A., Jermutus, L., Tiefenauer, L., and Pluckthun, A. (2000). Unbinding forces of single antibody-antigen complexes correlate with their thermal dissociation rates. *Proc. Natl Acad. Sci. USA* 97: 9972–9977.

Scott, W.W. and Bhushan, B. (2003). Use of phase imaging in atomic force microscopy for measure-ment of viscoelastic contrast in polymer nanocomposites and molecularly thick lubricant films. *Ultramicroscopy* 97: 151–169.

Sekatskii, S.K., Shubeita, G.T., and Dietler, G. (2000). Time-gated scanning near-field optical microscopy. *Appl. Phys. Lett.* 77: 2089–2091.

Senden, T.J. and Drummond, C.J. (1995). Surface chemistry and tip-sample interactions in atomicforce microscopy. *Colloids and Surfaces* 94.

Seong, G.H., Yanagida, Y., Aizawa, M., and Kobatake, E. (2002). Atomic force microscopy identification of transcription factor NFkappaB bound to streptavidin-pin-holding DNA probe. *Anal. Biochem.* 309: 241–247.

Shaw, J.E., Slade, A., and Yip, C.M. (2003). Simultaneous in situ total internal reflectance fluorescence/atomic force microscopy studies of DPPC/dPOPC microdomains in supported planar lipid bilayers. *J. Am. Chem. Soc.* 125: 111838–111839.

Shellenberger, K. and Logan, B.E. (2002). Effect of molecular scale roughness of glass beads on colloidal and bacterial deposition. *Environ. Sci. Technol.* 36: 184–189.

Sherrat, M.J., Holmes, D.F., Shuttleworth, C.A., and Kielty, C.M. (2004). Substrate-dependent morphology of supramolecular assemblies: fibrillin and type-IV collagen microfibrils. *Biophys. J.* 86: 3211–3222.

Shroff, S.G., Saner, D.R., and Lal, R. (1995). Dynamic micromechanical properties of cultured rat atrial myocytes measured by atomic force microscopy. *Am. J. Physiol.* 269: C286–C292.

Slade, A., Luh, J., Ho, S., and Yip, C.M. (2002). Single molecule imaging of supported planar lipid bilayer — reconstituted human insulin receptors by in situ scanning probe microscopy. *J. Struct. Biol.* 137: 283–291.

Smith, D.A. and Radford, S.E. (2000). Protein folding: pulling back the frontiers. *Curr. Biol.* 10: R662–R664.

Sommer, A.P. and Franke, R.P. (2002). Near-field optical analysis of living cells in vitro. *J. Proteome Res.* 1: 111–114.

Steinem, C., Galla, H.-J., and Janshoff, A. (2000). *Phys. Chem. Chem. Phys.* 2: 4580–4585.

Stenert, M., Döring, A., and Bandermann, F. (2004). Poly(methyl methacrylate)-block-polystyrene and polystyrene-block-poly (*n*-butyl acrylate) as compatibilizers in PMMA/PnBA blends. *e-Polymers* 15: 1–16.

Stroh, C.M., Ebner, A., Geretschlager, M., Freudenthaler, G., Kienberger, F., Kamruzzahan, A.S., Smith-Gill, S.J., Gruber, H.J., and Hinterdorfer, P. (2004). Simultaneous topography and recognition imaging using force microscopy. *Biophys. J.* 87: 1981–1990.

Strunz, T., Oroszlan, K., Schumakovitch, I., Guntherodt, H.J., and Hegner, M. (2000). Model energy landscapes and the force-induced dissociation of ligand-receptor bonds. *Biophys. J.* 79.

Suda, H., Sasaki, Y.C., Oishi, N., Hiraoka, N., and Sutoh, K. (1999). Elasticity of mutant myosin subfragment-1 arranged on a functional silver surface. *Biochem. Biophys. Res. Commun.* 261: 276–282.

Taatjes, D.J., Quinn, A.S., and Bovill, E.G. (1999). Imaging of collagen type III in fluid by atomic force microscopy. *Microsc. Res. Tech.* 44: 347–352.

Tahirov, T.H., Sato, K., Ichikawa-Iwata, E., Sasaki, M., Inoue-Bungo, T., Shiina, M., Kimura, K., Takata, S., Fujikawa, A., Morii, H., et al. (2002). Mechanism of c-Myb-C/EBP beta cooperation from separated sites on a promoter. *Cell* 108: 57–70.

Takeyasu, K., Omote, H., Nettikadan, S., Tokumasu, F., Iwamoto-Kihara, A., and Futai, M. (1996). Molecular imaging of *Escherichia coli* F0F1-ATPase in reconstituted membranes using atomic force microscopy. *FEBS Lett.* 392: 110–113.

Teng, H.H., Dove, P.M., Orme, C.A., and De Yoreo, J.J. (1998). Thermodynamics of calcite growth: baseline for understanding biomineral formation. *Science* 282: 724–727.

Thompson, J.B., Paloczi, G.T., Kindt, J.H., Michenfelder, M., Smith, B.L., Stucky, G., Morse, D.E., and Hansma, P.K. (2000). Direct observation of the transition from calcite to aragonite growth as induced by abalone shell proteins. *Biophys. J.* 79: 3307–3312.

Thomson, N.H., Smith, B.L., Almqvist, N., Schmitt, L., Kashlev, M., Kool, E.T., and Hansma, P.K. (1999). Oriented, active Escherichia coli RNA polymerase: an atomic force microscope study. *Biophys. J.* 76: 1024–1033.

Toikka, G. and Hayes, R.A. (1997). Direct measurement of colloidal forces between mica and silica in aqueous electrolyte. *J. Colloid Interface Sci.* 191: 102–109.

Tokumasu, F., Jin, A.J., and Dvorak, J.A. (2002). Lipid membrane phase behaviour elucidated in real time by controlled environment atomic force microscopy. *J. Electron Microsc. (Tokyo)* 51: 1–9.

Touhami, A., Nysten, B., and Dufrene, Y.F. (2003). Nanoscale mapping of the elasticity of microbial cells by atomic force microscopy. *Langmuir* 19: 1745–1751.

Trottier, M., Mat-Arip, Y., Zhang, C., Chen, C., Sheng, S., Shao, Z., and Guo, P. (2000). Probing the structure of monomers and dimers of the bacterial virus phi29 hexamer RNA complex by chemical modification. *Rna* 6: 1257–1266.

Tulpar, A., Subramaniam, V., and Ducker, W.A. (2001). Decay lengths in double-layer forces in solutions of partly associated ions. *Langmuir* 17: 8451–8454.

van der Werf, K.O., Putman, C.A., de Grooth, B.G., and Greve, J. (1994). Adhesion force imaging in air and liquid by adhesion mode atomic force microscopy. *Appl. Phys. Lett.* 65: 1195–1197.

van Duyl, B.Y., Ganchev, D., Chupin, V., de Kruijff, B., and Killian, J.A. (2003). Sphingomyelin is much more effective than saturated phosphatidylcholine in excluding unsaturated phosphatidylcholine from domains formed with cholesterol. *FEBS Lett.* 547: 101–106.

van Hulst, N.F., Veerman, J.A., Garcia-Parajo, M.F., and Kuipers, J. (2000). Analysis of individual (macro)molecules and proteins using near-field optics. *J. Chem. Phys.* 112: 7799–7810.

Van Landringham, M.R., Dagastine, R.R., Eduljee, R.F., McCullough, R.L., and Gillespie, J.W.J. (1999). Characterization of nanoscale property variations in polymer composite systems: Part 1 — Experimental results. *Composites Part A* 30.

Van Landringham, M.R., McKnight, S.H., Palmese, G.R., Bogetti, T.A., Eduljee, R.F., and Gillespie, J.W.J. (1997a). Characterization of interphase regions using atomic force microscopy. *Mat. Res. Soc. Symp. Proc.* 458: 313–318.

Van Landringham, M.R., McKnight, S.H., Palmese, G.R., Eduljee, R.F., Gillespie, J.W.J., and McCullough, R.L. (1997b). Relating polymer indentation behavior to elastic modulus using atomic force microscopy. *Mat. Res. Soc. Symp. Proc.* 440: 195–200.

Van Landringham, M.R., McKnight, S.H., Palmese, G.R., Huang, X., Bogetti, T.A., Eduljee, R.F., and Gillespie, J.W.J. (1997c). Nanoscale indentation of polymer systems using the atomic force microscope. *J. Adhesion* 64: 31–59.

Velegol, S.B. and Logan, B.E. (2002). Contributions of bacterial surface polymers, electrostatics, and cell elasticity to the shape of AFM force curves. *Langmuir* 18: 5256–5262.

Vesenka, J., Manne, S., Giberson, R., Marsh, T., and Henderson, E. (1993). Collidal gold particles as an incompressible atomic force microscope imaging standard for assessing the compressibility of biomolecules. *Biochem. J.* 65: 992–997.

Vinckier, A., Dumortier, C., Engelborghs, Y., and Hellemans, L. (1996). Dynamical and mechanical study of immobilized microtubules with atomic force microscopy. *J. Vac. Sci. Technol.* 14: 1427–1431.

Wadu-Mesthrige, K., Amro, N.A., and Liu, G.Y. (2000). Immobilization of proteins on self-assembled monolayers. *Scanning* 22: 380–388.

Wagner, P. (1998). Immobilization strategies for biological scanning probe microscopy. *FEBS Lett.* 430: 112–115.

Wakelin, S. and Bagshaw, C.R. (2003). A prism combination for near isotropic fluorescence excitation by total internal reflection. *J. Microsc.* 209: 143–148.

Walch, M., Ziegler, U., and Groscurth, P. (2000). Effect of streptolysin O on the microelasticity of human platelets analyzed by atomic force microscopy. *Ultramicroscopy* 82: 259–267.

Wang, Z., Zhou, C., Wang, C., Wan, L., Fang, X., and Bai, C. (2003). AFM and STM study of beta-amyloid aggregation on graphite. *Ultramicroscopy* 97: 73–79.

Ward, M.D. (2001). Bulk crystals to surfaces: combining X-ray diffraction and atomic force microscopy to probe the structure and formation of crystal interfaces. *Chem. Rev.* 2001: 1697–1725.

Watanabe, M., Kobayashi, M., Fujita, Y., Senga, K., Mizutani, H., Ueda, M., and Hoshino, T. (1997). Association of type VI collagen with D-periodic collagen fibrils in developing tail tendons of mice. *Arch. Histol. Cytol.* 60: 427–434.

Waugh, D.F., Thompson, R.E., and Weimer, R.J. (1950). Assay of insulin *in vitro* by fibril elongation and precipitation. *J. Biol. Chem.* 185: 85–95.

Weisenhorn, A.L., Khorsandi, M., Kasas, S., Gotzos, V., and Butt, H.-J. (1993). Deformation and height anomaly of soft surfaces studied with an AFM. *Nanotechnology* 4: 106–113.

Wen, H.B., Moradian-Oldak, J., Zhong, J.P., Greenspan, D.C., and Fincham, A.G. (2000). Effects of amelogenin on the transforming surface microstructures of Bioglass in a calcifying solution. *J. Biomed. Mater. Res.* 52: 762–773.

Wielert-Badt, S., Hinterdorfer, P., Gruber, H.J., Lin, J.T., Badt, D., Wimmer, B., Schindler, H., and Kinne, R.K. (2002). Single molecule recognition of protein binding epitopes in brush border membranes by force microscopy. *Biophys. J.* 82: 2767–2774.

Willemsen, O.H., Snel, M.M., van der Werf, K.O., de Grooth, B.G., Greve, J., Hinterdorfer, P., Gruber, H.J., Schindler, H., van Kooyk, Y., and Figdor, C.G. (1998). Simultaneous height and adhesion imaging of antibody-antigen interactions by atomic force microscopy. *Biophys. J.* 75: 2220–2228.

Williams, P.M., Fowler, S.B., Best, R.B., Toca-Herrera, J.L., Scott, K.A., Steward, A., and Clarke, J. (2003). Hidden complexity in the mechanical properties of titin. *Nature* 422: 446–449.

Winkler, R.G., Spatz, J.P., Sheiko, S., Moller, M., Reineker, P., and Marti, O. (1996). Imaging material properties by resonant tapping-force microscopy: a model investigation. *Phys. Rev. B* 54: 8908–8912.

Yang, D.S., Yip, C.M., Huang, T.H., Chakrabartty, A., and Fraser, P.E. (1999). Manipulating the amyloid-beta aggregation pathway with chemical chaperones. *J. Biol. Chem.* 274: 32970–32974.

Yang, G., Cecconi, C., Baase, W.A., Vetter, I.R., Breyer, W.A., Haack, J.A., Matthews, B.W., Dahlquist, F.W., and Bustamante, C. (2000). Solid-state synthesis and mechanical unfolding of polymers of T4 lysozyme. *Proc. Natl Acad. Sci. USA* 97: 139–144.

Yang, G., Woodhouse, K.A., and Yip, C.M. (2002). Substrate-facilitated assembly of elastin-like peptides: studies by variable-temperature *in situ* atomic force microscopy. *J. Am. Chem. Soc.* 124: 10648–10649.

Yau, S.T., Petsev, D.N., Thomas, B.R., and Vekilov, P.G. (2000). Molecular-level thermodynamic and kinetic parameters for the self-assembly of apoferritin molecules into crystals. *J. Mol. Biol.* 303: 667–678.

Yau, S.T., Thomas, B.R., Galkin, O., Gliko, O., and Vekilov, P.G. (2001). Molecular mechanisms of microheterogeneity-induced defect formation in ferritin crystallization. *Proteins* 43: 343–352.

Yau, S.T. and Vekilov, P.G. (2000). Quasi-planar nucleus structure in apoferritin crystallization. *Nature* 406: 494–497.

Yau, S.T. and Vekilov, P.G. (2001). Direct observation of nucleus structure and nucleation pathways in apoferritin crystallization. *J. Am. Chem. Soc.* 123: 1080–1089.

Yip, C.M., Brader, M.L., Frank, B.H., DeFelippis, M.R., and Ward, M.D. (2000). Structural studies of a crystalline insulin analog complex with protamine by atomic force microscopy. *Biophys. J.* 78: 466–473.

Yip, C.M., Darabie, A.A., and McLaurin, J. (2002). Abeta42-peptide assembly on lipid bilayers. *J. Mol. Biol.* 318: 97–107.

Yip, C.M. and McLaurin, J. (2001). Amyloid-beta peptide assembly: a critical step in fibrillogenesis and membrane disruption. *Biophys. J.* 80: 1359–1371.

Young, R., Ward, J., and Scire, F. (1971). The topografiner: an instrument for measuring surface microtopography. *Rev. Sci. Instr.* 43: 999.

Yuan, C., Chen, A., Kolb, P., and Moy, V.T. (2000). Energy landscape of streptavidin-biotin complexes measured by atomic force microscopy. *Biochemistry* 39: 10219–10223.

Yuan, C. and Johnston, L.J. (2001). Atomic force microscopy studies of ganglioside GM1 domains in phosphatidylcholine and phosphatidylcholine/cholesterol bilayers. *Biophys. J.* 81: 1059–1069.

Zhang, B. and Evans, J.S. (2001). Modeling AFM-induced PEVK extension and the reversible unfolding of Ig/FNIII domains in single and multiple titin molecules. *Biophys. J.* 80: 597–605.

Zhang, B., Wustman, B.A., Morse, D., and Evans, J.S. (2002). Model peptide studies of sequence regions in the elastomeric biomineralization protein, Lustrin A. I. The C-domain consensus-PG-, -NVNCT-motif. *Biopolymers* 63: 358–369.

Zhang, H., Grim, P.C.M., Vosch, T., Wiesler, U.-M., Berresheim, A.J., Mullen, K., and De Schryver, F.C. (2000a). Discrimination of dendrimer aggregates on mica based on adhesion force: a pulsed force mode atomic force microscopy study. *Langmuir* 16: 9294–9298.

Zhang, H., Grim, P.C.M., Vosch, T., Wiesler, U.-M., Berresheim, A.J., Mullen, K., and De Schryver, F.C. (2000b). Discrimination of dendrimer aggregates on mica based on adhesion force: a pulsed mode atomic force microscopy study. *Langmuir* 16: 9294–9298.

Zhang, J., Uchida, E., Yuama, Y., and Ikada, Y. (1997). Electrostatic interaction between ionic polymer grafted surfaces studied by atomic force microscopy. *J. Colloid Interface Sci.* 188: 431–438.

68

Parenteral Infusion Devices

68.1 Performance Criteria for IV Infusion Devices **68**-1
68.2 Flow through an IV Delivery System **68**-3
68.3 Intravenous Infusion Devices **68**-4
    Gravity Flow/Resistance Regulation • Volumetric Infusion
    Pumps • Controllers • Syringe Pumps
68.4 Managing Occlusions of the Delivery System **68**-8
68.5 Summary **68**-11
References **68**-11
Further Information **68**-11

Gregory I. Voss
Robert D. Butterfield
IVAC Corporation

The circulatory system is the body's primary pathway for both the distribution of oxygen and other nutrients and the removal of carbon dioxide and other waste products. Since the entire blood supply in a healthy adult completely circulates within 60 sec, substances introduced into the circulatory system are distributed rapidly. Thus intravenous (IV) and intraarterial access routes provide an effective pathway for the delivery of fluid, blood, and medicants to a patient's vital organs. Consequently, about 80% of hospitalized patients receive infusion therapy. Peripheral and central veins are used for the majority of infusions. Umbilical artery delivery (in neonates), enteral delivery of nutrients, and epidural delivery of anesthetics and analgesics comprise smaller patient populations. A variety of devices can be used to provide flow through an intravenous catheter. An intravenous delivery system typically consists of three major components (1) fluid or drug reservoir, (2) catheter system for transferring the fluid or drug from the reservoir into the vasculature through a venipuncture, and (3) device for regulation and/or generating flow (see Figure 68.1).

This chapter is separated into five sections. Section 68.1 describes the clinical needs associated with intravenous drug delivery that determine device performance criteria. Section 68.2 reviews the principles of flow through a tube; Section 68.3 introduces the underlying electromechanical principles for flow regulation and/or generation and their ability to meet the clinical performance criteria. Section 68.4 reviews complications associated with intravenous therapy, and Section 68.5 concludes with a short list of articles providing more detailed information.

68.1 Performance Criteria for IV Infusion Devices

The IV pathway provides an excellent route for continuous drug therapy. The ideal delivery system regulates drug concentration in the body to achieve and maintain a desired result. When the drug's effect

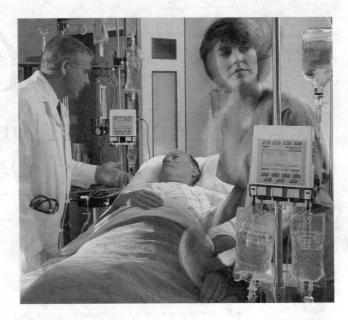

FIGURE 68.1   A typical IV infusion system.

cannot be monitored directly, it is frequently assumed that a specific blood concentration or infusion rate will achieve the therapeutic objective. Although underinfusion may not provide sufficient therapy, overinfusion can produce even more serious toxic side effects.

The therapeutic range and risks associated with under- and overinfusion are highly drug and patient dependent. Intravenous delivery of fluids and electrolytes often does not require very accurate regulation. Low-risk patients can generally tolerate well infusion rate variability of ±30% for fluids. In some situations, however, specifically for fluid-restricted patients, prolonged under- or overinfusion of fluids can compromise the patient's cardiovascular and renal systems.

The infusion of many drugs, especially potent cardioactive agents, requires high accuracy. For example, post-coronary-artery-bypass-graft patients commonly receive sodium nitroprusside to lower arterial blood pressure. Hypertension, associated with underinfusion, subjects the graft sutures to higher stress with an increased risk for internal bleeding. Hypotension associated with overinfusion can compromise the cardiovascular state of the patient. Nitroprusside's potency, short onset delay, and short half-life (30 to 180 sec) provide for very tight control, enabling the clinician to quickly respond to the many events that alter the patient's arterial pressure. The fast response of drugs such as nitroprusside creates a need for short-term flow uniformity as well as long-term accuracy.

The British Department of Health employs *Trumpet curves* in their Health Equipment Information reports to compare flow uniformity of infusion pumps. For a prescribed flow rate, the trumpet curve is the plot of the maximum and minimum measured percentage flow rate error as a function of the accumulation interval (Figure 68.2). Flow is measured gravimetrically in 30-sec blocks for 1 h. These blocks are summed to produce 120-sec, 300-sec, and other longer total accumulation intervals. Though the 120-sec window may not detect flow variations important in delivery of the fastest acting agents, the trumpet curve provides a helpful means for performance comparison among infusion devices. Additional statistical information such as standard deviations may be derived from the basic trumpet flow measurements.

The short half-life of certain pharmacologic agents and the clotting reaction time of blood during periods of stagnant flow require that fluid flow be maintained without significant interruption. Specifically, concern has been expressed in the literature that the infusion of sodium nitroprusside and other short

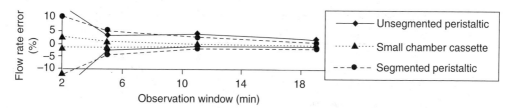

FIGURE 68.2 Trumpet curve for several representative large volume infusion pumps operated a 5 ml/h. Note that peristaltic pumps were designed for low risk patients.

half-life drugs occur without interruption exceeding 20 sec. Thus, minimization of false alarms and rapid detection of occlusions are important aspects of maintaining a constant vascular concentration. Accidental occlusions of the IV line due to improper positioning of stopcocks or clamps, kinked tubing, and clotted catheters are common.

Occlusions between pump and patient present a secondary complication in maintaining serum drug concentration. Until detected, the pump will infuse, storing fluid in the delivery set. When the occlusion is eliminated, the stored volume is delivered to the patient in a bolus. With concentrated pharmaceutic agents, this bolus can produce a large perturbation in the patient's status.

Occlusions of the pump intake also interrupt delivery. If detection is delayed, inadequate flow can result. During an intake occlusion, in some pump designs removal of the delivery set can produce abrupt aspiration of blood. This event may precipitate clotting and cause injury to the infusion site.

The common practice of delivering multiple drugs through a single venous access port produces an additional challenge to maintaining uniform drug concentration. Although some mixing will occur in the venous access catheter, fluid in the catheter more closely resembles a first-in/first-out digital queue: during delivery, drugs from the various infusion devices mix at the catheter input, an equivalent fluid volume discharges from the outlet. Rate changes and flow nonuniformity cause the mass flow of drugs at the outlet to differ from those at the input. Consider a venous access catheter with a volume of 2 ml and a total flow of 10 ml/h. Due to the digital queue phenomenon, an incremental change in the intake flow rate of an individual drug will not appear at the output for 12 min. In addition, changing flow rates for one drug will cause short-term marked swings in the delivery rate of drugs using the same access catheter. When the delay becomes significantly larger than the time constant for a drug that is titrated to a measurable patient response, titration becomes extremely difficult leading to large oscillations.

As discussed, the performance requirements for drug delivery vary with multiple factors: drug, fluid restriction, and patient risk. Thus the delivery of potent agents to fluid-restricted patients at risk require the highest performance standards defined by flow rate accuracy, flow rate uniformity, and ability to minimize risk of IV-site complications. These performance requirements need to be appropriately balanced with the device cost and the impact on clinician productivity.

68.2 Flow through an IV Delivery System

The physical properties associated with the flow of fluids through cylindrical tubes provide the foundation for understanding flow through a catheter into the vasculature. Hagen–Poiseuille's equation for laminar flow of a Newtonian fluid through a rigid tube states

$$Q = \pi \cdot r^4 \cdot \frac{(P_1 - P_2)}{8 \cdot \eta \cdot L} \tag{68.1}$$

where Q is the flow; P_1 and P_2 are the pressures at the inlet and outlet of the tube, respectively; L and r are the length and internal radius of the tube, respectively; and η is fluid viscosity. Although many drug delivery systems do not strictly meet the flow conditions for precise application of the laminar flow

TABLE 68.1 Resistance Measurements for Catheter Components Used for Infusion

Component	Length, cm	Flow Resistance, Fluid Ohm, mmHg/(l/h)
Standard administration set	91–213	4.3–5.3
Extension tube for CVP monitoring	15	15.5
19-gauge epidural catheter	91	290.4–497.1
18-gauge needle	6–9	14.1–17.9
23-gauge needle	2.5–9	165.2–344.0
25-gauge needle	1.5–4.0	525.1–1412.0
Vicra Quick-Cath Catheter 18-gauge	5	12.9
Extension set with 0.22 μm air-eliminating filter		623.0
0.2 μm filter		555.0

Note: Mean values are presented over a range of infusions (100, 200, and 300 ml/h) and sample size ($n = 10$).

equation, it does provide insight into the relationship between flow and pressure in a catheter. The fluid analog of Ohms Law describes the resistance to flow under constant flow conditions:

$$R = \frac{P_1 - P_2}{Q} \qquad (68.2)$$

Thus, resistance to flow through a tube correlates directly with catheter length and fluid viscosity and inversely with the fourth power of catheter diameter. For steady flow, the delivery system can be modeled as a series of resistors representing each component, including administration set, access catheter, and circulatory system. When dynamic aspects of the delivery system are considered, a more detailed model including catheter and venous compliance, fluid inertia, and turbulent flow is required. Flow resistance may be defined with units of mmHg/(l/h), so that 1 fluid ohm = 4.8×10^{-11} Pa sec/m^3. Studies determining flow resistance for several catheter components with distilled water for flow rates of 100, 200, and 300 ml/h appear in Table 68.1.

68.3 Intravenous Infusion Devices

From Hagen–Poiselluie's equation, two general approaches to intravenous infusion become apparent. First, a hydrostatic pressure gradient can be used with adjustment of delivery system resistance controlling flow rate. Complications such as partial obstructions result in reduced flow which may be detected by an automatic flow monitor. Second, a constant displacement flow source can be used. Now complications may be detected by monitoring elevated fluid pressure and/or flow resistance. At the risk of overgeneralization, the relative strengths of each approach will be presented.

68.3.1 Gravity Flow/Resistance Regulation

The simplest means for providing regulated flow employs gravity as the driving force with a roller clamp as controlled resistance. Placement of the fluid reservoir 60 to 100 cm above the patient's right atrium provides a hydrostatic pressure gradient P_h equal to 1.34 mmHg/cm of elevation. The modest physiologic mean pressure in the veins, P_v, minimally reduces the net hydrostatic pressure gradient. The equation for flow becomes

$$Q = \frac{P_h - P_v}{R_{mfr} + R_n} \qquad (68.3)$$

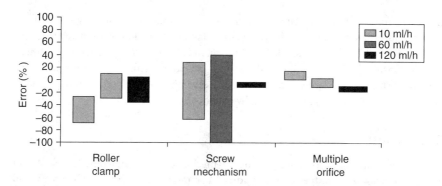

FIGURE 68.3   Drift in flow rate (mean ± standard deviation) over a 4-h period for three mechanical flow regulators at initial flow rates of 10, 60, and 120 ml/h with distilled water at constant hydrostatic pressure gradient.

where R_{mfr} and R_n are the resistance to flow through the mechanical flow regulator and the remainder of the delivery system, respectively. Replacing the variables with representative values for an infusion of 5% saline solution into a healthy adult at 100 ml/h yields

$$100 \text{ ml/h} = \frac{(68 - 8) \text{ mmHg}}{(550 + 50) \text{ mmHg/(l/h)}} \tag{68.4}$$

Gravity flow cannot be used for arterial infusions since the higher vascular pressure exceeds available hydrostatic pressure.

Flow stability in a gravity infusion system is subject to variations in hydrostatic and venous pressure as well as catheter resistance. However, the most important factor is the change in flow regulator resistance caused by viscoelastic creep of the tubing wall (see Figure 68.3). Caution must be used in assuming that a preset flow regulator setting will accurately provide a predetermined rate. The clinician typically estimates flow rate by counting the frequency of drops falling through an in-line drip-forming chamber, adjusting the clamp to obtain the desired drop rate. The cross-sectional area of the drip chamber orifice is the major determinant of drop volume. Various manufacturers provide minidrip sets designed for pediatric (e.g., 60 drops/ml) and regular sets designed for adult (10 to 20 drops/ml) patients. Tolerances on the drip chamber can cause a 3% error in minidrip sets and a 17% error in regular sets at 125 ml/h flow rate with 5% dextrose in water. Mean drop size for rapid rates increased by as much as 25% over the size of drops which form slowly. In addition, variation in the specific gravity and surface tension of fluids can provide an additional large source of drop size variability.

Some mechanical flow regulating devices incorporate the principle of a Starling resistor. In a Starling device, resistance is proportional to hydrostatic pressure gradient. Thus, the device provides a negative feedback mechanism to reduce flow variation as the available pressure gradient changes with time.

Mechanical flow regulators comprise the largest segment of intravenous infusion systems, providing the simplest means of operation. Patient transport is simple, since these devices require no electric power. Mechanical flow regulators are most useful where the patient is not fluid restricted and the acceptable therapeutic rate range of the drug is relatively wide with minimal risk of serious adverse sequelae. The most common use for these systems is the administration of fluids and electrolytes.

68.3.2 Volumetric Infusion Pumps

Active pumping infusion devices combine electronics with a mechanism to generate flow. These devices have higher performance standards than simple gravity flow regulators. The Association for the Advancement of Medical Instrumentation (AAMI) recommends that long-term rate accuracy for infusion pumps remain within ±10% of the set rate for general infusion and, for the more demanding applications, that long-term flow remain within ±5%. Such requirements typically extend to those agents with narrow therapeutic indices and/or low flow rates, such as the neonatal population or other fluid-restricted patients. The British Department of Health has established three main categories for hospital-based infusion devices: neonatal infusions, high-risk infusions, and low-risk infusions. Infusion control for neonates requires the highest performance standards, because their size severely restricts fluid volume. A fourth category, ambulatory infusion, pertains to pumps worn by patients.

68.3.3 Controllers

These devices automate the process of adjusting the mechanical flow regulator. The most common controllers utilize sensors to count the number of drops passing through the drip chamber to provide flow feedback for automatic rate adjustment. Flow rate accuracy remains limited by the rate and viscosity dependence of drop size. Delivery set motion associated with ambulation and improper angulation of the drip chamber can also hinder accurate rate detection.

An alternative to the drop counter is a volumetric metering chamber. A McGaw Corporation controller delivery set uses a rigid chamber divided by a flexible membrane. Instrument-controlled valves allow fluid to fill one chamber from the fluid reservoir, displacing the membrane driving the fluid from the second chamber toward the patient. When inlet and outlet valves reverse state, the second chamber is filled while the first chamber delivers to the patient. The frequency of state change determines the average flow rate. Volumetric accuracy demands primarily on the dimensional tolerances of the chamber. Although volumetric controllers may provide greater accuracy than drop-counting controllers, their disposables are inherently more complex, and maximum flow is still limited by head height and system resistance.

Beyond improvements in flow rate accuracy, controllers should provide an added level of patient safety by quickly detecting IV-site complications. The IVAC Corporation has developed a series of controllers employing pulsed modulated flow providing for monitoring of flow resistance as well as improved accuracy.

The maximum flow rate achieved by gravimetric based infusion systems can become limited by R_n and by concurrent infusion from other sources through the same catheter. In drop-counting devices, flow rate uniformity suffers at low flow rates from the discrete nature of the drop detector.

In contrast with infusion controllers, pumps generate flow by mechanized displacement of the contents of a volumetric chamber. Typical designs provide high flow rate accuracy and uniformity for a wide rate range (0.1 to 1000.0 ml/h) of infusion rates. Rate error correlates directly with effective chamber volume, which, in turn, depends on both instrument and disposable repeatability, precision, and stability under varying load. Stepper or servo-controlled dc motors are typically used to provide the driving force for the fluid. At low flow rates, dc motors usually operate in a discrete stepping mode. On average, each step propels a small quanta of fluid toward the patient. Flow rate uniformity therefore is a function of both the average volume per quanta and the variation in volume. Mechanism factors influencing rate uniformity include: stepping resolution, gearing and activator geometries, volumetric chamber coupling geometry, and chamber elasticity. When the quanta volume is not inherently uniform over the mechanism's cycle, software control has been used to compensate for the variation.

68.3.4 Syringe Pumps

These pumps employ a syringe as both reservoir and volumetric pumping chamber. A precision leadscrew is used to produce constant linear advancement of the syringe plunger. Except for those ambulatory systems that utilize specific microsyringes, pumps generally accept syringes ranging in size from 5 to 100 ml. Flow rate accuracy and uniformity are determined by both mechanism displacement characteristics and tolerance on the internal syringe diameter. Since syringe mechanisms can generate a specified linear travel with less than 1% error, the manufacturing tolerance on the internal cross-sectional area of the syringe largely determines flow rate accuracy. Although syringes can be manufactured to tighter tolerances, standard plastic syringes provide long-term accuracy of ±5%. Flow rate uniformity, however, can benefit

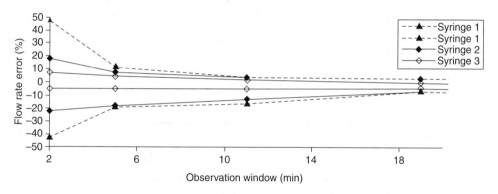

FIGURE 68.4   Effect of syringe type on Trumpet curve of a syringe pump at 1 ml/h.

from the ability to select syringe size (see Figure 68.4). Since many syringes have similar stroke length, diameter variation provides control of volume. Also the linear advancement per step is typically fixed. Therefore selection of a lower-volume syringe provides smaller-volume quanta. This allows tradeoffs among drug concentration, flow rate, and duration of flow per syringe. Slack in the gear train and drive shaft coupling as well as plunger slip cause rate inaccuracies during the initial stages of delivery (see Figure 68.5a).

Since the syringe volumes are typically much smaller than reservoirs used with other infusion devices, syringe pumps generally deliver drugs in either fluid-restricted environments or for short duration. With high-quality syringes, flow rate uniformity in syringe pumps is generally superior to that accomplished by other infusion pumps. With the drug reservoir enclosed within the device, syringe pumps manage patient transport well, including the operating room environment.

Cassette pumps conceptually mimic the piston type action of the syringe pump but provide an automated means of repeatedly emptying and refilling the cassette. The process of refilling the cassette in single piston devices requires an interruption in flow (see Figure 68.5b). The length of interruption relative to the drug's half-life determines the impact of the refill period on hemodynamic stability. To eliminate the interruption caused by refill, dual piston devices alternate refill and delivery states, providing nearly continuous output. Others implement cassettes with very small volumes which can refill in less than a second (see Figure 68.2). Tight control of the internal cross-sectional area of the pumping chamber provides exceptional flow rate accuracy. Manufacturers have recently developed remarkably small cassette pumps that can still generate the full spectrum of infusion rate (0.1 to 999.0 ml/h). These systems combine pumping chamber, inlet and outlet valving, pressure sensing, and air detection into a single complex component.

Peristaltic pumps operate on a short segment of the IV tubing. Peristaltic pumps can be separated into two subtypes. Rotary peristaltic mechanisms operate by compressing the pumping segment against the rotor housing with rollers mounted on the housing. With rotation, the rollers push fluid from the container through the tubing toward the patient. At least one of the rollers completely occludes the tubing against the housing at all times precluding free flow from the reservoir to the patient. During a portion of the revolution, two rollers trap fluid in the intervening pumping segment. The captured volume between the rollers determines volumetric accuracy. Linear peristaltic pumps hold the pumping segment in a channel pressed against a rigid backing plate. An array of cam-driven actuators sequentially occlude the segment starting with the section nearest the reservoir forcing fluid toward the patient with a sinusoidal wave action. In a typical design using uniform motor step intervals, a characteristic flow wave resembling a positively biased sine wave is produced (see Figure 68.5c).

Infusion pumps provide significant advantages over both manual flow regulators and controllers in several categories. Infusion pumps can provide accurate delivery over a wide range of infusion rates (0.1 to 999.0 ml/h). Neither elevated system resistance nor distal line pressure limit the maximum infusion rate. Infusion pumps can support a wider range of applications including arterial infusions, spinal and

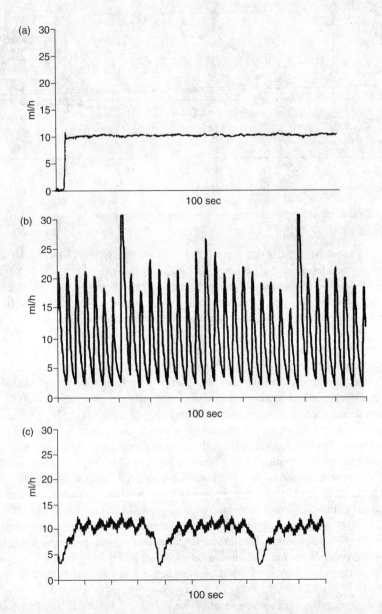

FIGURE 68.5   Continuous flow pattern for a representative, (a) syringe, (b) cassette, and (c) linear peristaltic pump at 10 ml/h.

epidural infusions, and infusions into pulmonary artery or central venous catheters. Flow rate accuracy of infusion pumps is highly dependent on the segment employed as the pumping chamber (see Figure 68.2). Incorporating special syringes or pumping segments can significantly improve flow rate accuracy (see Figure 68.6). Both manufacturing tolerances and segment material composition significantly dictate flow rate accuracy. Time- and temperature-related properties of the pumping segment further impact long-term drift in flow rate.

68.4   Managing Occlusions of the Delivery System

One of the most common problems in managing an IV delivery system is the rapid detection of occlusion in the delivery system. With a complete occlusion, the resistance to flow approaches infinity. In this condition,

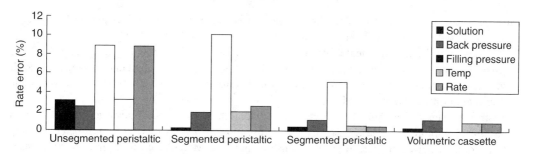

FIGURE 68.6 Impact of 5 variables on flow rate accuracy in 4 different infusion pumps. Variables tested included Solution: Distilled water and 25% dextrose in water; Back pressure: −100 and 300 mmHg; Pumping Segment Filling Pressure: −30 inches of water and +30 inches of water; Temperature: 10°C and 40°C; and Infusion rate: 5 ml/h and 500 ml/h. Note: first and second peristaltic mechanism qualified for low risk patients, while the third peristaltic device qualified for high-risk patients.

gravimetric-based devices cease to generate flow. Mechanical flow regulators have no mechanism for adverse event detection and thus must rely on the clinician to identify an occlusion as part of routine patient care. Electronic controllers sense the absence of flow and alarm in response to their inability to sustain the desired flow rate.

The problem of rapidly detecting an occlusion in an infusion pump is more complex. Upstream occlusions that occur between the fluid reservoir and the pumping mechanism impact the system quite differently than downstream occlusions which occur between the pump and the patient. When an occlusion occurs downstream from an infusion pump, the pump continues to propel fluid into the section of tubing between the pump and the occlusion. The time rate of pressure rise in that section increases in direct proportion to flow rate and inversely with tubing compliance (compliance, C, is the volume increase in a closed tube per mmHg pressure applied). The most common approach to detecting downstream occlusion requires a pressure transducer immediately below the pumping mechanism. These devices generate an alarm when either the mean pressure or rate of change in pressure exceeds a threshold. For pressure-limited designs, the time to downstream alarm (TTA) may be estimated as

$$\text{TTA} = \frac{P_{\text{alarm}} \cdot C_{\text{delivery-set}}}{\text{flow rate}} \qquad (68.5)$$

Using a representative tubing compliance of 1 μl/mmHg, flow rate of 1 ml/h, and a fixed alarm threshold set of 500 mmHg, the time to alarm becomes

$$\text{TTA} = \frac{500_{\text{mmHg}} \cdot 1000 \text{ ml/mmHg}}{1 \text{ ml/h}} = 30 \text{ min} \qquad (68.6)$$

where TTA is the time from occlusion to alarm detection. Pressure-based detection algorithms depend on accuracy and stability of the sensing system. Lowering the threshold on absolute or relative pressure for occlusion alarm reduces the TTA, but at the cost of increasing the likelihood of false alarms. Patient movement, patient-to-pump height variations, and other clinical circumstances can cause wide perturbations in line pressure. To optimize the balance between fast TTA and minimal false alarms, some infusion pumps allow the alarm threshold to be set by the clinician or be automatically shifted upward in response to alarms; other pumps attempt to optimize performance by varying pressure alarm thresholds with flow rate.

A second approach to detection of downstream occlusions uses motor torque as an indirect measure of the load seen by the pumping mechanism. Although this approach eliminates the need for a pressure sensor, it introduces additional sources for error including friction in the gear mechanism or pumping mechanism that requires additional safety margins to protect against false alarms. In syringe pumps, where the coefficient of static friction of the syringe bunge (rubber end of the syringe plunger) against the syringe wall can be substantial, occlusion detection can exceed 1 h at low flow rates.

Direct, continuous measurement of downstream flow resistance may provide a monitoring modality which overcomes the disadvantages of pressure-based alarm systems, especially at low infusion rates. Such a monitoring system would have the added advantage of performance unaffected by flow rate, hydrostatic pressure variations, and motion artifacts.

Upstream occlusions can cause large negative pressures as the pumping mechanism generates a vacuum on the upstream tubing segment. The tube may collapse and the vacuum may pull air through the tubing walls or form cavitation bubbles. A pressure sensor situated above the mechanism or a pressure sensor below the mechanism synchronized with filling of the pumping chamber can detect the vacuum associated with an upstream occlusion. Optical or ultrasound transducers, situated below the mechanism, can detect air bubbles in the catheter, and air-eliminating filters can remove air, preventing large air emboli from being introduced into the patient.

Some of the most serious complications of IV therapy occur at the venipuncture site; these include extravasation, postinfusion phlebitis (and thrombophlebitis), IV-related infections, ecchymosis, and hematomas. Other problems that do not occur as frequently include speed shock and allergic reactions.

Extravasation (or infiltration) is the inadvertent perfusion of infusate into the interstitial tissue. Reported percentage of patients to whom extravasation has occurred ranges from 10% to over 25%. Tissue damage does not occur frequently, but the consequences can be severe, including skin necrosis requiring significant plastic and reconstructive surgery and amputation of limbs. The frequency of extravasation injury correlates with age, state of consciousness, and venous circulation of the patient as well as the type, location, and placement of the intravenous cannula. Drugs that have high osmolality, vessicant properties, or the ability to induce ischemia correlate with frequency of extravasation injury. Neonatal and pediatric patients who possess limited communication skills, constantly move, and have small veins that are difficult to cannulate require superior vigilance to protect against extravasation.

Since interstitial tissue provides a greater resistance to fluid flow than the venous pathway, infusion devices with accurate and precise pressure monitoring systems have been used to detect small pressure increases due to extravasation. To successfully implement this technique requires diligence by the clinician, since patient movement, flow rate, catheter resistance, and venous pressure variations can obscure the small pressure variations resulting from the extravasation. Others have investigated the ability of a pumping mechanism to withdraw blood as indicative of problems in a patent line. The catheter tip, however, may be partially in and out of the vein such that infiltration occurs yet blood can be withdrawn from the patient. A vein might also collapse under negative pressure in a patent line without successful blood withdrawal. Techniques currently being investigated which monitor infusion impedance (resistance and compliance) show promise for assisting in the detection of extravasation.

When a catheter tip wedges into the internal lining of the vein wall, it is considered positional. With the fluid path restricted by the vein wall, increases in line resistance may indicate a positional catheter. With patient movement, for example wrist flexation, the catheter may move in and out of the positional state. Since a positional catheter is thought to be more prone toward extravasation than other catheters, early detection of a positional catheter and appropriate adjustment of catheter position may be helpful in reducing the frequency of extravasation.

Postinfusion phlebitis is acute inflammation of a vein used for IV infusion. The chief characteristic is a reddened area or red streak that follows the course of the vein with tenderness, warmth, and edema at the venipuncture site. The vein, which normally is very compliant, also hardens. Phlebitis positively correlates with infusion rate and with the infusion of vesicants.

Fluid overload and speed shock result from the accidental administration of a large fluid volume over a short interval. Speed shock associates more frequently with the delivery of potent medications, rather than fluids. These problems most commonly occur with manually regulated IV systems, which do not provide the safety features of instrumented lines. Many IV sets designed for instrumented operation will free-flow when the set is removed from the instrument without manual clamping. To protect against this possibility, some sets are automatically placed in the occluded state on disengagement. Although an apparent advantage, reliance on such automatic devices may create a false sense of security and lead to manual errors with sets not incorporating these features.

68.5 Summary

Intravenous infusion has become the mode of choice for delivery of a large class of fluids and drugs both in hospital and alternative care settings. Modern infusion devices provide the clinician with a wide array of choices for performing intravenous therapy. Selection of the appropriate device for a specified application requires understanding of drug pharmacology and pharmacokinetics, fluid mechanics, and device design and performance characteristics. Continuing improvements in performance, safety, and cost of these systems will allow even broader utilization of intravenous delivery in a variety of settings.

References

Association for the Advancement of Medical Instrumentation (1992). *Standard for Infusion Devices.* Arlington.

Bohony J. (1993). Nine common intravenous complications and what to do about them. *Am. J. Nursing* 10: 45.

British Department of Health (1990). *Evaluation of Infusion Pumps and Controllers.* HEI Report #198.

Glass P.S.A., Jacobs J.R., Reves J.G. (1991). Technology for continuous infusions in anesthesia. Continuous Infusions in Anesthesia. *Int. Anesthesiol. Clin.* 29: 39.

MacCara M. (1983). Extravasation: A hazard of intravenous therapy. *Drug Intell. Clin. Pharm.* 17: 713.

Further Information

Peter Glass provides a strong rationale for intravenous therapy including pharmacokinetic and pharmacodynamic bases for continuous delivery. Clinical complications around intravenous therapy are well summarized by MacCara [1983] and Bohony [1993]. The AAMI Standard for Infusion Devices provides a comprehensive means of evaluating infusion device technology, and the British Department of Health OHEI Report #198 provides a competitive analysis of pumps and controllers.

69

Clinical Laboratory: Separation and Spectral Methods

69.1	Separation Methods	69-1
69.2	Chromatographic Separations	69-2
69.3	Gas Chromatography	69-2
69.4	High-Performance Liquid Chromatography	69-3
69.5	Basis for Spectral Methods	69-4
69.6	Fluorometry	69-5
69.7	Flame Photometry	69-6
69.8	Atomic Absorption Spectroscopy	69-6
69.9	Turbidimetry and Nephelometry	69-7
	Defining Terms	69-7
	References	69-8

Richard L. Roa
Baylor University Medical Center

The purpose of the clinical laboratory is to analyze body fluids and tissues for specific substances of interest and to report the results in a form which is of value to clinicians in the diagnosis and treatment of disease. A large range of tests has been developed to achieve this purpose. Four terms commonly used to describe tests are **accuracy, precision, sensitivity,** and **specificity.** An accurate test, on average, yields true values. Precision is the ability of a test to produce identical results upon repeated trials. Sensitivity is a measure of how small an amount of substance can be measured. Specificity is the degree to which a test measures the substance of interest without being affected by other substances which may be present in greater amounts.

The first step in many laboratory tests is to separate the material of interest from other substances. This may be accomplished through extraction, filtration, and centrifugation. Another step is derivatization, in which the substance of interest is chemically altered through addition of reagents to change it into a substance which is easily measured. For example, one method for measuring glucose is to add otoluidine which, under proper conditions, forms a green-colored solution with an absorption maximum at 630 nm. Separation and derivatization both improve the specificity required of good tests.

69.1 Separation Methods

Centrifuges are used to separate materials on the basis of their relative densities. The most common use in the laboratory is the separation of cells and platelets from the liquid part of the blood. This requires a relative centrifugal force (RCF) of roughly 1000 g (1000 times the force of gravity) for a period of 10 min. Relative centrifugal force is a function of the speed of rotation and the distance of the sample from the center of rotation as stated in Equation 69.1

$$RCF = (1.12 \times 10^{-5}) \, r(rpm)^2 \tag{69.1}$$

where RCF is the relative centrifugal force in g, and r is the radius in cm.

Some mixtures require higher g-loads in order to achieve separation in a reasonable period of time. Special rotors contain the sample tubes inside a smooth container, which minimizes air resistance to allow faster rotational speeds. Refrigerated units maintain the samples at a cool temperature throughout long high-speed runs which could lead to sample heating due to air friction on the rotor. Ultracentrifuges operate at speeds on the order of 100,000 rpm and provide relative centrifugal forces of up to 600,000 g. These usually require vacuum pumps to remove the air which would otherwise retard the rotation and heat the rotor.

69.2   Chromatographic Separations

Chromatographic separations depend upon the different rates at which various substances moving in a stream (mobile phase) are retarded by a stationary material (stationary phase) as they pass over it. The mobile phase can be a volatilized sample transported by an inert carrier gas such as helium or a liquid transported by an organic solvent such as acetone. Stationary phases are quite diverse depending upon the separation being made, but most are contained within a long, thin tube (column). Liquid stationary phases may be used by coating them onto inert packing materials. When a sample is introduced into a chromatographic column, it is carried through it by the mobile phase. As it passes through the column, the substances which have greater affinity for the stationary phase fall behind those with less affinity. The separated substances may be detected as individual peaks by a suitable detector placed at the end of the chromatographic column.

69.3   Gas Chromatography

The most common instrumental chromatographic method used in the clinical laboratory is the gas–liquid chromatograph. In this system the mobile phase is a gas, and the stationary phase is a liquid coated onto either an inert support material, in the case of a packed column, or the inner walls of a very thin tube, in the case of a capillary column. Capillary columns have the greatest resolving power but cannot handle large sample quantities. The sample is injected into a small heated chamber at the beginning of the column, where it is volatilized if it is not already a gaseous sample. The sample is then carried through the column by an inert carrier gas, typically helium or nitrogen. The column is completely housed within an oven. Many gas chromatographs allow for the oven temperature to be programmed to slowly increase for a set time after the sample injection is made. This produces peaks which are spread more uniformly over time.

Four detection methods commonly used with gas chromatography are thermal conductivity, flame ionization, nitrogen/phosphorous, and mass spectrometry. The thermal conductivity detector takes advantage of variations in thermal conductivity between the carrier gas and the gas being measured. A heated filament immersed in the gas leaving the chromatographic column is part of a Wheatstone bridge circuit. Small variations in the conductivity of the gas cause changes in the resistance of the filament, which are recorded. The flame ionization detector measures the current between two plates with a voltage applied between them. When an organic material appears in the flame, ions which contribute to the current are formed. The NP detector, or nitrogen/phosphorous detector, is a modified flame ionization detector (see Figure 69.1) which is particularly sensitive to nitrogen- and phosphorous-containing compounds.

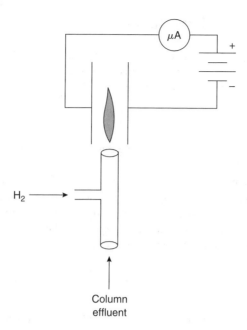

FIGURE 69.1 Flame ionization detector. Organic compounds in the column effluent are ionized in the flame, producing a current proportional to the amount of the compound present.

Mass spectrometry (MS) provides excellent sensitivity and selectivity. The concept behind these devices is that the volatilized sample molecules are broken into ionized fragments which are then passed through a mass analyzer that separates the fragments according to their mass/charge (m/z) ratios. A mass spectrum, which is a plot of the relative abundance of the various fragments versus m/z, is produced. The mass spectrum is characteristic of the molecule sampled. The mass analyzer most commonly used with gas chromatographs is the quadrupole detector, which consists of four rods that have dc and RF voltages applied to them. The m/z spectrum can be scanned by appropriate changes in the applied voltages. The detector operates in a manner similar to that of a photomultiplier tube except that the collision of the charged particles with the cathode begins the electron cascade, resulting in a measurable electric pulse for each charged particle captured. The MS must operate in a high vacuum, which requires good pumps and a porous barrier between the GC and MS that limits the amount of carrier gas entering the MS.

69.4 High-Performance Liquid Chromatography

In liquid chromatography, the mobile phase is liquid. High-performance liquid chromatography (HPLC) refers to systems which obtain excellent resolution in a reasonable time by forcing the mobile phase at high pressure through a long thin column. The most common pumps used are pistons driven by asymmetrical cams. By using two such pumps in parallel and operating out of phase, pressure fluctuations can be minimized. Typical pressures are 350–1500 psi, though the pressure may be as high as 10,000 psi. Flow rates are in the 1–10 ml/min range.

A common method for placing a sample onto the column is with a loop injector, consisting of a loop of tubing which is filled with the sample. By a rotation of the loop, it is brought in series with the column, and the sample is carried onto the column. A UV/visible spectrophotometer is often used as a detector for this method. A mercury arc lamp with the 254-nm emission isolated is useful for detection of aromatic compounds, while diode array detectors allow a complete spectrum from 190 to 600 nm in 10 msec. This provides for detection and identification of compounds as they come off the column. Fluorescent, electrochemical, and mass analyzer detectors are also used.

69.5   Basis for Spectral Methods

Spectral methods rely on the absorption or emission of electromagnetic radiation by the sample of interest. Electromagnetic radiation is often described in terms of frequency or wavelength. Wavelengths are those obtained in a vacuum and may be calculated with the formula

$$\lambda = c/\upsilon \tag{69.2}$$

where λ is the wavelength in meters, c the speed of light in vacuum (3×10^8 m/sec), and υ the frequency in Hz.

The frequency range of interest for most clinical laboratory work consists of the visible (390–780 nm) and the ultraviolet or UV (180–390 nm) ranges. Many substances absorb different wavelengths preferentially. When this occurs in the visible region, they are colored. In general, the color of a substance is the complement of the color it absorbs, for example, absorption in the blue produces a yellow color. For a given wavelength or bandwidth, transmittance is defined as

$$T = \frac{I_t}{I_i} \tag{69.3}$$

where T is the transmittance ratio (often expressed as %), I_i the incident light intensity, and I_t the transmitted light intensity. Absorbance is defined as

$$A = -\log_{10} 1/T \tag{69.4}$$

Under suitable conditions, the absorbance of a solution with an absorbing compound dissolved in it is proportional to the concentration of that compound as well as the path length of light through it. This relationship is expressed by Beer's law:

$$A = abc \tag{69.5}$$

where A is the absorbance, a the a constant, b the path length, and c the concentration.

A number of situations may cause deviations from Beer's law, such as high concentration or mixtures of compounds which absorb at the wavelength of interest. From an instrumental standpoint, the primary causes are stray light and excessive spectral bandwidth. Stray light refers to any light reaching the detector other than light from the desired pass-band which has passed through sample. Sources of stray light may include room light leaking into the detection chamber, scatter from the cuvette, and undesired **fluorescence**.

A typical spectrophotometer consists of a light source, some form of wavelength selection, and a detector for measuring the light transmitted through the samples. There is no single light source that covers the entire visible and UV spectrum. The source most commonly used for the visible part of the spectrum is the tungsten–halogen lamp, which provides continuous radiation over the range of 360 to 950 nm. The deuterium lamp has become the standard for much UV work. It covers the range from 220 to 360 nm. Instruments which cover the entire UV/visible range use both lamps with a means for switching from one lamp to the other at a wavelength of approximately 360 nm (Figure 69.2).

Wavelength selection is accomplished with filters, prisms, and diffraction gratings. Specially designed interference filters can provide bandwidths as small as 5 nm. These are useful for instruments which do not need to scan a range of wavelengths. Prisms produce a nonlinear dispersion of wavelengths with the longer wavelengths closer together than the shorter ones. Since the light must pass through the prism material, they must be made of quartz for UV work. Diffraction gratings are surfaces with 1000 to 3000 grooves/mm cut into them. They may be transmissive or reflective; the reflective ones are more popular since there is no attenuation of light by the material. They produce a linear dispersion. By proper selection of slit widths, pass bands of 0.1 nm are commonly achieved.

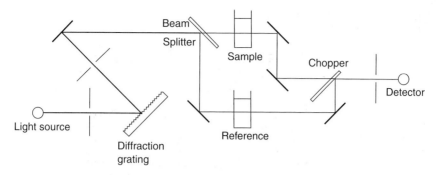

FIGURE 69.2 Dual-beam spectrophotometer. The diffraction grating is rotated to select the desired wavelength. The beam splitter consists of a half-silvered mirror which passes half the light while reflecting the other half. A rotating mirror with cut-out sections (chopper) alternately directs one beam and then the other to the detector.

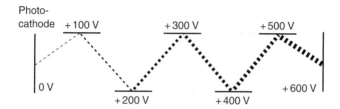

FIGURE 69.3 Photomultiplier tube. Incident photons cause the photocathode to emit electrons which collide with the first dynode which emits additional electrons. Multiple dynodes provide sufficient gain to produce an easily measurable electric pulse from a single photon.

The most common detector is the photomultiplier tube, which consists of a photosensitive cathode that emits electrons in proportion to the intensity of light striking it (Figure 69.3). A series of 10–15 dynodes, each at 50–100 V greater potential than the preceding one, produce an electron amplification of 4–6 per stage. Overall gains are typically a million or more. Photomultiplier tubes respond quickly and cover the entire spectral range. They require a high voltage supply and can be damaged if exposed to room light while the high voltage is applied.

69.6 Fluorometry

Certain molecules absorb a photon's energy and then emit a photon with less energy (longer wavelength). When the reemission occurs in less than 10^{-8} sec, the process is known as fluorescence. This physical process provides the means for assays which are 10 to 100 times as sensitive as those based on absorption measurements. This increase in sensitivity is largely because the light measured is all from the sample of interest. A dim light is easily measured against a black background, while it may be lost if added to an already bright background.

Fluorometers and spectrofluorometers are very similar to photometers and spectrophotometers but with two major differences. Fluorometers and spectrofluorometers use two monochrometers, one for excitation light and one for emitted light. By proper selection of the bandpass regions, all the light used to excite the sample can be blocked from the detector, assuring that the detector sees only fluorescence. The other difference is that the detector is aligned off-axis, commonly at 90°, from the excitation source. At this angle, scatter is minimal, which helps ensure a dark background for the measured fluorescence. Some spectrofluorometers use polarization filters both on the input and output light beams, which allows for fluorescence polarization studies (Figure 69.4). An intense light source in the visible-to-UV range is

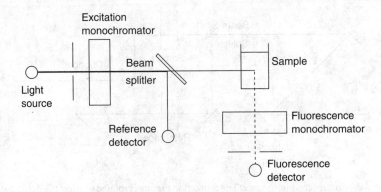

FIGURE 69.4   Spectrofluorometer. Fluorescence methods can be extremely sensitive to the low background interference. Since the detector is off-axis from the incident light and a second monochromator blocks light of wavelengths illuminating the sample, virtually no signal reaches the detector other than the desired fluorescence.

desirable. A common source is the xenon or mercury arc lamps, which provide a continuum of radiation over this range.

69.7   Flame Photometry

Flame photometry is used to measure sodium, potassium, and lithium in body fluids. When these elements are heated in a flame they emit characteristic wavelengths of light. The major emission lines are 589 nm (yellow) for sodium, 767 nm (violet) for potassium, and 671 nm (red) for lithium. An atomizer introduces a fine mist of the sample into a flame. For routine laboratory use, a propane and compressed air flame is adequate. High-quality interference filters with narrow pass bands are often used to isolate the major emission lines. The narrow band pass is necessary to maximize the signal-to-noise ratio. Since it is impossible to maintain stable aspiration, atomization, and flame characteristics, it is necessary to use an internal standard of known concentration while making measurements of unknowns. In this way the ratio of the unknown sample's emission to the internal standard's emission remains stable even as the total signal fluctuates. An internal standard is usually an element which is found in very low concentration in the sample fluid. By adding a high concentration of this element to the sample, its concentration can be known to a high degree of accuracy. Lithium, potassium, and cesium all may be used as internal standards depending upon the particular assay being conducted.

69.8   Atomic Absorption Spectroscopy

Atomic absorption spectroscopy is based on the fact that just as metal elements have unique emission lines, they have identical absorption lines when in a gaseous or dissociated state. The atomic absorption spectrometer takes advantage of these physical characteristics in a clever manner, producing an instrument with approximately 100 times the sensitivity of a flame photometer for similar elements. The sample is aspirated into a flame, where the majority of the atoms of the element being measured remain in the ground state, where they are capable of absorbing light at their characteristic wavelengths. An intense source of exactly these wavelengths is produced by a hollow cathode lamp. These lamps are constructed so that the cathode is made from the element to be measured, and the lamps are filled with a low pressure of argon or neon gas. When a current is passed through the lamp, metal atoms are sputtered off the cathode and collide with the argon or neon in the tube, producing emission of the characteristic wavelengths. A monochromator and photodetector complete the system.

Light reaching the detector is a combination of that which is emitted by the sample (undesirable) and light from the hollow cathode lamp which was not absorbed by the sample in the flame (desirable).

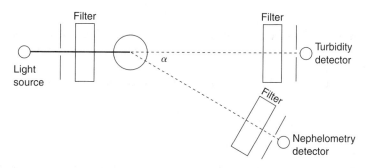

FIGURE 69.5 Nephelometer. Light scattered by large molecules is measured at an angle α away from the axis of incident light. The filters select the wavelength range desired and block undesired fluorescence. When $\alpha = 0$, the technique is known as turbidimetry.

By pulsing the light from the lamp either by directly pulsing the lamp or with a chopper, and using a detector which is sensitive to ac signals and insensitive to dc signals, the undesirable emission signal is eliminated. Each element to be measured requires a lamp with that element present in the cathode. Multielement lamps have been developed to minimize the number of lamps required. Atomic absorption spectrophotometers may be either single beam or double beam; the double-beam instruments have greater stability.

There are various flameless methods for atomic absorption spectroscopy in which the burner is replaced with a method for vaporizing the element of interest without a flame. The graphite furnace which heats the sample to 2700° consists of a hollow graphite tube which is heated by passing a large current through it. The sample is placed within the tube, and the light beam is passed through it while the sample is heated.

69.9 Turbidimetry and Nephelometry

Light scattering by particles in solution is directly proportional to both concentration and molecular weight of the particles. For small molecules the scattering is insignificant, but for proteins, immunoglobulins, immune complexes, and other large particles, light scattering can be an effective method for the detection and measurement of particle concentration. For a given wavelength λ of light and particle size d, scattering is described as Raleigh ($d < \lambda/10$), Raleigh-Debye ($d \acute{Y} \lambda$), or Mie ($d > 10\lambda$). For particles that are small compared to the wavelength, the scattering is equal in all directions. However, as the particle size becomes larger than the wavelength of light, it becomes preferentially scattered in the forward direction. Light-scattering techniques are widely used to detect the formation of antigen–antibody complexes in immunoassays.

When light scattering is measured by the attenuation of a beam of light through a solution, it is called **turbidimetry.** This is essentially the same as absorption measurements with a photometer except that a large pass-band is acceptable. When maximum sensitivity is required a different method is used — direct measurement of the scattered light with a detector placed at an angle to the central beam. This method is called **nephelometry.** A typical nephelometer will have a light source, filter, sample cuvette, and detector set at an angle to the incident beam (Figure 69.5).

Defining Terms

Accuracy: The degree to which the average value of repeated measurements approximate the true value being measured.

Fluorescence: Emission of light by an atom or molecule following absorption of a photon by greater energy. Emission normally occurs within 10^{-8} of absorption.

Nephelometry: Measurement of the amount of light scattered by particles suspended in a fluid.

Precision: A measure of test reproducibility.

Sensitivity: A measure of how small an amount or concentration of an analyte can be detected.
Specificity: A measure of how well a test detects the intended analyte without being "fooled" by other substances in the sample.
Turbidimetry: Measurement of the attenuation of a light beam due to light lost to scattering by particles suspended in a fluid.

References

[1] Burtis C.A. and Ashwood E.R. (Eds.) 1994. *Tietz Textbook of Clinical Chemistry*, 2nd ed., Philadelphia, W.B. Saunders.
[2] Hicks M.R., Haven M.C., and Schenken J.R. et al. (Eds.) 1987. *Laboratory Instrumentation*, 3rd ed., Philadelphia, Lippincott.
[3] Kaplan L.A. and Pesce A.J. (Eds.) 1989. *Clinical Chemistry: Theory, Analysis, and Correlation*, 2rd ed., St. Louis, Mosby.
[4] Tietz N.W. (Ed.) 1987. *Fundamentals of Clinical Chemistry*, 3rd ed., Philadelphia, W.B. Saunders.
[5] Ward J.M., Lehmann C.A., and Leiken A.M. 1994. *Clinical Laboratory Instrumentation and Automation: Principles, Applications, and Selection*, Philadelphia, W.B. Saunders.

70

Clinical Laboratory: Nonspectral Methods and Automation

70.1	Particle Counting and Identification	**70**-1
70.2	Electrochemical Methods	**70**-3
70.3	Ion-Specific Electrodes	**70**-4
70.4	Radioactive Methods	**70**-5
70.5	Coagulation Timers....................................	**70**-7
70.6	Osmometers...	**70**-7
70.7	Automation..	**70**-7
70.8	Trends in Laboratory Instrumentation................	**70**-8
	Defining Terms...	**70**-8
	References	**70**-9

Richard L. Roa
Baylor University Medical Center

70.1 Particle Counting and Identification

The Coulter principle was the first major advance in automating blood cell counts. The cells to be counted are drawn through a small aperture between two fluid compartments, and the electric impedance between the two compartments is monitored (see Figure 70.1). As cells pass through the aperture, the impedance increases in proportion to the volume of the cell, allowing large numbers of cells to be counted and sized rapidly. Red cells are counted by pulling diluted blood through the aperture. Since red cells greatly outnumber white cells, the contribution of white cells to the red cell count is usually neglected. White cells are counted by first destroying the red cells and using a more concentrated sample.

Modern cell counters using the Coulter principle often use **hydrodynamic focusing** to improve the performance of the instrument. A sheath fluid is introduced which flows along the outside of a channel with the sample stream inside it. By maintaining laminar flow conditions and narrowing the channel, the sample stream is focused into a very thin column with the cells in single file. This eliminates problems with cells flowing along the side of the aperture or sticking to it and minimizes problems with having more than one cell in the aperture at a time.

Flow cytometry is a method for characterizing, counting, and separating cells which are suspended in a fluid. The basic flow cytometer uses hydrodynamic focusing to produce a very thin stream of fluid containing cells moving in single file through a quartz flow chamber (Figure 70.2). The cells are characterized on the basis of their scattering and fluorescent properties. This simultaneous measurement of

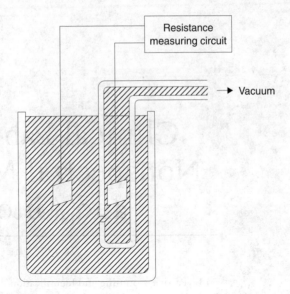

FIGURE 70.1 Coulter method. Blood cells are surrounded by an insulating membrane, which makes them non-conductive. The resistance of electrolyte-filled channel will increase slightly as cells flow through it. This resistance variation yields both the total number of cells which flow through the channel and the volume of each cell.

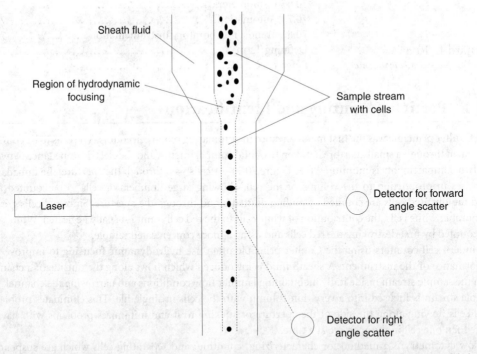

FIGURE 70.2 Flow cytometer. By combining hydrodynamic focusing, state-of-the-art optics, fluorescent labels, and high-speed computing, large numbers of cells can be characterized and sorted automatically.

scattering and fluorescence is accomplished with a sophisticated optical system that detects light from the sample both at the wavelength of the excitation source (scattering) as well as at longer wavelengths (fluorescence) at more than one angle. Analysis of these measurements produces parameters related to the cells' size, granularity, and natural or tagged fluorescence. High-pressure mercury or xenon arc lamps can be used as light sources, but the argon laser (488 nm) is the preferred source for high-performance instruments.

One of the more interesting features of this technology is that particular cells may be selected at rates that allow collection of quantities of particular cell types adequate for further chemical testing. This is accomplished by breaking the outgoing stream into a series of tiny droplets using piezoelectric vibration. By charging the stream of droplets and then using deflection plates controlled by the cell analyzer, the cells of interest can be diverted into collection vessels.

The development of monoclonal antibodies coupled with flow cytometry allows for quantitation of T and B cells to assess the status of the immune system as well as characterization of leukemias, lymphomas, and other disorders.

70.2 Electrochemical Methods

Electrochemical methods are increasingly popular in the clinical laboratory, for measurement not only of electrolytes, blood gases, and pH but also of simple compounds such as glucose. **Potentiometry** is a method in which a voltage is developed across electrochemical cells as shown in Figure 70.3. This voltage is measured with little or no current flow.

Ideally, one would like to measure all potentials between the reference solution in the indicator electrode and the test solution. Unfortunately there is no way to do that. Interface potentials develop across any metal-liquid boundary, across liquid junctions, and across the ion-selective membrane. The key to making potentiometric measurements is to ensure that all the potentials are constant and do not vary with the composition of the test solution except for the potential of interest across the ion-selective membrane. By maintaining the solutions within the electrodes constant, the potential between these solutions and the metal electrodes immersed in them is constant. The liquid junction is a structure which severely limits bulk flow of the solution but allows free passage of all ions between the solutions. The reference electrode commonly is filled with saturated KCl, which produces a small, constant liquid-junction potential. Thus, any change in the measured voltage (V) is due to a change in the ion concentration in the test solution for which the membrane is selective.

The potential which develops across an ion-selective membrane is given by the Nernst equation:

$$V = \left(\frac{RT}{zF}\right) \ln \frac{a_2}{a_1} \tag{70.1}$$

where R is the gas constant $= 8.314$ J/K mol, $T =$ the temperature in K, $z =$ the ionization number, $F =$ the Faraday constant $= 9.649 \times 10^4$ C/mol, $a_n =$ the activity of ion in solution n. When one of the

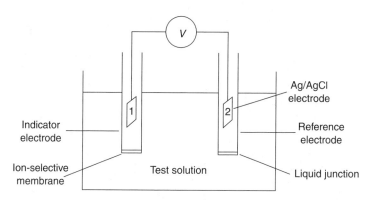

FIGURE 70.3   Electrochemical cell.

solutions is a reference solution, this equation can be rewritten in a convenient form as

$$V = V_0 + \frac{N}{z} \log_{10} a \tag{70.2}$$

where V_0 is the constant voltage due to reference solution and N the Nernst slope Ý 59 mV/decade at room temperature. The actual Nernst slope is usually slightly less than the theoretical value. Thus, the typical pH meter has two calibration controls. One adjusts the offset to account for the value of V_0, and the other adjusts the range to account for both temperature effects and deviations from the theoretical Nernst slope.

70.3   Ion-Specific Electrodes

Ion-selective electrodes use membranes which are permeable only to the ion being measured. To the extent that this can be done, the specificity of the electrode can be very high. One way of overcoming a lack of specificity for certain electrodes is to make multiple simultaneous measurement of several ions which include the most important interfering ones. A simple algorithm can then make corrections for the interfering effects. This technique is used in some commercial electrolyte analyzers. A partial list of the ions that can be measured with ion-selective electrodes includes H^+ (pH), Na^+, K^+, Li^+, Ca^{++}, Cl^-, F^-, NH_4^+, and CO_2.

NH_4^+, and CO_2 are both measured with a modified ion-selective electrode. They use a pH electrode modified with a thin layer of a solution (sodium bicarbonate for CO_2 and ammonium chloride for NH_4^+) whose pH varies depending on the concentration of ammonium ions or CO_2 it is equilibrated with. A thin membrane holds the solution against the pH glass electrode and provides for equilibration with the sample solution. Note that the CO_2 electrode in Figure 70.4 is a combination electrode. This means that both the reference and indicating electrodes have been combined into one unit. Most pH electrodes are made as combination electrodes.

The Clark electrode measures pO_2 by measuring the current developed by an electrode with an applied voltage rather than a voltage measurement. This is an example of **amperometry.** In this electrode a voltage

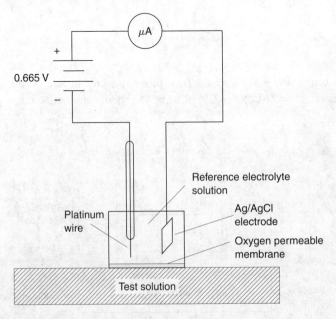

FIGURE 70.4   Clark electrode.

of approximately $-0.65\,V$ is applied to a platinum electrode relative to a Ag/AgCl electrode in an electrolyte solution. The reaction

$$O_2 + 2H^+ + 2e^- \rightarrow H_2O_2$$

proceeds at a rate proportional to the partial pressure of oxygen in the solution. The electrons involved in this reaction form a current which is proportional to the rate of the reaction and thus to the pO_2 in the solution.

70.4 Radioactive Methods

Isotopes are atoms which have identical atomic number (number of protons) but different atomic mass numbers (protons + neutrons). Since they have the same number of electrons in the neutral atom, they have identical chemical properties. This provides an ideal method for labeling molecules in a way that allows for detection at extremely low concentrations. Labeling with radioactive isotopes is extensively used in radioimmunoassays where the amount of antigen bound to specific antibodies is measured. The details of radioactive decay are complex, but for our purposes there are three types of emission from decaying nuclei: *alpha*, *beta*, and **gamma radiation**. Alpha particles are made up of two neutrons and two protons (helium nucleus). Alpha emitters are rarely used in the clinical laboratory. Beta emission consists of electrons or positrons emitted from the nucleus. They have a continuous range of energies up to a maximum value characteristic of the isotope. **Beta radiation** is highly interactive with matter and cannot penetrate very far in most materials. Gamma radiation is a high-energy form of electromagnetic radiation. This type of radiation may be continuous, discrete, or mixed depending on the details of the decay process. It has greater penetrating ability than beta radiation (see Figure 70.5).

The kinetic energy spectrum of emitted radiation is characteristic of the isotope. The energy is commonly measured in electron volts (eV). One electron volt is the energy acquired by an electron falling through a potential of 1 V. The isotopes commonly used in the clinical laboratory have energy spectra which range from 18 keV to 3.6 MeV.

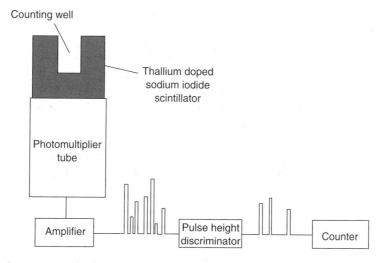

FIGURE 70.5 Gamma counted. The intensity of the light flash produced when a gamma photon interacts with a scintillator is proportional to the energy of the photon. The photomultiplier tube converts these light flashes into electric pulses which can be selected according to size (gamma energy) and counted.

The activity of a quantity of radioactive isotope is defined as the number of disintegrations per second which occur. The usual units are the curie (Ci), which is defined as 3.7×10^{10} dps, and the becquerel (Bq), defined as 1 dps. Specific activity for a given isotope is defined as activity per unit mass of the isotope.

The rate of decay for a given isotope is characterized by the decay constant λ, which is the proportion of the isotope which decays in unit time. Thus, the rate of loss of radioactive isotope is governed by the equation

$$\frac{dN}{dt} = -\lambda N \tag{70.3}$$

where N is the amount of radioactive isotope present at time t. The solution to this differential equation is:

$$N = N_0 e^{-\lambda t} \tag{70.4}$$

It can easily be shown that the amount of radioactive isotope present will be reduced by half after time

$$t_{1/2} = \frac{0.693}{\lambda} \tag{70.5}$$

This is known as the half-life for the isotope and can vary widely; for example, carbon-14 has a half-life of 5760 years, and iodine-131 has a half-life of 8.1 days.

The most common method for detection of radiation in the clinical laboratory is by **scintillation**. This is the conversion of radiation energy into photons in the visible or near-UV range. These are detected with photomultiplier tubes.

For gamma radiation, the scintillating crystal is made of sodium iodide doped with about 1% thallium, producing 20 to 30 photons for each electron-volt of energy absorbed. The photomultiplier tube and amplifier circuit produce voltage pulses proportional to the energy of the absorbed radiation. These voltage pulses are usually passed through a pulse-height analyzer which eliminates pulses outside a preset energy range (window). Multichannel analyzers can discriminate between two or more isotopes if they have well-separated energy maxima. There generally will be some spill down of counts from the higher-energy isotope into the lower-energy isotope's window, but this effect can be corrected with a simple algorithm. Multiple well detectors with up to 64 detectors in an array are available which increase the throughput for counting systems greatly. Counters using the sodium iodide crystal scintillator are referred to as gamma counters or well counters.

The lower energy and short penetration ability of beta particles requires a scintillator in direct contact with the decaying isotope. This is accomplished by dissolving or suspending the sample in a liquid fluor. Counters which use this technique are called beta counters or liquid scintillation counters.

Liquid scintillation counters use two photomultiplier tubes with a coincidence circuit that prevents counting of events seen by only one of the tubes. In this way, false counts due to chemiluminescence and noise in the phototube are greatly reduced. Quenching is a problem in all liquid scintillation counters. Quenching is any process which reduces the efficiency of the scintillation counting process, where efficiency is defined as

$$\text{Efficiency} = \text{counts per minute/decays per minute} \tag{70.6}$$

A number of techniques have been developed that automatically correct for quenching effects to produce estimates of true decays per minute from the raw counts. Currently there is a trend away from beta-emitting isotopic labels, but these assays are still used in many laboratories.

70.5 Coagulation Timers

Screening for and diagnosis of coagulation disorders is accomplished by assays that determine how long it takes for blood to clot following initiation of the clotting cascade by various reagents. A variety of instruments have been designed to automate this procedure. In addition to increasing the speed and throughput of such testing, these instruments improve the reproducibility of such tests. All the instruments provide precise introduction of reagents, accurate timing circuits, and temperature control. They differ in the method for detecting clot formation. One of the older methods still in use is to dip a small metal hook into the blood sample repeatedly and lift it a few millimeters above the surface. The electric resistance between the hook and the sample is measured, and when fibrin filaments form, they produce a conductive pathway which is detected as clot formation. Other systems detect the increase in viscosity due to fibrin formation or the scattering due to the large polymerized molecules formed. Absorption and fluorescence spectroscopy can also be used for clot detection.

70.6 Osmometers

The **colligative properties** of a solution are a function of the number of solute particles present regardless of size or identity. Increased solute concentration causes an increase in osmotic pressure and boiling point and a decrease in vapor pressure and freezing point. Measuring these changes provides information on the total solute concentration regardless of type. The most accurate and popular method used in clinical laboratories is the measurement of freezing point depression. With this method, the sample is supercooled to a few degrees below $0°C$ while being stirred gently. Freezing is then initiated by vigorous stirring. The heat of fusion quickly brings the solution to a slushy state where an equilibrium exists between ice and liquid, ensuring that the temperature is at the freezing point. This temperature is measured. A solute concentration of 1 osmol/kg water produces a freezing point depression of $1.858°C$. The measured temperature depression is easily calibrated in units of milliosmols/kg water.

The vapor pressure depression method has the advantage of smaller sample size. However, it is not as precise as the freezing point method and cannot measure the contribution of volatile solutes such as ethanol. This method is not used as widely as the freezing point depression method in clinical laboratories.

Osmolality of blood is primarily due to electrolytes such as Na^+ and Cl^-. Proteins with molecular weights of 30,000 or more atomic mass units (amu) contribute very little to total osmolality due to their smaller numbers (a single Na^+ ion contributes just as much to osmotic pressure as a large protein molecule). However, the contribution to osmolality made by proteins is of great interest when monitoring conditions leading to pulmonary edema. This value is known as colloid osmotic pressure, or oncotic pressure, and is measured with a membrane permeable to water and all molecules smaller than about 30,000 amu. By placing a reference saline solution on one side and the unknown sample on the other, an osmotic pressure is developed across the membrane. This pressure is measured with a pressure transducer and can be related to the true colloid osmotic pressure through a calibration procedure using known standards.

70.7 Automation

Improvements in technology coupled with increased demand for laboratory tests as well as pressures to reduce costs have led to the rapid development of highly automated laboratory instruments. Typical automated instruments contain mechanisms for measuring, mixing, and transport of samples and reagents, measurement systems, and one or more microprocessors to control the entire system. In addition to system control, the computer systems store calibration curves, match test results to specimen IDs, and generate reports. Automated instruments are dedicated to complete blood counts, coagulation studies, microbiology assays, and immunochemistry, as well as high-volume instruments used in clinical chemistry laboratories. The chemistry analyzers tend to fall into one of four classes: continuous flow, centrifugal, pack-based, and dry-slide-based systems. The continuous flow systems pass successive samples and reagents through a single set of tubing, where they are directed to appropriate mixing, dialyzing, and measuring stations. Carry-over from one sample to the next is minimized by the introduction of air bubbles and wash solution between samples.

Centrifugal analyzers use plastic rotors which serve as reservoirs for samples and reagents and also as cuvettes for optical measurements. Spinning the plastic rotor mixes, incubates, and transports the test solution into the cuvette portion of the rotor, where the optical measurements are made while the rotor is spinning.

Pack-based systems are those in which each test uses a special pack with the proper reagents and sample preservation devices built-in. The sample is automatically introduced into as many packs as tests required. The packs are then processed sequentially.

Dry chemistry analyzers use no liquid reagents. The reagents and other sample preparation methods are layered onto a slide. The liquid sample is placed on the slide, and after a period of time the color developed is read by reflectance photometry. Ion-selective electrodes have been incorporated into the same slide format.

There are a number of technological innovations found in many of the automated instruments. One innovation is the use of fiberoptic bundles to channel excitation energy toward the sample as well as transmitted, reflected, or emitted light away from the sample to the detectors. This provides a great deal of flexibility in instrument layout. Multiwavelength analysis using a spinning filter wheel or diode array detectors is commonly found. The computers associated with these instruments allow for innovative improvements in the assays. For instance, when many analytes are being analyzed from one sample, the interference effects of one analyte on the measurement of another can be predicted and corrected before the final report is printed.

70.8   Trends in Laboratory Instrumentation

Predicting the future direction of laboratory instrumentation is difficult, but there seem to be some clear trends. Decentralization of the laboratory functions will continue with more instruments being located in or around ICUs, operating rooms, emergency rooms, and physician offices. More electrochemistry-based tests will be developed. The flame photometer is already being replaced with ion-selective electrode methods. Instruments which analyze whole blood rather than **plasma** or **serum** will reduce the amount of time required for sample preparation and will further encourage testing away from the central laboratory. Dry reagent methods increasingly will replace wet chemistry methods. Radioimmunoassays will continue to decline with the increasing use of methods for performing immunoassays that do not rely upon radioisotopes such as enzyme-linked fluorescent assays.

Defining Terms

Alpha radiation: Particulate radiation consisting of a helium nucleus emitted from a decaying anucleus.

Amperometry: Measurements based on current flow produced in an electrochemical cell by an applied voltage.

Beta radiation: Particulate radiation consisting of an electron or positron emitted from a decaying nucleus.

Colligative properties: Physical properties that depend on the number of molecules present rather than on their individual properties.

Gamma radiation: Electromagnetic radiation emitted from an atom undergoing nuclear decay.

Hydrodynamic focusing: A process in which a fluid stream is first surrounded by a second fluid and then narrowed to a thin stream by a narrowing of the channel.

Isotopes: Atoms with the same number of protons but differing numbers of neutrons.

Plasma: The liquid portion of blood.

Potentiometry: Measurement of the potential produced by electrochemical cells under equilibrium conditions with no current flow.

Scintillation: The conversion of the kinetic energy of a charged particle or photon to a flash of light.

Serum: The liquid portion of blood remaining after clotting has occurred.

References

Burtis C.A. and Ashwood E.R. (Eds.) 1994. *Tietz Textbook of Clinical Chemistry*, 2nd ed., Philadelphia, Saunders Company.

Hicks M.R., Haven M.C., Schenken J.R. et al. (Eds.) 1987. *Laboratory Instrumentation*, 3rd ed., Philadelphia, Lippincott Company, 1987.

Kaplan L.A. and Pesce A.J. (Eds.) 1989. *Clinical Chemistry: Theory, Analysis, and Correlation*, 2nd ed., St. Louis, Mosby.

Tietz N.W. (Ed.). 1987. *Fundamentals of Clinical Chemistry*, 3rd ed., Philadelphia, W.B. Saunders.

Ward J.M., Lehmann C.A., and Leiken A.M. 1994. *Clinical Laboratory Instrumentation and Automation: Principles, Applications, and Selection*, Philadelphia, W.B. Saunders.

71

Noninvasive Optical Monitoring

71.1 Oximetry and Pulse Oximetry 71-2
    Background • Theory • Application and Future Directions
71.2 Nonpulsatile Spectroscopy 71-7
    Background • Cytochrome Spectroscopy • Near-Infrared
    Spectroscopy and Glucose Monitoring • Time-Resolved
    Spectroscopy
71.3 Conclusions 71-9
Defining Terms 71-9
References 71-9
Further Information 71-10

Ross Flewelling
Nellcor Incorporation

Optical measures of physiologic status are attractive because they can provide a simple, noninvasive, yet real-time assessment of medical condition. Noninvasive optical monitoring is taken here to mean the use of visible or near-infrared light to directly assess the internal physiologic status of a person without the need of extracting a blood of tissue sample or using a catheter. Liquid water strongly absorbs ultraviolet and infrared radiation, and thus these spectral regions are useful only for analyzing thin surface layers or respiratory gases, neither of which will be the subject of this review. Instead, it is the visible and near-infrared portions of the electromagnetic spectrum that provide a unique "optical window" into the human body, opening new vistas for noninvasive monitoring technologies.

Various molecules in the human body possess distinctive spectral absorption characteristics in the visible or near-infrared spectral regions and therefore make optical monitoring possible. The most strongly absorbing molecules at physiologic concentrations are the hemoglobins, myoglobins, **cytochromes**, melanins, carotenes, and bilirubin (see Figure 71.1 for some examples). Perhaps less appreciated are the less distinctive and weakly absorbing yet ubiquitous materials possessing spectral characteristics in the near-infrared: water, fat, proteins, and sugars. Simple optical methods are now available to quantitatively and noninvasively measure some of these compounds directly in intact tissue. The most successful methods to date have used hemoglobins to assess the oxygen content of blood, cytochromes to assess the respiratory status of cells, and possibly near-infrared to assess endogenous concentrations of metabolites, including glucose.

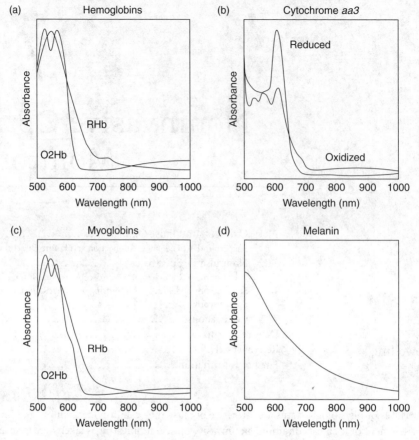

FIGURE 71.1 Absorption spectra of some endogenous biologic materials. (a) hemoglobins, (b) cytochrome *aa3*, (c) myoglobins, and (d) melanin.

71.1 Oximetry and Pulse Oximetry

Failure to provide adequate oxygen to tissues — **hypoxia** — can in a matter of minutes result in reduced work capacity of muscles, depressed mental activity, and ultimately cell death. It is therefore of considerable interest to reliably and accurately determine the amount of oxygen in blood or tissues. **Oximetry** is the determination of the oxygen content of blood of tissues, normally by optical means. In the clinical laboratory the oxygen content of whole blood can be determined by a bench-top cooximeter or blood gas analyzer. But the need for timely clinical information and the desire to minimize the inconvenience and cost of extracting a blood sample and later analyze it in the lab has led to the search for alternative noninvasive optical methods. Since the 1930s, attempts have been made to use multiple wavelengths of light to arrive at a complete spectral characterization of a tissue. These approaches, although somewhat successful, have remained of limited utility owing to the awkward instrumentation and unreliable results.

It was not until the invention of **pulse oximetry** in the 1970s and its commercial development and application in the 1980s that noninvasive oximetry became practical. Pulse oximetry is an extremely easy-to-use, noninvasive, and accurate measurement of real-time arterial oxygen saturation. Pulse oximetry is now used routinely in clinical practice, has become a standard of care in all U.S. operating rooms, and is increasingly used wherever critical patients are found. The explosive growth of this new technology and its considerable utility led John Severinghaus and Poul Astrup [1986] in an excellent historical review to conclude that pulse oximetry was "arguably the most significant technological advance ever made in monitoring the well-being and safety of patients during anesthesia, recovery and critical care."

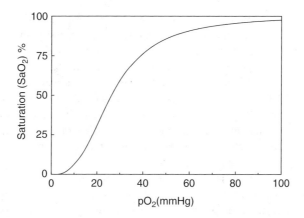

FIGURE 71.2 Hemoglobin oxygen dissociation curve showing the sigmoidal relationship between the partial pressure of oxygen and the oxygen saturation of blood. The curve is given approximately by %$SaO_2 = 100\%/[1+P_{50}/pO_2^n]$, with $n = 2.8$ and $P_{50} = 26$ mmHg.

71.1.1 Background

The partial pressure of oxygen (pO_2) in tissues need only be about 3 mmHg to support basic metabolic demands. This tissue level, however, requires capillary pO_2 to be near 40 mmHg, with a corresponding arterial pO_2 of about 95 mmHg. Most of the oxygen carried by blood is stored in red blood cells reversibly bound to hemoglobin molecules. Oxygen saturation (SaO_2) is defined as the percentage of hemoglobin-bound oxygen compared to the total amount of hemoglobin available for reversible oxygen binding. The relationship between the oxygen partial pressure in blood and the oxygen saturation of blood is given by the hemoglobin oxygen dissociation curve as shown in Figure 71.2. The higher the pO_2 in blood, the higher the SaO_2. But due to the highly cooperative binding of four oxygen molecules to each hemoglobin molecule, the oxygen binding curve is sigmoidal, and consequently the SaO_2 value is particularly sensitive to dangerously low pO_2 levels. With a normal arterial blood pO_2 above 90 mmHg, the oxygen saturation should be at least 95%, and a pulse oximeter can readily verify a safe oxygen level. If oxygen content falls, say to a pO_2 below 40 mmHg, metabolic needs may not be met, and the corresponding oxygen saturation will drop below 80%. Pulse oximetry therefore provides a direct measure of oxygen sufficiency and will alert the clinician to any danger of imminent hypoxia in a patient.

Although endogenous molecular oxygen is not optically observable, hemoglobin serves as an oxygen-sensitive "dye" such that when oxygen reversibly binds to the iron atom in the large heme prosthetic group, the electron distribution of the heme is shifted, producing a significant color change. The optical absorption of hemoglobin in its oxygenated and deoxygenated states is shown in Figure 71.1. Fully oxygenated blood absorbs strongly in the blue and appears bright red; deoxygenated blood absorbs through the visible region and is very dark (appearing blue when observed through tissue due to light scattering effects). Thus the optical absorption spectra of oxyhemaglobin (O_2Hb) and "reduced" deoxyhemoglobin (RHb) differ substantially, and this difference provides the basis for spectroscopic determinations of the proportion of the two hemoglobin states. In addition to these two normal functional hemoglobins, there are also **dysfunctional hemoglobins** — carboxyhemoglobin, methemoglobin, and sulhemoglobin — which are spectroscopically distinct but do not bind oxygen reversibly. Oxygen saturation is therefore defined in Equation 71.1 only in terms of the **functional saturation** with respect to O_2Hb and RHb:

$$S_aO_2 = \frac{O_2Hb}{RHb + O_2Hb} \times 100\% \tag{71.1}$$

Cooximeters are bench-top analyzers that accept whole blood samples and utilize four or more wavelengths of monochromatic light, typically between 500 and 650 nm, to spectroscopically determine the various individual hemoglobins in the sample. If a blood sample can be provided, this spectroscopic method is accurate and reliable. Attempts to make an equivalent quantitative analysis noninvasively through intact tissue have been fraught with difficulty. The problem has been to contend with the wide variation in scattering and nonspecific absorption properties of very complex heterogeneous tissue. One of the more successful approaches, marketed by Hewlett–Packard, used eight optical wavelengths transmitted through the pinna of the ear. In this approach a "bloodless" measurement is first obtained by squeezing as much blood as possible from an area of tissue; the arterial blood is then allowed to flow back, and the oxygen saturation is determined by analyzing the change in the spectral absorbance characteristics of the tissue. While this method works fairly well, it is cumbersome, operator dependent, and does not always work well on poorly perfused or highly pigmented subjects.

In the early 1970s, Takuo Aoyagi recognized that most of the interfering nonspecific tissue effects could be eliminated by utilizing only the change in the signal during an arterial pulse. Although an early prototype was built in Japan, it was not until the refinements in implementation and application by Biox (now Ohmeda) and Nellcor Incorporated in the 1980s that the technology became widely adopted as a safety monitor for critical care use.

71.1.2 Theory

Pulse oximetry is based on the fractional change in light transmission during an arterial pulse at two different wavelengths. In this method the fractional change in the signal is due only to the arterial blood itself, and therefore the complicated nonpulsatile and highly variable optical characteristics of tissue are eliminated. In a typical configuration, light at two different wavelengths illuminating one side of a finger will be detected on the other side, after having traversed the intervening vascular tissues (Figure 71.3). The transmission of light at each wavelength is a function of the thickness, color, and structure of the skin, tissue, bone, blood, and other material through which the light passes. The absorbance of light by a sample is defined as the negative logarithm of the ratio of the light intensity in the presence of the sample (I) to that without (I_0): $A = -\log(I/I_0)$. According to the **Beer–Lambert law,** the absorbance of a sample at a given wavelength with a molar absorptivity (ϵ) is directly proportional to both the concentration (c) and pathlength (l) of the absorbing material: $A = \epsilon cl$. (In actuality, biologic tissue is highly scattering, and the Beer–Lambert law is only approximately correct; see the references for further elaboration). Visible or near-infrared light passing through about one centimeter of tissue (e.g., a finger) will be attenuated by about one or two orders of magnitude for a typical emitter–detector geometry, corresponding to an effective optical density (OD) of 1 to 2 OD (the detected light intensity is decreased

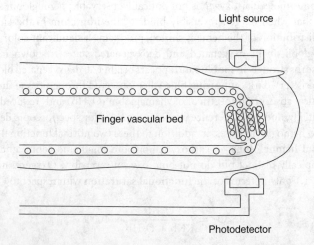

FIGURE 71.3 Typical pulse oximeter sensing configuration on a finger. Light at two different wavelengths is emitted by the source, diffusely scattered through the finger, and detected on the opposite side by a photodetector.

by one order of magnitude for each OD unit). Although hemoglobin in the blood is the single strongest absorbing molecule, most of the total attenuation is due to the scattering of light away from the detector by the highly heterogeneous tissue. Since human tissue contains about 7% blood, and since blood contains typically about 14 g/dL hemoglobin, the effective hemoglobin concentration in tissue is about 1 g/dL ($\sim$150 μM). At the wavelengths used for pulse oximetry (650–950 nm), the oxy- and deoxyhemoglobin molar absorptivities fall in the range of 100–1000 $M^{-1}cm^{-1}$, and consequently hemoglobin accounts for less than 0.2 OD of the total observed optical density. Of this amount, perhaps only 10% is pulsatile, and consequently pulse signals of only a few percent are ultimately measured, at times even one-tenth of this.

A mathematical model for pulse oximetry begins by considering light at two wavelengths, λ_1 and λ_2, passing through tissue and being detected at a distant location as in Figure 71.3. At each wavelength the total light attenuation is described by four different component absorbances: oxyhemoglobin in the blood (concentration c_o, molar absorptivity ϵ_o, and effective pathlength l_o), "reduced" deoxyhemoglobin in the blood (concentration c_r, molar absorptivity ϵ_r, and effective pathlength l_r), specific variable absorbances that are not from the arterial blood (concentration c_x, molar absorptivity ϵ_x, and effective pathlength l_x), and all other non-specific sources of optical attenuation, combined as A_y, which can include light scattering, geometric factors, and characteristics of the emitter and detector elements. The total absorbance at the two wavelengths can then be written:

$$\begin{cases} A_{\lambda_1} = \epsilon_{o_1} c_o l_o + \epsilon_{r_1} c_r l_r + \epsilon_{x_1} c_x l_x + A_{y_1} \\ A_{\lambda_2} = \epsilon_{o_2} c_o l_o + \epsilon_{r_2} c_r l_r + \epsilon_{x_2} c_x l_x + A_{y_2} \end{cases} \qquad (71.2)$$

The blood volume change due to the arterial pulse results in a modulation of the measured absorbances. By taking the time rate of change of the absorbances, the two last terms in each equation are effectively zero, since the concentration and effective pathlength of absorbing material outside the arterial blood do not change during a pulse [$d(c_x l_x)/dt = 0$], and all the nonspecific effects on light attenuation are also effectively invariant on the time scale of a cardiac cycle ($dA_y/dt = 0$). Since the extinction coefficients are constant, and the blood concentrations are constant on the time scale of a pulse, the time-dependent changes in the absorbances at the two wavelengths can be assigned entirely to the change in the blood pathlength (dl_o/dt and dl_r/dt). With the additional assumption that these two blood pathlength changes are equivalent (or more generally, their ratio is a constant), the ratio R of the time rate of change of the absorbance at wavelength 1 to that at wavelength 2 reduces to the following:

$$R = \frac{dA_{\lambda_1}/dt}{dA_{\lambda_2}/dt} = \frac{-d\log(I_1/I_o)/dt}{-d\log(I_2/I_o)/dt} = \frac{(\Delta I_1/I_1)}{(\Delta I_2/I_2)} = \frac{\epsilon_{o_1} c_o + \epsilon_{r_1} c_r}{\epsilon_{o_2} c_o + \epsilon_{r_2} c_r} \qquad (71.3)$$

Observing that functional oxygen saturation is given by $S = c_o/(c_o + c_r)$, and that $(1 - S) = c_r/(c_o + c_r)$, the oxygen saturation can then be written in terms of the ratio R as follows

$$S = \frac{\epsilon_{r1} - \epsilon_{r2} R}{(\epsilon_{r1} - \epsilon_{o1}) - (\epsilon_{r2} - \epsilon_{o2})R} \qquad (71.4)$$

Equation 71.4 provides the desired relationship between the experimentally determined ratio R and the clinically desired oxygen saturation S. In actual use, commonly available LEDs are used as the light sources, typically a red LED near 660 nm and a near-infrared LED selected in the range 890 to 950 nm. Such LEDs are not monochromatic light sources, typically with bandwidths between 20 and 50 nm, and therefore standard molar absorptivities for hemoglobin cannot be used directly in Equation 71.4. Further, the simple model presented above is only approximately true; for example, the two wavelengths do not necessarily have the exact same pathlength changes, and second-order scattering effects have been ignored. Consequently the relationship between S and R is instead determined empirically by fitting the clinical data to a generalized function of the form $S = (a - bR)/(c - dR)$. The final empirical calibration will ultimately depend on the details of an individual sensor design, but these variations can be determined

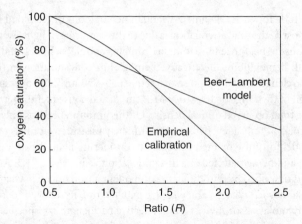

FIGURE 71.4 Relationship between the measured ratio of fractional changes in light intensity at two wavelengths, R, and the oxygen saturation S. Beer–Lambert model is from Equation 71.4 with $\epsilon_{o1} = 100$, $\epsilon_{o2} = 300$, $\epsilon_{r1} = 800$, and $\epsilon_{r2} = 200$. Empirical calibration is based on $\%S = 100\% \times (a - bR)/(c - dR)$ with $a = 1000$, $b = 550$, $c = 900$, and $d = 350$, with a linear extrapolation below 70%.

for each sensor and included in unique calibration parameters. A typical empirical calibration for R vs. S is shown in Figure 71.4, together with the curve that standard molar absorptivities would predict.

In this way the measurement of the ratio of the fractional change in signal intensity of the two LEDs is used along with the empirically determined calibration equation to obtain a beat-by-beat measurement of the arterial oxygen saturation in a perfused tissue — continuously, noninvasively, and to an accuracy of a few percent.

71.1.3 Application and Future Directions

Pulse oximetry is now routinely used in nearly all operating rooms and critical care areas in the United States and increasingly throughout the world. It has become so pervasive and useful that it is now being called the "fifth" vital sign (for an excellent review of practical aspects and clinical applications of the technology see Kelleher [1989]).

The principal advantages of pulse oximetry are that it provides continuous, accurate, and reliable monitoring of arterial oxygen saturation on nearly all patients, utilizing a variety of convenient sensors, reusable as well as disposable. Single-patient-use adhesive sensors can easily be applied to fingers for adults and children and to arms for legs or neonates. Surface reflectance sensors have also been developed based on the same principles and offer a wider choice for sensor location, though they tend to be less accurate and prone to more types of interference.

Limitations of pulse oximetry include sensitivity to high levels of optical or electric interference, errors due to high concentrations of dysfunctional hemoglobins (methemoglobin or carboxyhemoglobin) or interference from physiologic dyes (such as methylene blue). Other important factors, such as total hemoglobin content, fetal hemoglobin, or sickle cell trait, have little or no effect on the measurement except under extreme conditions. Performance can also be compromised by poor signal quality, as may occur for poorly perfused tissues with weak pulse amplitudes or by motion artifact.

Hardware and software advances continue to provide more sensitive signal detection and filtering capabilities, allowing pulse oximeters to work better on more ambulatory patients. Already some pulse oximeters incorporate ECG synchronization for improved signal processing. A pulse oximeter for use in labor and delivery is currently under active development by several research groups and companies. A likely implementation may include use of a reflectance surface sensor for the fetal head to monitor the adequacy of fetal oxygenation. This application is still in active development, and clinical utility remains to be demonstrated.

71.2 Nonpulsatile Spectroscopy

71.2.1 Background

Nonpulsatile optical spectroscopy has been used for more than half a century for noninvasive medical assessment, such as in the use of multiwavelength tissue analysis for oximetry and skin reflectance measurement for bilirubin assessment in jaundiced neonates. These early applications have found some limited use, but with modest impact. Recent investigations into new nonpulsatile spectroscopy methods for assessment of deep-tissue oxygenation (e.g., cerebral oxygen monitoring), for evaluation of respiratory status at the cellular level, and for the detection of other critical analytes, such as glucose, may yet prove more fruitful. The former applications have led to spectroscopic studies of cytochromes in tissues, and the latter has led to considerable work into new approaches in near-infrared analysis of intact tissues.

71.2.2 Cytochrome Spectroscopy

Cytochromes are electron-transporting, heme-containing proteins found in the inner membranes of mitochondria and are required in the process of oxidative phosphorylation to convert metabolites and oxygen into CO_2 and high-energy phosphates. In this metabolic process the cytochromes are reversibly oxidized and reduced, and consequently the oxidation–reduction states of cytochromes c and aa_3 in particular are direct measures of the respiratory condition of the cell. Changes in the absorption spectra of these molecules, particularly near 600 and 830 nm for cytochrome aa_3, accompany this shift. By monitoring these spectral changes, the cytochrome oxidation state in the tissues can be determined (see, e.g., Jöbsis [1977] and Jöbsis et al. [1977]). As with all nonpulsatile approaches, the difficulty is to remove the dependence of the measurements on the various nonspecific absorbing materials and highly variable scattering effects of the tissue. To date, instruments designed to measure cytochrome spectral changes can successfully track relative changes in brain oxygenation, but absolute quantitation has not yet been demonstrated.

71.2.3 Near-Infrared Spectroscopy and Glucose Monitoring

Near-infrared (NIR), the spectral region between 780 and 3000 nm, is characterized by broad and overlapping spectral peaks produced by the overtones and combinations of infrared vibrational modes. Figure 71.5 shows typical NIR absorption spectra of fat, water, and starch. Exploitation of this spectral region for *in vivo*

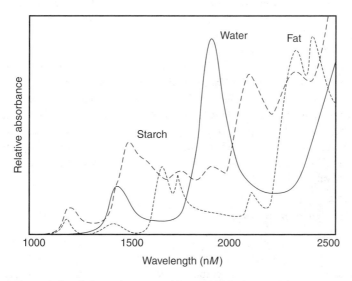

FIGURE 71.5 Typical near-infrared absorption spectra of several biologic materials.

analysis has been hindered by the same complexities of nonpulsatile tissue spectroscopy described above and is further confounded by the very broad and indistinct spectral features characteristic of the NIR. Despite these difficulties, NIR spectroscopy has garnered considerable attention, since it may enable the analysis of common analytes.

Karl Norris and coworkers pioneered the practical application of NIR spectroscopy, using it to evaluate water, fat, and sugar content of agricultural products (see Osborne et al. [1993] and Burns and Cuirczak [1992]). The further development of sophisticated **multivariate analysis** techniques, together with new scattering models (e.g., Kubelka–Munk theory) and high-performance instrumentation, further extended the application of NIR methods. Over the past decade, many research groups and companies have touted the use of NIR techniques for medical monitoring, such as for determining the relative fat, protein, and water content of tissue, and more recently for noninvasive glucose measurement. The body composition analyses are useful but crude and are mainly limited to applications in nutrition and sports medicine. Noninvasive glucose monitoring, however, is of considerable interest.

More than 2 million diabetics in the United States lance their fingers three to six times a day to obtain a drop of blood for chemical glucose determination. The ability of these individuals to control their glucose levels, and the quality of their life generally, would dramatically improve if a simple, noninvasive method for determining blood glucose levels could be developed. Among the noninvasive optical methods proposed for this purpose are optical rotation, NIR analysis, and Raman spectroscopy. The first two have received the most attention. Optical rotation methods aim to exploit the small optical rotation of polarized light by glucose. To measure physiologic glucose levels in a 1-cm thick sample to an accuracy of 25 mg/dL would require instrumentation that can reliably detect an optical rotation of at least 1 millidegree. Finding an appropriate *in vivo* optical path for such measurements has proved most difficult, with most approaches looking to use either the aqueous humor or the anterior chamber of the eye [Coté et al., 1992; Rabinovitch et al., 1982]. Although several groups have developed laboratory analyzers that can measure such a small effect, so far *in vivo* measurement has not been demonstrated, due both to unwanted scattering and optical activity of biomaterials in the optical path and to the inherent difficulty in developing a practical instrument with the required sensitivity.

NIR methods for noninvasive glucose determination are particularly attractive, although the task is formidable. Glucose has spectral characteristics near 1500 nm and in the 2000 to 2500 nm band where many other compounds also absorb, and the magnitude of the glucose absorbance in biologic samples is typically two orders of magnitude lower than those of water, fat, or protein. The normal detection limit for NIR spectroscopy is on the order of one part in 10^3, whereas a change of 25 mg/dL in glucose concentration corresponds to an absorbance change of 10^{-4} to 10^{-5}. In fact, the temperature dependence of the NIR absorption of water alone is at least an order of magnitude greater than the signal from glucose in solution. Indeed, some have suggested that the apparent glucose signature in complex NIR spectra may actually be the secondary effect of glucose on the water.

Sophisticated chemometric (particularly multivariate analysis) methods have been employed to try to extract the glucose signal out of the noise (for methods reviews see Martens and Næs [1989] and Haaland [1992]). Several groups have reported using multivariate techniques to quantitate glucose in whole blood samples, with encouraging results [Haaland et al., 1992]. And despite all theoretical disputations to the contrary, some groups claim the successful application of these multivariate analysis methods to noninvasive *in vivo* glucose determination in patients [Robinson et al., 1992]. Yet even with the many groups working in this area, much of the work remains unpublished, and few if any of the reports have been independently validated.

71.2.4 Time-Resolved Spectroscopy

The fundamental problem in making quantitative optical measurements through intact tissue is dealing with the complex scattering phenomena. This scattering makes it difficult to determine the effective pathlength for the light, and therefore attempts to use the Beer–Lambert law, or even to determine a consistent empirical calibration, continue to be thwarted. Application of new techniques in time-resolved spectroscopy may be able to tackle this problem. Thinking of light as a packet of photons, if a single packet from a light source is sent through tissue, then a distant receiver will detected a photon distribution over time — the photons least scattered arriving first and the photons most scattered arriving later. In principle, the first photons arriving at the detector passed directly through the tissue. For these first photons the distance between the emitter and the detector is fixed and known, and the Beer–Lambert law should apply, permitting determination of an *absolute* concentration for an absorbing component. The difficulty in this is, first, that the measurement time scale must be on the order of the photon transit time (subnanosec), and second, that the number of photons getting through without scattering will be extremely small, and therefore the detector must be exquisitely sensitive. Although these considerable technical problems have been overcome in the laboratory, their implementation in a practical instrument applied to a real subject remains to be demonstrated. This same approach is also being investigated for noninvasive optical imaging, since the unscattered photons should produce sharp images (see Chance et al. [1988], Chance [1991], and Yoo and Alfano [1989]).

71.3   Conclusions

The remarkable success of pulse oximetry has established noninvasive optical monitoring of vital physiologic functions as a modality of considerable value. Hardware and algorithm advances in pulse oximetry are beginning to broaden its use outside the traditional operating room and critical care areas. Other promising applications of noninvasive optical monitoring are emerging, such as for measuring deep tissue oxygen levels, determining cellular metabolic status, or for quantitative determination of other important physiologic parameters such as blood glucose. Although these latter applications are not yet practical, they may ultimately impact noninvasive clinical monitoring just as dramatically as pulse oximetry.

Defining Terms

Beer–Lambert law: Principle stating that the optical absorbance of a substance is proportional to both the concentration of the substance and the pathlength of the sample.

Cytochromes: Heme-containing proteins found in the membranes of mitochondria and required for oxidative phosphorylation, with characteristic optical absorbance spectra.

Dysfunctional hemoglobins: Those hemoglobin species that cannot reversibly bind oxygen (carboxyhemoglobin, methemoglobin, and sulfhemoglobin).

Functional saturation: The ratio of oxygenated hemoglobin to total nondysfunctional hemoglobins (oxyhemoglobin plus deoxyhemoglobin).

Hypoxia: Inadequate oxygen supply to tissues necessary to maintain metabolic activity.

Multivariate analysis: Empirical models developed to relate multiple spectral intensities from many calibration samples to known analyte concentrations, resulting in an optimal set of calibration parameters.

Oximetry: The determination of blood or tissue oxygen content, generally by optical means.

Pulse oximetry: The determination of functional oxygen saturation of pulsatile arterial blood by ratiometric measurement of tissue optical absorbance changes.

References

Burns, D.A. and Ciurczak, E.W. (Eds.). (1992). *Handbook of Near-Infrared Analysis.* New York, Marcel Dekker.

Chance, B. (1991). Optical method. *Annu. Rev. Biophys. Biophys. Chem.* 20: 1.

Chance, B., Leigh, J.S., Miyake, H. et al. (1988). Comparison of time-resolved and -unresolved measurements of deoxyhemoglobin in brain. *Proc. Natl Acad. Sci. USA* 85: 4971.

Coté G.L., Fox M.D., and Northrop, R.B. (1992). Noninvasive optical polarimetric glucose sensing using a true phase measurement technique. *IEEE Trans. Biomed. Eng.* 39: 752.

Haaland, D.M. (1992). Multivariate calibration methods applied to the quantitative analysis of infrared spectra. In P.C. Jurs (Ed.), *Computer-Enhanced Analytical Spectroscopy*, Vol. 3, pp. 1–30. New York, Plenum Press.

Haaland, D.M., Robinson, M.R., Koepp, G.W., et al. (1992). Reagentless near-infrared determination of glucose in whole blood using multivariate calibration. *Appl. Spectros.* 46: 1575.

Jöbsis, F.F. (1977). Noninvasive, infrared monitoring of cerebral and myocardial oxygen sufficiency and circulatory parameters. *Science* 198: 1264.

Jöbsis, F.F., Keizer, L.H., LaManna, J.C. et al. (1977). Reflectance spectrophotometry of cytochrome *aa*$_3$ *in vivo. J. Appl. Physiol.* 43: 858.

Kelleher, J.F. (1989). Pulse oximetry. *J. Clin. Monit.* 5: 37.

Martens, H. and Næs, T. (1989). *Multivariate Calibration.* New York, John Wiley & Sons.

Osborne, B.G., Fearn, T., and Hindle, P.H. (1993). *Practical NIR Spectroscopy with Applications in Food and Beverage Analysis.* Essex, England, Longman Scientific & Technical.

Payne, J.P. and Severinghaus, J.W. (Eds.). (1986). *Pulse Oximetry.* New York, Springer-Verlag.

Rabinovitch, B., March, W.F., and Adams, R.L. (1982). Noninvasive glucose monitoring of the aqueous humor of the eye: Part I. Measurement of very small optical rotations. *Diabetes Care* 5: 254.

Robinson, M.R., Eaton, R.P., Haaland, D.M. et al. (1992). Noninvasive glucose monitoring in diabetic patients: A preliminary evaluation. *Clin. Chem.* 38: 1618.

Severinghaus, J.W. and Astrup, P.B. (1986). History of blood gas analysis. VI. Oximetry. *J. Clin. Monit.* 2: 135.

Severinghaus, J.W. and Honda, Y. (1987a). History of blood gas analysis. VII. Pulse oximetry. *J. Clin. Monit.* 3: 135.

Severinghaus, J.W. and Honda, Y. (1987b). Pulse oximetry. *Int. Anesthesiol. Clin.* 25: 205.

Severinghaus, J.W. and Kelleher, J.F. (1992). Recent developments in pulse oximetry. *Anesthesiology* 76: 1018.

Tremper, K.K. and Barker, S.J. (1989). Pulse oximetry. *Anesthesiology* 70: 98.

Wukitsch, M.W., Petterson, M.T., Tobler, D.R. et al. (1988). Pulse oximetry: Analysis of theory, technology, and practice. *J. Clin. Monit.* 4: 290.

Yoo, K.M. and Alfano, R.R. (1989). Photon localization in a disordered multilayered system. *Phys. Rev. B* 39: 5806.

Further Information

Two collections of papers on pulse oximetry include a book edited by J.P. Payne and J.W. Severinghaus, *Pulse Oximetry* (New York, Springer-Verlag, 1986), and a journal collection — *International Anesthesiology Clinics* (25, 1987). For technical reviews of pulse oximetry, see J.A. Pologe's, 1987 "Pulse Oximetry" (*Int. Anesthesiol. Clin.* 25: 137), Kevin K. Tremper and Steven J. Barker's, 1989 "Pulse Oximetry" (*Anesthesiology* 70: 98), and Michael W. Wukitsch, Michael T. Patterson, David R. Tobler, and coworkers' 1988 "Pulse Oximetry: Analysis of Theory, Technology, and Practice" (*J. Clin. Monit.* 4: 290).

For a review of practical and clinical applications of pulse oximetry, see the excellent review by Joseph K. Kelleher (1989) and John Severinghaus and Joseph F. Kelleher (1992). John Severinghaus and Yoshiyuki Honda have written several excellent histories of pulse oximetry (1987a, 1987b).

For an overview of applied near-infrared spectroscopy, see Donald A. Burns and Emil W. Ciurczak (1992) and B.G. Osborne, T. Fearn, and P.H. Hindle (1993). For a good overview of multivariate methods, see Harald Martens and Tormod Næs (1989).

72

Medical Instruments and Devices Used in the Home

72.1 Scope of the Market for Home Medical Devices....... **72**-1
72.2 Unique Challenges to the Design and Implementation of High-Tech Homecare Devices **72**-3
The Device Must Provide a Positive Clinical Outcome • The Device Must Be Safe to Use • The Device Must Be Designed So That It *Will* Be Used
72.3 Infant Monitor Example **72**-6
72.4 Conclusions **72**-8
Defining Terms **72**-9
References **72**-9

Bruce R. Bowman
Edward Schuck
EdenTec Corporation

72.1 Scope of the Market for Home Medical Devices

The market for medical devices used in the home and alternative sites has increased dramatically in the last 10 years and has reached an overall estimated size of more than $1.6 billion [FIND/SVP, 1992]. In the past, hospitals have been thought of as the only places to treat sick patients. But with the major emphasis on reducing healthcare costs, increasing numbers of sicker patients move from hospitals to their homes. Treating sicker patients outside the hospital places additional challenges on medical device design and patient use. Equipment designed for hospital use can usually rely on trained clinical personnel to support the devices. Outside the hospital, the patient and/or family members must be able to use the equipment, requiring these devices to have a different set of design and safety features. This chapter will identify some of the major segments using medical devices in the home and discuss important design considerations associated with home use.

Table 72.1 outlines market segments where devices and products are used to treat patients outside the hospital [FIND/SVP, 1992]. The durable medical equipment market is the most established market providing aids for patients to improve access and mobility. These devices are usually not life supporting or sustaining, but in many cases they can make the difference in allowing a patient to be able to function outside a hospital or nursing or skilled facility. Other market segments listed employ generally more sophisticated solutions to clinical problems. These will be discussed by category of use.

The incontinence and ostomy area of products is one of the largest market segments and is growing in direct relationship to our aging society. Whereas sanitary pads and colostomy bags are not very "high-tech," well-designed aids can have a tremendous impact on the comfort and independence of these patients. Other solutions to incontinence are technically more sophisticated, such as use of electric stimulation of the **sphincter** muscles through an implanted device or a miniature stimulator inserted as an anal or vaginal plug to maintain continence [Wall et al., 1993].

Many forms of equipment are included in the Respiratory segment. These devices include those that maintain life support as well as those that monitor patients' respiratory function. These patients, with proper medical support, can function outside the hospital at a significant reduction in cost and increased patient comfort [Pierson, 1994]. One area of this segment, infant apnea monitors, provides parents or caregivers the cardio/respiratory status of an at-risk infant so that intervention (**CPR**, etc.) can be initiated if the baby has a life-threatening event. The infant monitor shown in Figure 72.1 is an example of a patient monitor designed for home use and will be discussed in more detail later in this chapter. Pulse oximetry

TABLE 72.1   Major Market Segments Outside Hospitals

Market segment	Estimated equipment size 1991	Device examples
Durable medical equipment	$373 M*	Specialty beds, wheelchairs, toilet aids, ambulatory aids
Incontinence and **ostomy** products	$600 M*	Sanitary pads, electrical stimulators, **colostomy** bags
Respiratory equipment	$180 M*	Oxygen therapy, portable ventilators, nasal CPAP, monitors, **apnea** monitors
Drug infusion, drug measurement	$300 M	Infusion pumps, access ports, patient-controlled analgesia (PCA), glucose measurement, implantable pumps
Pain control and functional stimulation	$140 M	**Transcutaneous electrical nerve stimulation (TENS), functional electrical nerve stimulation (FES)**

Source: FIND/SVP (1992). The Market for Home Care Products, a Market Intelligence Report. New York.

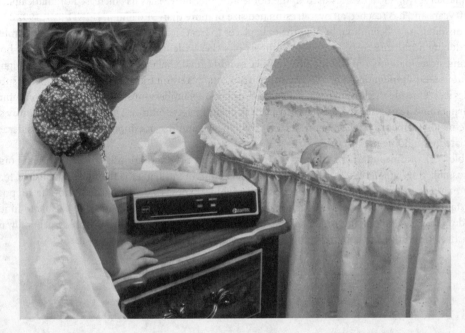

FIGURE 72.1   Infant apnea monitor used in a typical home setting. (Photo courtesy of EdenTec Corporation.)

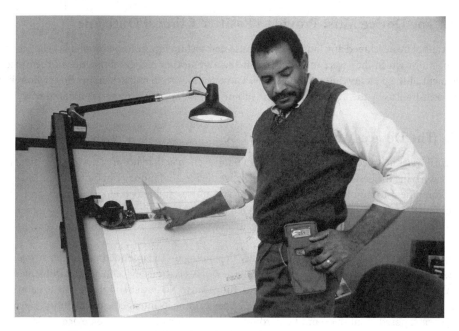

FIGURE 72.2   Portable drug pump used throughout the day. (Photo courtesy of Pharmacia Deltec Inc.)

monitors are also going home with patients. They are used to measure noninvasively the oxygen level of patients receiving supplemental oxygen or ventilator-dependent patients to determine if they are being properly ventilated.

Portable infusion pumps are an integral part of providing antibiotics, pain management, **chemotherapy**, and **parenteral** and **enteral nutrition**. The pump shown in Figure 72.2 is an example of technology that allows the patient to move about freely while receiving sometimes lengthy drug therapy. Implantable drug pumps are also available for special long-term therapy needs.

Pain control using electric stimulation in place of drug therapy continues to be an increasing market. The delivery of small electric impulses to block pain is continuing to gain medical acceptance for treatment outside the hospital setting. A different form of electric stimulation called functional electric stimulation (FES) applies short pulses of electric current to the nerves that control weak or paralyzed muscles. This topic is covered as a separate chapter in this book.

Growth of the homecare business has created problems in overall healthcare costs since a corresponding decrease in hospital utilization has not yet occurred. In the future, however, increased homecare will necessarily result in reassessment and downsizing in the corresponding hospital segment. There will be clear areas of growth and areas of consolidation in the new era of healthcare reform. It would appear, however, that homecare has a bright future of continued growth.

72.2   Unique Challenges to the Design and Implementation of High-Tech Homecare Devices

What are some of the unique requirements of devices that could allow more sophisticated equipment to go home with ordinary people of varied educational levels without compromising their care? Even though each type of clinical problem has different requirements for the equipment that must go home with the patient, certain common qualities must be inherent in most devices used in the home. Three areas to consider when equipment is used outside of the hospital are that the device (1) must provide a positive clinical outcome, (2) must be safe and easy to use, and (3) must be user-friendly enough so that it will be used.

72.2.1 The Device Must Provide a Positive Clinical Outcome

Devices cannot be developed any longer just because new technology becomes available. They must solve the problem for which they were intended and make a significant clinical difference in the outcome or management of the patient while saving money. These realities are being driven by those who reimburse for devices, as well as by the FDA as part of the submission for approval to market a new device.

72.2.2 The Device Must Be Safe to Use

Homecare devices may need to be even *more* reliable and even *safer* than hospital devices. We often think of hospitals as having the best quality and most expensive devices that money can buy. In addition to having the best equipment to monitor patients, hospitals have nurses and aids that keep an eye on patients so that equipment problems may be quickly discovered by the staff. A failure in the home may go unnoticed until it is too late. Thus systems for home use really need extra reliability with automatic backup systems and early warning signals.

Safety issues can take on a different significance depending on the intended use of the device. Certain safety issues are important regardless of whether the device is a critical device such as an implanted **cardiac pacemaker** or a noncritical device such as a bed-wetting alarm. No device should be able to cause harm to the patient regardless of how well or poorly it may be performing its intended clinical duties. Devices must be safe when exposed to all the typical environmental conditions to which the device could be exposed while being operated by the entire range of possible users of varied education and while exposed to siblings and other untrained friends or relatives. For instance, a bed-wetting alarm should not cause skin burns under the sensor if a glass of water spills on the control box. This type of safety issue must be addressed even when it significantly affects the final cost to the consumer.

Other safety issues are not obviously differentiated as to being actual safety issues or simply nuisances or inconveniences to the user. It is very important for the designer to properly define these issues; although some safety features can be included with little or no extra cost, other safety features may be very costly to implement. It may be a nuisance for the patient using a TENS pain control stimulator to have the device inadvertently turned off when its on/off switch is bumped while watching TV. In this case, the patient only experiences a momentary cessation of pain control until the unit is turned back on. But it could mean injuries or death to the same patient driving an automobile who becomes startled when his TENS unit inadvertently turns on and he causes an accident.

Reliability issues can also be mere inconveniences or major safety issues. Medical devices should be free of design and materials defects so that they can perform their intended functions reliably. Once again, reliability does not necessarily need to be expensive and often can be obtained with good design. Critical devices, that is, devices that could cause death or serious injury if they stopped operating properly, may need to have redundant systems for backup, which likely will increase cost.

72.2.3 The Device Must Be Designed So That It *Will* Be Used

A great deal of money is being spent in healthcare on devices for patients that end up not being used. There are numerous reasons for this happening including that the wrong device was prescribed for the patient's problem in the first place; the device works, but it has too many false alarms; the device often fails to operate properly; it is cumbersome to use or difficult to operate or too uncomfortable to wear.

72.2.3.1 Ease of Use

User-friendliness is one of the most important features in encouraging a device to be used. Technological sophistication may be just as necessary in areas that allow ease of use as in attaining accuracy and reliability in the device. The key is that the technologic sophistication be transparent to the user so that the device does not intimidate the user. Transparent features such as automatic calibration or automatic sensitivity adjustment may help allow successful use of a device that would otherwise be too complicated.

Notions of what makes a device easy to use, however, need to be thoroughly tested with the patient population intended for the device. Caution needs to be taken in defining what "simple" means to different people. A VCR may be simple to the designer because all features can be programmed with one button, but it may not be simple to users if they have to remember that it takes two long pushes and one short to get into the clock-setting program.

Convenience for the user is also extremely important in encouraging use of a device. Applications that require devices to be portable must certainly be light enough to be carried. Size is almost always important for anything that must fit within the average household. Either a device must be able to be left in place in the home or it must be easy to set up, clean, and put away. Equipment design can make the difference between the patient appropriately using the equipment or deciding that it is just too much hassle to bother.

72.2.3.2 Reliability

Users must also have confidence in the reliability of the device being used and must have confidence that if it is not working properly, the device will tell them that something is wrong. Frequent breakdowns or false alarms will result in frustration and ultimately in reduced compliance. Eventually patients will stop using the device altogether. Most often, reliability can be designed into a product with little or no extra cost in manufacturing, and everything that can be done at no cost to enhance reliability should be done. It is very important, however, to understand what level of additional reliability involving extra cost is necessary for product acceptance. Reliability can always be added by duplicated backup systems, but the market or application may not warrant such an approach. Critical devices which are implanted, such as cardiac pacemakers, have much greater reliability requirements, since they involve not only patient frustration but also safety.

72.2.3.3 Cost Reimbursement

Devices must be paid for before the patient can realize the opportunity to use new, effective equipment. Devices are usually paid for by one of two means. First, they are covered on an American Medical Association Current Procedural Terminology Code (**CPT-code**) which covers the medical, surgical, and diagnostic services provided by physicians. The CPT-codes are usually priced out by Medicare to establish a baseline reimbursement level. Private carriers usually establish a similar or different level of reimbursement based on regional or other considerations. Gaining new CPT-codes for new devices can take a great deal of time and effort. The second method is to cover the procedure and device under a **capitated fee** where the hospital is reimbursed a lump sum for a procedure including the device, hospital, homecare, and physician fees.

Every effort should be made to design devices to be low cost. Device cost is being scrutinized more and more by those who reimburse. It is easy to state, however, that a device needs to be inexpensive. Unfortunately the reality is that healthcare reforms and new regulations by the FDA are making medical devices more costly to develop, to obtain regulatory approvals for [FDA, 1993], and to manufacture.

72.2.3.4 Professional Medical Service Support

The more technically sophisticated a device is, the more crucial that homecare support and education be a part of a program. In fact, in many cases, such support and education are as important as the device itself.

Medical service can be offered by numerous homecare service companies. Typically these companies purchase the equipment instead of the patient, and a monthly fee is charged for use of the equipment along with all the necessary service. The homecare company then must obtain reimbursement from third-party payers. Some of the services offered by the homecare company include training on how to use the equipment, CPR training, transporting the equipment to the home, servicing/repairing equipment, monthly visits, and providing on-call service 24 h a day. The homecare provider must also be able to provide feedback to the treating physician on progress of the treatment. This feedback may include how well the equipment is working, the patient's medical status, and compliance of the patient.

72.3   Infant Monitor Example

Many infants are being monitored in the home using apnea monitors because they have been identified with breathing problems [Kelly, 1992]. These include newborn premature babies who have **apnea of prematurity** [Henderson-Smart, 1992; NIH, 1987], siblings of babies who have died of **sudden infant death syndrome (SIDS)** [Hunt, 1992; NIH, 1987], or infants who have had an **apparent life-threatening episode (ALTE)** related to lack of adequate respiration [Kahn et al., 1992; NIH, 1987]. Rather than keeping infants in the hospital for a problem that they may soon outgrow (1–6 months), doctors often discharge them from the hospital with an infant apnea monitor that measures the duration of breathing pauses and heart rate and sounds an alarm if either parameter crosses limits prescribed by the doctor.

Infant apnea monitors are among the most sophisticated devices used routinely in the home. These devices utilize microprocessor control, sophisticated breath-direction and artifact rejection firmware algorithms, and internal memory that keeps track of use of the device as well as recording occurrence of events and the physiologic waveforms associated with the events. The memory contents can be downloaded directly to computer or sent via modem remotely where a complete 45-day report can be provided to the referring physician (see Figure 72.3).

Most apnea monitors measure breathing effort through impedance pneumography. A small (100–200 μA) high-frequency (25–100 kHz) constant-current train of pulses is applied across the chest between a pair of electrodes. The voltage needed to drive the current is measured, and thereby the effective impedance between the electrodes can be calculated. Impedance across the chest increases as the chest expands and decreases as the chest contracts with each breath. The impedance change with each breath can be as low as 0.2 Ω on top of an electrode base impedance of 2000 Ω, creating some interesting signal-to-noise challenges. Furthermore, motion artifact and blood volume changes in the heart and chest can cause impedance changes of 0.6 Ω or more that can look just like breathing. Through the same pair of electrodes, heart rate is monitored by picking up the **electrocardiogram (ECG)** [AAMI, 1988].

Because the impedance technique basically measures the motion of the chest, this technique can only be used to monitor **central apnea** or lack of breathing effort. Another less common apnea in infants called **obstructive apnea** results when an obstruction of the airway blocks air from flowing in spite of breathing effort. Obstructive apnea cannot be monitored using impedance pneumography [Kelly, 1992].

There is a very broad socioeconomic and educational spectrum of parents or caregivers who may be monitoring their infants with an apnea monitor. This creates an incredible challenge for the design of the device so that it is easy enough to be used by a variety of caregivers. It also puts special requirements on the homecare service company that must be able to respond to these patients within a matter of minutes, 24 h a day.

The user-friendly monitor shown in Figure 72.1 uses a two-button operation, the on/off switch, and a reset switch. The visual alarm indicators are invisible behind a back-lit panel except when an actual alarm occurs. A word describing the alarm then appears. By not showing all nine possible alarm conditions unless an alarm occurs, parent confusion and anxiety is minimized. Numerous safety features are built into the unit, some of which are noticeable but many of which are internal to the operation of the monitor. One useful safety feature is the self-check. When the device is turned on, each alarm LED lights in sequence, and the unit beeps once indicating that the self-check was completed successfully. This gives users the opportunity to confirm that all the alarm visual indicators and the audible indicator are working and provides added confidence for users leaving their baby on the monitor. A dual-level battery alarm gives an early warning that the battery will soon need charging. The weak battery alarm allows users to reset the monitor and continue monitoring their babies for several more hours before depleting the battery to the charge battery level where the monitor must be attached to the ac battery charger/adapter. This allows parents the freedom to leave their homes for a few hours knowing that their child can continue to be monitored.

A multistage alarm reduces the risk of parents sleeping through an alarm. Most parents are sleep-deprived with a new baby. Consequently, it can be easy for parents in a nearby room to sleep through a monitor alarm even when the monitor sounds at 85 dB. A three-stage alarm helps to reduce this risk. After

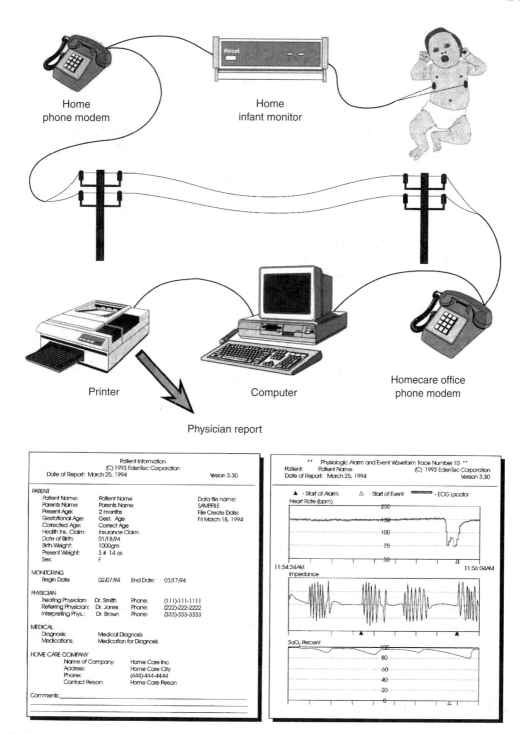

FIGURE 72.3 Infant apnea monitor with memory allows data to be sent by modem to generate physician report. (Drawing courtesy of EdenTec Corporation.)

10 sec of sounding at 1 beep/sec, the alarm switches to 3 beeps/sec for the next 10 sec. Finally, if an alarm has not resolved itself after 20 sec, the alarm switches to 6 beeps/sec. Each stage of alarm sounds more intense than the previous one and offers the chance of jolting parents out of even the deepest sleep.

The physician always prescribes what alarm settings should be used by the homecare service company when setting up the monitor. As a newborn matures, these settings may need to be adjusted. Sometimes the parents can be relied upon for making these setting changes. To allow both accessibility to these switches as well as to keep them safe from unauthorized tampering from a helping brother or sister, a special tamper-resistant-adjustment procedure is utilized. Two simultaneous actions are required in order to adjust the alarm limit settings. The reset button must be continually pressed on the front of the unit while changing settings on the back of the unit. Heart rate levels are set in beats per minute, and apnea duration is set in single-second increments. Rather than using easy-to-set push-button switches, "pen-set" switches are used which require a pen or other sharp implement to make the change. If the proper switch adjustment procedure is not followed, the monitor alarms continuously and displays a switch alarm until the settings are returned to their original settings. A similar technique is used for turning the monitor off. The reset button must first be pressed and then the on/off switch turned to the off position. Violation of this procedure will result in a switch alarm.

Other safety features are internal to the monitor and are transparent to the user. The monitor's alarm is designed to be normally on from the moment the device is turned on. Active circuitry controlled by the microprocessor turns the alarm off when there are no active alarm conditions. If anything hangs up the processor or if any of a number of components fail, the alarm will not turn off and will remain on in a fail-safe mode. This "alarm on unless turned off" technique is also used in a remote alarm unit for parents with their baby in a distant room. If a wire breakage occurs between the monitor and the remote alarm unit, or a connector pulls loose, or a component fails, the remote alarm no longer is turned off by the monitor and it alarms in a fail-safe condition.

Switches, connectors, and wires are prone to fail. One way to circumvent this potential safety issue is use of switches with a separate line for each possible setting. The monitor continuously polls every switch line of each switch element to check that "exactly" one switch position is making contact. This guards against misreading bad switch elements, a switch inadvertently being set between two positions, or a bad connector or cable. Violation of the "exactly one contact condition" results in a switch alarm.

It is difficult to manage an apnea monitoring program in rural areas where the monitoring family may be a hundred miles or more away from the homecare service company. There are numerous ways to become frustrated with the equipment and stop using the monitor. Therefore, simplicity of use and reliability are important. Storing occurrence of alarms and documenting compliance in internal memory in the monitor help the homecare service company and the remote family cope with the situation. The monitor shown in Figure 72.1 stores in digital memory the time, date, and duration of (1) each use of the monitor; (2) occurrence of all equipment alarms; and (3) all physiologic alarms including respiratory waveforms, heart rate, and ECG for up to a 45-day period. These data in the form of a report (see Figure 72.3) can be downloaded to a laptop PC or sent via modem to the homecare service company or directly to the physician.

72.4 Conclusions

Devices that can provide positive patient outcomes with reduced overall cost to the healthcare system while being safe, reliable, and user-friendly will succeed based on pending healthcare changes. Future technology in the areas of sensors, communications, and memory capabilities should continue to increase the potential effectiveness of homecare management programs by using increasingly sophisticated devices. The challenge for the medical device designer is to provide cost-effective, reliable, and easy-to-use solutions that can be readily adopted by the multidisciplinary aspects of homecare medicine while meeting FDA requirements.

Defining Terms

Apnea: Cessation of breathing. Apnea can be classified as **central, obstructive,** or mixed, which is a combination.

Apnea of prematurity: Apnea in which the incidence and severity increases with decreasing gestational age attributable to immaturity of the respiratory control system. The incidence has increased due to improved survival rates for very-low-birth-weight premature infants.

Apparent life-threatening episode (ALTE): An episode characterized by a combination of apnea, color change, muscle tone change, choking, or gagging. To the observer it may appear the infant has died.

Capitated fee: A fixed payment for *total* program services versus the more traditional fee for service in which each individual service is charged.

Cardiac pacemaker: A device that electrically stimulates the heart at a certain rate used in absence of normal function of the heart's sino-atrial node.

Central apnea: Apnea secondary to lack of respiratory or diaphragmatic effort.

Chemotherapy: Treatment of disease by chemical agents. Term popularly used when fighting cancer chemically.

Colostomy: The creation of a surgical hole as an alternative opening of the colon.

CPR (cardiopulmonary resuscitation): Artificially replacing heart and respiration function through rhythmic pressure on the chest.

CPT-code (current procedural terminology code): A code used to describe specific procedures/tests developed by the AMA.

Electrocardiogram (ECG): The electric potential recorded across the chest due to depolarization of the heart muscle with each heartbeat.

Enteral nutrition: Chemical nutrition injected intestinally.

Food and Drug Administration (FDA): Federal agency that oversees and regulates foods, drugs, and medical devices.

Functional electrical stimulation (FES): Electric stimulation of peripheral nerves or muscles to gain functional, purposeful control over partially or fully paralyzed muscles.

Incontinence: Loss of voluntary control of the bowel or bladder.

Obstructive apnea: Apnea in which the effort to breath continues but airflow ceases due to obstruction or collapse of the airway.

Ostomy: Surgical procedure that alters the bladder or bowel to eliminate through an artificial passage.

Parenteral nutrition: Chemical nutrition injected subcutaneously, intramuscular, intrasternally, or intravenously.

Sphincter: A band of muscle fibers that constricts or closes an orifice.

Sudden infant death syndrome (SIDS): The sudden death of an infant which is unexplained by history or postmortem exam.

Transcutaneous electrical nerve stimulation (TENS): Electrical stimulation of sensory nerve fibers resulting in control of pain.

References

AAMI (1988). Association for the Advancement of Medical Instrumentation Technical Information Report. Apnea Monitoring by Means of Thoracic Impedance Pneumography, Arlington, Virg.

FDA (November 1993). Reviewers Guidance for Premarket Notification Submissions (Draft), Anesthesiology and Respiratory Device Branch, Division of Cardiovascular, Respiratory, and Neurological Devices. Food and Drug Administration. Washington, DC.

FIND/SVP (1992). The Market for Home Care Products, a Market Intelligence Report. New York.

Henderson-Smart D.J. 1992. Apnea of prematurity. In R. Beckerman, R. Brouillette, and C. Hunt (Eds.), *Respiratory Control Disorders in Infants and Children*, pp. 161–177, Baltimore, Williams and Wilkins.

Hunt C.E. (1992). Sudden infant death syndrome. In R. Beckerman, R. Brouillette, and C. Hunt (Eds.), *Respiratory Control Disorders in Infants and Children*, pp. 190–211, Baltimore, Williams and Wilkins.

Kahn A., Rebuffat E., Franco P., et al. (1992). Apparent life-threatening events and apnea of infancy. In R. Beckerman, R. Brouillette, and C. Hunt (Eds.), *Respiratory Control Disorders in Infants and Children*, pp 178–189, Baltimore, Williams and Wilkins.

Kelly D.H. (1992). Home monitoring. In R. Beckerman, R. Brouillette, and C. Hunt (Eds.), *Respiratory Control Disorders in Infants and Children*, pp. 400–412, Baltimore, Williams and Wilkins.

NIH (1987). Infantile Apnea and Home Monitoring Report of NIH Consensus Development Conference, US Department of Health and Human Services, NIH publication 87-2905.

Pierson D.J. (1994). Controversies in home respiratory care: Conference summary. *Respir. Care* 39: 294.

Wall L.L., Norton P.A., and Dehancey J.O.L. 1993. *Practical Urology*, Baltimore, Williams and Wilkins.

73

Virtual Instrumentation: Applications in Biomedical Engineering

73.1 Overview **73**-1
   A Revolution — Graphical Programming and Virtual Instrumentation
73.2 Virtual Instrumentation and Biomedical Engineering **73**-2
   Example 1: BioBench™ — A Virtual Instrument Application for Data Acquisition and Analysis of Physiological Signals • Example 2: A Cardiovascular Pressure-Dimension Analysis System
73.3 Summary **73**-7
References **73**-8

Eric Rosow
Hartford Hospital
Premise Development Corporation

Joseph Adam
Premise Development Corporation

73.1 Overview

73.1.1 A Revolution — Graphical Programming and Virtual Instrumentation

Over the last decade, the graphical programming revolution has empowered engineers to develop customized systems, the same way the spreadsheet has empowered business managers to analyze financial data. This software technology has resulted in another type of revolution — the virtual instrumentation revolution, which is rapidly changing the instrumentation industry by driving down costs without sacrificing quality.

Virtual Instrumentation can be defined as:

A layer of software and/or hardware added to a general-purpose computer in such a fashion that users can interact with the computer as though it were their own custom-designed traditional electronic instrument.

Today, computers can serve as the engine for instrumentation. Virtual instruments utilize the open architecture of industry-standard computers to provide the processing, memory, and display capabilities; while the off-the-shelf, inexpensive interface boards plugged into an open bus, standardized communications bus provides the vehicle for the instrument's capabilities. As a result, the open architecture of PCs and workstations allow the functionality of virtual instruments to be user defined. In addition, the processing power of virtual instruments is much greater than stand-alone instruments. This advantage will continue to accelerate due to the rapid technology evolution of PCs and workstations that results from the huge investments made in this industry.

The major benefits of virtual instrumentation include increased performance and reduced costs. In addition, because the user controls the technology through software, the flexibility of virtual instrumentation is unmatched by traditional instrumentation. The modular, hierarchical programming environment of virtual instrumentation is inherently reusable and reconfigurable.

73.2   Virtual Instrumentation and Biomedical Engineering

Virtual Instrumentation applications have encompassed nearly every industry including the telecommunications, automotive, semiconductor, and biomedical industries. In the fields of health care and biomedical engineering, virtual instrumentation has empowered developers and end-users to conceive of, develop, and implement a wide variety of research-based biomedical applications and executive information tools. These applications fall into several categories including: clinical research, equipment testing and quality assurance, data management, and performance improvement.

In a collaborative approach, physicians, researchers, and biomedical and software engineers at Hartford Hospital (Hartford, CT) and Premise Development Corporation (Avon, CT) have developed various data acquisition and analysis systems that successfully integrate virtual instrumentation principles in a wide variety of environments. These include:

- "The EndoTester™," a patented quality assurance system for fiberoptic endoscopes
- A Non-Invasive Pulmonary Diffusion and Cardiac Output Measurement System
- A Cardiovascular Pressure-Dimension Analysis System
- "BioBench™," a powerful turnkey application for physiological data acquisition and analysis
- "PIVIT™," a Performance Indicator Virtual Instrument Toolkit to manage and forecast financial data
- A "Virtual Intelligence Program" to manage the discrete components within the continuum of care "BabySave™," an analysis and feedback system for apnea interruption via vibratory stimulation

This chapter will describe several of these applications and describe how they have allowed clinicians and researchers to gain new insights, discover relationships that may not have been obvious, and test and model hypotheses based on acquired data sets. In some cases, these applications have been developed into commercial products to address test and measurement needs at other healthcare facilities throughout the world.

73.2.1   Example 1: BioBench™ — A Virtual Instrument Application for Data Acquisition and Analysis of Physiological Signals

The biomedical industry is an industry that relies heavily on the ability to acquire, analyze, and display large quantities of data. Whether researching disease mechanisms and treatments by monitoring and storing physiological signals, researching the effects of various drugs interactions, or teaching students in labs where students study physiological signs and symptoms, it was clear that there existed a strong demand for a flexible, easy-to-use, and cost-effective tool. In a collaborative approach, biomedical engineers, software engineers and clinicians, and researchers created a suite of virtual instruments called BioBench™.

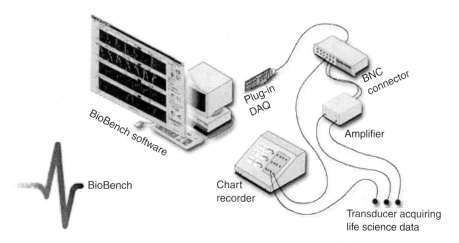

FIGURE 73.1 A typical biomedical application using BioBench. (Courtesy of National Instruments.)

BioBench™ (National Instruments, Austin, TX) is a new software application designed for physiological data acquisition and analysis. It was built with LabVIEW™, the world's leading software development environment for data acquisition, analysis, and presentation.[1] Coupled with National Instruments data acquisition (DAQ) boards, BioBench integrates the PC with data acquisition for the life sciences market.

Many biologists and physiologists have made major investments over time in data acquisition hardware built before the advent of modern PCs. While these scientists cannot afford to throw out their investment in this equipment, they recognize that computers and the concept of virtual instrumentation yield tremendous benefits in terms of data analysis, storage, and presentation. In many cases, traditional medical instrumentation may be too expensive to acquire and maintain. As a result, researchers and scientists are opting to create their own PC-based data monitoring systems in the form of virtual instruments.

Other life scientists, who are just beginning to assemble laboratory equipment, face the daunting task of selecting hardware and software needed for their application. Many manufacturers for the life sciences field focus their efforts on the acquisition of raw signals and converting these signals into measurable linear voltages. They do not concentrate on digitizing signals or the analysis and display of data on the PC. BioBench™ is a low-cost turnkey package that requires no programming. BioBench is compatible with any isolation amplifier or monitoring instrument that provides an analog output signal. The user can acquire and analyze data immediately because BioBench automatically recognizes and controls the National Instruments DAQ hardware, minimizing configuration headaches.

Some of the advantages of PC-Based Data Monitoring include:

- Easy-to-use-software applications
- Large memory and the PCI bus
- Powerful processing capabilities
- Simplified customization and development
- More data storage and faster data transfer
- More efficient data analysis

Figure 73.1 illustrates a typical setup of a data acquisition experiment using BioBench. BioBench also features pull-down menus through which the user can configure devices. Therefore, those who have made large capital investments can easily migrate their existing equipment into the computer age. Integrating a combination of old and new physiological instruments from a variety of manufacturers is an important and straightforward procedure. In fact, within the clinical and research setting, it is a common requirement

---

[1]BioBench™ was developed for National Instruments (Austin, TX) by Premise Development Corporation (Avon, CT).

to be able to acquire multiple physiological signals from a variety of medical devices and instruments which do not necessarily communicate with each other. Often times, this situation is compounded by the fact that end-users would like to be able to view and analyze an entire waveform and not just an average value. In order to accomplish this, the end-user must acquire multiple channels of data at a relatively high sampling rate and have the ability to manage many large data files. BioBench can collect up to 16 channels simultaneously at a sampling rate of 1000 Hz per channel. Files are stored in an efficient binary format which significantly reduces the amount of hard disk and memory requirements of the PC. During data acquisition, a number of features are available to the end-user. These features include:

Data Logging: Logging can be enabled prior to or during an acquisition. The application will either prompt the user for a descriptive filename or it can be configured to automatically assign a filename for each acquisition. Turning the data logging option on and off creates a log data event record that can be inspected in any of the analysis views of BioBench.

Event Logging: The capacity to associate and recognize user commands associated with a data file may be of significant value. BioBench has been designed to provide this capability by automatically logging user-defined events, stimulus events, and file logging events. With user-defined events, the user can easily enter and associate date and time-stamped notes with user actions or specific subsets of data. Stimulus events are also data and time-stamped and provide the user information about whether a stimulus has been turned on or off. File logging events note when data has been logged to disk. All of these types of events are stored with the raw data when logging data to file and they can be searched for when analyzing data.

Alarming: To alert the user about specific data values and thresholds, BioBench incorporates user-defined alarms for each signal which is displayed. Alarms appear on the user interface during data acquisition and notify the user that an alarm condition has occurred.

Figure 73.2 is an example of the Data Acquisition mode of BioBench. Once data has been acquired, BioBench can employ a wide array of easy-to-use analysis features. The user has the choice of importing recently acquired data or opening a data file that had been previously acquired for comparison or teaching

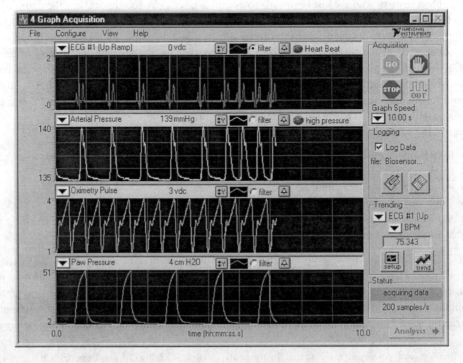

FIGURE 73.2 BioBench acquisition mode with alarms enabled.

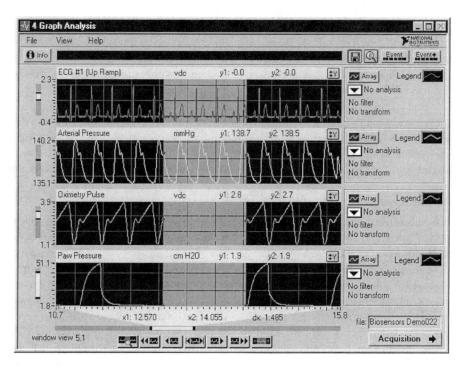

FIGURE 73.3 BioBench analysis mode.

purposes. Once a data set has been selected and opened, BioBench allows the user to simply select and highlight a region of interest and choose the analysis options to perform a specific routine.

BioBench implements a wide array of scalar and array analyses. For example, scalar analysis tools will determine the minimum, maximum, mean, integral, and slope of a selected data set, while the array analysis tools can employ Fast Fourier Transforms (FFTs), peak detection, histograms, and X vs. Y plots.

The ability to compare multiple data files is very important in analysis and BioBench allows the user to open an unlimited number of data files for simultaneous comparison and analysis. All data files can be scanned using BioBench's search tools in which the user can search for particular events that are associated with areas of interest. In addition, BioBench allows the user to employ filters and transformations to their data sets and all logged data can be easily exported to a spreadsheet or database for further analysis. Finally, any signal acquired with BioBench can be played back, thus taking lab experience into the classroom. Figure 73.3 illustrates the analysis features of BioBench.

73.2.2 Example 2: A Cardiovascular Pressure-Dimension Analysis System

73.2.2.1 Introduction

The intrinsic contractility of the heart muscle (myocardium) is the single most important determinant of prognosis in virtually all diseases affecting the heart (e.g., coronary artery disease, valvular heart disease, and cardiomyopathy). Furthermore, it is clinically important to be able to evaluate and track myocardial function in other situations, including chemotherapy (where cardiac dysfunction may be a side effect of treatment) and liver disease (where cardiac dysfunction may complicate the disease).

The most commonly used measure of cardiac performance is the ejection fraction. Although it does provide some measure of intrinsic myocardial performance, it is also heavily influenced by other factors such as heart rate and loading conditions (i.e., the amount of blood returning to the heart and the pressure against which the heart ejects blood).

Better indices of myocardial function based on the relationship between pressure and volume throughout the cardiac cycle (pressure–volume loops) exist. However, these methods have been limited because they require the ability to track ventricular volume continuously during rapidly changing loading conditions. While there are many techniques to measure volume under steady state situations, or at end-diastole and end-systole (the basis of ejection fraction determinations), few have the potential to record volume during changing loading conditions.

Echocardiography can provide online images of the heart with high temporal resolution (typically 30 frames/sec). Since echocardiography is radiation-free and has no identifiable toxicity, it is ideally suited to pressure–volume analyses. Until recently however, its use for this purpose has been limited by the need for manual tracing of the endocardial borders, an extremely tedious and time-consuming endeavor.

73.2.2.2 The System

Biomedical and software engineers at Premise Development Corporation (Avon, CT), in collaboration with physicians and researchers at Hartford Hospital, have developed a sophisticated research application called the "Cardiovascular Pressure-Dimension Analysis (CPDA) System." The CPDA system acquires echocardiographic volume and area information from the acoustic quantification (AQ) port, in conjunction with vetricular pressure(s) and ECG signals to rapidly perform pressure–volume and pressure–area analyses. This fully automated system allows cardiologists and researchers to perform online pressure–dimension and stroke work analyses during routine cardiac catheterizations and open-heart surgery. The system has been designed to work with standard computer hardware. Analog signals for ECG, pressure, and area/volume (AQ) are connected to a standard BNC terminal board. Automated calibration routines ensure that each signal is properly scaled and allows the user to immediately collect and analyze pressure–dimension relationships.

The CPDA can acquire up to 16 channels of data simultaneously. Typically, only three physiological parameters, ECG, pressure, and the AQ signals are collected using standard data acquisition hardware. In addition, the software is capable of running on multiple operating systems including Macintosh, Windows 95/98/NT, and Solaris. The CPDA also takes advantage of the latest hardware developments and form-factors and can be used with either a desktop or a laptop computer.

The development of an automated, online method of tracing endocardial borders (Hewlett–Packard's AQ Technology) (Hewlett–Packard Medical Products Group, Andover, MA) has provided a method for rapid online area and volume determinations. Figure 73.4 illustrates this AQ signal from a Hewlett–Packard

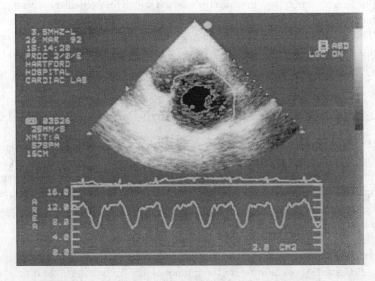

FIGURE 73.4 The Acoustic Quantification (AQ) signal. (Courtesy of Hewlett–Packard.)

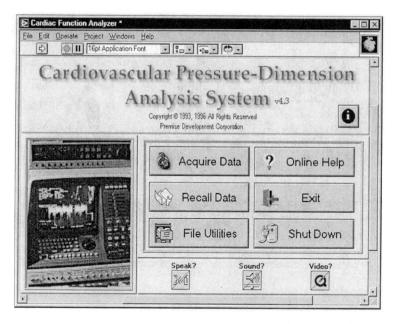

FIGURE 73.5 Cardiovascular pressure-dimension analysis main menu.

Sonos Ultrasound Machine. This signal is available as an analog voltage (-1 to $+1$ V) through the Sonos Dataport option (BNC connector).

73.2.2.3 Data Acquisition and Analysis

Upon launching this application, the user is presented with a dialog box that reviews the license agreement and limited warranty. Next, the Main Menu is displayed, allowing the user to select from one of six options as shown in Figure 73.5.

73.2.2.4 Clinical Significance

Several important relationships can be derived from this system. Specifically, a parameter called the *End-Systolic Pressure–Volume Relationship (ESPVR)* describes the line of best fit through the peak-ratio (maximum pressure with respect to minimum volume) coordinates from a series of pressure–volume loops generated under varying loading conditions. The slope of this line has been shown to be a sensitive index of myocardial contractility that is independent of loading conditions. In addition, several other analyses, including *time varying elastance* (E_{max}) and *stroke work*, are calculated. Time-varying elastance is measured by determining the maximum slope of a regression line through a series of isochronic pressure–volume coordinates. Stroke work is calculated by quantifying the area of each pressure–volume loop. Statistical parameters are also calculated and displayed for each set of data. Figure 73.7 illustrates the pressure–dimension loops and each of the calculated parameters along with the various analysis options. Finally, the user has the ability to export data sets into spreadsheet and database files and export graphs and indicators into third-party presentation software packages such as Microsoft PowerPoint®.

73.3 Summary

Virtual Instrumentation allows the development and implementation of innovative and cost-effective biomedical applications and information management solutions. As the healthcare industry continues to respond to the growing trends of managed care and capitation, it is imperative for clinically useful, cost-effective technologies to be developed and utilized. As application needs will surely continue to change,

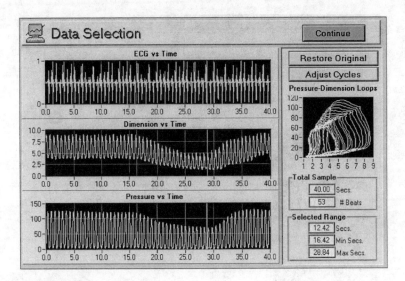

FIGURE 73.6   The data selection front panel.

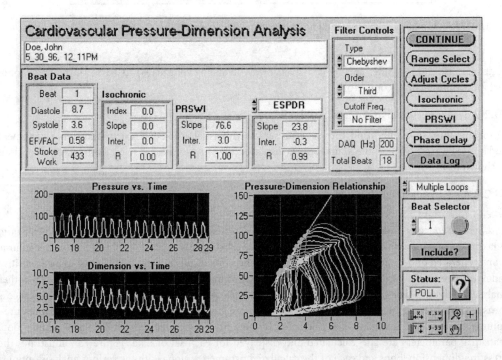

FIGURE 73.7   The cardiac cycle analysis front panel.

virtual instrumentation systems will continue to offer users flexible and powerful solutions without requiring new equipment or traditional instruments.

References

[1] 1. Fisher, J.P., Mikan, J.S., Rosow, E., Nagle, J., Fram, D.B., Maffucci, L.M., McKay, R.G., and Gillam, L.D., "Pressure-Dimension Analysis of Regional Left Ventricular Performance Using

Echocardiographic Automatic Boundary Detection: Validation in an Animal Model of Inotropic Modulation," *J. Am. Coll. Cardiol.* 19, 262A, 1992.

[2] Fisher, J.P., McKay, R.G., Mikan, J.S., Rosow, E., Nagle, J., Mitchel, J.F., Kiernan, F.J., Hirst, J.A., Primiano, C.A., Fram, D.B., and Gillam, L.D., Hartford Hospital and University of Connecticut, Hartford, CT, *"Human Left Ventricular Pressure–Area and Pressure–Volume Analysis Using Echocardiographic Automatic Boundary Detection." 65th Scientific Session of the American Heart Association* (11/92).

[3] Fisher, J.P., Mitchel, J.F., Rosow, E., Mikan, J.S., Nagle, J., Kiernan, F.J., Hirst, J.A., Primiano, and Gillam, L.D., Hartford Hospital and University of Connecticut, Hartford, CT, *"Evaluation of Left Ventricular Diastolic Pressure–Area Relations with Echocardiographic Automatic Boundary Detection," 65th Scientific Session of the American Heart Association* (11/92).

[4] Fisher, J.P., McKay, R.G., Mikan, J.S., Rosow, E., Nagle, J., Mitchel, J.F., Fram, D.B., and Gillam, L.D., Hartford Hospital, *"A Comparison of Echocardiographic Methods of Evaluating Regional LV Systolic Function: Fractional Area Change vs. the End-Systolic Pressure–Area Relation." 65th Scientific Session of the American Heart Association* (11/92).

[5] Fisher, J.P., McKay, R.G., Rosow, E. Mikan, J. Nagle, J. Hirst, J.A., Fram, D.B., and Gillam, L.D., *"On-Line Derivation of Human Left Ventricular Pressure–Volume Loops and Load Independent Indices of Contractility Using Echocardiography with Automatic Boundary Detection-A Clinical Reality." Circulation* 88, I–304, 1993.

[6] Fisher, J.P., Chen, C., Krupowies, N., Li Li, Kiernan, F.J., Fram, D.B., Rosow, E., Adam, J., and Gillam, L.D., *"Comparison of Mechanical and Pharmacologic Methods of Altering Loading Conditions to Determine End-Systolic Indices of Left Ventricle Function." Circulation* 90, 1–494, 1994.

[7] Fisher, J.P., Martin, J., Day, F.P., Rosow, E., Adam, J., Chen, C., and Gillam, L.D. "Validation of a Less Invasive Method for Determining Preload Recruitable Stroke Work Derived with Echocardiographic Automatic Boundary Detection." *Circulation* 92, 1–278, 1995.

[8] Fontes, M.L., Adam, J., Rosow, E., Mathew, J., and DeGraff, A.C. "Non-Invasive Cardiopulmonary Function Assessment System," *J. Clin. Monit.* 13, 413, 1997.

[9] Johnson, G.W., *LabVIEW Graphical Programming: Practical Applications in Instrumentation and Control,* 2nd ed., McGraw-Hill, New York, 1997.

[10] Mathew, J.P., Adam, J., Rosow, E., Fontes, M.L., Davis, L., Barash, P.G., and Gillam, L., "Cardiovascular Pressure-Dimension Analysis System," *J. Clin. Monit.* 13, 423, 1997.

[11] National Instruments. Measurement and Automation Catalog, National Instruments, Austin, TX, 1999.

[12] Rosow, E. "Technology and Sensors," Presented at the *United States Olympic Committee's Sports Equipment and Technology Conference,* Colorado Springs, CO; November 19–23, 1992.

[13] Rosow, E. "Biomedical Applications using LabVIEW," Presented at the *New England Society of Clinical Engineering, Sturbridge,* MA, November 14, 1993.

[14] Rosow, E., Adam, J.S., Nagle, J., Fisher, J.P., and Gillam, L.D. Premise Development Corporation, Avon, CT and Hartford Hospital, Hartford, CT, "A Cardiac Analysis System: LabVIEW and Acoustic Quantification (AQ)," Presented at the *Association for the Advancement of Medical Instrumentation* in Washington, D.C., May 21–25, 1994.

VII

Clinical Engineering

Yadin David
Texas Children's Hospital

74 Clinical Engineering: Evolution of a Discipline
Joseph D. Bronzino **74**-1

75 Management and Assessment of Medical Technology
Yadin David, Thomas M. Judd **75**-1

76 Risk Factors, Safety, and Management of Medical Equipment
Michael L. Gullikson **76**-1

77 Clinical Engineering Program Indicators
Dennis D. Autio, Robert L. Morris **77**-1

78 Quality of Improvement and Team Building
Joseph P. McClain **78**-1

79 A Standards Primer for Clinical Engineers
Alvin Wald **79**-1

80 Regulatory and Assessment Agencies
Mark E. Bruley, Vivian H. Coates **80**-1

81 Applications of Virtual Instruments in Health Care
Eric Rosow, Joseph Adam **81**-1

O VER THE PAST 100 YEARS, the health care system's dependence on medical technology for the delivery of its services has grown continuously. To some extent, all professional care providers depend on technology, be it in the area of preventive medicine, diagnosis, therapeutic care, rehabilitation, administration, or health-related education and training. Medical technology enables practitioners to intervene through integrated interactions with their patients in a cost-effective, efficient, and safe manner. As a result, the field of clinical engineering has emerged as the discipline of biomedical engineering that fulfills the need to manage the deployment of medical technology and to integrate it appropriately with desired clinical practices.

The healthcare delivery system presents a very complex environment where facilities, equipment, materials, and a full range of human interventions are involved. It is in this clinical environment that patients of various ages and conditions, trained staff, and the wide variety of medical technology converge. This complex mix of interactions may lead to unacceptable risk when programs for monitoring, controlling, improving, and educating all entities involved are not appropriately integrated by qualified professionals.

This section of clinical engineering focuses on the methodology for administering critical engineering services that vary from facilitation of innovation and technology transfer to the performance of technology assessment and operations support and on the management tools with which today's clinical engineer needs to be familiar. With increased awareness of the value obtained by these services, new career opportunities are created for clinical engineers.

In addition to highlighting the important roles that clinical engineers serve in many areas, the section focuses on those areas of the clinical engineering field that enhance the understanding of the "bigger picture." With such an understanding, the participation in and contribution by clinical engineers to this enlarged scope can be fully realized. The adoption of the tools described here will enable clinical engineers to fulfill their new role in the evolving health care delivery system.

All the authors in this section recognize this opportunity and here recognized for volunteering their talent and time so that others can excel as well.

74

Clinical Engineering: Evolution of a Discipline

74.1 Who Is a Clinical Engineer? **74**-1
74.2 Evolution of Clinical Engineering **74**-1
74.3 Hospital Organization and the Role of Clinical
      Engineering **74**-3
      Governing Board (Trustees) • Hospital Administration
74.4 Clinical Engineering Programs **74**-4
      Major Functions of a Clinical Engineering Department
Defining Terms **74**-7
References **74**-7
Further Reading **74**-7

Joseph D. Bronzino
Trinity College

74.1 Who Is a Clinical Engineer?

As discussed in the introduction to this *Handbook*, biomedical engineers apply the concepts, knowledge, and techniques of virtually all engineering disciplines to solve specific problems in the biosphere, that is, the realm of biology and medicine. When biomedical engineers work within a hospital or clinic, they are more appropriately called *clinical engineers*. But what exactly is the definition of the term *clinical engineer*? For the purposes of this handbook, a *clinical engineer* is defined as an engineer who has graduated from an accredited academic program in engineering or who is licensed as a professional engineer or engineer-in-training and is engaged in the application of scientific and technological knowledge developed through engineering education and subsequent professional experience within the health care environment in support of clinical activities. Furthermore, clinical environment means that portion of the health care system in which patient care is delivered, and clinical activities include direct patient care, research, teaching, and public service activities intended to enhance patient care.

74.2 Evolution of Clinical Engineering

Engineers were first encouraged to enter the clinical scene during the late 1960s in response to concerns about patient safety as well as the rapid proliferation of clinical equipment, especially in academic medical centers. In the process, a new engineering discipline — clinical engineering — evolved to provide the technological support necessary to meet these new needs. During the 1970s, a major expansion of clinical engineering occurred, primarily due to the following events:

- The Veterans' Administration (VA), convinced that clinical engineers were vital to the overall operation of the VA hospital system, divided the country into biomedical engineering districts, with a chief biomedical engineer overseeing all engineering activities in the hospitals in that district.
- Throughout the United States, clinical engineering departments were established in most of the large medical centers and hospitals and in some smaller clinical facilities with at least 300 beds.
- Clinical engineers were hired in increasing numbers to help these facilities use existing technology and incorporate new technology.

Having entered the hospital environment, routine electrical safety inspections exposed the clinical engineer to all types of patient equipment that was not being maintained properly. It soon became obvious that electrical safety failures represented only a small part of the overall problem posed by the presence of medical equipment in the clinical environment. The equipment was neither totally understood nor properly maintained. Simple visual inspections often revealed broken knobs, frayed wires, and even evidence of liquid spills. Investigating further, it was found that many devices did not perform in accordance with manufacturers' specifications and were not maintained in accordance with manufacturers' recommendations. In short, electrical safety problems were only the tip of the iceberg. The entrance of clinical engineers into the hospital environment changed these conditions for the better. By the mid-1970s, complete performance inspections before and after use became the norm, and sensible inspection procedures were developed. In the process, clinical engineering departments became the logical support center for all medical technologies and became responsible for all the biomedical instruments and systems used in hospitals, the training of medical personnel in equipment use and safety, and the design, selection, and use of technology to deliver safe and effective health care.

With increased involvement in many facets of hospital/clinic activities, clinical engineers now play a multifaceted role (Figure 74.1). They must interface successfully with many "clients," including clinical staff, hospital administrators, regulatory agencies, etc., to ensure that the medical equipment within the hospital is used safely and effectively.

Today, hospitals that have established centralized clinical engineering departments to meet these responsibilities use clinical engineers to provide the hospital administration with an objective option of equipment function, purchase, application, overall system analysis, and preventive maintenance policies.

Some hospital administrators have learned that with the in-house availability of such talent and expertise, the hospital is in a far better position to make more effective use of its technological resources [Bronzino, 1992]. By providing health professionals with needed assurance of safety, reliability, and efficiency in using new and innovative equipment, clinical engineers can readily identify poor-quality and ineffective equipment, thereby resulting in faster, more appropriate utilization of new medical equipment. Typical pursuits of clinical engineers, therefore, include:

- Supervision of a hospital clinical engineering department that includes clinical engineers and biomedical equipment technicians (BMETs)
- Prepurchase evaluation and planning for new medical technology
- Design, modification, or repair of sophisticated medical instruments or systems
- Cost-effective management of a medical equipment calibration and repair service
- Supervision of the safety and performance testing of medical equipment performed by BMETs
- Inspection of all incoming equipment (i.e., both new and returning repairs)
- Establishment of performance benchmarks for all equipment
- Medical equipment inventory control
- Coordination of outside engineering and technical services performed by vendors

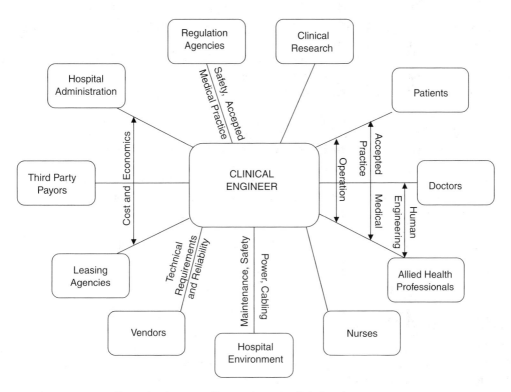

FIGURE 74.1 Diagram illustrating the range of interactions of a clinical engineer.

- Training of medical personnel in the safe and effective use of medical devices and systems
- Clinical applications engineering, such as custom modification of medical devices for clinical research, evaluation of new noninvasive monitoring systems, etc.
- Biomedical computer support
- Input to the design of clinical facilities where medical technology is used, for example, operating rooms (ORs), intensive care units, etc.
- Development and implementation of documentation protocols required by external accreditation and licensing agencies

Clinical engineers thus provide extensive engineering services for the clinical staff and, in recent years, have been increasingly accepted as valuable team members by physicians, nurses, and other clinical professionals. Furthermore, the acceptance of clinical engineers in the hospital setting has led to different types of engineering–medicine interactions, which in turn have improved health care delivery.

74.3 Hospital Organization and the Role of Clinical Engineering

In the hospital, management organization has evolved into a diffuse authority structure that is commonly referred to as the *triad model*. The three primary components are the governing board (trustees), hospital administration (CEO and administrative staff), and the medical staff organization. The role of the governing board and the chief executive officer are briefly discussed below to provide some insight regarding their individual responsibilities and their interrelationship.

74.3.1 Governing Board (Trustees)

The **Joint Commission on the Accreditation of Healthcare Organizations (JCAHO)** summarizes the major duties of the governing board as "adopting by-laws in accordance with its legal accountability and its responsibility to the patient." The governing body, therefore, requires both medical and paramedical departments to monitor and evaluate the quality of patient care, which is a critical success factor in hospitals today. To meet this goal, the governing board essentially is responsible for establishing the mission statement and defining the specific goals and objectives that the institution must satisfy. Therefore, the trustees are involved in the following functions:

- Establishing the policies of the institution
- Providing equipment and facilities to conduct patient care
- Ensuring that proper professional standards are defined and maintained (i.e., providing quality assurance)
- Coordinating professional interests with administrative, financial, and community needs
- Providing adequate financing by securing sufficient income and managing the control of expenditures
- Providing a safe environment
- Selecting qualified administrators, medical staff, and other professionals to manage the hospital

In practice, the trustees select a hospital chief administrator who develops a plan of action that is in concert with the overall goals of the institution.

74.3.2 Hospital Administration

The hospital administrator, the chief executive officer of the medical enterprise, has a function similar to that of the chief executive officer of any corporation. The administrator represents the governing board in carrying out the day-to-day operations to reflect the broad policy formulated by the trustees. The duties of the administrator are summarized as follows:

- Preparing a plan for accomplishing the institutional objectives, as approved by the board.
- Selecting medical chiefs and department directors to set standards in their respective fields.
- Submitting for board approval an annual budget reflecting both expenditures and income projections.
- Maintaining all physical properties (plant and equipment) in safe operating condition.
- Representing the hospital in its relationships with the community and health agencies.
- Submitting to the board annual reports that describe the nature and volume of the services delivered during the past year, including appropriate financial data and any special reports that may be requested by the board.

In addition to these administrative responsibilities, the chief administrator is charged with controlling cost, complying with a multitude of governmental regulations, and ensuring that the hospital conforms to professional norms, which include guidelines for the care and safety of patients.

74.4 Clinical Engineering Programs

In many hospitals, administrators have established clinical engineering departments to manage effectively all the technological resources, especially those relating to medical equipment, that are necessary for providing patient care. The primary objective of these departments is to provide a broad-based engineering program that addresses all aspects of medical instrumentation and systems support.

Figure 74.2 illustrates the organizational chart of the medical support services division of a typical major medical facility. Note that within this organizational structure, the director of clinical engineering reports directly to the vice-president of medical support services. This administrative relationship is extremely important because it recognizes the important role clinical engineering departments play in delivering quality care. It should be noted, however, that in other common organizational structures, clinical engineering services may fall under the category of "facilities," "materials management," or even just

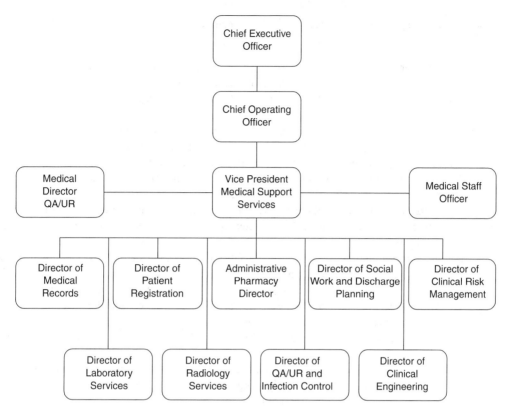

FIGURE 74.2 Organizational chart of medical support services division for a typical major medical facility. This organizational structure points out the critical interrelationship between the clinical engineering department and the other primary services provided by the medical facility.

"support services." Clinical engineers also can work directly with clinical departments, thereby bypassing much of the hospital hierarchy. In this situation, clinical departments can offer the clinical engineer both the chance for intense specialization and, at the same time, the opportunity to develop personal relationships with specific clinicians based on mutual concerns and interests.

Once the hospital administration appoints a qualified individual as director of clinical engineering, the person usually functions at the department-head level in the organizational structure of the institution and is provided with sufficient authority and resources to perform the duties efficiently and in accordance with professional norms. To understand the extent of these duties, consider the job title for "clinical engineering director" as defined by the World Health Organization [Issakov et al., 1990]:

General Statement. The clinical engineering director, by his or her education and experience, acts as a manager and technical director of the clinical engineering department. The individual designs and directs the design of equipment modifications that may correct design deficiencies or enhance the clinical performance of medical equipment. The individual may also supervise the implementation of those design modifications. The education and experience that the director possesses enables him or her to analyze complex medical or laboratory equipment for purposes of defining corrective maintenance and developing appropriate preventive maintenance or performance assurance protocols. The clinical engineering director works with nursing and medical staff to analyze new medical equipment needs and participates in both the prepurchase planning process and the incoming testing process. The individual also participates in the equipment management process through involvement in the system development, implementation, maintenance, and modification processes.

Duties and Responsibilities. The director of clinical engineering has a wide range of duties and responsibilities. For example, this individual:

- Works with medical and nursing staff in the development of technical and performance specifications for equipment requirements in the medical mission.
- Once equipment is specified and the purchase order developed, generates appropriate testing of the new equipment.
- Does complete performance analysis on complex medical or laboratory equipment and summarizes results in brief, concise, easy-to-understand terms for the purposes of recommending corrective action or for developing appropriate preventive maintenance and performance assurance protocols.
- Designs and implements modifications that permit enhanced operational capability. May supervise the maintenance or modification as it is performed by others.
- Must know the relevant codes and standards related to the hospital environment and the performance assurance activities. (Examples in the United States are NFPA 99, UL 544, and JCAHO, and internationally, IEC-TC 62.)
- Is responsible for obtaining the engineering specifications (systems definitions) for systems that are considered unusual or one-of-a-kind and are not commercially available.
- Supervises in-service maintenance technicians as they work on codes and standards and on preventive maintenance, performance assurance, corrective maintenance, and modification of new and existing patient care and laboratory equipment.
- Supervises parts and supply purchase activities and develops program policies and procedures for same.
- Sets departmental goals, develops budgets and policy, prepares and analyzes management reports to monitor department activity, and manages and organizes the department to implement them.
- Teaches measurement, calibration, and standardization techniques that promote optimal performance.
- In equipment-related duties, works closely with maintenance and medical personnel. Communicates orally and in writing with medical, maintenance, and administrative professionals. Develops written procedures and recommendations for administrative and technical personnel.

Minimum Qualifications. A bachelor's degree (4 years) in an electrical or electronics program or its equivalent is required (preferably with a clinical or biomedical adjunct). A master's degree is desirable. A minimum of 3 years' experience as a clinical engineer and 2 years in a progressively responsible supervisory capacity is needed. Additional qualifications are as follows:

- Must have some business knowledge and management skills that enable him or her to participate in budgeting, cost accounting, personnel management, behavioral counseling, job description development, and interviewing for hiring or firing purposes. Knowledge and experience in the use of microcomputers are desirable.
- Must be able to use conventional electronic trouble-shooting instruments such as multimeters, function generators, oscillators, and oscilloscopes. Should be able to use conventional machine shop equipment such as drill presses, grinders, belt sanders, brakes, and standard hand tools.
- Must possess or be able to acquire knowledge of the techniques, theories, and characteristics of materials, drafting, and fabrication techniques in conjunction with chemistry, anatomy, physiology, optics, mechanics, and hospital procedures.
- Clinical engineering certification or professional engineering registration is required.

74.4.1 Major Functions of a Clinical Engineering Department

It should be clear by the preceding job description that clinical engineers are first and foremost engineering professionals. However, as a result of the wide-ranging scope of interrelationships within the medical setting, the duties and responsibilities of clinical engineering directors are extremely diversified. Yet a common thread is provided by the very nature of the technology they manage. Directors of clinical engineering departments are usually involved in the following core functions:

Technology Management: Developing, implementing, and directing equipment management programs. Specific tasks include accepting and installing new equipment, establishing preventive maintenance and repair programs, and managing the inventory of medical instrumentation. Issues such as cost-effective use and quality assurance are integral parts of any *technology management* program. The director advises the hospital administrator of the budgetary, personnel, space, and test equipment requirements necessary to support this equipment management program.

Risk management: Evaluating and taking appropriate action on incidents attributed to equipment malfunctions or misuse. For example, the clinical engineering director is responsible for summarizing the technological significance of each incident and documenting the findings of the investigation. He or she then submits a report to the appropriate hospital authority and, according to the Safe Medical Devices Act of 1990, to the device manufacturer, the Food and Drug Administration (FDA), or both.

Technology assessment: Evaluating and selecting new equipment. The director must be proactive in the evaluation of new requests for capital equipment expenditures, providing hospital administrators and clinical staff with an in-depth appraisal of the benefits/advantages of candidate equipment. Furthermore, the process of **technology assessment** for all equipment used in the hospital should be an ongoing activity.

Facilities design and project management: Assisting in the design of new or renovated clinical facilities that house specific medical technologies. This includes operating rooms, imaging facilities, and radiology treatment centers.

Training: Establish and deliver instructional modules for clinical engineering staff as well as clinical staff on the operation of medical equipment.

In the future, it is anticipated that clinical engineering departments will provide assistance in the application and management of many other technologies that support patient care, including computer support (which includes the development of virtual instrumentation), telecommunications, and facilities operations.

Defining Terms

JCAHO, Joint Commission on the Accreditation of Healthcare Organizations: The accrediting body responsible for checking compliance of a hospital with approved rules and regulations regarding the delivery of health care.

Technology assessment: Involves an evaluation of the safety, efficiency, and cost-effectiveness, as well as consideration of the social, legal, and ethical effects, of medical technology.

References

Bronzino J.D. 1992. *Management of Medical Technology: A Primer for Clinical Engineers*. Boston, Butter-worth.

ICC. 1991. International Certification Commission's Definition of a Clinical Engineer, International Certification Commission Fact Sheet. Arlington, VA, ICC.

Issakov A., Mallouppas A., and McKie J. 1990. Manpower development for a healthcare technical service. Report of the World Health Organization, WHO/SHS/NHP/90.4.

Further Reading

1. Journals: *Journal of Clinical Engineering and Journal of Medical Engineering and Physics, Biomedical Instrumentation and Technology.*

75

Management and Assessment of Medical Technology

75.1 The Health Care Delivery System **75**-2
Major Health Care Trends and Directions • System Pressures
• The Technology Manager's Responsibility

75.2 Strategic Technology Planning **75**-3
Strategic Planning Process • Clinical and Technology
Strategic Plan • Technology Strategic Planning Process

75.3 Technology Assessment **75**-5
Prerequisites for Technology Assessment • Technology
Assessment Process

75.4 Equipment Assets Management **75**-8
Equipment Management Process • Technology Management
Activities • Case Study: A Focus on Medical Imaging

75.5 Equipment Acquisition and Deployment **75**-10
Process of Acquiring Technology • Acquisition Process
Strategies • Clinical Team Requirements

Defining Terms **75**-12

References **75**-15

Yadin David
Texas Children's Hospital

Thomas M. Judd
Kaiser Permanente

As medical technology continues to evolve, so does its impact on patient outcome, hospital operations, and financial efficiency. The ability to plan for this evolution and its subsequent implications has become a major challenge in most decisions of health care organizations and their related industries. Therefore, there is a need to adequately plan for and apply those management tools which optimize the deployment of medical technology and the facilities that house it. Successful management of the technology and facilities will ensure a good match between the needs and the capabilities of staff and technology, respectively. While different types and sizes of hospitals will consider various strategies of actions, they all share the need to manage efficient utilization of their limited resources and its monitoring. Technology is one of these resources, and while it is frequently cited as the culprit behind cost increases, the well-managed technology program contribute to a significant containment of the cost of providing quality patient care. Clinical engineer's skills and expertise are needed to facilitate the adoption of an objective methodology for implantation of a program that will match the hospital's needs and operational conditions. Whereas both the knowledge and practice patterns of management in general are well organized in today's literature, the management of the health care delivery system and that of medical technology in the clinical environment has not yet reached that same high level. However, as we begin to understand the relationship between the methods and information that guide the decision-making processes regarding the management of medical technology that are being deployed in this highly complex environment, the role of the qualified clinical engineer becomes more valuable. This is achieved by reformulating the technology management process, which starts with the strategic planning process, continues with the **technology assessment** process, leads to the equipment planning and procurement processes, and finally ends with the assets management process. Definition of terms used in this chapter are provided at the end of the chapter.

75.1 The Health Care Delivery System

Societal demands on the health care delivery system revolve around cost, technology, and expectations. To respond effectively, the delivery system must identify its goals, select and define its priorities, and then wisely allocate its limited resources. For most organizations, this means that they must acquire only appropriate technologies and manage what they have already more effectively. To improve performance and reduce costs, the delivery system must recognize and respond to the key dynamics in which it operates, must shape and mold its planing efforts around several existing health care trends and directions, and must respond proactively and positively to the pressures of its environment. These issues and the technology manager's response are outlined here (1) technology's positive impact on care quality and effectiveness, (2) an unacceptable rise in national spending for health care services, (3) a changing mix of how Americans are insured for health care, (4) increases in health insurance premiums for which **appropriate technology** application is a strong limiting factor, (5) a changing mix of health care services and settings in which care is delivered, and (6) growing pressures related to technology for hospital capital spending and budgets.

75.1.1 Major Health Care Trends and Directions

The major trends and directions in health care include (1) changing location and design of treatment areas, (2) evolving benefits, coverages, and choices, (3) extreme pressures to manage costs, (4) treating of more acutely ill older patients and the prematurely born, (5) changing job structures and demand for skilled labor, (6) the need to maintain a strong cash flow to support construction, equipment, and information system developments, (7) increased competition on all sides, (8) requirement for information systems that effectively integrate clinical and business issues, (9) changing reimbursement policies that reduce new purchases and lead to the expectation for extended equipment life cycles, (10) internal **technology planning and management programs** to guide decision making, (11) technology planning teams to coordinate adsorption of new and replacement technologies, as well as to suggest delivery system changes, and (12) equipment maintenance costs that are emerging as a significant expense item under great administrative scrutiny.

75.1.2 System Pressures

System pressures include (1) society's expectations — highest quality care at the lowest reasonable price, where quality is a function of personnel, facilities, technology, and clinical procedures offered; (2) economic conditions — driven often by reimbursement criteria; (3) legal-pressures — resulting primarily from malpractice issues and dealing with rule-intensive "government" clients; (4) regulatory — multistate delivery systems with increased management complexity, or heavily regulated medical device industries facing free-market competition, or hospitals facing the Safe Medical Devices Act reporting requirements and credentialling requirements; (5) ethics — deciding who gets care and when; and (6) technology pressures — organizations having enough capabilities to meet community needs and to compete successfully in their marketplaces.

75.1.3   The Technology Manager's Responsibility

Technology managers should (1) become deeply involved and committed to technology planning and management programs in their system, often involving the need for greater personal responsibilities and expanded credentials, (2) understand how the factors above impact their organization and how technology can be used to improve outcomes, reduce costs, and improve quality of life for patients, (3) educate other health care professionals about how to demonstrate the value of individual technologies through involving financial, engineering, **quality of care**, and management perspective, and (4) assemble a team of care-givers with sufficient broad clinical expertise and administrators with planning and financial expertise to contribute their knowledge to the assessment process [1].

75.2   Strategic Technology Planning

75.2.1   Strategic Planning Process

Leading health care organizations have begun to combine **strategic technology planning** with other tech-nology management activities in program that effectively integrate new technologies with their existingly technology base. This has resulted in high-quality care at a reasonable cost. Among those who have been its leading catalysts, ECRI (formerly the Emergency Care Research Institute) is known for artic-ulating this program [2] and encouraging its proliferation initially among regional health care systems and now for single or multihospital systems as well [3]. Key components of the program include clin-ical strategic-planning, technology strategic planning, technology assessment, interaction with capital budgeting, acquisition and deployment, resource (or equipment assets) management, and monitoring and evaluation. A proper technology strategic plan is derived from and supports as well-defined clinical strategic plan [4].

75.2.2   Clinical and Technology Strategic Plan

Usually considered long-range and continually evolving, a clinical strategic plan is updated annually. For a given year, the program begins when key hospital participants, through the strategic planning process, assess what clinical services the hospital should be offering in its referral area. They take into account health care trends, demographic and market share data, and space and facilities plans. They analyze their facility's strengths and weaknesses, goals and objectives, competition, and existing technology base. The outcome of this process is a clinical strategic plan that establishes the organization's vision for the year and referral area needs and the hospital's objectives in meeting them.

It is not possible to adequately complete a clinical strategic plan without engaging in the process of strategic technology planning. A key role for technology managers is to assist their organizations throughout the combined clinical and technology strategic planning processes by matching available technical capabilities, both existing and new, with clinical requirements. To accomplish this, technology managers must understand why their institution's values and mission are set as they are, pursue their institution's strategic plans through that knowledge, and plan in a way that effectively allocates limited resources. Although a technology manager may not be assigned to develop an institution's overall strategic plan, he or she must understand and believe it in order to offer good input for hospital management. In providing this input, a technology manager should determine a plan for evaluating the present state of the hospital's technological deployment, assist in providing a review of emerging technological innovations and their possible impact on the hospital, articulate justifications and provisions for adoption of new technologies or enhancement of existing ones, visit research and laboratories and exhibit areas at major medical and scientific meetings to view new technologies, and be familiar with the institution and its equipment users' abilities to assimilate new technology.

The past decade has shown a trend toward increased legislation in support of more federal regulations in health care. These and other pressures will require that additional or replacement medical technology be well anticipated and justified. As a rationale for technology adoption, the Texas Children's Hospital focuses on the issues of clinical necessity, management support, and market preference. Addressing the issue of clinical necessity, the hospital considers the technology's comparison against medical standard of care, its impact on the level of care and quality of life, its improvement on intervention's accuracy and **safety**, its impact on the rate of recovery, the needs or desires of the community, and the change in service volume or focus. On the issue of management support, the hospital estimates if the technology will create a more effective care plan and decision-making process, improve operational efficiency in the current service programs, decrease liability exposure, increase compliance with regulations, reduce workload and dependence on user skill level ameliorate departmental support, or enhance clinical proficiency. Weighting the issue of market preference, the hospital contemplate if it will improve access to care, increase customer convenience and satisfaction, enhance the organization's image and market share, decrease the cost of adoption and ownership, or provide a return on its investment.

75.2.3 Technology Strategic Planning Process

When the annual clinical strategic planning process has started and hospital leaders have begun to analyze or reaffirm what clinical services they want to offer to the community, the hospital can then conduct efficient technology strategic planning. Key elements of this planning involve (1) performing an initial audit of existing technologies, (2) conducting a technology assessment for new and emerging technologies for fit with current or desired clinical services, (3) planning for replacement and selection of new technologies, (4) setting priorities for technology acquisition, and (5) developing processes to implement equipment acquisition and monitor ongoing utilization. "Increasingly, hospitals are designating a senior manager (e.g., an administrator, the director of planning, the director of clinical engineering) to take the responsibility for technology assessment and planning. That person should have the primary responsibility for developing the strategic technology plan with the help of key physicians, department managers, and senior executives" [2].

Hospitals can form a medical technology advisory committee (MTAC), overseen by the designated senior manager and consisting of the types of members mentioned above, to conduct the strategic technology planning process and to annually recommend technology priorities to the hospital strategic planning committee and capital budget committee. It is especially important to involve physicians and nurses in this process.

In the initial technology audit, each major clinical service or product line must be analyzed to determine how well the existing technology base supports it. The audit can be conducted along service lines (radiology, cardiology, surgery) or technology function (e.g., imaging, therapeutic, diagnostic) by a team of designated physicians, department heads, and technology managers. The team should begin by developing a complete hospital-wide assets inventory, including the quantity and quality of equipment. The team should compare the existing technology base against known and evolving standards-of-care information, patient outcome data, and known equipment problems. Next, the team should collect and examine information on technology utilization to assess its appropriate use, the opportunities for improvement, and the risk level. After reviewing the technology users' education needs as they relate to the application and servicing of medical equipment, the team should credential users for competence in the application of new technologies. Also, the auditing team should keep up with published clinical protocols and practice guidelines using available health care **standards** directories and utilize clinical outcome data for quality-assurance and risk-management program feedback [5].

While it is not expected that every hospital has all the required expertise in-house to conduct the initial technology audit or ongoing technology assessment, the execution of this planning process is sufficiently critical for a hospital's success that outside expertise should be obtained when necessary. The audit allows for the gathering of information about the status of the existing technology base and enhances the capability of the medical technology advisory committee to assess the impact of new and emerging technologies on their major clinical services.

All the information collected from the technology audit results and technology assessments is used in developing budget strategies. Budgeting is part of strategic technology planning in that a 2- to 5-year long-range capital spending plan should be created. This is in addition to the annual capital budget preparation that takes into account 1 year at a time. The MTAC, as able and appropriate, provides key information regarding capital budget requests and makes recommendations to the capital budget committee each year. The MTAC recommends priorities for replacement as well as new and emerging technologies that over a period of several years guides that acquisition that provides the desired service developments or enhancements. Priorities are recommended on the basis of need, risk, cost (acquisition, operational and maintenance), utilization, and fit with the clinical strategic plan.

75.3 Technology Assessment

As medical technology continues to evolve, so does its impact on patient outcome, hospital operations, and financial resources. The ability to manage this evolution and its subsequent implications has become a major challenge for all health care organizations. Successful management of technology will ensure a good match between needs and capabilities and between staff and technology. To be successful, an ongoing technology assessment process must be an integral part of an ongoing technology planning and management program at the hospital, addressing the needs of the patient, the user, and the support team. This facilitates better equipment planning and utilization of the hospital's resources. The manager who is knowledgeable about his or her organization's culture, equipment users' needs, the environment within which equipment will be applied, equipment engineering, and emerging technological capabilities will be successful in proficiently implementing and managing technological changes [6].

It is in the technology assessment process that the clinical engineering/technology manager professional needs to wear two hats: that of the manager and that of the engineer. This is a unique position, requiring expertise and detailed preparation, that allows one to be a key leader and contributor to the decision-making process of the medical technology advisory committee (MTAC).

The MTAC uses an ad hoc team approach to conduct technology assessment of selected services and technologies throughout the year. The ad hoc teams may incorporate representatives of equipment users, equipment service providers, physicians, purchasing agents, reimbursement mangers, representatives of administration, and other members from the institution as applicable.

75.3.1 Prerequisites for Technology Assessment

Medical technology is a major strategic factor in positioning and creating a positive community perception of the hospital. Exciting new biomedical devices and systems are continually being introduced. And they are introduced at a time when the pressure on hospitals to contain expenditures is mounting. Therefore, forecasting the deployment of medical technology and the capacity to continually evaluate its impact on the hospital require that the hospital be willing to provide the support for such a program. (*Note*: Many organizations are aware of the principle that an in-house "champion" is needed in order to provide for the leadership that continually and objectively plans ahead. The champion and the program being "championed" may use additional in-house or independent expertise as needed. To get focused attention on the technology assessment function and this program in larger, academically affiliated and government hospitals, the position of a chief technology officer is being created.) Traditionally, executives rely on their staff to produce objective analyses of the hospital's technological needs. Without such analyses, executives may approve purchasing decisions of sophisticated biomedical equipment only to discover later that some needs or expected features were not included with this installation, that those features are not yet approved for delivery, or that the installation has not been adequately planned.

Many hospitals perform technology assessment activities to project needs for new assets and to better manage existing assets. Because the task is complex, an interdisciplinary approach and a cooperative attitude among the assessment team leadership is required. The ability to integrate information from disciplines such as clinical, technical, financial, administrative, and facility in a timely and objective manner is critical to the success of the assessment. This chapter emphasizes how technology assessment fits within a technology planning and management program and recognizes the importance of corporate skills forecasting medical equipment changes and determining the impact of changes on the hospital's market position. Within the technology planning and management program, the focus on capital assets management of medical equipment should not lead to the exclusion of accessories, supplies, and the disposables also required.

Medical equipment has a life cycle that can be identified as (1) the innovation phase, which includes the concept, basic and applies research, and development, and (2) the adoption phase, which begins with the clinical studies, through diffusion, and then widespread use. These phases are different from each other in the scope of professional skills involved, their impact on patient care, compliance with regulatory requirements, and the extent of the required operational support. In evaluating the applicability of a device or a system for use in the hospital, it is important to note in which phase of its life cycle the equipment currently resides.

75.3.2 Technology Assessment Process

More and more hospitals are faced with the difficult phenomenon of a capital equipment requests list that is much larger than the capital budget allocation. The most difficult decision, then, is the one that matches clinical needs with the financial capability. In doing so, the following questions are often raised: How do we avoid costly technology mistakes? How do we wisely target capital dollars for technology? How do we avoid medical staff conflicts as they relate to technology? How do we control equipment-related risks? and How do we maximize the useful life of the equipment or systems while minimizing the cost ownership? A hospital's clinical engineering department can assist in providing the right answers to these questions.

Technology assessment is a component of technology planning that begins with the analysis of the hospital's existing technology base. It is easy to perceive then that technology assessment, rather than an equipment comparison, is a new major function for a clinical engineering department [7]. It is important that clinical engineers be well prepared for the challenge. They must have a full understanding of the mission of their particular hospitals, a familiarity with the health care delivery system, and the cooperation of hospital administrators and the medical staff. To aid in the technology assessment process, clinical engineers need to utilize the following tools (1) access to national database services, directories, and libraries, (2) visits to scientific and clinical exhibits, (3) a network with key industry contacts, and (4) a relationship with peers throughout the country [8].

The need for clinical engineering involvement in the technology assessment process becomes evident when recently purchased equipment or its functions are underutilized, users have ongoing problems with equipment, equipment maintenance costs become excessive, the hospital is unable to comply with standards or guidelines (i.e., JCAHO requirements) for equipment management, a high percentage of equipment is awaiting repair, or training for equipment operators is inefficient due to shortage of allied health professionals. A deeper look at the symptoms behind these problems would likely reveal a lack of a central clearinghouse to collect, index, and monitor all technology-related information for future planning purposes, the absence of procedures for identifying emerging technologies for potential acquisition, the lack of a systematic plan for conducting technology assessment, resulting in an ability to maximize the benefits from deployment of available technology, the inability to benefit from the organization's own previous experience with a particular type of technology, the random replacement of medical technologies rather than a systematic plan based on a set of well-developed criteria, and the lack of integration of technology acquisition into the strategic and capital planning of the hospital.

To address these issues, efforts to develop a technology microassessment process were initiated at one leading private hospital with the following objectives (1) accumulate information on medical equipment, (2) facilitate systematic planning, (3) create an administrative structure supporting the assessment process and its methodology, (4) monitor the replacement of outdated technology, and (5) improve the capital budget process by focusing on long-term needs relative to the acquisition of medical equipment [9].

The process, in general, and the collection of up-to-date pertinent information, in particular, require the expenditure of certain resources and the active participation of designated hospital staff in networks providing technology assessment information. For example, corporate membership in organizations and societies that provide such information needs to be considered, as well as subscriptions to certain computerized database and printed sources [10].

At the example hospital, and MTAC was formed to conduct technology assessment. It was chaired by the director of clinical engineering. Other managers from equipment user departments usually serve as the MTAC's designated technical coordinators for specific task forces. Once the committee accepted a request from an individual user, it identified other users that might have an interest in that equipment or system and authorized the technical coordinator to assemble a task force consisting of users identified by the MTAC. This task force then took responsibility for the establishment of performance criteria that would be used during this particular assessment. The task force also should answer the questions of effectiveness, safety, and **cost-effectiveness** as they relate to the particular assessment. During any specific period, there may be multiple task forces, each focusing on a specific equipment investigation.

The task force technical coordinator cooperates with the material management department in conducting a market survey, in obtaining the specified equipment for evaluation purposes, and in scheduling vendor-provided in-service training. The coordinator also confers with clinical staff to determine if they have experience with the equipment and the maturity level of the equipment under assessment. After establishment of a task force, the MTACs technical coordinator is responsible for analyzing the clinical experiences associated with the use of this equipment, for setting evaluation objectives, and for devising appropriate technical tests in accord with recommendations from the task force. Only equipment that successfully passes the technical tests will proceed to a clinical trial. During the clinical trial, a task force-appointed clinical coordinator collects and reports a summary of experiences gained. The technical coordinator then combines the results from both the technical tests and the clinical trial into a summary report for MTAC review and approval. In this role, the clinical engineer/technical coordinator serves as a multidisciplinary professional, bridging the gap between the clinical and technical needs of the hospital. To complete the process, financial staff representatives review the protocol.

The technology assessment process at this example hospital begins with a department or individual filling out two forms (1) a request for review (RR) form and (2) a capital asset request (CAR) form. These forms are submitted to the hospital's product standards committee, which determines if an assessment process is to be initiated, and the priority for its completion. It also determines if a previously established standard for this equipment already exists (if the hospital is already using such a technology) — if so, an assessment is not needed.

On the RR, the originator delineates the rationale for acquiring the medical device. For example, the originator must tell how the item will improve quality of patient care, who will be its primary user, and how it will improve ease of use. On the CAR, the originator describes the item, estimates its cost, and provides purchase justification. The CAR is then routed to the capital budget office for review. During this process, the optimal financing method for acquisition is determined. If funding is secured, the CAR is routed to the material management department, where, together with the RR, it will be processed. The rationale for having the RR accompany the CAR is to ensure that financial information is included as part of the assessment process. The CAR is the tool by which the purchasing department initiates a market survey and later sends product requests for bid. Any request for evaluation that is received without a CAR or any CAR involving medical equipment that is received without a request for evaluation is returned to the originator without action. Both forms are then sent to the clinical engineering department, where a designated technical coordinator will analyze the requested technology maturity level and results of clinical experience with its use, review trends, and prioritize various manufactures' presentations for MTAC review.

Both forms must be sent to the MTAC if the item requested is not currently used by the hospital or if it does not conform to previously adopted hospital standards. The MTAC has the authority to recommend either acceptance or rejection of any request for review, based on a consensus of its members. A task force consisting of potential equipment users will determine the "must have" equipment functions, review the impact of the various equipment configurations, and plan technical and clinical evaluations.

If the request is approved by the MTAC, the requested technology or equipment will be evaluated using technical and performance standards. Upon completion of the review, a recommendation is returned to the hospital's products standard committee, which reviews the results of the technology assessment, determines whether the particular product is suitable as a hospital standard, and decides if it should be purchased. If approved, the request to purchase will be reviewed by the capital budget committee (CBC) to determine if the required expenditure meets with available financial resources and if or when it may be feasible to make the purchase. To ensure coordination of the technology assessment program, the chairman of the MTAC also serves as a permanent member of the hospital's CBC. In this way, there is a planned integration between technology assessment and budget decisions.

75.4 Equipment Assets Management

An accountable, systemic approach will ensure that cost-effective, efficacious, safe, and appropriate equipment is available to meet the demands of quality patient care. Such an approach requires that existing medical equipment resources be managed and that the resulting management strategies have measurable outputs that are monitored and evaluated. Technology managers/clinical engineers are well positioned to organize and lead this function. It is assumed that cost accounting is managed and monitored by the health care organization's financial group.

75.4.1 Equipment Management Process

Through traditional assets management strategies, medical equipment can be comprehensively managed by clinical engineering personnel. First, the management should consider a full range of strategies for equipment technical support. Plans may include use of a combination of equipment service providers such as manufacturers, third-party service groups, shared services, and hospital-based (in-house) engineers and biomedical equipment technicians (BMETs). All these service providers should be under the general responsibility of the technology manager to ensure optimal equipment performance through comprehensive and ongoing best-value equipment service. After obtaining a complete hospital medical equipment inventory (noting both original manufacturer and typical service provider), the management should conduct a thorough analysis of hospital accounts payable records for at least the past 2 years, compiling all service reports and preventative maintenance-related costs from all possible sources. The manager then should document in-house and external provider equipment service costs, extent of maintenance coverage for each inventory time, equipment-user operating schedule, quality of maintenance coverage for each item, appropriateness of the service provider, and reasonable maintenance costs. Next, he or she should establish an effective equipment technical support process. With an accurate inventory and best-value service providers identified, service agreements/contracts should be negotiated with external providers using prepared terms and conditions, including a log-in system. There should be an in-house clinical engineering staff ensuring ongoing external provider cost control utilizing several tools. By asking the right technical questions and establishing friendly relationships with staff, the manager will be able to handle service purchase orders (POs) by determining if equipment is worth repairing and obtaining exchange prices for parts. The staff should handle service reports to review them for accuracy and proper use of the log-in system. They also should match invoices with the service reports to verify opportunities and review service histories to look for symptoms such as need for user training, repeated problems, run-on calls billed months apart, or evidence of defective or worn-out equipment. The manager should take responsibility for emergency equipment rentals. Finally, the manager should develop, implement, and monitor all the service performance criteria.

To optimize technology management programs, clinical engineers should be willing to assume responsibilities for technology planning and management in all related areas. They should develop policies and procedures for their hospital's management program. With life-cycle costs determined for key high-risk or high-cost devices, they should evaluate methods to provide additional cost savings in equipment operation and maintenance. They should be involved with computer networking systems within the hospital. As computer technology applications increase, the requirements to review technology-related information in a number of hospital locations will increase. They should determine what environmental conditions and facility changes are required to accommodate new technologies or changes in standards and guidelines. Lastly, they should use documentation of equipment performance and maintenance costs along with their knowledge of current clinical practices to assist other hospital personnel in determining the best time and process for planning equipment replacement [11].

75.4.2 Technology Management Activities

A clinical engineering department, through outstanding performance in traditional equipment management, will win its hospital's support and will be asked to be involved in a full range of technology management activities. The department should start an equipment control program that encompasses routine performance testing, inspection, periodic and preventive maintenance, on-demand repair services, incidents investigation, and actions on recalls and hazards. The department should have multidisciplinary involvement in equipment acquisition and replacement decisions, development of new services, and planning of new construction and major renovations, including intensive participation by clinical engineering, materials management, and finance. The department also should initiate programs for training all users of patient care equipment, quality improvement (QI), as it relates to technology use, and technology-related **risk management** [12].

75.4.3 Case Study: A Focus on Medical Imaging

In the mid-1980s, a large private multihospital system contemplated the startup of a corporate clinical engineering program. The directors recognized that involvement in a diagnostic imaging equipment service would be key to the economic success of the program. They further recognized that maintenance cost reductions would have to be balanced with achieving equal or increased quality of care in the utilization of that equipment.

Programs startup was in the summer of 1987 in 3 hospitals that were geographically close. Within the first year, clinical engineering operations began in 11 hospitals in 3 regions over a two-state area. By the fall of 1990, the program included 7 regions and 21 hospitals in a five-state area. The regions were organized, typically, into teams including a regional manager and 10 service providers, serving 3 to 4 hospitals, whose average size was 225 beds. Although the staffs were stationed at the hospitals, some specialists traveled between sites in the region to provide equipment service. Service providers included individuals specializing in the areas of diagnostic imaging (x-ray and computed tomography [CT]), clinical laboratory, general biomedical instrumentation, and respiratory therapy.

At the end of the first 18 months, the program documented over $1 million in savings for the initial 11 hospitals, a 23% reduction from the previous annual service costs. Over 63% of these savings were attributable to "in-house" service x-ray and CT scanner equipment. The mix of equipment maintained by 11 imagining service providers — from a total staff of 30 — included approximately 75% of the radiology systems of any kind found in the hospitals and 5 models of CT scanners from the three different manufacturers.

At the end of 3 years in 1990, program-wide savings had exceeded 30% of previous costs for participating hospitals. Within the imaging areas of the hospitals, savings approached and sometimes exceed 50% of initial service costs. The 30 imaging service providers — out of a total staff of 62 — had increased their coverage of radiology equipment to over 95%, had increased involvement with CT to include nine models from five different manufacturers, and had begun in-house work in other key imaging modalities.

Tracking the financial performance of the initial 11 hospitals over the first 3 years of the program yields the following composite example: a hospital of 225 beds was found to have equipment service costs of $540,000 prior to program startup. Sixty-three percent of these initial costs (or $340,000) was for the maintenance of the hospital's x-ray and CT scanner systems. Three years later, annual service costs for this equipment were cut in half, to approximately $170,000. That represents a 31% reduction in hospital-wide costs due to the imaging service alone.

This corporate clinical engineering operation is, in effect, a large in-house program serving many hospitals that all have common ownership. The multihospital corporation has significant purchasing power in the medical device marketplace and provides central oversight of the larger capital expenditures for its hospitals. The combination of the parent organization's leverage and the program's commitment to serve only hospitals in the corporation facilitated the development of positive relationships with medical device manufacturers. Most of the manufacturers did not see the program as competition but rather as a potentially helpful ally in the future marketing and sales of their equipment and systems. What staff provided these results? All service providers were either medical imaging industry or military trained. All were experienced at troubleshooting electronic subsystems to component level, as necessary. Typically, these individuals had prior experience on the manufacture's models of equipment under their coverage. Most regional managers had prior industry, third party, or in-house imaging service management experience. Each service provider had the test equipment necessary for day-to-day duties. Each individual could expect at least 2 weeks of annual service training to keep appropriate skills current. Desired service training could be acquired in a timely manner from manufactures and third-party organizations. Spare or replacement parts inventory was minimal because of the program's ability to get parts from manufacturers and other sources either locally or shipped in overnight.

As quality indicators for the program, the management measured user satisfaction, equipment downtime, documentation of technical staff service training, types of user equipment errors and their effect on patient outcomes, and regular attention to hospital technology problems. User satisfaction surveys indicated a high degree of confidence in the program service providers by imaging department mangers. Problems relating to technical, management, communication, and financial issues did occur regularly, but the regional manager ensured that they were resolved in a timely manner. Faster response to daily imaging equipment problems, typically by on-site service providers, coupled with regular preventive maintenance (PM) according to established procedures led to reduced equipment downtime. PM and repair service histories were captured in a computer documentation system that also tracked service times, costs, and user errors and their effects. Assisting the safety committee became easier with ability to draw a wide variety of information quickly from the program's documenting system.

Early success in imaging equipment led to the opportunity to do some additional value-added projects such as the moving and reinstallation of x-ray rooms that preserved exiting assets and opened up valuable space for installation of newer equipment and upgrades of CT scanner systems. The parent organization came to realize that these technology management activities could potentially have a greater financial and quality impact on the hospital's health care delivery than equipment management. In the example of one CT upgrade (which was completed over two weekends with no downtime), there was a positive financial impact in excess of $600,000 and improved quality of care by allowing faster off-line diagnosis of patient scans. However, opportunity for this kind of contribution would never have occurred without the strong base of a successful equipment management program staffed with qualified individuals who receive ongoing training.

75.5   Equipment Acquisition and Deployment

75.5.1   Process of Acquiring Technology

Typically, medical device systems will emerge from the strategic technology planning and technology assessment processes as required and budgeted needs. At acquisition time, a needs analysis should be conducted, reaffirming clinical needs and device intended applications. The "request for review" documentation from the assessment process or capital budget request and incremental financial analysis from the planning process may provide appropriate justification information, and a capital asset request (CAR) form should be completed [13]. Materials management and clinical engineering personnel should ensure that this item is a candidate for centralized and coordinated acquisition of similar equipment with other hospital departments. Typical hospital prepurchase evaluation guidelines include an analysis of needs and development of a specification list, formation of a vendor list and requesting proposals, analyzing proposals and site planning, evaluating samples, selecting finalists, making the award, delivery and installation, and acceptance testing. Formal request for proposals (RFPs) from potential equipment vendors are required for intended acquisitions whose initial or life-cycle cost exceeds a certain threshold, that is, $100,000. Finally, the purchase takes place, wherein final equipment negotiations are conducted and purchase documents are prepared, including a purchase order.

75.5.2 Acquisition Process Strategies

The cost-of-ownership concept can be used when considering what factors to include in cost comparisons of competing medical devices. Cost of ownership encompasses all the direct and indirect expenses associated with medical equipment over its lifetime [4]. It expresses the cost factors of medical equipment for both the initial price of the equipment (which typically includes the equipment, its installation, and initial training cost) and over the long term. Long-term costs include ongoing training, equipment service, supplies, connectivity, upgrades, and other costs. Health care organizations are just beginning to account for a full range of cost-of-ownership factors in their technology assessment and acquisition processes, such as acquisition costs, operating costs, and maintenance costs (installation, supplies, downtime, training, spare parts, test equipment and tools, and depreciation). It is estimated that the purchase price represents only 20% of the life-cycle cost of ownership.

When conducting needs analysis, actual utilization information form the organization's existing same or similar devices can be very helpful. One leading private multihospital system has implemented the following approach to measuring and developing relevant management feedback concerning equipment utilization. It is conducting equipment utilization review for replacement planning, for ongoing accountability of equipment use, and to provide input before more equipment is purchased. This private system attempts to match product to its intended function and to measure daily (if necessary) the equipment's actual utilization. The tools they use include knowing their hospital's entire installed base of certain kinds of equipment, that is, imaging systems. Utilization assumptions for each hospital and its clinical procedural mix are made. Equipment functional requirements to meet the demands of the clinical procedures are also taken into account.

Life-cycle cost analysis is a tool used during technology planning, assessment, or acquisition "either to compare high-cost, alternative means for providing a service or to determine whether a single project or technology has a positive or negative economic value. The strength of the life-cycle cost analysis is that it examines the cash flow impact of an alternative over its entire life, instead of focusing solely on initial capital investments" [4].

"Life-cycle cost analysis facilitates comparisons between projects or technologies with large initial cash outlays and those with level outlays and inflows over time. It is most applicable to complex, high-cost choices among alternative technologies, new service, and different means for providing a given service. Life-cycle cost analysis is particularly useful for decisions that are too complex and ambiguous for experience and subjective judgment alone. It also helps decision makers perceive and include costs that often are hidden or ignored, and that may otherwise invalidate results" [11].

"Perhaps the most powerful life-cycle cost technique is net present value (NPV) analysis, which explicitly accounts for inflation and foregone investment opportunities by expressing future cash flows in present dollars" [11].

Examples where LCC and NPV analysis prove very helpful are in deciding whether to replace/rebuild or buy/lease medical imaging equipment. The kinds of costs captured in life-cycle cost analysis, include decision-making costs, planning agency/certificate of need costs (if applicable), financing, initial capital investment costs including facility changes, life-cycle maintenance and repairs costs, personnel costs, and other (reimbursement consequences, resale, etc.).

One of the best strategies to ensure that a desired technology is truly of value to the hospital is to conduct a careful analysis in preparation for its assimilation into hospital operations. The process of equipment prepurchase evaluation provides information that can be used to screen unacceptable performance by either the vendor or the equipment before it becomes a hospital problem.

Once the vendor has responded to informal requests or formal RFPs, the clinical engineering department should be responsible for evaluating the technical response, while the materials management department should devaluate the financial responses.

In translating clinical needs into a specification list, key features or "must have" attributes of the desired device are identified. In practice, clinical engineering and materials management should develop a "must have" list and an extras list. The extras list contains features that may tip the decision in favor of one vendor, all other factors being even. These specification lists are sent to the vendor and are effective in a self-elimination process that results in a time savings for the hospital. Once the "must have" attributes have been satisfied, the remaining candidate devices are evaluated technically, and the extras are considered. This is accomplished by assigning a weighting factor (i.e., 0 to 5) to denote the relative importance of each of the desired attributes. The relative ability of each device to meet the defined requirements is then rated [14].

One strategy that strengthens the acquisition process is the conditions-of-sale document. This multifaceted document integrates equipment specifications, performance, installation requirements, and follow-up services. The conditions-of-sale document ensures that negotiations are completed before a purchase order is delivered and each participant is in agreement about the product to be delivered. As a document of compliance, the conditions-of-sale document specifies the codes and standards having jurisdiction over that equipment. This may include provisions for future modification of the equipment, compliance with standards under development, compliance with national codes, and provision for software upgrades.

Standard purchase orders that include the conditions of sale for medical equipment are usually used to initiate the order. At the time the order is placed, clinical engineering is notified of the order. In addition to current facility conditions, the management must address installation and approval requirements, responsibilities, and timetable; payment, assignment, and cancellation; software requirements and updates; documentation; clinical and technical training; acceptance testing (hospital facility and vendor); warranty, spare parts, and service; and price protection.

All medical equipment must be inspected and tested before it is placed into service regardless of whether it is purchased, leased, rented, or borrowed by the hospital. In any hospital, clinical engineering should receive immediate notification if a very large device or system is delivered directly into another department (e.g., imaging or cardiology) for installation. Clinical engineering should be required to sign off on all purchase orders for devices after installation and validation of satisfactory operation. Ideally, the warranty period on new equipment should not begin until installation and acceptance testing are completed. It is not uncommon for a hospital to lose several months of free parts and service by the manufacturer when new equipment is, for some reason, not installed immediately after delivery.

75.5.3 Clinical Team Requirements

During the technology assessment and acquisition processes, clinical decision makers analyze the following criteria concerning proposed technology acquisitions, specifically as they relate to clinical team requirements: ability of staff to assimilate the technology, medical staff satisfaction (short term and long term), impact on staffing (numbers, functions), projected utilization, ongoing related supplies required, effect on delivery of care and outcomes (convenience, safety, or standard of care), result of what is written in the clinical practice guidelines, credentialling of staff required, clinical staff initial and ongoing training required, and the effect on existing technology in the department or on other services/departments.

Defining Terms

Appropriate technology [14]: A term used initially in developing countries, referring to selecting medical equipment that can "appropriately" satisfy the following constraints: funding shortages, insufficient numbers of trained personnel, lack of technical support, inadequate supplies of consumables/accessories, unreliable water and power utilities/supplies, and lack of operating and maintenance manuals. In the context of this chapter, appropriate technology selection must take into consideration local health needs and disease prevalence, the need for local capability of equipment maintenance, and availability of resources for ongoing operational and technical support.

Clinical engineers/biomedical engineers: As we began describing the issues with the management of medical technology, it became obvious that some of the terms are being used interchangeably in the literature. For example, the terms engineers, clinical engineers, biomedical equipment technicians, equipment managers, and health care engineers are frequently used. For clarification, in this chapter we will refer to clinical engineers and the clinical engineering department as a representative group for all these terms.

Cost-effectiveness [14]: A mixture of quantitative and qualitative considerations. It includes the health priorities of the country or region at the macro assessment level and the community needs at the institution micro assessment level. Product life-cycle cost analysis (which, in turn, includes initial purchase price, shipping, renovations, installation, supplies, associated disposables, cost per use, and similar quantitative measures) is a critical analysis measure. Life-cycle cost also takes into account staff training, ease of use, service, and many other cost factors. But experience and judgement about the relative importance of features and the ability to fulfill the intended purpose also contribute critical information to the cost-effectiveness equation.

Equipment acquisition and deployment: Medical device systems and products typically emerge from the strategic technology planning process as "required and budgeted" needs. The process that follows, which ends with equipment acceptance testing and placement into general use, is known as the equipment acquisition and deployment process.

Health care technology: Health care technology includes the devices, equipment, systems, software, supplies, pharmaceuticals, biotechnologies, and medical and surgical procedures used in the prevention, diagnosis, and treatment of disease in humans, for their rehabilitation, and for assistive purposes. In short, technology is broadly defined as encompassing virtually all the human interventions intended to cope with disease and disabilities, short of spiritual alternatives. This chapter focuses on medical equipment products (devices, systems, and software) rather than pharmaceuticals, biotechnologies, or procedures [14]. The concept of technology also encompasses the facilities that house both patients and products. Facilities cover a wide spectrum — from the modern hospital on one end to the mobile imaging trailer on the other.

Quality of care (QA) and quality of improvement (QI): Quality assurance (QA) and Quality improvement (QI) are formal sets of activities to measure the quality of care provided; these usually include a process for selecting, monitoring, and applying corrective measures. The 1994 Joint Commission on the Accreditation of Healthcare Organizations (JCAHO) standards require hospital QA, programs to focus on patient outcomes as a primary reference. JCAHO standards for plant, technology, and safety management (PTSM), in turn, require certain equipment management practices and QA or QI activities. Identified QI deficiencies may influence equipment planning, and QI audits may increase awareness of technology overuse or under utilization.

Risk management: Risk management is a program that helps the hospital avoid the possibility of risks, minimize liability exposure, and stay compliant with regulatory reporting requirements. JCAHO PTSM standards require minimum technology-based risk-management activities. These include clinical engineering's determination of technology-related incidents with follow-up steps to prevent recurrences and evaluation and documentation of the effectiveness of these steps.

Safety: Safety is the condition of being safe from danger, injury, or damage. It is judgment about the acceptability of risk in a specified situation (e.g., for a given medical problem) by a provider with specified training at a specified type of facility equipment.

Standards [14]: A wide variety of formal standards and guidelines related to health care technology now exists. Some standards apply to design, development, and manufacturing practices for devices, software, and pharmaceuticals; some are related to the construction and operation of a health care facility; some are safety and performance requirements for certain classes of technologies, such as standards related to radiation or electrical safety; and others relate to performance, or even construction specifications, for specific types of technologies. Other standards and guidelines deal with administrative, medical, and surgical procedures and the training of clinical personnel. Standards and guidelines are produced and adopted by government agencies, international organizations, and professional and specialty organizations and societies. ECRI's Healthcare Standards Directory lists over 20,000 individual standards and guidelines produced by over 600 organizations and agencies from North America alone.

Strategic technology planning: Strategic technology planning encompasses both technologies new to the hospital and replacements for existing equipment that are to be acquired over several quarters. Acquisitions can be proposed for reasons related to safety, standard-of-care issues, and age or obsolescence of existing equipment. Acquisitions also can be proposed to consolidate several service area, expand a service area to reduce cost of service, or add a new service area.

Strategic technology planning optimizes the way the hospital's capital resources contribute to its mission. It encourages choosing new technologies that are cost-effective, and it also allows the hospital to be competitive in offering state-of-the-art services. Strategic technology planning works for a single department, product line, or clinical service. It can be limited to one or several high-priority areas. It also can be used for an entire multihospital system or geographic region [2].

Technology assessment: Assessment of medical technology is any process used for examining and reporting properties of medical technology used in health care, such as safety, efficacy, feasibility, and indications for use, cost, and cost-effectiveness, as well as social, economic, and ethical consequences, whether intended or unintended [15]. A primary technology assessment is one that seeks new, previously nonexistent data through research, typically employing long-term clinical studies of the type described below. A secondary technology assessment is usually based on published data, interviews, questionnaires, and other information-gathering methods rather than original research that creates new, basic data.

In technology assessment, there are six basic objectives that the clinical engineering department should have in mind. First, there should be ongoing monitoring of developments concerning new and emerging technologies. For new technologies, there should be an assessment of the clinical efficacy, safety, and cost/benefit ratio, including their effects on established technologies. There should be an evaluation of the short- and long-term costs and benefits of alternate approaches to managing specific clinical conditions. The appropriateness of existing technologies and their clinical uses should be estimated, while outmoded technologies should be identified and eliminated from their duplicative uses. The department should rate specific technology-based interventions in terms of improved overall value (quality and outcomes) to patients, providers, and payers. Finally, the department should facilitate a continuous uniformity between needs, offerings, and capabilities [16].

The locally based (hospital or hospital group) technology assessment described in this chapter is a process of secondary assessment that attempts to judge whether a certain medical equipment/product can be assimilated into the local operational environment.

Technology diffusion [14]: The process by which a technology is spread over time in a social system. The progression of technology diffusion can be described in four stages. The emerging or applied research stage occurs around the time of initial clinical testing. In the new stage, the technology has passed the phase of clinical trials but is not yet in widespread use. During the established stage, the technology is considered by providers to be a standard approach to a particular condition and diffuses into general use. Finally, in the obsolete/outmoded stage, the technology is superseded by another and is demonstrated to be ineffective or harmful.

Technology life cycle: Technology has a life cycle — a process by which technology is created, tested, applied, and replaced or abandoned. Since the life cycle varies from basic research and innovation to obsolescence and abatement, it is critical to know the maturity of a technology prior to making decisions regarding its adoption. Technology forecast assessment of pending technological changes are the investigative tools that support systematic and rational decisions about the utilization of a given institution's technological capabilities.

Technology planning and management [16]: Technology planning and management are an accountable, systematic approach to ensuring that cost-effective, efficacious, appropriate, and safe equipment is available to meet the demands of quality patient care and allow an institution to remain competitive. Elements include in-house service management, management and analysis of equipment external service providers, involvement in the equipment acquisition process, involvement of appropriate hospital personnel in facility planning and design, involvement in reducing technology-related patient and staff incidents, training equipment users, reviewing equipment replacement needs, and ongoing assessment of emerging technologies [2].

References

[1] ECRI. Healthcare Technology Assessment Curriculum. Philadelphia, August 1992.

[2] Banata H.D. Institute of Medicine. Assessing Medical Technologies. Washington, National Academy Press, 1985.

[3] Lumsdon K. Beyond technology assessment: balancing strategy needs, strategy. *Hospitals* 15: 25, 1992.

[4] ECRI. Capital, Competition, and Constraints: Managing Healthcare in the 1990s. A Guide for Hospital Executives. Philadelphia, 1992.

[5] Berkowtiz D.A. and Solomon R.P. Providers may be missing opportunities to improve patient outcomes. *Costs, Outcomes Measure Manage* May–June: 7, 1991.

[6] ECRI. Regional Healthcare Technology Planning and Management Program. Philadelphia, 1990.

[7] Sprague G.R. Managing technology assessment and acquisition. *Health Exec.* 6: 26, 1988.

[8] David Y. Technology-related decision-making issues in hospitals. In *IEEE Engineering in Medicine and Biology Society. Proceedings of the 11th Annual International Conference*, 1989.

[9] Wagner M. Promoting hospitals high-tech equipment. *Mod. Healthcare* 46, 1989.

[10] David Y. *Medical Technology 2001. CPA Healthcare Conference*, 1992.

[11] ECRI. Special Report on Technology Management, Health Technology. Philadelphia, 1989.

[12] ECRI. Special Report on Devices and Dollars, Philadelphia, 1988.

[13] Gullikson M.L., David Y., and Brady M.H. An automated risk management tool. JCAHO, Plant, Technology and Safety Management Review, PTSM Series, no. 2, 1993.

[14] David Y., Judd T., and ECRI. Special Report on Devices and Dollars, Philadelphia, 1988. Medical Technology Management, SpaceLabs Medical, Inc., Redmond, WA, 1993.

[15] Bronzino J.D. (ed). *Management of Medical Technology: A Primer for Clinical Engineers.* Stoneham, MA, Butterworth, 1992.

[16] David Y. *Risk Measurement For Managing Medical Technology. Conference Proceedings*, PERM-IT 1997, Australia.

76

Risk Factors, Safety, and Management of Medical Equipment

76.1 Risk Management: A Definition **76**-1
76.2 Risk Management: Historical Perspective **76**-2
76.3 Risk Management: Strategies........................... **76**-4
76.4 Risk Management: Application **76**-11
76.5 Case Studies **76**-13
76.6 Conclusions **76**-14
References **76**-15

Michael L. Gullikson
Texas Children's Hospital

76.1 Risk Management: A Definition

Inherent in the definition of risk management is the implication that the hospital environment cannot be made risk-free. In fact, the nature of medical equipment — to invasively or noninvasively perform diagnostic, therapeutic, corrective, or monitoring intervention on behalf of the patient — implies that risk is present. Therefore, a standard of acceptable risk must be established that defines manageable risk in a real-time economic environment.

Unfortunately, a preexistent, quantitative standard does not exist in terms of, for instance, mean time before failure (MTBF), number of repairs or repair redos per equipment item, or cost of maintenance that provides a universal yardstick for risk management of medical equipment. Sufficient clinical management of risk must be in place that can utilize safeguards, preventive maintenance, and failure analysis information to minimize the occurrence of injury or death to patient or employee or property damage. Therefore, a process must be put in place that will permit analysis of information and modification of the preceding factors to continuously move the medical equipment program to a more stable level of manageable risk.

Risk factors that require management can be illustrated by the example of the "double-edge" sword concept of technology (see Figure 76.1). The front edge of the sword represents the cutting edge of technology and its beneficial characteristics: increased quality, greater availability of technology, timeliness of test results and treatment, and so on. The back edge of the sword represents those liabilities which must be addressed to effectively manage risk: the hidden costs discussed in the next paragraph, our dependence on technology, incompatibility of equipment, and so on [1].

For example, the purchase and installation of a major medical equipment item may only represent 20% of the lifetime cost of the equipment [2]. If the operational budget of a nursing floor does not include

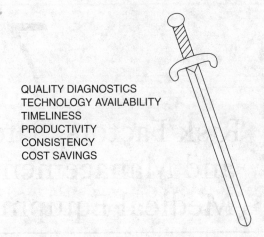

QUALITY DIAGNOSTICS
TECHNOLOGY AVAILABILITY
TIMELINESS
PRODUCTIVITY
CONSISTENCY
COST SAVINGS

HIDDEN COSTS
MULTIPLE OPTIONS
NEW SKILLS/RETRAINING
BUILT-IN OBSOLESCENCE
TECHNOLOGY
    DEPENDENCE
NON-STANDARDIZATION
INCOMPATIBILITY
TECHNICAL LANGUAGE

FIGURE 76.1   Double-edged sword concept of risk management.

the other 80% of the equipment costs, the budget constraints may require cutbacks where they appear to minimally affect direct patient care. Preventive maintenance, software upgrades that address "glitches," or overhaul requirements may be seen as unaffordable luxuries. Gradual equipment deterioration without maintenance may bring the safety level below an acceptable level of manageable risk.

Since economic factors as well as those of safety must be considered, a balanced approach to risk management that incorporates all aspects of the medical equipment lifecycle must be considered.

The operational flowchart in Figure 76.2 describe the concept of medical equipment life-cycle management from the clinical engineering department viewpoint. The flowchart includes planning, evaluation, and initial purchase documentation requirements. The condition of sale, for example, ensures that technical manuals, training, replacement parts, etc. are received so that all medical equipment might be fully supported in-house after the warranty period. Introduction to the preventive maintenance program, unscheduled maintenance procedures, and retirement justification must be part of the process. Institutional-wide cooperation with the life-cycle concept requires education and patience to convince health care providers of the team approach to managing medical equipment technology.

This balanced approach requires communication and comprehensive planning by a health care team responsible for evaluation of new and shared technology within the organization. A medical technology evaluation committee (see Figure 76.3), composed of representatives from administration, medical staff, nursing, safety department, biomedical engineering, and various services, can be an effective platform for the integration of technology and health care. Risk containment is practiced as the committee reviews not only the benefits of new technology but also the technical and clinical liabilities and provides a 6-month followup study to measure the effectiveness of the selection process. The history of risk management in medical equipment management provides helpful insight into its current status and future direction.

76.2   Risk Management: Historical Perspective

Historically, risk management of medical equipment was the responsibility of the clinical engineer (Figure 76.4). The engineer selected medical equipment based on individual clinical department consultations and established preventive maintenance (PM) programs based on manufacturer's recommendation and clinical experience. The clinical engineer reviewed the documentation and "spot-checked" equipment used in the hospital. The clinical engineer met with biomedical supervisors and technicians to discuss PM completion and to resolve repair problems. The clinical engineer then attempted to analyze failure information to avoid repeat failure.

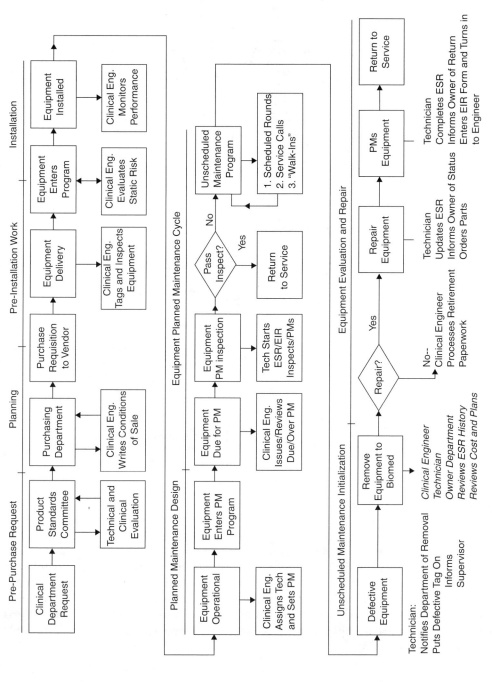

FIGURE 76.2 Biomedical engineering equipment management system (BEEMS).

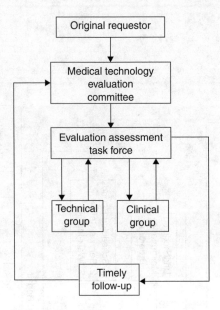

FIGURE 76.3 Medical technology evaluation committee.

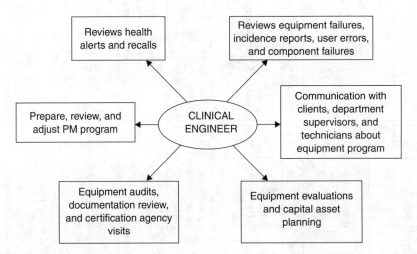

FIGURE 76.4 Operational flowchart.

However, greater public awareness of safety issues, increasing equipment density at the bed-side, more sophisticated software-driven medical equipment, and financial considerations have made it more difficult for the clinical engineer to singularly handle risk issues. In addition, the synergistic interactions of various medical systems operating in proximity to one another have added another dimension to the risk formula. It is not only necessary for health care institutions to manage risk using a team approach, but it is also becoming apparent that the clinical engineer requires more technology-intensive tools to effectively contribute to the team effort [3].

76.3 Risk Management: Strategies

Reactive risk management is an outgrowth of the historical attitude in medical equipment management that risk is an anomaly that surfaces in the form of a failure. If the failure is analyzed and proper operational

100 Medical Equipment Operator Error
101 Medical Equipment Failure
102 Medical Equipment Physical Damage
103 Reported Patient Injury
104 Reported Employee Injury
105 Medical Equipment Failed PM
108 Medical Equipment MBA

FIGURE 76.5 Failure codes.

procedures, user in-services, and increased maintenance are supplied, the problem will disappear and personnel can return to their normal work. When the next failure occurs, the algorithm is repeated. If the same equipment fails, the algorithm is applied more intensely. This is a useful but not comprehensive component of risk management in the hospital. In fact, the traditional methods of predicting the reliability of electronic equipment from field failure data have not been very effective [4]. The health care environment, as previously mentioned, inherently contains risk that must be maintained at a manageable level. A reactive tool cannot provide direction to a risk-management program, but it can provide feedback as to its efficiency.

The engine of the reactive risk-management tool is a set of failure codes (see Figure 76.5) that flag certain anomalous conditions in the medical equipment management program. If operator training needs are able to be identified, then codes 100, 102, 104, and 108 (MBA equipment returned within 9 days for a subsequent repair) may be useful. If technician difficulties in handling equipment problems are of concern, then 108 may be of interest. The key is to develop failure codes not in an attempt to define all possible anomaly modalities but for those which can clearly be defined and provide unambiguous direction for the correction process. Also, the failure codes should be linked to equipment type, manufacturer/model, technician service group, hospital, and clinical department. Again, when the data are analyzed, will the result be provided to an administrator, engineer, clinical departmental director, or safety department? This should determine the format in which the failure codes are presented.

A report intended for the clinical engineer might be formatted as in Figure 76.6. It would consist of two parts, sorted by equipment type and clinical department (not shown). The engineer's report shows the failure code activity for various types of equipment and the distribution of those failure codes in clinical departments.

Additionally, fast data-analysis techniques introduced by NASA permit the survey of large quantities of information in a three-dimensional display [5] (Figure 76.7). This approach permits viewing time-variable changes from month to month and failure concentration in specific departments and equipment types.

The importance of the format for failure modality presentation is critical to its usefulness and acceptance by health care professionals. For instance, a safety director requests the clinical engineer to provide a list of equipment that, having failed, could have potentially harmed a patient or employee. The safety director is asking the clinical engineer for a clinical judgment based on clinical as well as technical factors. This is beyond the scope of responsibility and expertise of the clinical engineer. However, the request can be addressed indirectly. The safety director's request can be addressed in two steps first, providing a list of high-risk equipment (assessed when the medical equipment is entered into the equipment inventory) and, second, a clinical judgment based on equipment failure mode, patient condition, and so on. The flowchart in Figure 76.8 provides the safety director with useful information but does not require the clinical engineer to make an unqualified clinical judgment. If the "failed PM" failure code were selected from the list of high-risk medical equipment requiring repair, the failure would be identified by the technician during routine preventive maintenance and most likely the clinician still would find the equipment clinically efficacious. This condition is a "high risk, soft failure" or a high-risk equipment item whose failure is least likely to cause injury. If the "failed PM" code were not used, the clinician would question the clinical

Source	Failed PM	Fall in Items	% Fail	Reported Fail-OK	Physical Damage	Patient Injury	Employee Injury	Back Again	Equip. Fail	Equip. Count	% Fail
10514											
PULMONARY INSTR TEXAS CHILDREN'S HOSP											
1 NON-TAGGED EQUIPMENT	0		0.00	1	5				14		0.00
1280 THERMOMETER, ELECTRONIC	2		0.00						1	99	1.01
1292 RADIANT WARMER, INFANT	1		0.00						3	63	4.76
1306 INCUBATOR, NEONATAL	0	2	0.00		7				9	56	16.07
1307 INCUBATOR, TRANSPORT, NEONATAL	9	3	33.33		1			1*	4	9	44.44
1320 PHOTOTHERAPHY UNIT, NEONATAL	4		0.00						2	28	7.14
1321 INFUSION PUMP	35		0.00	15	9			3*	34	514	6.61
1357 SUCTION, VAC POWERED, BODY FLUID	0		0.00						4	358	1.12
1384 EXAMINATION LIGHT, AC-POWERED	11		0.00	1				1*	1	47	2.13
1447 CARDIAC MONITOR W/ RATE ALARM	0		0.00		1				1		0.00
1567 SURGICAL NERVE STIMULATOR /LOC	0		0.00						2	15	13.33
1624 OTOSCOPE	73		0.00						1	101	0.99
1675 OXYGEN GAS ANALYZER	0		0.00						3	44	6.82
1681 SPIROMETER DIAGNOSTIC	0		0.00						1	8	12.50
1703 AIRWAY PRESSURE MONITOR	1		0.00					1*	7	9	77.78
1735 BREATHING GAS MIXER	13		0.00					1*	4	38	10.53
1749 HYPO/HYPERTHERMIA DEVICE	1		0.00						1	3	33.33
1762 NEBULIZER	25		0.00						1	56	1.79
1787 VENTILATOR CONTINUOUS	96	7	7.29		1			1*	11	99	11.11
1788 VENTILATOR NONCONTINUOUS	1		0.00		1				3	27	11.11
2014 HEMODIALYSIS SYSTEM ACCESSORIE	0		0.00						3	1	300.00
2051 PERITONEAL DIALYSIS SYS & ACC	4		0.00						1	5	20.00
2484 SPECTROPHOTOMETER, MASS	0		0.00						2	3	66.67
2695 POWERED SUCTION PUMP	16		0.00		1			1*	1	32	3.13
5028 PH METER	0		0.00		1				1	4	25.00
5035 COMPUTER & PERIPHERALS	0		0.00						3	18	16.67
5081 OXYGEN MONITOR	0		0.00	3					15	102	14.71
5082 RESPIRATION ANALYZER	1		0.00		1				1	5	20.00
5097 EXAM TABLE	75		0.00						1	86	1.16
5113 PRINTER	2		0.00						1	12	8.33
5126 ADDRESSOGRAPH	2		0.00						4	1	400.00
9102 STADIOMETER	0		0.00						1	8	12.50
17211 ANESTHESIA MONITOR	23		0.00						2	23	8.70
90063 POWER SUPPLY, PORTABLE	20		0.00						1	25	4.00
Total for TEXAS CHILDREN'S HOSP	415	12		20	28			9	144	1899	

FIGURE 76.6 Engineer's failure analysis report.

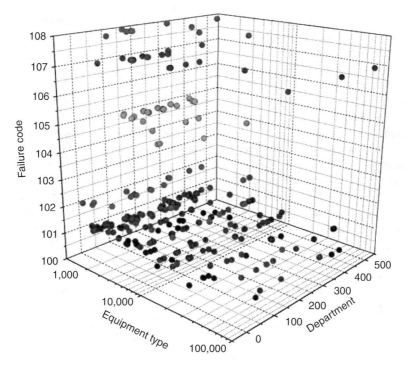

FIGURE 76.7 Failure code analysis using a 3D display.

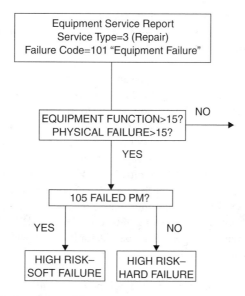

FIGURE 76.8 High-risk medical equipment failures.

efficacy of the medical equipment item, and the greater potential for injury would be identified by "high risk, hard failure." Monitoring the distribution of high-risk equipment in these two categories assists the safety director in managing risk.

Obviously, a more forward-looking tool is needed to take advantage of the failure codes and the plethora of equipment information available in a clinical engineering department. This proactive tool should use failure codes, historical information, the "expert" knowledge of the clinical engineer, and the baseline of an established "manageable risk" environment (perhaps not optimal but stable).

The overall components and process flow for a proactive risk-management tool [6] are presented in Figure 76.9. It consists of a two-component static risk factor, a two-component dynamic risk factor, and two "shaping" or feedback loops.

The static risk factor classifies new equipment by a generic equipment type: defibrilator, electrocardiograph, pulse oximeter, etc. When equipment is introduced into the equipment database, it is assigned to two different static risk (Figure 76.10) categories [7]. The first is the equipment function that defines the application and environment in which the equipment item will operate. The degree of interaction with the patient is also taken into account. For example, a therapeutic device would have a higher risk assignment than a monitoring or diagnostic device. The second component of the static risk factor is the physical risk category. It defines the worst-cases scenario in the event of equipment malfunction. The correlation between equipment function and physical risk on many items might make the two categories appear redundant. However, there are sufficient equipment types where there is not the case. A scale of 1–25 is assigned to each risk category. The larger number is assigned to devices demonstrating greater risk because of their function or the consequences of device failure. The 1–25 scale is an arbitrary assignment, since a validated scale of risk factors for medical equipment, as previously described, is nonexistent. The risk points assigned to the equipment from these two categories are algebraically summed and designated the static risk factor. This value remains with the equipment type and the individual items within that equipment type permanently. Only if the equipment is used in a clinically variant way or relocated to a functionally different environment would this assignment be reviewed and changed.

The dynamic component (Figure 76.11) of the risk-management tool consists or two parts. The first is a maintenance requirement category that is divided into 25 equally spaced divisions, ranked by least (1) to greatest (25) average manhours per device per year. These divisions are scaled by the maintenance hours for the equipment type requiring the greatest amount of maintenance attention. The amount of nonplanned (repair) manhours from the previous 12 months of service reports is totaled for each equipment type. Since this is maintenance work on failed equipment items, it correlates with the risk associated with that equipment type.

If the maintenance hours of an equipment type are observed to change to the point of placing it in a different maintenance category, a flag notifies the clinical engineer to review the equipment-type category. The engineer may increase the PM schedule to compensate for the higher unplanned maintenance hours. If the engineer believes the system "overacted," a "no" decision adjusts a scaling factor by a −5%. Progressively, the algorithm is "shaped" for the equipment maintenance program in that particular institution. However, to ensure that critical changes in the average manhours per device for each equipment type is not missed during the shaping period, the system is initialized. This is accomplished by increasing the average manhours per device for each equipment type to within 5% of the next higher maintenance requirement division. Thus the system is sensitized to variations in maintenance requirements.

The baseline is now established for evaluating individual device risk. Variations in the maintenance requirement hours for any particular equipment type will, for the most part, only occur over a substantial period of time. For this reason, the maintenance requirement category is designated a "slow" dynamic risk element.

The second dynamic element assigns weighted risk points to individual equipment items for each unique risk occurrence. An occurrence is defined as when the device:

- Exceeds the American Hospital Association Useful Life Table for Medical Equipment or exceeds the historical MTBF for that manufacturer and model
- Injures a patient or employee
- Functionally fails or fails to pass a PM inspection
- Is returned for repair or returned for rerepair within 9 days of a previous repair occurrence
- Misses a planned maintenance inspection

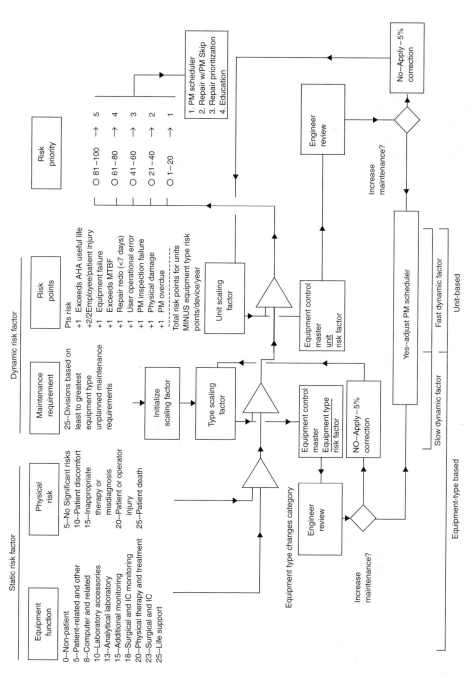

FIGURE 76.9 Biomedical engineering risk-management tool.

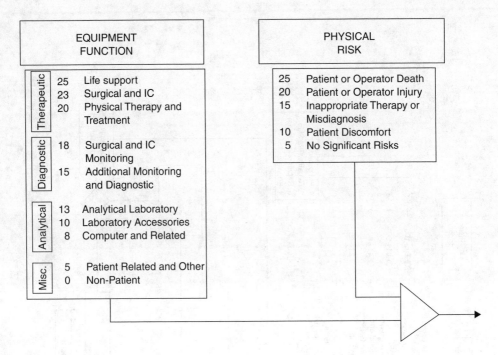

FIGURE 76.10   Static risk components.

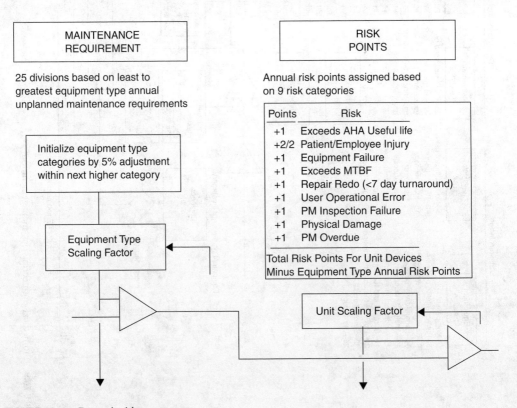

FIGURE 76.11   Dynamic risk components.

- Is subjected to physical damage
- Was reported to have failed but the problem was determined to be a user operational error

Their risk occurrences include the failure codes previously described. Although many other risk occurrences could be defined, these nine occurrences have been historically effective in managing equipment risk. The risk points for each piece or equipment are algebraically summed over the previous year. Since the yearly total is a moving window, the risk points will not continue to accumulate but will reflect a recent historical average risk. The risk points for each equipment type are also calculated. This provides a baseline to measure the relative risk of devices within an equipment type. The average risk points for the equipment type are subtracted from those for each piece of equipment within the equipment type. If the device has a negative risk point value, the device's risk is less than the average device in the equipment type. If positive, then the device has higher risk than the average device. This positive or negative factor is algebraically summed to the risk values from the equipment function, physical risk, and maintenance requirements. The annual risk points for an individual piece of equipment might change quickly over several months. For this reason, this is the "fast" component of the dynamic risk factor.

The concept of risk has now been quantified in term of equipment function, physical risk, maintenance requirements, and risk occurrences. The total risk count for each device then places it in one of five risk priority groups that are based on the sum of risk points. These groups are then applied in various ways to determine repair triage, PM triage, educational and in-service requirements and test equipment/parts, etc. in the equipment management program.

Correlation between the placement of individual devices in each risk priority group and the levels of planned maintenance previously assigned by the clinical engineer have shown that the proactive risk-management tool calculates a similar maintenance schedule as manually planned by the clinical engineer. In other words, the proactive risk-management tool algorithm places equipment items in a risk priority group commensurate with the greater or lesser maintenance as currently applied in the equipment maintenance program.

As previously mentioned, the four categories and the 1 to 25 risk levels within each category are arbitrary because a "gold standard" for risk management is nonexistent. Therefore, the clinical engineer is given input into the dynamic components making up the risk factor to "shape the system" based on the equipment's maintenance history and the clinical engineer's experience. Since the idea of a safe medical equipment program involves "judgment about the acceptability of risk in a specified situation" [8], this experience is a necessary component of the risk-assessment tool for a specific health care setting.

In the same manner, the system tracks the unit device's assigned risk priority group. If the risk points for a device change sufficiently to place it in a different group, it is flagged for review. Again, the clinical engineer reviews the particular equipment item and decides if corrective action is prudent. Otherwise, the system reduces the scaling factor by 5%. Over a period of time, the system will be "formed" to what is acceptable risk and what deserves closer scrutiny.

76.4   Risk Management: Application

The information can be made available to the clinical engineer in the form of a risk assessment report (see Figure 76.12). The report lists individual devices by property tag number (equipment control number), manufacturer, model, and equipment type. Assigned values for equipment function and physical risk are constant for each equipment type. The maintenance sensitizing factor enables the clinical engineer to control the algorithm's response to the maintenance level of an entire equipment type. These factors combine to produce the slow risk factor (equipment function + physical risk + maintenance requirements). The unit risk points are multiplied for the unit scaling factor, which allows the clinical engineer to control the algorithm's response to static and dynamic risk components on individual pieces of equipment. This number is then added to the slow risk factor to determine the risk factor for each item. The last two columns are the risk priority that the automated system has assigned and the PM level set by the clinical

Equip. Control Number	Manuf.	Model	Equipment Type	Equip. Func.	Phys. Risk	Maint. Avg. Requir	Hours	Maint. Sensitiz. Factor	Slow Risk Factor	Unit Risk Points	Unit Scaling Factor	Risk Factor	Risk Priority	Equip. Type Priority
Manager:														
			PHYSIOLOGICAL GROUP											
17407	322	4000A	NIBP SYSTEM	18	15	1	1.66	1.78	38	6.62	1.00	41	3	2
17412	322	4000A	NIBP SYSTEM	18	15	1	1.66	1.78	38	6.62	1.00	41	3	2
17424	322	4000A	NIBP SYSTEM	18	15	1	1.66	1.78	38	6.62	1.00	41	3	2
17431	322	4000A	NIBP SYSTEM	18	15	1	1.66	1.78	38	6.62	1.00	41	3	2
15609	65	BW5	BLOOD & PLMA WARMING DEVICE	5	5	1	2.51	1.17	14	10.64	1.00	22	2	1
3538	167	7370000	HR/RESP MONITOR	18	15	1	0.10	29.47	35	8.69	1.00	43	3	2
3543	167	7370000	HR/RESP MONITOR	18	15	1	0.10	29.47	35	7.69	1.00	42	3	2
15315	167	7370000	HR/RESP MONITOR	18	15	1	0.10	29.47	35	7.69	1.00	42	3	2
17761	167	7370000	HR/RESP MONITOR	18	15	1	0.10	29.47	35	6.69	1.00	41	3	2
18382	574	N100C	PULSE OXIMETER	18	15	1	0.70	4.21	35	7.54	1.00	42	3	2
180476	574	N100C	PULSE OXIMETER	18	15	1	0.70	4.21	35	7.54	1.00	42	3	2
16685	167	7275217	2 CHAN CHART REC	18	15	1	0.42	7.02	37	6.83	1.00	41	3	2

FIGURE 76.12 Engineer's risk-assessment report.

engineer. This report provides the clinical engineer with information about medical equipment that reflects a higher than normal risk factor for the equipment type to which it belongs.

The proactive risk management tool can be used to individually schedule medical equipment devices for PM based on risk assessment. For example, why should newer patient monitors be maintained at the same maintenance level as older units if the risk can be demonstrated to be less? The tool is used as well to prioritize the planned maintenance program. For instance, assume a PM cycle every 17 weeks is started on January 1 for a duration of 1 week. Equipment not currently available for PM can be inspected at a later time as a function of the risk priority group for that device. In other words, an equipment item with a risk priority of 2, which is moderately low, would not be overdue for 2/5 of the time between the current and the next PM start date or until the thirteenth week after the start of a PM cycle of 17 weeks. The technicians can complete more critical overdue equipment first and move on to less critical equipment later.

Additionally, since PM is performed with every equipment repair, is it always necessary to perform the following planned PM? Assume for a moment that unscheduled maintenance was performed 10 weeks into the 17 weeks between the two PM periods discussed above. IF the equipment has a higher risk priority of the three, four, or five, the equipment is PMed as scheduled in April. However, if a lower equipment risk priority of one or two is indicated, the planned maintenance is skipped in April and resumed in July. The intent of this application is to reduce maintenance costs, preserve departmental resources, and minimize the war and tear on equipment during testing.

Historically, equipment awaiting service has been placed in the equipment holding area and inspected on a first in, first out (FIFO) basis when a technician is available. A client's request to expedite the equipment repair was the singular reason for changing the work priority schedule. The proactive risk-management tool can prioritize the equipment awaiting repair, putting the critical equipment back into service more quickly, subject to the clinical engineer's review.

76.5 Case Studies

Several examples are presented of the proactive risk-assessment tool used to evaluate the performance of medical equipment within a program.

The ventilators in Figure 76.13 show a decreasing unit risk factor for higher equipment tag numbers. Since devices are put into service with ascending tag numbers and these devices are known to have

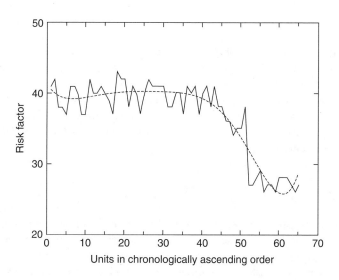

FIGURE 76.13 Ventilator with time-dependent risk characteristics.

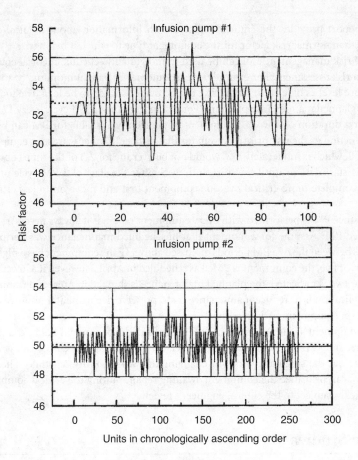

FIGURE 76.14   Time-independent risk characteristics infusion pump #1.

been purchased over a period of time, the x-axis represents a chronological progression. The ventilator risk factor is decreasing for newer units and could be attributable to better maintenance technique or manufacturer design improvements. This device is said to have a time-dependent risk factor.

A final illustration uses two generations of infusion pumps from the same manufacturer. Figure 76.14 shows the older vintage pump as Infusion Pump 1 and the newer version as Infusion Pump 2. A linear regression line for the first pump establishes the average risk factor as 53 with a standard deviation of 2.02 for the 93 pumps in the analysis. The second pump, a newer version of the first, had an average risk factor of 50 with a standard deviation of 1.38 for 261 pumps. Both pumps have relatively time-independent risk factors. The proactive risk-management tool reveals that this particular brand of infusion pump in the present maintenance program is stable over time and the newer pump has reduced risk and variability of risk between individual units. Again, this could be attributable to tighter manufacturing control or improvements in the maintenance program.

76.6   Conclusions

In summary, superior risk assessment within a medical equipment management program requires better communication, teamwork, and information analysis and distribution among all health care providers. Individually, the clinical engineer cannot provide all the necessary components for managing risk in the health care environment. Using historical information to only address equipment-related problems, after an incident, is not sufficient. The use of a proactive risk-management tool is necessary.

The clinical engineer can use this tool to deploy technical resources in a cost-effective manner. In addition to the direct economic benefits, safety is enhanced as problem equipment is identified and monitored more frequently. The integration of a proactive risk-assessment tool into the equipment management program can more accurately bring to focus technical resources in the health care environment.

References

[1] Gullikson M.L. (1994). Biotechnology Procurement and Maintenance II: Technology Risk Management. *Proceedings of the 3rd Annual International Pediatric Colloquium*, Houston, TX.

[2] David Y. (1992). Medical Technology 2001. *Health Care Conference*, Texas Society of Certified Public Accountants, San Antonio, TX.

[3] Gullikson M.L. (1993). An Automated Risk Management Tool. Plant, Technology, and Safety Management Series, Joint Commission on the Accreditation of Healthcare Facilities (JCAHO) Monograph 2.

[4] Pecht M.L. and Nash F.R. (1994). Predicting the reliability of electronic equipment. *Proceedings of the IEEE* 82: 990.

[5] Gullikson M.L. and David Y. (1993). Risk-Based Equipment Management Systems. *Proceedings of the 9th National Conference on Medical Technology Management*, American Society for Hospital Engineering of the American Hospital Association (AHA), New York, Orleans, LA.

[6] Gullikson M.L. (1992). Biomedical Equipment Maintenance System. *Proceedings of the 27th Annual Meeting and Exposition, Hospital and Medical Industry Computerized Maintenance Systems*, Association for the Advancement of Medical Instrumentation (AAMI), Anaheim, CA.

[7] Fennigkoh L. (1989). Clinical Equipment Management. Plant, Technology, and Safety Management Monograph 2.

[8] David Y. and Judd T. (1993). *Medical Technology Management*, Biophysical Measurement Series. Spacelabs Medical, Inc., Redmond, WA.

77

Clinical Engineering Program Indicators

77.1	Department Philosophy	**77-2**
	Monitoring Internal Operations • Process for Quality Improvement • External Comparisons	
77.2	Standard Database	**77-3**
77.3	Measurement Indicators	**77-4**
77.4	Indicator Management Process	**77-5**
77.5	Indicator Example 1: Productivity Monitors	**77-7**
77.6	Indicator Example 2: Patient Monitors IPM	**77-8**
	Completion Time	
77.7	Summary	**77-8**
References		**77-9**

Dennis D. Autio
Robert L. Morris
Dybonics, Inc.

The role, organization, and structure of clinical engineering departments in the modern health care environment continue to evolve. During the past 10 years, the rate of change has increased considerably faster than mere evolution due to fundamental changes in the management and organization of health care. Rapid, significant changes in the health care sector are occurring in the United States and in nearly every country. The underlying drive is primarily economic, the recognition that resources are finite.

Indicators are essential for survival of organizations and are absolutely necessary for effective management of change. Clinical engineering departments are not exceptions to this rule. In the past, most clinical engineering departments were task-driven and their existence justified by the tasks performed. Perhaps the most significant change occurring in clinical engineering practice today is the philosophical shift to a more business-oriented, cost-justified, bottom-line-focused approach than has been generally the case in the past.

Changes in the health care delivery system will dictate that clinical engineering departments justify their performance and existence on the same basis as any business, the performance of specific functions at a high quality level and at a competitive cost. Clinical engineering management philosophy must change from a purely task-driven methodology to one that includes the economics of department performance. Indicators need to be developed to measure this performance. Indicator data will need to be collected and analyzed. The data and indicators must be objective and defensible. If it cannot be measured, it cannot be managed effectively.

Indicators are used to measure performance and function in three major areas. Indicators should be used as internal measurements and monitors of the performance provided by individuals, teams, and the department. These essentially measure what was done and how it was done. Indicators are essential during quality improvement and are used to monitor and improve a process. A third important type of program indicator is the benchmark. It is common knowledge that successful businesses will continue to use benchmarks, even though differing terminology will be used. A business cannot improve its competitive position unless it knows where it stands compared with similar organizations and businesses.

Different indicators may be necessary depending on the end purpose. Some indicators may be able to measure internal operations, quality improvement, and external benchmarks. Others will have a more restricted application.

It is important to realize that a single indicator is insufficient to provide the information on which to base significant decisions. Multiple indicators are necessary to provide cross-checks and verification. An example might be to look at the profit margin of a business. Even if the profit margin per sale is 100%, the business will not be successful if there are few sales. Looking at single indicators of gross or net profit will correct this deficiency but will not provide sufficient information to point the way to improvements in operations.

77.1 Department Philosophy

A successful clinical engineering department must define its mission, vision, and goals as related to the facility's mission. A mission statement should identify what the clinical engineering department does for the organization. A vision statement identifies the direction and future of the department and must incorporate the vision statement of the parent organization. Department goals are then identified and developed to meet the mission and vision statements for the department and organization. The goals must be specific and attainable. The identification of goals will be incomplete without at least implied indicators. Integrating the mission statement, vision statement, and goals together provides the clinical engineering department management with the direction and constraints necessary for effective planning.

Clinical engineering managers must carefully integrate mission, vision, and goal information to develop a strategic plan for the department. Since available means are always limited, the manager must carefully assess the needs of the organization and available resources, set appropriate priorities, and determine available options. The scope of specific clinical engineering services to be provided can include maintenance, equipment management, and technology management activities. Once the scope of services is defined, strategies can be developed for implementation. Appropriate program indicators must then be developed to document, monitor, and manage the services to be provided. Once effective indicators are implemented, they can be used to monitor internal operations and quality-improvement processes and complete comparisons with external organizations.

77.1.1 Monitoring Internal Operations

Indicators may be used to provide an objective, accurate measurement of the different services provided in the department. These can measure specific individual, team, and departmental performance parameters. Typical indicators might include simple tallies of the quantity or level of effort for each activity, productivity (quantify/effort), percentage of time spent performing each activity, percentage of scheduled IPMs (inspection and preventive maintenance procedures) completed within the scheduled period, mean time per job by activity, repair jobs not completed within 30 days, parts order for greater than 60 days, etc.

77.1.2 Process for Quality Improvement

When program indicators are used in a quality-improvement process, an additional step is required. Expectations must be quantified in terms of the indicators used. Quantified expectations result in the establishment of a threshold value for the indicator that will precipitate further analysis of the process. Indicators combined with expectations (threshold values of the indicators) identify the opportunities for program improvement. Periodic monitoring to determine if a program indicator is below (or above, depending on whether you are measuring successes or failures) the established threshold will provide a flag to whether the process or performance is within acceptable limits. If it is outside acceptable limits for the indicator, a problem has been identified. Further analysis may be required to better define the problem. Possible program indicators for quality improvement might include the number of repairs completed within 24 or 48 h, the number of callbacks for repairs, the number of repair problems caused by user error, the percentage of hazard notifications reviewed and acted on within a given time frame, meeting time targets for generating specification, evaluation or acceptance of new equipment, etc.

An example might be a weekly status update of the percentage of scheduled IPMs completed. Assume that the department has implemented a process in which a group of scheduled IPMs must be completed within 8 weeks. The expectation is that 12% of the scheduled IPMs will be completed each week. The indicator is the percentage of IPMs completed. The threshold value of the indicator is 12% per week increase in the percentage of IPMs completed. To monitor this, the number of IPMs that were completed must be tallied, divided by the total number scheduled, and multiplied by 100 to determine the percentage completed. If the number of completed IPMs is less than projected, then further analysis would be required to identify the source of the problem and determine solutions to correct it. If the percentage of completed IPMs were equal to or greater than the threshold or target, then no action would be required.

77.1.3 External Comparisons

Much important and useful information can be obtained by carefully comparing one clinical engineering program with others. This type of comparison is highly valued by most hospital administrators. It can be helpful in determining performance relative to competitors. External indicators or benchmarks can identify specific areas of activity in need of improvement. They offer insights when consideration is being given to expanding into new areas of support. Great care must be taken when comparing services provided by clinical engineering departments located in different facilities. There are number of factors that must be included in making such comparisons; otherwise, the results can be misleading or misinterpreted. It is important that the definition of the specific indicators used be well understood, and great care must be taken to ensure that the comparison utilizes comparable information before interpreting the comparisons. Failure to understand the details and nature of the comparison and just using the numbers directly will likely result in inappropriate actions by managers and administrators. The process of analysis and explanation of differences in benchmark values between a clinical engineering department and a competitor (often referred to as gap analysis) can lead to increased insight into department operations and target areas for improvements.

Possible external indicators could be the labor cost per hour, the labor cost per repair, the total cost per repair, the cost per bed supported, the number of devices per bed supported, percentage of time devoted to repairs vs. IPMs vs. consultation, cost of support as a percentage of the acquisition value of capital inventory, etc.

77.2 Standard Database

> In God we trust . . . all others bring data!
>
> —*Florida Power and Light*

Evaluation of indicators requires the collection, storage, and analysis of data from which the indicators can be derived. A standard set of data elements must be defined. Fortunately, one only has to look at commercially available equipment management systems to determine the most common data elements used. Indeed, most of the high-end software systems have more data elements than many clinical engineering departments are willing to collect. These standard data elements must be carefully defined and understood. This is especially important if the data will later be used for comparisons with other organizations. Different departments often have different definitions for the same data element. It is crucial that the data collected be accurate and complete. The members of the clinical engineering department must be trained to properly gather, document, and enter the data into the database. It makes no conceptual difference if the database is maintained on paper or using computers. Computers and their databases are ubiquitous and so much easier to use that usually more data elements are collected when computerized systems are used. The effort required for analysis is less and the level of sophistication of the analytical tools that can be used is higher with computerized systems.

The clinical engineering department must consistently gather and enter data into the database. The database becomes the practical definition of the services and work performed by the department. This standardized database allows rapid, retrospective analysis of the data to determine specific indicators identifying problems and assist in developing solutions for implementation. A minimum database should allow the gathering and storage of the following data:

In-House Labor. This consists of three elements: the number of hours spent providing a particular service, the associated labor rate, and the identity of the individual providing the service. The labor cost is not the hourly rate the technician is paid multiplied by the number of hours spent performing the service. It should include the associated indirect costs, such as benefits, space, utilities, test equipment, and tools, along with training, administrative overhead, and many other hidden costs. A simple, straightforward approach to determine an hourly labor rate for a department is to take the total budget of the department and subtract parts' costs, service contract costs, and amounts paid to outside vendors. Divide the resulting amount by the total hours spent providing services as determined from the database. This will provide an average hourly rate for the department.

Vendor Labor. This should include hours spent and rate, travel, and zone charges and any perdiem costs associated with the vendor supplied service.

Parts. Complete information on parts is important for any retrospective study of services provided. This information is similar for both in-house and vendor-provided service. It should include the part number, a description of the part, and its cost, including any shipping.

Timeless. It is important to include a number of time stamps in the data. These should include the date the request was received, data assigned, and date completed.

Problem Identification. Both a code for rapid computer searching and classification and a free text comment identifying the nature of the problem and description of service provided are important. The number of codes should be kept to as few as possible. Detailed classification schemes usually end up with significant inaccuracies due to differing interpretations of the fine gradations in classifications.

Equipment Identification. Developing an accurate equipment history depends on reliable means of identifying the equipment. This usually includes a department- and/or facility-assigned unique identification number as well as the manufacturer, vendor, model, and serial number. Identification numbers provided by asset management are often inadequate to allow tracking of interchangeable modules or important items with a value less than a given amount. Acquisition cost is a useful data element.

Service Requester. The database should include elements allowing identification of the department, person, telephone number, cost center, and location of the service requester.

77.3 Measurement Indicators

Clinical engineering departments must gather objective, quantifiable data in order to assess ongoing performance, identify new quality-improvement opportunities, and monitor the effect of improvement action plans. Since resources are limited and everything cannot be measured, certain selection criteria must be implemented to identify the most significant opportunities for indicators. High-volume, high-risk, or problem-prone processes require frequent monitoring of indicators. A new indicator may be developed after analysis of ongoing measurements or feedback from other processes. Customer feedback and surveys often can provide information leading to the development of new indicators. Department management, in consultation with the quality-management department, typically determines what indicators will be monitored on an ongoing basis. The indicators and resulting analysis are fed back to individuals and work teams for review and improvement of their daily work activities. Teams may develop new indicators during their analysis and implementation of solutions to quality-improvement opportunities.

An indicator is an objective, quantitative measurement of an outcome or process that relates to performance quality. The event being assessed can be either desirable or undesirable. It is objective in that the same measurement can be obtained by different observers. This indicator represents quantitative, measured data that are gathered for further analysis. Indicators can assess many different aspects of quality, including accessibility, appropriateness, continuity, customer satisfaction, effectiveness, efficacy, efficiency, safety, and timeliness.

A program indicator has attributes that determine its utility as a performance measure. The reliability and variability of the indicator are distinct but related characteristics. An indicator is reliable if the same measurement can be obtained by different observers. A valid indicator is one that can identify opportunities for quality improvement. As indicators evolve, their reliability and validity should improve to the highest level possible.

An indicator can specify a part of a process to be measured or the outcome of that process. An outcome indicator assesses the results of a process. Examples include the percentage of uncompleted, scheduled IPMs, or the number of uncompleted equipment repairs not completed within 30 days. A process indicator assesses an important and discrete activity that is carried out during the process. An example would be the number of anesthesia machines in which the scheduled IPM failed or the number of equipment repairs awaiting parts that are uncompleted within 30 days.

Indicators also can be classified as sentinel event indicators and aggregate data indicators. A performance measurement of an individual event that triggers further analysis is called a sentinel-event indicator. These are often undesirable events that do not occur often. These are often related to safety issues and do not lend themselves easily to quality-improvement opportunities. An example may include equipment failures that result in a patient injury.

An aggregate data indicator is a performance measurement based on collecting data involving many events. These events occur frequently and can be presented as a continuous variable indicator or as rate-based indicators. A continuous variable indicator is a measurement where the value can fall anywhere along a continuous scale. Examples could be the number of IPMs scheduled during a particular month or the number of repair requests received during a week. A rate-based variable indicator is the value of a measurement that is expressed as a proportion or a ratio. Examples could be the percentage of IPMs completed each month or the percentage of repairs completed within one workday.

General indicators should be developed to provide a baseline monitoring of the department's performance. They also should provide a cross-check for other indicators. These indicators can be developed to respond to a perceived need within a department or to solve a specific problem.

77.4 Indicator Management Process

The process to develop, monitor, analyze, and manage indicators is shown in Figure 77.1. The different steps in this process include defining the indicator, establishing the threshold, monitoring the indicator, evaluating the indicator, identifying quality-improvement opportunities, and implementing action plans.

Define Indicator. The definition of the indicator to be monitored must be carefully developed. This process includes at least five steps. The event or outcome to be measured must be described. Define any specific terms that are used. Categorize the indicator (sentinel event or rate-based, process or outcome, desirable or undesirable). The purpose for this indicator must be defined, as well as how it is used in specifying and assessing the particular process or outcome.

Establish Threshold. A threshold is a specific data point that identifies the need for the department to respond to the indicator to determine why the threshold was reached. Sentinel-event indicator thresholds are set at zero. Rate indicator thresholds are more complex to define because they may require expert

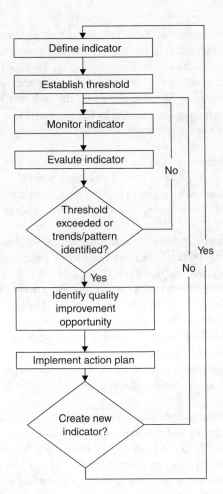

FIGURE 77.1 Indicator management process.

consensus or definition of the department's objectives. Thresholds must be identified, including the process used to set the specific level.

Monitor Indicator.   Once the indicator is defined, the data-acquisition process identifies the data sources and data elements. As these data are gathered, they must be validated for accuracy and completeness. Multiple indicators can be used for data validation and cross-checking. The use of a computerized database allows rapid access to the data. A database management tool allows quick sorting and organization of the data. Once gathered, the data must be presented in a format suitable for evaluation. Graphic presentation of data allows rapid visual analysis for thresholds, trends, and patterns.

Evaluate Indicator.   The evaluation process analyze and reports the information. This process includes comparing the information with established thresholds and analyzing for any trends or patterns. A trend is the general direction the indicator measurement takes over a period of time and may be desirable or undesirable. A pattern is a grouping or distribution of indicator measurements. A pattern analysis is often triggered when thresholds are crossed or trends identified. Additional indicator information is often required. If an indictor threshold has not been reached, no further action may be necessary, other than continuing to monitor this indicator. The department also may decide to improve its performance level by changing the threshold.

  Factors may be present leading to variation of the indicator data. These factors may include failure of the technology to perform properly, failure of the operators to use the technology properly, and failure of the organization to provide the necessary resources to implement this technology properly. Further analysis of these factors may lead to quality-improvement activities later.

Identify Quality-Improvement Opportunity. A quality-improvement opportunity may present itself if an indicator threshold is reached, a trend is identified, or a pattern is recognized. Additional information is then needed to further define the process and improvement opportunities. The first step in the process is to identify a team. This team must be given the necessary resources to complete this project, a timetable to be followed, and an opportunity to periodically update management on the status of the project. The initial phase of the project will analyze the process and establish the scope and definition of the problem. Once the problem is defined, possible solutions can be identified and analyzed for potential implementation. A specific solution to the problem is then selected. The solution may include modifying existing indictors or thresholds to more appropriate values, modifying steps to improve existing processes, or establishing new goals for the department.

Implement Action Plan. An action plan is necessary to identify how the quality-improvement solution will be implemented. This includes defining the different tasks to be performed, the order in which they will be addressed, who will perform each task, and how this improvement will be monitored. Appropriate resources must again be identified and a timetable developed prior to implementation. Once the action plan is implemented, the indicators are monitored and evaluated to verify appropriate changes in the process. New indicators and thresholds may need to be developed to monitor the solution.

77.5   Indicator Example 1: Productivity Monitors

Define Indicator. Monitor the productivity of technical personnel, teams, and the department. Productivity is defined as the total number of documented service support hours compared with the total number of hours available. This is a desirable rate-based outcome indicator. Provide feedback to technical staff and hospital administration regarding utilization of available time for department support activities.

Establish Threshold. At least 50% of available technician time will be spent providing equipment maintenance support services (revolving equipment problems and scheduled IPMs). At least 25% of available technician time will be spent providing equipment management support services (installations, acceptance testing, incoming inspections, equipment inventory database management, hazard notification review).

Monitor Indicator. Data will be gathered every 4 weeks from the equipment work order history database. A trend analysis will be performed with data available from previously monitored 4-week intervals. These data will consist of hours worked on completed and uncompleted jobs during the past 4-week interval.

Technical staff available hours is calculated for the 4-week interval. The base time available is 160 h (40 h/week × 4 week) per individual. Add to this any overtime worked during the interval. Then subtract any holidays, sick days, and vacation days within the interval.

CJHOURS: Hours worked on completed jobs during the interval
UJHOURS: Hours worked on uncompleted jobs during the interval
AHOURS: Total hours available during the 4-week interval

$$\text{Productivity} = (\text{CJHOURS} + \text{UJHOURS})/\text{AHOURS}$$

Evaluate Indicator. The indicator will be compared with the threshold, and the information will be provided to the individual. The individual team member data can be summed for team review. The data from multiple teams can be summed and reviewed by the department. Historical indicator information will be utilized to determine trends and patterns.

Quality-Improvement Process. If the threshold is not met, a trend is identified, or a pattern is observed, a quality-improvement opportunity exists. A team could be formed to review the indicator, examine the process that the indicator measured, define the problem encountered, identify ways to solve the problem, and select a solution. An action plan will then be developed to implement this solution.

Implement Action Plan.   During implementation of the action plan, appropriate indicators will be used to monitor the effectiveness of the action plan.

77.6   Indicator Example 2: Patient Monitors IPM

77.6.1   Completion Time

Define Indicator.   Compare the mean to complete an IPM for different models of patient monitors. Different manufacturers of patient monitors have different IPM requirements. Identify the most timely process to support this equipment.

Establish Threshold.   The difference between the mean time to complete an IPM for different models of patient monitors will not be greater than 30% of the lesser time.

Monitor Indicator.   Determine the mean time to complete an IPM for each model of patient monitor. Calculate the percentage difference between the mean time for each model and the model with the least mean time.

Evaluate Indicator.   The mean time to complete IPMs was compared between the patient monitors, and the maximum difference noted was 46%. A pattern also was identified in which all IPMs for that one particular monitor averaged 15 min longer than those of other vendors.

Quality-Improvement Process.   A team was formed to address this problem. Analysis of individual IPM procedures revealed that manufacturer X requires the case to be removed to access internal filters. Performing an IPM for each monitor required moving and replacing 15 screws for each of the 46 monitors. The team evaluated this process and identified that 5 min could be saved from each IPM if an electric screwdriver was utilized.

Implement Action Plan.   Electric screwdrivers were purchased and provided for use by the technician. The completion of one IPM cycle for the 46 monitors would pay for two electric screwdrivers and provide 4 h of productive time for additional work. Actual savings were greater because this equipment could be used in the course of daily work.

77.7   Summary

In the ever-changing world of health care, clinical engineering departments are frequently being evaluated based on their contribution to the corporate bottom line. For many departments, this will require difficult and painful changes in management philosophy. Administrators are demanding quantitative measures of performance and value. To provide the appropriate quantitative documentation required by corporate managers, a clinical engineering a manager must collect available data that are reliable and accurate. Without such data, analysis is valueless. Indicators are the first step in reducing the data to meaningful information that can be easily monitored and analyzed. The indicators can then be used to determine department performance and identify opportunities for quality improvement.

Program indicators have been used for many years. What must change for clinical engineering departments is a conscious evaluation and systematic use of indicators. One traditional indicator of clinical engineering department success is whether the department's budget is approved or not. Unfortunately, approval of the budget as an indicator, while valuable, does not address the issue of predicting long-term survival, measuring program and quality improvements, or allowing frequent evaluation and changes.

There should be monitored indicators for every significant operational aspect of the department. Common areas where program indicators can be applied include monitoring interval department activities, quality-improvement processes, and benchmarking. Initially, simple indicators should be developed. The complexity and number of indicators should change as experience and needs demand.

The use of program indicators is absolutely essential if a clinical engineering departments is to survive. Program and survival are now determined by the contribution of the department to the bottom line of the parent organization. Indicators must be developed and utilized to determine the current contribution of the clinical engineering department to the organization. Effective utilization and management of program indicators will ensure future department contributions.

References

AAMI. 1993. Management Information Report MIR 1: Design of Clinical Engineering Quality Assurance Risk Management Programs. Arlington, VA, Association for the Advancement of Medical Instrumentation.

AAMI. 1993. Management Information Report MIR 2: Guideline for Establishing and Administering Medical Instrumentation Maintenance Programs. Arlington, VA, Association for the Advancement of Medical Instrumentation.

AAMI. 1994. Management Information Report MIR 3: Computerized Maintenance Management Systems for Clinical Engineering. Arlington, VA, Association for the Advancement of Medical Instrumentation.

Bauld T.J. 1987. Productivity: standard terminology and definitions. *J. Clin. Eng.* 12: 139.

Betts W.F. 1989. Using productivity measures in clinical engineering departments. *Biomed. Instrum. Technol.* 23: 120.

Bronzino J.D. 1992. *Management of Medical Technology: A Primer for Clinical Engineers.* Stoneham, MA, Butterworth-Heinemann.

Coopers and Lybrand International, AFSM. 1994. Benchmarking Impacting the Boston Line. Fort Myers, FL, Association for Services Management International.

David Y. and Judd T.M. 1993. Risk management and quality improvement. In *Medical Technology Management*, pp. 72–75. Redmond, WA, SpaceLab Medical.

David Y. and Rohe D. 1986. Clinical engineering program productivity and measurement. *J. Clin. Eng.* 11: 435.

Downs K.J. and McKinney W.D. 1991. Clinical engineering workload analysis: a proposal for standardization. *Biomed. Instrum. Technol.* 25: 101.

Fennigkoh L. 1986. ASHE Technical Document No 055880: medical equipment maintenance performance measures. Chicago, American Society for Hospital Engineers.

Furst E. 1986. Productivity and cost-effectiveness of clinical engineering. *J. Clin. Eng.* 11: 105.

Gordon G.J. 1995. Breakthrough management — a new model for hospital technical services. Arlington, VA, Association for the Advancement of Medical Instrumentation.

Hertz E. 1990. Developing quality indicators for a clinical engineering department. In *Plant, Technology and Safety Management Series: Measuring Quality in PTSM*. Chicago, Joint Commission on Accreditation of Healthcare Organizations.

JCAHO. 1990. Primer on Indicator Development and Application, Measuring Quality in Health Care. Oakbrook, IL, Joint Commission on Accreditation of Healthcare Organizations.

JCAHO. 1994. Framework for improving performance. Oakbrook, IL, Joint Commission on Accreditation of Healthcare Organizations.

Keil O.R. 1989. The challenge of building quality into clinical engineering programs. *Biomed. Instrum. Technol.* 23: 354.

Lodge D.A. 1991. Productivity, efficiency, and effectiveness in the management of healthcare technology: an incentive pay proposal. *J. Clin. Eng.* 16: 29.

Mahachek A.R. 1987. Management and control of clinical engineering productivity: a case study. *J. Clin. Eng.* 12: 127.

Mahachek A.R. 1989. Productivity measurement. Taking the first steps. *Biomed. Instrum. Technol.* 23: 16.

Selsky D.B. et al. 1991. Biomedical equipment information management for the next generation. *Biomed. Instrum. Technol.* 25: 24.

Sherwood M.K. 1991. Quality assurance in biomedical or clinical engineering. *J. Clin. Eng.* 16: 479.

Stiefel R.H. 1991. Creating a quality measurement system for clinical engineering. *Biomed. Instrum. Technol.* 25: 17.

78

Quality of Improvement and Team Building

78.1 Deming's 14 Points **78**-2
78.2 Zero Defects **78**-2
78.3 TQM (Total Quality Management)..................... **78**-3
78.4 CQI (Continuous Quality Improvement) **78**-3
78.5 Tools Used for Quality Improvement **78**-4
    Cause-and-Effect or Ishikawa Chart • Control Chart • Flowchart • Histogram • Pareto Chart • The Plan-Do-Check-Act or Shewhart Cycle
78.6 Quality Performance Indicators (QPI) **78**-8
78.7 Teams **78**-9
    Process Action Teams (PAT) • Transition Management Team (TMT) • Quality Improvement Project Team (QIPT) • Executive Steering Committee (ESC) • Quality Management Board (QMB)
78.8 Process Improvement Model........................... **78**-10
    Problem-Solving Model
78.9 Summary **78**-11
    PARADES — Seven Dimensions of Quality • Quality Has a Monetary Value!
References **78**-12

Joseph P. McClain
Walter Reed Army Medical Center

In today's complex health care environment, quality improvement and team building must go hand in hand. This is especially true for Clinical Engineers and Biomedical Equipment Technicians as the diversity of the field increases and technology moves so rapidly that no one can know all that needs to be known without the help of others. Therefore, it is important that we work together to ensure quality improvement. Ken Blachard, the author of the One Minute Manager series, has made the statement that "all of us are smarter than any one of us" — a synergy that evolves from working together.

Throughout this chapter we will look closely at defining quality and the methods for continuously improving quality, such as collecting data, interpreting indicators, and team building. All this will be put together, enabling us to make decisions based on scientific deciphering of indicators.

Quality is defined as conformance to customer or user requirements. If a product or service does what it is supposed to do, it is said to have high quality. If the product or service fails its mission, it is said to be low quality. Dr. W. Edward Demings, who is known to many as the "father of quality," defined it as surpassing customer needs and expectations throughout the life of the product or service.

Dr. Demings, a trained statistician by profession, formed his theories on quality during World War II while teaching industry how to use statistical methods to improve the quality of military production. After the war, he focused on meeting customer or consumer needs and acted as a consultant to Japanese organizations to change consumers' perceptions that "Made in Japan" meant junk. Dr. Demings predicted that people would be demanding Japanese products in just 5 years, if they used his methods. However, it only took 4, and the rest is history.

78.1 Deming's 14 Points

1. Create constancy of purpose toward improvement of product and service, with an aim to become competitive and to stay in business and provide jobs
2. Adopt the new philosophy. We are in a new economic age. Western management must awaken and lead for change
3. Cease dependence on inspection to achieve quality. Eliminate the needs for mass inspection by first building in quality
4. Improve constantly and forever the system of production and service to improve quality and productivity and thus constantly decrease costs
5. Institute training on the job
6. Institute leadership: The goal is to help people, machines, and gadgets to do a better job
7. Drive out fear so that everyone may work effectively for the organization
8. Break down barriers between departments
9. Eliminate slogans, exhortations, and targets for the workforce
10. Eliminate work standards (quota) on the factory floor
11. Substitute leadership: Eliminate management by objective, by numbers, and numerical goals
12. Remove barriers that rob the hourly worker of the right to pride of workmanship
13. Institute a vigorous program of education and self-improvement
14. Encourage everyone in the company to work toward accomplishing transformation. Transformation is everyone's job

78.2 Zero Defects

Another well-known quality theory, called zero defects (ZD), was established by Philip Crosby. It got results for a variety of reasons. The main reasons are as follows:

1. *A strict and specific management standard.* Management, including the supervisory staff, do not use vague phrases to explain what it wants. It made the quality standard very clear: Do it the right way from the start. As Philip Crosby said, "What standard would you set on how many babies nurses are allowed to drop?"
2. *Complete commitment of everyone.* Interestingly, Crosby denies that ZD was a motivational program. But ZD worked because everyone got deeply into the act. Everyone was encouraged to spot problems, detect errors, and prescribe ways and means for their removal. This commitment is best illustrated by the ZD pledge: "I freely pledge myself to make a constant, conscious effort to do my job right the first time, recognizing that my individual contribution is a vital part of the overall effort."
3. *Removal of actions and conditions that cause errors.* Philip Crosby claimed that at ITT, where he was vice-president for quality, 90% of all error causes could be acted on and fully removed by

first-line supervision. In other words, top management must do its part to improve conditions, but supervisors and employees should handle problems directly. Errors, malfunctions, and/or variances can best be corrected where the rubber hits the road — at the source.

78.3   TQM (Total Quality Management)

The most recent quality theory that has found fame is called TQM (Total Quality Management). It is a strategic, integrated management system for achieving customer satisfaction which involves all managers and employees and uses quantitative methods to continuously improve an organization's processes. Total Quality Management is a term coined in 1985 by the Naval Air Systems Command to describe its management approach to quality improvement. Simply put, TQM is a management approach to long-term success through customer satisfaction. TQM includes the following three principles (1) achieving customer satisfaction, (2) making continuous improvement, and (3) giving everyone responsibility. TQM includes eight practices. These practices are (1) focus on the customer, (2) effective and renewed communications, (3) reliance on standards and measures, (4) commitment to training, (5) top management support and direction, (6) employee involvement, (7) rewards and recognition, and (8) long-term commitment.

78.4   CQI (Continuous Quality Improvement)

Step 8 of the total quality management practices leads us to the quality concept coined by the Joint Commission On Accreditation of Healthcare Organizations and widely used by most health care agencies. It is called CQI (Continuous Quality Management). The principles of CQI are as follows:

Unity of Purpose

- Unity is established throughout the organization with a clear and widely understood vision
- Environment nurtures total commitment from all employees
- Rewards go beyond benefits and salaries to the belief that "We are family" and "We do excellent work"

Looking for Faults in the Systems

- Eighty percent of an organization's failures are the fault of management-controlled systems
- Workers can control fewer than 20% of the problems
- Focus on rigorous improvement of every system, and cease blaming individuals for problems (the 80/20 rule of J.M. Juran and the nineteenth-century economist Vilfredo Pareto)

Customer Focus

- Start with the customer
- The goal is to meet or exceed customer needs and give lasting value to the customer
- Positive returns will follow as customers boast of the company's quality and service

Obsession with Quality

- Everyone's job
- Quality is relentlessly pursued through products and services that delight the customer
- Efficient and effective methods of execution

Recognizing the Structure in Work

- All work has structure
- Structure may be hidden behind workflow inefficiency
- Structure can be studied, measured, analyzed, and improved

Freedom Through Control

- There is control, yet freedom exists by eliminating micromanagement
- Employees standardize processes and communicate the benefits of standardization
- Employees reduce variation in the way work is done
- Freedom comes as changes occur resulting in time to spend on developing improved processes, discovering new markets, and adding other methods to increase productivity

Continued Education and Training

- Everyone is constantly learning
- Educational opportunities are made available to employees
- Greater job mastery is gained and capabilities are broadened

Philosophical Issues on Training

- Training must stay tuned to current technology
- Funding must be made available to ensure that proper training can be attained
- Test, measurement, and diagnostic equipment germane to the mission must be procured and technicians trained on its proper use, calibration, and service
- Creativity must be used to obtain training when funding is scarce
  - Include training in equipment procurement process
  - Contact manufacturer or education facility to bring training to the institution
  - Use local facilities to acquire training, thus eliminating travel cost
  - Allow employees to attend professional seminars where a multitude of training is available

Teamwork

- Old rivalries and distrust are eliminated
- Barriers are overcome
- Teamwork, commitment to the team concept, and partnerships are the focus
- Employee empowerment is critical in the CQI philosophy and means that employees have the authority to make well-reasoned, data-based decisions. In essence, they are entrusted with the legal power to change processes through a rational, scientific approach

Continuous quality improvement is a means for tapping knowledge and creativity, applying participative problem solving, finding and eliminating problems that prevent quality, eliminating waste, instilling pride, and increasing teamwork. Further it is a means for creating an atmosphere of innovation for continued and permanent quality improvement. Continuous quality improvement as outlined by the Joint Commission on Accreditation of Healthcare Organizations is designed to improve the work processes within and across organizations.

78.5   Tools Used for Quality Improvement

The tools listed on the following pages will assist in developing quality programs, collecting data, and assessing performance indicators within the organization. These tools include several of the most frequently used and most of the seven tools of quality. The seven tools of quality are tools that help health care organizations understand their processes in order to improve them. The tools are the cause-and-effect diagram, check sheet, control chart, flowchart, histogram, Pareto chart, and scatter diagram. Additional tools shown are the Shewhart cycle (PDCA process) and the bar chart. The Clinical Engineering Manager must access the situation and determine which tool will work best for his/her situational needs.

Two of the seven tools of quality discussed above are not illustrated. These are the scatter diagram and the check sheet. The scatter diagram is a graphic technique to analyze the relationship between two variations and the check sheet is simple data-recording device. The check sheet is custom designed by the

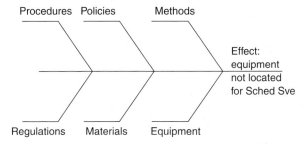

FIGURE 78.1 Cause-and-effect or Ishikawa chart.

user, which facilitates interpretation of the results. Most Biomedical Equipment Technicians use the check sheet on a daily basis when performing preventive maintenance, calibration, or electrical safety checks.

78.5.1 Cause-and-Effect or Ishikawa Chart

This is a tool for analyzing process dispersion (Figure 78.1). The process was developed by Dr. Karou Ishikawa and is also known as the fishbone diagram because the diagram resembles a fish skeleton. The diagram illustrates the main causes and subcauses leading to an effect. The cause-and-effect diagram is one of the seven tools of quality.

The following is an overview of the process:

1. Used in group problem solving as a brainstorming tool to explore and display the possible causes of a particular problem
2. The effect (problem, concern, or opportunity) that is being investigated is stated on the right side, while the contributing causes are grouped in component categories through group brainstorming on the left side
3. This is an extremely effective tool for focusing a group brainstorming session
4. Basic components include environment, methods (measurement), people, money information, materials, supplies, capital equipment, and intangibles

78.5.2 Control Chart

A control chart is a graphic representation of a characteristic of a process showing plotted values of some statistic gathered from that characteristic and one or two control limits (Figure 78.2). It has two basic uses:

1. As a judgment to determine if the process is in control
2. As an aid in achieving and maintaining statistical control

(This chart was used by Dr. W.A. Shewhart for a continuing test of statistical significance.) A control chart is a chart with a baseline, frequently in time order, on which measurement or counts are represented by points that are connected by a straight line with an upper and lower limit. The control chart is one of the seven tools of quality.

78.5.3 Flowchart

A flowchart is a pictorial representation showing all the steps of a process (Figure 78.3). Flowcharts provide excellent documentation of a program and can be a useful tool for examining how various steps in a process are related to each other. Flowcharting uses easily recognizable symbols to represent the type of processing performed. The flowchart is one of the seven tools of quality.

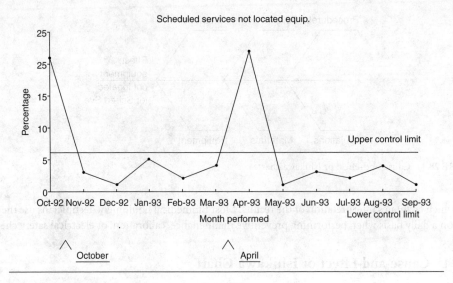

FIGURE 78.2   Control chart.

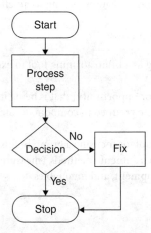

FIGURE 78.3   Flowchart.

78.5.4 Histogram

A graphic summary of variation in a set of data is a histogram (Figure 78.4). The pictorial nature of the histogram lets people see patterns that are difficult to see in a simple table of numbers. The histogram is one of the seven tools of quality.

78.5.5 Pareto Chart

A Pareto chart is a special form of vertical bar graph that helps us to determine which problems to solve and in what order (Figure 78.5). It is based on the Pareto principle, which was first developed by J.M. Juran in 1950. The principle, named after the nineteenth-century economist Vilfredo Pareto, suggests that most effects come from relatively few causes; that is, 80% of the effects come from 20% of the possible causes.

Doing a Pareto chart, based on either check sheets or other forms of data collection, helps us direct our attention and efforts to truly important problems. We will generally gain more by working on the tallest bar than tackling the smaller bars. The Pareto chart is one of the seven tools of quality.

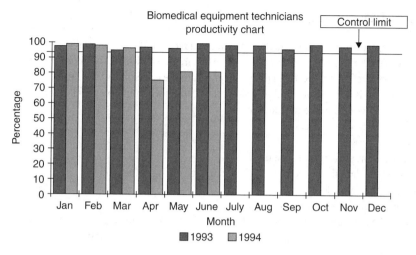

FIGURE 78.4 Histogram.

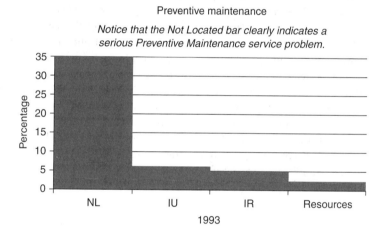

FIGURE 78.5 Pareto chart.

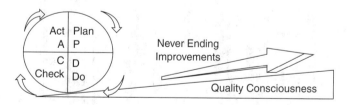

FIGURE 78.6 The Shewhart cycle.

78.5.6 The Plan-Do-Check-Act or Shewhart Cycle

This is a four-step process for quality improvement that is sometimes referred to as the Deming cycle (Figure 78.6). One of the consistent requirements of the cycle is the long-term commitment required. The Shewhart cycle or PDCA cycle is outlined here and has had overwhelming success when used properly. It is also a very handy tool to use in understanding the quality cycle process. The results of the cycle are studied to determine what was learned, what can be predicted, and appropriate changes to be implemented.

78.6   Quality Performance Indicators (QPI)

An indicator is something that suggests the existence of a fact, condition, or quality — an omen (a sign of future good or evil). It can be considered as evidence of a manifestation or symptom of an incipient failure or problem. Therefore, quality performance indicators are measurements that can be used to ensure that quality performance is continuous and will allow us to know when incipient failures are starting so that we may take corrective and preventive actions.

QPI analysis is a five-step process:

Step 1: Decide what performance we need to track
Step 2: Decide the data that need to be collected to track this performance
Step 3: Collect the data
Step 4: Establish limits, a parameter, or control points
Step 5: Utilize BME (management by exception) — where a performance exceeds the established control limits, it is indicating a quality performance failure, and corrective action must be taken to correct the problem

In the preceding section, there were several examples of QPIs. In the Pareto chart, the NL = not located, IU = in use, IR = in repair. The chart indicates that during the year 1994, 35% of the equipment could not be located to perform preventive maintenance services. This indicator tells us that we could eventually have a serious safety problem that could impact on patient care, and if not corrected, it could prevent the health care facility from meeting accreditation requirements. In the control chart example, an upper control limit of 6% "not located equipment" is established as acceptable in any one month. However, this upper control limit is exceeded during the months of April and October. This QPI could assist the clinical and Biomedical Equipment Manager in narrowing the problem down to a 2-month period. The histogram example established a lower control limit for productivity at 93%. However, productivity started to drop off in May, June, and July. This QPI tells the manager that something has happened that is jeopardizing the performance of his or her organization. Other performance indicators have been established graphically in Figure 78.7 and Figure 78.8. See if you can determine what the indicators are and what the possible cause might be. You may wish to use these tools to establish QPI tracking germane to your own organization.

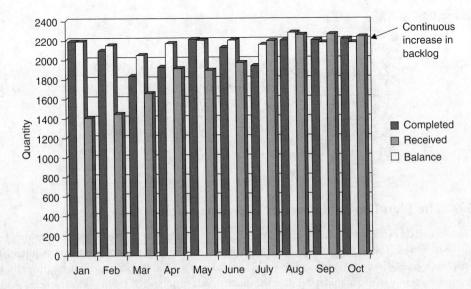

FIGURE 78.7   Sample repair service report.

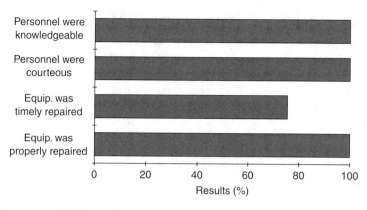

FIGURE 78.8 Customer satisfaction survey. August–September 1994.

78.7 Teams

A team is a formal group of persons organized by the company to work together to accomplish certain goals and objectives. Normally, when teams are used in quality improvement programs, they are designed to achieve the organization's vision. The organization's vision is a statement of the desired end state of the organization articulated and deployed by the executive leadership. Organizational visions are inspiring, clear, challenging, reasonable, and empowering. Effective visions honor the past, while they prepare for the future. The following are types of teams that are being used in health care facilities today. Some of the names may not be common, but their definitions are very similar if not commensurate.

78.7.1 Process Action Teams (PAT)

Process action teams are composed of those who are involved in the process being investigated. The members of a PAT are often chosen by their respective managers. The primary consideration for PAT membership is knowledge about the operations of the organization and consequently the process being studied. The main function of a PAT is the performance of an improvement project. Hence customers are often invited to participate on the team. PATs use basic statistical and other tools to analyze a process and identify potential areas for improvement. PATs report their findings to an Executive Steering Committee or some other type of quality management improving group. ("A problem well defined is half solved." John Dewey, American philosopher and educator; 1859–1952.)

78.7.2 Transition Management Team (TMT)

The transition management team (see *Harvard Business Review,* November–December 1993, pp. 109–118) is normally used for a major organizational change such as restructuring or reengineering. The TMT can be initiated due to the findings of a PAT, where it has been indicated that the process is severely broken and unsalvageable. The TMT is not a new layer of bureaucracy or a job for fading executives. The TMT oversees the large-scale corporate change effort. It makes sure that all change initiatives fit together. It is made up of 8 to 12 highly talented leaders who commit all their time making the transition a reality. The team members and what they are trying to accomplish must be accepted by the power structure of the organization. For the duration of the change process, they are the CEO's version of the National Guard. The CEO should be able to say, "I can sleep well tonight, the TMT is managing this." In setting up a TMT, organizations should adopt a fail–safe approach: Create a position to oversee the emotional and behavioral issues unless you can prove with confidence that you do not need one.

78.7.3 Quality Improvement Project Team (QIPT)

A quality improvement project team can be initiated due to the findings of a PAT, where it has been indicated that the process is broken. The main agenda of the QIPT is to improve the work process that managers have identified as important to change. The team studies this process methodically to find permanent solutions to problems. To do this, members can use many of the tools described in this chapter and in many other publications on quality and quality improvement available from schools, bookstores, and private organizations.

78.7.4 Executive Steering Committee (ESC)

This is an executive-level team composed of the Chief Executive Officer (CEO) of the organization and the executive staff that reports directly to the CEO. Whereas an organization may have numerous QMBs, PATs, and QIPTs, it has only one ESC. The ESC identifies strategic goals for organizational quality improvement efforts. It obtains information from customers to identify major product and service requirements. It is through the identification of these major requirements that quality goals for the organization are defined. Using this information, the ESC lists, prioritizes, and determines how to measure the organization's goals for quality improvement. The ESC develops the organization's improvement plan and manages the execution of that plan to ensure that improvement goals are achieved.

78.7.5 Quality Management Board (QMB)

This is a permanent cross-functional team made up of top and midlevel managers who are jointly responsible for a specific product, service, or process. The structure of the board intended to improve communication and cooperation by providing vertical and horizontal "links" throughout the organization.

78.8 Process Improvement Model

This process is following the Joint Commission on the Accreditation of Healthcare Organizations' Quality Cube, a method of assessing the quality of the organization.

Plan:

1. Identify the process to be monitored
2. Select important functions and dimensions of performance applicable to the process identified
3. Design a tool for collection of data

Measure (Under this heading, you will document how, when, and where data was collected):

1. Collect data
2. Select the appropriate tool to deliver your data (charts, graphs, tables, etc.)

Assess (Document findings under this heading):

1. Interpret data collected
2. Design and implement change
   - Redesign the process or tool if necessary
   - If no changes are necessary, then you have successfully used the Process Improvement pathway

Improvement (Document details here):

1. Set in place the process to gain and continue the improvement

Outcome (Document all changes here):

1. Positive changes made to improve quality of care based on Performance Improvement Activity

78.8.1 Problem-Solving Model

The FOCUS-PDCA/PMAIO Process Improvement Model is a statistical-based quality control method for improving processes. This approach to problem-solving could be used by all Process Action Teams to ensure uniformity within an organization. FOCUS-PDCA/PMAIO is as follows:

F — Find a process to improve.
O — Organize a team that knows the process.
C — Clarify current knowledge of the process.
U — Understand the cause or variations.
S — Select the process to improve.
P — Plan the improvement. P — Plan
D — Do the improvement (pilot test). M — Measure
C — Check the results of the improvement. A — Assess
A — Act to hold the gain. I — Improve
O — Outcome

78.9   Summary

Although quality can be simply defined as conformity to customer or user requirements, it has many dimensions. Seven of them are described here (1) performance, (2) aesthetics, (3) reliability (how dependably it performs), (4) availability (there when you need it), (5) durability (how long it lasts), (6) extras or features (supplementary items), and (7) serviceability (how easy it is to get serviced). The word PARADES can help you remember this.

78.9.1 PARADES — Seven Dimensions of Quality

1. *Performance*: A product or service that performs its intended function well scores high on this dimension of quality
2. *Aesthetics*: A product or service that has a favorable appearance, sound, taste, or smell is perceived to be of good quality
3. *Reliability*: Reliability, or dependability, is such an important part of product quality that quality-control engineers are sometimes referred to as reliability engineers
4. *Availability*: A product or service that is there when you need it
5. *Durability*: Durability can be defined as the amount of use one gets from a product before it no longer functions properly and replacement seems more feasible than constant repair
6. *Extras*: Feature or characteristics about a product or service that supplements its basic functioning (i.e., remote control dialing on a television)
7. *Serviceability*: Speed, courtesy, competence, and ease of repair are all important quality factors

78.9.2 Quality Has a Monetary Value!

Good quality often pays for itself, while poor quality is expensive in both measurable costs and hidden costs. The hidden costs include loss of goodwill, including loss of repeat business and badmouthing of the firm. High quality goods and services often carry a higher selling price than do those of low quality. This information is evidenced by several reports in the Wall Street Journal, Forbes Magazine, Money Magazine, Business Week Magazine, etc. A good example is the turnaround of Japanese product sales using quality methodologies outlined in The Deming Guide to Quality and Competitive Position, by Howard S. and Shelly J. Gitlow. As Dr. Demings has stated, quality improvement must be continuous!

Quality is never an accident; it has always the result of intelligent energy.

John Ruskin, 1819–1900, English art critic and historian
Seven Lamps of Architecture

References

Bittel L.R. 1985. *Every Supervisor Should Know*, 5th ed., pp. 455–456. New York, Gregg Division/ McGraw-Hill.

DuBrin A.J. 1994. *Essentials of Management*, 3rd ed. Cleveland, South-Western Publishing Co.

Duck J.D. 1993. Managing change — the art of balancing. *Harvard Business Review*, November–December 1993, pp. 109–118.

Gitlow H.S. and Gitlow S.J. 1987. *The Deming Guide to Quality and Competitive Position*. Englewood Cliffs, NJ, Prentice-Hall.

Goal/QPC. 1988. *The Memory Jogger. A Pocket Guide of Tools for Continuous Improvement*. Massachusetts, Goal/QPC.

Ishikawa K. 1991. *Guide to Quality Control*. New York, Quality Resources (Asian Productivity Organization, Tokyo, Japan).

Joint Commission on Accreditation of Healthcare Organizations — Comprehensive Accreditation Manual for Hospitals — Official Handbook, Library of Congress Number 96-076721, 1998, Oakbrook Terrace, Illinois 60181.

Juran J.M. 1979. *Quality Control Handbook*, 3rd ed. New York, McGraw-Hill.

Katzenbach J.R. and Smith D.K. 1994. *The Wisdom of Teams*. New York, Harper Business. A Division of Harper Collins Publishers.

Mizuno S. 1988. *Management for Quality Improvement. The Seven New QC Tools*. Boston, Productivity Press.

Sholters P.R. 1993. *The Team Handbook. How to Use Teams to Improve Quality*. Madison, WI, Joiner Associates, Inc.

Walton M. 1986. *The Deming Management Method*. New York, Putnam Publishing Group.

79

A Standards Primer
for Clinical Engineers

79.1 Introduction... **79**-1
79.2 Definitions **79**-2
79.3 Standards for Clinical Engineering **79**-3
79.4 A Hierarchy of Standards............................. **79**-3
79.5 Medical Devices.. **79**-5
79.6 International Standards **79**-7
79.7 Compliance with Standards........................... **79**-9
79.8 Limitations of Standards **79**-9
       Noncompliance with a Standard • Standards and the Law •
       Incorporation and Revision • Safety • Liability •
       Inhibition • *Ex Post Facto* • Costs
79.9 Conclusions **79**-12
References **79**-12

Alvin Wald
Columbia University

79.1 Introduction

The development, understanding, and use of standards is an important component of a clinical engineer's activities. Whether involved in industry, a health care facility, governmental affairs, or commercial enterprise, one way or another, the clinical engineer will find that standards are a significant aspect of professional activities. With the increasing emphasis on health care cost containment and efficiency, coupled with the continued emphasis on patient outcome, standards must be viewed both as a mechanism to reduce expenses and as another mechanism to provide quality patient care. In any case, standards must be addressed in their own right, in terms of technical, economic, and legal implications.

It is important for the clinical engineer to understand fully how standards are developed, how they are used, and most importantly, how they affect the entire spectrum of health related matters. Standards exist that address systems (protection of the electrical power distribution system from faults), individuals (means to reduce potential electric shock hazards), and protection of the environment (disposal of deleterious waste substances).

From a larger perspective, standards have existed since biblical times. In the Book of Genesis (Chap. 6, ver. 14), Noah is given a construction standard by God, "Make thee an ark of gopher wood; rooms shalt thou make in the ark, and shalt pitch it within and without with pitch." Standards for weights and measures have played an important role in bringing together human societies through trade and commerce. The earliest record of a standard for length comes from ancient Egypt, in Dynasty IV (ca. 3000 BC). This length was the royal cubit, 20.620 in. (52.379 cm), as used in construction of the Great Pyramid.

The importance of standards to society is illustrated in the Magna Carta, presented by the English barons to King John in 1215 on the field at Runnymede. Article 35 states:

> There shall be standard measures of wine, beer, and corn — the London quarter — throughout the whole of our kingdom, and a standard width of dyed, russet and halberject cloth — two ells within the selvedges; and there shall be standard weights also.

The principles of this article appear in the English Tower system for weight and capacity, set in 1266 by the assize of Bread and Ale Act:

> An English penny called a sterling, round and without any clipping, shall weigh thirty-two wheatcorns in the midst of the ear; and twenty ounces a pound: and eight pounds do make a gallon of wine, and eight gallons of wine do make a bushell, which is the eighth part of a quarter.

In the United States, a noteworthy use of standards occurred after the Boston fire of 1689. With the aim of rapid rebuilding of the city, the town fathers specified that all bricks used in construction were to be $9 \times 4 \times 4$ in. An example of standardization to promote uniformity in manufacturing practices was the contract for 10,000 muskets awarded to Eli Whitney by President Thomas Jefferson in 1800. The apocryphal story is that Eli Whitney (better known to generations of grammar school children for his invention of the cotton gin) assembled a large number of each musket part, had one of each part randomly selected, and then assembled a complete working musket. This method of production, the complete interchangeability of assembly parts, came to be known as the "armory method," replacing hand crafting, which at that time had been the prevailing method of manufacturing throughout the world.

79.2   Definitions

A most general definition of a standard is given by Rowe (1983). "A standard is a multi-party agreement for establishing an arbitrary criterion for reference." Each word used in the definition by Rowe corresponds to a specific characteristic that helps to define the concept of a standard. Multi means more than one party, organization, group, government, agency, or individual. Agreement means that the concerned parties have come to some mutually agreed upon understanding of the issues involved and of ways to resolve them. This understanding has been confirmed via some mechanism such as unanimity, consensus, ballot, or other means that has been specified. Establishing defines the purpose of the agreement — to create the standard and carry forth its provisions.

Arbitrary emphasizes an understanding by the parties that there are no absolute criteria in creating the standard. Rather, the conditions and values chosen are based on the most appropriate knowledge and conditions available at the time the standard was established. Criterions are those features and conditions that the parties to the agreement have chosen as the basis for the standard. Not all issues may be addressed, but only those deemed, for whatever reasons, suitable for inclusion.

A different type of definition of a standard is given in The United States Office of Management and Budget Circular A-119:

> . . . a prescribed set of rules, conditions, or requirements concerned with the definition of terms; classification of components; delineation of procedures; specifications of materials, performance, design, or operations; or measurement of quality and quantity in describing materials, products, systems, services, or practices.

A code is a compilation of standards relating to a particular area of concern, that is, a collection of standards. For example, local government health codes contain standards relating to providing of health care to members of the community. A regulation is an organization's way of specifying that some particular standard must be adhered to. Standards, codes, and regulations may or may not have legal implications, depending on whether the promulgating organization is governmental or private.

79.3 Standards for Clinical Engineering

There is a continually growing body of standards that affect health care facilities, and hence clinical engineering. The practitioner of health care technology must constantly search out, evaluate, and apply appropriate standards. The means to reconcile the conflicts of technology, cost considerations, the different jurisdictions involved, and the implementation of the various standards is not necessarily apparent. One technique that addresses these concerns and has proven to yield a consistent practical approach is a structured framework of the various levels of standards. This hierarchy of standards is a conceptual model that the clinical engineer can use to evaluate and apply to the various requirements that exist in the procurement and use of health care technology.

Standards have different purposes, depending on their particular applications. A hierarchy of standards can be used to delineate those conditions for which a particular standard applies. There are four basic categories, any one or all of which may be in simultaneous operation:

1. Local or proprietary standards (perhaps more properly called regulations) are developed to meet the internal needs of a particular organization
2. Common interest standards serve to provide uniformity of product or service throughout an industry or profession
3. Consensus standards are agreements amongst interested participants to address an area of mutual concern
4. Regulatory standards are mandated by an authority having jurisdiction to define a particular aspect of concern

In addition, there are two categories of standards adherence (1) voluntary standards, which carry no inherent power of enforcement, but provide a reference point of mutual understanding, and (2) mandatory standards, which are incumbent upon those to whom the standard is addressed, and enforceable by the authority having jurisdiction.

The hierarchy of standards model can aid the clinical engineer in the efficient and proper use of standards. More importantly, it can provide standards developers, users, and the authorities having jurisdiction in these matters with a structure by which standards can be effectively developed, recognized, and used to the mutual benefit of all.

79.4 A Hierarchy of Standards

Local, or proprietary standards, are developed for what might be called internal use. An organization that wishes to regulate and control certain of its own activities issues its own standards. Thus, the standard is local in the sense that it is applied in a specific venue, and it is proprietary in that it is the creation of a completely independent administration. For example, an organization may standardize on a single type of an electrocardiograph monitor. This standardization can refer to a specific brand or model, or to specific functional or operational features. In a more formal sense, a local standard may often be referred to as an institutional Policy and Procedure. The policy portion is the why of it; the procedure portion is the how. It must be kept in mind that standards of this type that are too restrictive will limit innovation and progress, in that they cannot readily adapt to novel conditions. On the other hand, good local standards contribute to lower costs, operational efficiency, and a sense of coherence within the organization.

Sometimes, local standards may originate from requirements of a higher level of regulation. For example, the Joint Commission for Accreditation of Healthcare Organizations (JCAHO) (formerly the Joint Commission for Hospital Accreditation (JCAH), a voluntary organization (but an organization that hospitals belong to for various reasons, for example, accreditation, reimbursement, approval of training programs), does not set standards for what or how equipment should be used. Rather, the JCAHO requires that each hospital set its own standards on how equipment is selected, used, and maintained. To monitor compliance with this requirement, the JCAHO inspects whether the hospital follows its own standards. In one sense, the most damaging evidence that can be adduced against an organization (or an individual) is that it (he) did not follow its (his) own standards.

Common interest standards are based on a need recognized by a group of interested parties, which will further their own interests, individually or collectively. Such standards are generally accepted by affected interests without being made mandatory by an authority; hence they are one type of voluntary standard. These standards are often developed by trade or professional organizations to promote uniformity in a product or process. This type of standard may have no inducement to adherence except for the benefits to the individual participants. For example, if you manufacture a kitchen cabinet that is not of standard size, it will not fit into the majority of kitchens and thus it will not sell. Uniformity of screw threads is another example of how a product can be manufactured and used by diverse parties, and yet be absolutely interchangeable. More recently, various information transfer standards allow the interchange of computer-based information amongst different types of instruments and computers.

Consensus standards are those that have been developed and accepted in accordance with certain well defined criteria so as to assure that all points of view have been considered. Sometimes, the adjective "consensus" is used as a modifier for a "voluntary standard." Used in this context, consensus implies that all interested parties have been consulted and have come to a general agreement on the provisions of the standard. The development of a consensus standard follows an almost ritualistic procedure to insure that fairness and due process are maintained. There are various independent voluntary and professional organizations that sponsor and develop standards on a consensus basis (see below). Each such organization has its own particular rules and procedures to make sure that there is a true consensus in developing a standard.

In the medical products field, standards are sometimes difficult to implement because of the independent nature of manufacturers and their high level of competition. A somewhat successful standards story is the adoption of the DIN configuration for ECG lead-cable connection by the Association for the Advancement of Medical Instrumentation (AAMI). The impetus for this standard was the accidental electrocution of several children brought about by use of the previous industry standard lead connection (a bare metal pin, as opposed to the new recessed socket). Most (but not all) manufacturers of ECG leads and cables now adhere to this standard. Agreement on this matter is in sharp contrast to the inability of the health care manufacturing industry to implement a standard for ECG cable connectors. Even though a standard was written, the physical configuration of the connector is not necessarily used by manufacturers in production, nor is it demanded by medical users in purchasing. Each manufacturer uses a different connector, leading to numerous problems in supply and incompatibility for users. This is an example of a voluntary standard, which for whatever reasons, is effectively ignored by all interested parties.

However, even though there have been some failures in standardization of product features, there has also been significant progress in generating performance and test standards for medical devices. A number of independent organizations sponsor development of standards for medical devices. For example, the American Society for Testing and Materials (ASTM) has developed, "Standard Specification for Minimum Performance and Safety Requirements for Components and Systems of Anesthesia Gas Machines (F1161-88)." Even though there is no statutory law that requires it, manufacturers no longer produce, and thus hospitals can no longer purchase anesthesia machines without the built-in safety features specified in this standard. AAMI has sponsored numerous standards that relate to performance of specific medical devices, such as defibrillators, electrosurgical instruments, and electronic sphygmomanometers. These standards are compiled in the AAMI publication, "Essential Standards for Biomedical Equipment Safety and Performance." The National Fire Protection Association (NFPA) publishes "Standard for Health Care Facilities (NFPA 99)," which covers a wide range of safety issues relating to facilities. Included are sections that deal with electricity and electrical systems, central gas and vacuum supplies, and environmental conditions. Special areas such as anesthetizing locations, laboratories, and hyperbaric facilities are addressed separately. Mandatory standards have the force of law or other authority having jurisdiction.

Mandatory standards imply that some authority has made them obligatory. Mandatory standards can be written by the authority having jurisdiction, or they can be adapted from documents prepared by others as proprietary or consensus standards. The authority having jurisdiction can be a local hospital or even a department within the hospital, a professional society, a municipal or state government, or an agency of the federal government that has regulatory powers.

In the United States, hospitals are generally regulated by a local city or county authority, and/or by the state. These authorities set standards in the form of health codes or regulations, which have the force of law. Often, these local bodies consider the requirements of a voluntary group, the Joint Commission for Accreditation of Healthcare Organizations, in their accreditation and regulatory processes.

American National Standards. The tradition in the United States is that of voluntary standards. However, once a standard is adopted by an organization, it can be taken one step further. The American National Standards Institute (ANSI) is a private, nongovernment, voluntary organization that acts as a coordinating body for standards development and recognition in the United States. If the development process for a standard meets the ANSI criteria of open deliberation of legitimate concerns, with all interested parties coming to a voluntary consensus, then the developers can apply (but are not required) to have their standard designated as an American National Standard. Such a designation does not make a standard any more legitimate, but it does offer some recognition as to the process by which it has been developed. ANSI also acts as a clearing house for standards development, so as to avoid duplication of effort by various groups that might be concerned with the same issues. ANSI is also involved as a U.S. coordinating body for many international standards activities.

An excellent source that lists existing standards and standards generating organizations, both nationally and internationally, along with some of the workings of the FDA (see below), is the "Medical Device Industry Fact Book" [Allen, 1996].

79.5 Medical Devices

On the national level, oversight is generally restricted to medical devices, and not on operational matters. Federal jurisdiction of medical devices falls under the purview of the Department of Health and Human Services, Public Health Service, Food and Drug Administration (FDA), Center for Devices and Radiological Health. Under federal law, medical devices are regulated under the "Medical Device Amendments of 1976" and the "Radiation Control for Health and Safety Act of 1968." Additional regulatory authorization is provided by the "Safe Medical Devices Act of 1990," the "Medical Device Amendments of 1992," the "FDA Reform and Enhancement Act of 1996," and the "Food and Drug Administration Modernization Act of 1997."

A medical device is defined by Section 201 of the Federal Food, Drug, and Cosmetic Act (as amended), as an:

instrument, apparatus, implement, machine, contrivance, implant, *in vitro* reagent, or other similar or related article including any component, part, or accessory which is:
recognized in the official National Formulary, or the United States Pharmacopeia, or any supplement to them;
intended for use in the diagnosis of disease or other conditions, or in the care, mitigation, treatment, or prevention of disease, in man or other animals, or
intended to affect the structure of any function of the body of man or other animals; and which does not achieve its primary intended purposes through chemical action within or on the body of man . . . and which is not dependent upon being metabolized for the achievement of its primary intended purposes.

The major thrust of the FDA has been in the oversight of the manufacture of medical devices, with specific requirements based on categories of perceived risks. The 1976 Act (Section 513) establishes three classes of medical devices intended for human use:

Class I. General controls regulate devices for which controls other than performance standards or premarket approvals are sufficient to assure safety and effectiveness. Such controls include regulations that (1) prohibit adulterated or misbranded devices; (2) require domestic device manufacturers and initial distributors to register their establishments and list their devices; (3) grant FDA authority to ban certain devices; (4) provide for notification of risks and of repair, replacement, or refund; (5) restrict the sale, distribution, or use of certain devices; and (6) govern Good Manufacturing Practices, records, and reports, and inspections. These minimum requirements apply also to Class II and Class III devices.

Class II. Performance Standards apply to devices for which general controls alone do not provide reasonable assurance of safety and efficacy, and for which existing information is sufficient to establish a performance standard that provides this assurance. Class II devices must comply not only with general controls, but also with an applicable standard developed under Section 514 of the Act. Until performance standards are developed by regulation, only general controls apply.

Class III. Premarket Approval applies to devices for which general controls do not suffice or for which insufficient information is available to write a performance standard to provide reasonable assurance of safety and effectiveness. Also, devices which are used to support or sustain human life or to prevent impairment of human health, devices implanted in the body, and devices which present a potentially unreasonable risk of illness or injury. New Class III devices, those not "substantially equivalent" to a device on the market prior to enactment (May 28, 1976), must have approved Premarket Approval Applications (Section 510 k).

Exact specifications for General Controls and Good Manufacturing Practices (GMP) are defined in various FDA documents. Aspects of General Controls include yearly manufacturer registration, device listing, and premarket approval. General Controls are also used to regulate adulteration, misbranding and labeling, banned devices, and restricted devices. Good Manufacturing Practices include concerns of organization and personnel; buildings and equipment; controls for components, processes, packaging, and labeling; device holding, distribution, and installation; manufacturing records; product evaluation; complaint handling; and a quality assurance program. Design controls for GMP were introduced in 1996. They were motivated by the FDA's desire to harmonize its requirements with those of a proposed international standard (ISO 13485). Factors that need to be addressed include planning, input and output requirements, review, verification and validation, transfer to production, and change procedures, all contained in a history file for each device. Device tracking is typically required for Class III life-sustaining and implant devices, as well as postmarket surveillance for products introduced starting in 1991.

Other categories of medical devices include combination devices, in which a device may incorporate drugs or biologicals. Combination devices are controlled via intercenter arrangements implemented by the FDA.

Transitional devices refer to devices that were regulated as drugs, prior to the enactment of the Medical Device Amendments Act of 1976. These devices were automatically placed into Class III, but may be transferred to Class I or II.

A custom device may be ordered by a physician for his/her own use or for a specific patient. These devices are not generally available, and cannot be labeled or advertised for commercial distribution.

An investigational device is one that is undergoing clinical trials prior to premarket clearance. If the device presents a significant risk to the patient, an Investigational Device Exemption must be approved by the FDA. Information must be provided regarding the device description and intended use, the origins of the device, the investigational protocol, and proof of oversight by an Institutional Review Board to insure informed patient consent. Special compassionate or emergency use for a nonapproved device or for a nonapproved use can be obtained from the FDA under special circumstances, such as when there is no other hope for the patient.

Adverse Events. The Safe Medical Devices Act of 1990 included a provision by which both users and manufacturers (and distributors) of medical devices are required to report adverse patient events that may be related to a medical device. Manufacturers must report to the FDA if a device (a) may have caused or contributed to a death or serious injury, or (b) malfunctioned in such a way as would be likely to cause or contribute to a death or serious injury if the malfunction were to reoccur. Device users are required to notify the device manufacturer of reportable incidents, and must also notify the FDA in case of a device-related death. In addition, the FDA established a voluntary program for reporting device problems that may not have caused an untoward patient event, but which may have the potential for such an occurrence under altered circumstances.

New devices. As part of the General Controls requirements, the FDA must be notified prior to marketing any new (or modifying an existing) device for patient use. This premarket notification, called the 510(k) process after the relevant section in the Medical Device Amendments Act, allows the FDA to review the device for safety and efficacy.

There are two broad categories that a device can fall into. A device that was marketed prior to May 28, 1976 (the date that the Medical Device Amendments became effective) can continue to be sold. Also, a product that is "substantially equivalent" to a preamendment device can likewise be marketed. However, the FDA may require a premarket approval application for any Class III device (see below). Thus, these preamendment devices and their equivalents are approved by "grandfathering." (Premarket notification to the FDA is still required to assure safety and efficacy). Of course, the question of substantial equivalency is open to an infinite number of interpretations. From the manufacturer's perspective, such a designation allows marketing the device without a much more laborious and expensive premarket approval process.

A new device that the FDA finds is not substantially equivalent to a premarket device is automatically placed into Class III. This category includes devices that provide functions or work through principles not present in preamendment devices. Before marketing, this type of device requires a Premarket Approval Application by the manufacturer, followed by an extensive review by the FDA. (However, the FDA can reclassify such devices into Class I or II, obviating the need for premarket approval.) The review includes scientific and clinical evaluation of the application by the FDA and by a Medical Advisory Committee (composed of outside consultants). In addition, the FDA looks at the manufacturing and control processes to assure that all appropriate regulatory requirements are being adhered to. Clinical (use of real patients) trials are often required for Class III devices in order to provide evidence of safety and efficacy. To carry out such trials, an Investigational Device Exemption must be issued by the FDA.

The Food and Drug Administration Modernization Act of 1997, which amends section 514 of the Food, Drug, and Cosmetic Act, has made significant changes in the above regulations. These changes greatly simplify and accelerate the entire regulatory process. For example, the law exempts from premarket notification Class I devices that are not intended for a use that is of substantial importance in preventing impairment of human health, or that do not present a potential unreasonable risk of illness or injury. Almost 600 Class I generic devices have been so classified by the agency. In addition, the FDA will specify those Class II devices for which a 510(k) submission will also not be required.

Several other regulatory changes have been introduced by the FDA to simplify and speed up the approval process. So-called "third party" experts will be allowed to conduct the initial review of all Class I and low-to-intermediate risk Class II devices. Previously, the FDA was authorized to create standards for medical devices. The new legislation allows the FDA to recognize and use all or parts of various appropriate domestic and internationally recognized consensus standards that address aspects of safety and effectiveness relevant to medical devices.

79.6 International Standards

Most sovereign nations have their own internal agencies to establish and enforce standards. However, in our present world of international cooperation and trade, standards are tending towards uniformity across national boundaries. This internationalization of standards is especially true since formation of the European Common Market. The aim here is to harmonize the standards of individual nations by promulgating directives for medical devices that address "Essential Requirements" [Freeman, 1993] (see below). Standards in other areas of the world (Asia, Eastern Europe) are much more fragmented, with each country specifying regulations for its own manufactured and imported medical devices.

There are two major international standards generating organizations, both based in Europe, the International Electrotechnical Commission (IEC) and the International Organization for Standardization (ISO). Nations throughout the world participate in the activities of these organizations.

The International Electrotechnical Commission (IEC), founded in 1906, oversees, on an international level, all matters relating to standards for electrical and electronic items. Membership in the IEC is held by a National Committee for each nation. The United States National Committee (USNC) for IEC was founded in 1907, and since 1931 has been affiliated with ANSI. USNC has its members representatives from professional societies, trade associations, testing laboratories, government entities, other organizations, and individual experts. The USNC appoints a technical advisor and a technical advisory group for each IEC Committee and Subcommittee to help develop a unified United States position. These advisory groups are drawn from groups that are involved in the development of related U.S. national standards.

Standards are developed by Technical Committees (TC), Subcommittees (SC), and Working Groups (WG). IEC TC 62, "Electrical Equipment in Medical Practice," is of particular interest here. One of the basic standards of this Technical Committee is document 601-1, "Safety of Medical Electrical Equipment, Part 1: General Requirements for Safety," 2nd Edition (1988) and its Amendment 1 (1991), along with Document 601-1-1, "Safety Requirements for Medical Electrical Systems" (1992).

The International Organization for Standardization (ISO) oversees aspects of device standards other than those related to electrotechnology. This organization was formed in 1946 with a membership comprised of the national standards organizations of 26 countries. There are currently some 90 nations as members. The purpose of the ISO is to "facilitate international exchange of goods and services and to develop mutual cooperation in intellectual, scientific, technological, and economic ability." ISO addresses all aspects of standards except for electrical and electronic issues, which are the purview of the International Electrotechnical Commission. ANSI has been the official United States representative to ISO since its inception. For each Committee or Subcommittee of the ISO in which ANSI participates, a U.S. Technical Advisory Group (TAG) is formed. The administrator of the TAG is, typically, that same U.S. organization that is developing the parallel U.S. standard.

Technical Committees (TC) of the ISO concentrate on specific areas of interest. There are Technical Committees, Subcommittees, Working Groups, and Study Groups. One of the member national standards organizations serves as the Secretariat for each of these technical bodies.

One standard of particular relevancy to manufacturers throughout the world is ISO 9000. This standard was specifically developed to assure a total quality management program that can be both universally recognized and applied to any manufacturing process. It does not address any particular product or process, but is concerned with structure and oversight of how processes are developed, implemented, monitored, and documented. An independent audit must be passed by any organization to obtain ISO 9000 registration. Many individual nations and manufacturers have adopted this standard and require that any product that they purchase be from a source that is ISO 9000 compliant.

The European Union was, in effect, created by the Single Europe Act (EC-92), as a region "without internal frontiers in which the free movement of goods, persons, and capital is ensured." For various products and classes of products, the European Commission issues directives with regard to safety and other requirements, along with the means for assessing conformity to these directives. Products that comply with the appropriate directives can then carry the CE mark. EU member states ratify these directives into national law.

Two directives related to medical devices are the Medical Devices Directive (MDD), enacted in 1993 (mandatory as of June 15,1998), and the Active Implanted Medical Devices Directive (AIMDD), effective since 1995. Safety is the primary concern of this system, and as in the United States, there are three classes of risk. These risks are based on what and for how long the device touches, and its effects. Safety issues include electrical, mechanical, thermal, radiation, and labeling. Voluntary standards that address these issues are formulated by the European Committee for Standardization (CEN) and the European Committee for Electrotechnical Standardization (CENELEC).

79.7   Compliance with Standards

Standards that were originally developed on a voluntary basis may take on mandatory aspects. Standards that were developed to meet one particular need may be used to satisfy other needs as well. Standards will be enforced and adhered to if they meet the needs of those who are affected by them. For example, consider a standard for safety and performance for a defibrillator. For the manufacturer, acceptance and sales are a major consideration in both the domestic and international markets. People responsible for specifying, selecting, and purchasing equipment may insist on adherence to the standard so as to guarantee safety and performance. The user, physician, or other health care professional, will expect the instrument to have certain operational and performance characteristics to meet medical needs. Hospital personnel want a certain minimum degree of equipment uniformity for ease of training and maintenance. The hospital's insurance company and risk manager want equipment that meets or exceeds recognized safety standards. Third party payers, that is private insurance companies or government agencies, insist on equipment that is safe, efficacious, and cost effective. Accreditation agencies, such as local health agencies or professional societies, often require equipment to meet certain standards. More basically, patients, workers, and society as a whole have an inherent right to fundamental safety. Finally, in our litigatious society, there is always the threat of civil action in the case of an untoward event in which a "non-standard," albeit "safe," instrument was involved. Thus, even though no one has stated "this standard must be followed," it is highly unlikely that any person or organization will have the temerity to manufacture, specify, or buy an instrument that does not "meet the standard."

Another example of how standards become compulsory is via accreditation organizations. The Joint Commission for Accreditation of Healthcare Organizations has various standards (requirements). This organization is a private body that hospitals voluntarily accept as an accrediting agent. However, various health insurance organizations, governmental organizations, and physician specialty boards for resident education use accreditation by the JCAHO as a touchstone for quality of activities. Thus, an insurance company might not pay for care in a hospital that is not accredited, or a specialty board might not recognize resident training in such an institution. Thus, the requirements of the JCAHO, in effect, become mandatory standards for health care organizations.

A third means by which voluntary standards can become mandatory is by incorporation. Existing standards can be incorporated into a higher level of standards or codes. For example, various state and local governments incorporate standards developed by voluntary organizations, such as the National Fire Protection Association, into their own building and health codes. These standards then become, in effect, mandatory government regulations, and have the force of (civil) law. In addition, as discussed above, the FDA will now recognize voluntary standards developed by recognized organizations.

79.8   Limitations of Standards

Standards are generated to meet the expectations of society. They are developed by organizations and individuals to meet a variety of specific needs, with the general goals of promoting safety and efficiency. However, as with all human activities, problems with the interpretation and use of standards do occur. Engineering judgment is often required to help provide answers. Thus, the clinical engineer must consider the limits of standards, a boundary that is not clear and is constantly shifting. Yet clinical engineers must always employ the highest levels of engineering principles and practices. Some of the limitations and questions of standards and their use will be discussed below.

79.8.1   Noncompliance with a Standard

Sooner or later, it is likely that a clinical engineer will either be directly involved with or become aware of deviation from an accepted standard. The violation may be trivial, with no noticeable effect, or there may be serious consequences. In the former case, either the whole incident may be ignored, or nothing more may be necessary than a report that is filed away, or the incident can trigger some sort of corrective action. In the latter case, there may be major repercussions involving investigation, censure, tort issues, or legal actions. In any event, lack of knowledge about the standard is not a convincing defense. Anyone who is in a position that requires knowledge about a standard should be fully cognizant of all aspects of that standard. In particular, one should know the provisions of the standard, how they are to be enforced, and the potential risks of noncompliance. Nonetheless, noncompliance with a standard, in whole or in part, may be necessary to prevent a greater risk or to increase a potential benefit to the patient. For example, when no other recourse is available, it would be defensible to use an electromagnet condemned for irreparable excessive leakage current to locate a foreign body in the eye of an injured person, and thus save the patient's vision. Even if the use of this device resulted in a physical injury or equipment damage, the potential benefit to the patient is a compelling argument for use of the noncompliant device. In such a case, one should be aware of and prepared to act on the possible hazard (excessive electrical current, here). A general disclaimer making allowance for emergency situations is often included in policy statements relating to use of a standard. Drastic conditions require drastic methods.

79.8.2 Standards and the Law

Standards mandated by a government body are not what is called "black letter law," that is a law actually entered into a criminal or civil code. Standards are typically not adopted in the same manner as laws, that is, they are not approved by a legislative body, ratified by an elected executive, and sanctioned by the courts. The usual course for a mandated standard is via a legislative body enacting a law that establishes or assigns to an executive agency the authority to regulate the concerned activities. This agency, under the control of the executive branch of government, then issues standards that follow the mandate of its enabling legislation. If conflicts arise, in addition to purely legal considerations, the judiciary must interpret the intent of the legislation in comparison with its execution. This type of law falls under civil rather than criminal application.

The penalty for noncompliance with a standard may not be criminal or even civil prosecution. Instead, there are administrative methods of enforcement, as well as more subtle yet powerful methods of coercion. The state has the power (and the duty) to regulate matters of public interest. Thus, the state can withhold or withdraw permits for construction, occupancy, or use. Possibly more effective, the state can withhold means of finance or payments to violators of its regulations. Individuals injured by failure to abide by a standard may sue for damages in civil proceedings. However, it must be recognized that criminal prosecution is possible when the violations are most egregious, leading to human injury or large financial losses.

79.8.3 Incorporation and Revision

Because of advances in technology and increases in societal expectations, standards are typically revised periodically. For example, the National Fire Protection Association revises and reissues its "Standard for Health Care Facilities" (NFPA 99) every three years. Other organizations follow a five year cycle of review, revision, and reissue of standards. These voluntary standards, developed in good faith, may be adapted by governmental agencies and made mandatory, as discussed above. When a standard is incorporated into a legislative code, it is generally referenced as to a particular version and date. It is not always the case that a newer version of the standard is more restrictive. For example, ever since 1984, the National Fire Protection Association "Standard for Health Care Facilities" (NFPA 99) does not require the installation of isolated power systems (isolation transformers and line isolation monitors) in anesthetizing locations that do not use flammable anesthetic agents, or in areas that are not classified as wet locations. A previous version of this standard, "Standard for the Use of Inhalation Anesthetics (Flammable and Nonflammable)," (NFPA 56A-1978) did require isolated power. However, many State Hospital Codes have incorporated, by name and date, the provisions of the older standard, NFPA 56A. Thus, isolated power may still be required, by code, in new construction of all anesthetizing locations, despite the absence of this requirement in the latest version of the standard that addresses this issue. In such a case, the organization having jurisdiction in the matter must be petitioned to remedy this conflict between new and old versions of the standard.

79.8.4 Safety

The primary purpose of standards in clinical practice is to assure the safety of patient, operator, and bystanders. However, it must be fully appreciated that there is no such thing as absolute safety. The more safety features and regulations attached to a device, the less useful and the more cumbersome and costly may be its actual use. In the development, interpretation, and use of a standard, there are questions that must be asked: What is possible? What is acceptable? What is reasonable? Who will benefit? What is the cost? Who will pay?

No one can deny that medical devices should be made as safe as possible, but some risk will always remain. In our practical world, absolute safety is a myth. Many medical procedures involve risk to the patient. The prudent physician or medical technologist will recognize the possible dangers of the equipment and take appropriate measures to reduce the risk to a minimum. Some instruments and procedures are inherently more dangerous than others. The physician must make a judgment, based on his/her own professional knowledge and experience, as well as on the expectations of society, whether using a particular device is less of a risk than using an alternative device or doing nothing. Standards will help — but they do not guarantee complete safety, a cure, or legal and societal approval.

79.8.5 Liability

Individuals who serve on committees that develop standards, as well as organizations involved in such activities, are justifiably concerned with their legal position in the event that a lawsuit is instituted as a result of a standard that they helped to bring forth. Issues involved in such a suit may include restraint of trade, in case of commercial matters, or to liability for injury due to acts of commission or of omission. Organizations that sponsor standards or that appoint representatives to standards developing groups often have insurance for such activities. Independent standards committees and individual members of any standards committees may or may not be covered by insurance for participation in these activities. Although in recent times only one organization and no individual has been found liable for damages caused by improper use of standards (see following paragraph), even the possibility of being named in a lawsuit can intimidate even the most self-confident "expert." Thus, it is not at all unusual for an individual who is asked to serve on a standards development committee first to inquire as to liability insurance coverage. Organizations that develop standards or appoint representatives also take pains to insure that all of their procedures are carefully followed and documented so as to demonstrate fairness and prudence.

The dark side of standards is the implication that individuals or groups may unduly influence a standard to meet a personal objective, for example, to dominate sales in a particular market. If standards are developed or interpreted unfairly, or if they give an unfair advantage to one segment, then restraint of trade charges can be made. This is why standards to be deemed consensus must be developed in a completely open and fair manner. Organizations that sponsor standards that violate this precept can be held responsible. In 1982, the United States Supreme Court, in the Hydrolevel Case [Perry, 1982], ruled that the American Society of Mechanical Engineers was guilty of antitrust activities because of the way some of its members, acting as a committee to interpret one of its standards, issued an opinion that limited competition in sales so as to unfairly benefit their own employers. This case remains a singular reminder that standards development and use must be inherently fair.

79.8.6 Inhibition

Another charge against standards is that they inhibit innovation and limit progress [Flink, 1984]. Ideally, standards should be written to satisfy minimum, yet sufficient, requirements for safety, performance, and efficacy. Improvements or innovations would still be permitted so long as the basic standard is followed. From a device users point of view, a standard that is excessively restrictive may limit the scope of permissible professional activities. If it is necessary to abrogate a standard in order to accommodate a new idea or to extend an existing situation, then the choice is to try to have the standard changed, which may be very time consuming, or to act in violation of the standard and accept the accompanying risks and censure.

79.8.7 *Ex Post Facto*

A question continually arises as to what to do about old equipment (procedures, policies, facilities, etc.) when a new standard is issued or an old standard is revised so that existing items become obsolete. One approach, perhaps the simplest, is to do nothing. The philosophy here being that the old equipment was acquired in good faith and conformed to the then existing standards. As long as that equipment is usable and safe, there is no necessity to replace it. Another approach is to upgrade the existing equipment to meet the new standard. However, such modification may be technically impractical or financially prohibitive. Finally, one can simply throw out all of the existing equipment (or sell it to a second-hand dealer, or use the parts for maintenance) and buy everything new. This approach would bring a smile of delight from the manufacturer and a scream of outrage from the hospital administrator. Usually what is done is a compromise, incorporating various aspects of these different approaches.

79.8.8 Costs

Standards cost both time and money to propose, develop, promulgate, and maintain. Perhaps the greatest hindrance to more participation in standards activities by interested individuals is the lack of funds to attend meetings where the issues are discussed and decisions are made. Unfortunately, but nonetheless true, organizations that can afford to sponsor individuals to attend such meetings have considerable influence in the development of that standard. On the other hand, those organizations that do have a vital interest in a standard should have an appropriate say in its development. A consensus of all interested parties tempers the undue influence of any single participant. From another viewpoint, standards increase the costs of manufacturing devices, carrying out procedures, and administering policies. This incremental cost is, in turn, passed on to the purchaser of the goods or services. Whether or not the increased cost justifies the benefits of the standard is not always apparent. It is impossible to realistically quantify the costs of accidents that did not happen or the confusion that was avoided by adhering to a particular standard. However, it cannot be denied that standards have made a valuable contribution to progress, in the broadest sense of that word.

79.9   Conclusions

Standards are just like any other human activity, they can be well used or a burden. The danger of standards is that they will take on a life of their own; and rather than serve a genuine need will exist only as a justification of their own importance. This view is expressed in the provocative and iconoclastic book by Bruner and Leonard [1989], and in particular in their Chapter 9, *"Codes and Standards: Who Makes the Rules?"* However, the raison d'être of standards is to do good. It is incumbent upon clinical engineers, not only to understand how to apply standards properly, but also how to introduce, modify, and retire standards as conditions change. Furthermore, the limitations of standards must be recognized in order to realize their maximum benefit. No standard can replace diligence, knowledge, and a genuine concern for doing the right thing.

References

Allen, A. (ed.) 1996. *Medical Device Industry Fact Book*, 3rd ed. Canon Communications, Santa Monica, CA.

American Society for Testing and Materials (ASTM). 1916. Race Street, Philadelphia, PA 19103.

Association for the Advancement of Medical Instrumentation (AAMI) 3330 Washington Boulevard, Suite 400, Arlington, VA 22201.

Bruner, J.M.R. and Leonard, P.F. 1989. *Electricity, Safety and the Patient*, Year Book Medical Publishers, Chicago.

Flink, R. 1984. Standards: Resource or Constraint? *IEEE Eng. Med. Biol. Mag.*, 3: 14–16.

Food and Drug Administration, Center for Devices and Radiological Health, 5600 Fishers Lane, Rockville, MD 20857. URL: http://www.fda.gov/.

Freeman, M. 1993. The EC Medical Devices Directives, *IEEE Eng. Med. Biol. Mag.*, 12: 79–80.

International Organization for Standardization (ISO), Central Secretariat, 1 rue de Varembe, Case postale 56, CH 1211, Geneva 20, Switzerland. URL: http://www.iso.ch/index.html.

International Electrotechnical Commission (IEC), Central Office, 3 rue de Varembé, P. O. Box 131, CH-1211, Geneva 20, Switzerland. URL: http://www.iec.ch/.

Joint Commission for Accreditation of Healthcare organizations (JCAHO) 1 Renaissance Boulevard, Oakbrook, IL 60181.

National Fire Protection Association (NFPA) Batterymarch Park, Quincy, MA 02269.

Perry, T.S. 1982. Antirust Ruling Chills Standards Setting, *IEEE Spectrum*, 19: 52–54.

Rowe, W.D. 1983. Design and Performance Standards. In *Medical Devices: Measurements, Quality Assurance, and Standards*, C.A. Caceres, H.T. Yolken, R.J. Jones, and H.R. Piehler (eds.), pp. 29–40. American Society for Testing and Materials, Philadelphia, PA.

80

Regulatory and Assessment Agencies

Mark E. Bruley
Vivian H. Coates
ECRI

80.1   Regulatory Agencies....................................... **80**-1
80.2   Technology Assessment Agencies **80**-4
References **80**-10
Further Information **80**-10

Effective management and development of clinical and biomedical engineering departments (hereafter called clinical engineering departments) in hospitals requires a basic knowledge of relevant regulatory and technology assessment agencies. Regulatory agencies set standards of performance and record keeping for the departments and the technology for which they are responsible. Technology assessment agencies are information resources for what should be an ever expanding role of the clinical engineer in the technology decision-making processes of the hospital's administration.

This chapter presents an overview of regulatory and technology assessment agencies in the United States, Canada, Europe, and Australia that are germane to clinical engineering. Due to the extremely large number of such agencies and information resources, we have chosen to focus on those of greatest relevance and/or informational value. The reader is directed to the references and sources of further information presented at the end of the chapter.

80.1   Regulatory Agencies

Within the healthcare field, there are over 38,000 applicable standards, clinical practice guidelines, laws, and regulations [ECRI, 1999]. Voluntary standards are promulgated by more than 800 organizations; mandatory standards by more than 300 state and federal agencies. Many of these organizations and agencies issue guidelines that are relevant to the vast range of healthcare technologies within the responsibility of clinical engineering departments. Although many of these agencies also regulate the manufacture and clinical use of healthcare technology, such regulations are not directly germane to the management of a clinical department and are not presented.

For the clinical engineer, many agencies promulgate regulations and standards in the areas of, for example, electrical safety, fire safety, technology management, occupational safety, radiology and nuclear medicine, clinical laboratories, infection control, anesthesia and respiratory equipment, power distribution, and medical gas systems. In the United States medical device problem reporting is also regulated by many state agencies and by the U.S. Food and Drug Administration (FDA) via its MEDWATCH program. It is important to note that, at present, the only direct regulatory authority that the FDA has over U.S. hospitals is in the reporting of medical device related accidents that result in serious injury or death.

Chapter 80 discusses in detail many of the specific agency citations. Presented below are the names and addresses of the primary agencies whose codes, standards, and regulations have the most direct bearing on clinical engineering and technology management:

American Hospital Association
1 North Franklin
Chicago, IL 60606
(312) 422-3000
Website: www.aha.org

American College of Radiology
1891 Preston White Drive
Reston, VA 22091
(703) 648-8900
Website: www.acr.org

American National Standards Institute
11 West 42nd Street
13th Floor, New York, NY 10036
(212) 642-4900
Website: www.ansi.org

American Society for Hospital Engineering
840 North Lake Shore Drive
Chicago, IL 60611
(312) 280 5223
Website: www.ashe.org

American Society for Testing and Materials
1916 Race Street
Philadelphia, PA 19103
(215) 299-5400
Website: www.astm.org

Association for the Advancement of
  Medical Instrumentation
3330 Washington Boulevard
Suite 400, Arlington, VA 22201
(703) 525-4890
Website: www.aami.org

Australian Institute of Health and Welfare
GPO Box 570
Canberra, ACT 2601
Australia, (61) 06-243-5092
Website: www.aihw.gov.au

British Standards Institution
2 Park Street
London, W1A 2BS
United Kingdom
(44) 071-629-9000
Website: www.bsi.org.uk

Canadian Healthcare Association
17 York Street
Ottawa, ON K1N 9J6
Canada, (613) 241-8005
Website: www.canadian-healthcare.org

CSA International
178 Rexdale Boulevard
Etobicoke, ON M9W 1R3
Canada, (416) 747-4000
Website: www.csa-international.org

Center for Devices and Radiological Health
Food and Drug Administration
9200 Corporate Boulevard
Rockville, MD 20850
(301) 443-4690
Website: www.fda.gov/cdrh

Compressed Gas Association, Inc.
1725 Jefferson Davis Highway
Suite 1004, Arlington, VA 22202
(703) 412-0900

ECRI
5200 Butler Pike
Plymouth Meeting, PA 19462
(610) 825-6000; (610) 834-1275 (fax)
Websites: www.ecri.org; www.ecriy2k.org
www.mdsr.ecri.org

Environmental Health Directorate
Health Protection Branch
Health Canada
Environmental Health Centre
19th Floor, Jeanne Mance Building
Tunney's Pasture
Ottawa, ON K1A 0L2 Canada
(613) 957-3143
Website: www.hc-sc.gc.ca/hpb/index_e.html

Therapeutic Products Programme
Health Canada
Holland Cross, Tower B
2nd Floor, 1600 Scott Street
Address Locator #3102D1
Ottawa, ON K1A 1B6
(613) 954-0288
Website: www.hc-sc.gc.ca/hpb-dgps/therapeut

Food and Drug Administration
MEDWATCH, FDA Medical Products
Reporting Program
5600 Fishers Lane
Rockville, MD 20857-9787
(800) 332-1088
Website: www.fda.gov/cdrh/mdr.html

Institute of Electrical and Electronics Engineers
445 Hoes Lane
P.O. Box 1331
Piscataway, NJ 08850-1331
(732) 562-3800
Website: www.standards.ieee.org

International Electrotechnical Commission
Box 131
3 rue de Varembe, CH 1211
Geneva 20, Switzerland
(41) 022-919-0211
Website: www.iec.ch

International Organization for
 Standardization
1 rue de Varembe
Case postale 56, CH 1211
Geneva 20
Switzerland
(41) 022-749-0111
Website: www.iso.ch

Joint Commission on Accreditation
 of Healthcare Organizations
1 Renaissance Boulevard
Oakbrook Terrace, IL 60181
(630) 792-5600
Website: www.jcaho.org

Medical Devices Agency
Department of Health
Room 1209, Hannibal House
Elephant and Castle
London, SE1 6TQ
United Kingdom
(44) 171-972-8143
Website: www.medical-devices.gov.uk

National Council on Radiation
 Protection and Measurements
7910 Woodmont Avenue, Suite 800
Bethesda, MD 20814
(310) 657-2652
Website: www.ncrp.com

National Fire Protection Association
1 Batterymarch Park
PO Box 9101
Quincy, MA 02269-9101
(617) 770-3000
Website: www.nfpa.org

Nuclear Regulatory Commission
11555 Rockville Pike, Rockville
MD 20852, (301) 492-7000
Website: www.nrc.gov

Occupational Safety and Health Administration
US Department of Labor
Office of Information and Consumer Affairs
200 Constitution Avenue, NW
Room N3647, Washington, DC 20210
(202) 219-8151
Website: www.osha.gov

ORKI
National Institute for Hospital and
 Medical Engineering
Budapest dios arok 3, H-1125
Hungary, (33) 1-156-1522

Radiation Protection Branch
Environmental Health Directorate
Health Canada, 775 Brookfield Road
Ottawa, ON K1A 1C1
Website: www.hc-sc.gc.ca/ehp/ehd/rpb

Russian Scientific and Research Institute
Russian Public Health Ministry
EKRAN, 3 Kasatkina Street
Moscow, Russia 129301
(44) 071-405-3474

Society of Nuclear Medicine, Inc.
1850 Samuel Morse Drive
Reston, VA 20190-5316, (703) 708-9000
Website: www.snm.org

Standards Association of Australia
PO Box 1055, Strathfield
NSW 2135, Australia
(61) 02-9746-4700
Website: www.standards.org.au

Therapeutic Goods Administration
PO Box 100, Wooden, ACT 2606
Australia, (61) 2-6232-8610
Website: www.health.gov.au/tga

Underwriters Laboratories, Inc.
333 Pfingsten Road
Northbrook, IL 60062-2096
(847) 272-8800
Website: www.ul.com

VTT, Technical Research Center of Finland
Postbox 316
SF-33101 Tampere 10
Finland, (358) 31-163300
Website: www.vti.fi

80.2 Technology Assessment Agencies

Technology assessment is the practical process of determining the value of a new or emerging technology in and of itself or against existing or competing technologies using safety, efficacy, effectiveness, outcome, risk management, strategic, financial, and competitive criteria. Technology assessment also considers ethics and law as well as health priorities and cost-effectiveness compared to competing technologies. A "technology" is defined as devices, equipment, related software, drugs, biotechnologies, procedures, and therapies; and systems used to diagnose or treat patients. The processes of technology assessment are discussed in detail in Chapter 76.

Technology assessment is not the same as technology acquisition/procurement or technology planning. The latter two are processes for determining equipment vendors, soliciting bids, and systematically determining a hospital's technology related needs based on strategic, financial, risk management, and clinical criteria. The informational needs differ greatly between technology assessment and the acquisition/procurement or planning processes. This section focuses on the resources applicable to technology assessment.

Worldwide, there are nearly 400 organizations (private, academic, and governmental), providing technology assessment information, databases, or consulting services. Some are strictly information clearing houses, some perform technology assessment, and some do both. For those that perform assessments, the quality of the information generated varies greatly from superficial studies to in-depth, well referenced analytical reports. In 1997, the U.S. Agency for Health Care Policy and Research (AHCPR) designated 12 "Evidence-Based Practice Centers" (EPC) to undertake major technology assessment studies on a contract basis. Each of these EPCs are noted in the list below and general descriptions of each center may be viewed on the internet at the AHCPR Website http://www.ahcpr.gov/clinic/epc/.

Language limitations are a significant issue. In the ultimate analysis, the ability to undertake technology assessment requires assimilating vast amounts of information, most of which exists only in the English language. Technology assessment studies published by the International Society for Technology Assessment in Health Care (ISTAHC), by the World Health Organization, and other umbrella organizations are generally in English. The new International Health Technology Assessment database being developed by ECRI in conjunction with the U.S. National Library of Medicine contains more than 30,000 citations to technology assessments and related documents.

Below are the names, mailing addresses, and Internet Website addresses of some of the most prominent organizations undertaking technology assessment studies:

Agence Nationale pour le Develeppement
de l'Evaluation Medicale
159 Rue Nationale
Paris 75013
France
(33) 42-16-7272
Website: www.upml.fr/andem/andem.htm

Agencia de Evaluacion de
 Technologias Sanitarias
Ministerio de Sanidad y Consumo
Instituto de Salud Carlos III, AETS
Sinesio Delgado 6, 28029 Madrid
Spain, (34) 1-323-4359
Website: www.isciii.es/aets

Agence Nationale pour
le Develeppement
de l'Evaluation Medicale
159 Rue Nationale
Paris 75013
France
(33) 42-16-7272
Website: www.upml.fr/andem/andem.htm

Alberta Heritage Foundation for
Medical Research
125 Manulife Place
10180-101 Street
Edmonton, AB T5J 345
(403) 423-5727
Website: www.ahfmr.ab.ca

American Association of Preferred
Provider Organizations
601 13th Street, NW
Suite 370 South
Washington, DC 20005
(202) 347-7600

American Academy of Neurology
1080 Montreal Avenue
St. Paul, MN 55116-2791
(612) 695-2716
Website: www.aan.com

American College of Obstetricians
and Gynecologists
409 12th Street, SW
Washington, DC 20024
(202) 863-2518
Website: www.acog.org

Australian Institute of
Health and Welfare
GPO Box 570
Canberra, ACT 2601
Australia
(61) 06-243-5092
Website: www.aihw.gov.au

Battelle Medical Technology
Assessment and Policy
Research Center (MEDTAP)
901 D Street, SW
Washington, DC 20024
(202) 479-0500
Website: www.battelle.org

Blue Cross and Blue Shield Association
Technology Evaluation Center
225 N Michigan Avenue
Chicago, IL 60601-7680
(312) 297-5530
(312) 297-6080 (publications)
Website: www.bluecares.com/new/clinical
(An EPC of AHCPR)

British Columbia Office of Health
Technology Assessment
Centre for Health Services & Policy Research,
University of British Columbia
429-2194 Health Sciences Mall
Vancouver, BC V6T 1Z3
Canada, (604) 822-7049
Website: www.chspr.ubc.ca

British Institute of Radiology
36 Portland Place
London, W1N 4AT
United Kingdom
(44) 171-580-4085
Website: www.bir.org.uk

Canadian Coordinating Office for
Health Technology Assessment
110-955 Green Valley Crescent
Ottawa ON K2C 3V4
Canada, (613) 226-2553
Website: www.ccohta.ca

Canadian Healthcare Association
17 York Street
Ottawa, ON K1N 9J6
Canada, (613) 241-8005
Website: www.canadian-healthcare.org

Catalan Agency for Health
Technology Assessment
Travessera de les Corts 131-159
Pavello Avenue
Maria, 08028 Barcelona
Spain, (34) 93-227-29-00
Website: www.aatm.es

Centre for Health Economics
University of York
York Y01 5DD
United Kingdom
(44) 01904-433718
Website: www.york.ac.uk

Center for Medical
  Technology Assessment
Linköping University
5183 Linköping, Box 1026 (551-11)
Sweden, (46) 13-281-000

Center for Practice and Technology
  Assessment Agency for Health
  Care Policy and Research (AHCPR)
6010 Executive Boulevard, Suite 300
Rockville, MD 20852
(301) 594-4015
Website: www.ahcpr.gov

Committee for Evaluation and Diffusion
  of Innovative Technologies
3 Avenue Victoria
Paris 75004, France
(33) 1-40-273-109

Conseil d'evaluation des technologies
de la sante du Quebec
201 Cremazie Boulevard East
Bur 1.01, Montreal
PQ H2M 1L2, Canada
(514) 873-2563
Website: www.msss.gouv.qc.ca

Danish Hospital Institute
Landermaerket 10
Copenhagen K
Denmark DK1119
(45) 33-11-5777

Danish Medical Research Council
Bredgade 43
1260 Copenhagen
Denmark
(45) 33-92-9700

Danish National Board of Health
Amaliegade 13, PO Box 2020
Copenhagen K, Denmark DK1012
(45) 35-26-5400

Duke Center for Clinical Health
  Policy Research
Duke University Medical Center
2200 West Main Street, Suite 320
Durham, NC 27705
(919) 286-3399
Website: www.clinipol.mc.duke.edu
(An EPC of AHCPR)

ECRI
5200 Butler Pike
Plymouth Meeting, PA 19462
(610) 825-6000
(610) 834-1275 fax
Websites: www.ecri.org
www.ecriy2k.org
www.mdsr.ecri.org
(An EPC of AHCPR)

Finnish Office for Health Care
  Technology Assessment
PO Box 220
FIN-00531 Helsinki
Finland, (35) 89-3967-2296
Website: www.stakes.fi/finohta

Frost and Sullivan, Inc.
106 Fulton Street
New York, NY 10038-2786
(212) 233-1080
Website: www.frost.com

Health Council of
  the Netherlands
PO Box 1236
2280 CE, Rijswijk
The Netherlands
(31) 70-340-7520

Health Services Directorate
  Strategies and Systems for Health
Health Promotion
Health Promotion and Programs Branch
Health Canada
1915B Tunney's Pasture
Ottawa, ON K1A 1B4
Canada, (613) 954-8629
Website: www.hc-sc.gc.ca/hppb/hpol

Health Technology Advisory Committee
121 East 7th Place, Suite 400
PO Box 64975
St. Paul, MN 55164-6358
(612) 282-6358

Hong Kong Institute of Engineers
9/F Island Centre
No. 1 Great George Street
Causeway Bay
Hong Kong

Institute for Clinical PET
7100-A Manchester Boulevard
Suite 300
Alexandria, VA 22310
(703) 924-6650
Website: www.icpet.org

Institute for Clinical
  Systems Integration
8009 34th Avenue South
Minneapolis, MN 55425
(612) 883-7999
Website: www.icsi.org

Institute for Health Policy Analysis
8401 Colesville Road, Suite 500
Silver Spring, MD 20910
(301) 565-4216

Institute of Medicine (U.S.)
National Academy of Sciences
2101 Constitution Avenue, NW
Washington, DC 20418
(202) 334-2352
Website: www.nas.edu/iom

International Network of Agencies for
  Health Technology Assessment
c/o SBU, Box 16158
S-103 24 Stockholm
Sweden, (46) 08-611-1913
Website: www.sbu.se/sbu-site/links/inahta

Johns Hopkins Evidence-based
  Practice Center
The Johns Hopkins
  Medical Institutions
2020 E Monument Street, Suite 2-600
Baltimore, MD 21205-2223
(410) 955-6953
Website: www.jhsph.edu/Departments/Epi/
(An EPC of AHCPR)

McMaster University Evidence-based
Practice Center
1200 Main Street West, Room 3H7
Hamilton, ON L8N 3Z5
Canada
(905) 525-9140 ext. 22520
Website: http://hiru.mcmaster.ca.epc/
(An EPC of AHCPR)

Medical Alley
1550 Utica Avenue, South
Suite 725
Minneapolis, MN 55416
(612) 542-3077
Website: www.medicalalley.org

Medical Devices Agency
Department of Health
Room 1209
Hannibal House
Elephant and Castle
London, SE1 6TQ
United Kingdom
(44) 171-972-8143
Website: www.medical-devices.gov.uk

Medical Technology Practice
  Patterns Institute
4733 Bethesda Avenue, Suite 510
Bethesda, MD 20814
(301) 652-4005
Website: www.mtppi.org

MEDTAP International
7101 Wisconsin Avenue, Suite 600
Bethesda MD 20814
(301) 654-9729
Website: www.medtap.com

MetaWorks, Inc.
470 Atlantic Avenue
Boston, MA 02210
(617) 368-3573 ext. 206
Website: www.metawork.com
(An EPC of AHCPR)

National Institute of
  Nursing Research, NIH
31 Center Drive
Room 5B10. MSC 2178
Bethesda, MD 20892-2178
(301) 496-0207
Website: www.nih.gov/ninr

National Commission on
  Quality Assurance
2000 L Street NW, Suite 500
Washington. DC 20036
(202) 955-3500
Website: www.ncqa.org

National Committee of Clinical
  Laboratory Standards (NCCLS)
940 West Valley Road, Suite 1400
Wayne, PA 19087-1898
(610) 688-0100
Website: www.nccls.org

National Coordinating Center for
  Health Technology Assessment
Boldrewood (Mailpoint 728)
Univ of Southampton SO16 7PX
United Kingdom, (44) 170-359-5642
Website: www.soton.ac.uk/~hta/address.htm

National Health and Medical Research Council
GPO Box 9848
Canberra, ACT Australia
(61) 06-289-7019

New England Medical Center
Center for Clinical Evidence Synthesis
Division of Clinical Research
750 Washington Street, Box 63
Boston, MA 02111
(617) 636-5133
Website: www.nemc.org/medicine/ccr/cces.htm
(An EPC of AHCPR)

New York State Department of Health
Tower Building, Empire State Plaza
Albany, NY 12237
(518) 474-7354
Website: www.health.state.ny.us

NHS Centre for Reviews and Dissemination
University of York
York Y01 5DD, United Kingdom
(44) 01-904-433634
Website: www.york.ac.uk

Office of Medical Applications of Research
NIH Consensus Program Information Service
PO Box 2577, Kensington
MD 20891, (301) 231-8083
Website: odp.od.nih.gov/consensus

Ontario Ministry of Health
Hepburn Block
80 Grosvenor Street
10th Floor
Toronto, ON M7A 2C4
(416) 327-4377

Oregon Health Sciences University
Division of Medical Informatics
  and Outcomes Research
3181 SW Sam Jackson Park Road
Portland, OR 97201-3098
(503) 494-4277
Website: www.ohsu.edu/epc
(An EPC of AHCPR)

Pan American Health Organization
525 23rd Street NW
Washington, DC 20037-2895
(202) 974-3222
Website: www.paho.org

Physician Payment Review
  Commission (PPRC)
2120 L Street NW, Suite 510
Washington, DC 20037
(202) 653-7220

Prudential Insurance Company
  of America Health Care Operations and
  Research Division
56 N Livingston Avenue
Roseland, NJ 07068
(201) 716-3870

Research Triangle Institute
3040 Cornwallis Road
PO Box 12194
Research Triangle Park, NC 27709-2194
(919) 541-6512
(919) 541-7480
Website: www.rti.org/epc/
(An EPC of AHCPR)

San Antonio Evidence-based Practice Center
University of Texas Health Sciences Center
Department of Medicine
7703 Floyd Curl Drive
San Antonio, TX 78284-7879
(210) 617-5190
Website: www.uthscsa.edu/
(An EPC of AHCPR)

Saskatchewan Health
Acute and Emergency
  Services Branch
3475 Albert Street
Regina, SK S4S 6X6
(306) 787-3656

Scottish Health Purchasing
  Information Centre
Summerfield House
2 Eday Road
Aberdeen AB15 6RE
Scotland
United Kingdom
(44) 0-1224-663-456 ext. 75246
Website: www.nahat.net/shpic

Servicio de Evaluacion de
  Technologias Sanitarias
Duque de Wellington 2
E01010 Vitoria-Gasteiz
Spain, (94) 518-9250
E-mail: osteba-san@ej-gv.es

Society of Critical Care Medicine
8101 E Kaiser Boulevard
Suite 300
Anaheim, CA 92808-2259
(714) 282-6000
Website: www.sccm.org

Swedish Council on Technology
  Assessment in Health Care
Box 16158
S-103 24 Stockholm
Sweden
(46) 08-611-1913
Website: www.sbu.se

Southern California EPC-RAND
1700 Main Street
Santa Monica, CA 90401
(310) 393-0411 ext. 6669
Website: www.rand.org/organization/health/epc/
(An EPC of AHCPR)

Swiss Institute for Public
  Health Technology Programme
Pfrundweg 14
CH-5001 Aarau
Switzerland
(41) 064-247-161

TNO Prevention and Health
PO Box 2215
2301 CE Leiden
The Netherlands
(31) 71-518-1818
Website: www.tno.n1/instit/pg/index.html

University HealthSystem Consortium
2001 Spring Road, Suite 700
Oak Brook, IL 60523
(630) 954-1700
Website: www.uhc.edu

University of Leeds
School of Public Health
30 Hyde Terrace
Leeds L52 9LN
United Kingdom
Website: www.leeds.ac.uk

USCF-Stanford University EPC
University of California
San Francisco
505 Parnassus Avenue
Room M-1490, Box 0132
San Francisco, CA 94143-0132
(415) 476-2564
Website: www.stanford.edu/group/epc/
(An EPC of AHCPR)

U.S. Office of Technology
  Assessment (former address)
600 Pennsylvania Avenue SE
Washington, DC 20003
Note: OTA closed on 29 Sep, 1995.
However, documents can be
  accessed via the internet at
  www.wws.princeton.edu/§ota/html2/cong.html
Also a complete set of
OTA publications is
available on CD-ROM; contact
the U.S. Government Printing Office
(www.gpo.gov) for more information

Veterans Administration
Technology Assessment Program
VA Medical Center (152M)
150 S Huntington Avenue
Building 4
Boston, MA 02130
(617) 278-4469
Website: www.va.gov/resdev

Voluntary Hospitals of America, Inc.
220 East Boulevard
Irving, TX 75014
(214) 830-0000

Wessex Institute of Health Research
   and Development
Boldrewood Medical School
Bassett Crescent East
Highfield, Southampton SO16 7PX
United Kingdom
(44) 01-703-595-661
Website: www.soton.ac.uk/~wi/index.html

World Health Organization
Distribution Sales, CH 1211
Geneva 27, Switzerland 2476
(41) 22-791-2111
Website: www.who.ch
Note: Publications are also available from the
   WHO Publications Center, USA,
   at (518) 436-9686.

References

ECRI. *Healthcare Standards Official Directory.* ECRI, Plymouth Meeting, PA, 1999.

Eddy D.M. *A Manual for Assessing Health Practices & Designing Practice Policies: The Explicit Approach.* American College of Physicians, Philadelphia, PA, 1992.

Goodman C., Ed. *Medical Technology Assessment Directory.* National Academy Press, Washington, DC, 1988.

Marcaccio K.Y., ed. *Gale Directory of Databases. Volume 1: Online Databases.* Gale Research International, London, 1993.

van Nimwegen Chr., ed. *International List of Reports on Comparative Evaluations of Medical Devices.* TNO Centre for Medical Technology, Leiden, the Netherlands, 1993.

Further Information

A comprehensive listing of healthcare standards and the issuing organizations is presented in the Healthcare Standards Directory published by ECRI. The Directory is well organized by keywords, organizations and their standards, federal and state laws, legislation and regulations, and contains a complete index of names and addresses.

The International Health Technology Assessment database is produced by ECRI. A portion of the database is also available in the U.S. National Library of Medicine's new database called HealthSTAR. Internet access to HealthSTAR is through Website address http://igm.nlm.nih.gov. A description of the database may be found at http://www.nlm.nih.gov/pubs/factsheets/healthstar.html.

81

Applications of Virtual Instruments in Health Care

Eric Rosow
Hartford Hospital
Premise Development Corporation

Joseph Adam
Premise Development Corporation

81.1 Applications of Virtual Instruments in Health Care .. **81**-1
Example Application #1: The EndoTester™ — A Virtual
Instrument-Based Quality Control and Technology
Assessment System for Surgical Video Systems • Example
Application #2: PIVIT™ — Performance Indicator
Virtual Instrument Toolkit • Trending, Relationships, and
Interactive Alarms • Data Modeling • Medical Equipment
Risk Criteria • Peer Performance Reviews
References **81**-9

81.1 Applications of Virtual Instruments in Health Care

Virtual Instrumentation (which was previously defined in Chapter 73, *"Virtual Instrumentation: Applications in Biomedical Engineering"*) allows organizations to effectively harness the power of the PC to access, analyze, and share information throughout the organization. With vast amounts of data available from increasingly sophisticated enterprise-level data sources, potentially useful information is often left hidden due to a lack of useful tools. Virtual instruments can employ a wide array of technologies such as multidimensional analyses and Statistical Process Control (SPC) tools to detect patterns, trends, causalities, and discontinuities to derive knowledge and make informed decisions.

Today's enterprises create vast amounts of raw data and recent advances in storage technology, coupled with the desire to use this data competitively, has caused a data glut in many organizations. The healthcare industry in particular is one that generates a tremendous amount of data. Tools such as databases and spreadsheets certainly help manage and analyze this data; however databases, while ideal for extracting data are generally not suited for graphing and analysis. Spreadsheets, on the other hand, are ideal for analyzing and graphing data, but this can often be a cumbersome process when working with multiple data files. Virtual instruments empower the user to leverage the best of both worlds by creating a suite of user-defined applications which allow the end-user to convert vast amounts of data into information which is ultimately transformed into knowledge to enable better decision making.

This chapter will discuss several virtual instrument applications and tools that have been developed to meet the specific needs of healthcare organizations. Particular attention will be placed on the use of quality control and "performance indicators" which provide the ability to trend and forecast various metrics. The use of SPC within virtual instruments will also be demonstrated. Finally, a nontraditional application of virtual instrumentation will be presented in which a "peer review" application has been developed to allow members of an organization to actively participate in the Employee Performance Review process.

81.1.1 Example Application #1: The EndoTester™ — A Virtual Instrument-Based Quality Control and Technology Assessment System for Surgical Video Systems

The use of endoscopic surgery is growing, in large part because it is generally safer and less expensive than conventional surgery, and patients tend to require less time in a hospital after endoscopic surgery. Industry experts conservatively estimate that about 4 million minimally invasive procedures were performed in 1996. As endoscopic surgery becomes more common, there is an increasing need to accurately evaluate the performance characteristics of endoscopes and their peripheral components.

The assessment of the optical performance of laparoscopes and video systems is often difficult in the clinical setting. The surgeon depends on a high quality image to perform minimally invasive surgery, yet assurance of proper function of the equipment by biomedical engineering staff is not always straightforward. Many variables in both patient and equipment may result in a poor image. Equipment variables, which may degrade image quality, include problems with the endoscope, either with optics or light transmission. The light cable is another source of uncertainty as a result of optical loss from damaged fibers. Malfunctions of the charge coupled device (CCD) video camera are yet another source of poor image quality. Cleanliness of the equipment, especially lens surfaces on the endoscope (both proximal and distal ends) are particularly common problems. Patient variables make the objective assessment of image quality more difficult. Large operative fields and bleeding at the operative site are just two examples of patient factors that may affect image quality.

The evaluation of new video endoscopic equipment is also difficult because of the lack of objective standards for performance. Purchasers of equipment are forced to make an essentially subjective decision about image quality. By employing virtual instrumentation, a collaborative team of biomedical engineers, software engineers, physicians, nurses, and technicians at Hartford Hospital (Hartford, CT) and Premise Development Corporation (Avon, CT) have developed an instrument, the EndoTester™, with integrated software to quantify the optical properties of both rigid and flexible fiberoptic endoscopes. This easy-to-use optical evaluation system allows objective measurement of endoscopic performance prior to equipment purchase and in routine clinical use as part of a program of prospective maintenance.

The EndoTester™ was designed and fabricated to perform a wide array of quantitative tests and measurements. Some of these tests include (1) Relative light loss, (2) Reflective symmetry, (3) Lighted (good) fibers, (4) Geometric distortion, and (5) Modulation transfer function (MTF). Each series of tests is associated with a specific endoscope to allow for trending and easy comparison of successive measurements.

Specific information about each endoscope (i.e., manufacturer, diameter, length, tip angle, department/unit, control number, and operator), the reason for the test (i.e., quality control, pre/post repair, etc.), and any problems associated with the scope are also documented through the electronic record. In addition, all the quantitative measurements from each test are automatically appended to the electronic record for life-cycle performance analysis.

Figure 81.1 and Figure 81.2 illustrate how information about the fiberoptic bundle of an endoscope can be displayed and measured. This provides a record of the pattern of lighted optical fibers for the endoscope under test. The number of lighted pixels will depend on the endoscope's dimensions, the distal end geometry, and the number of failed optical fibers. New fiber damage to an endoscope will be apparent by comparison of the lighted fiber pictures (and histogram profiles) from successive tests. Statistical data is also available to calculate the percentage of working fibers in a given endoscope.

In addition to the two-dimensional profile of lighted fibers, this pattern (and all other image patterns) can also be displayed in the form of a three-dimensional contour plot. This interactive graph may be viewed from a variety of viewpoints in that the user can vary the elevation, rotation, size, and perspective controls.

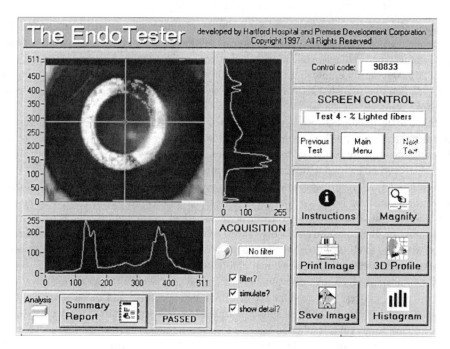

FIGURE 81.1 Endoscope tip reflection.

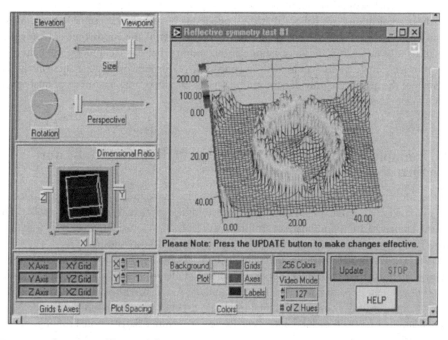

FIGURE 81.2 Endoscope profiling module.

Figure 81.2 illustrates how test images for a specific scope can be profiled over time (i.e., days, months, years) to identify degrading performance. This profile is also useful to validate repair procedures by comparing test images before and after the repair.

The EndoTester™ has many applications. In general, the most useful application is the ability to objectively measure an endoscope's performance prior to purchase, and in routine clinical use as part of a program of prospective maintenance. Measuring parameters of scope performance can facilitate equipment purchase. Vendor claims of instrument capabilities can be validated as a part of the negotiation process. Commercially available evaluation systems (for original equipment manufacturers) can cost upward of $50,000, yet by employing the benefits of virtual instrumentation and a standard PC, an affordable, yet highly accurate test system for rigid and flexible fiberoptic endoscopes can now be obtained by clinical institutions.

In addition to technology assessment applications, the adoption of disposable endoscopes raises another potential use for the EndoTester™. Disposable scopes are estimated to have a life of 20 to 30 procedures. However, there is no easy way to determine exactly when a scope should be "thrown away." The EndoTester™ could be used to define this end-point.

The greatest potential for this system is as part of a program of preventive maintenance. Currently, in most operating rooms, endoscopes are removed from service and sent for repair when they fail in clinical use. This causes operative delay with attendant risk to the patient and an increase in cost to the institution. The problem is difficult because an endoscope may be adequate in one procedure but fail in the next which is more exacting due to clinical variables such as large patient size or bleeding. Objective assessment of endoscope function with the EndoTester™ may eliminate some of these problems.

Equally as important, an endoscope evaluation system will also allow institutions to ensure value from providers of repair services. The need for repair can be better defined and the adequacy of the repair verified when service is completed. This ability becomes especially important as the explosive growth of minimally invasive surgery has resulted in the creation of a significant market for endoscope repairs and service. Endoscope repair costs vary widely throughout the industry with costs ranging from $500 to 1500 or more per repair. Inappropriate or incomplete repairs can result in extending surgical time by requiring the surgeon to "switch scopes" (in some cases several times) during a surgical procedure.

Given these applications, we believe that the EndoTester™ can play an important role in reducing unnecessary costs, while at the same time improving the quality of the endoscopic equipment and the outcome of its utilization. It is the sincere hope of the authors that this technology will help to provide accurate, affordable and easy-to-acquire data on endoscope performance characteristics which clearly are to the benefit of the healthcare provider, the ethical service providers, manufacturers of quality products, the payers, and, of course, the patient.

81.1.2 Example Application #2: PIVIT™ — Performance Indicator Virtual Instrument Toolkit

Most of the information management examples presented in this chapter are part of an application suite called PIVIT™. PIVIT is an acronym for "Performance Indicator Virtual Instrument Toolkit" and is an easy-to-use data acquisition and analysis product. PIVIT was developed specifically in response to the wide array of information and analysis needs throughout the healthcare setting.

The PIVIT applies virtual instrument technology to assess, analyze, and forecast clinical, operational, and financial performance indicators. Some examples include applications which profile institutional indicators (i.e., patient days, discharges, percent occupancy, ALOS, revenues, expenses, etc.), and departmental indicators (i.e., salary, nonsalary, total expenses, expense per equivalent discharge, DRGs, etc.). Other applications of PIVIT include 360° Peer Review, Customer Satisfaction Profiling, and Medical Equipment Risk Assessment.

The PIVIT can access data from multiple data sources. Virtually any parameter can be easily accessed and displayed from standard spreadsheet and database applications (i.e., Microsoft Access, Excel, Sybase, Oracle, etc.) using Microsoft's Open Database Connectivity (ODBC) technology. Furthermore, multiple parameters can be profiled and compared in real-time with any other parameter via interactive polar plots and three-dimensional displays. In addition to real-time profiling, other analyses such as SPC can be employed to view large data sets in a graphical format. SPC has been applied successfully for decades to help companies reduce variability in manufacturing processes. These SPC tools range from Pareto graphs

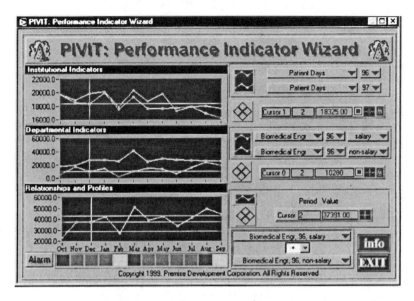

FIGURE 81.3   PIVIT™ — Performance Indicator Wizard displays institutional and departmental indicators.

to Run and Control charts. Although it will not be possible to describe all of these applications, several examples are provided below to illustrate the power of PIVIT.

81.1.3   Trending, Relationships, and Interactive Alarms

Figure 81.3 illustrates a virtual instrument that interactively accesses institutional and department specific indicators and profiles them for comparison. Data sets can be acquired directly from standard spreadsheet and database applications (i.e., Microsoft Access®, Excel®, Sybase®, Oracle®, etc.). This capability has proven to be quite valuable with respect to quickly accessing and viewing large sets of data. Typically, multiple data sets contained within a spreadsheet or database had to be selected and then a new chart of this data had to be created. Using PIVIT, the user simply selects the desired parameter from any one of the pull-down menus and this data set is instantly graphed and compared to any other data set.

Interactive "threshold cursors" dynamically highlight when a parameter is over and/or under a specific target. Displayed parameters can also be ratios of any measured value, for example, "Expense per Equivalent Discharge" or "Revenue to Expense Ratio." The indicator color will change based on how far the data value exceeds the threshold value (i.e., from green to yellow to red). If multiple thresholds are exceeded, then the entire background of the screen (normally gray) will change to red to alert the user of an extreme condition.

Finally, multimedia has been employed by PIVIT to alert designated personnel with an audio message from the personal computer or by sending an automated message via e-mail, fax, pager, or mobile phone.

The PIVIT also has the ability to profile historical trends and project future values. Forecasts can be based on user-defined history (i.e., "Months for Regression"), the type of regression (i.e., linear, exponential, or polynomial), the number of days, months, or years to forecast, and if any offset should be applied to the forecast. These features allow the user to create an unlimited number of "what if" scenarios and allow only the desired range of data to be applied to a forecast. In addition to the graphical display of data values, historical and projected tables are also provided. These embedded tables look and function very much like a standard spreadsheet.

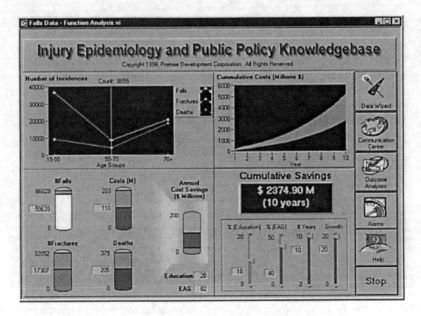

FIGURE 81.4   Injury epidemiology and public policy knowledgebase.

81.1.4 Data Modeling

Figure 81.4 illustrates another example of how virtual instrumentation can be applied to financial modeling and forecasting. This example graphically profiles the annual morbidity, mortality, and cost associated with falls within the state of Connecticut. Such an instrument has proved to be an extremely effective modeling tool due to its ability to interactively highlight relationships and assumptions, and to project the cost and/or savings of employing educational and other interventional programs.

Virtual instruments such as these are not only useful with respect to modeling and forecasting, but perhaps more importantly, they become a "knowledgebase" in which interventions and the efficacy of these interventions can be statistically proven. In addition, virtual instruments can employ standard technologies such as Dynamic Data Exchange (DDE), ActiveX, or TCP/IP to transfer data to commonly used software applications such as Microsoft Access® or Microsoft Excel®. In this way, virtual instruments can measure and graph multiple signals while at the same time send this data to another application which could reside on the network or across the Internet.

Another module of the PIVIT application is called the "Communications Center." This module can be used to simply create and print a report or it can be used to send e-mail, faxes, messages to a pager, or even leave voice-mail messages. This is a powerful feature in that information can be easily and efficiently distributed to both individuals and groups in real-time.

Additionally, Microsoft Agent® technology can be used to pop-up an animated help tool to communicate a message, indicate an alarm condition, or can be used to help the user solve a problem or point out a discrepancy that may have otherwise gone unnoticed. Agents employ a "text-to-speech" algorithm to actually "speak" an analysis or alarm directly to the user or recipient of the message. In this way, on-line help and user support can also be provided in multiple languages.

In addition to real-time profiling of various parameters, more advanced analyses such as SPC can be employed to view large data sets in a graphical format. SPC has been applied successfully for decades to help companies reduce variability in manufacturing processes. It is the opinion of this author that SPC has enormous applications throughout healthcare. For example, Figure 81.5 shows how Pareto analysis can be applied to a sample trauma database of over 12,000 records. The Pareto chart may be frequency or percentage depending on front panel selection and the user can select from a variety of different parameters by clicking on the "pull-down" menu. This menu can be configured to automatically display each database

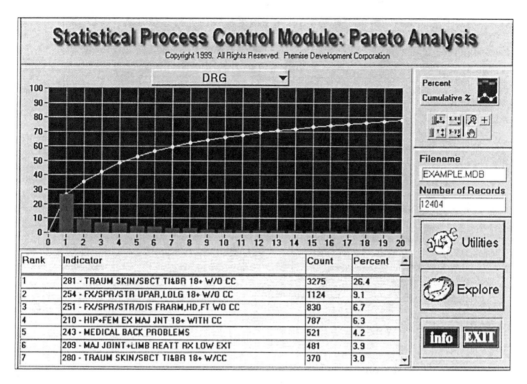

FIGURE 81.5   Statistical process control — Pareto analysis of a sample trauma registry.

field directly from the database. In this example, various database fields (i.e., DRG, Principal Diagnosis, Town, Payer, etc.) can be selected for Pareto analysis. Other SPC tools include run charts, control charts, and process capability distributions.

81.1.5   Medical Equipment Risk Criteria

Figure 81.6 illustrates a virtual instrument application which demonstrates how four "static" risk categories (and their corresponding values) are used to determine the inclusion of clinical equipment in the Medical Equipment Management Program at Hartford Hospital. Each risk category includes specific sub-categories that are assigned points, which when added together according to the formula listed below, yield a total score which ranges from 4 to 25.

Considering these scores, the equipment is categorized into five priority levels (High, Medium, Low, Grey List, and Non-Inclusion into the Medical Equipment Management Program). The four static risk categories are:

Equipment function (EF): Stratifies the various functional categories (i.e., therapeutic, diagnostic, analytical, and miscellaneous) of equipment. This category has "point scores" which range from 1 (miscellaneous, non-patient related devices) to 10 (therapeutic, life support devices)

Physical risk (PR): Lists the "worst case scenario" of physical risk potential to either the patient or the operator of the equipment. This category has "point scores" which range from 1 (no significant identified risk) to 5 (potential for patient and/or operator death)

Environmental use classification (EC): Lists the primary equipment area in which the equipment is used and has "point scores" which range from 1 (non-patient care areas) to 5 (anesthetizing locations)

Preventive maintenance requirements (MR): Describes the level and frequency of required maintenance and has "point scores" which range from 1 (not required) to 5 (monthly maintenance)

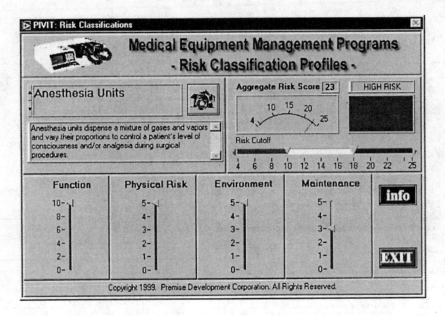

FIGURE 81.6   Medical equipment risk classification profiler.

The aggregate static risk score is calculated as follows:

$$\text{Aggregate Risk Score} = EF + PR + EC + MR \tag{81.1}$$

Using the criteria's system described above, clinical equipment is categorized according to the following priority of testing and degree of risk:

High risk: Equipment that scores between and including 18 to 25 points on the criteria's evaluation system. This equipment is assigned the highest risk for testing, calibration, and repair

Medium risk: Equipment that scores between and including 15 to 17 points on the criteria's evaluation system

Low risk: Equipment that scores between and including 12 to 14 points on the criteria's evaluation system

Hazard surveillance (gray): Equipment that scores between and including 6 and 11 points on the criteria's evaluation system is visually inspected on an annual basis during the hospital hazard surveillance rounds

Medical equipment management program deletion: Medical equipment and devices that pose little risk and scores less than 6 points may be deleted from the management program as well as the clinical equipment inventory

Future versions of this application will also consider "dynamic" risk factors such as: user error, mean-time-between failure (MTBF), device failure within 30 days of a preventive maintenance or repair, and the number of years beyond the American Hospital Association's recommended useful life

81.1.6   Peer Performance Reviews

The virtual instrument shown in Figure 81.7 has been designed to easily acquire and compile performance information with respect to institution-wide competencies. It has been created to allow every member of a team or department to participate in the evaluation of a co-worker (360° peer review). Upon running the application, the user is presented with a "Sign-In" screen where he or she enters their username and password. The application is divided into three components. The first (top section) profiles the employee

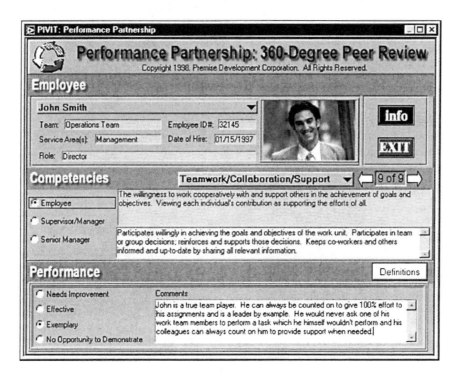

FIGURE 81.7   Performance reviews using virtual instrumentation.

and relevant service information. The second (middle section) indicates each competency as defined for employees, managers, and senior managers. The last (bottom) section allows the reviewer to evaluate performance by selecting one of four "radio buttons" and also provide specific comments related to each competency. This information is then compiled (with other reviewers) as real-time feedback.

References

[1] American Society for Quality Control. American National Standard. Definitions, Symbols, Forumulas, and Tables for Control Charts, 1987.

[2] Breyfogle, F.W. *Statistical Methods for Testing, Development and Manufacturing*, John Wiley & Sons, New York, 1982.

[3] Carey, R.G. and Lloyd, R.C. *Measuring Quality Improvement in Healthcare: A Guide to Statistical Process Control Applications*, 1995.

[4] Fennigkow, L. and Lagerman, B. Medical Equipment Management. 1997 EC/PTSM Series/No. 1; Joint Commission on Accreditation of Hospital Organizations, 1997, pp. 47–54.

[5] Frost & Sullivan Market Intelligence, file 765, The Dialog Corporation, Worldwide Headquarters, 2440 W. El Camino Real, Mountain View, CA 94040.

[6] Inglis, A. *Video Engineering*, McGraw Hill, New York, 1993.

[7] Kutzner J., Hightower L., and Pruitt C. Measurement and Testing of CCD Sensors and Cameras, *SMPTE Journal*, 325–327, 1992.

[8] Measurement of Resolution of Camera Systems, *IEEE Standard* 208, 1995.

[9] Medical Device Register 1997, Volume 2, Montvale NJ, Medical Economics Data Production Company, 1997.

[10] Montgomery, D.C. *Introduction to Statistical Quality Control*, 2nd ed., John Wiley & Sons, New York, 1992.

[11] Rosow, E. Virtual Instrumentation Applications with BioSensors, presented at the *Biomedical Engineering Consortium for Connecticut (BEACON) Biosensor Symposium*, Trinity College, Hartford, CT, October 2, 1998.

[12] Rosow, E., Adam, J., and Beatrice, F. The EndoTester': A Virtual Instrument Endoscope Evaluation System for Fiberoptic Endoscopes, *Biomedical Instrumentation and Technology*, 480–487, September/October 1998.

[13] Surgical Video Systems, *Health Devices*, 24, 428–457, 1995.

[14] Walker, B. *Optical Engineering Fundamentals*, McGraw Hill, New York, 1995.

[15] Wheeler, D.J. and Chambers, D.S. *Understanding Statistical Process Control*, 2nd ed., SPC Press, 1992.

VIII

Ethical Issues Associated with the Use of Medical Technology

Subrata Saha
Clemson University

Joseph D. Bronzino
Trinity College/Biomedical Engineering Alliance for Connecticut (BEACON)

82 Beneficence, Nonmaleficence, and Medical Technology
Joseph D. Bronzino **82**-1

83 Ethical Issues Related to Clinical Research
Joseph D. Bronzino **83**-1

BIOMEDICAL ENGINEERING IS RESPONSIBLE for many of the recent advances in modern medicine. These development have led to new treatment modalities that have significantly improved not only medical care, but the quality of life for many patients in our society. However, along with such positive outcomes new ethical dilemmas and challenges have also emerged. These include (1) involvement of humans in clinical research, (2) definition of death and the issue of euthanasia, (3) animal experimentation and human trials for new medical devices, (4) patient access to sophisticated and high cost medical technology, (5) regulation of new biomaterials and devices. With these issues in mind, this section discusses some of these topics. The first chapter focuses on the concept of professional ethics and its importance to the practicing biomedical engineer. The second chapter deals with the role medical technology has played in the definition of death and the dilemmas posed by advocates of euthanasia. The third chapter focuses on the use of animals and humans in research and clinical experimentation. The final chapter addresses the issue of regulating the use of devices, materials, etc. in the care of patients.

Since the space allocated in the handbook is limited, a complete discussion of many ethical dilemmas encountered by practicing biomedical engineers is beyond the scope of this section. Therefore, it is our sincere hope that the readers of this handbook will further explore these ideas from other texts and articles, some of which are references at the end of the chapter. Clearly, a course on biomedical ethics should be an essential component of any bioengineering curriculum.

With new developments in biotechnology and genetic engineering, we need to ask ourselves not only if we can do it, but also "should it be done?" As professional engineers we also have an obligation to educate the public and other regulatory agencies regarding the social implications of such new developments. It is our hope that the topics covered in this can provide an impetus for further discussion of the ethical issues and challenges faced by the bioengineer during the course of his/her professional life.

82

Beneficence, Nonmaleficence, and Medical Technology

82.1 Defining Death: A Moral Dilemma Posed by
      Medical Technology **82**-2
82.2 Euthanasia **82**-3
      Active vs. Passive Euthanasia • Involuntary and
      Nonvoluntary Euthanasia • Should Voluntary Euthanasia Be
      Legalized?

Joseph D. Bronzino
Trinity College

References **82**-8
Further Information **82**-8

Two moral norms have remained relatively *constant across* the various moral codes and oaths that have been formulated for health-care deliverers since the beginning of Western medicine in classical Greek civilization, namely beneficence — the provision of benefits — and nonmaleficence — the avoidance of doing harm. These norms are traced back to a body of writings from classical antiquity known as the *Hippocratic Corpus.* Although these writings are associated with the name of Hippocrates, the acknowledged founder of Western medicine, medical historians remain uncertain whether any, including the *Hippocratic Oath,* were actually his work. Although portions of the Corpus are believed to have been authored during the 6th century B.C., other portions are believed to have been written as late as the beginning of the Christian Era. Medical historians agree, though, that many of the specific moral directives of the *Corpus* represent neither the actual practices nor the moral ideals of the majority of physicians of ancient Greece and Rome.

Nonetheless, the general injunction, *"As to disease, make a habit of two things — to help or, at least, to do no harm,"* was accepted as a fundamental medical ethical norm by at least some ancient physicians. With the decline of Hellenistic civilization and the rise of Christianity, beneficence and nonmaleficence became increasingly accepted as the fundamental principles of morally sound medical practice. Although beneficence and nonmaleficence were regarded merely as concomitant to the craft of medicine in classical Greece and Rome, the emphasis upon compassion and the brotherhood of humankind, central to Christianity, *increasingly made* these norms the only acceptable motives for medical practice. Even today the provision of benefits and the avoidance of doing harm are stressed just as much in virtually all contemporary Western codes of conduct for health professionals as they were in the oaths and codes that guided the health-care providers of past centuries.

Traditionally, the ethics of medical care have given greater prominence to nonmaleficence than to beneficence. This priority was grounded in the fact that, historically, medicine's capacity to do harm far exceeded its capacity to protect and restore health. Providers of health care possessed many treatments that posed clear and genuine risks to patients but that offered little prospect of benefit. Truly effective therapies were all too rare. In this context, it is surely rational to give substantially higher priority to avoiding harm than to providing benefits.

The advent of modern science changed matters dramatically. Knowledge acquired in laboratories, tested in clinics, and verified by statistical methods has increasingly dictated the practices of medicine. This *ongoing alliance* between medicine and science became a critical source of the plethora of technologies that now pervades medical care. The impressive increases in therapeutic, preventive, and rehabilitative capabilities that these technologies have provided have pushed beneficence to the forefront of medical morality. Some have even gone so far as to hold that the old medical ethic of *"Above all, do no harm"* should be superseded by the new ethic that *"The patient deserves the best."* However, the rapid advances in medical technology capabilities have also produced great uncertainty as to what is most beneficial or least harmful for the patient. In other words, along with increases in ability to be beneficent, medicine's technology has generated much debate about what actually counts as beneficent or nonmaleficent treatment. To illustrate this point, let us turn to several specific moral issues posed by the use of medical technology [Bronzino, 1992, 1999].

82.1 Defining Death: A Moral Dilemma Posed by Medical Technology

Supportive and resuscitative devices, such as the respirator, found in the typical modern intensive care unit provide a useful starting point for illustrating how technology has rendered medical morality more complex and problematic. Devices of this kind allow clinicians to sustain respiration and circulation in patients who have suffered massive brain damage and total permanent loss of brain *function*. These technologies force us to ask: precisely when does a human life end? When is a human being indeed dead? This is not the straightforward factual matter it may appear to be. All of the relevant facts may show that the patient's brain has suffered injury grave enough to destroy its functioning forever. The facts may show that such an individual's circulation and respiration would permanently cease without artificial support. Yet these facts do not determine whether treating such an individual as a corpse is morally appropriate. To know this, it is necessary to know or perhaps to decide on those features of living persons that are essential to their status as "living persons." It is necessary to know or decide which human qualities, if irreparably lost, make an individual identical in all morally relevant respects to a corpse. Once those qualities have been specified, deciding whether total and irreparable loss of brain function constitutes death becomes a straightforward factual matter. Then, it would simply have to be determined if such loss itself deprives the individual of those qualities. If it does, the individual is morally identical to a corpse. If not, then the individual must be regarded and treated as a living person.

The traditional criterion of death has been irreparable cessation of heart beat, respiration, and blood pressure. This criterion would have been quickly met by anyone suffering massive trauma to the brain prior to the development of modern supportive technology. Such technology allows indefinite artificial maintenance of circulation and respiration and, thus, forestalls what once was an inevitable consequence of severe brain injury. The existence and use of such technology therefore challenges the traditional criterion of death and forces us to consider whether continued respiration and circulation are in themselves sufficient to distinguish a living individual from a corpse. Indeed, total and irreparable loss of brain function, referred to as "brainstem death," "whole brain death," and, simply, "brain death," has been widely accepted as the legal standard for death. By this standard, an individual in a state of brain death is legally indistinguishable from a corpse and may be legally treated as one even though respiratory and circulatory functions may be sustained through the intervention of technology. Many take this legal standard to be the morally appropriate one, noting that once destruction of the brain stem has occurred, the brain *cannot function* at all, and the body's regulatory mechanisms will fail unless artificially sustained. Thus, mechanical sustenance of an individual in a state of brain death is merely postponement of the inevitable and sustains nothing of the personality, character, or consciousness of the individual. It is merely the mechanical intervention that differentiates such an individual from a corpse and a mechanically ventilated corpse is a corpse nonetheless.

Even with a consensus that brainstem death is death and thus that an individual in such a state is indeed a corpse, hard cases remain. Consider the case of an individual in a persistent vegetative state, the condition known as "neocortical death." Although severe brain injury has been suffered, enough brain function remains to make mechanical *sustenance* of respiration and circulation unnecessary. In a persistent vegetative state, an individual exhibits no purposeful response to external stimuli and no evidence of self-awareness. The eyes may open periodically and the individual may exhibit sleep–wake cycles. Some patients even yawn, make chewing motions, or swallow spontaneously. Unlike the complete unresponsiveness of individuals in a state of brainstem death, a variety of simple and complex responses can be elicited from an individual in a persistent vegetative state. Nonetheless, the chances that such an individual will regain consciousness virtually do not exist. Artificial feeding, kidney dialysis, and the like make it possible to sustain an individual in a state of neocortical death for decades. This sort of condition and the issues it raises were exemplified by the famous case of Karen Ann Quinlan. James Rachels [1986] provided the following description of the situation created by Quinlan's condition:

> In April 1975, this young woman ceased breathing for at least two 15-min periods, for reasons that were never made clear. As a result, she suffered severe brain damage, and, in the words of the attending physicians, was reduced to a "chronic vegetative state" in which she "no longer had any cognitive function." Accepting the doctors' judgment that there was no hope of recovery, her parents sought permission from the courts to disconnect the respirator that was keeping her alive in the intensive care unit of a New Jersey hospital.
>
> The trial court, and then the Supreme Court of New Jersey, agreed that Karen's respirator could be removed. So it was disconnected. However, the nurse in charge of her care in the Catholic hospital opposed this decision and, anticipating it, had begun to wean her from the respirator so that by the time it was disconnected she could remain alive without it. So Karen did not die. Karen remained alive for ten additional years. In June 1985, she finally died of acute pneumonia. Antibiotics, which would have fought the pneumonia, were not given.

If brainstem death is death, is neocortical death also death? Again, the issue is not a straightforward factual matter. For, it too, is a matter of specifying which features of living individuals distinguish them from corpses and so make treatment of them as corpses morally impermissible. Irreparable cessation of respiration and circulation, the classical criterion for death, would entail that an individual in a persistent vegetative state is not a corpse and so, morally speaking, must not be treated as one. The brainstem death criterion for death would also entail that a person in a state of neocortical death is not yet a corpse. On this criterion, what is crucial is that brain damage be severe enough to cause failure of the body's regulatory mechanisms.

Is an individual in a state of neocortical death any less in possession of the characteristics that distinguish the living from cadavers than one whose respiration and circulation are mechanically maintained? Of course, it is a matter of what the relevant characteristics are, and it is a matter that society must decide. It is not one that can be settled by greater medical information or more powerful medical devices. Until society decides, it will not be clear what would count as beneficent or nonmaleficent treatment of an individual in a state of neocortical death.

82.2 Euthanasia

A long-standing issue in medical ethics, which has been made more pressing by medical technology, is euthanasia, the deliberate termination of an individual's life for the individual's own good. Is such an act ever a permissible use of medical resources? Consider an individual in a persistent vegetative state. On the assumption that such a state is not death, withdrawing life support would be a deliberate termination of a human life. Here a critical issue is whether the quality of a human life can be so low or so great a liability to the individual that deliberately taking action to hasten death or at least not to postpone death is morally defensible. Can the quality of a human life be so low that the value of extending its quantity is totally negated? If so, then Western medicine's traditional commitment to providing benefits and avoiding harm would seem to make cessation of life support a moral requirement in such a case.

Consider the following hypothetical version of the kind of case that actually confronts contemporary patients, their families, health-care workers, and society as a whole. Suppose a middle-aged man suffers a brain hemorrhage and loses consciousness as a result of a ruptured aneurysm. Suppose that he never regains consciousness and is hospitalized in a state of neocortical death, a chronic vegetative state. He is maintained by a surgically implanted gastronomy tube that drips liquid nourishment from a plastic bag directly into his stomach. The care of this individual takes $7\frac{1}{2}$ of nursing time daily and includes (1) shaving, (2) oral hygiene, (3) grooming, (4) attending to his bowels and bladder, and so forth.

Suppose further that his wife undertakes legal action to force his care givers to end all medical treatment, including nutrition and hydration, so that complete bodily death of her husband will occur, She presents a preponderance of evidence to the court to show that her husband would have wanted this result in these circumstances.

The central moral issue raised by this sort of case is whether the quality of the individual's life is sufficiently compromised by neocortical death to make intentioned termination of that life morally permissible. While alive, he made it clear to both family and friends that he would prefer to be allowed to die rather than be mechanically maintained in a condition of irretrievable loss of consciousness. Deciding whether the judgment in such a case should be allowed requires deciding which capacities and qualities make life worth living, which qualities are sufficient to endow it with value worth sustaining, and whether their absence justifies deliberate termination of a life, at least when this would be the wish of the individual in question. Without this decision, the traditional norms of medical ethics, beneficence and nonmaleficence, provide no guidance. Without this decision, it cannot be determined whether termination of life support is a benefit or a harm to the patient.

An even more difficult type of case was provided by the case of Elizabeth Bouvia. Bouvia, who had been a lifelong quadriplegic sufferer of cerebral palsy, was often in pain, completely dependent upon others, and spent all of her time bedridden. Bouvia, after deciding that she did not wish to continue such a life, entered Riverside General Hospital in California. She desired to be kept comfortable while starving to death. Although she remained adamant during her hospitalization, Bouvia's requests were denied by hospital officials with the legal sanction of the courts.

Many who might believe that neocortical death renders the quality of life sufficiently low to justify termination of life support, especially when this agrees with the individual's desires, would not arrive at this conclusion in a case like Bouvia's. Whereas neocortical death completely destroys consciousness and makes purposive interaction with the individual's environment impossible, Bouvia was fully aware and mentally alert. She had previously been married and had even acquired a college education. Televised interviews with her portrayed a very intelligent person who had great skill in presenting persuasive arguments to support her wish not to have her life continued by artificial means of nutrition. Nonetheless, she judged her life to be of such low quality that she should be allowed to choose to deliberately starve to death. Before the existence of life support technology, maintenance of her life against her will might not have been possible at all and at least would have been far more difficult.

Should Elizabeth Bouvia's judgment have been accepted? Her case is more difficult than the care of a patient in a chronic vegetative state because, unlike such an *individual, she* was able to engage in meaningful interaction with her environment. Regarding an individual who cannot speak or otherwise meaningfully interact with others as nothing more than living matter, as a "human vegetable," is not especially difficult. Seeing Bouvia this way is not easy. Her awareness, intelligence, mental acuity, and ability to interact with others means that although her life is one of discomfort, indignity, and complete dependence, she is not a mere "human vegetable."

Despite the differences between Bouvia's situation and that of someone in a state of neocortical death, the same issue is posed. Can the quality of an individual's life be so low that deliberate termination is morally justifiable? How that question is answered is a matter of what level of quality of life, if any, is taken to be sufficiently low to justify deliberately acting to end it or deliberately failing to end it. If there is such a level, the conclusion that it is not always beneficent or even nonmaleficent to use life-support technology must be accepted.

Another important issue here is the respect for individual autonomy. For the cases of Bouvia and the hypothetical instance of neocortical death discussed earlier, both concern voluntary euthanasia, that is, euthanasia voluntarily requested by the patient. A long-standing commitment, vigorously defended by various schools of thought in Western moral philosophy, is the notion that competent adults should be free to conduct their lives as they please as long as they do not impose undeserved harm on others. Does this commitment entail a right to die? Some clearly believe that it does. If one owns anything at all, surely one owns one's life. In the two cases discussed earlier, neither individual sought to impose undeserved harm on anyone else, nor would satisfaction of their wish to die do so. What justification can there be then for not allowing their desires to be fulfilled?

One plausible answer is based upon the very respect of individual autonomy at issue here. A necessary condition, in some views, of respect for autonomy is the willingness to take whatever measures are necessary to protect it, including measures that restrict autonomy. An autonomy-respecting reason offered against laws that prevent even competent adults from voluntarily entering lifelong slavery is that such an exercise of autonomy is self-defeating and has the consequence of undermining autonomy altogether. Same token, an individual who acts to end his own life thereby exercises his autonomy in a manner that places it in jeopardy of permanent loss. Many would regard this as justification for using the coercive force of the law to prevent suicide. This line of thought does not fit the case of an individual in a persistent vegetative state because his/her autonomy has been destroyed by the circumstances that rendered him/her neocortically dead. It does fit Bouvia's case though. Her actions indicate that she is fully competent and her efforts to use medical care to prevent the otherwise inevitable pain of starvation is itself an exercise of her autonomy. Yet, if allowed to succeed, those very efforts would destroy her autonomy as they destroy her. On this reasoning, her case is a perfect instance of limitation of autonomy being justified by respect for autonomy and of one where, even against the wishes of a competent patient, the life-saving power of medical technology should be used.

82.2.1 Active vs. Passive Euthanasia

Discussions of the morality of euthanasia often distinguish active from passive euthanasia in light of the distinction made between killing a person and letting a person die, a distinction that rests upon the difference between an act of commission and an act of omission. When failure to take steps that could effectively forestall death results in an individual's demise, the resultant death is an act of omission and a case of letting a person die. When a death is the result of doing something to hasten the end of a person's life (e.g., giving a lethal injection), that death is caused by an act of commission and is a case of killing a person. When a person is allowed to die, death is a result of an act of omission, and the motive is the person's own good, the omission is an instance of passive euthanasia. When a person is killed, death is the result of an act of commission, and the motive is the person's own good, the commission is an instance of active euthanasia.

Does the difference between passive and active euthanasia, which reduces to a difference in how death comes about, make any moral difference? It does in the view of the American Medical Association. In a statement adopted on December 4, 1973, the House of Delegates of the American Medical Association asserted the following [Rachels, 1978]:

The intentional termination of the life of one human being by another — mercy killing — is contrary to that for which the medical profession stands and is contrary to the policy of the American Medical Association (AMA).

The cessation of extraordinary means to prolong the life of the body where there is irrefutable evidence that biological death is imminent is the decision of the patient and immediate family. The advice of the physician would be freely available to the patient and immediate family.

In response to this position, Rachels [1978, 1986] answered with the following:

The AMA policy statement isolates the crucial issue very well, the crucial issue is "intentional termination of the life of one human being by another." But after identifying this issue and forbidding "mercy killing," the statement goes on to deny that the cessation of treatment is the intentional termination of a life. This is where the mistake comes in, for what is the cessation of treatment in those circumstances (where the intention is to release the patient from continued suffering), if it is not "the intentional termination of the life of one human being by another?"

As Rachels correctly argued, when steps that could keep an individual alive are omitted for the person's own good, this omission is as much the intentional termination of life as taking active measures to cause death. Not placing a patient on a respirator due to a desire not to prolong suffering is an act intended to end life as much as the administration of a lethal injection. In many instances the main difference between the two cases is that the latter would release the individual from his pain and suffering more quickly than the former. Dying can take time and involve considerable pain even if nothing is done to prolong life. Active killing can be done in a manner that causes death painlessly and instantly. This difference certainly does not render killing, in this context, morally worse than letting a person die. In so far as the motivation is merciful (as it must be if the case is to be a genuine instance of euthanasia) because the individual is released more quickly from a life that is disvalued than otherwise, the difference between killing and letting one die may provide support for active euthanasia. According to Rachels, the common rejoinder to this argument is the following:

The important difference between active and passive euthanasia is that in passive euthanasia the doctor does not do anything to bring about the patient's death. The doctor does nothing and the patient dies of whatever ills already afflict him. In active euthanasia, however, the doctor does something to bring about the patient's death: he kills the person. The doctor who gives the patient with cancer a lethal injection has himself caused his patient's death; whereas if he merely ceases treatment, the cancer is the cause of death.

According to this rejoinder, in active euthanasia someone must do something to bring about the patient's death, and in passive euthanasia the patient's death is caused by illness rather than by anyone's conduct. Surely this is mistaken. Suppose a physician deliberately decides not to treat a patient who has a routinely curable ailment and the patient dies. Suppose further that the physician were to attempt to exonerate himself by saying, "I did nothing. The patient's death was the result of illness. I was not the cause of death." Under current legal and moral norms, such a response would have no credibility. As Rachels noted, *"it would be no defense at all for him to insist that he didn't do anything. He would have done something very serious indeed, for he let his patient die."*

The physician would be blameworthy for the patient's death as surely as if he had actively killed him. If causing death is justifiable under a given set of circumstances, whether it is done by allowing death to occur or by actively causing death is morally irrelevant. If causing someone to die is not justifiable under a given set of circumstances, whether it is done by allowing death to occur or by actively causing death is also morally irrelevant. Accordingly, if voluntary passive euthanasia is morally justifiable in the light of the duty of beneficence, so is voluntary active euthanasia. Indeed, given that the benefit to be achieved is more quickly realized by means of active euthanasia, it may be preferable to passive euthanasia in some cases.

82.2.2 Involuntary and Nonvoluntary Euthanasia

An act of euthanasia is involuntary if it hastens the individual's death for his own good but against his wishes. To take such a course would be to destroy a life that is valued by its possessor. Therefore, it is no different in any morally relevant way from unjustifiable homicide. There are only two legitimate reasons for hastening an innocent person's death against his will: self-defense and saving the lives of a larger number of other innocent persons. Involuntary euthanasia does not fit either of these justifications. By definition, it is done for the good of the person who is euthanized and for self-defense or saving innocent others.

No act that qualifies as involuntary euthanasia can be morally justifiable. Hastening a person's death for his own good is an instance of non-voluntary euthanasia when the individual is incapable of agreeing or disagreeing. Suppose it is clear that a particular person is sufficiently self-conscious to be regarded a person but cannot make his wishes known. Suppose also that he is suffering from the kind of ailment that, in the eyes of many persons, makes one's life unendurable. Would hastening his death be permissible? It would be if there were substantial evidence that he has given prior consent. This person may have told friends and relatives that under certain circumstances efforts to prolong his life should not be undertaken or continued. He might have recorded his wishes in the form of a Living Will (as shown in the box) or on audio or videotape. Where this kind of substantial evidence of prior consent exists, the decision to hasten death would be morally justified. A case of this scenario would be virtually a case of voluntary euthanasia.

But what about an instance in which such evidence is not available? Suppose the person at issue has never had the capacity for competent consent or dissent from decisions concerning his life. It simply cannot be known what value the individual would place on his life in his present condition of illness. What should be done is a matter of what is taken to be the greater evil — mistakenly ending the life of an innocent person for whom that life has value or mistakenly forcing him to endure a life that he radically disvalues.

To My Family, My Physician, My Clergyman, and My Lawyer:

If the time comes when I can no longer take part in decisions about my own future, let this statement stand as testament of my wishes: If there is no reasonable expectation of my recovery from physical or mental disability. I, _____, request that I be allowed to die and not be kept alive by artificial means or heroic measures. Death is as much a reality as birth, growth, maturity, and old age — it is the one certainty. I do not fear death as much as I fear the indiginity of deterioration, dependence, and hopeless pain. I ask that drugs be mercifully administered to me for the terminal suffering even if they hasten the moment of death.

This request is made after careful consideration. Although this document is not legally binding, you who care for me will, I hope, feel morally bound to follow its mandate. I recognize that it places a heavy burden of responsibility upon you, and it is with the intention of sharing that responsibility and of mitigating any feelings of guild that this statement is made.

Signed:_____
Date: _____

Witnessed by:
_____
_____

Living Will statutes have been passed in at least 35 states and the District of Columbia. For a Living Will to be a legally binding document, the person signing it must be of sound mind at the time the will is made and shown not to have altered his opinion in the interim between the signing and his illness. The witnesses must not be able to benefit from the individual's death.

82.2.3 Should Voluntary Euthanasia Be Legalized?

Recent events have raised the question: "Should voluntary euthanasia be legalized?" Some argue that even if voluntary euthanasia is morally justifiable, it should be prohibited by social policy nonetheless. According to this position, the problem with voluntary euthanasia is its impact on society as a whole. In other words, the overall disutility of allowing voluntary euthanasia outweighs the good it could do for its beneficiaries. The central moral concern is that legalized euthanasia would eventually erode respect for human life and ultimately become a policy under which "socially undesirable" persons would have their deaths hastened (by omission or commission). The experience of Nazi Germany is often cited in support of this fear. What began there as a policy of euthanasia soon became one of eliminating individuals deemed racially inferior or otherwise undesirable. The worry, of course, is that what happened there can happen here as well. If social policy encompasses efforts to hasten the deaths of people, respect for human life in general is eroded and all sorts of abuses become socially acceptable, or so the argument goes.

No one can provide an absolute guarantee that the experience of Nazi Germany would not be repeated, but there is reason to believe that its likelihood is negligible. The medical moral duty of beneficence justifies only voluntary euthanasia. It justifies hastening an individual's death only for the individual's benefit and only with the individual's consent. To kill or refuse to save people judged socially undesirable is not to engage in euthanasia at all and violates the medical moral duty of nonmaleficence. As long as only voluntary euthanasia is legalized, and it is clear that involuntary euthanasia is not and should never be, no degeneration of the policy need occur. Furthermore, such degeneration is not likely to occur if the beneficent nature of voluntary euthanasia is clearly distinguished from the maleficent nature of involuntary euthanasia and any policy of exterminating the socially undesirable. Euthanasia decisions must be scrutinized carefully and regulated strictly to ensure that only voluntary cases occur, and severe penalties must be established to deter abuse.

References

Bronzino, J.D. Chapter 190. Beneficence, Nonmaleficence and Technological Progress. *The Biomedical Engineering Handbook*. CRC Press, Boca Raton, Fl, 1995; 2000.

Bronzino, J.D. Chapter 10. Medical and Ethical Issues in Clinical Engineering Practice. *Management of Medical Technology*. Butterworth, 1992.

Bronzino, J.D. Chapter 20. Moral and Ethical Issues Associated with Medical Technology. *Introduction to Biomedical Engineering*. Academic Press, New York, 1999.

Rachels, J. "Active and Passive Euthanasia," In *Moral Problems*, 3rd ed., Rachels, J. (Ed.), Harper and Row, New York, 1978.

Rachels, J. *Ethics at the End of Life: Euthanasia and Morality*, Oxford University Press, Oxford, 1986.

Further Information

Dubler, N.N. and Nimmons D. *Ethics on Call*. Harmony Books, New York, 1992.

Jonsen, A.R. *The New Medicine and the Old Ethics*, Harvard University Press, Cambridge, MA, 1990.

Seebauer, E.G. and Barry R.L. *Fundamentals of Ethics for Scientists and Engineers*, Oxford University Press, Oxford, 2001.

83

Ethical Issues Related to Clinical Research

83.1   Introduction.. **83**-1
83.2   Ethical Issues in Feasibility Studies **83**-2
83.3   Ethical Issues in Emergency Use **83**-4
83.4   Ethical Issues in Treatment Use **83**-5
83.5   The Safe Medical Devices Act **83**-6
References **83**-6
Further Reading... **83**-6

Joseph D. Bronzino
Trinity College

83.1   Introduction

The Medical Device Amendment of 1976, and its updated 1990 version, requires approval from the Food and Drug Administration (FDA) before new devices are marketed and imposes requirements for the clinical investigation of new medical devices on human subjects. Although the statute makes interstate commerce of an unapproved new medical device generally unlawful, it provides an exception to allow interstate distribution of unapproved devices in order to conduct clinical research on human subjects. This investigational device exemption (IDE) can be obtained by submitting to the FDA *"a protocol for the proposed clinical testing of the device, reports of prior investigations of the device, certification that the study has been approved by a local institutional review board, and an assurance that informed consent will be obtained from each human subject"* [Bronzino et al., 1990a,b; Bronzino 1992; 1995; 1999; 2000].

With respect to clinical research on humans, the FDA distinguishes devices into two categories: devices that pose significant risk and those that involve insignificant risk. Examples of the former included orthopedic implants, artificial hearts, and infusion pumps. Examples of the latter include various dental devices and daily-wear contact lenses. Clinical research involving a significant risk device cannot begin until an institutional review board (IRB) has approved both the protocol and the informed consent form and the FDA itself has given permission. This requirement to submit an IDE application to the FDA is waived in the case of clinical research where the risk posed is insignificant. In this case, the FDA requires only that approval from an IRB be obtained certifying that the device in question poses only insignificant risk. In deciding whether to approve a proposed clinical investigation of a new device, the IRB and the FDA must determine the following:

1. Risks to subjects are minimized
2. Risks to subjects are reasonable in relation to the anticipated benefit and knowledge to be gained

3. Subject selection is equitable
4. Informed consent materials and procedures are adequate
5. Provisions for monitoring the study and protecting patient information are acceptable

The FDA allows unapproved medical devices to be used without an IDE in three types of situations: emergency use, treatment use, and feasibility studies. However, in each instance there are specific ethical issues.

83.2 Ethical Issues in Feasibility Studies

Manufacturers seeking more flexibility in conducting investigations in the early developmental stages of a device have submitted a petition to the FDA, requesting that certain limited investigations of significant risk devices be subject to abbreviated IDE requirements. In a feasibility study, or "limited investigation," human research on a new device would take place at a single institution and involve no more than ten human subjects. *The sponsor of a limited investigation would be required to submit to the FDA a "Notice of Limited Investigation," which would include a description of the device,* a *summary of the purpose of the investigation, the protocol, a sample of the informed consent form, and a certification of approval by the responsible IRB. In certain circumstances, the FDA could require additional information, or require the submission of a full IDE application, or suspend the investigation* [Bronzino et al., 1990a,b].

Investigations of this kind would be limited to certain circumstances (1) investigations of new uses of existing devices, (2) investigations involving temporary or permanent implants during the early developmental stages, and (3) investigations involving modification of an existing device.

To comprehend adequately the ethical issues posed by clinical use of unapproved medical devices outside the context of an IDE, it is necessary to utilize the distinctions between practice, nonvalidated practice, and research elaborated in the previous pages. How do those definitions apply to feasibility studies?

Clearly, the goal of this sort of study, that is, generalizable knowledge, makes it an issue of research rather than practice. Manufacturers seek to determine the performance of a device with respect to a particular patient population in an effort to gain information about its efficacy and safety. Such information would be important in determining whether further studies (animal or human) need to be conducted, whether the device needs modification before further use, and the like. The main difference between use of an unapproved device in a feasibility study and use under the terms of an IDE is that the former would be subject to significantly less intensive FDA review than the latter. This, in turn, means that the responsibility for ensuring that use of the device is ethically sound would fall primarily to the IRB of the institution conducting the study.

The ethical concerns posed here are best comprehended with a clear understanding of what justifies research. Ultimately, no matter how much basic research and animal experimentation has been conducted on a given device, the risks and benefits it poses for humans cannot be adequately determined until it is actually used on humans.

The benefits of research on humans lie primarily in the knowledge that is yielded and the generalizable information that is provided. This information is crucial to medical science's ability to generate new modes and instrumentalities of medical treatment that are both efficacious and safe. Accordingly, for necessary but insufficient condition for experimentation to be ethically sound, it must be scientifically sound [Capron, 1978, 1986].

Although scientific soundness is a necessary condition of ethically acceptable research on humans, it is not of and by itself sufficient. Indeed, it is widely recognized that the primary ethical concern posed by such investigation is the use of one person by another to gather knowledge or other benefits where these benefits may only partly or not at all accrue to the first person. In other words, the human subjects of such research are at risk of being mere research resources, as having value only for the ends of the research. Research upon human beings runs the risk of failing to respect them as people. The notion that human beings are not mere things but entities whose value is inherent rather than wholly instrumental is one of the most widely held norms of contemporary Western society. That is, human beings are not valuable wholly or solely for the uses to which they can be put. They are valuable simply by being the kinds of entities they are. To treat them as such is to respect them as people.

Respecting individuals as people is generally agreed to entail two requirements in the context of biomedical experimentation. First, since what is most generally taken to make human beings people is their autonomy — their ability to make rational choices for themselves — treating individuals as people means respecting that autonomy. This requirement is met by ensuring that no competent person is subjected to any clinical intervention without first giving voluntary and informed consent. Second, respect for people means that the physician will not subject a human to unnecessary risks and will minimize the risks to patients in required procedures.

Much of the ethical importance of the scrutiny that the FDA imposes upon use of unapproved medical devices in the context of an IDE derives from these two conditions of ethically sound research. The central ethical concern posed by use of medical devices in a feasibility study is that the decreased degree of FDA scrutiny will increase the likelihood that either or both of these conditions will not be met. This possibility may be especially great because many manufacturers of medical devices are, after all, commercial enterprises, companies that are motivated to generate profit and thus to get their devices to market as soon as possible with as little delay and cost as possible. These self-interested motives are likely, at times, to conflict with the requirements of ethically sound research and thus to induce manufacturers to fail (often unwittingly) to meet these requirements. Note that profit is not the only motive that might induce manufacturers to contravene the requirements of ethically sound research on humans. A manufacturer may sincerely believe that its product offers great benefit to many people or to a population of especially needy people and so from this utterly altruistic motive may be prompted to take shortcuts that compromise the quality of the research. Whether the consequences being sought by the research are desired for reasons of self-interest, altruism, or both, the ethical issue is the same. Research subjects may be placed at risk of being treated as mere objects rather than as people.

What about the circumstances under which feasibility studies would take place? Are these not sufficiently different from the "normal" circumstances of research to warrant reduced FDA scrutiny? As noted earlier, manufacturers seek to be allowed to engage in feasibility studies in order to investigate new uses of existing devices, to investigate temporary or permanent implants during the early developmental stages, and to investigate modifications to an existing device. As also noted earlier, a feasibility study would take place at only one institution and would involve no more than ten human subjects. Given these circumstances, is the sort of research that is likely to occur in a feasibility study less likely to be scientifically unsound or to fail to respect people in the way that normal research upon humans does in "normal" circumstances?

Such research would be done on a very small subject pool, and the harm of any ethical lapses would likely affect fewer people than if such lapses occurred under more usual research circumstances. Yet even if the harm done is limited to a failure to respect the ten or fewer subjects in a single feasibility study, the harm would still be ethically wrong. To wrong ten or fewer people is not as bad as to wrong in the same way more than ten people but it is to engage in wrongdoing nonetheless. In either case, individuals are reduced to the status of mere research resources and their dignity as people is not properly respected.

Are ethical lapses more likely to occur in feasibility studies than in studies that take place within the requirements of an IDE? Although nothing in the preceding discussion provides a definitive answer to this question, it is a question to which the FDA should give high priority in deciding whether to allow this type of exception to IDE use of unapproved medical devices. The answer to this question might be quite different when the device at issue is a temporary or permanent implant than when it is an already approved device being put to new uses or modified in some way. Whatever the contemplated use under the feasibility studies mechanism, the FDA would be ethically advised not to allow this kind of exception to IDE use of an unapproved device without a reasonably high level of certainty that research subjects would not be placed in greater jeopardy than in "normal" research circumstances.

83.3 Ethical Issues in Emergency Use

What about the mechanism for avoiding the rigors of an IDE for emergency use?

The FDA has authorized emergency use where an unapproved device offers the only alternative for saving the life of a dying patient, but an IDE has not yet been approved for the device or its use, or an IDE has been approved but the physician who wishes to use the device is not an investigator under the IDE [Bronzino et al., 1990a,b].

Because the purpose of emergency use of an unapproved device is to attempt to save a dying patient's life under circumstances where no other alternative is at hand, this sort of use constitutes practice rather than research. Its aim is primarily benefit to the patient rather than provision of new and generalizable information. Because this sort of use occurs prior to the completion of clinical investigation of the device, it constitutes a nonvalidated practice. What does this mean?

First, it means that while the aim of the use is to save the life of the patient, the nature and likelihood of the potential benefits and risks engendered by use of the device are far more speculative than in the sort of clinical intervention that constitutes validated practice. In validated practice, thorough investigation, including preclinical studies, animal studies, and studies on human subjects of a device has established its efficacy and safety. The clinician thus has a well-founded basis upon which to judge the benefits and risks such an intervention poses for his patients.

It is precisely this basis that is lacking in the case of a nonvalidated practice. Does this mean that emergency use of an unapproved device should be regarded as immoral? This conclusion would follow only if there were no basis upon which to make an assessment of the risks and benefits of the use of the device. The FDA requires that a physician who engages in emergency use of an unapproved device must *"have substantial reason to believe that benefits will exist. This means that there should be a body of preclinical and animal tests allowing a prediction of the benefit to a human patient."*

Thus, although the benefits and risks posed by use of the device are highly speculative, they are not entirely speculative. Although the only way to validate a new technology is to engage in research on humans at some point, not all nonvalidated technologies are equal. Some will be largely uninvestigated, and assessment of their risks and benefits will be wholly or almost wholly speculative. Others will at least have the support of preclinical and animal tests. Although this is not sufficient support for incorporating use of a device into regular clinical practice, it may however represent sufficient support to justify use in the desperate circumstances at issue in emergency situations. Desperate circumstances can justify desperate actions, but desperate actions are not the same as reckless actions, hence the ethical soundness of the FDA's requirement that emergency use be supported by solid results from preclinical and animal tests of the unapproved device.

A second requirement that the FDA imposes on emergency use of unapproved devices is the expectation that physicians *"exercise reasonable foresight with respect to potential emergencies and make appropriate arrangements under the IDE procedures. Thus, a physician should not 'create' an emergency in order to circumvent IRB review and avoid requesting the sponsor's authorization of the unapproved use of a device."*

From a Kantian point of view, which is concerned with protecting the dignity of people, it is a particularly important requirement to create an emergency in order to avoid FDA regulations, which prevent the patient being treated as a mere resource whose value is reducible to a service of the clinician's goals. Hence, the FDA is quite correct to insist that emergencies are circumstances that reasonable foresight would not anticipate.

Also especially important here is the nature of the patient's consent. Individuals facing death are especially vulnerable to exploitation and deserve greater measures for their protection than might otherwise be necessary. One such measure would be to ensure that the patient, or his legitimate proxy, knows the highly speculative nature of the intervention being offered. That is, to ensure that it is clearly understood that the clinician's estimation of the intervention's risks and benefits is far less solidly grounded than in the case of validated practices. The patient's consent must be based upon an awareness that the particular device has not undergone complete and rigorous testing on humans and that estimations of its potential are based wholly upon preclinical and animal studies. Above all the patient must not be led to believe that there is complete understanding of the risks and benefits of the intervention. Another important point here is to ensure that the patient is aware that the options he is facing are not simply life or death but may include life of a severely impaired quality, and therefore that even if his life is saved, it may be a life of significant impairment. Although desperate circumstance may legitimize desperate actions, the decision to take such actions must rest upon the informed and voluntary consent of the patient, especially when he/she is an especially vulnerable patient.

It is important here for a clinician involved in emergency use of an unapproved device to recognize that these activities constitute a form of nonvalidated practice and not research. Hence, the primary obligation is to the well being of the patient. The patient enters into the relationship with the clinician with the same trust that accompanies any normal clinical situation. To treat this sort of intervention as if it were an instance of research and hence justified by its benefits to science and society would be to abuse this trust.

83.4   Ethical Issues in Treatment Use

The FDA has adopted regulations authorizing the use of investigational new drugs in certain circumstances — where a patient has not responded to approved therapies. This "treatment use" of unapproved new drugs is not limited to life-threatening emergency situations, but rather is also available to treat "serious" diseases or conditions.

The FDA has not approved treatment use of unapproved medical devices, but it is possible that a manufacturer could obtain such approval by establishing a specific protocol for this kind of use within the context of an IDE.

The criteria for treatment use of unapproved medical devices would be similar to criteria for treatment use of investigational drugs (1) the device is intended to treat a serious or life-threatening disease or condition, (2) there is no comparable or satisfactory alternative product available to treat that condition, (3) the device is under an IDE, or has received an IDE exemption, or all clinical trials have been completed and the device is awaiting approval, and (4) the sponsor is actively pursuing marketing approval of the investigational device. The treatment use protocol would be submitted as part of the IDE, and would describe the intended use of the device, the rationale for use of the device, the available alternatives and why the investigational product is preferred, the criteria for patient selection, the measures to monitor the use of the device and to minimize risk, and technical information that is relevant to the safety and effectiveness of the device for the intended treatment purpose.

Were the FDA to approve treatment use of unapproved medical devices, what ethical issues would be posed? First, because such use is premised on the failure of validated interventions to improve the patient's condition adequately, it is a form of practice rather than research. Second, since the device involved in an instance of treatment use is unapproved, such use would constitute nonvalidated practice. As such, like emergency use, it should be subject to the FDA's requirement that prior preclinical tests and animal studies have been conducted that provide substantial reason to believe that patient benefit will result. As with emergency use, although this does not prevent assessment of the intervention's benefits and risks from being highly speculative, it does prevent assessment from being totally speculative. Here too, although desperate circumstances can justify desperate action, they do not justify reckless action. Unlike emergency use, the circumstances of treatment use involve serious impairment of health rather than the threat of premature death. Hence, an issue that must be considered is how serious such impairment must be to justify resorting to an intervention whose risks and benefits have not been solidly established.

In cases of emergency use, the FDA requires that physicians not use this exception to an IDE to avoid requirements that would otherwise be in place. This particular requirement would be obviated in instances of treatment use by the requirement that a protocol for such use be previously addressed within an IDE.

As with emergency use of unapproved devices, the patients involved in treatment use would be particularly vulnerable patients. Although they are not dying, they are facing serious medical conditions and are thereby likely to be less able to avoid exploitation than patients under less desperate circumstances.

Consequently, it is especially important that patients be informed of the speculative nature of the intervention and of the possibility that treatment may result in little or no benefit to them.

83.5 The Safe Medical Devices Act

On November 28, 1991, the Safe Medical Devices Act of 1990 (Public Law 101-629) went into effect. This regulation requires a wide range of healthcare institutions, including hospitals, ambulatory-surgical facilities, nursing homes, and outpatient treatment facilities, to report information that "reasonably suggests" the likelihood that the death, serious injury, or serious illness of a patient at that facility has been caused or contributed to by a medical device. When a death is devicerelated, a report must be made directly to the FDA *and* to the manufacturer of the device. When a serious illness or injury is device related, a report must be made to the manufacturer *or to* the FDA in cases where the manufacturer is not known. In addition, summaries of previously submitted reports must be submitted to the FDA on a semiannual basis. Prior to this regulation, such reporting was voluntary. This new regulation was designed to enhance the FDA's ability to quickly learn about problems related to medical devices. It also supplements the medical device reporting (MDR) regulations promulgated in 1984. MDR regulations require that reports of device-related deaths and serious injuries be submitted to the FDA by manufacturers and importers. The new law extends this requirement to users of medical devices along with manufacturers and importers. This act represents a significant step forward in protecting patients exposed to medical devices.

References

Bronzino, J.D. "Medical and Ethical Issues in Clinical Engineering Practice," *Management of Medical Technology.* Butterworth, Chapter 10, 1992.

Bronzino, J.D. "Moral and Ethical Issues Associated with Medical Technology," *Introduction to Biomedical Engineering. Academic Press,* Chapter 20, 1999.

Bronzino, J.D. "Regulation of Medical Device Innovation," *The Biomedical Engineering Handbook.* CRC Press, Chapter 192, 1995; 2000.

Bronzino, J.D., Flannery, E.J., and Wade, M.L. "Legal and Ethical Issues in the Regulation and Development of Engineering Achievements in Medical Technology," Part I *IEEE Engineering in Medicine and Biology,* 1990a.

Bronzino, J.D., Flannery, E.J., and Wade, M.L. "Legal and Ethical Issues in the Regulation and Development of Engineering Achievements in Medical Technology," Part II *IEEE Engineering in Medicine and Biology,* 1990b.

Capron, A. "Human Experimentation: Basic Issues," *The Encyclopedia of Bioethics* Vol. II. The Free Press, Glencoe, II. 1978.

Capron, A. "Human Experimentation," (J.P. Childress et al., eds.) University Publications of America, 1986.

Further Reading

1. Dubler, N.N. and Nimmons, D. *Ethics on Call.* Harmony Books, New York, 1992.
2. Jonsen, A.R. *The New Medicine and the Old Ethics.* Harvard University Press, Cambridge, MA, 1990.

Index

Note: Page numbers in *italics* refer to illustrations.

A

Abbott/MediSense Sof-Tact
meter, in blood glucose
monitoring, **66**-7
Abdominal cooling, *21-14*
Abnormal VEP, *7–6*
Abstract bolometer detector
structure, *37-6*
AC coupled instrumentation
amplifier designs, *52-7*
Accelerator-produced
radionuclides, **16**-2–**16**-4
Accelerometers
in biomedical sensors,
46-8–**46**-9
fundamental structure, *46-8*
Acoustic beam focusing and
steering, using a phased
array, *14-3*
Acoustic impedance, **14**-2, **14**-14
Acquisition process strategies, in
medical technology
management and
assessment, **75**-11–**75**-12
Acquisition, digital biomedical
signal acquisition,
2-2–**2**-6
Active dynamic thermal, *see* ADT
Active electrodes, in
electrosurgical devices,
63-6
Active shimming approach, in
magnetic field
homogeneity, **12**-15
Acute muscle injuries, **31**-4
Adaptive filtering, in biomedical
signals, *1-19*, **1**-18–**1**-21
ADC (analog-to-digital
convertor), **10**-15

ADT (active dynamic thermal)
IR-imaging, **22**-2, **22**-14
and TT, **22**-3–**22**-6, *22-9*
Adult respiratory distress
syndrome, *see* ARDS
Advanced thermal image
processing, **28**-1–**28**-12
in classification, **28**-9–**28**-12
first order thermal signatures,
histogram-based,
28-3–**28**-5
second order statistical
parameters in,
28-5–**28**-7
wavelet transformation in,
28-8–**28**-9
AEC (automatic exposure
control), **10**-30
AEDs (automatic external
defibrillators), **57**-6–**57**-8
Affine class
Affine class kernels and
constraints, *4-15*
of TFRs, **4**-14–**4**-15
Affinity chromatography, *51-8*
AFM, *see* SPM
Ahmed N., **3**-4
Ahn C.B., **15**-4
Ahn Y., **14**-33
Air, in anesthesia, **62**-3
Alarms, in anesthesia delivery
essentials, **62**-11
Aliasing, **12**-5
Allen R.B., **7**-6
ALOPEX process, **7**-4
'Alternate site testing', in blood
glucose monitoring,
66-6–**66**-8
Alveoli types, *60-9*
Amalric D., **25**-9, **25**-11, **26**-6

Amalu W., **25**-6
American Society for Testing and
Materials, *see* ASTM
Ammer K., **31**-8–**31**-9, **31**-11
Amperometric transduction, **50**-7
Amplitude zone time epoch
coding, *see* AZTEC
Analog-to-digital convertor, *see*
ADC
Analytical models, in non-AI
decision making, **44**-2
Anatomical imaging and medical
image fusion, using VR
technology, **18**-11–**18**-13
Anbar M., **26**-7, **36**-2
Anesthesia
anesthesia delivery essentials,
62-1–**62**-12
anesthesia machine, *62-5–62-7*
computer-aided record
keeping in, **62**-11
delivery system function
monitoring,
62-8–**62**-10
depth monitoring, **62**-10
gases during, *62-3–62-7*
gases used in, physical
properties, *62-4*
and humidification, **62**-8
simulation in, **62**-11
Angelsen B., **14**-24
Anger camera detector design,
13-6
'Angiogenesis', **27**-3
Angiographic systems, x-rays for,
10-8–18
ANNs (artificial neural networks)
analysis, **24**-11–**24**-12
in non-AI decision making,
44-8

ANOVA test, *32*-7
Antiscatter grid, **10**-7
  in mammography,
      10-27–**10**-28
Aorta, blood velocity
      measurement in, **14**-28
Aoyagi T., **49**-8, **71**-4
Apnea detection, by BEI
      measurements, **53**-4–**53**-5
AQ (acoustic quantification)
      signal, *73*-6
Architecture/construction, VR
      applications in, **18**-6
ARDS (adult respiratory distress
      syndrome), **23**-19
Array transducers, scanning with,
      14-2–**14**-5, *see also*
      individual entries
Array-element
  complex electrical impedance,
      14-11
  configurations and acoustic
      beam scanned region,
      14-5
  radiation pattern of, *14-9*
Arrhythmia analysis, wavelets in,
      5-17–**5**-18
Arrhythmia therapy, in
      implantable defibrillators,
      58-4–**58**-5
Arterial buckling application,
      55-3
Arterial inflow and venous
      outflow measurement,
      53-5
Arterial tonometry, **55**-10
Arteriovenous anastamoses, *see*
      AVA
Artifact, in CT, **11**-13
  and reconstruction error,
      11-13–**11**-14
Artificial Neural Networks, *see*
      ANNs
Arzbaecher R.C., **55**-8
ASC X12N standards, in health
      care information
      infrastructure, **42**-3
ASTM (American Society for
      Testing and Materials),
      42-3–**42**-4
Astrup P.B., **71**-2
Asymmetric analysis, in breast
      cancer detection,
      27-4–**27**-12
  asymmetry identification using
      supervised learning,
      27-11–**27**-12
  automatic segmentation in,
      27-4–**27**-8
  edge image generation in, **27**-5
  feature extraction in,
      27-11–**27**-12
  Hough transform for edge
      linking, **27**-5–**27**-6

Asymmetric warfare and
      bioterrorism, **45**-2–**45**-3
Asymmetry analysis, in breast
      cancer detection,
      27-1–**27**-13
Asymmetry identification by
      unsupervised learning,
      27-8–**27**-10
Asynchronous transfer mode, *see*
      ATM
ATM (asynchronous transfer
      mode), and public
      switched network, **9**-2
Atomic absorption spectroscopy,
      in clinical laboratory,
      69-6–**69**-7
Atomic force microscopy, *see*
      SPM
ATR (automatic target
      recognition), in medical
      infrared imaging, **19**-7
Atrial fibrillation, **54**-11, **58**-5
Attenuation
  compensation for, **13**-22
  of ultrasonic signals,
      14-17–**14**-18
Auscultatory method, **55**-5–**55**-6
Austria, medical infrared imaging
      advances in, **19**-4
Autobipolar mode, in
      electrosurgical devices,
      63-8
Automatic exposure control, *see*
      AEC
Automatic external defibrillators,
      see AEDs
Automatic kilovoltage control, in
      mammography, **10**-30
Automatic target recognition, *see*
      ATR
Automation, in clinical
      laboratory, **70**-7–**70**-8
AVA (arteriovenous
      anastamoses), **21**-3–**21**-4
AVM (arteriovenous
      malformation), MRI
      image, *16-8*
AZTEC (amplitude zone time
      epoch coding) method,
      3-3
  of an ECG waveform, *3–3*

B

Babic S.H., **44**-3
Backpropagation, *see* BP
Backscatter, **14**-16
Bacon P.A., **31**-3
Bandpass filter, *5–6*, *54–4*
Banson M.B., **15**-7
Barber W., **14**-33
Bartlett M.S., **2**-19
Bartnik E.A., **4**-19

Barton S.P., **22**-6
Baseband signal system
      architecture, *14-32*
Basic needle electrode, **47**-8
Baxt W.B., **7**-8
Bayer GLUCOMETER
      ENCORE^{TM} test strip, in
      blood glucose
      monitoring, **66**-4
Bayesian approach/analysis
  facial tissue delineation using,
      29-2–**29**-6, *see also*
      Facial tissue delineation
  in non-AI decision making,
      44-5–**44**-6
BCDDP (breast cancer detection
      and demonstration
      project), **25**-12–**25**-14,
      26-3–**26**-5, *see also*
      Pre-BCDDP;
      Post-BCDDP
  study design in, **25**-13
  personnel and protocol
      violations in, **25**-14
BCM (Bienenstock, Cooper, and
      Munro) neurons, **7**-6
Beam blanking, in X-ray
      projection angiography,
      10-14
Beam shaping on tissues optics,
      64-9
BEEMS (biomedical engineering
      equipment management
      system), **76**-3
Beer–Lambert law, and pulse
      oximetry, **71**-4
Behavioral evaluation and
      intervention, using VR
      technology, **18**-16–**18**-17
BEI (bioelectric impedance)
      measurements, **53**-1–**53**-8
  and ECG, *53-4*
  measurement methods,
      53-1–**53**-3
  modeling and formula
      development,
      53-3–**53**-4
Bell J., **7**-4
Belliveau J.W., **12**-22
Bender–Blau autofluoroscope,
      13-5
Beneficence, nonmaleficence, and
      medical technology,
      82-1–**82**-8
Benign and malignant breast
      diseases, TTM evaluation
      results, *23-15*
Bertram C.D., **14**-36
Bi-lateral vein thrombosis, *32-5*
Binding forces, in SPM,
      67-10–**67**-14
  coupled imaging in, **1**-2
  mechanical properties, **1**-2
Bioacoustic signals, **1**-2

Bioanalytic sensors, **50**-1–**50**-10
BioBench^{TM}, virtual instrument,
    73-2–**73**-5
  acquisition mode with alarms
    enabled, *73-4*
  analysis mode, *73-5*
  biomedical application, *73-3*
Biochemical reactions
    classification, and sensor
    design and development,
    50-1–**50**-2
Biochemical signals, 1-3
Bioelectric impedance, *see* BEI
Bioelectric signals, 1-2, **47**-2–**47**-4
  sensed by biopotential
    electrodes, *47-2*
'Bioheat equation', **21**-4
Bioimpedance signals, 1-2
Bioinformatics partnership of
    nurses and engineers,
    43-7–**43**-9
Biologic tissue
  absorption in, **64**-2–**64**-3
  scattering in, **64**-2
  UV–IR laser radiation on,
    64-2–**64**-3
Biological sensors for diagnostics,
    51-1–**51**-12
Biological tissue
  optical properties, **30**-2–**30**-4
  photon migration models in,
    30-6–**30**-9
  thermal properties of,
    22-3–**22**-6
Biomagnetic signals, 1-2–1-3
Biomechanical signals, 1-3
Biomedical applications, of TFRs,
    4-17–**4**-20
Biomedical emergencies and
    medical informatics,
    45-1–**45**-9
Biomedical engineering
  risk-management tool in, *76-9*
  virtual instrumentation
    applications in,
    73-1–**73**-8
Biomedical lasers, **64**-1–**64**-11
  applications, *64-11*
  features, **64**-9
  laser beam delivery systems,
    64-7–**64**-11
  operating principles, *64-10*
Biomedical measurements,
    practical electrodes for,
    47-5–**47**-11
Biomedical sensors
  accelerometers in **46**-8–**46**-9
  classification, **V**-*2*
  description, **46**-2–**46**-15
  Doppler ultrasound in,
    46-7–**46**-8
  flow measurement in,
    46-11–**46**-12

  fluid dynamic variables
    measurement in,
    46-9–**46**-13
  magnetic induction in, **46**-7
  physical measurements of,
    46-1–**46**-17
  pressure measurement in,
    46-9–**46**-11
  velocity measurement in,
    46-7–**46**-8
Biomedical signal processing
  and networked multimedia
    Communications,
    9-1–**9**-3
  complexity, scaling, and
    fractals in, **8**-1–**8**-10
  decomposition, **5**-7–**5**-10
  HOS in, **6**-11–**6**-13
  neural networks in, **7**-1–**7**-11
  wavelet (time-scale) analysis
    in, **5**-1–**5**-23
Biomedical signals, *1-4, see also*
    individual entries
  amplitudes and spectral ranges
    of, *52-5*
  classification, 1-3–1-5
  data windows in, 1-11–1-12
  frequency-domain analysis,
    1-2–1-22
  optimal filtering in, 1-16–1-18
  origin and dynamic
    characteristics,
    1-2–1-22
  origin, 1-2–1-3
  signal enhancement, 1-15–1-16
  spectral estimation in,
    1-13–1-15
  time-domain coding of,
    3-2–**3**-4
  time-frequency signal
    representations for,
    4-1–**4**-20
Biomedicine, radionuclides in,
    16-3–16-4
Biometrics, **29**-1–**29**-14
Biomolecular interactions
    probing, using SPM,
    67-1–**67**-14
Biooptical signals, 1-3
Biopotential amplifiers,
    52-1–**52**-14
  and surge protection,
    52-9–**52**-10
  basic amplifier requirements,
    52-1–**52**-5
  dynamic range and recovery of,
    52-10–**52**-11
  input guarding of, **52**-10
  instrumentation amplifier,
    52-5–**52**-7
  interferences in, **52**-4–**52**-5
  main stages of, *52-3*
  special circuits in, **52**-5–**52**-9

Biopotential electrodes,
    47-1–**47**-12
  biomedical applications,
    47-11–**47**-12
  electric characteristics,
    47-4–**47**-5
  equivalent circuit, *47-5*
Biopotential measurement, *47-3*
Biopotentials measurement
    configuration, *52-2*
Biosignals, *see* Biomedical signals
Bioterrorism and asymmetric
    warfare, **45**-2–**45**-3
Bipolar mode, in electrosurgical
    devices, **63**-4
Birdcage resonator, *12-18*
Black body calibration source,
    33-5
Black R.D., **15**-6
Black-box approach, **2**-19
Blackman–Tukey method, of
    spectral estimation, 1-13
Blatties C.M. **24**-5
Blend, **63**-4
Blood flow measurement,
    using ultrasound,
    14-22–**14**-29
  clinical applications and their
    requirements,
    14-27–**14**-29
  color flow mapping in,
    14-25–**14**-26
  data acquisition system of,
    14-23–**14**-24
  fundamental concepts,
    14-22–**14**-29
  in aorta, **14**-28
  in cardiology, **14**-28
  in peripheral arteries,
    14-28–**14**-29
  intervening medium in, **14**-24
  operating environment in,
    14-23
  single sample volume
    doppler instruments
    for, **14**-25
  target scattering medium of,
    14-24
  ultrasonic flow estimation
    systems in,
    14-24–**14**-26
  velocity estimation techniques
    in, **14**-29–**14**-36, *see*
    also separate entry
Blood flow reduction, and
    objective thermography,
    21-8–**21**-11
Blood gases, **49**-9–**49**-12
Blood glucose monitoring,
    66-1–**66**-9
  colorimetric test strips and
    optical reflectance
    meters development in,
    66-2–**66**-5

Blood glucose monitoring
(*continued*)
electrochemical strips
emergence, in blood
glucose monitoring,
66-5–**66**-6
medicine and historical
methods, **66**-2
user interactions
improvements and
alternate site testing in,
66-6–**66**-8
Blood oxygenation, **12**-22
blood velocity estimation
blood velocity profiles, **14**-27
operating environment, *14-23*
using a cross-correlation
estimator, *14-35*
using the wideband MLE,
14-36
Blood volume changes images,
using EIT, **17**-11
Bloom R.W., **18**-17
Body composition
measurements, using BEI,
53-7
Body temperature
linear regression line, *24-10*
measurements types,
34-2–**34**-3
vs. skin temperature (eye
region), **24**-3–**24**-5
Body-surface biopotential
electrodes, **47**-6–**47**-8
BOLD (blood oxygenation level
dependent), **12**-*22*
Bonnefous O., **14**-35
Boone K., **17**-5
Bornzin G.A., **49**-7, **26**-6
Bottomley L.A., **67**-4
Bourland H., **7**-6
Bowman H.F., **22**-6
BP (backpropagation), **7**-1–**7**-2
Brachial plexus paresis, **31**-9
bradyarrhythmias, **54**-2
'Brain death', **82**-2
Brain-inflow problem, **12**-28
Brain–vein problem, **12**-28
Breast cancer detection, *see also*
BCDDP
asymmetric analysis in,
27-4–**27**-12
breast cancer detection
imaging, *19-6*
breast cancer multi-imaging
detection strategy, **26**-*8*
current status, **25**-15–**25**-16
in Ville Marie
multi-disciplinary
breast center,
26-7–**26**-24
IR imaging in, *26-11*

using thermal infrared images
by asymmetry analysis,
27-1–**27**-13
Breast cancer, early breast cancer
TTM in, **23**-3–**23**-7
thermal–electric analog for,
23-3–**23**-4
heat source depth estimation
using TTM in,
23-4–**23**-5
experimental results and
analysis, **23**-5–**23**-7
Breast cancer, *see also* breast
tumor
detection, *see separate entry*
digital high-resolution
functional infrared
imaging to,
26-14–**26**-20
early breast cancer, *see separate
entry*
early detection, **27**-4
image processing and medical
applications, **19**-7
medical infrared imaging in,
19-5–**19**-8
sensor technology in,
19-7–**19**-8
website and database in, **19**-7
Breast
breast cancer, *see separate entry*
breast lumps, **26**-12
breast nodule, **26**-17
breast thermographs with
malignant tumor, **28**-5
dense breast, **10**-32
endocrine logical triple images,
23-14
FCD diagnosis in, *26-18*
functional infrared imaging, of
past, present and
future, **26**-1–**26**-28
healthy breast thermographs,
28-*4*
infrared imaging, *see* Infrared
breast imaging
thermal images of the breast,
28-2–**28**-3, **28**-*11*
vascular asymmetry in, *26-18*,
26-21–26-25
Breast disease examination
with TTM, **23**-12–**23**-16
Breast tumor, **30**-*12*
2-D optical image, *30-11*
Breath delivery control, in
mechanical ventilation,
61-6–**61**-10
Breathing circuits, in anesthesia
delivery essentials,
62-7–**62**-8
Brody W., **14**-34–35
Brown B.H., **17**-5, **17**-9–**17**-10
Brown M.L., **4**-19
Brugada P., **7**-7

Bruha I., **7**-2
Bulgrin J.R.,19
Burke J.C., **18**-15
Burn fields, thermal conductivity
distribution
reconstruction, *22-23*
Burn wound, first day after the
accident, *22-13*
burned skin thickness, *22-20*
Burns D.A., **71**-8
Burns P.N., **14**-37

C

Caldwell C.W., **47**-9
Calorimetric, thermometric, and
pyroelectric transducers,
50-5–**50**-6
Camera technology, emerging
and future, **19**-11
Canada, medical infrared
imaging advances in, **19**-3
Cancer cells and Human body,
metabolic activity,
27-2–**27**-3
Capacitive sensors, **46**-6
Carbon dioxide, in anesthesia,
62-4
Carbon-filled elastomer dry
electrode, *47-7*
Carbonization, **63**-2
Cardiac cycle analysis front panel,
73-8
Cardiac measurements, using
BEI, **53**-5–**53**-7
Cardiac output measurement,
56-1–**56**-10
Cardiac signal processing,
5-11–**5**-18
Cardiac surgery, **22**-22–**22**-25
in vivo experiments on pigs,
22-22–**22**-25
Cardilogy, *see also individual
entries*
blood velocity measurement
in, **14**-28
neural networks in, **7**-7–**7**-11
Cardiovascular
pressure-dimension
analysis system,
73-5–**73**-7
clinical significance, **73**-7
data acquisition and analysis,
73-7
and fluid dynamics,
14-26–**14**-27
Cardioversion, **57**-1
Cardis C., **26**-6
Carotid arteries, **14**-28
Carotid occlusal disease
assessment, with infrared
thermography, **34**-4

Carpal Tunnel Syndrome, *see* CTS
Carson P.L., 14-37
Carter G.C., 14-35
Catheter components resistance measurements, *68-4*
catheter or probe electrode, *47-9*
Causal modeling, in non-AI decision making, 44-7–44-8
Causal probabilistic network, *see* CPN
Cause-and-effect, *78*-5
   in quality improvement, **78**-5
CCD (charge-coupled device), **10**-12–**10**-13
CDSS (clinical decision support system), 41-3–**41**-5
   CDSS hurdles, 41-6
   knowledge server in, 41-3–**41**-5
   knowledge sources in, 41-4
   MLM in, 41-4
   nomenclature, 41-4–**41**-5
Cellular automata, 8-3, 8-10
Cellular force measurement, **65**-5–**65**-9
   membrane wrinkling in, **65**-6–**65**-7
   techniques, **65**-6
Cellular mechanics, **65**-2–**65**-4
   instrumentation, **65**-1–**65**-10
   scaling laws in, **65**-4–**65**-5
Cellular processes sensors, **51**-10–**51**-11
Central Nervous System
   complexity theory in model development of, 8-9
   stimulators, 59-10
Centrifugal analyzers, in nonspectral methods and automation, 70-8
Cerebellar stimulation, 59-10
Cerebrovascular accident, *see* CVA
CERESPECT brain SPECT system, 13-15
Chang L.T., **13**-22
Chaos, **8**-10
   dynamics at the edge of, **8**-5–**8**-6
Charge-coupled device, *see* CCD
Chato J.C., **21**-4
Chemical sensors, 50-1, *50*-8
Chemical-shift imaging, *see* CSI
Chen J.D.Z., 4-19
Chen M.M., **21**-4
Cheney M.D., **17**-8
China, medical infrared imaging advances in, 19-3–**19**-4
Cho Y.E., 31-7
Cho Z.H., **15**-4, **13**-13
Choi–Williams exponential distribution, *see* CWD

Chromatography
   in clinical laboratory, **69**-2
   for proteins and enzymes measurement, 51-7
'Chronic inflammation of bone', 31-3
Chronic patient monitoring electrodes, 47-6–**47**-8
Chughtai M.S., 26-2
Ciurczak E.W., 71-8
Clark electrode, 70-4
Clark R.P., 36-2
Clark type of oxygen sensor, 48-1
Classical thermogram, *22*-20
Clearance measurement, in cutaneous circulation measurement technique, 21-6
Clement R.M., **33**-12
Clinical and technology strategic plan, in medical technology management and assessment, 75-3–**75**-4
Clinical data representations (Codes), in health care information infrastructure, 42-5–**42**-6
Clinical decision support system, *see* CDSS
Clinical defibrillators, 57-3–**57**-5
Clinical engineering, *see also individual entries*
   Clinical engineering programs, 74-4–**74**-7
   evolution, 74-1–**74**-7
   hospital organization, 74-3–**74**-4
Clinical engineering program indicators, 77-1–**77**-9
   department philosophy, 77-2–**77**-3
   external comparisons in, 77-3
   indicator management process, 77-5–**77**-7
   internal operations monitoring in, 77-2
   measurement indicators, 77-4–**77**-5
   patient monitors IPM, 77-8
   productivity monitors, 77-7–**77**-8
   quality improvement process in, 77-2–**77**-3
   standard database for, 77-3–**77**-4
Clinical engineers standards primer, 79-1–**79**-12
   costs, 79-12
   definitions, 79-2–**79**-3
   ex post facto, 79-12
   in medical devices, 79-5–**79**-7
   incorporation and revision, **79**-10

inhibition, 79-11–**79**-12
international standards, **79**-7–**79**-8
and the law, 79-10
liability, 79-11
limitations, 79-9–**79**-12
safety, 79-11
standards compliance, 79-9
Clinical information systems framework, 43-7
Clinical Laboratory, separation and spectral methods, **69**-1–**69**-8
   atomic absorption spectroscopy, **69**-6–**69**-7
   chromatographic separations, **69**-2
   flame photometry, **69**-6
   fluorometry, **69**-5–**69**-6
   gas chromatography, **69**-2–**69**-3
   high-performance liquid chromatography, **69**-3
   nonspectral methods and automation in, **70**-1–**70**-9, *see also separate entry*
   separation methods, **69**-1–**69**-2
Clinical research, ethical issues in, 83-1–836
Closed circuit circle breathing system, *62*-7
Cloutier G., 4-20
Clutter signal, in ultrasound, 14-24
CMOS circuit technology, 54-3
CMRR (common mode rejection ratio), 52-2–**52**-3
Coagulation, 63-2
   in nonspectral methods and automation, 70-7
Coaxial needle electrode, *47*-9
Cohen's class, of TFRs, 4-11–**4**-14
Coiled wire electrode, *47*-9
Cold war NDMS structure, 45-4
Cole K.S., **17**-2
Cole R.H., **17**-2
Collateral damage analysis, using thermal imaging, 33-5–**33**-6
Collins A.J., 31-2–**31**-3, 36-1
Collision algorithms, and VR technology, 18-8
Color Doppler energy (CDE), 14-37
Color flow mapping, in blood flow measurement, 14-25–**14**-26
Colorimetric test strips and optical reflectance meters development, blood glucose monitoring, 66-2–**66**-5

Common mode rejection ratio, *see* CMRR

Common thermocouples, *46-15*

Communications standards, in health care information infrastructure, **42**-3–**42**-5

Compensation
for attenuation, **13**-22
for collimator–detector response, **13**-23–**13**-24
for scatter, **13**-23

Complex dynamics, in biomedical signals, **8**-2–**8**-6

Complex regional pain syndrome, *see* CRPS

Complexity, *see also* Complexity theory
and scaling, and fractals, in biomedical signals, **8**-1–**8**-10
self-organized criticality in, **8**-4–**8**-5

Complexity theory, in Central Nervous System model development, **8**-9

Compression device, in mammography, **10**-27

Computed Tomography, *see* CT

Computer laser scanning sample sequences, *33-13*

Computer-aided design, VR applications in, **18**-6

Computer-based patient records, *see* CPR

Computerized laser scanning, **33**-11–**33**-15

Conduction anesthesia, **62**-2

Conductivity/capacitance electrochemical sensors, **48**-1–**48**-3

Conductometric transducers, **50**-7–**50**-8

Confidentiality, data security, and authentication, in health care information infrastructure, **42**-6

Congestive heart failure, **54**-11

Contact mode imaging, in SPM, **67**-3

Content and structure standards, in health care information infrastructure, **42**-5

Continuous and pulsed IR–visible laser radiation effects, **64**-5–**64**-6

Continuous positive airway pressure, *see* CPAP

Continuous quality improvement, *see* CQI

Continuous vascular unloading, **55**-8–**55**-9

Continuous wavelet transform, *see* CWT

Control chart, *78-6*
in quality improvement, **78**-5

Conventional and bioterrorist attacks, *45-3*

Cook L.P., **7**-4

Cormack A.M., **11**-11

Coulter method, *70-2*
in particle counting and identification, **70**-1

CPAP (Continuous Positive Airway Pressure) in spontaneous mode, **61**-5–**61**-6, *61-6*

CPN (causal probabilistic network), **44**-7

CPR (Computer-based patient records), **41**-1–**41**-15
clinical decision support system in, *see* CDSS
data quality, **41**-14
driving forces for, **41**-9–**41**-11
extended uses, **41**-11
federal programs, **41**-11–**41**-12
patient safety, **41**-9–**41**-10
private sector initiatives, **41**-9
quality of care in, **41**-10–**41**-11
rising healthcare spending, **41**-10
rising healthcare spending, **41**-10–**41**-11
scientific evidence, **41**-5–**41**-7, *see also individual entry*
security issue, **41**-13–**41**-14
standards issue, **41**-12–**41**-13
varying state requirements, **41**-14–**41**-15

CPT (current procedural terminology), **42**-5–**42**-6, **72**-5

CQI (continuous quality improvement), **78**-3

Critical phenomena
criticality, **8**-10
magnetism as, **8**-3–**8**-4
phase transitions as, **8**-3

Crosby P., **78**-2

Crowe J.A., **4**-19

CRPS (Complex regional pain syndrome), **31**-9–**31**-11

CsI (cesium iodide), as modern image intensifier, **10**-11

CSI (chemical-shift imaging), **12**-31
and contrast mechanism in magnetic resonance microscopy, **15**-3
general methodology, **12**-31–**12**-33
practical utility, **12**-33–**12**-37
theory and practice, **12**-31–**12**-38

CT (computed tomography)
imaging, **11**-1–**11**-12
of abdomen, *11-2*
of brain, *11-2*
of chest showing lungs, *11-2*
computer systems used in, **11**-9
data-acquisition geometries in, **11**-2–**11**-4, *see also separate entry*
data-acquisition system in, **11**-8–**11**-9
gas ionization detectors in, **11**-8
of head showing orbits, *11-2*
instrumentation, **11**-1–**11**-12
patient dose considerations in, **11**-9
reconstruction principles in, **11**-13–16, *see also separate entry*
solid-state detectors in, **11**-8
and TTM, performance comparison, *23-21*
x-ray detectors in, **11**-7–**11**-8
x-ray source in, **11**-5–**11**-7
x-ray system in, **11**-4–**11**-9

CT dose index, *see* CTDI

CT scanner installation, *11-2*

CTDI (CT dose index), **11**-9, *11-10*

CTS (Carpal tunnel syndrome), **31**-8

Cuff pressure during oscillometric blood pressure measurement, *55-6*

Curie P., **14**-1

Curry G.R., **14**-26

Curvilinear arrays, **14**-4

Cutaneous circulation measurement techniques, **21**-5–**21**-7
clearance measurement in, **21**-6
cutaneous nerves distribution to the hand, *21-12*
Doppler measurement in, **21**-6
dyes and stains in, **21**-5
procedures, **21**-5
thermal skin measurement, **21**-6–**21**-7

CVA (Cerebrovascular accident), **34**-4

CWD (Choi–Williams exponential distribution), **4**-18

CWT (Continuous Wavelet Transform), **5**-2–**5**-7

Cyclic voltammetry, **48**-5

Cyclotrons, in PET, **16**-2

Cytochrome spectroscopy, **71**-7
cytochrome *aa3* absorption spectra, *71-2*

Cytoskeleton, **65**-2

Czerny V., **31**-3

D

DAD (directional anisotropic diffusion), 29-7
Danesh A., 67-6
Dariell P.J., 2-19
DAS (data aquistion system), in medical diagnostics, 11-2, 11-8, 22-9
Dassen W.R.M., 7-1
Data visualization, VR applications in, 18-6
Data-acquisition geometries, in CT, 11-11-2–11-11-4
 fifth generation scanning electron beam, 11-4
 first generation parallel-beam geometry, 11-3
 fourth generation fan beam, fixed detectors, 11-4
 second generation fan beam, multiple detectors, 11-3
 spiral/helical scanning in, 11-4
 third generation fan beam, rotating detectors, 11-4
DataGlove^TM, a VR control device, 18-3, 18-3, 18-13
DataSuit^TM for ergonomic and sports medicine applications, 18-5, 18-3–18-5, 18-13
Davies J., 31-4
Dayhoff J.E., 7-2
DCT (discrete cosine transform), 3-4
De Calcina-Goff, M., 36-2
DeBossan M.C., 7-1
Decision theoretic models, in non-AI decision making, 44-2–44-3
Deep brain stimulation, 59-10
Deep inferior epigastric perforator, see DIEP
Deep tissue structure, near-infrared quantitative imaging of, 30-2–30-15
Defibrillation mechanism, 57-2–57-3
 clinical defibrillators, 57-3–57-5
 defibrillator safety, 57-8
 trapezoidal wave defibrillator, 57-5
Defibrillator, 57-1, see also Defibrillation mechanism; External defibrillators
 block diagram, 57-4
Defining death, 82-2–82-3
Delahanty D.D., 35-1
Deming's 14 points, for quality improvement, 78-2
Demings W.E., 78-2
Demography, and informatics and nursing, 43-2

Dempster A., 44-6
Dempster–Shafer theory, 44-6
Dentistry, infrared imaging to, 34-1–34-5
Depth of field, see DOF
Derivative high-pass filter, 2-15
Derivative oscillometry, 55-7, 55-7–55-8
 experimental evaluation, 55-8
Dermatology, laser applications in, 33-6–33-8, 33-10
Dermatome patterns of horses and other animal species, 35-3–35-4
Desiccation, 63-2
Detector arrays, see also individual entries
 and Infrared detectors, 37-1–37-25
Detector materials, 37-7–37-12
Detector modulation transfer function, 10–15
Detector readout challenges, to infrared detectors, 37-17
Detector readouts, 37-12–37-14, see also individual entries
 readout evolution, 37-13–37-14
Detre J., 12-22–23, 12-25
DFT and its sampled signal, 1–11
Diabetes, medical devices in, see Blood glucose monitoring
Diagnostic sensors, for proteins and enzymes measurement, 51-1–51-7
Diagnostics industry, and biological sensors, 51-1
DICOM (digital imaging and communications), 42-4–42-5
DIEP (deep inferior epigastric perforator) flap, 21-15
Differential imaging, in EIT, 17-8–17-9
Differential pulse code modulation, see DPCM
Digital angiography, 10-15–10-17
 image storage in, 1-7
Digital biomedical signals acquisition and processing, 2-1–2-22
 compression of, 3-1–3-11
Digital electronics, and biopotential amplifiers, 52-13
Digital filter, 2-6
Digital high-resolution functional infrared imaging, to breast cancer, 26-14–26-20
Digital image processor, 10-15–10-17

Digital imaging and communications, see DICOM
Digital imaging technology, 10-8
Digital mammography, 10-31–10-34, 10-32–10-33, 26-25
Digital signal, acquisition procedure, 2-2
Digital subtraction angiography, see DSA
Dilhuydy M.H., 25-11
Dilution curve, 56-1
 obscured by recirculation, 56-5
Dimensional noise, in infrared camera characterization, 38-3–38-5
Directional anisotropic diffusion, see DAD
Disaster management paradigms, 45-3–45-5
Disaster response paradigms, 45-5–45-6
Discrete cosine transform, see DCT
Discrete signals, 1-9–1-11
Discrete wavelet transform, 5-7
Dispersive electrodes, in electrosurgical devices, 63-6
Displacement sensors, 46-3
Disposable electrode, 47-7
Disposable finger probe, of a noninvasive pulse oximeter, 49-9
Distributed relaxation processes, 8-8
Distributed stimulators, 59-10–59-11
DNA extraction and amplification technologies, 51-8–51-9
DNA/RNA probes, 51-9–51-10
Dodd G.D., 25-12, 26-3
DOF (depth of field), 39-10–39-11
Doppler measurement, in cutaneous circulation measurement technique, 21-6
Doppler ultrasound signal, 4-20
 in biomedical sensors, 46-7–46-8
'Doppler' systems, for blood flow measurement, using ultrasound, 14-25
DPCM (differential pulse code modulation), data compression by, 3-2–3-3
DPW (dual photopeak window) method, 13-23
Dry chemistry analyzers, in nonspectral methods and automation, 70-8

Dry electrodes, **47**-8
Dry spirometer, **60**-5
'Dry' heat exchange, **24**-5
Drzewiecki G.M., **55**-3, **55**-7, **55**-12
DSA (digital subtraction angiography), **10**-8, **10**-16
DSM (Diagnostic and Statistical Manual of Mental Disorders), **42**-5
Dual photopeak window, *see* DPW
Dual-beam spectrophotometer, *69*-5
Ductal carcinoma in the left breast, *23*-7
Dundee thermal imaging system, *33*-6
Dye lasers, **64**-6, **64**-10
Dynamic IR-thermography, for perforating vessels, **21**-14–**21**-15
Dynamic range, in infrared camera characterization, **38**-6–**38**-8
Dynamic systems, **8**-5–**8**-6
Dysfunctional hemoglobins, **71**-3

E

Early CRPS after radius fracture, *31-10*
ECG
    compression via parameter extraction, **3**-3–**3**-4
    ECG cycle, detail and coarse components, *5–16*
    ECG signal, *2-14*
    late potentials analysis in, **5**-14–**5**-17
Echo planar trajectory, *12-6*
Echocardiography, **73**-5–**73**-7
Echo-planar imaging, *see* EPI
ECT (emission computed tomographic) method, **13**-10
Eddy D.M., **44**-5
Edwards R.Q., **13**-13
EEG (Electroencephalographic) signals
    power spectrum, *2-4*
    and seizures, **5**-21
EF (ejection fraction)
    in cardiac output measurement, **56**-7–**56**-10
    measurement, using saline method, *56-9*
Effective healthcare information infrastructure
    barriers to creation, **43**-9–**43**-11

creation opportunities, **43**-10–**43**-11
EIT (Electrical impedance tomography), **17**-1–**17**-12
    applications to gastrointestinal system study, **17**-10
    applications to respiratory system study, **17**-10
    data collection in, **17**-5–**17**-6
    differential imaging in, **17**-8–**17**-9
    electrical impedance of tissue, **17**-1
    existing systems performance, **17**-6
    image reconstruction in, **17**-6–**17**-9
    impedance distribution determination in, **17**-3–**17**-10
    multifrequency measurements in, **17**-10
    optimal current patterns in, **17**-7–**17**-8
    single-step reconstruction in, **17**-8
    three-dimensional imaging in, **17**-8
Ejection fraction, *see* EF
Elam D., **30**-16
Electric conductivity mechanism in the body, **47**-2–**47**-4
Electrical impedance tomography, *see* EIT
Electrical impedance, and transducers, **14**-9–**14**-14
Electrical matching networks, in transducers, **14**-5
Electrochemical methods, in nonspectral methods and automation, **70**-3–**70**-4
Electrochemical sensors, **48**-1–**48**-6
    conductivity/capacitance electrochemical sensors, **48**-1–**48**-3
Electrochemical strips emergence, in blood glucose monitoring, **66**-5–**66**-6
Electrochemical transducers, **50**-7–**50**-8
Electrodes, *see also individual entries*
    for chronic patient monitoring, **47**-6–**47**-8
    using microelectronic technology, **47**-11
Electroencephalographic signals, *see* EEG
Electromagnetic flow sensor, **46**-17
Electromagnetic flowmeter structure, *46-11*

Electromagnets and permanent magnets, **12**-12–**12**-13
Electronic health record system core functions, *41-3*
Electronics challenges, to infrared detectors, **37**-16–**37**-17
Electrophoresis, for proteins and enzymes measurement, **51**-6–**51**-7
Electrosurgery, **63**-1–**63**-8
Electrosurgical devices, **63**-1–**63**-8
    recent developments, **63**-8
ELISA (enzyme linked immunosorbent assay), **51**-4
    steps in, *51-5*
Elliott R.L., **25**-7
Ellipsometry, **50**-7
Embree P.M., **14**-35
Emergency use, ethical issues in, **83**-4–**83**-5
Emergent global behavior, **8**-10
EMG, *1-16*
Emission computed tomographic, *see* ECT
Emissivity corrected temperature, **30**-16–**30**-17
Endoscope profiling module, *81-3*
Endoscope tip reflection, *81-3*
Endoscopic sinus surgery, *see* ESS
EndoTester^{TM} assessment system, **81**-2–**81**-4
End-systolic pressure–volume relationship, *see* ESPVR
Energized surgery, thermal imaging during, **33**-4–**33**-6
Energy-weighted acquisition, *see* EWA
Engel B., **31**-9
Engel J.-M., **36**-1
Enthesopathies, **31**-4
Entrance skin exposure, *see* ESE
Enzyme linked immunosorbent assay, *see* ELISA
EP (evoked potential), *2-18*
EPI (echo-planar imaging), **12**-6, **12**-19
    in MRI system, **12**-22
Epicardial ICD systems, *58-2*
Epilepsy burst, *5–21*
Epoxy encapsulation, in implantable stimulators, **59**-6
Equipment acquisition and deployment, in medical technology management and assessment, **75**-10–**75**-12

Equipment assets management, in medical technology management and assessment, 75-8–75-10

Equivalent frequency response, for the signal-averaging procedure, *2-17*

Er:YAG laser, 64-10

Ergonomics
in anesthesia delivery essentials, 62-11
rehabilitation, and disabilities studies, using VR technology, 18-13–18-15

ERI (electivereplacement indicators), 54-6

ERV (expiratory reserve volume), 60-1

ESC (executive steering committee), 78-10

ESE (entrance skin exposure), 10-21

ESPVR (end-systolic pressure–volume relationship), 73-7

ESS (endoscopic sinus surgery) Simulator, 18-9

ESU (electrosurgical unit), *63-3–63-4*
design, 63-4–63-6
hazards, 63-6–63-8

Ethical issues
in clinical research, 83-1–83-6
defining death, 82-2–82-3
in emergency use, 83-4–83-5
in feasibility studies, 83-2–83-3
and medical technology, 82-1–82-6
in treatment use, 83-5–83-6

Euthanasia, 82-3–82-5
active vs. passive euthanasia, 82-5–82-6
involuntary and nonvoluntary euthanasia, 82-6–82-7
voluntary euthanasia legalization, 82-7–82-8

Evanescent wave spectroscopy, 49-5–49-6, 67-13–67-14

Evans blue dye, in cutaneous circulation measurement technique, 21-5

Evoked potentials, in neurological signal processing, 5-18–5-19

EWA (energy-weighted acquisition) technique, 13-23

Executive steering committee, *see* ESC

Expiratory pressure control in mandatory mode, in mechanical ventilation, 61-9

Expiratory reserve volume, *see* ERV

External defibrillators, 57-1–57-8
electrodes in, 57-5–57-6
synchronization in, 57-6

Extracorporeal measurement, 49-9–49-10

Extravasation, in intravenous infusion devices, 68-10

F

Face recognition system architecture, *29-2*

Face recognition/detection, in thermal infrared, *29-1–29-14, see also individual entries*

Facial feature extraction, in thermal infrared, *29-6–29-13*

Facial nerve, 31-9

Facial tissue delineation, using a Bayesian approach, *29-2–29-6*
inference, *29-5–29-6*
initialization, *29-4–29-5*

Fan beam
fixed detectors, in CT, 11-4
multiple detectors, in CT, 11-3
rotating detectors, in CT, 11-4

Fast Fourier transform, *see* FFT

Fast spin echo, *see* FSE

FBP (filtered backprojection), as image reconstruction method, 13-20

FDE (finite derivative estimator), in blood flow measurement, 14-34–14-35

Feasibility studies, ethical issues in, 83-2–83-3

Feig S.A., 23-16, 26-3

Fesolution and field of view, *see* FOV

FEV (forced expiratory volume), 60-2

Fever, 24-5–24-6
fever monitoring devices, IR imagers as, 24-1–24-19
FEV*t* (timed forced expiratory volume) and FVC (forced vital capacity), *60-3*

FFT (fast Fourier transform), 12-18

Fiber optic antigen-antibody sensor, *49-13*

Fiber optic blood gas catheter, *49-10*

Fiber optic sensor tips, *49-5*

Fiber optical catheter for SvO_2/HCT measurement, *49-8*

Fibrillation mechanism, 57-1–57-2

Fibroglandular tissue, 10-20–10-22, 10-32

Fibromyalgia, 31-6

Fick method, 56-5–56-7

FID (free induction decay), 12-31

Fifth-generation ultrafast CT system, *11-6*

Filtered backprojection, *see* FBP

Filters, *see individual entries*

Finite derivative estimator, *see* FDE

FIR (functional infrared imaging) of the breast, past, present and future, 26-1–26-28
in clinical applications, 32-1–32-13
and IIR filters, 2-10–2-11

First responders, 45-1–45-9

Flame ionization detection method, 69-3
in clinical laboratory, 69-2–69-3

Flame photometry, in clinical laboratory, 69-6

Flandrin P., 4-20

Flashlamp pumped pulsed dye laser, 64-9

Flexible diaphragm tonometry, 55-10–55-12
design and concept, *55-11*

FLIR (forward looking infrared) systems, 20-3

Florescin dye, in cutaneous circulation measurement technique, 21-5

Flow cytometry, 51-10–51-11, *51-12*, 70-1, *70-2*

Flow measurement, in biomedical sensors, 46-11–46-12

Flowchart, *78-6*
in quality improvement, 78-5–78-6

Fluid dynamics
and the cardiovascular system, 14-26–14-27
fluid dynamic variables measurement, in biomedical sensors, 46-9–46-13

fluorescence affinity sensor for glucose measurement, *49-13*

Fluorescent Screens, 10-28–10-29

Fluorine-18, as PET, 16-6

Fluorometry, in clinical laboratory, 69-5–69-6

fMRI mapping, **12**-22–29,
see also Functional brain
mapping
fMRI cerebral blood flow(CBF)
index, of a low-flow
brain tumor, *12-27*
large vessel problems reduction
techniques in, **12**-28
mechanism of, **12**-24–**12**-28
of motor cortex for
preoperative planning,
12-26
of the primary visual cortex
(V1), *12-23*–*12-24*
problem and artifacts in, **12**-28
Focal spot, **10**-3, **10**-9,
10-15–**10**-16,
10-23–**10**-27, **11**-5–**11**-7,
11-13, **64**-9
Force spectroscopy, **67**-8–**67**-10
Force, in biomedical sensors, **46**-9
Forced expiratory volume, *see*
FEV
Forced vital capacity, *see* FVC
Forward looking infrared, *see*
FLIR
Foster S.G., **14**-35
Four-electrode impedance
measurement technique,
53-2
Fourth-generation CT gantry,
11-3–*11-5*
FOV (resolution and field of
view), **12**-5
Fractals
fractal measures, **8**-7–**8**-8
fractal preliminaries, in scaling
theories, **8**-6–**8**-7
mathematical and natural
fractals, **8**-7
multifractals, **8**-8–**8**-9
Fractional brownian motion,
8-10
Fraser S.E., **15**-11
FRC (functional residual
capacity), **60**-1
measurement,
nitrogen-washout
method for, **60**-7–**60**-9
measurement,
nitrogen-washout
method for, **60**-7–**60**-9
Free induction decay, *see* FID
Frequency-domain analysis,
1-7–**1**-9
Frequency-domain data
compression methods,
3-4–**3**-5
Frincu M.C., **67**-6

Fringing fields, in magnetic field
homogeneity, **12**-15
Fry D.I., **60**-7
FSE (fast spin echo) technique,
12-18
Fujimasa I., **36**-2
Fulguration, **63**-4
Functional brain mapping,
advances in, **12**-23–**12**-24
Functional electrical stimulation,
59-1–**59**-2
Functional infrared imaging, *see*
FIR
Functional MRI, *see* fMRI
Functional residual capacity, *see*
FRC
FVC (Forced vital capacity), **60**-2

G

Gain detector, in infrared camera
and optics, **39**-6–**39**-7
nonuniformity calibration,
39-7
Gallium aluminum (GaAlAs)
lasers, **64**-6
Gamagami P., **25**-8, **26**-7
Gamma ray detection, **13**-2, *70-5*
Gas blending and vaporization
system, during anesthesia,
62-5–**62**-7
Gas chromatography technique,
in clinical laboratory,
69-2–**69**-3
Gas ionization detector arrays,
11-8
Gas scavenging systems, in
anesthesia delivery
essentials, **62**-8
Gas-filled lasers, **64**-6
Gaskell P., **21**-3
GasStat^TM extracorporeal
system, **49**-9–**49**-10
Gastrointestinal system study,
using EIT, **17**-10
Gautherie M., **25**-9–**25**-12, **26**-6
Gautheriehe M., **23**-16
Geddes L.A., **47**-5, **55**-4
Gel electrophoresis, **51**-6–**51**-7,
51-7
Gene array, *51-10*
Gene chip arrays, **51**-9
Generalized detector system, *13-7*
Generator-produced
radionuclides, **16**-5
Generic bioanalytic sensor, *50-2*
George J.R., **35**-1
Germany, medical infrared
imaging advances in, **19**-4
Gershon-Cohen J., **25**-8, **26**-2
Gerstein G.L., **7**-3
Glucose monitoring, landmarks
in, *66-2*

Glucose sensors, **49**-12–**49**-13
Goble J., **17**-8
Golfer Elbow, **31**-4
Goodman P.H., **36**-1
Governing board (Trustees), in
hospital organization,
74-3–**74**-4
Gradient coils, in MRI scanners,
12-15–**12**-17
Graphical programming and
virtual instrumentation,
73-1–**73**-2
Grating lobes, **14**-15
Gravitational clustering method,
7-3
Greenleaf W.J., **18**-13
Greig G, **29**-7
Gros C., **25**-9–**25**-10, **25**-12, **26**-6
Guidi A.J., **26**-7
Gulevich S.J., **31**-9
Guo S., **67**-6
Guo Z., **4**-20

H

Haberman J., **25**-9, **25**-14, **26**-2
Hair follicle, oblique laser
illumination, *33-15*
Hand skin
heat transport efficiency in,
21-8
median nerve block in,
21-11–**21**-12
Handley R.S., **26**-2, **27**-1
Haptics, and VR technology, **18**-5
Hardy J., **20**-3, **30**-16
Hardy J.D., **34**-2, **36**-3
Harris A.K., **65**-5, **65**-7
Hatle L., **14**-24
Head J.F., **25**-7
Head related transfer function,
see HRTF
Head-mounted display, *see* HMD
Health care delivery system,
75-2–**75**-3
technology manager's
responsibility in,
75-3
Health care information
infrastructure standards,
42-1–**42**-8
clinical data representations
(Codes) in, **42**-5–**42**-6
communications standards,
42-3–**42**-5
confidentiality, data security,
and authentication in,
42-6
content and structure
standards, **42**-5
identifier standards, **42**-2–**42**-3
International standards in,
42-7

quality indicators and data sets in, **42**-7
standards coordination and promotion organizations in, **42**-7–**42**-8
Health care, virtual instruments applications in, **81**-1–**81**-9
Health Level Seven, *see* HL7
Healthcare Information and Management Systems Society, *see* HIMSS
Heart thermograms, *22-24*
Heart, M-mode imaging, *14-18*
Heat transfers
   formulation, **23**-8–**23**-9
   modeling equations for microcirculation, **21**-4–**21**-5
   skin blood flow regulation for, **21**-3–**21**-4
Heat transport efficiency, in hand skin, **21**-8
Hedén B., **7**-8
Heilig M., **18**-5
Hein I., **14**-35
Heir R.M., **49**-7
Helium, in anesthesia, **62**-4
Helmholtz pair, **12**-14
Helstrom C.W., **14**-35
Hemoglobin oxygen dissociation curve, *71-3*
Hemoglobins absorption spectra, *71-2*
Hendin O., **18**-12
Hendrick R.E., **10**-31
Hermetic packaging, in implantable stimulators, **59**-6
Herschel J., **20**-2
Herschel W., **20**-2
HgCdTe alloy detectors, spectral response curves, *37-8*
Higher-order spectral analysis, *see* HOS
High-pass spatial filtration, **10**-17
High-risk medical equipment failures, *76-7*
High-tech homecare devices, design and implementation challenges, **72**-3–**72**-5
High-time-bandwidth signals, in blood flow measurement, **14**-36
HIMSS (healthcare information and management systems society), **41**-9
Hippocratic oath, **82**-1
HIS (hospital information systems)
   data acquisition, **40**-3–**40**-4
   function and state, **40**-1–**40**-7

HIS interoperability and connectivity, federal initiatives, **41**-7–**41**-9
patient admission, transfer, and discharge functions, **40**-4
patient database strategies for, **40**-2–**40**-3
patient evaluation, **40**-4–**40**-5
patient management, **40**-5–**40**-7
HL7 (Health Level Seven), **42**-4
HMD (head-mounted display), in VR technology, **18**-4
HMM (Markov model), **7**-6
Ho:YAG (Holmium:YAG) laser, **64**-9
Hobbins W.B., **31**-8
HOCM (hypertrophic obstructive cardiomyopathy), **54**-2
Hoffman R., **25**-8
Hoffman R.M., **31**-7
Hollander J.L., **31**-2
Holmes K.R., **21**-4
Holt J.P., **56**-7
Home medical devices, **72**-1–**72**-9, *see also* High-tech homecare devices
Horner's syndrome, **35**-4
Horvath S.M., **31**-2
HOS (Higher-order spectra), **6**-1–**6**-4, **6**-7
   in biomedical signal processing, **6**-11–**6**-13
   definitions and properties, **6**-2–**6**-4
   HOS computation from real data, *see separate entry*
   linear processes in, **6**-6–**6**-8, *see also separate entry*
   nonlinear processes in, **6**-8–**6**-11
HOS computation from real data, **6**-4–**6**-6
   direct method in, **6**-5–**6**-6
   indirect method in, **6**-4–**6**-5
Hospital administration, **74**-4
Hospital information systems, *see* HIS
Hough transform based image segmentation, *27-6*
Hounsfield G.N., **11**-11-1, **11**-11-3, **11**-11-11
HPLC (high-performance liquid chromatography), in clinical laboratory, **69**-3
HRTF (head related transfer function), in VR technology, **18**-4
human blood and melanin, spectral absorption curves, *33-9*

Human body
   and cancer cells, metabolic activity, **27**-2–**27**-3
   heat exchange in, **24**-5, *24-6*
   temperature measurement in, **27**-2
Human tissues, specific conductance values for, *17-2*
Human-in-the-loop (HITL), **38**-2
Humidification, and anesthesia, **62**-8
Hunter I.A., **7**-7
Hybrid cascode amplifier, **63**-5
Hybrid detector array structure, **37**-12
Hybrid multichannel ECG coding, **3**-6–**3**-10
Hydrosun® irradiator, **21**-8
Hyperbolic class of TFRs, **4**-15–**4**-16
Hyperhidrosis palmaris, **21**-11
Hypoxia, **71**-2

I

IAN (inferior alveolar nerve) deficit assessment, with Infrared thermography, **34**-4
IC (inspiratory capacity), **60**-1
ICD (implantable cardioverter defibrillator), **58**-1–**58**-8
ICG (indocyanine green) dye, in cutaneous circulation measurement technique, **21**-5
Identifier standards, in health care information infrastructure, **42**-2–**42**-3
IEEE (Institute of Electrical and Electronics Engineers, Inc.), **42**-4–**42**-5
IFOV (instantaneous field of view), **39**-8–**39**-9
IJAT (implantable joint angle transducer), **59**-11
IJAT (joint angle transducer), *59-12*
Image detection, in x-ray, **10**-4–**10**-7
   digital systems in, **10**-6–**10**-7
   screen film combinations, **10**-4
   x-ray image intensifiers with televisions, **10**-4–**10**-6
Image formation, in mammography **10**-21–**10**-22
Image intensifier-based digital angiographic and cine imaging system, *10-9*
Image morphology, **29**-8–**29**-13

τ-Image technique, disease stage quantification using, **32**-2–**32**-5
Immunoassays, **51**-3–**51**-4
Immunofluorescence, *65*-4
Immunosensors, **49**-13–**49**-14
Impedance cardiographic waveforms, *53*-6
Impedance distribution determination, in EIT, **17**-3–**17**-10
Impedance spectroscopy, **53**-7
Implantable cardiac pacemakers, **54**-1–**54**-12
    clinical outcomes and cost implications in, **54**-10–**54**-11
    indications to implant, **54**-2–**54**-3
    leads in, **54**-7–**54**-9
    programmers in, **54**-9
    system operation in, **54**-9–**54**-10
Implantable cardioverter defibrillator, *see* ICD
Implantable defibrillators, **58**-1–**58**-8, *58*-6
    arrhythmia detection in, **58**-4–**58**-5
    arrhythmia therapy in, **58**-5–**58**-6
    electrode systems, **58**-2–**58**-4
    follow-up in, **58**-7
    implantable monitoring in, **58**-6–**58**-7
    pulse generators in, **58**-1–**58**-2
Implantable electrodes with attached lead wires, *58*-8
Implantable electronics packaging, **59**-6–**59**-7
Implantable joint angle transducer, *see* IJAT
Implantable neuromuscular stimulators, **59**-3–**59**-6
    data processing, **59**-5
    data retrieval in, **59**-5
    output stage in, **59**-5–**59**-6
    power supply in, **59**-4–**59**-5
    receiving circuit in, **59**-3–**59**-4
Implantable pacing leads, **54**-5–**54**-7
Implantable stimulators, for neuromuscular control, **59**-1–**59**-12
    in clinical use, **59**-9–**59**-10
    future, **59**-10–**59**-11
    implantable stimulation parameters, **59**-2–**59**-3
    leads and electrodes in, **59**-7
    safety issues, **59**-7–**59**-9
Implantable transducer-generated and physiological signals sensing, **59**-11

Implanted FES hand grasp system, *59*-4
IMRR (isolation mode rejection ratio), **52**-8
In vitro tissue study, in TTM, **23**-7–**23**-12
    experimental design and results, **23**-10–**23**-11
    method, **23**-8–**23**-9
    surface temperature distribution and internal heat source size of, **23**-7–**23**-12
Indicator management process, **77**-6
    in clinical engineering program, **77**-5–**77**-7
Indicator recirculation, in cardiac output measurement, **56**-4–**56**-5
Indicator-dilution method, *56*-2
    in cardiac output measurement, **56**-1–**56**-5
    for ejection fraction, **56**-7–**56**-10
Indicator-mediated transducers, **49**-4–**49**-5
Indocyanine green, *see* ICG
Inductance sensors, **46**-5–**46**-6
Infant apnea monitors, **72**-2, *72*-2, **72**-6–**72**-8
Inferior alveolar nerve, *see* IAN
Inflammation, **31**-2–**31**-3
Inflammatory spondylarthropathy, *31*-5
Influence diagrams, in non-AI decision making, **44**-3
Informatics and nursing, **43**-1–**43**-13, *see also* Nursing informatics
Information systems in patient care benefits, **43**-8–**43**-9
Infrared breast imaging, **25**-1–**25**-17
    equipment considerations, **25**-3
    fundamentals, **25**-2–**25**-7
    future advancements, **25**-16–**25**-17
    image interpretation, **25**-6–**25**-7
    imaging process, **25**-4–**25**-5
    in cancer detection, **25**-8–**25**-10
    laboratory and patient preparation protocols, **25**-3–**25**-4
    and mammography, **25**-14–**25**-15
    and pathology, **25**-7–**25**-8
    as a prognostic indicator, **25**-11–**25**-12
    as a risk indicator, **25**-10–**25**-11

Infrared camera and optics
    depth of field, **39**-10–**39**-11
    gain detector in, **39**-6–**39**-7, *see also individual entries*
    infrared optical considerations, **39**-8–**39**-9
    for medical applications, **39**-1–**39**-14
    operational considerations, **39**-7–**39**-8
    reflective optics, **39**-13–**39**-14
    resolution, **39**-8–**39**-9
    selecting optical materials, **39**-11–**39**-14
    spectral requirement in, **39**-10–**39**-11
Infrared camera characterization, **38**-1–**38**-9
    dimensional noise in, **38**-3–**38**-5
    dynamic range in, **38**-6–**38**-8
    MRT in, **38**-8–**38**-9
    MTF in, **38**-8
    Pixel size in, **38**-9
    spatial resolution in, **38**-9
Infrared detectors, technical challenges for, **37**-14–**37**-24
    detector readout challenges, **37**-17
    electronics challenges, **37**-16–**37**-17
Infrared detectors and detector arrays, **37**-1–**37**-25
    optics challenges, **37**-17–**37**-18
    third-generation cooled imagers, challenges for, **37**-18–**37**-24, *see also separate entry*
Infrared facial thermography, abnormal facial conditions demonstration, **34**-3–**34**-5
Infrared imaging
    of an abdominal skin flap during breast reconstruction surgery, *21*-16
    and breast cancer detection, **26**-7–**26**-14, *26*-11
    for breast screening, *19*-2
    for cancer research, *19*-3
    to dentistry, **34**-1–**34**-5
    as fever monitoring devices, **24**-1–**24**-19
    linear regression analysis, **24**-9–**24**-10
    in medicine, standard procedures for, **36**-1–**36**-9
IR materials transmission range, *39*-12
    pathophysiology, **24**-3–**24**-7

ROC (Receiver Operating Curve) analysis, 24-10–24-11
study design, 24-7–24-9
for tissue characterization and function, 30-1–30-20
in veterinary medicine, 35-1–35-7
Infrared optical materials, 39-12
infrared photon detectors, quantum efficiencies comparison, 37-11
Infrared sensor calibration, 39-4–39-5
Infrared thermal monitoring of disease processes, 30-15–30-20
temperature calibration in, 30-17–30-18
Infrared thermographic monitoring, see ITM 33-6–33-7
Infrared-nondestructive testing (IR-NDT), see ADT IR-imaging
Injury epidemiology and public policy knowledge base, 81-6
Inman D.P., 18-14
Inspiratory capacity, see IC
Instantaneous field of view, see IFOV
Institute of Electrical and Electronics Engineers Inc, see IEEE
Instrumentation amplifiers for biomedical applications, 52-6
providing input guarding, 52-10
Instrumented clothing, in VR technology, 18-3
Intermittent contact mode imaging, in SPM, 67-4
Internal electrodes, 47-9
'Internal milieu' maintenance, 62-1–62-2
Internal operations monitoring, in clinical engineering program, 77-2
International classification of diseases (ICD) codes, 42-5
International standards, in health care information infrastructure, 42-7
Intracavitary and intratissue electrodes, 47-8–47-10
Intrator N., 7-6
Intravascular catheters, 49-10
Intravascular fiber optic SvO_2 catheters, 49-7–49-8
Intravascular ultrasonic imaging, 14-37

Intravenous infusion devices, 68-4–68-8
controllers in, 68-6
gravity flow/resistance regulation, 68-4–68-5
syringe pumps, 68-6–68-8
volumetric infusion pumps, 68-5–68-6
Ion-specific electrodes, in nonspectral methods and automation, 70-4–70-5
IR imagers, see Infrared imaging
Isaacson D., 17-7–17-8
Isard H.J., 26-6
Ischemia, and QRS complex analysis, 5-11–5-14
Ishikawa chart, 78-5
in quality improvement, 78-5
Isolation amplifier and patient safety, 52-7–52-9
equivalent circuit, 52-8
Isolation mode rejection ratio, see IMRR
Italy, medical infrared imaging advances in, 19-5
ITM (Infrared thermographic monitoring), 21-13, 24-6–24-7, 33-6–33-7
and ADT and TT, 22-3–22-6
carotid occlusal disease assessment with, 34-4
IAN deficit assessment with, 34-4
and laser Doppler mapping, of skin blood flow, 21-12–21-14
in pathophysiology, 24-6–24-7
in perforating vessel highlighting, 21-14–21-15
in skin blood flow measurement, 21-12–21-14
skin temperatures by, 21-11–21-12
TMJ disorders assessment in, 34-4
Ito M., 18-12
Ives D.J.G., 47-4

J

Jacobs R.E., 15-11
Jacques S.L., 14-1
Janz G.I., 47-4
Japan, medical infrared imaging advances in, 19-4
Jeong J., 4-20
Johnson J.M., 32-11
Johnston M.E., 41-5
Jones C.H., 25-10, 26-2

Jones D.L., 4-19, 30-16
Juran J.M., 78-6

K

Kadambe S., 4-19
Kaewlium A., 4-19
Kaluzinski K., 14-33
Kanam C.A., 7-6
Kaposi's Sarcoma (KS), 30-18–30-20
Kaposi's sarcoma associated herpesvirus, see KSHV
Karhunen–Loeve Transform, see KLT
Karplus M., 67-11
Karrakchou M., 5-11
Kasai C., 14-33
k-edge filters, 10-27
Kelly R., 55-2
Kennedy R.S., 14-30
Kenney W.L., 32-11
Keyserlingk J.R., 25-12, 25-15–25-16, 27-4
Kidney transplantation, 21-15
Kim Y.S., 31-7
Kinematic viscosity, 14-27
Kinoshita T., 33-6
KLT (Karhunen–Loeve transform), 3-4
Knapp C.H., 14-35
Knutson J.S., 47-9
Korea, medical infrared imaging advances in, 19-4
Korotkoff N., 55-5
Kostis J.B., 7-9
Kowalewski T., 67-6
Kreuger M., 18-5
Kristoffersen K., 14-35
KSHV (Kaposi's sarcoma associated herpesvirus), 30-18
k-th power class, of TFR, 4-16–4-17
Kuhl D.E., 13-13
Kwong K.K., 12-22

L

LABC (locally advanced breast cancer), 26-14
Laboratory Instrumentation trends, 70-8
Laine A., 4-19
Lamson R., 18-17
Lanigan S.W., 33-11
LANs (local area networks), 9-2
Larsson S.A., 13-15
Laser depilation, 33-14–33-15
Laser light and tissue, interaction effects, 33-9

Laser light passage within skin layers, *33*-8

Laser positioning, thermographic results, 33-11

Laser therapy
  characteristics, *33*-8, *33*-10
  in dermatology, *33*-10

Lasers, *see also individual entries*
  applications, in dermatology, 33-6–*33*-8
  general description and operation, 64-6–**64**-7
  laser therapy, *see separate entry*
  optimization, 33-9–*33*-11

Laser-tissue interactions, 33-8–**33**-9

Late potentials, in ECG, 5-14–**5**-17

Lathan C., **18**-11

Lauterbur P.C., **15**-7

Lawson R.N., **26**-2

LDA (linear discriminant analysis), **28**-2, 28-10–**28**-12

Lead Collimation, *13*-3

Lead–zirconate–titanate, *see* PZT

Lean C.L., **15**-3

Leandro J., **29**-9

Leaning M.S., **44**-2

Ledley R.S., **44**-1

Less J.R., **14**-37

Levi L., **64**-7–**64**-8

Li C., **4**-19

Life-cycle cost analysis, in medical technology management and assessment, **75**-11

Lin Z.Y., **4**-19

Linear and angular displacement sensors, 46-2–**46**-5
  strain gauge in, 46-3–**46**-5

Linear phase FIR filters, impulse response, *2*-11

Linear phased arrays, 14-2, 14-4

Linear processes, in HOS, 6-6–8
  nonparametric methods in, **6**-7
  parametric methods in, **6**-8

Linear regression analysis, 24-9–24-10, 24-12–**24**-15

Linear sequential arrays, **14**-4

Linear sweep voltammetry, **48**-5

Linear transformer, in Hybrid multichannel ECG coding, 3-7

Linear variable differential transformer, *see* LVDT

Linear-array transducers, **14**-2–**14**-11

Linked predictive NNs, *see* LPNNs

Liquid crystal sensors, **20**-2

Liquid metal strain gauges, **46**-16

LMS adaptive noise canceler, 1-19–1-21, *1*-20

Lobular carcinoma in the left breast, *23*-6

Local area networks, *see* LANs

Logan B.E., **1**-3

London R.E., **55**-5

London S.B., **55**-5

Long wavelength infrared, *see* LWIR

Longbotham H, **4**-19

Lookup tables, *see* LUTs

Loupas T. **14**-33

low-pass filters, *2*-13

Low-pass temporal filtration, **10**-17

LPNNs (linked predictive NNs), 7-5

LROI (linear region of interest), in collateral damage, 33-5–**33**-6

Lübbers D.W., **49**-9, **49**-11

Ludsted L.B., **44**-1

Lung volumes, 60-1, *60*-2

LUTs (Lookup tables), **10**-15

LVDT (linear variable differential transformer), **46**-6

LWIR (long wave infrared) sensors, 19-10–**19**-11, **37**-7–**37**-12

M

Madhavan G.P., **7**-2

Magnetic field gradient coils, 15-8–**15**-9

Magnetic field homogeneity, 12-14–**12**-15

Magnetic Induction, in biomedical sensors, **46**-7

Magnetic resonance imaging, *see* MRI

Magnetic resonance spectroscopy, *see* MRS

Magnetism, as critical phenomena, 8-3–**8**-4

Magnetization, *see also individual entries*
  relaxation of, **12**-7

Maier J., **7**-4

Major health care trends and directions, **75**-2

Malik J., **29**-8

Mallat S., **5**-9

Mammography, 10-19–**10**-30
  and infrared imaging, 25-14–**25**-15
  and ultrasound and TTM, in breast disease examination, 23-12–**23**-16
  antiscatter grid in, 10-27–**10**-28
  compression device in, **10**-27
  definition, **10**-19

  digital mammography, 10-31–**10**-34
  equipment for, 10-22–**10**-30
  film emulsion for, **10**-29
  film processing in, 10-29–**10**-30
  image formation, 10-21–**10**-22
  image receptor in, 10-28–**10**-30
  mammographic image acquisition process, *10*-20
  mammographic quality control minimum test frequencies, *10*-31
  mammographic screen-film image receptor, *10*-28–*10*-29
  mammography machine, *10*-23
  noise and dose in, **10**-30
  principles, **10**-20
  quality control in, 10-30–**10**-31
  stereotactic biopsy devices in, **10**-31
  x-ray beam filtration in, 10-26–**10**-27
  x-ray source in, 10-24–**10**-26

Mandatory and spontaneous breath delivery control structure, **61**-7

Mandatory ventilation, 61-4–**61**-5

Mandatory volume controlled inspiratory flow delivery, in mechanical ventilation, 61-7–**61**-8

Marey E.J., 55-3, 55-6

Mariel L., **26**-6

Marker channel diagram, for ECG strip interpretation, *54*-10

Markle D.R., **49**-11

Markov model, *see* HMM

Marks R.M., **22**-6

MAS (motion analysis software), **18**-13

Mass spectrometry
  in clinical laboratory, 69-2–**69**-3
  for proteins and enzymes measurement, 51-4–**51**-6

Mass spectrophotometry, *51*-6

Matched filter, in biomedical signals, **1**-18

Max M.L., **18**-15

Maximum voluntary ventilation, *see* MVV

McCoy M.D., **35**-2

McCulloch J., **31**-7

McDicken W.N., **14**-33

Mean glandular dose, *see* MGD

Measurement indicators, in clinical engineering program, 77-4–77-5

Mechanical ventilation, 61-1–61-10, *see also individual entries*

ventilation modes, 61-3–61-6

Median nerve block in the hand, 21-11–21-12

Medical data interchange standard, *see* MEDIX

Medical devices, and clinical engineers standards primer, 79-5–79-7

Medical diagnostics, quantitative active dynamic thermal IR-imaging and thermal tomography in, 22-1–22-26

Medical education, modeling, and nonsurgical training, VR applications in, 18-10–18-11

Medical equipment

risk classification profiler, *81*-8

risk criteria, 81-7–81-8

risk factors, safety, and management, 76-1–76-15

Medical imaging, 75-9–75-10

Medical informatics and biomedical emergencies, 45-1–45-9

as advanced technologies, 45-8–45-9

and emergency response, 45-6–45-8

Medical infrared imaging, advances in, 19-1–19-13

in Austria, 19-4

in breast cancer, 19-5–19-8, *see also separate entry*

in China, 19-3–19-4

in Germany, 19-4

in Italy, 19-5

in Japan, 19-4

in Korea, 19-4

in Poland, 19-5

in United Kingdom, 19-4

in United States of America and Canada, 19-3

worldwide use, 19-3–19-5

Medical instruments and devices at home, *see* Home medical devices

Medical logic module, *see* MLM

Medical technology management and assessment, 75-1–75-15

acquisition process strategies, 75-11–75-12

equipment acquisition and deployment in, 75-10–75-12

moral dilemma of, 82-2–82-3

strategic technology planning in, 75-3–75-5

Medium wavelength infrared, *see* MWIR

MEDIX (medical data interchange standard), 42-4

Meehl R., 44-1

MEI-guided therapy, *12*-20

Meindl J., 14-34–14-35

Meisner M., 18-17

Melanin absorption spectra, *71*-2

Membrane protein structure and assemblies, in SPM crystallography, 67-7–67-8

MEMS (microelectromechanical systems) technology, 46-8–46-9

Mendelson Y., 49-7

Merla A., 32-2, 32-6, 32-9, 32-11–32-12

Merril J.R., 18-9

MES (myoelectric signals), 7-2

Message format standards, in health care information infrastructure, 42-3–42-4

Metabolic activity, of human body and cancer cells, 27-2–27-3

metal cup EEG electrode, 47-7

metal plate electrode, 47-6, *47*-7

Metallic resistance thermometers, 46-13

Metherall P., 17-6, 17-8–17-9

Method of Korotkoff, 55-5–55-6

MGD (mean glandular dose), 10-21

Micro-cantilever force sensors, 65-8–65-9

Microcirculation, heat transfer modeling equations for, 21-4–21-5

Microelectrodes, *47*-10, 47-10–47-11

Microelectromechanical systems technology, *see* MEMS

Microelectronic technology, 47-11

Microelectronics applications, in sensor fabrication, 50-8–50-10

Microstimulator, *59*-11

Mid-IR laser radiation effects, in biomedical lasers, 64-4

Military, VR applications in, 18-6

Miller I.D., *64*-3

Milton J.G., 4-19

Miniature silicon pressure sensors, 46-17

Minimum mean squares error, *see* MMSE

Minimum resolvable temperature, *see* MRT

Mirrored articulated arm characteristics, in biomedical laser beam delivery systems, 64-8

MIST-VR laparoscopic simulator, 18-9

MLM (medical logic module) in CPR

MMSE (minimum mean squares error), 13-21

MMT (molybdenum target tube), and mammography, 23-12

Modulation transfer function, *see* MTF

Molybdenum target spectrum, *10*-26

Molybdenum target tube, *see* MMT

Monitored anesthesia care, 62-2

Monopolar mode, in electrosurgical devices, 63-2–63-4

Moody E.B., 7-2

Moore G.P., 7-4

Morlet D., 4-19

Morlet's wavelet, 5-4

Moskowitz M., 25-9, 26-5–26-6

Motion analysis software, *see* MAS

Moubarak I., 55-10

MR microscopy, radiofrequency coils in, 15-7

MRI

acquisition and processing in, 12-1–12-9

chemical-shift imaging, *see separate entry*

contrast mechanisms of, *12*-7, 12-7–12-8

current trends, 12-19

digital data processing in, 12-18

fast imaging in, 12-6

functional MRI, *see* fMRI

fundamentals, 12-2–12-7

gradient coils in, 12-15–12-17

hardware/instrumentation in, 12-9–12-15

MRI imaging, digital and analog domains, *12*-10

MRI instrumentation fundamentals, 12-10–12-11

MRI response to photic stimulation, *12*-29

MRI scanner, *12*-11

perspective, 12-5

radiofrequency (RF) coils, in MRI scanners, 12-17–12-18

SNR considerations in, 12-5

MRI (*continued*)
  k-space analysis of data
      acquisition in,
      12-3–12-7
  2D imaging in, 12-4
MRS (magnetic resonance
      spectroscopy), 12-31,
      15-1–15-11
  applications, 15-9–15-11
  basic principles, 15-2–15-3
  image contrast in, 15-3
  instrumentation, 15-6–15-9
  magnetic field gradient coils in,
      15-8–15-9
  radiofrequency coils in,
      15-7–15-8
  resolution limits of, 15-4–15-6,
      see also separate entry
  spatial encoding and decoding
      in, 15-2–15-3
MRT (minimum resolvable
      temperature), in infrared
      camera characterization,
      38-8–38-9
MTD (maximum tumor
      dimension), *26-23*
MTF (modulation transfer
      function), 10-3
  in Infrared camera
      characterization, 38-8
Multichannel ECG data
      compression scheme
      block diagram, *3–6*
Multichannel implantable
      stimulator telemeter,
      59-7
Multifractals, 8-8–8-9
Multimedia, *see* Networked
      multimedia
      communications
Multineuronal activity analysis,
      7-2–7-3
Multiresolution theory, 5-7–5-10
Multiresolution wavelet
      transform,
      implementation, 5-10
Muscle spasm and injury,
      31-4
Muscle tissue thermal properties,
      22-5
Muscular lesion, *32-2, 32-4*
Musculoskeletal injuries,
      35-5–35-6
Mutual inductance, 46-5
MVV (maximum voluntary
      ventilation), 60-2
MWIR (medium wave infrared)
      sensors, 19-10–19-11,
      37-7–37-12
Myocardial Ischemia, QRS
      complex analysis,
      5-11–5-14
Myoelectric signals, *see* MES

Myoglobins absorption spectra,
      71-2
Myosin, in cellular mechanics,
      65-3

N

Nadal J., 7
Narrowband estimation
      techniques, in blood flow
      measurement,
      14-32–14-35
  autocorrelator in, 14-33–14-34
  autoregressive estimation (AR)
      in, 14-33
  classic Doppler estimation in,
      14-32–14-33
  finite derivative estimator
      (FDE), 14-34–14-35
NASPE/NPEG Code, *54-11*
NDA (nonlinear discriminant
      analysis), 28-9
NDMS transformation, 45-4
Needle electrode, *47-9*
Negative-pressure ventilators,
      61-2, *61-2*
Nelson H.A., 35-1
Neo-angiogenesis, in patients
      with advanced breast
      cancer, 26-14–26-20
Nephelometry, 69-7, *69-7*
Nerve entrapment syndrome,
      31-6–31-9
NETD (noise equivalent
      temperature difference),
      38-5–38-6
Networked multimedia
      communications, *see also*
      Wireless communication
  and biomedical signal
      processing, 9-1–9-3
Neurectomies, 35-4
Neurological signal processing,
      5-18–5-21
Neurology, NNs in, 7-11
Neuromuscular control,
      implantable stimulators
      for, 59-1–59-12
Newtonian mathematics, 8-2–8-3
NIR (near-infrared spectroscopy)
      and glucose monitoring, in
      noninvasive optical
      monitoring, 71-7–71-8
NIR absorption spectra
  of biologic materials, *71-7,
      72-2*
NIR laser radiation effects, in
      biomedical lasers,
      64-4–64-5
NIR quantitative imaging, of
      deep tissue structure,
      30-2–30-15

measurable quantities and
      experimental
      techniques, 30-4–30-6
Nitrogen washout curve, *60-8*
Nitrogen/phosphorous detection
      method, in clinical
      laboratory, 69-2–69-3
Nitrogen-washout technique
      equipment arrangement,
      60-7
Nitrous oxide, in anesthesia,
      62-3–62-4
NMR (nuclear magnetic
      resonance), 12-2–12-3
NNs (Neural networks), 7-1
      Neural networks, *see* NNs
  in biomedical signal
      processing, 7-1–7-11
  in Cardiology, 7-7–7-11
  in neurology, 7-11
  in sensory waveform analysis,
      7-2–7-5
  in speech recognition, 7-5–7-7
Noise equivalent temperature
      difference, *see* NETD
Non-AI decision making,
      44-1–44-8
  analytical models in, 44-2
  ANNs in, 44-8
  Bayesian analysis in, 44-5–44-6
  causal modeling in, 44-7–44-8
  clinical algorithms, in decision
      theoretic models,
      44-2–44-3
  database search in, 44-4
  decision theoretic models,
      44-2–44-3
  decision trees in, 44-3
  influence diagrams in, 44-3
  regression analysis, 44-4
  statistical models, 44-4–44-8
  statistical pattern analysis, 44-4
  syntactic pattern analysis in,
      44-6–44-7
Noncontact mode imaging, in
      SPM, 67-3
Noninvasive arterial blood
      pressure and mechanics,
      55-1–55-14
  long-term sampling methods
      in, 55-2–55-8
Noninvasive arterial mechanics,
      55-12–55-14
Noninvasive cerebral oximetry,
      49-9
Noninvasive optical monitoring,
      71-1–71-9
Noninvasive pulse oximetry,
      49-8–49-9
  disposable finger probe in,
      49-9
Nonlinear discriminant analysis,
      see NDA

Nonpulsatile spectroscopy, in
noninvasive optical
monitoring, 71-7–71-9
Nonspectral methods and
automation, in clinical
laboratory, 70-1–70-9
coagulation timers in, 70-7
electrochemical methods,
70-3–70-4
ion-specific electrodes in,
70-4–70-5
particle counting and
identification,
70-1–70-3
potentiometry methods, 70-3
radioactive methods,
70-5–70-7
Nonstationary signals,
segmentation in
biomedical signals,
1-21–1-22
Norberg I., 1-1
Normal infrared facial
thermography, 34-3
Norris K., 71-8
Nowicki A., 14-26
Nuclear magnetic resonance, see
NMR
Nuclear magnetism, 12-9
Nuclear medicine imaging
process, conventional,
13-11
Nuclear medicine, 13-1–13-26
ancillary electronic equipment
for detection in,
13-7–13-8
choices in, 13-1–13-3
detector configurations,
13-4–13-6
detectors in, 13-2
instrumentation, 13-1–13-10
photon radiation detection in,
13-3–13-4
planar imaging applications
and economics in,
13-8–13-9
SPECT in, see separate entry
Nuclear reactor-produced radio
nuclides, 16-2
Nucleic acids measurement
sensors, 51-7–51-10
Nursing informatics, 43-1–43-13,
see also individual entries
and engineering specialties,
bridging, 43-7–43-9
clinical information systems in,
43-6–43-7
definition, 43-3–43-4
nursing informatics groups,
43-3–43-4
research and development
needs, 43-11–43-13
roles expansion, 43-3

standards in vocabularies and
data sets, 43-5–43-6
Nursing process, 43-4–43-5
ethics and regulation in,
43-4–43-5
Nyboer J., 53-1, 53-3
Nyirjesy I., 26-6

O

O'Brien W.D., 14-35
O₂ uptake measurement, using
water-sealed spirometer,
56-6, 60-4–60-5
Object under test, see OUT
Objective thermography,
21-7–21-17
blood flow reduction effect on,
21-8–21-11
Obstructive apnea, 72-6
Occlusive cuff mechanics,
55-3–55-5
Oesterhelt D., 67-11
Offenbacher H., 49-11
Ogawa S., 12-22
Okamura T., 18-12
Olfaction, and VR technology,
18-5
Oliver R., 30-16
1.5D arrays, 14-4
1/f process, 8-8, 8-10
ONE TOUCH® test strip, in
blood glucose
monitoring, 66-3–66-4
One-dimensional signal
representations, 4-2
Operation, theory of, 63-2
Opitz N., 49-9, 49-11
Optical distributor, 10–10
Optical fiber sensors, 49-4
Optical fibers, 49-3–49-5
critical reflection and
propagation within,
64-8
probe configurations in, 49-4
transmission characteristics,
64-7–64-8
Optical sensors, 49-1–49-14
and signal processing, 49-3
applications, 49-7–14
general principles, 49-5–49-7
instrumentation, 49-2–49-3
light source, 49-2
optical elements, 49-2
Photodetectors, 49-3
Optical, optoelectronic
transducers, 50-6–50-7
Optics challenges, to infrared
detectors, 37-17–37-18
Optimal filtering, 7-2
in biomedical signals,
1-16–1-18
Orthogonal wavelets, 5-7–5-10

Oscillometry, 55-6–55-7, see also
Derivative oscillometry
Osheim D.L., 35-1
Osmometers, in nonspectral
methods and automation,
70-7
Osteoarthritis examination, in
thermography, 35-5
OUT (object under test), in TT,
22-3
Ovarian blood flow, flow map
and Doppler spectrum,
14-25
Oximetry, 49-7–49-8, see also
individual entries
and pulse oximetry, 71-2–71-6
Oxygen, in anesthesia, 62-3
Oyama H., 18-13

P

Pacemakers, see Implantable
cardiac pacemakers
Paci E., 67-11
Pack-based systems, in
nonspectral methods and
automation, 70-8
Paget J., 31-3–31-4
Paget's disease of bone, 31-3–31-4
Pahlm O., 7-8
Pain management, 62-2
Pallás-Areny R.A., 52-6
PARADES (seven dimensions of
quality), 78-11
Parallel-beam geometry, in CT,
11-3
Parenteral infusion devices,
68-1–68-11, see also IV
Infusion devices;
Intravenous infusion
devices
delivery system occlusions
management in,
68-8–68-11
Pareto analysis, 78-7
in quality improvement, 78-6
of a sample trauma registry,
81-7
Parisky H.R., 26-7
Parisky Y.R., 25-10
Park S. 14-33
Parker P.B., 7-1
Parker S.H., 10-31
Parsons J., 18-12
Particle counting and
identification, in
nonspectral methods and
automation, 70-1–70-3
Passive isolation amplifier, 52-12,
52-11–52-12
Passive shimming approach, in
Magnetic field
homogeneity, 12-15

PAT (process action teams), **78**-9

Patient circuit, **61**-3

Patient identifiers, in health care information infrastructure, **42**-2

Patient monitoring, during anesthesia, **62**-10–**62**-12

Patient monitors IPM, in clinical engineering program, **77**-8

Patient position and image capture, in thermal images variability sources, **36**-4–**36**-6

ambient temperature control in, **36**-5

field of view in, **36**-6

positions for imaging in, **36**-6

pre-imaging equilibration in, **36**-5–**36**-6

thermal imaging location in, **36**-5

Patient temperature control, during anesthesia, **62**-10

Patil K.D., **30**-16

Patterson B., **30**-13

Patterson R.P., **53**-5, **53**-7

PCA (principal-components analysis), **7**-7, **28**-2–**28**-3

PCNs (personal communications networks), **9**-2

PCO_2 sensors, **49**-11

PEEP (positive end expiratory pressure), **61**-4–**61**-6

Penaz J., **55**-8

Pennes H.H., **21**-4, **23**-8

Percolation

percolation network, **8**-5

as phase transition model, **8**-4

Percutaneous stimulation, **59**-2

Perforating vessels, dynamic IR-thermography for, **21**-14–**21**-15

Periarthropathia of the shoulder, **31**-5–**31**-6

Periodogram, in spectral estimation, **1**-14

Peripheral arteries, blood velocity measurement in, **14**-28–**14**-29

Peripheral blood flow, measurement using BEI, **53**-5

Peripheral nerves, **31**-6–**31**-9

peripheral nerve paresis, **31**-9

peripheral nerve stimulators, **59**-9–**59**-10

Peripheral neuro-vascular thermography, **35**-4

Peristaltic pumps, in intravenous infusion devices, **68**-7

Permanent magnet, *12-12*

and electromagnets, **12**-12–**12**-13

Perona P., **29**-7

Peroneal nerve, **31**-9

Personal communications networks, *see* PCNs

Personalized medicine, **51**-11–**51**-12

Pesque P., **14**-35

PET (positron-emission tomography), **16**-1–**16**-16

instrumentation, **16**-7–**16**-16

PET detectors, **16**-8–**16**-11

PET radionuclides, **16**-5–**16**-6

PET theory, **16**-8

physical factors affecting resolution of, **16**-11–**16**-13

random coincidences in, **16**-13

resolution evolution, *16-12*

resolution, *16-11*

sensitivity, **16**-14

statistical properties of, **16**-15–**16**-16

tomographic reconstruction, **16**-13–**16**-14

Peterson J.I., **49**-10

PF (Peak flow), **60**-2

P_H sensors, **49**-10–**49**-11

Phan F., **7**-7

Phase transitions

as critical phenomena, **8**-3

percolation as model for, **8**-4

Phased arrays, focusing and steering with, **14**-3–**14**-4

Phased-array transducer, designing, **14**-11–**14**-14

array dimensions choice in, **14**-11–**14**-12

Philips W, **3**-5

Phillips B., **30**-5

Photoconductive detectors, *37-2*, **37**-2–**37**-3

Photomultiplier tube (PMT), **13**-7, **69**-5

Photon attenuation, **13**-12–**13**-13

Photon detectors, **37**-1–**37**-6

photon detectors readouts, **37**-12–**37**-13

Photon migration in tissue, **30**-2, **30**-6–**30**-9

Photon radiation detection, in nuclear medicine, **13**-3–**13**-4

Photonics, **9**-3

Photoplethysmograph, **55**-9

Photostimulable phosphors, **10**-6

Photovoltaic detectors, **37**-3–**37**-6

detector structure, *37-3–37-4*

Physical measurements, of biomedical sensors, **46**-1–**46**-17

Physical sensors, biomedical applications, *46-16*, **46**-16–**46**-17

Physiologic dead space, **60**-9–**60**-10

Physiological signals analysis, using BioBench^{TM}, **73**-2–**73**-5

Picard D., **19**

Piezoelectric transducer, **14**-14, **50**-7

equivalent circuit, *14-10*

Pilla J., **55**-12

Pisano E.D., **25**-15

Piston-shaped transducers, **14**-2

PITAC (President's information technology advisory committee), **41**-8–**41**-9

PIVIT^{TM} assessment system, *81-5*, **81**-4–**81**-6

Pixel size, in Infrared camera characterization, **38**-9

Planar imaging, in nuclear medicine, **13**-8–**13**-9

Planck's blackbody radiation curves, *39-2*

Plan-do-check-act, in quality improvement, **78**-7

Plethysmography, **21**-5–**21**-6

PMT, **13**-2–**13**-8, **13**-11, **13**-15, **51**-11–**51**-12

in the Anger camera, **13**-6

Pneumonia, nonsymmetrical temperature distribution for, *28-2*

Pneumotachographs, **60**-5–**60**-7, *60-6*

PO_2 sensors, **49**-11–**49**-12

Pogue B.W., **30**-13

Poiseuille flow, **14**-26

Poland, medical infrared imaging advances in, **19**-5

Polanyi M.L., **49**-7

Poles and zeroes geometry, *2-10*

Polhemus tracker, in VR technology, **18**-11

Polymerase chain reaction, *51-9*

Polyvinylidene difluoride, *see* PVDF

Pordy L, **3**-10

Porta J.D., **20**-2

Portable infusion pumps, as home medical device, **72**-3

Port-Wine Stain, *see* PWS

Position sensitive photodetector, *see* PSPD

Positive end expiratory pressure, *see* PEEP

Positive-pressure ventilators, **61**-2–**61**-3, *61-3*

Positron-Emission Tomography, *see* PET

Post-BCDDP, **26**-5–**26**-7

Postinfusion phlebitis, **68**-10

Potentiometric sensors, **48**-3–**48**-4

Potentiometric transduction, **50**-7
Potentiometry methods, in nonspectral methods and automation, **70**-3
Power law and 1/f processes, **8**-8
PPT (pulse phase thermography), **22**-14
    synthetic pictures calculation, *22-16*
Practical electrodes, for biomedical measurements, **47**-5–**47**-11
Pre- BCDDP, **26**-2–**26**-3
Pre-operative chemohormonotherapy-induced changes, in breast cancer, **26**-14–**26**-20
Preprocessor, in hybrid multichannel ECG coding, **3**-7
President's information technology advisory committee, *see* PITAC
Pressure controlled inspiratory flow delivery, in mechanical ventilation, **61**-9
Pressure controlled ventilation, **61**-4
Pressure measurement, in biomedical sensors, **46**-9–**46**-11
Pressure support
    pressure support spontaneous breath delivery, *61-6*
    in spontaneous mode, **61**-6
Price R., **14**-30
Principal-components analysis, *see* PCA
Probe electrode, **47**-8
Problem-solving model, in quality improvement, **78**-11
Process action teams, *see* PAT
Process improvement model, in quality improvement, **78**-10–**78**-11
Product and supply labeling identifiers, in health care information infrastructure, **42**-2
Productivity monitors, in clinical engineering program, **77**-7–**77**-8
Protein aggregation and fibril formation, in SPM crystallography, **67**-6–**67**-7
Proteins and enzymes measurement, using diagnostic sensors, **51**-1–**51**-7

Provider identifiers, in health care information infrastructure, **42**-2
PRT (platinum resistance thermometer), **33**-3–**33**-4
Pseudo-WD, *see* PWD
PSPD (position sensitive photodetector), **67**-3
Public entertainment, VR applications in, **18**-6
Public switched network, and asynchronous transfer mode, **9**-2
Pulmonary function tests, **60**-1–**60**-9
    dynamic tests, **60**-2–**60**-5
Pulse dynamics methods, **55**-8–12
Pulse generators, **54**-3–**54**-7
    internal view, *54-3*
    output circuit in, **54**-5
    power source for, **54**-6–**54**-7
    sensing circuit in, **54**-3–**54**-5
    telemetry circuit, **54**-6
    timing circuit, **54**-6
Pulse oximeter sensors, **49**-8, **71**-2–**71**-6
    on a finger, *71-4*
Pulse phase thermography, *see* PPT
Pulse sensors, **55**-9–**55**-10
Pulsed force mode imaging, in SPM, **67**-10
Pulsed thermography, **22**-13
Pulsed-progressive fluoroscopy, **10**-14
pulsed-progressive mode, image acquisition using, *10–14*
Pulse-echo Doppler processing, **14**-32
Purohit R.C., **35**-2, **35**-6
PVDF (polyvinylidene difluoride), as transducers, **14**-2
PWD (pseudo-WD), **4**-17
PWS (port-wine stain), **33**-13–**33**-14
Pyroelectric heat flow transducers, **50**-5
PZT (lead–zirconate–titanate) ceramic material, as transducer, **14**-2

Q

QIPT (quality improvement project team), **78**-10
QMB (quality management board), **78**-10
QPC (quadratic phase coupling), **6**-11
QPI (quality performance indicators), **78**-8–**78**-9

QRS complex, **2**-12–**2**-13, **3**-3, **3**-10
    analysis, under myocardial ischemia, **5**-11–**5**-14
    in ECG signals, **4**-18–**4**-19
    in late potential analysis, **5**-14–**5**-17
    in neural networks, **7**-7
Q-switched Ruby ($Cr:Al_2O_3$) laser, **64**-9
Quadratic phase coupling, *see* QPC
Quality improvement and team building, **78**-1–**78**-12
    teams, **78**-9–**78**-10
Quality Improvement Project Team, *see* QIPT
Quality improvement tools, **78**-4–**78**-7
Quality indicators and data sets, in health care information infrastructure, **42**-7
Quality management board, *see* QMB
Quality performance indicators, *see* QPI
Quality, monetary value of, **78**-11–**78**-12
Quantitative active dynamic thermal IR-imaging and thermal tomography, in medical diagnostics, **22**-1–**22**-26
Quantitative fluorescence imaging and spectroscopy, **30**-12–**30**-15
Quantization effects, in digital biomedical signal acquisition, **2**-4–**2**-6
Quantum detection efficiency, **10**-7
Quantum well infrared photodetectors, *see* QWIPs
QWIP detectors, **37**-9–**37**-10, **37**-8–**37**-12

R

Raab A., **67**-11
Rachels J., **82**-6
Radiation dose, in nuclear medicine, **13**-2
Radiculopathy, **31**-7
Radioactive methods, in nonspectral methods and automation, **70**-5–**70**-7
Radiofrequency (RF) coils, in MRI scanners, **12**-17–**12**-18
Radionuclides, *see also individual entries*
    in biomedicine, *16-3–16-4*

Radiopharmaceuticals, **16**-1–**16**-6

Ramon F., **7**-4

Rastegar S., **64**-3

Rate-adaptive pulse generators, **54**-3

Raynaud's phenomenon, *see* RP

Real impedance transducer, *14-12*

Real low-pass filter, amplitude response, *2-11*

Receiver operating curve, *see* ROC

Recessed electrode, *47-7*

'Recognition imaging', **67**-11

Recognition reactions and receptor processes classification, **50**-2, *50-3–50-5*

Reconstruction principles, in CT, **11**-13–**11**-16
image processing in, **11**-13–**11**-14
projection data to image in, **11**-14–**11**-15

Reduced interference distribution, *see* RID

Reference electrodes, **48**-5–**48**-6

Reflectance-based test strip, in glucose monitoring, *66-3*

Reflection, **14**-26
critical reflection, in optical fiber, *64-8*
endoscope tip reflection, *81-3*

Reflective optics, **39**-13–**39**-14

Regulatory and assessment agencies, **80**-1–**80**-10

Reid J.M., **14**-26

REL (resting expiratory level), **60**-1

Reliability, in anesthesia delivery system, **62**-11–**62**-12

Relief of pain, and anesthesia, **62**-1–**62**-2

Renormalization, **8**-10

Reperfusion of transplanted tissue, **21**-15

Resister–capacitor–inductor defibrillator, *57-5*

Resistive magnets, **12**-13

Resolution limits
digital resolution limit, **15**-5
intrinsic resolution limit, **15**-4–**15**-5
of magnetic resonance microscopy, **15**-4–**15**-6
practical resolution limit, **15**-5–**15**-6

Respiration monitoring, by BEI measurements, **53**-4–**53**-5

Respiration, **60**-1–**60**-10, *see also* Respiration monitoring

Respiratory system study, using EIT, **17**-10

Resting expiratory level, *see* REL

Reswick J.B., *47-9*

RF coils, in MR microscopy, **15**-7–**15**-8

RF Electrosurgery, **33**-4–**33**-5

RID (reduced interference distribution), **4**-18

Right breast cancer, right partial mastectomy, radiation, and chemotherapy for, *26-27*

Ring E.F.J., **21**-4, **31**-2–**31**-4, **36**-1–**36**-2

Rinia H.A., **67**-7

Rioul O., **5**-2, **5**-7

Risk factors, safety, and management, of medical equipment, **76**-1–**76**-15

Risk management
application, **76**-11–**76**-13
case studies, **76**-13–**76**-14
definition, **76**-1–**76**-2
double-edged sword concept of, *76-2*
historical perspective, **76**-2–**76**-4
strategies, **76**-4–**76**-11

ROC (receiver operating curve) analysis, **24**-10–**24**-11, **24**-15–**24**-16, *24-13–*, *24-18*

Roche Accu-Chek® Easy™ test strip, in blood glucose monitoring, **66**-4

Roche Accu-Chek® Instant™ strip, in blood glucose monitoring, **66**-4

Roddie I.C., **21**-3

Rolland J.P., **18**-12

Rosenberg R.D., **25**-14

Rosenblatt F., **7**-3

Rothbaum B.O., **18**-17

Rovetta A., **18**-16

Rowe W.D., **79**-2

RP (Raynaud's phenomenon), **32**-5–**32**-8

Rudimentary night vision systems, **20**-2

R-wave time interval technique, **55**-8

RWT(random walk theory)
in breast quantitative spectroscopy, **30**-9–**30**-12

S

Safe medical devices act, **83**-6

Saidi S.L., **30**-3

Saillant P.A., **4**-20

Saline method of ejection fraction measurement, *56-9*

Salmon M., **21**-5

Sampling theorem, in digital biomedical signal acquisition, **2**-2–**2**-4

Sapiro G., **29**-7

SARS
CT and TTM in, *23-21*
diagnosis using CT and TTM, **23**-17–**23**-19
diagnosis using CT and TTM, comparison, **23**-21–**23**-22
diagnosis, using TTM, **23**-16–**23**-22
dynamic evolution imaging in, **23**-20
initial stage image characterization, **23**-20
outbreak, **24**-1–**24**-2
pathology, **23**-17
progressive stage imaging characterization, **23**-20
recovery stage image characterization, **23**-20
result analysis and performance comparison, **23**-19–**23**-22
SARS-CoV infection, **23**-16–**23**-22
SARS-CoV infection stages, *23-17*
study design, **23**-19

Savage L.I., **44**-1, **44**-5

SBC (subband coding), **3**-8–**3**-10
and wavelet transform, **3**-5–**3**-6

Scaling theories, **8**-6–**8**-9
fractal preliminaries in, **8**-6–**8**-7

Scalogram, **4**-18

Scanning electron beam scanners, in CT, **11**-4

Scanning tunneling microscope, *see* STM

Schiff S.J., **4**-19

Schlieren Photography, **20**-2

Schnitt S.J., **26**-7

Schultz J.S., **49**-12

Scientific evidence, in CPR, **41**-5–**41**-7
evaluation, **41**-6
incentives in, **41**-6
patient care processes in, **41**-5–**41**-6
research databases, **41**-6–**41**-7

Scoliosis treatment, in peripheral nerve stimulators, **59**-10

Scrotum thermography, **35**-6

Second-order statistics, *see* SOS

Second-order Volterra system, *6–10*

Seitz W.R., **49**-11

Self-organized criticality, in complexity, **8**-4–**8**-5

Semiconductor technology, and
    biomedical sensors
    pressure measurement,
    46-10
Senger S., **18**-12
Senhadji L., **5**-6
Sensing circuit, in pulse
    generators, **54**-3–**54**-5
Sensors, *see also individual entries*
    design and development, and
        biochemical reactions
        classification,
        50-1–**50**-2
    detection means and
        conversion phenomena
        in, *50*-6
    fabrication, microelectronics
        applications in,
        50-8–**50**-10
    for nucleic acids measurement,
        51-7–**51**-10
    in breast cancer, **19**-7–**19**-8
    medical applications,
        19-7–**19**-8
Separation and spectral methods,
    in clinical laboratory,
    69-1–**69**-8
    basis for spectral methods,
        69-4–**69**-5
September 11 attacks, **45**-1–**45**-2
Seven dimensions of quality, *see*
    PARADES
Severe acute respiratory
    syndrome, *see* SARS
Severinghaus J.W., **71**-2
Shafer G., **44**-6
Sharir T., **55**-8
Shepp L.A., **11**-13–**11**-14
Sheth D., **55**-3
Shewhart cycle, in quality
    improvement, **78**-7, *78*-7
Short Time Fourier Transform,
    see STFT
Short wavelength infrared, *see*
    SWIR
Signal PRocessing In The
    Element, *see* SPRITE
Signal processing
    in biomedicine, **2**-6–**2**-22, *see
        also individual entry*
    design criteria in, **2**-11
    digital filters, **2**-6–**2**-12
    signal averaging, **2**-12–**2**-18
Signals, *see also individual entries*
    amplitude spectrum of, *1*-10
    classification, *1*-5
    in the time and frequency
        domains, *1*-8
    time-series model for, *1*-14
Signal-to-noise ratio, *see* SNR
Silicon chip accelerometer, *46*-9
Silipo R., **7**-8
Silverman L., **60**-7
Silver–silver electrodes, *47*-4

Silverstein, **18**-12
Simple backprojection, as image
    reconstruction method,
    13-19–**13**-20
Simple spirometer, *60*-4
Simulated EEG, adaptive
    segmentation of, *1*-22
Singer A.J., **22**-18–**22**-19
Single molecule force
    spectroscopy, **67**-9
Single nucleotide polymorphism,
    see SNP
Single-photon emission
    computed tomography,
    see SPECT
Site-of-care identifiers, in health
    care information
    infrastructure, **42**-2
Sjogren's syndrome (SS), in
    quantitative fluorescence
    imaging, **30**-12
Skeletal and neuromuscular
    systems diseases, thermal
    imaging, **31**-1–**31**-11
Skin anatomy, *22*-19
Skin and skin-surface
    temperature
    measurement, **34**-2
Skin blood flow
    infrared-thermography and
        laser Doppler mapping
        of, **21**-12–**21**-14
    regulation, for heat transfers,
        21-3–**21**-4
Skin burns, **22**-19–**22**-22
    in vivo experiments on pigs,
        22-19–**22**-22
Skin electrodes, *47*-7
Skin of the hand, heat transport
    efficiency in, **21**-8
Skin temperature analysis
    during exercise, **32**-11–**32**-13
    in response to stress, **21**-2–**21**-3
Slip rings, *11*-6
Smoothed PWD, *see* SPWD
SNOM/NSOM, in SPM, **67**-13
'Snow-plow' effect in SPM, **67**-4
SNP (Single nucleotide
    polymorphism), **51**-10
SNP detection, by primer
    extension method,
    51-11
SNR (signal-to-noise ratio), **17**-8,
    22-13, **37**-3, **37**-14–**37**-22
    and evoked potentials, **5**-18
    and linear-array transducer
        performance, **14**-5,
        14-9, **14**-14, **14**-24,
        14-36
    in MR microscopy, **15**-5–**15**-11
    in MRI, **12**-5–**12**-7, **12**-11,
        12-19
Soft tissue Rheumatism,
    31-4–**31**-6

Solid-state lasers, **64**-6
Sonic and ultrasonic sensors,
    46-6–**46**-7
Sophisticated chemometric
    methods, in noninvasive
    optical monitoring, **71**-8
Sort-time Fourier transform, *see*
    STFT
SOS (second-order statistics),
    6-12–**6**-13
Spatial resolution, in Infrared
    camera characterization,
    38-9
SPECT (single-photon emission
    computed tomography),
    13-10–**13**-26
    algorithms for image
        reconstruction from
        projections in,
        13-19–**13**-21
    analytical reconstruction
        algorithms in,
        13-20–**13**-21
    and image reconstruction
        problem, **13**-17–**13**-19
    basic principles, **13**-10–**13**-13
    camera-based SPECT systems,
        13-14–**13**-15, *13*-15
    compensation methods in,
        13-22–**13**-24
    imaging process of,
        13-11–**13**-12
    instrumentation, **13**-13–**13**-17
    iterative reconstruction
        algorithms in, **13**-21
    multidetector SPECT system,
        13-13–**13**-14
    multidetector-based, *13*-14
    novel SPECT system designs,
        13-15–**13**-16, *13*-16
    phantom SPECT study, *13*-25
    physical and instrumentation
        that affect, **13**-12–**13**-13
    reconstruction methods in,
        13-17–**13**-24
    sample SPECT images,
        13-24–**13**-25
    special collimator designs for,
        13-16–**13**-17
SPECT imaging process,
    13-11–**13**-12
Spectral methods, in clinical
    laboratory, *see also
        individual entries*
    in biomedical signals,
        1-13–**1**-15
    parametric estimators in,
        2-19–**2**-21
    in signal processing, **2**-18–**2**-22
Spectrofluorometer, **69**-6
Spectrogram, and TFRs, **4**-17–18
Spectrophotometry, **51**-2–**51**-3
    principle, *51*-3

Speech recognition, neural networks in, 7-5–7-7

Spin echo, **12**-2

Spin–lattice relaxation, in magnetization, **12**-7

Spin–spin relaxation, in magnetization, **12**-7

Spin-warp imaging technique, **12**-15

Spiral scanning, *11-7*

Spiral/helical scanning, in CT, **11**-4

Spitalier J., **25**-9–**25**-11

SPM (scanning probe microscopy), biomolecular interactions probing, **67**-1–**67**-14
  applications, **67**-4–**67**-5
  basics, **67**-2–**67**-3
  crystallography, **67**-5–**67**-8
  force volume maps, **67**-9–**67**-10
  imaging mechanisms, **67**-3–**67**-5

Spontaneous breath delivery control, in mechanical ventilation, **61**-9–**61**-10

Spontaneous ventilation, **61**-5–**61**-6

Sports medicine injury, 21-15–21-16

Sprains and strains, **31**-4

SPRITE (Signal PRocessing In The Element) detector, **20**-3

SPWD (smoothed PWD), **4**-17

Standard database, for clinical engineering program indicators, **77**-3–**77**-4

Standards coordination and promotion organizations, in health care information infrastructure, **42**-7–**42**-8

Standards hierarchy, **79**-3–**79**-5

Stark A., **25**-9, **26**-5

Static field magnets, **12**-11–**12**-15

Static risk components, *76-10*

Stekettee J., **30**-16

Stereotactic biopsy devices, **10**-31

Stern Y., **7**-11

Sterns E., **26**-6

Steroid elution electrode, *54-8*

STFT (short-time Fourier transform), **1**-12–**1**-13, **1**-21, **5**-2, **5**-6–**5**-7, **5**-14

Stimulation pulses to excitable tissue delivery technology, **59**-2

STM (scanning tunneling microscope), **67**-3

Stochastic signals, **1**-5–**1**-7

Strategic technology planning, in medical technology management and assessment, **75**-3–**75**-5

Stress, and skin thermal properties, 21-2–21-3

Strickland D., **18**-15

Stroke, *see* CVA

Stromberg B., **35**-1

Strus J., **55**-1

Subband Coding, *see* SBC

Suction electrode for ECG, *47-7*

Superconducting magnets, **12**-13, *12-13–12-14*

Superficial blood vessels morphological reconstruction, **29**-7–**29**-13
  image morphology, **29**-8–**29**-13
  top hat segmentation, **29**-11
  white top-hat segmentation, **29**-12

SureStep™ test strips, in blood glucose monitoring, **66**-3–**66**-4

Surface or transcutaneous stimulation, **59**-2

Surface plasmon resonance, **49**-6–**49**-7

Surgical training and surgical planning, VR applications in, **18**-7–**18**-10

Suzuki N., **18**-12

SWIR (short wavelength infrared), 37-7–37-12

Syntactic pattern analysis, in non-AI decision making, **44**-6–**44**-7

Syringe pumps, in intravenous infusion devices, **68**-6–**68**-8

System pressures, in health care delivery system, **75**-2

T

Taffinder, **18**-9

Takahashi Y., **31**-7

Team building, and quality improvement, **78**-1–**78**-12

Technology acquiring process, in medical technology management and assessment, **75**-10–**75**-11

Technology assessment agencies, **80**-2–**80**-10
  name and addresses of, **80**-4–**80**-10

Technology assessment, in medical technology management and assessment, **75**-5–**75**-8
  prerequisites, **75**-5–**75**-6

Technology strategic planning process, in medical technology management and assessment, **75**-4–**75**-5

Telemedicine, **41**-7

Telemetry circuit, in pulse generators, **54**-6

Telesurgery and telemedicine, **18**-15–**18**-16

Telethermography, and varicocele, 32-9

Temperature calibration, in infrared thermal monitoring, 30-17–30-18

Temperature sensors, **46**-12–**46**-13
  properties, *46-12*

Temperature, importance, 34-1–34-2

Temporal point spread function, *see* TPSF

Temporomandibular Joint, *see* TMJ

Tennis elbow, 31-4, *31-5*

Test strips, in blood glucose monitoring, **66**-2–**66**-5, *see also individual entries*

Tested object, *see* TO

Testes thermography, **35**-6

TFR(time-frequency signal representation), *4-4–4-16*
  Affine class, **4**-14-4-15
  biomedical applications of, **4**-17–**4**-20
  classes, **4**-3–**4**-17
  Cohen's class, **4**-11–**4**-14
  desirable properties of, **4**-2–**4**-3
  hyperbolic class of, **4**-15–**4**-16
  kth power class of, **4**-16–**4**-17

Thakor N.V., **4**-19

Thermal conductivity detection method, in clinical laboratory, **69**-2–**69**-3

Thermal detectors, 37-6–37-7
  thermal detector readouts, 37-13

Thermal dilution method, in cardiac output measurement, **56**-2–**56**-4

Thermal images variability sources, 36-3–36-9
  camera initialization, 36-4
  camera systems, standards, and calibration, 36-3–36-4
  image analysis, 36-8
  image exchange in, 36-8–36-9
  image presentation, 36-9
  image processing in, 36-8

imaging system, **36**-3–**36**-4
information protocols and
        resources, **36**-6–**36**-8
mounting the imager, **36**-4
patient position and image
        capture, *see separate
        entry*
temperature reference, **36**-4
Thermal imaging systems, for
        medical applications,
        19-8–**19**-12
accuracy, **36**-2
in breast cancer detection,
        27-1–**27**-13
collateral damage analysis
        using, **33**-5–**33**-6
definition, **36**-2–**36**-3
during energized surgery,
        33-4–**33**-6
dynamic range in, **19**-9
energized systems in,
        33-2–**33**-3
face recognition, in,
        29-1–**29**-14
facial feature extraction in,
        29-6–**29**-13
instrument calibration,
        33-3–**33**-4
precision, **36**-2–**36**-3
resolution and sensitivity in,
        19-9–**19**-10
responsiveness, **36**-3
single Band imagers in,
        19-10–**19**-11
in skeletal and neuromuscular
        systems diseases,
        31-1–**31**-11
in surgery, *33*-3
temperature calibration in,
        19-10
Thermal models
and equivalent/synthetic
        parameters, **22**-7–**22**-8
Thermal radiation theory, Physics
        of, **24**-2–**24**-3
Thermal signals, physiology of,
        21-1–**21**-18, *see also*
        Cutaneous circulation
        measurement Techniques;
        Heat transfers; Objective
        thermography; Skin
        thermal properties
heat transport efficiency, in
        hand skin, **21**-8
of perforating vessels,
        21-14–**21**-15
of skin blood flow,
        21-12–**21**-14
and sports medicine injury,
        21-15–**21**-16
thermal skin measurement,
        21-6–**21**-7
and transplanted tissue
        reperfusion, **21**-15

Thermal skin measurement,
        21-6–**21**-7
Thermal texture mapping, *see*
        TTM
Thermal time constant
        representation, *22-22*
Thermal–electric analog, for
        breast cancer diagnosis,
        23-3–**23**-4
Thermistors, **46**-13–**46**-14, *46-14*
Thermocouples, **46**-14–**46**-15
Thermodilution method, *56*-3
'Thermogram', **20**-2
Thermograms reliability
        standards, **35**-2–**35**-3
Thermographic nondestructive
        testing, *see* TNDT
Thermography
    diagnostic applications, **34**-3
    of the testes and scrotum in
        mammalian species,
        35-6
Thermometry and thermal
        imaging in medicine,
        historical development,
        20-1–**20**-4
Thin-film electrode, *47-7*, **47**-8
Third-generation cooled imagers,
        challenges for,
        37-18–**37**-24
    cost challenges, **37**-19
    dynamic range and sensitivity
        constraints as,
        37-21–**37**-23
    high frame rate operation as,
        37-23–**37**-24
    higher operating temperature
        as, **37**-24
    performance challenges,
        37-21–**37**-24
    sensor format and packaging
        issues as, **37**-19–**37**-20
    temperature cycling fatigue as,
        37-20–**37**-21
    two-color pixel designs as,
        37-19
Thomassin L., **25**-10
Thoracic outlet syndrome, *see*
        TOS
Threatt B., **25**-9, **26**-5
Three-dimensional imaging, in
        EIT, **17**-8
3D noise model, **38**-3
3D spatialized sound, in VR
        technology, **18**-4
Thrombolytic therapy,
        reperfusion detection
        during, **5**-14
Thrombosis detection using BEI,
        53-5
Tidal volume, *see* TV
Tierney W.M., **41**-5

Time–frequency distributions of
        the vector magnitude of
        two ECG leads, *5–14*
Time-frequency signal
        representations, for
        biomedical signals,
        4-1–**4**-20
Time-resolved spectroscopy, in
        noninvasive optical
        monitoring, **71**-8–**71**-9
Time-series analysis methods, in
        spectral estimation, **1**-14
Timing circuit, in pulse
        generators, **54**-6
TIRF (total internal reflection
        fluorescence microscopy),
        67-13–**67**-14
Tissue characterization and
        function, and infrared
        imaging, **30**-1–**30**-20
Tissue impedance, Cole-Cole
        model, *17*-2
Tissue transplantation, **21**-15
Tissues, *see also individual entries*
    electrical impedance of, **17**-1
    conduction in human tissues,
        17-1–**17**-3
Titterington D.M., **44**-4
TMJ (temporomandibular joint)
        disorders assessment, with
        infrared thermography,
        34-4
TMT (transition management
        team), **78**-9
TNDT (thermographic
        nondestructive testing),
        see ADT IR-imaging
TO (tested object), in IRT, ADT
        and TT, **22**-9–**22**-10
Togawa T., **30**-16
Tomography, *see individual
        entries*
TOS (thoracic outlet syndrome),
        31-7–**31**-8
Total internal reflection
        fluorescence microscopy,
        see TIRF
Total quality management, *see*
        TQM
TPSF (temporal point spread
        function), **30**-5–**30**-6
TQM (total quality
        management), **78**-3
Traction force microscopy,
        65-7–**65**-8
Trahey G.E., **14**-35
Transducers, **14**-1–**14**-15, *see also
        individual entries*
    acoustic backing and matching
        layers impact, **14**-12
    array transducers, scanning
        with **14**-2–**14**-5
    array-element configurations
        in, **14**-4–**14**-5

Transducers (*continued*)
  axial resolution in, **14**-7
  electric impedance impact on,
    14-9–**14**-11
  electrical impedance matching,
    14-13–**14**-14
  linear-array transducer
    performance,
    14-5–**14**-11
  phased arrays, **14**-3–**14**-4
  radiation pattern of,
    14-7
  transducer materials,
    14-2
Transduction processes
  classification, by detection
    methods, **50**-2–**50**-8
Transform domain signals,
  compression, **3**-8
z-Transform
  in digital filters, 7
  transfer function in, **2**-7–**2**-10
Transition management team, *see*
  TMT
Transplanted tissue reperfusion,
  21-15
Transverse gradient coil, *12-16*
Trapezoidal wave defibrillator,
  57-5, *57*-5
Treatment use, ethical issues in,
  83-5–**83**-6
Triad model, in clinical
    engineering, **74**-3–**74**-4
TT (thermal tomography)
  data and image processing
    procedures in,
    22-12–**22**-17
  experiments and applications,
    22-17–**22**-25
  and IRT and ADT, **22**-3–**22**-6
  measurement equipment in,
    22-11–**22**-12
  measurement procedures in,
    22-8–10
  organization of experiments
    in, **22**-17–**22**-19
  and quantitative active
    dynamic thermal
    IR-imaging, in medical
    diagnostics,
    22-1–**22**-26
TTM (Thermal Texture Maps),
    23-1–**23**-26, *see also* TTM
    slicing
  and Chi-square test results,
    23-24
  and mammography and
    ultrasound, in breast
    disease examination,
    23-12–**23**-16
  and MMT, benign bumps,
    23-14
  and MMT, malignant bumps,
    23-14

  and MMT, ultrasound, and
    pathological results,
    correlation rate
    comparison, *23*-13
  concept, theory, and
    applications,
    23-1–**23**-26
  development status, **23**-2–**23**-3
  existing problems and
    expectations, **23**-3
  in breast diseases
    differentiation, **23**-16
  in early breast cancer
    application, **23**-3–**23**-7
  in early breast cancer
    diagnosis, **23**-3–**23**-7,
    see also separate entry
  in SARS diagnosis,
    23-16–**23**-22
  in vitro tissue study in,
    23-7–**23**-12, *see also*
    separate entry
  mechanism, **23**-15
  medical evaluation of,
    23-1–**23**-3
  SARS diagnosis using,
    23-17–**23**-19,
    23-21–**23**-22
  trilogy-imaging characteristics
    on, and malignancies,
    23-22–**23**-24
TTM slicing
  of lung TB condition, *23*-18
  of normal case, *23*-18
  of SARS patient, *23*-18
  of SARS patient, *23*-19
Tumor angiogenesis, *26*-9
Tumor thermal image, *28*-8
Tumor vascularity, **14**-37
Tungsten and molybdenum
    target x-ray spectra
    comparison, *10*-26
Turbidimetry, **69**-7
Turner R., **12**-22
Turner T.A., **35**-2
Turning point ECG compression
    method, **3**-3
Tuteur F.B., 19
TV (tidal volume), **60**-1
2D FT (two-dimensional Fourier
    transform imaging), **12**-4,
    12-4
2D Imaging, *13*-18
  in MRI, **12**-4
2D Phased-arrays, **14**-4
Two-dimensional Fourier
    transform imaging, *see*
    2D FT
Two-dimensional spin-echo CSI
    sequence, with CHESS for
    proton study, *12*-36
Tyack P.L., **4**-20

U

Uematsu S., **31**-7, **36**-1
Ultrasonic Doppler flowmeter
    structure, *46*-12
Ultrasonic flow estimation
    systems, in blood flow
    measurement,
    14-24–**14**-26
Ultrasonic imaging, **6**-11
  attenuation of ultrasonic
    signals, **14**-17–**14**-18
  economic advantages of,
    14-20–**14**-21
  fundamentals, **14**-17–**14**-20
Ultrasound contrast agents,
    14-37
Ultrasound, **14**-1–**14**-38, *see also*
    Ultrasonic imaging
  blood flow measurement
    using, **14**-22–**14**-29, *see*
    also separate entry
  and mammography and TTM,
    in breast disease
    examination,
    23-12–**23**-16
UltraTrainer, in VR technology,
    18-11
'Umbrella' electrode array,
    47-9
UMLS (unified medical language
    system), **42**-6
Unbonded strain gauge pressure
    sensor structure, *46*-10
Uncooled infrared detector
    challenges, **37**-14–**37**-16
Uncooled microbolometer pixel
    structures, *37*-13
United Kingdom, medical
    infrared imaging advances
    in, **19**-4
United States of America, medical
    infrared imaging advances
    in, **19**-3
Upscanning, in X-ray projection
    angiography, **10**-14
Useki H., **26**-6
UV laser radiation effects, **64**-5
UV–IR laser radiation interaction
    and effects, on biologic
    tissues, **64**-2–**64**-3
UV–IR laser radiation
    penetration and effects,
    on biologic tissues,
    64-3–**64**-4

V

Vagal stimulation, **59**-10
Van duyl B.Y., **67**-7
Van Trees H.L., **14**-30, **14**-35
Variable reluctance sensor,
    46-2–**46**-6

Variable time and frequency resolution, in wavelet (time-scale) analysis, 5-2–5-7

Varicocele, diagnosis follow-up of the treatment, 32-8–32-11

Vascular injuries, 35-5

Vascular unloading principle, 55-2–55-3

Vascularization, 27-3

Vasculature treatment types, 33-14

Veitch A.R., 64-3

Velocity estimation techniques, in blood flow measurement, 14-29–14-36
  classic theory of, 14-30–14-32
  clutter echoes in, 14-30
  in biomedical sensors, 46-7–46-8
  narrowband estimation, 14-32–14-35, see also separate entry
  wideband estimation techniques, see separate entry

Venous occlusion plethysmography, see VOP

Venous system compliance measurement using BEI, 53-5

Ventricular tachycardia diagnosis, 5-19

VEPs (Visual evoked potentials), 7-2–7-5

Verreault E, 4-19

Veterinary medicine, infrared imaging in, 35-1–35-7

Vetterli M., 5-2, 5-7

Ville Marie Infrared (IR) grading scale, 26-10
  modified Ville Marie Infrared scoring scale, 26-20

Ville Marie multi-disciplinary breast center, breast cancer monitoring and detection experience, 26-7–26-24

Virtual instrumentation, 81-1–81-9, 81-9
  and graphical programming, 73-1–73-2
  applications, in biomedical engineering, 73-1–73-8
  data modeling in, 81-6–81-7
  peer performance reviews, 81-8–81-9
  trending, relationships, and interactive alarms in, 81-5–81-6

Virtual reality modeling language, see VRML

Visible-range laser radiation effects, in biomedical lasers, 64-5

Visual evoked potentials, see VEPs

Vital organ function maintenance, 62-1–62-2

VMET, 18-10–18-11

Volatile anesthetic agents, physical properties, 62-4

Voltammetric sensors, 48-3–48-5

Volume controlled ventilation, 61-4

Volumetric infusion pumps, in intravenous infusion devices, 68-5–68-6

VOP (venous occlusion plethysmography), 21-5–21-7

VR (Virtual Reality) technology, 18-2
  anatomical imaging and medical image fusion, 18-11–18-13
  current status, 18-6–18-7
  as disability solution, 18-7
  instrumented clothing, 18-3
  medical applications, 18-1–18-17, see also individual entries
  overview, 18-2–18-5, 18-7–18-17
  VR application examples, 18-5–18-6
  VR Interface Technology, 18-4–18-5
  VR-based rehabilitation workstation, 18-4

VRML (virtual reality modeling language), 18-12

Vurek G.G., 49-11

W

Wallace J.D., 23-16, 25-12, 26-3

Wasner G., 31-9

Water-sealed spirometer, 60-2–60-4
  O$_2$ uptake.measurement using, 60-4–60-5

Watmough J., 30-16

Wavelet (time-scale) analysis applications, 5-11–5-18
  in biomedical signal processing, 5-1–5-23

Wavelet or subband coding, 3-5–3-6

Wavelet transformation
  in advanced thermal image processing, 28-8–28-9
  wavelet transform squared magnitude, 4-18

Way S., 25-9

WD (Wigner distribution), 4-17

Weaver J.B., 4-20

Website and database, in breast cancer, 19-7

Webster J.G., 52-6

Weghorst S., 18-9

Welch D.P., 2-19

Werbos P., 7-1

Wesseling K.H., 55-9

Whistler S.J., 55-4

White D.N., 14-26

Whittenberger J., 60-7

Wideband estimation techniques, in blood flow measurements, 14-35–14-36
  cross-correlation estimator in, 14-35
  WMLE in, 14-35–14-36

Widmalm W.E., 4-19

Wiener filter, in biomedical signals, 1-16–1-18

Wigner–Ville distribution, see WVD

Williams K., 26-2

Williams K.L., 20-3, 27-1, 30-16

Williams W.J., 4-20

Wireless communication/network, 9-2–9-3, see also Networked multimedia Communications

WMLE (wideband maximum likelihood estimator), in blood flow measurement, 14-35–14-36

Wolfbeis O.S., 49-11, 49-12

'Wrinkle stiffness', 65-7

Wunderlich C., 20-1

WVD (Wigner–Ville distribution), 5-6

X

X-ray image intensifier, 10–5

X-ray linear attenuation coefficients, 11-11
  of breast, 10-22

X-ray projection angiography, 10-8–10-18
  beam blanking in, 10-14
  digital angiography, 10-15–10-17
  film in, 10-10–10-11
  image formation in, 10-10–10-15
  image intensifier/video camera in, 10-11–10-12
  optical distributor in, 10-12
  progressive scanning in, 10-13–10-14
  upscanning in, 10-14
  video system in, 10-12–10-15

X-ray projection angiography
(*continued*)
x-ray generation in,
10-9–**10**-10
x-ray projection image, *10–20*
X-Ray, **10**-1–**10**-34, *see also
individual entries*
image detection in, **10**-4, *see
also separate entry*
mammography in,
10-19–**10**-30, *see also
individual entry*

production, **10**-2–**10**-4
x-ray equipment, **10**-1–**10**-7
x-ray generator, **10**-3–**10**-4
x-ray tube, **10**-2–**10**-3, *10–2*

Y

Yamakoshi K., **55**-9
Yi C., **7**-8
Yoshiya I., **49**-8
Young R., **67**-2

Z

Zahner D., **7**-11
Zaveri H.P., **4**-19
Zero defects, in quality
improvement, **78**-2–**78**-3
Z-gradient coil, *12-16*
Zhang H.Y., **31**-7
Zhang M., **7**-11
Zheng C., **4**-19
Zhou Z., **15**-7
Zhujun Z., **49**-11
Zontak A., **32**-11